a *Lange medical* book

Medical Immunology

ninth edition

Edited by

Daniel P. Stites, MD
Professor and Chairman
Department of Laboratory Medicine
University of California, San Francisco

Abba I. Terr, MD
Clinical Professor of Medicine
Stanford University School of Medicine
Stanford, California

Tristram G. Parslow, MD, PhD
Professor of Pathology
and of Microbiology and Immunology
University of California, San Francisco

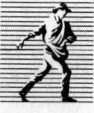

APPLETON & LANGE
Stamford, Connecticut

Notice: The authors and the publisher of this volume have taken care to make certain that the doses of drugs and schedules of treatment are correct and compatible with the standards generally accepted at the time of publication. Nevertheless, as new information becomes available, changes in treatment and in the use of drugs become necessary. The reader is advised to carefully consult the instruction and information material included in the package insert of each drug or therapeutic agent before administration. This advice is especially important when using, administering, or recommending new or infrequently used drugs. The authors and publisher disclaim all responsibility for any liability, loss, injury, or damage incurred as a consequence, directly or indirectly, of the use and application of any of the contents of this volume.

ISSN 0891-2076

ISBN 0-8385-0586-4

9 780838 505861   90000

Acquisitions Editor: John Butler
Production Service: Rainbow Graphics, Inc.
Associate Art Manager: Maggie Belis Darrow
Designer: Libby Schmitz

PRINTED IN THE UNITED STATES OF AMERICA

Table of Contents

Authors vii

Preface xi

History of Immunology 1
David W. Talmage, MD

SECTION I. BASIC IMMUNOLOGY _____

1. Fundamentals of Blood Cell Biology 9
   Clifford Lowell, MD, PhD

2. Innate Immunity 25
   Tristram G. Parslow, MD, PhD, & Dorothy F. Bainton, MD

3. Lymphocytes & Lymphoid Tissues 43
   Tristram G. Parslow, MD, PhD

4. The Immune Response 63
   Tristram G. Parslow, MD, PhD

5. Immunogens, Antigens, & Vaccines 74
   Tristram G. Parslow, MD, PhD

6. Antigen Presentation & the Major Histocompatibility Complex 83
   Frances M. Brodsky, DPhil

7. Immunoglobulins & Immunoglobulin Genes 95
   Tristram G. Parslow, MD, PhD

8. B-Cell Development & the Humoral Immune Response 115
   Anthony L. DeFranco, PhD

9. T Lymphocytes & Natural Killer Cells 130
   John B. Imboden, MD

10. Cytokines 146
    Joost J. Oppenheim, MD, & Francis W. Ruscetti, PhD

11. Complement & Kinin 169
    Michael M. Frank, MD

12. Inflammation 182
    Abba I. Terr, MD

13. The Mucosal Immune System 196
    Warren Strober, MD, & Ivan J. Fuss, MD

SECTION II. IMMUNOLOGIC LABORATORY TESTS

14. **Clinical Laboratory Methods for Detection of Antigens & Antibodies** **211**
    *Daniel P. Stites, MD, R.P. Channing Rodgers, MD,
    James D. Folds, PhD, & John Schmitz, PhD*

15. **Clinical Laboratory Methods for Detection of Cellular Immunity** **254**
    Daniel P. Stites, MD, James D. Folds, PhD, & John Schmitz, PhD

16. **Blood Banking & Immunohematology** **275**
    *Maurene Viele, MD, Elizabeth Donegan, MD,
    & Edith L. Bossom, SBB*

17. **Histocompatibility Testing** **286**
    Beth W. Colombe, PhD

18. **Molecular Genetic Techniques for Clinical Analysis of the Immune System** **309**
    Tristram G. Parslow, MD, PhD

19. **Laboratory Evaluation of Immune Competence** **319**
    Daniel P. Stites, MD, James D. Folds, PhD, & John Schmitz, PhD

SECTION III. CLINICAL IMMUNOLOGY

20. **Mechanisms of Immunodeficiency** **327**
    Arthur J. Ammann, MD, & E. Richard Stiehm, MD

21. **Antibody (B-Cell) Immunodeficiency Disorders** **332**
    Arthur J. Ammann, MD, & E. Richard Stiehm, MD

22. **T-Cell Immunodeficiency Disorders** **345**
    Arthur J. Ammann, MD, & E. Richard Stiehm, MD

23. **Combined Antibody (B-Cell) & Cellular (T-Cell) Immunodeficiency Disorders** **352**
    E. Richard Stiehm, MD, & Arthur J. Ammann, MD

24. **Phagocytic Dysfunction Diseases** **364**
    E. Richard Stiehm, MD, & Arthur J. Ammann, MD

25. **Complement Deficiencies** **371**
    Michael M. Frank, MD

26. **Mechanisms of Hypersensitivity** **376**
    Abba I. Terr, MD

27. **The Atopic Diseases** **389**
    Abba I. Terr, MD

28. **Anaphylaxis & Urticaria** **409**
    Abba I. Terr, MD

29. **Immune-Complex Allergic Diseases** **419**
    Abba I. Terr, MD

30. **Cell-Mediated Hypersensitivity Diseases** **425**
    Abba I. Terr, MD

31. **Drug Allergy** **433**
H. James Wedner, MD

32. **Mechanisms of Disordered Immune Regulation** **444**
Cornelia M. Weyand, MD, PhD, & Jörg J. Goronzy, MD, PhD

33. **Rheumatic Diseases** **456**
Kenneth E. Sack, MD, & Kenneth H. Fye, MD

34. **Endocrine Diseases** **480**
James R. Baker, Jr., MD

35. **Hematologic Diseases** **493**
J. Vivian Wells, MD, FRACP, FRCPA, & James P. Isbister, FRACP, FRCPA

36. **Cardiac & Vascular Diseases** **513**
Thomas R. Cupps, MD

37. **Gastrointestinal, Hepatobiliary, & Orodental Diseases** **528**
Stephen P. James, MD, Warren Strober, MD,
& John S. Greenspan, BDS, PhD, FRCPath

38. **Renal Diseases** **549**
Curtis B. Wilson, MD, Lili Feng, MD, & David M. Ward, MB, ChB, FRCP

39. **Immune-Mediated Dermatologic Diseases** **564**
Neil J. Korman, MD, PhD, Sanford M. Goldstein, MD, & Bruce U. Wintroub, MD

40. **Neurologic Diseases** **579**
Hillel S. Panitch, MD, Paul S. Fishman, MD, PhD, & Christopher T. Bever, Jr., MD

41. **Eye Diseases** **591**
Mitchell H. Friedlaender, MD, & G. Richard O'Connor, MD

42. **Respiratory Diseases** **599**
John F. Fieselmann, MD, & Hal B. Richerson, MD

43. **Reproduction & the Immune System** **613**
Karen Palmore Beckerman, MD

44. **Mechanisms of Tumor Immunology** **631**
Philip D. Greenberg, MD

45. **Cancer in the Immunocompromised Host** **640**
John L. Ziegler, MD

46. **Neoplasms of the Immune System** **651**
Susan K. Atwater, MD

47. **Mechanisms of Immunity to Infection** **678**
John Mills, MD

48. **Bacterial Diseases** **684**
John L. Ryan, MD, PhD

49. **Viral Infections** **694**
John Mills, MD

50. **Fungal Diseases** **706**
Thomas F. Patterson, MD, & David J. Drutz, MD

51. **Parasitic Diseases** **725**
James McKerrow, MD, PhD

52. **Spirochetal Diseases** 739
Charles S. Pavia, PhD, & David J. Drutz, MD

53. **Virus Infections of the Immune System** 748
Suzanne Crowe, MBBS, FRACP, & John Mills, MD

SECTION IV. IMMUNOLOGIC THERAPY

54. **Immunologic Therapy** 766
Abba I. Terr, MD

55. **Immunization** 772
Moses Grossman, MD

56. **Allergy Desensitization** 796
Abba I. Terr, MD

57. **Clinical Transplantation** 802
Marvin R. Garovoy, MD, Peter Stock, MD, Fraser Keith, MD, & Charles Linker, MD

58. **Immunosuppressive Therapy** 827
Alan Winkelstein, MD

59. **Immunomodulators** 846
Lawrence R. Hennessey, MD, & James R. Baker, Jr., MD

60. **Anti-Inflammatory Drugs** 852
James S. Goodwin, MD

Appendices

The CD Classification of Hematopoietic Cell Surface Markers 862

Glossary of Symbols Used in Illustrations 864

Index 867

The Authors

Arthur J. Ammann, MD
Director, Ariel Project for the Prevention of HIV Transmission from Mother to Infant; Chairman, Health Advisory Board Pediatric AIDS Foundation; Adjunct Professor, Pediatric Immunology, University of California, San Francisco.

Susan K. Atwater, MD
Assistant Professor, Clinical Laboratory Medicine, University of California, San Francisco.

Dorothy F. Bainton, MD
Professor of Pathology, Office of the Vice Chancellor for Academic Affairs, University of California, San Francisco.

James R. Baker, Jr., MD
Associate Professor, Internal Medicine and Pathology, Chief, Division of Allergy, University of Michigan, Ann Arbor.

Karen Palmore Beckerman, MD
Assistant Professor, University of California, San Francisco; Chief of Obstetrics, San Francisco General Hospital.

Christopher T. Bever, Jr., MD
Associate Professor of Neurology, University of Maryland at Baltimore.

Edith L. Bossom, SBB
Former Supervisor, Blood Bank, University of California, San Francisco.

Frances M. Brodsky, D. Phil.
Professor, The G. W. Hooper Foundation, Department of Microbiology and Immunology, School of Medicine; Departments of Biopharmaceutical Sciences and Pharmaceutical Chemistry, School of Pharmacy, University of California, San Francisco.

Beth W. Colombe, PhD
Associate Director, Immunogenetics and Transplantation Laboratory, Department of Surgery, University of California, San Francisco.

Suzanne Crowe, MBBS, FRACP
Head, AIDS Pathogenesis Research Unit, MacFarlane Burnet Centre and Staff Physician, Fairfield Hospital, Melbourne, Australia.

Thomas R. Cupps, MD
Associate Professor of Medicine, Georgetown University Medical Center, Washington, DC.

Anthony L. DeFranco, PhD
Professor, Department of Microbiology and Immunology, University of California, San Francisco.

Elizabeth Donegan, MD
Associate Professor of Clinical Laboratory Medicine, Pathology, Microbiology, and Immunology, University of California, San Francisco.

David J. Drutz, MD
Clinical Professor of Medicine, Seton Hall University, School of Graduate Medicine; Adjunct Professor of Microbiology and Immunology, Temple University Medical School, Philadelphia.

Lili Feng, MD
Assistant Member, Department of Immunology, The Scripps Research Institute, La Jolla, California.

John F. Fieselmann, MD
Associate Profesor, Division of Pulmonary Diseases, Department of Internal Medicine, University of Iowa College of Medicine and University of Iowa Hospitals, Iowa City, Iowa.

Paul S. Fishman, MD, PhD
Associate Professor of Neurology, University of Maryland School of Medicine, Baltimore, Maryland.

James D. Folds, PhD
Professor of Pathology and Laboratory Medicine, McLendon Clinical Laboratory, University of North Carolina Hospital, Chapel Hill.

Michael M. Frank, MD
Samuel L. Katz Professor and Chairman of Pediatrics; Professor of Immunology and Medicine, Duke University Medical Center, Durham, North Carolina.

Mitchell H. Friedlaender, MD
Director, Cornea and Refractive Surgery, Scripps Clinic and Research Foundation, La Jolla, California.

Ivan J. Fuss, MD
Senior Staff Research Fellow, Mucosal Immunology Section, National Institute of Allergy and Infectious Diseases, National Institutes of Health, Bethesda, Maryland.

Kenneth H. Fye, MD, FACP, FACR
Clinical Professor of Medicine, University of California, San Francisco.

Marvin R. Garovoy, MD
Professor of Surgery and Medicine; Director, Immunogenetics and Transplantation Laboratory, University of California, San Francisco.

James S. Goodwin, MD
George and Cynthia Mitchell Distinguished Professor; Director, UTMB Center on Aging, The University of Texas Medical Branch, Galveston, Texas.

Jorg J. Goronzy, MD, PhD
Associate Professor of Medicine, Mayo Clinic, Rochester, Minnesota.

Philip D. Greenberg, MD
Professor of Medicine and Immunology, University of Washington; Member, Fred Hutchinson Cancer Research Center, Seattle, Washington.

John Greenspan, BSc, BDS, PhD, FRCPath
Professor and Chair, Department of Stomatology; Director, Oral AIDS Center and UCSF AIDS Specimen Bank, School of Dentistry; Professor, Department of Pathology; Director, UCSF AIDS Clinical Research Center, School of Medicine, University of California, San Francisco.

Moses Grossman, MD
Professor Emeritus of Pediatrics, University of California, San Francisco.

Lawrence R. Hennessey, MD
Assistant Clinical Professor, Michigan State University College of Human Medicine, Okemos, Michigan.

John B. Imboden, MD
Associate Professor of Medicine, University of California, San Francisco.

James P. Isbister, FRACP, FRCPA
Head, Department of Hematology, Royal North Shore Hospital of Sydney, St. Leonards, New South Wales, Australia.

Stephen P. James, MD
Professor of Medicine; Head, Division of Gastroenterology, University of Maryland, Baltimore.

Fraser Keith, MD
Associate Clinical Professor, University of California, San Francisco.

Charles Linker, MD
Clinical Professor of Medicine; Director, Adult Leukemia and Bone Marrow Transplant Program, University of California, San Francisco.

Neil J. Korman, MD, PhD
Assistant Professor of Dermatology, Case Western Reserve University, Cleveland, Ohio.

Clifford Lowell, MD, PhD
Assistant Professor, Department of Laboratory Medicine, University of California, San Francisco.

James McKerrow, MD, PhD
Professor, Departments of Pathology and Pharmaceutical Chemistry, Veterans Administration Medical Center, San Francisco, California.

John Mills, BS, MD, FACP, FRACP
Director, MacFarlane Burnet Centre for Medical Research; Professor of Microbiology, Melbourne and Monash Universities, Fairfield, Victoria, Australia.

G. Richard O'Connor, MD
Professor Emeritus, Department of Ophthalmology, University of California, San Francisco.

Joost J. Oppenheim, MD
Chief, Laboratory of Immunoregulation, National Cancer Institute, Frederick, Maryland.

Hillel S. Panitch, MD
Professor of Neurology, University of Maryland School of Medicine and VA Medical Center, Baltimore, Maryland.

Thomas F. Patterson, MD
Associate Professor of Medicine, The University of Texas Health Science Center, San Antonio, Texas.

Charles S. Pavia, PhD
Associate Professor of Microbiology, New York College of Osteopathic Medicine; Director, NYCOM Immunodiagnostic Laboratory, Old Westbury, New York.

Hal B. Richerson, MD
Professor, Division of Allergy-Immunology, Department of Internal Medicine, University of Iowa College of Medicine and University of Iowa Hospitals, Iowa City, Iowa.

R. P. Channing Rodgers, MD
National Library of Medicine, National Institutes of Health, Bethesda, Maryland.

Francis W. Ruscetti, PhD
Chief, Laboratory of Leukocyte Biology, DBS, NCI-FCRDC, Frederick, Maryland.

John L. Ryan, MD, PhD
Vice President, Clinical Development, Genetics Institute, Inc., Cambridge, Massachusetts.

Kenneth E. Sack, MD
Professor of Clinical Medicine; Director of Clinical Programs in Rheumatology, University of California, San Francisco.

John Schmitz, PhD
Clinical Assistant Professor of Microbiology Immunology, University of North Carolina Hospitals, Clinical Microbiology Immunology Laboratories, Chapel Hill.

E. Richard Stiehm, MD
Professor, Department of Pediatrics, UCLA School of Medicine, Los Angeles.

Peter Stock, MD
Transplantation Service, University of California, San Francisco.

Warren Strober, MD
Head, Mucosal Immunity Section, National Institute of Allergy and Infectious Diseases, National Institutes of Health, Bethesda, Maryland.

David W. Talmage, MD
Distinguished Professor, University of Colorado, Health Sciences Center, Denver.

Maurene Viele, MD
Assistant Professor, Department of Laboratory Medicine; Assistant Director, Transfusion Medicine, University of California, San Francisco.

David M. Ward, MB, ChB, FRCP
Professor of Clinical Medicine, Chief of Clinical Nephrology, Director of Dialysis and Pheresis Programs, University of California, San Diego.

H. James Wedner, MD
Professor of Medicine, Washington University School of Medicine, St. Louis, Missouri.

J. Vivian Wells, MD, FRACP, FRCPA, FACP
Senior Staff Specialist; Director, Clinical Immunology, Royal North Shore Hospital, St. Leonards, NSW, Australia.

Cornelia M. Weyand, MD, PhD
Associate Professor of Medicine, Mayo Medical School; Associate Professor of Immunology, Mayo Graduate School; Consultant, Department of Medicine, Division of Rheumatology, Mayo Clinic, Rochester, Minnesota.

Curtis B. Wilson, MD
Member, Department of Immunology, The Scripps Research Institute, La Jolla, California.

Alan Winkelstein, MD
Professor of Medicine, Hematology/Bone Marrow Transplant, University of Pittsburgh Medical Center, Pittsburgh, Pennsylvania.

Bruce U. Wintroub, MD
Executive Vice Dean, Professor of Dermatology, School of Medicine, University of California, San Francisco.

John L. Ziegler, MD
Professor, Department of Medicine, University of California, San Francisco.

Preface

The current edition bears a new title—*Medical Immunology*. We have made this change from *Basic & Clinical Immunology* after eight successful editions during a 20-year period. We believe that the new title more accurately reflects the emphasis of the book on human fundamental and clinical immunology and should serve as a better indication of its subject matter for potential readers.

The 9th edition of *Medical Immunology* continues the tradition of a popular textbook for health-care students and practitioners. It is designed to be a comprehensive treatise on immunology, accessible to the student and practitioner alike.

We recognize that immunology is a difficult subject because of its intrinsic complexity and vast array of new information, which accumulates at accelerating rates. The many authors and the editors of the book have made every effort to write in a readable style without sacrificing essential details.

Key features of the 9th edition are as follows:

- The first section has been extensively updated and revised under the guidance of Dr. Tristram Parslow. A new chapter, Fundamentals of Blood Cell Biology, has been added as an introduction to the cells of immunity.
- The book focuses mainly on human immunology. Nevertheless, results of critical experiments with animal models are included when they help explain human physiology or pathology.
- A new system of colored illustrations has been introduced. Attention to detail in the numerous figures is provided to clarify the sometimes confusing nature of various cells and processes in the immune system.
- Included for easy reference are an appendix that lists the most important CD (clusters of differentiation) cell markers and a key to the symbols used throughout the book.
- The sections and chapters are organized to emphasize a logical progression from normal immune function to laboratory abnormalities to, eventually, clinical diseases.

The book comprises four sections, including Basic Immunology, Immunologic Laboratory Tests, Clinical Immunology, and Immunologic Therapy.

Section I, Basic Immunology, is a concise but thorough overview of the science of immunology. Designed to be both authoritative and accessible, it can serve as either a textbook for introductory courses or a state-of-the-art review and reference source for practicing physicians, immunologists, and scientists from other fields. The section opens with a new chapter that reviews the key molecular processes governing intercellular communication, signal transduction, mitosis, and cell death as they apply to blood cell biology. Chapter 2 offers an expanded discussion of innate immunity, emphasizing the roles of phagocytic cells in host defense. This is followed, in Chapters 3 through 13, by detailed explorations of lymphocyte biology; antigen presentation; humoral, cellular, and mucosal immune responses; inflammation; complement; and the cytokines. The expert authors of each chapter (several of whom are new for this edition) have worked to ensure timely and complete coverage of each topic, as well as a clear, logical presentation that will benefit readers encountering this material for the first time. Major themes are revisited with increasing sophistication in successive chapters, and a list of references is presented at the end of each chapter for readers wishing to explore these subjects further. Our goal has been to present an engaging, well-integrated distillation of current knowledge in immunobiology as a basis for modern clinical practice and as a means for staying abreast of future advances in this fast-moving field.

Section II, Immunologic Laboratory Tests, provides a bridge between basic immunology and the clinical sections that follow. Extensive descriptions of traditional immunochemical and cellular immunologic laboratory tests are given. The section emphasizes both clinical laboratory evaluation of patients with immune disorders and tests that use immunologic analytic procedures. Important areas of immunogenetics, histocompatibility, immunohematology, and blood banking are discussed. An entire chapter emphasizes the important new and developing area of molecular immunology testing. A brief chapter on the evaluation of immune competence in patients ends this section.

Section III, Clinical Immunology, encompasses broad areas of clinical practice in categories based on mechanisms of disease production. The chapters on Immunodeficiency Diseases emphasize, in particular, the congenital diseases with up-to-date information about genetic defects. The category of Allergic Diseases is divided into chapters on the basis of the underlying immunologic pathogenesis. Disordered Immune Regulation covers this large and heterogeneous group of diseases by organ systems, as in previous editions. Neoplasms of the Immune System is an overview of the salient immune-related features of leukemias and lymphomas and their relationship to the normal immune system. The final category, Immunity to Infection, comprehensively covers the primary role of the human immune system in protection against the deleterious effects of living pathogens.

Section IV, Immunologic Therapy, is a pharmacopoeia of drugs and other treatment modalities currently used in immunologic diseases. This section also discusses various strategies for manipulation of the immune system to treat other diseases, particularly infections and cancer. Such methods include immunization, immune suppression, and immune modulation.

ACKNOWLEDGMENTS

The editors are deeply grateful to John Dolan for his expertise and advice during the preparation of this 9th edition. The meticulous editing skills of Linda Davoli and the artistic illustrations of Linda F. Harris and Shirley Bortoli, who also introduced color to the art, greatly enhance the text. We would like to thank Dr. Steve Rosen and Dr. Richard Locksley of UCSF for their helpful discussions on some of the chapters in Section I. Finally, the authors and editors are indebted to the editorial staff of Appleton & Lange, particularly Deborah Feher, Maggie Darrow, Chris Langan, and Joann Allen, for their efforts and patience.

Recommendations about diagnosis and treatment of disease are based on the best scientific and clinical information currently available. These are intended, however, as guidance to the clinician and not necessarily as recommendations for specific cases. Furthermore, we recognize that we may have overlooked errors despite our best efforts. We would be grateful if our readers would point these out so that they may be corrected in the next edition.

Daniel P. Stites, MD
Abba I. Terr, MD
Tristram G. Parslow, MD, PhD

San Francisco
March 1997

History of Immunology

David W. Talmage, MD

THE ORIGIN OF IMMUNOLOGY

Immunology began as a branch of microbiology; it grew out of the study of infectious diseases and the body's responses to them. The concepts of contagion and the germ theory of disease are attributed to Girolamo Fracastoro, a colleague of Copernicus at the University of Padua, who wrote in 1546 that "Contagion is an infection that passes from one thing to another . . . The infection is precisely similar in both the carrier and the receiver of the contagion . . . The term is more correctly used when infection originates in very small imperceptible particles." Fracastoro's conclusions were remarkable because they were contrary to the philosophy of his time in that he postulated the existence of germs that were too small to be seen. He was a practical physician who gave more credence to his own observations than to traditional beliefs.

It was more than two centuries later that another physician, Edward Jenner, extended the concept of contagion to a study of the immunity produced in the host. This was the beginning of immunology. Jenner, a country doctor in Gloucestershire, England, noted in 1798 that a pustular disease of the hooves of horses called "the grease" was frequently carried by farm workers to the nipples of cows, where it was picked up by milkmaids. "Inflamed spots now begin to appear on the hands of the domestics employed in milking, and sometimes on the wrists . . . but what renders the Cowpox virus so extremely singular, is, that the person who has been thus affected is for ever after secure from the infection of Small Pox; neither exposure to the variolous effluvia, nor the insertion of the matter into the skin, producing this distemper."

Jenner was unclear about the nature of the infectious agent of cowpox and its relation to smallpox, but he reported 16 cases of resistance to smallpox in farm workers who had recovered from cowpox. He described how he deliberately inserted matter "taken from a sore on the hand of a dairymaid, on the 14th of May, 1796, into the arm of the boy by means of two superficial incisions, barely penetrating the cutis, each about half an inch long." Two months later, Jenner inoculated the same 8-year-old boy with matter from a smallpox patient, a dangerous but accepted procedure called **variolation.** The boy developed only a small sore at the site of inoculation, however. His exposure to the mild disease cowpox had made him immune to the deadly disease smallpox. In this manner Jenner began the science of immunology, the study of the body's response to foreign substances.

Immunology has always been dependent on technology, particularly lens-making and microscopy. Eyeglasses were introduced into Europe in the 14th century (perhaps by Marco Polo), and telescopes were used by Galileo in 1609 to discover the moons of Jupiter. Useful microscopes, however, were not available until the middle of the 19th century. After that, progress in microbiology was rapid. In 1850, Casimir Davaine reported that he could see anthrax bacilli in the blood of infected sheep. In 1858, Alfred Russel Wallace and Charles Darwin jointly submitted reports proposing evolution through natural selection, and in the same year, Louis Pasteur demonstrated to the French wine industry that fermentation was due to a living microorganism. In 1864, Pasteur disproved the theory of spontaneous generation; in 1867, Joseph Lister introduced aseptic surgery; and in 1871, DNA was discovered by Johann Miescher. Anthrax was first transmitted from in vitro culture to animals by Robert Koch in 1876, thus fulfilling **Koch's postulates,** which he had said were required to prove that the bacteria caused the disease. Between 1879 and 1881, Pasteur developed the first three attenuated vaccines (after cowpox); these were for chicken cholera, anthrax, and rabies.

Bacteriology and histology were recognized as established scientific fields during this period. The gonococcus, the first human pathogen, was isolated in 1879 by Albert Neisser, and 10 other pathogens were isolated in the next decade. Of particular importance to immunology was the isolation of the diphtheria bacillus by Theodor Klebs and Friederich Löffler in 1883; this led to the production of the first defined antigen, diphtheria toxin, by Emile Roux and A. J. E. Yersin in 1888. In that same year, the first antibodies, serum bactericidins, were reported by George Nuttall, and Pasteur recognized that nonliving substances as well as living organisms could induce immunity. This led to the discovery of antitoxins by Emil von Behring and Shibasaburo Kitasato in 1890 and later to the development of toxoids for diphtheria and tetanus.

CELLULAR VERSUS HUMORAL IMMUNITY

In 1883, Elie Metchnikoff observed the phagocytosis of fungal spores by leukocytes and advanced the idea that immunity was due primarily to white blood cells. This provoked an intense controversy with the advocates of **humoral immunity.** The discovery of complement in 1894 by Jules Bordet and **precipitins** in 1897 by Rudolf Kraus appeared to favor the humoral side of the controversy. Paul Ehrlich's side chain theory, proposed in 1898, was an attempt to harmonize the two views. According to Ehrlich, cells possessed on their surfaces a wide variety of side chains (we would call them antigen receptors) that were used to bring nutrients into the cell. When toxic substances blocked one of these side chains through an accidental affinity, the cell responded by making large numbers of that particular side chain, some of which spilled out into the blood and functioned as circulating antibodies.

In 1903, Sir Almoth Wright reported that antibodies could aid in the process of phagocytosis, thus effectively settling the controversy over cellular versus humoral community. Wright called these antibodies "opsonins." This followed the practice of labeling antibodies according to their observed action, for example, agglutinins, precipitins, hemolysins, and bactericidins.

It was gradually realized that antibodies could have deleterious as well as beneficial effects and could produce hypersensitivity. The term "anaphylaxis" was coined by Charles Richet and Paul Portier in 1902 to denote the frequently lethal state of shock induced by a second injection of antigen. The term "allergy" was introduced by Clemens von Pirquet in 1906 to denote the positive reaction to a scratch test with tuberculin in individuals infected with tuberculosis.

THE PERIOD OF SEROLOGY

Blood group antigens and their corresponding agglutinins were discovered by Karl Landsteiner in 1900. This led to the ability to give blood transfusions without provoking reactions. Landsteiner was a dominant figure in immunology for 40 years, developing the concept of the antigenic determinant and demonstrating the exquisite specificity of antibodies for chemically defined haptens, a term he applied to simple chemicals that could bind to antibodies but were by themselves incapable of stimulating antibody formation. Landsteiner rejected Ehrlich's side chain theory because he was able to make antibodies against a seemingly infinite number of different substances, synthetic as well as natural.

In 1901, Bordet and Octave Gengou introduced the complement fixation test, which became a standard diagnostic test in the hospital laboratory. The word "immunology" first appeared in the *Index Medicus* in 1910, and the *Journal of Immunology* began publication in 1916. The first 30 years of the Journal were devoted almost exclusively to a study of serologic reactions.

Landsteiner's book, *The Specificity of Serological Reactions,* was published in German in 1933 and in English in 1936. P. Marrack's text, *The Chemistry of Antigens and Antibodies,* was published in 1935. Antibodies were viewed as being formed directly on antigens, which functioned as templates, in a theory published by Friedrich Breinl and Felix Haurowitz in 1930. In 1939, Arne Wilhelm Tiselius and Elvin Kabat showed that antibodies were gamma globulins, and in 1940, L. Pauling proposed the variable-folding theory of antibody formation. According to Pauling's theory, gamma globulin peptides are folded into a complementary configuration in the presence of antigen. This fit the "unitarian" view of antibodies generally accepted at that time, which held that all antibodies were the same except for their specificity.

Immunochemistry was a natural outgrowth of this chemical approach to immunology. The quantitative precipitin test was developed by M. Heidelberger, Edward Kendall, and Kabat and was used to study the structure of polysaccharide antigens.

THE REBIRTH OF CELLULAR IMMUNOLOGY

Two events of 1941–1942 heralded the rediscovery of the cell by immunologists. Albert Coons demonstrated the presence of antigens and antibodies inside cells by the new technique of **immunofluorescence,** and Merrill Chase and Landsteiner reported that delayed hypersensitivity could be transferred by cells but not by serum. The very next year (1943) O. T. Avery, C. M. MacCleod, and M. McCarty reported that DNA was responsible for the transfer of hereditary traits in bacteria.

In 1945, Ray Owen discovered blood chimeras in cattle twins, and in 1948, Astrid Fagraeus showed that antibodies were made in plasma cells. In 1949,

Macfarlane Burnet and Frank Fenner published their adaptive enzyme theory of antibody formation, which again established immunology as a biologic science. They also proposed the "self-marker" concept, which was the first formal explanation of self-tolerance.

In 1953, Rupert Billingham, Leslie Brent, and Peter Medawar demonstrated acquired immunologic tolerance in bone marrow chimeras in mice injected with allogeneic bone marrow at or before birth. In that same year, James Watson and Francis Crick described the double helix of DNA. The close association in the development of immunology and molecular biology is illustrated by these two discoveries. Two years later, Niels Jerne proposed his natural selection theory of antibody formation, in which randomly diversified gamma globulin molecules were thought to replicate after binding to injected antigen. Jerne's theory explained the known facts of immunology of that time, such as immunologic memory and the logarithmic rate of rise of antibody. This theory was incompatible, however, with the new concepts of cellular and molecular biology. Within 2 years, two new theories of antibody production were proposed, the first by David Talmage and the second by Burnet. Both theories substituted randomly diversified cells for randomly diversified gamma globulin molecules and proposed that the interaction of antigen with receptors on the cell surface stimulated antibody production and the replication of the selected cell.

After more than 30 years, the cell selection theory and the name given to it by Burnet—**clonal selection**—have become part of the established dogma of immunology. This theory has been confirmed by numerous experiments and was popularized in 1975 by the development of Georges Köhler and Cesar Milstein of the technique of producing monoclonal antibodies.

Cellular immunology reached its zenith in 1966 with the discovery by Henry Claman, E. A. Chaperon, and R. F. Triplett of the presence and cooperation of **B cells** and **T cells.** Since that time, the study of the development, specificity, and activation of B cells and T cells has occupied the energy of a great many immunologists.

THE ADVENT OF MOLECULAR IMMUNOLOGY

By 1959, the field of protein chemistry had reached the point at which it was possible to analyze the structure of the antibody molecule in detail. In that same year, the three fragments of immunoglobulins—two Fabs and one Fc—were separated by Rodney Porter, and the heavy and light chains were separated by Gerald Edelman. The discovery of common and variable regions by F. Putnam and by N. Hilschmann and L. Craig came in 1965. Edelman and colleagues reported the first complete amino acid sequence of an immunoglobulin molecule in 1969.

The 1960s and 1970s saw similar advances in the identification, separation, and characterization of other molecules important to the immune system, such as complement components, interleukins, and cell receptors. These studies were greatly enhanced by the application of monoclonal antibody technology, which allowed sensitive and specific identification and isolation of many such molecules.

The first monoclonal antibody identifying a T-cell subset (OKT4, now called CD4) was described by Patrick Kung and associates in 1979. The elusive T-cell receptor was finally isolated in 1982–1983 by James Allison and colleagues and Kathryn Haskins and associates. The steps required for antigen processing and presentation and the chemical reactions required for lymphocyte activation by antigen were also elucidated.

IMMUNOGENETICS & GENETIC ENGINEERING

The major histocompatibility antigens were discovered by P. A. Gorer in 1936, but it was not until 1968 that Hugh McDevitt and Marvin Tyan showed that immune response genes were linked to the genes of the major histocompatibility complex. Six years later, Peter Doherty and Rolf Zinkernagel reported that the recognition of antigen by T cells was restricted by major histocompatibility complex molecules. During this time, the technology of recombinant DNA was developed. This led to the demonstration of immunoglobulin gene rearrangement by Susumu Tonegawa in 1978 and the production of transgenic mice by Jon Gordon and colleagues in 1980. The identification of genes for the T-cell receptor by Mark Davis and Tak Mak and coworkers came in 1984.

It is too early to tell where the revolution in genetics will go. History may mark as important the decision of the National Institutes of Health to create the human genome project. Although far from complete, the project has already led to numerous important findings.

IMMUNOLOGY TIME LINE

1798   Edward Jenner
        Cowpox vaccination.

1880   Louis Pasteur
        Attenuated vaccines.

1883   Elie I. I. Metchnikoff
        Phagocytic theory.

1888   P. P. Emile Roux and A. E. J. Yersin
        Bacterial toxins.

1888   George H. F. Nuttall
        Bactericidal antibodies.

1890   Robert Koch
        Hypersensitivity.

1890   Emil A. von Behring and Shibasaburo
        Kitasato
        Diphtheria antitoxin.

1894   Jules J. B. V. Bordet
        Complement.

1897   Rudolf Kraus
        Precipitins.

1898   Paul Ehrlich
        Side chain theory.

1900   Karl Landsteiner
        Blood group antigens and antibodies.

1902   Charles R. Richet and Paul J. Portier
        Anaphylaxis.

1903   Almoth E. Wright
        Opsonins.

1905   Clemens P. von Pirquet and Bela Schick
        Serum sickness.

1906   Clemens P. von Pirquet
        Allergy.

1930   Friedrich Breinl and Felix Haurowitz
        Template theory.

1939   Arne Wilhelm Tiselius and Elvin A. Kabat
        Identity of antibodies with gamma globulins.

1941   Albert H. Coons et al
        Immunofluorescence.

1942   Karl Landsteiner and Merrill W. Chase
        *Transfer of delayed-type hypersensitivity
        with cells.*

1945   Ray D. Owen
        Chimeras in bovine twins.

1948   Astrid E. Fagraeus
        Antibodies in plasma cells.

1949   F. Macfarlane Burnet and Frank Fenner
        Adaptive enzyme theory.

1953   Rupert E. Billingham, Leslie Brent, and Peter
        B. Medawar
        Bone marrow chimeras in mice.

1955   Niels K. Jerne
        Natural selection theory.

1957   David W. Talmage and F. Macfarlane Burnet
        Cell selection theories.

1959   Rodney R. Porter and Gerald M. Edelman
        Structure of antibodies.

1966   Henry N. Claman et al
        Cooperation of T and B cells.

1968   Hugh O. McDevitt and Marvin L. Tyan
        *Linkage of immune response genes to major
        histocompatibility complex genes.*

1974   Peter C. Doherty and Rolf M. Zinkernagel
        T-cell restriction.

1975   Cesar Milstein and Georges J. F. Köhler
        Monoclonal antibodies.

1978   Susumu Tonegawa
        Immunoglobulin gene rearrangement.

1979   Patrick Kung, Gideon Goldstein, Ellis
        Reinherz, and Stuart Schlossman
        *Monoclonal antibody to CD4 marker on T
        cells.*

1980   Jon W. Gordon et al
        Transgenic mice.

1983   James Allison, Kathryn Haskins et al
        T-cell receptor isolation.

1984   Mark Davis et al and Tak Mak et al
        T-cell receptor genes.

NOBEL PRIZE WINNERS
IN IMMUNOLOGY

1901   EMIL ADOLF von BEHRING for his work
        on serum therapy, especially application
        against diphtheria.

1905   ROBERT KOCH for his investigations and
        discoveries in relation to tuberculosis.

1908   PAUL EHRLICH and ELIE METCH-
        NIKOFF for their work on immunity.

1913   CHARLES ROBERT RICHET for his work
        on anaphylaxis.

1919 JULES BORDET for his discoveries relating to immunity, particularly complement.

1928 CHARLES JULES HENRI NICOLLE for his work on typhus.

1930 KARL LANDSTEINER for his discovery of human blood groups.

1960 FRANK MACFARLANE BURNET and PETER BRIAN MEDAWAR for their discovery of acquired immunologic tolerance.

1972 GERALD MAURICE EDELMAN and RODNEY ROBERT PORTER for their discoveries concerning the chemical structure of antibodies.

1977 ROSALYN YALOW for the development of radioimmunoassays of peptide hormones.

1980 BARUJ BENACERRAF, JEAN DAUSSET, and GEORGE DAVIS SNELL for their discoveries concerning genetically determined structures on the cell surface that regulate immunologic reactions.

1984 NIELS K. JERNE, GEORGES F. KÖHLER, and CESAR MILSTEIN for theories concerning the specificity in development and control of the immune system and the discovery of the principle for production of monoclonal antibodies.

1987 SUSUMU TONEGAWA for his discovery of the genetic principle for generation of antibody diversity.

1990 JOSEPH E. MURRAY and E. DONNALL THOMAS for their work on human organ and cell transplantation.

SUMMARY

Immunology began as a study of the response of the whole animal to infection. Over the years, it has become progressively more basic, passing through phases of emphasis on serology, cellular immunology, molecular immunology, and immunogenetics. At the same time, immunology has grown to encompass many fields, such as allergy, clinical immunology, immunochemistry, immunopathology, immunopharmacology, tumor immunology, and transplantation. Thus, it has always provided an excellent mix of fundamental and applied science.

Immunology has always depended on and stimulated the application of technology, such as the use of microscopy, electrophoresis, radiolabeling, immunofluorescence, recombinant DNA, and transgenic mice. In general, immunology has not become an inbred discipline but has maintained close associations with many other fields of medical science. From a base in microbiology, immunologists have spread out into all of the basic and clinical departments.

REFERENCES

Alexander HL: The history of allergy. In: *Immunological Diseases.* Samter M (editor). Little Brown, 1965.

Allison JP et al: Tumor specific antigen of murine T-lymphoma defined with monoclonal antibody. *J Immunol* 1982;**129**:2293.

Billingham RE, et al: Actively acquired tolerance of foreign cells. *Nature* 1953;**172**:603.

Bordet J: *Traite de L'Immunité dans les Maladies infectieuses,* 2nd ed. Masson, 1937.

Brack C et al: A complete immunoglobulin gene is created by somatic recombination. *Cell* 1978;**15**:1.

Burnet FM: A modification of Jerne's theory of antibody production using the concept of clonal selection. *Aust J Sci* 1957;**20**:67.

Burnet FM, Fenner F: *The Production of Antibodies.* Macmillan (Melbourne), 1949.

Claman HN et al: Thymus-marrow cell combination. Synergism in antibody production. *Proc Soc Exp Biol Med* 1966;**122**:1167.

Coons AH et al: Immunological properties of an antibody containing a fluorescent group. *Proc Soc Exp Biol Med* 1941;**47**:200.

Doherty PC, Zinkernagel RM: T-cell mediated immunopathology in viral infections. *Transplant Rev* 1974;**19**:89.

Dubos R: *The Unseen World.* Rockefeller Univ Press, 1962.

Edelman GM: Dissociation of gamma globulin. *J Am Chem Soc* 1959;**81**:3155.

Ehrlich P: On immunity with special reference to cell life. *Proc R Soc London Ser B* 1900;**66**:424.

Fagraeus A: The plasma cellular reaction and its relation to the formation of antibodies in vitro. *J Immunol* 1948;**58**:1.

Foster WD: *A History of Medical Bacteriology and Immunology.* Heineman, 1970.

Gay FP: Immunology, a medical science developed through animal experimentation. *J Am Med Assoc* 1911;**56**:578.

Gordon JW et al: Genetic transformation of mouse embryos by microinjection of purified DNA. *Proc Natl Acad Sci USA* 1980;**77**:7380.

Haskins K et al: The major histocompatibility complex restricted antigen receptor on T cells. I. Isolation with a monoclonal antibody. *J Exp Med* 1983;**157**:1149.

Hedrick SM et al: Isolation of cDNA clones encoding T

cell-specific membrane-associated proteins. *Nature* 1984;**308**:149.

Jerne NK: The natural selection theory of antibody formation. *Proc Natl Acad Sci USA* 1955;**41**:849.

Köhler G, Milstein C: Continuous culture of fused cells secreting antibody of predefined specificity. *Nature* 1975;**256**:495.

Kung PC et al: Monoclonal antibodies defining distinctive human T cell antigens. *Science* 1979;**206**:347.

Landsteiner K: *The Specificity of Serological Reactions.* Thomas, 1936; reissued by Dover, 1962.

Landsteiner K, Chase MW: Experiments on transfer of cutaneous sensitivity to simple compounds. *Proc Soc Exp Biol Med* 1942;**49**:688.

McDevitt HO, Tyan ML: Transfer of response by spleen cells and linkage to the major histocompatibility (H-2) locus. *J Exp Med* 1968;**128**:1.

Parrish HJ: *A History of Immunization.* E & S Livingstone, 1965.

Parrish HJ: *Victory with Vaccines.* E & S Livingstone, 1968.

Pauling L: A theory of the structure and process of formation of antibodies. *J Am Chem Soc* 1940;**62**:2643.

Porter RR: The hydrolysis of rabbit gamma globulin and antibodies with crystalline papain. *Biochem J* 1959;**73**:119.

Talmage DW: Allergy and immunology. *Ann Rev Med* 1957;**8**:239.

Talmage DW: A century of progress: Beyond molecular immunology. *J Immunol* 1988;**141**(Suppl):S5.

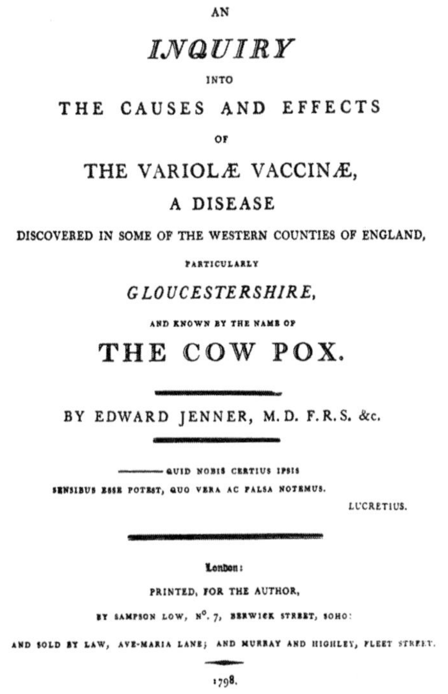

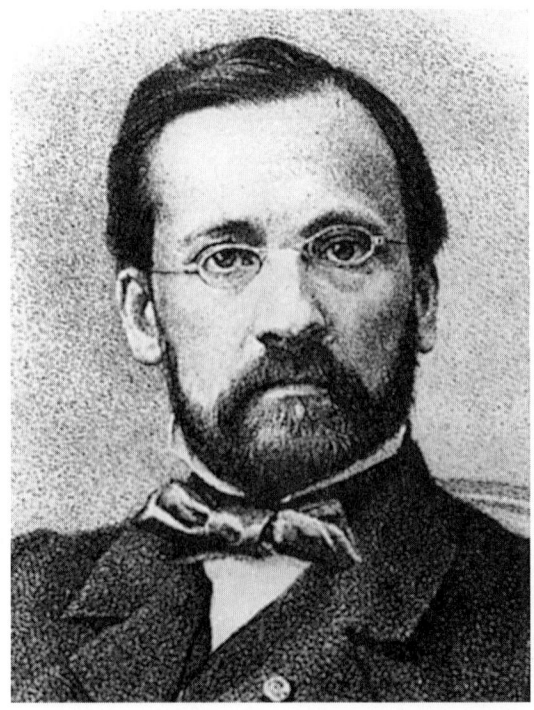

AN

INQUIRY

INTO

THE CAUSES AND EFFECTS

OF

THE VARIOLÆ VACCINÆ,

A DISEASE

DISCOVERED IN SOME OF THE WESTERN COUNTIES OF ENGLAND,

PARTICULARLY

GLOUCESTERSHIRE,

AND KNOWN BY THE NAME OF

THE COW POX.

BY EDWARD JENNER, M.D. F.R.S. &c.

——— QUID NOBIS CERTIUS IPSIS
SENSIBUS ESSE POTEST, QUO VERA AC FALSA NOTEMUS.
LUCRETIUS.

London:

PRINTED, FOR THE AUTHOR,

BY SAMPSON LOW, N°. 7, BERWICK STREET, SOHO:

AND SOLD BY LAW, AVE-MARIA LANE; AND MURRAY AND HIGHLEY, FLEET STREET.

1798.

Figure 1. Face plate from first edition (1798) of Jenner's inquiry into the Causes and Effects of . . . the Cow Pox.

Figure 2. Louis Pasteur (1822–1895). (Courtesy of the Museum of the Pasteur Institute, Paris.)

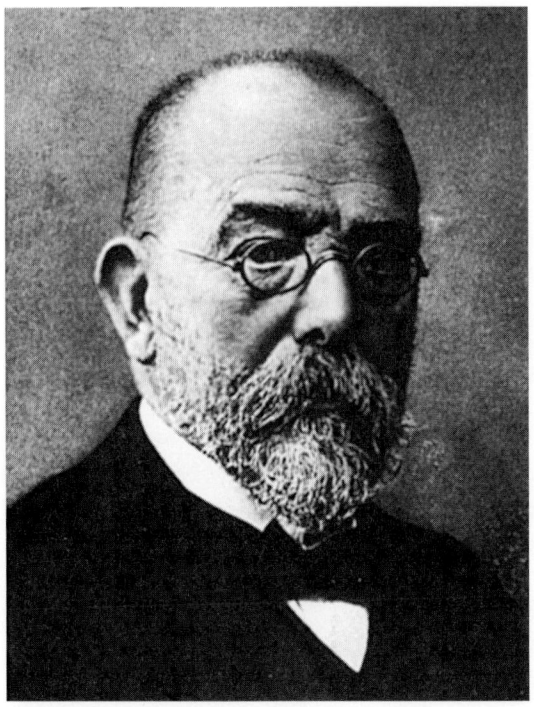

Figure 3. Robert Koch (1843–1910). (Courtesy of the Museum of the Pasteur Institute, Paris.)

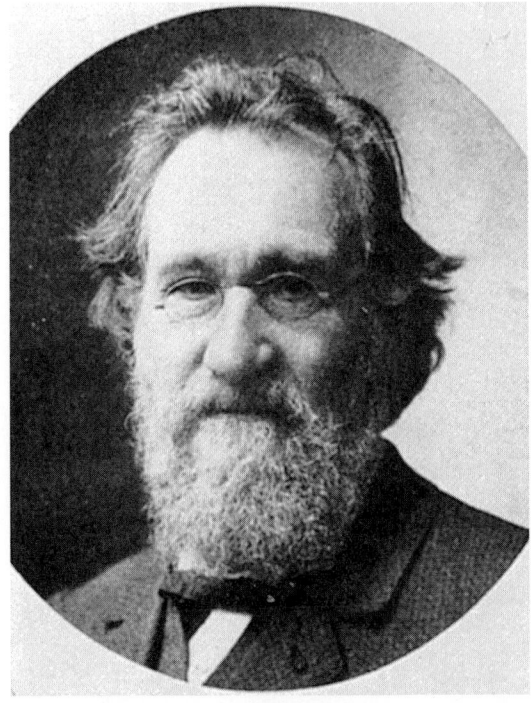

Figure 4. Elie Metchnikoff (1845–1916). (Courtesy of the Rare Book Library, the University of Texas Medical Branch, Galveston.)

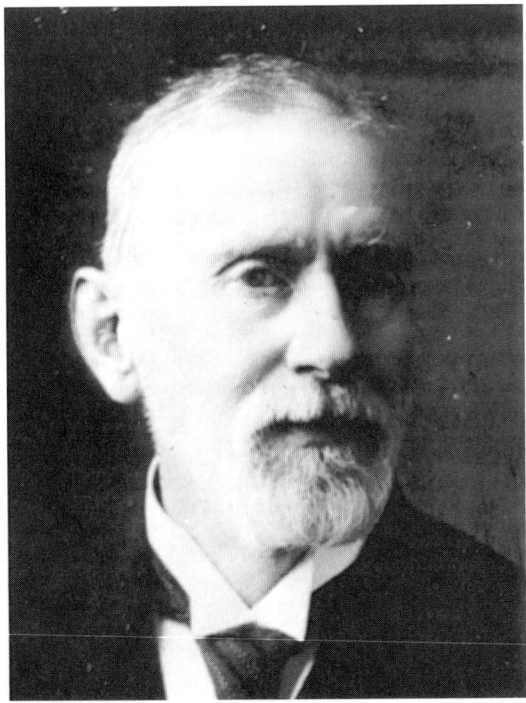

Figure 5. Paul Ehrlich (1854–1915). (Courtesy of the Museum of the Pasteur Institute, Paris.)

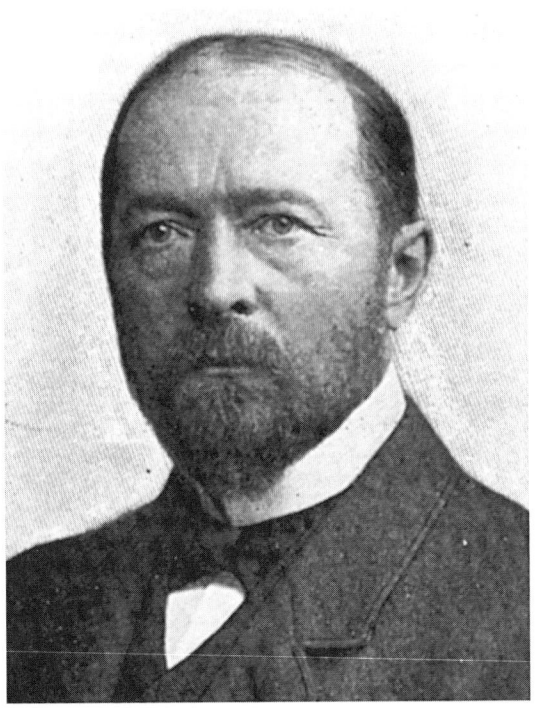

Figure 6. Emil von Behring (1854–1917). (Courtesy of the Museum of the Pasteur Institute, Paris.)

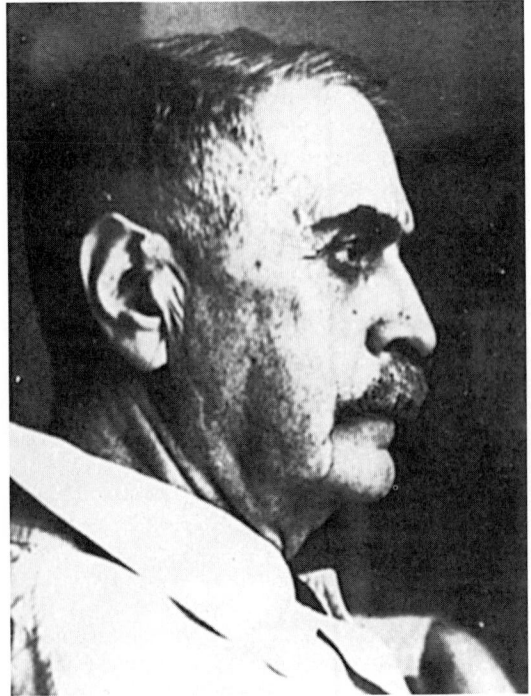

Figure 7. Karl Landsteiner (1868–1943). (Courtesy of the Museum of the Pasteur Institute, Paris.)

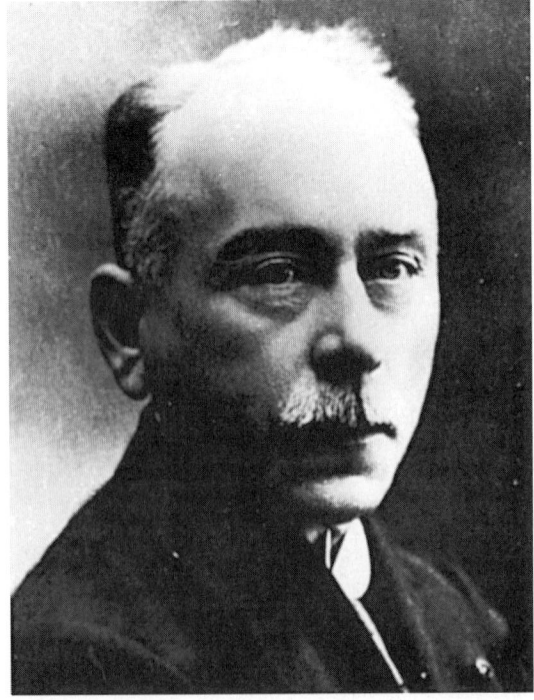

Figure 8. Jules Bordet (1870–1961). (Courtesy of the Museum of the Pasteur Institute, Paris.)

Section I.
Basic Immunology

Fundamentals of Blood Cell Biology

1

Clifford Lowell, MD, PhD

Immunology is the study of the ways in which the body defends itself from infectious agents and other foreign substances in its environment. Broadly defined, the field encompasses many layers of defense, including physical barriers like the skin, protective chemical substances in the blood and tissue fluids, and the physiologic reactions of tissues to injury or infection. But by far the most elaborate, dynamic, and effective defense strategies are carried out by cells that have evolved specialized abilities to recognize and eliminate potentially injurious substances. Some of these defensive cells circulate continually through the body in search of foreign invaders; others are stationary sentinels that lie in wait in solid tissues or at body surfaces. Because of their central roles in host defense, these cells are the major focus of contemporary immunology and are the principal subjects of this book.

Virtually all of the specialized defensive cells have two things in common: they all spend at least part of their lives in the bloodstream, and they are all ultimately derived from cells produced in the bone marrow. We therefore begin, in this chapter, by considering the processes involved in cell formation and maturation in the bone marrow—one of the most prolific sites of cell replication in the human body, and one that is indispensible for health and even for survival. This provides an opportunity to introduce many of the individual cell types that are involved in host defense, as well as several types of regulatory factors that govern their lives. We will also examine the fundamental molecular mechanisms by which cells receive signals from their environments and how these signals control whether cells proliferate, migrate, and carry out specific functions, and even when they die.

HEMATOPOIESIS

Origins of Cells in the Blood & Bone Marrow

The process by which blood cells grow, divide, and differentiate in the bone marrow is called **hematopoiesis.** Three general classes of cells are produced: (1) red blood cells (erythrocytes), responsible for oxygen transport; (2) platelets, responsible for the control of bleeding; and (3) white blood cells **(leukocytes),** the vast majority of which are involved in host defense. All three classes are ultimately derived from a pool of pleuripotent **hematopoietic stem cells (HSCs),** which reside in the marrow and have the unique ability to give rise to all of the different mature blood cell types, under the appropriate conditions. The HSCs are **self-renewing** cells: when they proliferate, at least some of their daughter cells remain as HSCs, so that the pool of stem cells does not become depleted.

The other daughters of HSCs, however, can each commit to any of several alternative differentiation pathways that lead to the production of one or more specific types of blood cells (Fig 1–1). A typical pathway involves several cycles of cell division (five or more) and proceeds in stages, with cells at each stage progressively acquiring features of one particular mature cell type while losing the capacity to form any others. Because progression along these pathways is coupled to cell division, the more mature forms greatly outnumber their less differentiated precursors. As the cells differentiate, however, their capacity for replication and self-renewal declines. Indeed, most types of hematopoietic cells lose replicative capacity altogether by the time they are fully mature, and so are said to be **terminally differentiated.** Thus, in general, the less differentiated cells

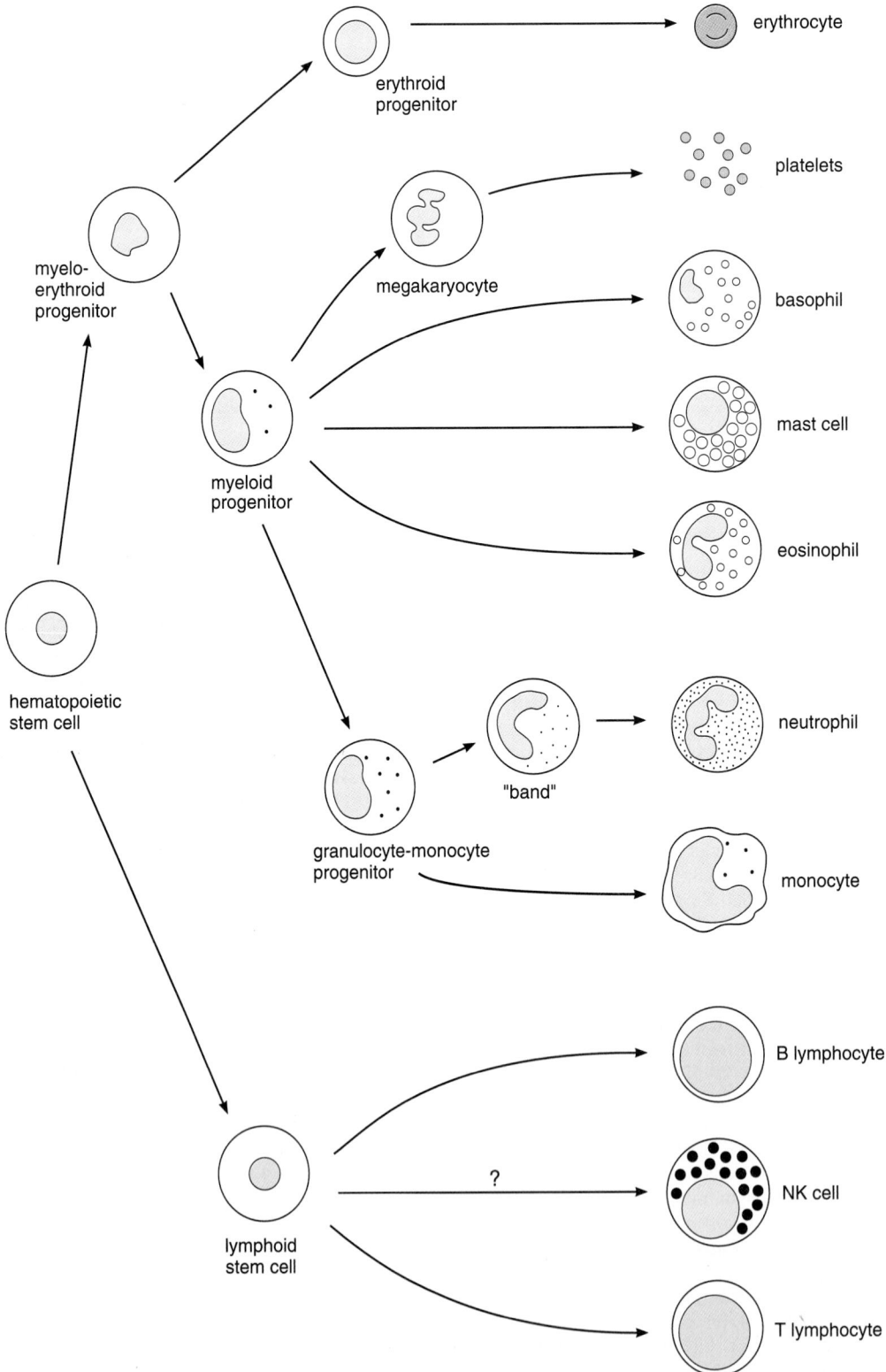

Figure 1–1. Schematic overview of hematopoiesis, emphasizing the erythroid, myeloid, and lymphoid pathways. This highly simplified depiction omits many recognized intermediate cell types in each pathway. All of the cells shown here develop to maturity in the bone marrow except T lymphocytes, which develop from marrow-derived progenitors that migrate to the thymus (see Chapter 3). A common lymphoid stem cell is believed to exist but has not yet been isolated. The histogenesis of natural killer (NK) cells is unknown.

in a given pathway are rare but replicate actively, whereas the mature cells are more numerous but mitotically inert.

The progeny of HSCs initially commit to one of three main alternative differentiation pathways (or **lineages**) that yield erythrocytes, lymphocytes, or myeloid cells, respectively. The most primitive cells in each lineage, called **lineage-committed progenitors,** cannot be identified morphologically; however, their existence and some of their properties can be inferred from their ability to generate particular types of mature cells in biologic assay systems (see later on). Erythrocyte development is outside the scope of this book and will not be considered further, but both myeloid cells and lymphocytes are critical to host defense. The mature cells of the myeloid lineage* include neutrophils, monocytes, mast cells, eosinophils, basophils, and megakaryocytes (the cells that produce platelets). All these cells descend from a common myeloid progenitor through a series of intermediate stages, only one of which—the granulocyte–monocyte progenitor, a precursor to both neutrophils and monocytes—is shown in Figure 1–1. Mature cells of the lymphocyte lineage include B lymphocytes, T lymphocytes, and possibly also natural killer (NK) cells; the development and functions of these three cell types is discussed in great detail in later chapters. Altogether, the myeloid and lymphocyte lineages account for roughly 60% and 15% of all marrow cells, respectively, the remainder being erythroid precursors.

Vast numbers of mature blood cells are produced daily in the marrow, but the rate of production of each cell type is precisely controlled and responsive to physiologic demands. For example, production of leukocytes often increases markedly during systemic infections, whereas red cell production can rise as a reaction to anemia. In addition, many mature leukocytes, particularly neutrophils, are stored in the marrow before being released into the bloodstream. This storage pool, which normally accounts for 10–20% of all marrow cells, provides a reservoir of mature defensive cells that can be mobilized rapidly in times of need. Thus, bone marrow hematopoiesis is precisely controlled at several levels, in order to (1) maintain an available pool of HSCs; (2) regulate the commitment, proliferation, and differentiation of cells at all stages of each hematopoietic pathway; and (3) modulate the activity of each pathway in response to physiologic demands. As we shall see, much of this regulation is achieved through physical interactions of the hematopoietic cells with other cells and with soluble factors in the surrounding tissues.

Ontogeny of Hematopoiesis

HSCs arise in the mesoderm of the yolk sac during the first weeks of embryonic life (Fig 1–2). Within 2 months following conception, most HSCs have migrated to the fetal liver, and it is here that the bulk of hematopoiesis occurs during fetal development. Most embryonic and fetal hematopoiesis is devoted to the production of red cells; platelet production first becomes apparent at 3 months of gestation, and leukocytes do not appear until the fifth month. Later in gestation, HSCs begin to colonize the developing bone marrow cavities throughout the skeleton, which contain a network of epithelial cells (called the **bone marrow stroma**) that provide the necessary environment for growth and differentiation of HSC and their progeny. By birth, virtually all of the marrow space is occupied by developing hematopoietic cells, giving the newborn child about the same hematopoietic capacity as his or her adult parents. Hematopoietic activity in the long bones then declines with age, so that after puberty hematopoiesis it is largely confined to the axial skeleton—the pelvis, sternum, ribs, vertebrae, and skull. If the bone marrow is injured by infection or malignancy, however, hematopoiesis can resume in the liver and spleen of an adult to maintain the supply of blood cells.

Hematopoietic Cell Growth & Differentiation

Our understanding of hematopoiesis has advanced greatly in recent years with the isolation and characterization of HSCs and the identification of many of the factors that influence the production and differen-

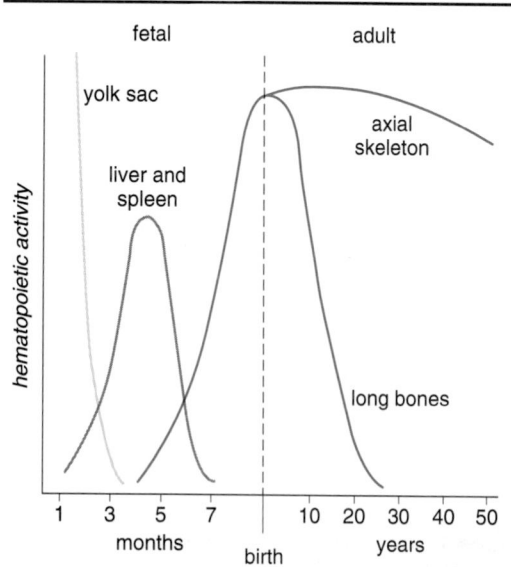

Figure 1–2. Tissue localization of hematopoiesis at various phases of prenatal and postnatal development in humans.

---

* The term *myeloid* means "of the bone marrow." As a group, cells of the myeloid lineage are the most abundant cells in the marrow.

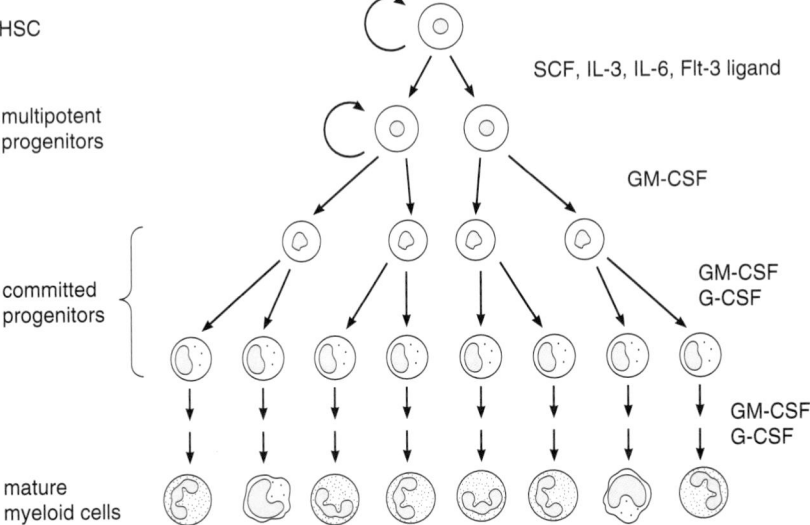

Figure 1–3. Proliferation and differentiation of cells in the myeloid lineage. Early cells are capable of self-renewal and proliferation; later cells are committed to differentiation only. Cytokines required for survival and progression through each stage are indicated at the right. Abbreviations: SCF = stem cell factor; IL = interleukin; G-CSF = granulocyte colony-stimulating factor; GM-CSF = granulocyte–monocyte colony–stimulating factor.

tiation of lineage-committed progenitors (Fig 1–3). HSCs are defined in theory by their abilities to self-renew throughout life and to give rise to committed progenitors that can differentiate along all of the possible hematopoietic lineages. They were first purified from mice as a tiny subpopulation of marrow cells that could completely reconstitute the bone marrows of other mice, whose own marrows had been destroyed by inherited mutations or by radiation. Although similar experiments cannot, of course, be done with human beings, presumptive human HSCs have since been identified that, under certain conditions, are able to repopulate the marrows of mice.

Human HSCs can be distinguished from other marrow cells by a characteristic protein, called **CD34,** expressed on their surface membranes. This is one of a large number of proteins that are each referred to by the initials **CD** (which stands for **cluster of differentiation**) followed by a unique identifying number. This CD system of nomenclature was originally developed for membrane proteins or protein complexes that could be identified by their physical properties (such as molecular weight) or by other means, but whose biologic functions had not yet been determined. Most CD proteins are not related to one another, either structurally or functionally. The CD nomenclature is most often used for proteins expressed on hematopoietic cells, although several of the proteins that carry CD designations are also expressed on one or more nonhematopoietic cell types.

Human HSCs characteristically express CD34 but do not express a different protein called CD38; hence, they are said to be CD34+CD38–. They are small, morphologically undistinguished cells, with round nuclei and scant cytoplasm, and are thought to comprise no more than 0.01% of all cells in the marrow. Surprisingly, although HSCs have enormous capacity for proliferation, most are mitotically inactive much of the time (in the terminology of the cell cycle, they are in a resting state called G_0, as will be discussed later). When removed from the body and cultured in vitro, however, HSCs can be induced to proliferate by treating them with large doses of certain hormonal factors, called **cytokines,** which are present in the marrow environment. The cytokines are a diverse family of polypeptide hormones that can be secreted individually by cells of one or more types and that each have specific effects on the growth, differentiation, or functions of other cells. There are several different classes of cytokines (see Chapter 10); most of those that are known to regulate hematopoiesis belong to subgroups called the **colony-stimulating factors (CSFs)** or the **interleukins.** The cytokines that can promote HSC growth in vitro include interleukin-3 (IL-3), granulocyte–monocyte colony-stimulating factor (GM-CSF), and a third cytokine called stem cell factor (SCF). It is believed that these and other cytokines, which are secreted by marrow stromal and hematopoietic cells, help regulate HSC proliferation in the bone marrow. Interestingly, HSC proliferation in vitro often produces lineage-committed progenitors and mature blood cells, confirming the linkage between proliferation and differentiation of these cells.

At any given moment, most mature blood cells of all types that are present in the circulation are descendants of a single HSC. This remarkable conclusion, termed the **clonal succession** model, emerged from studies in mice whose marrow cells had been genetically tagged in such a way that the progeny of any individual HSC could be distinguished from those of any other (Fig 1–4). Serial samples of hematopoietic cells taken from these animals revealed that most mature cells in any one sample were derived from the same HSC but that these cells disappeared over time

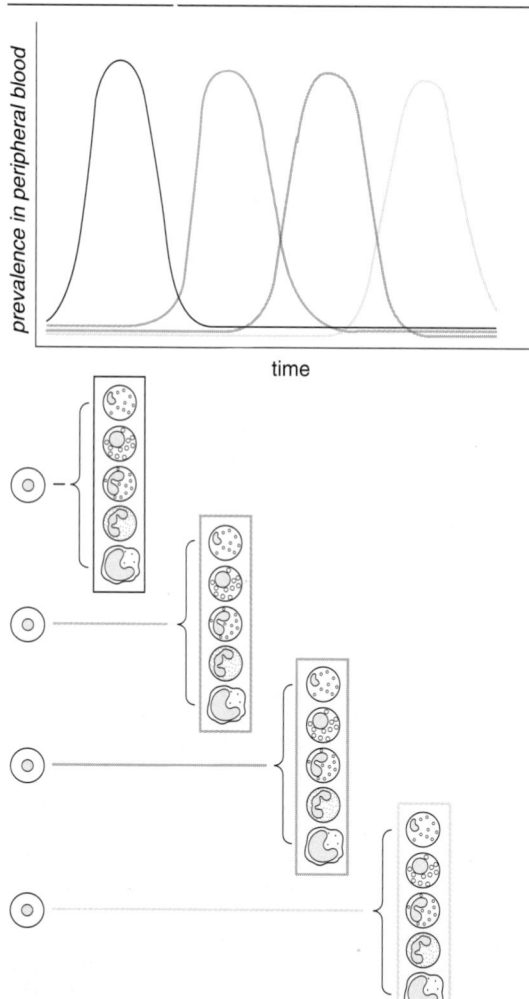

prevalence in peripheral blood

time

HSCs

Figure 1–4. Clonal derivation of peripheral blood cells from individual hematopoietic stem cells (HSCs). In this schematic illustration, most mature cells of all types in the circulation at any given moment are derived from a single HSC recruited from a preexisting pool. (Based on lineage-marking studies by Lemischka IR et al: Developmental potential and dynamic behavior of hematopoietic stem cells. Cell 1986;45:917.)

and were replaced by the progeny of a different HSC. This suggests that the constant overall rate of cell production in the marrow actually results from successive waves of proliferation, as individual HSCs become activated asynchronously, replicate prodigiously to yield mature progeny of all lineages, and then subside.

The factors that control the successive activation of HSCs, and that determine whether an individual HSC daughter cell will commit to differentiation, are presently unknown. A more complete understanding of these and other elements of HSC biology could be extremely valuable for clinical medicine, because of the potential that human HSCs could be propagated in vitro and used to restore hematopoiesis in individuals whose bone marrow has been damaged by disease or by the cytotoxic agents used to treat cancer. Moreover, if methods can be perfected for introducing exogenous genes into HSCs, these cells offer a very appealing target for **gene therapy** approaches to genetic and malignant disease.

Lineage-committed progenitors, the offspring of HSCs, are defined as those cells whose progeny include some, but not all, mature blood cell types. They are often subclassified as either "fully committed progenitors," which give rise to only one particular cell type, or "multipotent progenitors," which can generate two or more. An example of the latter is the granulocyte–monocyte progenitor, which gives rise to both neutrophils and monocytes (see Fig 1–1). Because such progenitors grow readily in tissue culture, they are comparatively easy to study experimentally, and it is from such cultures that most of our knowledge of human progenitor cells has been gained. For example, when a mixed population of bone marrow cells is cultured as a suspension in agar or some other semisolid medium, in the presence of specific cytokines, a few grow to produce small multicellular colonies composed of one or more mature cell types. Such experiments are called *colony-forming assays,* and the progenitors themselves are often referred to as **colony-forming units (CFUs).** Using these assays, individual cytokines have been shown to promote the growth of specific types of progenitors: for example, a CSF called erythropoietin (EPO) enhances production of erythrocyte colonies; interleukin-5 (IL-5) favors colonies of eosinophils; and GM-CSF promotes colonies containing both neutrophils and macrophages (from either HSCs or mixed marrow populations).

Progenitors of all types together account for fewer than 1% of marrow cells, and fully committed progenitors are more abundant than the multipotent forms. Though comparatively rare, these marrow progenitors are the cells that give rise to the various common forms of cancer known as **leukemias**—malignant populations of leukocytes, usually from a particular hematopoietic lineage, that flood the marrow cavities and peripheral blood and that result from excessive proliferation of the progeny from a single founder cell. Most mature cell types in the marrow, despite their greater abundance, cannot give rise to leukemias, in part because they have lost the ability to proliferate.

CELLULAR INTERACTIONS IN THE BONE MARROW

Though it is commonly imagined that hematopoiesis takes place in a liquid environment resembling the blood, with progenitors responding mainly to soluble hormone-like cytokines, this is in fact not the case at all. It is much more accurate to think of the bone marrow as a solid tissue in which different types of hematopoietic cells develop in physically different locations. These microenvironments are visible in histologic sections of bone marrow, which reveal a patchwork of microscopic foci, each devoted to the production of a particular cell type (Fig 1–5). The bone marrow microenvironment is set up and maintained by bone marrow stromal cells. Within each microenvironment, contact of cells with one another or with proteins and other substances that make up the **extracellular matrix (ECM)** greatly facilitates cell division and differentiation.

The physiology of these marrow microenvironments can be studied in artificial systems, called long-term bone marrow cultures (LTBMCs), in which hematopoietic progenitor cells are grown in combination with marrow stromal cells, ECM components, and other factors. The conditions of these cultures can be optimized to support sustained growth and differentiation of either myeloid or lymphoid cells. Studies of such cultures have demonstrated that hematopoiesis depends not only on specific cytokines but also on a group of cell surface macromolecules, known as **adhesion molecules,** that allow different cell types to adhere stably to one another or to the ECM. Among the primary types of adhesive molecules on hematopoietic progenitor cells are the integrins, the selectins, and various forms of CD44. Each of these classes recognizes and binds specific ligands that are present either on the bone marrow stromal cells or in the ECM (Table 1–1).

The **integrins** are a group of heterodimeric proteins, each composed of α-chain and β-chain polypeptides. There are over 15 different integrin α chains and 7 β chains, and these can associate in various combinations to produce dimers with distinct binding properties that are expressed on different cell types. For example, hematopoietic progenitors express primarily $\alpha4\beta1$ and $\alpha5\beta1$ dimers. The integrins bind a variety of ECM proteins, as well as nonintegrin adhesion molecules such as vascular cell adhesion molecule 1 (**VCAM-1**) found on the stromal cell surface. These interactions allow progenitors to bind tightly to

the marrow stroma and are responsible for sequestering progenitor cells in the appropriate marrow microenvironments. When baboons are injected with reagents that interfere with binding by the integrin $\beta1$ chain, for example, large numbers of hematopoietic progenitors are released from the marrow into the peripheral circulation. Contact of an integrin with its ligand also transmits a signal into the integrin-expressing cell, and this signal can directly stimulate its growth or other activities. Consequently, reagents that block ligand binding by integrin $\alpha4$ or $\beta1$ chains in vitro cause progenitors not only to dissociate from the stroma but also to cease proliferation. $\beta1$ integrins have also been implicated in directing migration of HSCs from the yolk sac mesenchyme into the fetal liver during embryogenesis and, subsequently, of HSCs from the fetal liver to the bone marrow.

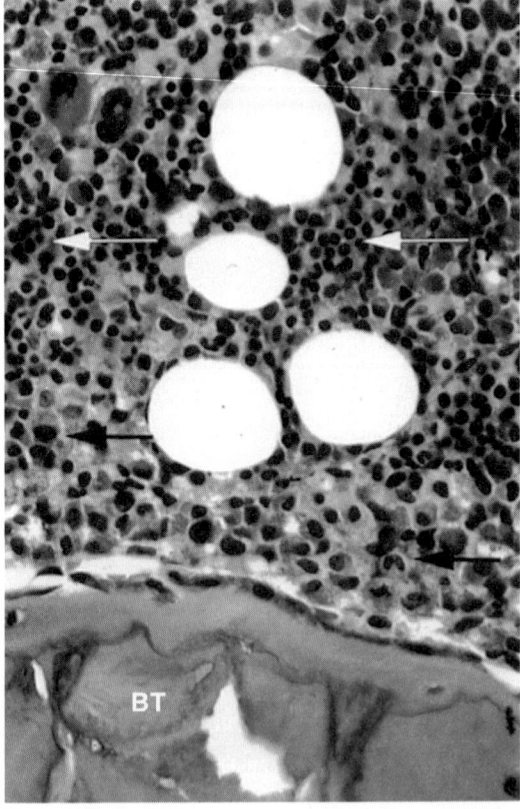

A

Figure 1–5. Bone marrow microenvironments. **A:** Regional variations in hematopoietic activity as demonstrated by histology. This section through a portion of a marrow cavity, stained with hematoxylin and eosin, shows a zone of predominantly myeloid cells (filled arrows) that is flanked on one side by a bone trabeculum (BT), and on the other by a zone of predominantly erythroid cells (open arrows). (Contributed by Susan Atwater.) *(Continued)*

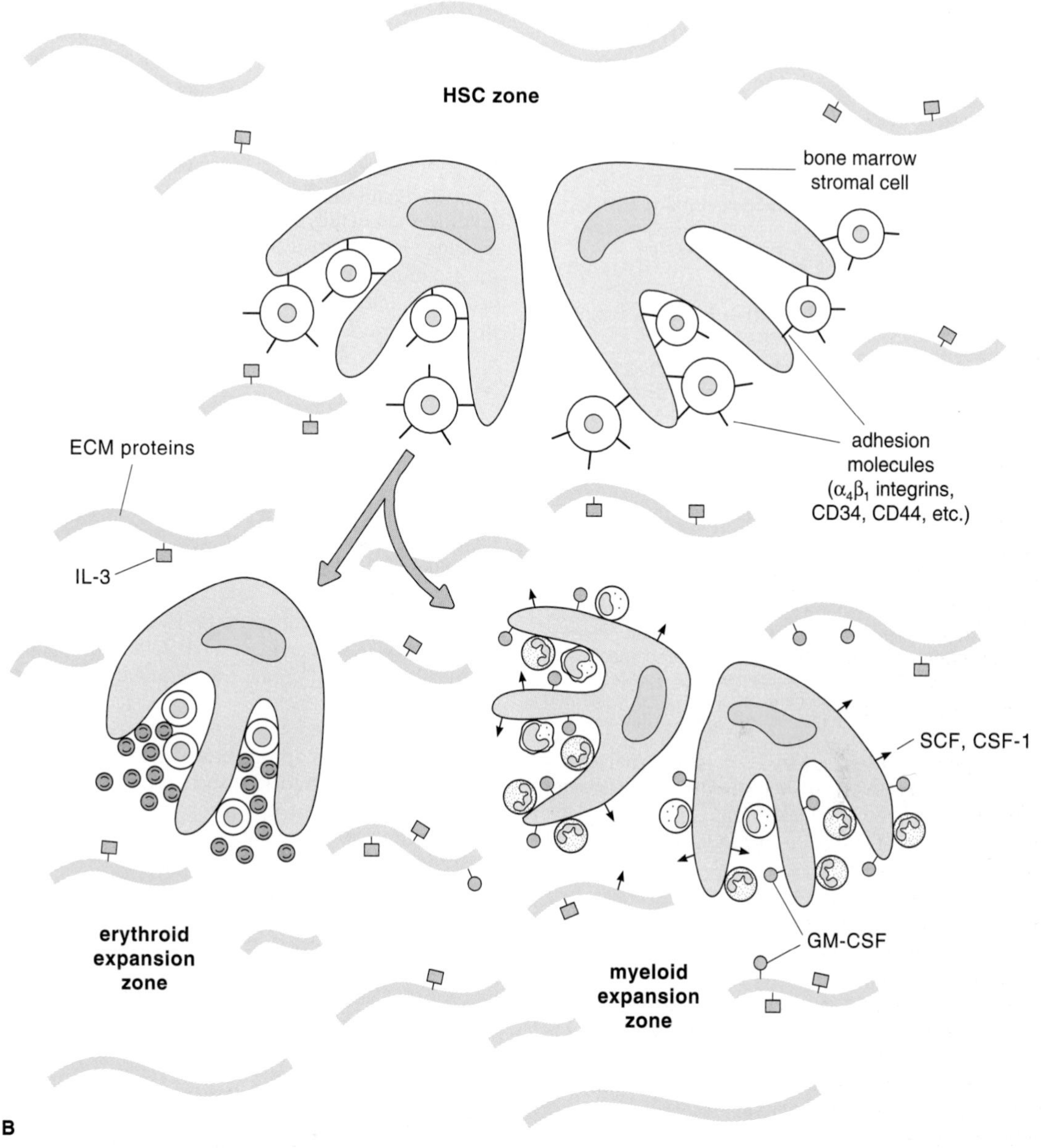

Figure 1–5 *(Continued)*. **B:** Model for the establishment of marrow microenvironments. Self-renewing pleuripotent hematopoietic stem cells (HSC), as well as lineage-committed progenitors, are localized to marrow niches based on the expression of specific surface adhesion molecules, such as integrins, CD34, and CD44. Different regions of the marrow serve as niches for myeloid or erythroid cell expansion based on expression of cell surface-bound cytokines (such as CSF-1 or SCF-1) on stromal cells or because of localized deposition of such cytokines in the extracellular matrix (ECM).

The **selectins** are a class of adhesion proteins that recognize specific oligosaccharide residues displayed on cell surface glycoproteins called **mucins.** The term *mucin* refers to any heavily glycosylated protein composed of an elongated polypeptide backbone containing many serine and threonine residues that serve as attachment sites for carbohydrate side chains. The se-

lectins bind primarily to sugar residues in the mucin side chains, though features of the polypeptide backbone may also contribute to recognition. One example of a mucin is the HSC surface marker CD34, which serves as a major ligand for L-selectin, a selectin found on all mature leukocytes. Marrow progenitor cells and stroma express various combinations of se-

Table 1–1. Selected adhesion proteins and their ligands.

Adhesion Protein	Principal Ligands
Integrins	ECM and cell surface proteins.
β1 family	
α1β1, α2β1, α6β1	Collagens, laminin.
α4β1, α5β1	Fibronectin, collagen, laminin, VCAM-1.
β2 family	
αLβ2	Fibrinogen, ICAM-1, ICAM-2.
αMβ2	Fibrinogen, ICAM-1, complement protein C3b.
αXβ2	Fibrinogen.
β3 family	
αvβ3	Vitronectin, thrombospondin, osteopontin.
Selectins[1]	Carbohydrate residues found on various cell surface mucins and other macromolecules.
L-selectin	CD34, GlyCAM-1, MAdCAM-1, and others.
E-selectin	CLA[2]
P-selectin	PSGL-1.
CD44[3]	Hyaluronic acid, collagen, fibronectin.

Abbreviations: ECM = extracellular matrix; VCAM-1 = vascular cell adhesion molecule 1; ICAM-1, -2 = intracellular adhesion molecules 1 and 2; GlyCAM-1 = glycosylated cell adhesion molecule 1; PSGL-1 = P-selectin glycoprotein ligand 1.
[1] The selectin ligands listed here are the major mucins and other macromolecules that carry the specific carbohydrate modifications recognized by each selectin and that serve as its main physiologic ligands in vivo.
[2] CLA denotes an incompletely characterized family of surface proteins on cutaneous lymphocytes.
[3] Multiple isoforms of CD44, with varying affinities for different ligands, are produced by alternative mRNA splicing.

lectins and mucins, which mediate cell–cell interactions between them. The importance of these carbohydrate-mediated interactions is illustrated by the finding that addition of synthetic oligosaccharides (which would competitively interfere with binding) to LTBMCs strongly inhibits hematopoietic cell division and differentiation. Selectins also play a critical role in the migration of hematopoietic cells from one body site to another, as will be discussed in Chapters 2 and 3.

The cell surface protein **CD44** can exist in a variety of alternative forms that differ in their extracellular ligand-binding regions (and hence in their binding specificities) as a result of alternative RNA splicing. Hematopoietic progenitor cells express the most truncated form of CD44, which binds hyaluronic acid, an abundant glycosaminoglycan found in the ECM. Compounds that interfere with this binding block hematopoietic cell proliferation in LTBMCs.

Thus, a wide variety of adhesive interactions, both of the cell–cell and cell–ECM variety, are critical for hematopoiesis. Abnormal interactions between hematopoietic progenitors and ECM components or stromal cells can be observed in many diseases that involve abnormal hematopoiesis. For example, the malignant cells in certain types of leukemias, particularly those arising from myeloid cells, often show significantly reduced adhesion to ECM proteins and stromal cells. Conversely, stromal cells from patients with leukemia often produce abnormal cytokines and ECM protein components.

Besides providing the appropriate adhesive and ECM molecules for progenitor cells, bone marrow stromal cells also synthesize and express a host of cytokines needed for hemotopoietic proliferation (Table 1–2). Some of these are not only secreted but also expressed as membrane-bound proteins that remain attached to the surface of the stromal cell. Much evidence suggests that these membrane-bound cytokines may have much greater biologic activity on hematopoietic progenitors than the secreted forms, presumably because the effective concentration of the cytokine is much higher on the stromal cell surface. In

Table 1–2. Major lineage-specific effects of the hematopoietic cytokines.[1]

Progenitors Affected	Cytokine	Principal Source
Multilineage		
Erythroid, myeloid, megakaryocyte	IL-3	Activated T lymphocytes.
Myeloid, megakaryocyte	GM-CSF	Stromal cells, activated macrophages.
Lineage-Restricted		
Granulocyte	G-CSF	Stromal cells, activated macrophages.
Monocyte	M-CSF (= CSF-1)	Stromal cells, endothelial cells, activated macrophages.
Eosinophils	IL-5	Activated T lymphocytes, mast cells.
Erythroid	EPO	Kidney epithelium.
Megakaryocyte	TPO	Stromal cells, liver
Lymphoid	IL-2	Activated T lymphocytes.
Synergistic		
All lineages	SCF	Stromal cells, endothelial cells, hepatocytes.
	IL-6	Fibroblasts, endothelial cells, stromal cells, activated macrophages.
	IL-1	Virtually all cell types.
	Flt-3 ligand	Stromal cells.

[1] Properties of most of these cytokines are considered in detail in Chapter 10.

addition, the strong adhesive contacts between the two cell types prolong the much weaker interaction between a membrane-bound cytokine and its receptor on the hematopoietic cell. In a similar fashion, IL-3, GM-CSF, and several other cytokines bind tightly to glycosaminoglycans and other components of the ECM, which immobilizes them, increases their local concentrations, and maximizes their availability to hematopoietic cells. Localized secretion of cytokines from stromal cells into the ECM may have a role in delineating specific microenvironments within the bone marrow.

HEMATOPOIETIC CYTOKINES & THEIR RECEPTORS

Cytokine Effects on Hematopoiesis

Hematopoietic progenitors depend on a variety of cytokines to control their growth and differentiation. These include several different types of CSFs and interleukins that each act on specific cell types to promote or inhibit particular types of responses. Detailed discussions of individual cytokines are presented in Chapter 10; for the present, we focus on general principles of cytokine action as illustrated in their effects on hematopoiesis.

In general terms, cytokines that influence hematopoiesis can be divided into three categories (see Table 1–2): those that act on multipotent progenitors, those that act on lineage-committed progenitors, and those that have little effect by themselves but dramatically augment or inhibit the effects of the preceding cytokines. These divisions are not absolute, however, and many cytokines could appropriately be assigned to more than one category. For example, GM-CSF supports proliferation of both multipotential progenitors and precursors committed to monocyte formation. Certain cytokines can also substitute for one another: for example, large doses of either IL-3 or GM-CSF can sustain HSC proliferation in vitro. Thus, it is important to recognize that the effects of cytokines often are redundant or overlap one another. In addition, many cytokines that influence hematopoiesis also can affect the functions of fully differentiated blood cells. GM-CSF, for example, is an important regulator of the defensive activities of mature neutrophils (see Chapter 2). Similarly, interleukin-2 (IL-2) promotes not only the development of lymphocytes but also many of their protective functions (see Chapters 3 and 4).

In light of these complexities, it is best to view the cytokines as acting in a cooperative, interactive network. This makes it difficult (and sometimes misleading) to assign unique roles to any individual cytokine, particularly in the intact host. Nevertheless, hints to the predominant effects of cytokines have been obtained from experiments in which animals are genetically altered to lack a particular cytokine. In most cases, these studies show that the absence of one or several cytokines has minimal effect on blood cell development but often a more pronounced effect on mature leukocyte function. For example, mice deficient in GM-CSF show only minor decreases in myeloid cell production, but the neutrophils they produce are dysfunctional.

Though it was long believed that specific cytokines acted by inducing HSCs and progenitors to differentiate along a certain pathway, the weight of evidence currently favors another view. It now appears instead that each cell is intrinsically predisposed toward one lineage or another (apparently choosing among them at random) but is unable to proliferate, or even survive, unless the cytokines appropriate to that lineage are present. In other words, cytokines do not direct cells into a particular pathway but instead act as lineage-specific growth and survival factors. Thus, when progenitor cells are deprived of an essential cytokine, they not only cease growing but often die—actively committing suicide through a process called **apoptosis** (see later discussion). On the other hand, progenitors that have been genetically manipulated so that they cannot undergo apoptosis continue growing and differentiating along a particular lineage even when the cytokine is withdrawn, implying that the differentiative fate of each cell is intrinsically programmed. These findings also illustrate the importance of cell death in hematopoiesis, as discussed later on.

Cytokine Receptors & Signal Transduction

The overlapping functions of cytokines largely reflect the properties of the cell surface receptors to which they bind. All cytokine receptors function as multiprotein complexes made up of two or more integral membrane polypeptides, called subunits (Fig 1–6). A typical subunit polypeptide has an extracellular domain that participates in cytokine binding, a transmembrane region, and an intracellular domain (also called a cytoplasmic tail) involved in **signal transduction**—the molecular events that transmit signals to the cell interior and induce specific cellular responses when the receptor binds its appropriate cytokine ligand. Some receptors (such as EPO-R) function as homodimers of a single type of subunit; others (eg, GM-CSFR) function as heterodimers, and still others (eg, IL-2R) as heterotrimers. In general, although the preformed subunits are present on the cell surface at all times, they do not assemble into a complete receptor complex until the appropriate cytokine is bound. It is this ligand-dependent assembly of the receptor complex that initiates the intracellular events in signal transduction.

Most cytokine receptors belong to a family of proteins called the **hematopoietin receptor family.** Members of this family all have a number of features in common, including extracellular domains that share common amino acid residues at key positions and that fold into a similar three-dimensional struc-

receptor tyrosine kinase family   **hematopoietin receptor family**

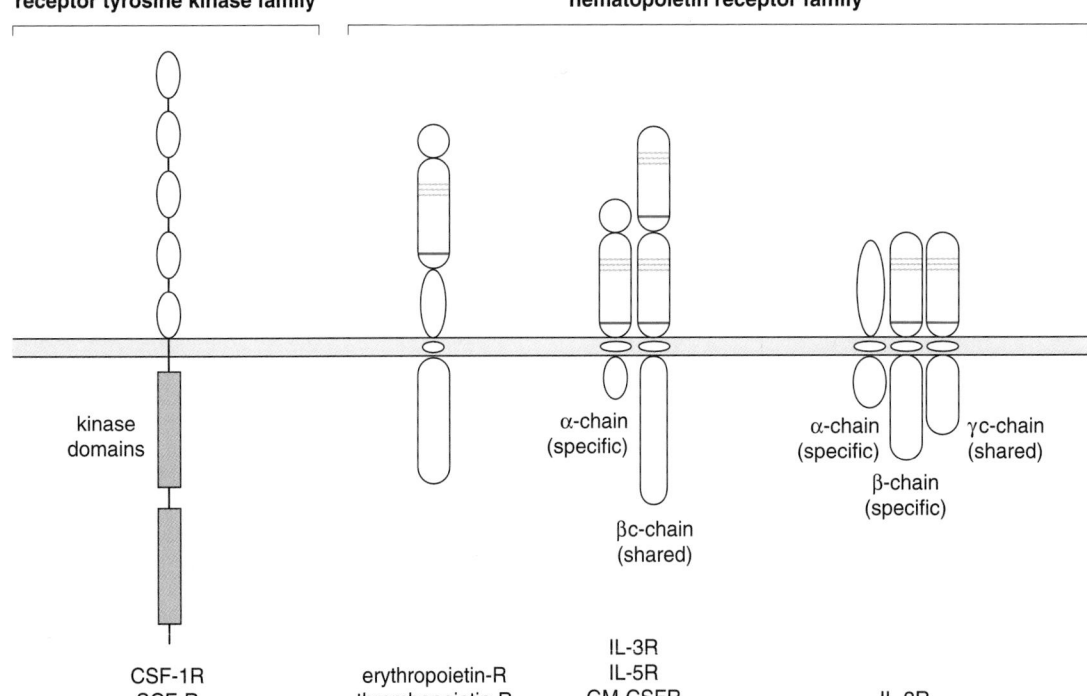

kinase
domains

CSF-1R
SCF-R

erythropoietin-R
thrombopoietin-R

α-chain
(specific)

βc-chain
(shared)

IL-3R
IL-5R
GM-CSFR

α-chain
(specific)

β-chain
(specific)

γc-chain
(shared)

IL-2R

Figure 1–6. Cytokine receptor families. The receptor tyrosine kinase family is characterized by the presence of tyrosine kinase domains (shaded boxes) within the intracellular portion of the receptor protein. Hematopoietin receptors lack tyrosine kinase domains, but their extracellular regions share conserved cysteine residues (thick lines) and the sequence motif TrpSerXTrpSer (narrow lines), where X is any amino acid. Hematopoietin receptors can be composed of one, two, or three polypeptide chains. Examples of each receptor type are listed at bottom.

ture composed of 14 antiparallel β strands. Each receptor consists of an α chain and a β chain; the α chain determines the specificity of cytokine binding, but the β chain is also required for maximal binding affinity. Trimeric receptors, such as IL-2R, may also include a γ subunit. As shown in Figure 1–6, many of these receptors share subunits; for example, IL-3R, IL-5R, and GM-CSFR all utilize a common β chain. These shared subunits are in part responsible for the overlapping functions of many cytokines, as they allow receptors with different ligand specificities to trigger identical signaling events inside a cell.

Attached noncovalently to the cytoplasmic tail of most hematopoietin receptor subunits is a cytoplasmic enzyme with **protein tyrosine kinase (PTK)** activity—that is, a protein with the ability to catalyze phosphorylation of tyrosine residues in other proteins. Phosphorylation, either at tyrosine or at serines and threonines, is a common mechanism of regulating protein function; indeed, many of the PTKs must themselves be phosphorylated before they can become active. When a cytokine binds, the component subunits of its receptor are brought into physical proximity with one another, along with their associated PTKs in the cytoplasm. Clustering of the PTKs allows

these enzymes to phosphorylate and activate one another, as well as other proteins in the cytoplasm. This PTK activation is the first step in cytoplasmic signal transduction by all known cytokine receptors. Interestingly, the few cytokine receptors (CSF-1R and SCF-R) that do not belong to the hematopoietin receptor family use a slightly different strategy to achieve the same result: the subunits of these receptors have intrinsic PTK enzymatic activity in their cytoplasmic domains, and these **receptor PTKs** become activated in a similar manner when the subunits are brought together. In each case, ligand binding causes the cytokine receptor subunits to associate with one another, which triggers PTK activity in the cytoplasm and initiates signal transduction. As we will see in later chapters, this same principle also applies to many other types of cell surface receptors.

The sequences of events that occur following PTK activation and lead to specific cellular responses vary among different cytokines, receptors, and cell types and are not well understood in most cases. Perhaps the best characterized signaling pathways are those that affect cell proliferation or modulate the transcription of particular genes. Following the onset of PTK activity, many such signals are commonly transmitted to the nucleus through two primary pathways, called

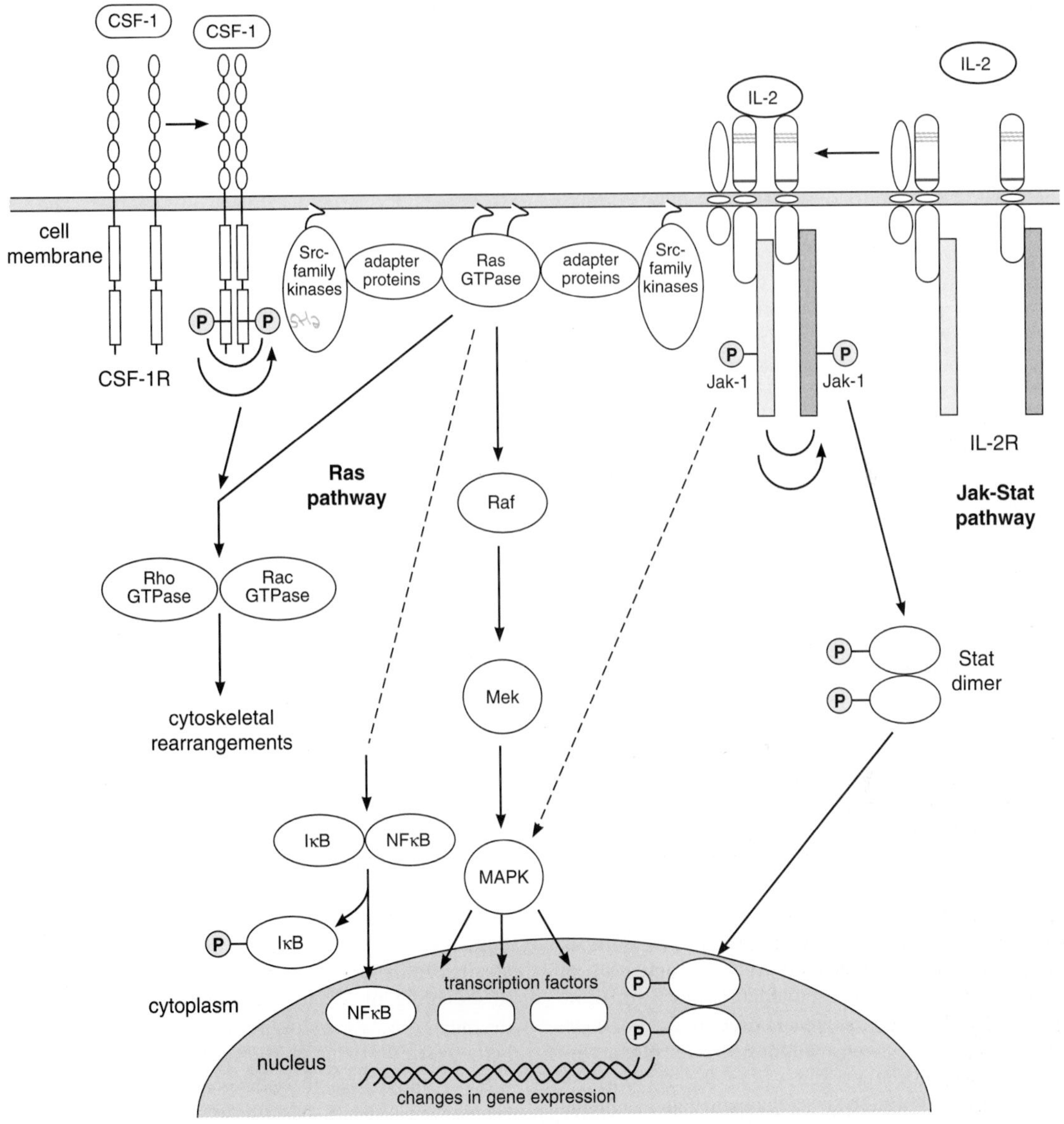

Figure 1–7. The Ras-dependent and Jak/Stat pathways of intracellular signal transduction. In each case, ligand binding to cell surface receptors causes oligomerization and activation of the associated tyrosine kinases (arrows). In the Ras pathway, signals communicated through Src-family kinases and a variety of adapter proteins (such as Grb-2, not shown) serve to activate the GTPase protein Ras, which is anchored to the inner aspect of the plasma membrane by fatty acyl groups (wavy lines). Ras signaling then proceeds through sequential activation of several other kinases (Raf, Mek, and MAPK), and ultimately leads to phosphorylation of transcription factors in the nucleus. The Ras pathway can also lead to cytoskeletal rearrangements by activating two other GTPases called Rho and Rac, and can activate the transcription factor NFκB by phosphorylating its cytoplasmic inhibitor, IκB. Jak/Stat signaling is initiated by phosphorylation of cytoplasmic Stat proteins, which causes these proteins to dimerize, translocate into the nucleus, and regulate gene expression by binding to DNA.

the Ras-dependent pathway and the Jak-Stat pathway (Fig 1–7).

The Ras-Dependent Signaling Pathway

The Ras-dependent pathway can be triggered by a variety of cytokine receptors, as well as by certain adhesion molecules and by many other surface receptors when they contact appropriate ligands. Signaling in this pathway can be initiated by cytosolic proteins called **Src-family kinases,** so named because they bear regions of sequence homology to the oncoprotein Src. These Src-like kinases contain specialized protein domains, termed **SH2 domains** (for Src-homology region 2), that enable them to bind other proteins containing phosphorylated tyrosine residues. When a cytokine receptor binds ligand, subunits of the receptor become phosphorylated and can immediately be bound by a Src-family kinase. This interaction leads to the binding of other cytoplasmic proteins, so that a multicomponent signaling complex forms on the inner aspect of the cell membrane. This complex then activates proteins of the **Ras** family, each of which has intrinsic GTPase activity. The cleavage of guanosine triphosphate (GTP) to guanosine diphosphate (GDP) by Ras-family proteins induces a structural change that somehow triggers activation of the Raf kinase. This, in turn, activates protein kinases called Mek and mitosis-associated protein kinase **(MAPK),** which phosphorylate and activate each other in sequence. Once activated, MAPK migrates into the nucleus, where it phosphorylates transcriptional regulatory proteins that control specific genes. Among the effects of MAPK activation are enhanced cell proliferation (see later discussion), gene activation, and changes in cytoskeletal organization that promote migration and function of hematopoietic cells.

The Ras pathway is actually much more complicated than the foregoing explanation would suggest. For example, there are at least three different forms of MAPK that are expressed by various tissues. The activities of individual Ras-pathway components can also be either enhanced or inhibited by other signaling factors in the cells. In addition, signaling through the Ras pathway also can affect cell functions independently of MAPK. One important example is the regulation of a transcription factor, called nuclear factor kappa B **(NFκB),** which controls the activities of many genes involved in hematopoietic cell function. NFκB must enter the nucleus in order to act but is ordinarily retained in the cytoplasm by its interaction with a cytoplasmic protein called the inhibitor of NFκB **(IκB).** Through a mechanism that is not yet known but that does not involve MAPK, activation of the Ras pathway leads to phosphorylation of IκB, which, in turn, allows NFκB to dissociate from IκB, enter the nucleus, and activate its target genes. Through this pathway, NFκB mediates many effects of cytokines on gene expression, including many of the lymphocyte genes involved in host defense. Recent evidence indicates that the steroid hormones called **glucocorticoids,** which are widely used in clinical medicine to inhibit lymphocyte-mediated defense reactions, produce their effects at least in part by enhancing synthesis of IκB and thereby inhibiting NFκB.

The Jak/Stat Signaling Pathway

Perhaps the most exciting recent advance in the cytokine signaling field has been the elucidation of the Jak/Stat pathway. The Janus kinase **(Jak)** family consists of four known enzymes (Jak1, Jak2, Jak3, and Tyk2), each of which associates specifically with the cytoplasmic tails of one or more cytokine receptor subunits. For example, IL-2R associates with both Jak1 and Jak3, which bind its α and γ subunits, respectively. Cytokine binding brings the receptor subunits together and allows the associated Jak proteins to phosphorylate and activate one another. The primary substrates of the activated Jaks are a family of transcription factors called the **Stat** (for signal transducers and activators of transcription) proteins. The Stat proteins contain SH2 domains and so are recruited to the vicinity of an activated receptor when its kinases become active. As a consequence, the Stat factors become phosphorylated, which causes them to dimerize and then translocate into the nucleus, where they act directly to promote expression of specific genes. There are at least six known Stat proteins (called Stat1–Stat6), each of which acts on different genes. There is no evidence that any individual Jak acts preferentially on a particular Stat. Therefore, the genes that are activated in response to a given cytokine are determined mainly by the combination of receptor subunits and Stat factors expressed by the responding cell. It is tempting to envision that one of the earliest events in lineage commitment by a hematopoietic progenitor may be expression of receptor subunits and Stat proteins that enable it to respond to lineage-specific cytokines. Cross-communication between the Ras-dependent pathway and the Jak/Stat pathway may also occur, as recent evidence suggests that Stats may also be phosphorylated by the MAPK proteins.

The redundancy of cytokine function therefore reflects the fact that different cytokines bind to structurally similar receptors that activate the same types of signaling molecules. This explains why absence of one or a few cytokines has minimal effect on hematopoiesis in vivo. By contrast, since many cytokines signal through common receptor subunits and signaling pathways, one might predict that loss of a particular subunit or signaling kinase would have a much more profound effect. This is indeed the case: in mice that carry mutations in Jak3, and in both humans and mice with mutations in the IL-2R γ chain, these genetic defects impair signaling by many cytokines simultaneously and result in profound deficits in hematopoiesis and in cellular defense functions.

CONTROL OF CELL PROLIFERATION & SURVIVAL

The Cell Cycle

One ultimate effect of many cytokines, ECM proteins, and cell–cell interactions is to influence the rate at which hematopoietic cells divide. The sequence of events that occurs in a cell during each round of mitosis is called the **cell cycle** and is traditionally di-

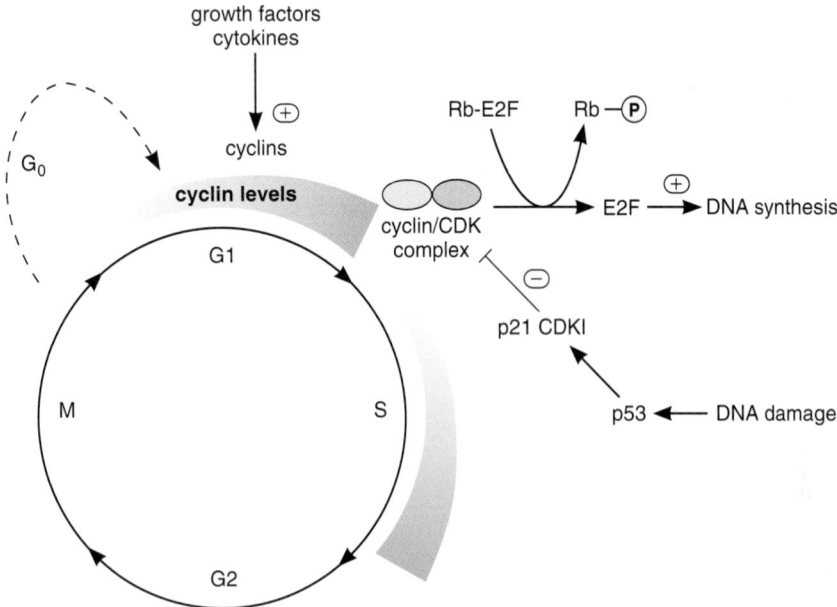

Figure 1–8. The cell cycle. This simplified depiction illustrates a few of the molecular factors that influence the G1/S transition. Abbreviations: CDK = cyclin-dependent kinase; CDKI = CDK inhibitor; sharp arrowheads = activation; blunt arrowheads = inhibition.

vided into four phases (Fig 1–8), designated G_1, S (when DNA synthesis occurs), G_2, and M (mitosis, when the cell actually divides). Cells that have ceased dividing (temporarily or permanently) are said to be in a resting phase called G_0. The ordered progression from one phase to the next is coordinated by a complex set of proteins, and the cellular signals that control cell division do so by modulating the activities of those proteins.

Cell cycle regulation takes place mainly at the transition points, or boundaries, between the different phases. Each of these boundaries serves as a **checkpoint:** specific requirements (such as completion of DNA synthesis or DNA repair) must be met before a cell can transition through the checkpoint from one phase to the next. In mammals, most variation in cell cycle timing is due to variation in the length of G_1, and the G_1/S checkpoint is tightly regulated. There are three main classes of proteins directly involved in checkpoint regulation: (1) the **cyclins,** whose levels rise and fall in specific phases of the cycle; (2) the cyclin-dependent kinases **(CDKs),** a class of serine–threonine kinases that regulate cyclin activity by phosphorylation; and (3) the CDK inhibitors **(CDKIs),** which inactivate the CDKs.

There are at least seven different cyclins and CDKs, each operative at different phases of the cycle. The intracellular levels of specific cyclins are in part responsive to external stimuli: for example, CSF-1 acts on cells of the monocyte lineage to increase expression of cyclins required for progression through the G_1/S checkpoint. As cyclin levels increase during a given phase, they form a complex with the corresponding CDKs; this activates the CDKs, which then phosphorylate other substrates that allow checkpoint progression. In hematopoietic cells, for example, one of the predominant species that accumulates during G_1 is the cyclinD/CDK6 complex, whose primary substrate is the nuclear retinoblastoma (Rb) protein. Rb ordinarily exists as a complex with transcription factors of the E2F family. When the cyclinD/CDK6 complex hyperphosphorylates Rb, the E2F proteins dissociate from it and instead bind and activate specific genes, such as those encoding DNA polymerase and thymidine synthetase, which are required for DNA synthesis and, hence, for entry into the S phase.

Other signals can inhibit cell cycle progression by inducing CDKIs. The CDKIs are small molecules, named after their molecular weights, which bind and inhibit specific cyclin/CDK complexes. In hematopoietic cells, for example, the cytokine called transforming growth factor beta (TGFβ) induces expression of CDKIs called p15 and p18, which inactivate the cyclinD/CDK6 complex and prevent entry into the S phase.

Progression through G1 is also marked by the accumulation of other transcription factors, including the proteins Fos, Jun, and **c-Myc,** which presumably act on other genes required for DNA replication. Like the E2F proteins, several of these factors are regulated by association with other proteins. For example, c-Myc must dimerize with another protein, called Max, in order to bind DNA and promote gene expression; however, Max can instead form dimers with other proteins that antagonize Myc/Max activity and slow cell cycle progression. Thus, a critical balance of cyclin/CDK and transcription factor activities is required for progression from G_1 to S. If this balance is not achieved, the cell stops dividing and either enters the G_0 resting state or dies through apoptosis (see later discussion). In some circumstances, the G_0 state is maintained by high-level expression of CDKIs.

A number of other factors can also inhibit progression through the G_1/S boundary. One of the most important is DNA damage, which occurs to some degree under normal conditions but is greatly enhanced by ultraviolet or gamma irradiation and by many of the chemotherapeutic agents used to treat cancer. The integrity of chromosomal DNA is continually monitored through an unknown mechanism that involves a protein called **p53.** When DNA damage is present, p53 directly induces a CDKI called p21, which blocks G_1/S progression until the damage is repaired. This process helps ensure that mutations caused by the damage will not be replicated and passed on to daughter cells. Cells with mutations in p53 manifest extreme genomic instability (ie, they accumulate numerous mutations) and are highly prone to becoming malignant. Indeed, p53 mutations are an important factor in the development of a wide variety of human cancers.

Physiologic Cell Death (Apoptosis)

Under some conditions, cells respond to environmental or internal signals by committing suicide—a phenomenon known as physiologic (or programmed) cell death. Such programmed deaths are extremely common in many cell types, and in fact are essential for maintaining stable cell populations by ensuring that the rate of new cell production is balanced by an equal rate of cell death. This is particularly true in the hematopoietic system, where vast numbers of new cells are generated each day, but programmed deaths are also critical for shaping and maintaining other tissues, such as in resorption of the tail bud and finger webs during embryogenesis, in selecting neural connections, and in regression of the mammary epithelium after lactation. Cellular suicide also has a defensive function: cells that are infected by a virus or other intracellular pathogen may kill themselves—often after having been instructed to do so by other host cells—which helps limit spread of the infection.

In all of these settings, programmed cell death occurs through a process called **apoptosis.** A cell undergoing apoptosis shows characteristic morphologic changes: over the course of several hours, it shrinks overall as its nucleus and cytoplasm become com-pacted; surface features such as microvilli disappear; fragments of cytoplasm pinch off from the surface (a phenomenon called blebbing); the nuclear chromatin condenses; and cellular endonucleases cleave the chromosomal DNA into segments. Ultimately, the cell disintegrates into small fragments (called apoptotic bodies) that are quickly engulfed and digested by adjacent cells. The stereotypical nature of these changes suggests that apoptosis occurs through a common biochemical pathway that can be activated in many (or all) mammalian cell types.

Though the sequence of intracellular events responsible for apoptosis is not yet completely known, several biochemical changes have been implicated in the process. Perhaps most important is the activation of a small group of cellular cysteine proteinases called **caspases,** whose prototype is the interleukin-1β-converting enzyme (**ICE,** also known as caspase-1). Caspase family members, of which at least ten are known in humans, ordinarily exist as inactive pro-enzymes but can be activated by proteolytic cleavage; once active, they can digest numerous protein substrates and also proteolytically activate one another. Caspases virtually always become activated during apoptosis and, though it is not yet clear which caspases and caspase substrates are most critical, their activity appears to be required for the apoptotic response. Consistent with that view, certain viruses produce specific caspase inhibitors which enable them to prevent infected cells from undergoing apoptosis. Among the known caspase targets are the nuclear lamins, which are intermediate filament proteins that organize chromatin structure; cleavage of lamins by these proteinases may be one mechanism of initiating the nuclear breakdown that is characteristic of apoptosis. In addition to proteinase activation, some apoptotic cells show evidence of oxidative injury caused by reactive oxygen species, which are by-products of aerobic metabolism; however, it is not clear whether such injury is essential to the apoptotic process. Similarly, although DNA fragmentation is considered a hallmark of apoptosis, both the identity of the cellular endonucleases involved and their relationship to cell death remain controversial.

Among the most critical intracellular factors controlling the apoptotic response are the members of a family of cytoplasmic proteins related to the human oncoprotein **Bcl2** (see Chapter 7). Members of the Bcl2 family have been identified in mammalian cells, viruses, and other organisms (Table 1–3). Most are integral membrane proteins that associate with organelles throughout the cytoplasm, including the endoplasmic reticulum, mitochondria, outer nuclear envelope, and inner plasma membrane. All Bcl2 family members share conserved amino acid sequences and tend to dimerize with themselves and with one another. Remarkably, however, they fall into two classes with opposite biologic effects: when expressed individually within cells, some of these pro-

Table 1–3. Proteins of the Bcl2 family.[1]

Inhibit Apoptosis	Promote Apoptosis
Bcl2	Bax
BclX$_L$	BclX$_S$
Mcl-1	Bak
A-1	Bik
Bhrf-I (Epstein-Barr virus)	Bad
p35 (Baculovirus)	
Ced-9 (Nematode)	

[1] Each of these proteins is expressed by mammalian cells unless otherwise indicated. BclX$_L$ and BclX$_S$ are alternatively spliced products from a single gene.

teins (such as Bax) actively induce or promote apoptosis, whereas others (such as Bcl2) inhibit apoptosis, making cells resistant to an assortment of stimuli that would otherwise trigger cell death. These two classes of proteins antagonize each other (perhaps by forming mixed heterodimers), so that the overall tendency of a cell to undergo apoptosis appears to be determined by the relative levels at which it expresses proteins of each class.

The biochemical mechanisms by which Bcl2 and related proteins promote or inhibit apoptosis are not known. It appears, however, that some cytokines regulate apoptosis by inducing or inhibiting expression of Bcl2 family members. For example, withdrawal of a particular cytokine may lead to reduced Bcl2 expression in some hematopoietic progenitors, leaving these cells vulnerable to the unopposed effects of Bax. Certain viruses also manipulate expression of these proteins: for example, the Epstein-Barr virus not only encodes a Bcl2-like protein of its own but also specifically activates expression of cellular Bcl2,

thereby preventing the infected cell from committing apoptosis. In addition, apoptosis in hematopoietic cells is closely tied to the cell cycle. Many cytokine-dependent hematopoietic cells must pass through the G_1 phase of the cell cycle before commencing apoptosis following cytokine withdrawal. In the process, these cells accumulate G_1-specific proteins such as c-Myc, which may, paradoxically, have a role in initiating cell death under these conditions. Another critical cell cycle regulator, p53, is also directly linked to apoptosis: if the DNA damage that triggers p53-dependent cell cycle arrest (see earlier discussion) cannot be repaired in a timely manner, p53 acts to initiate apoptosis (possibly by inducing Bax) and thereby eliminates the damaged cell for the benefit of the host.

CONCLUSION

The regulation of hematopoiesis reflects the individual and combined effects of soluble factors and direct cell–cell interactions in the marrow. By activating specific signal transduction pathways inside the developing cells, these external stimuli modulate the activities of transcription factors, cell cycle regulatory factors, and other intracellular proteins that determine whether a cell will proliferate, differentiate, or die. Mechanisms such as these are essential for controlling not only blood cell production but also the defensive functions carried out by mature blood cells. Hence, many of the themes that have been outlined here will be encountered again in subsequent chapters.

REFERENCES

HEMATOPOIESIS & HEMATOPOIETIC STEM CELLS
Levitt D, Mertelsmann R (editors): *Hematopoietic Stem Cells: Biology and Therapeutic Applications.* Marcel Dekker, 1995.
Ogawa M: Differentiation and proliferation of hematopoietic stem cells. *Blood* 1993;**81**:2844.
Uchida N et al: Heterogeneity of hematopoietic stem cells. *Curr Opin Immunol* 1993;**5**:177.

CYTOKINES & SIGNAL TRANSDUCTION
Ihle JN: Signal transducers and activators of transcription. *Cell* 1996;**84**:331.
Ivashkiv LB: Cytokines and STATs: How can signals achieve specificity? *Immunity* 1995;**3**:1.
Kishimoto T et al: Interleukin-6 family of cytokines and gp130. *Blood* 1995;**86**:1243.
Metcalf D: Implications of the polyfunctionality of hemopoietic regulators. *Stem Cells* 1994;**12**:259.

Paulson RF, Berstein A: Receptor tyrosine kinases and the regulation of hematopoiesis. *Semin Immunol* 1995;**7**:267.
Sachs L, Lotem J: The network of hematopoietic cytokines. *Proc Soc Exp Biol Med* 1994;**206**:170.
Sato N, Miyajima A: Multimeric cytokine receptors: Common versus specific functions. *Curr Opin Cell Biol* 1994;**6**:174.

BONE MARROW STROMA
Clark BR, Keating A: Biology of bone marrow stroma. *Ann NY Acad Sci* 1995;**770**:70.
Simmons P et al: Potential adhesion mechanisms for localization of haemopoietic progenitors to bone marrow stroma. *Leukemia Lymphoma* 1994;**12**:353.
Verfaillie et al: Role of bone matrix in normal and abnormal hematopoieis. *Crit Rev Oncol Hematol* 1994;**16**:210.
Whetton AD, Dexter TM: Influence of growth factors and

substrates on differentiation of hematopoietic stem cells. *Curr Opin Cell Biol* 1993;**5:**1044.

CELL CYCLE CONTROL

Hirama T, Koeffler HP: Role of the cyclin-dependent kinase inhibitors in the development of cancer. *Blood* 1995;**86:**841.

Stein GS et al: Molecular mechanisms mediating control of cell cycle and cell growth. *Exp Hematol* 1995;**23:**1053.

Weinberg RA: The retinoblastoma protein and cell cycle control. *Cell* 1995;**81:**323.

APOPTOSIS

Cotter TG et al: Cell death in the myeloid lineage. *Immunol Rev* 1994;**142:**93.

Hockenberry DM: bcl-2, a novel regulator of cell death. *Bioessays* 1995;**17:**631.

Meikrantz W, Schlegel R: Apoptosis and the cell cycle. *J Cell Biochem* 1995;**58:**160.

Squier MKT et al: Apoptosis in leukocytes. *J Leukocyte Biol* 1995;**57:**2.

White E: Life, death, and the pursuit of apoptosis. *Genes Dev* 1996;**10:**1.

Innate Immunity

2

Tristram G. Parslow, MD, PhD, & Dorothy F. Bainton, MD

The human body has many ways of protecting itself. The first line of defense is provided by mechanical barriers, such as the skin, which cover body surfaces and physically prevent microorganisms and other potentially injurious agents from entering the tissues beneath. In addition to being physically impervious, these barriers often have other specialized features that help them repel foreign invaders. For example, lactic acid and other substances in sweat maintain the surface of the epidermis at an acidic pH, which helps prevent colonization by bacteria and other organisms. Similarly, the more delicate epithelia lining the respiratory and digestive tracts are bathed in a protective layer of mucus, which can trap, dissolve, and sweep away foreign substances. Though mechanical barriers such as these are relatively constant, they often can be enhanced to some degree in times of need: a chronically irritated epidermis may thicken to form a callus, and the respiratory tract's efforts to cleanse itself by copious mucus production are familiar to anyone who has suffered from a cold or "hay fever" allergy. The importance of these physical defenses becomes most evident in people who lack them: for example, burn patients are at greatly increased risk for many types of infections, owing to loss of the cutaneous barrier.

Should any **pathogen** (that is, any microorganism with the potential to cause tissue injury or disease) succeed in breaching the surface barriers and enter the body, it encounters a panoply of additional factors that guard the inner tissues. Some are soluble proteins or other macromolecules that circulate in the blood and extracellular fluid, making them inhospitable to foreign invaders. Others are specialized cells endowed with the ability to recognize, sequester, and eliminate various types of organisms or harmful substances. Traditionally, these defensive factors have been categorized into two more-or-less distinct functional systems, based on the type of resistance (immunity) they confer against particular pathogens. **Innate** (or **natural**) **immunity** refers to any inborn resistance that is present the first time a pathogen is encountered; it does not require prior exposure and is not modified significantly by repeated exposures to the pathogen over the life of an individual. **Acquired immunity** refers to resistance that is weak or absent on first exposure but that increases dramatically with subsequent exposures to the same specific pathogen.

The innate and acquired immune systems are each made up of numerous soluble factors and diverse cell types that have specific roles to play in host defense. Both systems are essential for health; they usually act in concert and depend to a great extent on each other for maximal effectiveness. Nor are they entirely separate: the actions of one system frequently are able to influence the other, and certain individual cell types or proteins are pivotal to the workings of both systems. Of the two, the acquired immune system has received much more attention in recent years, because of its greater complexity and elegance and because of the predominant role it plays in human health and disease. In fact, most contemporary usage of the terms *immunology, immune response,* and so on refers primarily to the acquired immune system. That same emphasis will be apparent in this book, as most subsequent chapters focus on the cells and proteins that mediate acquired immunity. It is useful, nevertheless, to begin by describing the capabilities and limitations of the innate immune system, to understand how it functions as a guardian of the body, and to consider why this system alone cannot provide a sufficient defense against many types of pathogens.

SOLUBLE PROTEINS OF INNATE IMMUNITY

The body's innate resistance to many pathogens is provided by enzymes and other proteins in the blood and tissue fluids. Most proteins of this type have features in common that are also characteristic of the innate immune system as a whole. First, these proteins are continually expressed throughout life, regardless of whether or not their protective effects are needed at a given moment. Second, though many of these proteins can be produced in increased quantities in times of need, their qualitative properties (such as substrate specificity) do not change: the molecular characteristics of these proteins have been established through species evolution, are genetically determined, and are fixed at birth, so that they do not vary during an individual's lifetime. Third, although these proteins carry out highly specific functions at the molecular level, they recognize targets or substrates that are found on a wide range of different microorganisms, which enables them to provide relatively nonspecific protection against a broad array of pathogens.

Antimicrobial Enzymes & Binding Proteins

A few of the best known soluble mediators of innate immunity are listed in Table 2–1, along with the types of target molecules they recognize. As is apparent from this list, proteins of the innate immune system generally recognize and attack pathogenic organisms by virtue of particular carbohydrate or lipid molecules they express, which are not found in the normal host. This strategy is highly efficient, as it enables the innate system to immediately recognize many pathogens as chemically foreign even if they have never been encountered before. It also helps minimize the risk that these proteins might inadvertantly attack host tissues. The use of a carbohydrate- and lipid-based recognition system is also a key feature that distinguishes the innate from the acquired immune system, because, as we shall see in later chapters, the acquired immune system recognizes

Table 2–1. Some soluble proteins of the innate immune system.

Protein	Major Microbial Targets	Effects
Lysozyme	Peptidoglycan of bacterial cell walls.	Digestion of cell wall.
Mannose-binding protein	High-mannose glycoproteins and glycolipids.	Opsonization; complement activation.
C-reactive protein	Polysaccharides and phosphorylcholine on microbial surfaces.	Opsonization; complement activation.
Serum amyloid protein P	Carbohydrates in cell walls.	Opsonization.
LPS-binding protein	LPS	Promotes LPS binding to CD14.
Soluble CD14	LPS	Promotes LPS binding by host cells.
Complement protein C3	Covalent binding to carbohydrates and proteins on microbial surfaces.	Opsonization; complement activation; many other effects.

Abbreviations: LPS = bacterial lipopolysaccharide.

pathogens mainly by the specific proteins they express.

Some of the soluble mediators of innate immunity are enzymes that can directly injure or kill microbial pathogens. An example is **lysozyme,** an endoglycosidase found in human saliva, mucus, tears, and other secretions, which attacks the protective cell wall encasing every bacterial cell. Lysozyme acts by digesting the peptidoglycan—a meshwork formed by long carbohydrate chains of alternating N-acetylmuramic acid and N-acetylglucosamine residues, cross-linked covalently by short oligopeptide sidechains—which is a major constituent of all bacterial cell walls but is not found in mammalian tissues. By cleaving the linkages between carbohydrate residues in the peptidoglycan, lysozyme weakens the cell wall and leaves bacteria vulnerable to killing by osmotic lysis.

Many other soluble factors bind preferentially to pathogens but have no enzymatic activity of their own. For example, a serum protein known as **mannose-binding protein** binds residues of the sugar mannose, which are commonly found at the exposed ends of glycoprotein or glycolipid side chains on the surfaces of bacteria, viruses, and parasites. (Although mammalian glycoproteins also contain mannose residues, these are usually present in smaller amounts and masked by other carbohydrates added to the side chain termini, and so are not accessible for binding.) Similarly, **serum amyloid protein P** and the human **C-reactive protein** each bind a subset of carbohydrate or lipid determinants found on many different types of bacteria. Binding of these proteins has little direct effect on a pathogen but greatly increases the efficiency with which it is captured and destroyed by certain host cells, through a phenomenon called opsonization (see later section).

A unique bacterial surface product that is an especially favored target for immune recognition is **lipopolysaccharide (LPS).** This macromolecule is found only in the outer lipid bilayer that surrounds the cell walls of gram-negative bacteria, such as *Neisseria, Salmonella,* and *Escherichia coli.* Each molecule of LPS consists of a core carbohydrate linked to a phospholipid (called lipid A) anchored in the bilayer, and to a long polysaccharide chain (called the O side chain) that extends outward from the bacterial surface (Fig 2–1). The sequence of sugars making up the O side chain is species-specific and highly variable, even within a single bacterial genus: for example, there are over 1000 known variants in *Salmonella.* The core carbohydrate and lipid A, by contrast, are essentially invariant and serve as the target for binding by two human serum proteins, called **LPS-binding protein** and **soluble CD14.** The complexes that these proteins form with LPS on a bacterial surface are readily recognized, in turn, by receptors on endothelial cells, neutrophils, monocytes, and other human cell types, which facilitates binding and destruction of gram-negative bacteria by these cells.

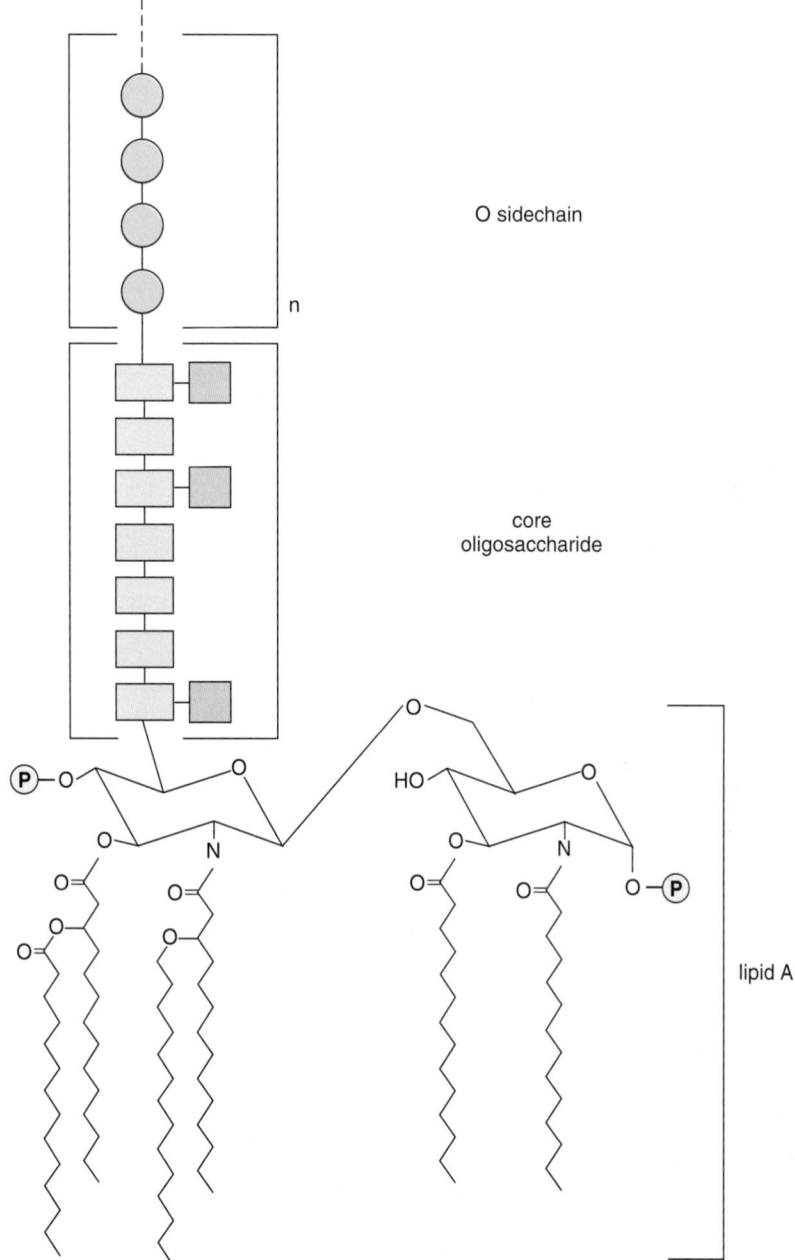

O sidechain

core
oligosaccharide

lipid A

Figure 2–1. Structure of lipopolysaccharide (LPS) from gram-negative bacteria. Lipid A contains two residues of phosphorylated glucosamine bearing six O- and N-linked saturated fatty acids, and accounts for half the lipids in the outer lipid bilayer. The core oligosaccharide is composed of 10 sugar residues. The O antigen comprises 25–50 repeating tetrasaccharide units, and its sequence varies widely among bacterial strains. Total mass of the LPS unit is about 10,000 d.

At the same time, binding of the LPS complexes to cell surface receptors transmits signals that can lead to powerful physiologic changes in host cells. For example, LPS binding induces many types of cells to secrete various cytokines, and these cytokines, in turn, are responsible for triggering a wide array of other immunologic phenomena that we will encounter later in this book.

The Complement Cascade

An especially elaborate and important type of innate antimicrobial defense is provided by a group of

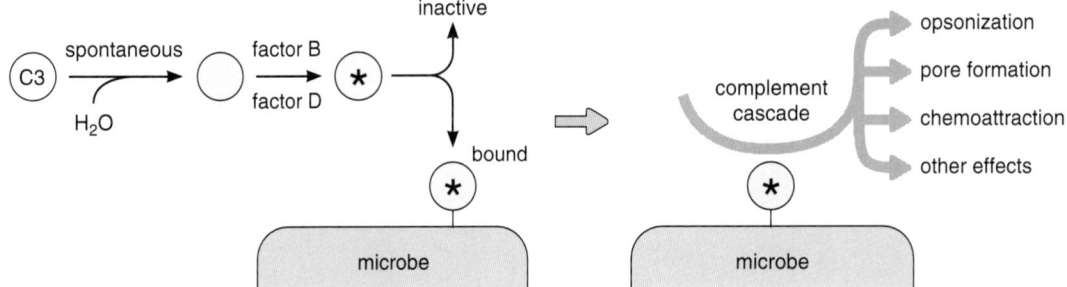

Figure 2–2. Complement activation through the alternative pathway. For details, see Chapter 11.

serum proteins that together make up the **complement** pathway. This group comprises more than two dozen different soluble proteins, called complement factors, or components, most of which have latent proteinase activity. As a rule, each of the proteinases becomes active when proteolytically cleaved, and then catalyzes cleavage and activation of a different complement component. These cleavages occur in a defined sequence, with each activated protein activating many copies of the next component, so that the reactions proceed in a self-amplifying cascade. When complement becomes activated on the surface of a pathogen, it leads to four distinct types of protective effects: some of the complement components assemble into pores that create holes in the microbial surface membrane; others coat the organism and enhance its killing by host cells through opsonization; others act as chemoattractants for various leukocytes; and still others bind to receptors on nearby host cells and trigger other types of defensive reactions that will be described later. Because it plays a key role in many aspects of immunity, the complement cascade is considered in great detail in Chapter 11. In the present discussion, we consider only a very simplified outline of its contributions to the innate defense against pathogens.

Complement can become activated through two distinct routes, both of which involve activation of a complement protein called C3, a fairly abundant protein with a normal serum concentration of roughly 1 g/L. The "classic" pathway uses proteins from the acquired immune system to activate C3, but the **"alternative" pathway** (Fig 2–2) requires only complement proteins and so constitutes a type of innate immunity. The alternative pathway depends on the fact that, under normal conditions, a small proportion of C3 molecules in the serum are continually becoming activated due to spontaneous hydrolysis. These activated C3 proteins can interact with two other serum complement components (factors B and D) to form a highly reactive, extremely short-lived species capable of bonding covalently to virtually any protein or carbohydrate molecule in its vicinity. With a half-life of

only 0.1 ms, this active C3 derivative cannot diffuse far from its site of formation before decaying to an inactive form. If during this time it encounters an appropriate molecule on a cell surface, however, the C3 derivative binds and is stabilized and can then act on other complement proteins in the surrounding serum to trigger the entire complement cascade.

Human cells express on their surfaces a number of complement-inhibitory proteins whose function is to inactivate immediately any molecule of this C3 species that attaches itself to the cell; in this way, human cells protect themselves from the effects of spontaneously activated C3. Many pathogens, however, lack such protection; when such organisms enter the bloodstream, their surfaces quickly become coated with the active C3 species, triggering localized complement activation. Thus, many pathogens directly activate serum complement through the alternative pathway, which results in perforation of their surface membranes, enhanced killing by host defensive cells, leukocyte chemoattraction, and the activation of many other types of defensive reactions in the surrounding tissues.

The Acute-Phase Response

With the exception of C3, most soluble mediators of innate immunity are found in relatively small amounts in the serum under normal conditions. The concentrations of several of these proteins, however, can increase as much as 1000-fold during serious infections, as part of a coordinated protective reaction called the hepatic **acute-phase response.** In this response, the liver temporarily increases its synthesis of more than a dozen different serum proteins that participate in antimicrobial defense, including complement factors C3 and B, the mannose-binding protein, C-reactive protein, serum amyloid protein P, and others. The response occurs when hepatocytes are exposed to certain cytokines—interleukin-6 **(IL-6),** as well as **IL-1** or tumor necrosis factor **(TNF)**—released locally or into the bloodstream by other host cells. Interestingly, one of the most potent inducers of these cytokines, and hence of the acute-phase response, is bacterial LPS. The acute-phase response can thus be viewed as a primitive, nonspecific defensive reaction, mediated by the liver, which serves to intensify some aspects of innate immunity when a pathogen is present.

VASCULAR & ENDOTHELIAL RESPONSES TO INJURY OR INFECTION

Dilatation & Permeability of Microscopic Vessels

Though blood vessels are not ordinarily considered part of the immune system, they react in characteristic ways to injury or infection, and these reactions are critical to the body's innate defenses. Virtually any type of insult to a solid tissue—whether by blunt trauma, thermal or chemical burn, laceration, microbial infection, or myriad other causes—is likely to be followed by a rapid dilatation of small blood vessels in and around the injured tissues (Fig 2–3). This vascular response (called **vasodilatation**) can occur within minutes after an acute injury; primarily involves arterioles, capillaries, and venules; and leads to an initial increase in local blood flow at the injured site. As the vessels dilate, endothelial cells lining some of the vessels actively retract away from one another to create temporary, microscopic gaps in the endothelial lining. Endothelial retraction occurs only in the smallest venules (often called **postcapillary venules**), which are thin-walled vessels that have lumenal diameters of 20–60 μm (Table 2–2). Retraction results in **increased permeability** of the venule wall, allowing protein-rich fluid from the plasma to leak

Table 2–2. Physical and hydrodynamic properties of human blood vessels.

Vessel Type	Wall Thickness (μm)	Lumen Diameter (μm)	Total Cross-Sectional Area (cm²)	Mean Flow Velocity (mm/s)
Aorta	2,000	25,000	5	185
Artery	1,000	4,000	20	42
Arteriole	20	30	400	2
Capillary	1	5	4,500	0.2
Venule[1]	2	20	4,000	0.2
Vein	500	5,000	40	21
Vena cava	1,500	30,000	18	46

Source: Modified from data in Ganong WF: *Review of Medical Physiology,* 17th ed. Appleton & Lange, 1995, for a resting, supine person with cardiac output of 5.0 L/min.
[1] All venules have a thin wall and low flow rate. The smallest venules (called postcapillary venules, with lumen diameters of 20–60 μm) also have endothelium specialized to retract and express leukocyte adhesion proteins when activated (see text).

out through the gaps, traverse the endothelial basement membrane, and flow into the extracellular space of the surrounding tissue. The leakage of fluid, in turn, creates a condition of stasis within the venules, as densely packed blood cells accumulate within the distended lumens and their rate of flow along the length of the vessels is decreased.

The vasodilatation induced by an injury results in part from a spinal reflex: pain receptors stimulated by the injury transmit signals along sensory nerves to the spinal cord, where they act on motor neurons to cause relaxation of arteriolar smooth muscles at the injured site. Even if the neurons are cut, however, vasodilata-

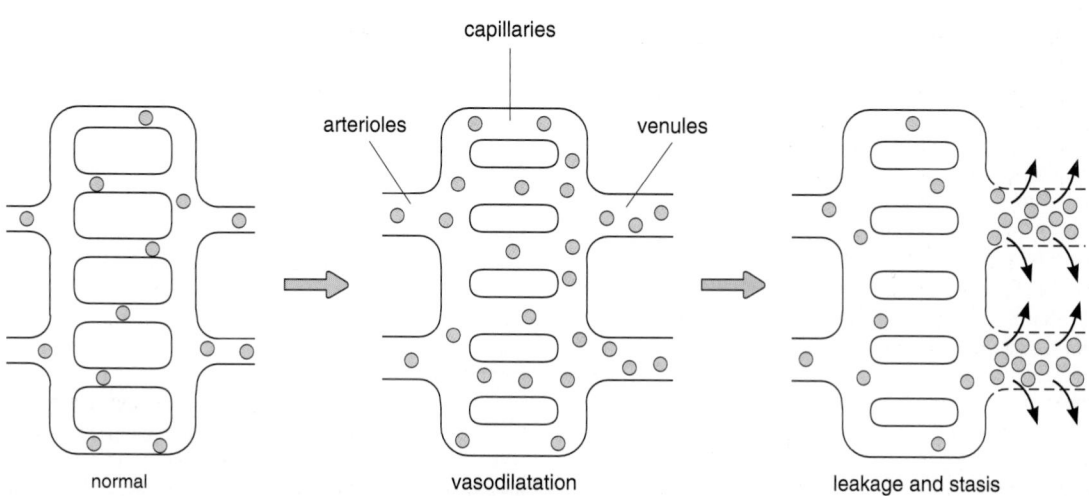

Figure 2–3. Vasodilatation and vascular leakage. Vasodilatation affects arterioles, capillaries, and venules. Leakage results from endothelial retraction that occurs only in postcapillary venules.

Table 2–3. Vasoactive mediators.[1]

Induce Vasodilatation
   Histamine
   Prostaglandins (especially PGD_2)
   Nitric oxide[2]

Enhance Vascular Permeability
   Histamine
   Prostaglandins (especially PGD_2)
   Leukotrienes (especially LTC_4, LTD_4, and LTE_4)
   Platelet-activating factor
   Bradykinin

---

[1] For detailed discussions of individual mediators, see Chapters 11 and 12.
[2] Nitric oxide directly dilates large, but not small, blood vessels; however, it also dilates small vessels indirectly by stimulating the release of histamine and other mediators.

tion and vascular leakage still occur, though to a somewhat lesser degree. This neural-independent component of the vascular response is triggered by low-molecular-weight molecules, called **vasoactive mediators,** that are produced at the injured site and act directly on the local vasculature (Table 2–3). An assortment of such mediators have been identified (see Chapter 12). One of the best studied is **histamine,** an amino acid metabolite stored in large amounts by cells called **mast cells,** which reside in connective tissues throughout the body. Within seconds after various physical or chemical stimuli (including contact with some activated complement proteins), mast cells can discharge histamine into the surrounding tissues, where it acts as a potent vasodilator and increases venular permeability. Similar effects are produced by certain **prostaglandins**—members of a class of mediators derived from cell membrane lipids, which can be secreted inducibly by many cell types, including mast cells.

In most cases, vasodilatation and increased vascular permeability are reversible responses whose extent and duration depend on the nature, severity, and type of injury sustained. Together, they are largely responsible for the clinical findings of redness (**erythema**), warmth, and swelling that accompany nearly all types of solid tissue injuries. These physiologic changes benefit the host in several ways. For example, the enhanced local blood supply helps improve delivery of oxygen, platelets, and clotting factors to the injured site, which in turn helps stabilize damaged tissues and facilitates wound healing and repair. Moreover, the vascular fluid that leaks into the tissues can immediately dilute or dissolve harmful substances in the tissues, and carries with it many of the antimicrobial proteins from the serum, thereby helping to deliver innate, nonspecific defensive factors rapidly to the site where they are needed.

Endothelial Activation & Enhanced Leukocyte Adhesion

The most important consequence of the vascular response, however, is that it promotes contact between blood leukocytes and the venular endothelium. Under normal conditions of flow, blood cells tend to be drawn toward the center of a vessel lumen, where frictional resistance with the wall is minimized and the flow rate is highest. When a vessel dilates and its average flow rate diminishes, the cells within it collide more frequently and at lower velocities against the endothelial lining. In the distended, leaky venules of an injured tissue, these random collisions have special significance because the endothelial cells express specific surface molecules that can bind passing leukocytes on contact.

The properties of endothelial cells normally vary among organs and among different types and sizes of blood vessels. The cells lining postcapillary venules, in particular, are uniquely adapted to express high levels of certain surface adhesion molecules when the surrounding tissue is distressed. The most critical of these molecules include two members of the selectin family of carbohydrate-binding proteins (called **E-selectin** and **P-selectin**), as well as intracellular adhesion molecule 1 (**ICAM-1**) and vascular cell adhesion molecule 1 (**VCAM-1**), which each can bind specific integrins on other cells (see Chapter 1). Endothelial cells express these proteins as part of a process called **endothelial cell activation,** which occurs when they detect factors in their environment that signify a nearby injury or infection (Table 2–4). Some of these activating factors (such as LPS) are microbial constituents, others are by-products of the blood-clotting or complement cascades, and still others (such as histamine, IL-1, and TNF) are released from various types of host cells during defensive responses. Induction of most endothelial adhesion proteins requires several hours of stimulation to allow for synthesis of the appropriate mRNAs and protein, but a few can be induced within minutes: for example, endothelial cells constitutively harbor P-selectin on the membranes of intracytoplasmic secretory vesicles called Weibel-Palade bodies; when the cell is stimu-

Table 2–4. Major adhesion proteins induced on activated endothelial cells.

Adhesion Protein	Kinetics[1]	Major Inducers
P-selectin	Rapid (min)	Thrombin Histamine Complement derivatives Peroxide
E-selectin	Slow (h)	Interleukin-1 Tumor necrosis factor LPS
ICAM-1, VCAM-1	Slow (h)	Interleukin-1 Tumor necrosis factor Interferon gamma LPS

Abbreviations: ICAM = intercellular adhesion molecule; VCAM = vascular cell adhesion molecule; LPS = lipopolysaccharide.
[1] Kinetics of appearance of binding activity after activating stimulus.

lated appropriately, these organelles quickly fuse with the plasma membrane, transferring P-selectin onto the cell surface. Each endothelial adhesion protein has an affinity for surface molecules expressed by one or more types of leukocytes (see Table 2–4). Thus, the postcapillary venules in a distressed tissue not only are dilated and leaky but also are lined by activated endothelial cells that have markedly increased affinity for leukocytes. As we shall see in the following section, binding of leukocytes onto the endothelium is the first, essential step in attracting these defensive cells to the site of an injury or infection.

THE PHAGOCYTES

Although virtually all types of leukocytes contribute to host defense, three types play especially preeminent roles (Table 2–5). Two of these—the **neutrophils** and the **monocyte–macrophage** series—are phagocytic cells, which act primarily by engulfing and digesting bacteria, cellular debris, and other particulate matter. The third group, comprising the **lymphocytes** and their relatives, has little phagocytic capacity but instead carries out a host of other pro-

tective reactions that are known collectively as **immune responses.** Lymphocytes are critical for all aspects of acquired immunity, and their properties will be considered at length in later chapters. The phagocytes, on the other hand, may act in cooperation with lymphocytes but also are able to recognize and kill many pathogens directly, and so constitute the most important cellular effectors of the innate immune system.

Neutrophils

Neutrophils make up an army of more-or-less identical circulating phagocytes that are poised to respond quickly and in vast numbers wherever tissue injury has occurred. The mature cells, which are also known as segmented neutrophils (segs) or polymorphonuclear leukocytes (polys, or PMNs), can easily be identified by their characteristic multilobed nucleus and by the abundant storage granules in their cytoplasm (Fig 2–4). These granules store bactericidal agents and lysosomal enzymes until they are needed to kill and digest an ingested microorganism. Synthesis of the granule proteins, and their incorporation into granules, occurs as immature neutrophil precursors develop in the bone marrow. The mature neutrophil contains three chemically distinct granule types,

Table 2–5. Properties of three major human cell lineages involved in host defense.[1]

	Neutrophils	Monocyte–Macrophages	Lymphocytes[2]
Primary effector function	Phagocytosis	Phagocytosis	Varies
Cytoplasmic granules	Many	Moderate	Few
Can synthesize new membrane or secretory proteins	Very limited	Yes	Yes
Terminally differentiated	Yes	Usually	No
Principal normal location	Blood and marrow	All tissues	Lymphoid tissues
Immunoregulatory cytokine production	No[3]	Yes	Yes
Antigen presentation[4]	No	Yes	Yes

[1] The properties as listed apply to the mature cells of each lineage.
[2] Several distinct subtypes of lymphocytes have been described, and their functional properties differ widely (see Chapter 3). Properties shown are those of B and α/β T lymphocytes.
[3] Except certain chemokines (see Chapter 10).
[4] To helper T lymphocytes (see Chapter 4).

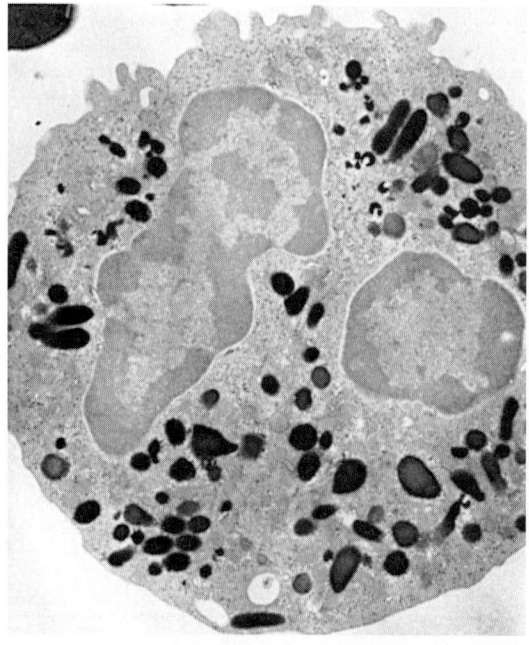

Figure 2–4. Electron micrograph of a human neutrophil. The single elongated nucleus is constricted at multiple sites to form segments, only two of which appear in this section. The cytoplasm contains numerous storage granules that differ in appearance and enzyme content; the myeloperoxidase-containing (azurophilic) granules are stained darkly in this preparation. Note the absence of rough endoplasmic reticulum.

which appear at different stages of maturation (Table 2–6). The azurophilic (or primary) granules are formed early during the promyelocyte stage and are known to contain an antibacterial enzyme, called myeloperoxidase, as well as numerous lysosomal enzymes and other proteins. The specific (or secondary) granules are formed later during the myelocyte stage and contain the soluble antibacterial proteins lysozyme and lactoferrin, as well as several important membrane receptors but lack myeloperoxidase. Gelatinase-containing granules are formed last, at the metamyelocyte stage. Thus, each neutrophil contains a diverse armamentarium of preformed antimicrobial proteins. Immature neutrophils precursors have a well-developed rough endoplasmic reticulum and Golgi apparatus that are used to synthesize the granules, but those organelles disappear or are greatly diminished as the cells mature, leaving the fully developed neutrophil with very limited ability to produce new secretory or membrane proteins. The mature neutrophil is also terminally differentiated—that is, it lacks the ability to replicate by cell division.

Neutrophils grow to full maturity in the bone marrow and are usually retained in the marrow for an additional 5 days as part of a large reserve pool. They then are released into the bloodstream, where they normally constitute one half to two thirds of all circulating white blood cells. An adult has approximately 50 billion neutrophils in the circulation at all times, each of which is programmed to die by apoptosis less than 12 hours, on average, after entering the blood. Thus, the marrow must produce vast numbers of neutrophils each day in order to maintain a stable circulating population. To meet this demand, roughly 60%

of all marrow hematopoietic activity is devoted to neutrophil production, as compared with only 20–30% that is devoted to erythrocyte formation.

Once released from the marrow, neutrophils normally circulate continuously in the blood throughout their brief lives. If their journey carries them into a site of injury or infection, however, the cells rapidly adhere to the endothelium of local postcapillary venules, migrate through the vessel walls, and invade into the affected tissues, where they may accumulate in vast numbers. As is true for all leukocytes, the process by which neutrophils adhere to a vessel wall is called **margination** and occurs in three phases (Fig 2–5). The first, **selectin-mediated phase** begins when a neutrophil collides with the vessel wall, allowing P-selectin and and E-selectin molecules on activated endothelial cells to bind neutrophil surface mucins that bear the appropriate carbohydrate side chains. At the same time, **L-selectin,** which is expressed constitutively on neutrophils (as well as on all other leukocytes), binds to its own set of target mucins on the activated endothelial surface. Together, these three types of selectins establish the initial adhesive contact between the neutrophil and the vessel wall. The selectins and their mucin ligands are elongated molecules and are often located at the tips of microvilli, which enhances their accessibility for binding. In contrast to other types of adhesion molecules, selectins bond tightly to their ligands in less than a millisecond, so that even momentary contact can tether a moving neutrophil firmly to the wall. Because this tethering involves only a few bonds at a time, however, and because the individual bonds dissociate after no more than a few seconds, the neutrophil continues to roll or

Table 2–6. Representative contents of human neutrophil granules.

	Azurophilic Granules	Specific Granules	Gelatinase Granules
Soluble Proteins			
Microbicidal proteins	Myeloperoxidase Lysozyme Defensins	Lysozyme	
Other enzymes	Lysosomal acid hydrolases Elastase Cathepsin G Proteinase 3 Azurocidin	Collagenase Gelatinase	Gelatinase
Other proteins		Lactoferrin β_2-microglobulin Vitamin B_{12}-binding protein	
Membrane Proteins			
Receptors for:		Complement proteins (CR3) Chemokines N-formyl peptides Laminin Vitronectin	Complement proteins (CR1) Immunoglobulin (FcγRIII)
Other proteins	CD63	Mac-1 (CD11b/CD18)	Mac-1 (CD11b/CD18)

Abbreviations: CR = complement receptor; FcγRIII = type-3 Fc receptor specific for immunoglobulin G (see Chapter 7). Mac-1 is an integrin composed of the CD11b and CD18 chains.

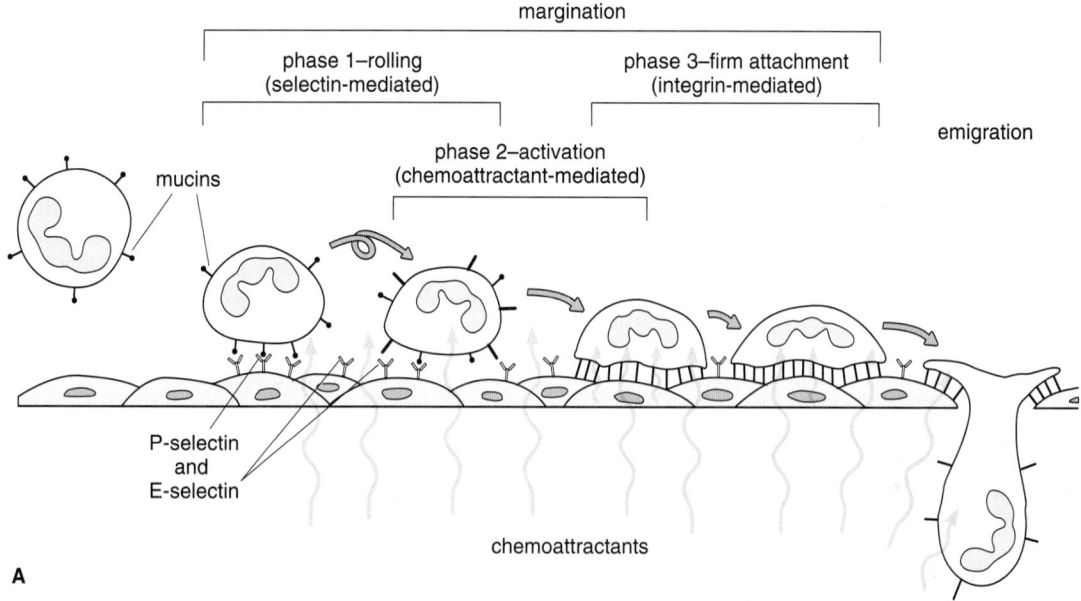

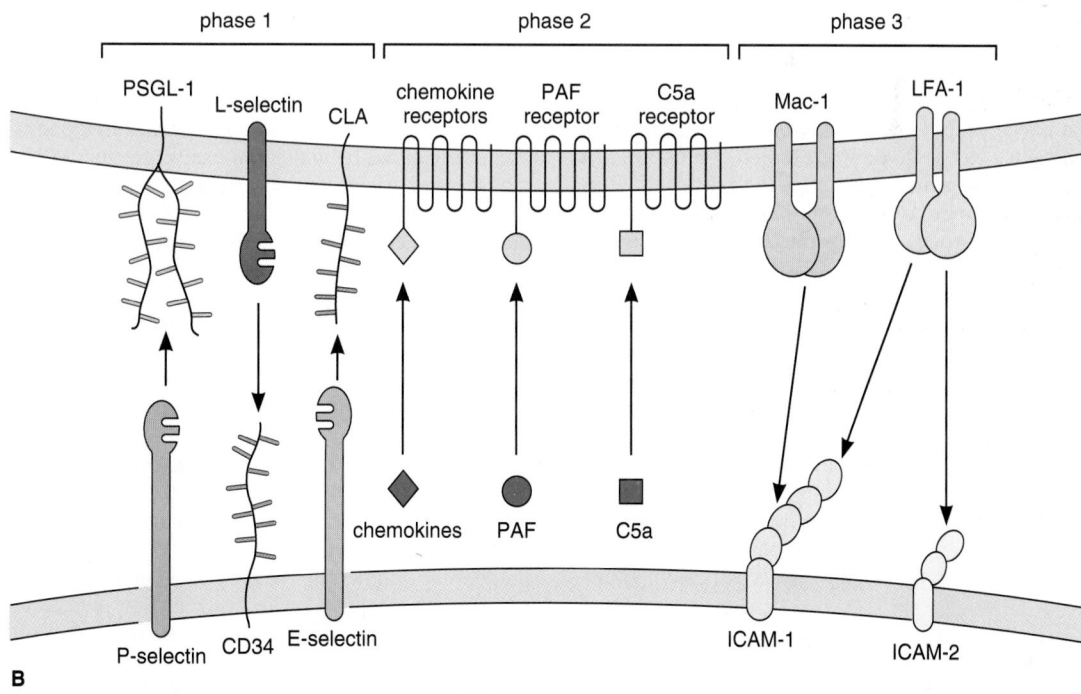

Figure 2–5. Neutrophil margination and emigration. **A:** Leukocyte adhesion to activated endothelium occurs in three over-lapping phases, each mediated by a particular class of molecules. **B:** Molecular interactions in the three phases of neutrophil adhesion. Representative surface molecules on the neutrophil **(above)** and endothelial cell **(below)** are shown with their corresponding ligands. Similar interactions also mediate endothelial binding by other leukocytes, though the specific molecules involved may vary. **Abbreviations:** PSGL-1 = P-selectin glycoprotein ligand; CLA = cutaneous lymphocyte antigen; PAF = platelet-activating factor; C5a = complement derivative 5a (see Chapter 11). (Modified and redrawn, with permission, from Springer TA, *Annu Rev Physiol* 1995;**57:**827.)

skip intermittently along the vessel wall during this phase, under the force of the flowing blood.

Selectin-mediated rolling of a neutrophil along the venule wall increases the cell's exposure to a diverse group of substances, known collectively as **leukocyte chemotactic factors** (Table 2–7), which may either be expressed by activated endothelium or diffuse into the blood from the injured tissue. These factors bind to receptors on the neutrophil surface and trigger the second, **activation phase** of endothelial binding. In general, the chemotactic factors are substances that signify the presence of an injury rather than its exact cause. Many are host-derived molecules that are produced either directly as a result of tissue damage or indirectly by the host response to it; these include fragments of fibrin or collagen (as might be generated in a wound), soluble factors released by activated platelets or mast cells, and certain by-products of the complement cascade. Others are unique products of bacterial metabolism, the most notable of which are peptides containing **N-formylmethionine** residues. This modified amino acid is present at the amino termini of proteins from most types of bacteria but is not found in proteins of human origin; it therefore serves as a telltale sign that bacteria are present in a host tissue. An especially important class of chemotactic factors is the group of cytokines known as **chemokines,** which can be secreted by activated endothelial cells and by other cell types in response to tissue distress and which each act selectively on particular types of leukocytes. Though they are soluble proteins, the chemokines tend to adhere to the surfaces of endothelial cells and also to the extracellular matrix, forming a gradient of concentrations through the tissues with its peak at the site of injury.

Each leukocyte chemotactic factor is recognized by a specific receptor on the leukocyte surface. Despite the diversity of their ligands, all of these receptors belong to the **7-transmembrane** receptor family, a very large group of receptors that each consist of a single polypeptide threaded across the plasma membrane seven times. Every neutrophil carries a host of receptors for different chemotactic factors. Contact with even minute amounts of such a factor, either dissolved in the blood or bound to the endothelial surface, triggers dramatic changes in the surface adhesion properties of the neutrophil. The most important effect of the chemotactic factors is to induce changes in the conformations of **integrins** on the leukocyte surface, enabling them to bind specific glycoprotein ligands on the endothelium. For example, exposure of a neutrophil to either N-formylmethionyl peptides or certain chemokines unmasks the binding activities of integrins called **Mac-1** and leukocyte functional antigen 1 (**LFA-1**), which can each then bind to ICAM-1 on an activated endothelial cell. These latter changes initiate the final, **integrin-mediated phase** of margination (see Fig 2–5). Though integrin-mediated interactions develop relatively slowly (evolving over the course of a few minutes), they lead to stable, long-lasting molecular contacts that prevent further movement of the neutrophil and cause it to flatten out against the endothelium.

Once attached, neutrophils actively insinuate themselves between endothelial cells to migrate out of the venule and into the adjacent tissue in a process termed **emigration.** The neutrophils then travel by ameboid motion up the concentration gradient of chemotactic factors until they arrive at the focus of injury or infection. Emigration and chemotaxis are facilitated in part by binding of neutrophil surface integrins to fibronectin and other components of the extracellular matrix.

On arrival at an injured site, neutrophils immediately begin the process of engulfing any bacteria, cellular debris, or foreign particulate matter in the area. The mechanisms by which these cells are able to recognize such a wide range of target particles are not fully understood. Some types of targets, such as unencapsulated bacteria, carbon particles, or polystyrene beads, are probably recognized by virtue of nonspecific surface properties such as hydrophobicity. Others may fortuitously carry particular oligosaccharides or other chemical features that are recognized by receptors on the neutrophil surface. Individual macromolecules, or submicroscopic particles such as viruses, that bind an individual receptor may be taken into the cell through **receptor-mediated endocytosis,** but larger (>100 nm diameter), multivalent particles, such as bacteria, undergo **phagocytosis,** which is thought to occur through a progressive "zippering" process in which increasing numbers of receptors on the cell surface membrane come into contact with the particle surface until it is completely engulfed (Fig 2–6).

Many types of particles, including most species of encapsulated bacteria, do not interact effectively with any cellular receptor, and hence cannot be phagocytized directly. Phagocytosis of such particles can occur, however, when their surfaces are coated with certain host-derived proteins. Proteins that have this ability to enhance phagocytosis are known as **opsonins.** Many different human proteins function as opsonins (for examples, see Table 2–1), but by far the most important are the complement derivatives and a

Table 2–7. Major leukocyte chemotactic factors.

Endogenous
  Fibrin fragments
  Collagen fragments
  Complement derivatives (especially C5a)
  Chemokines
  Platelet-activating factor (PAF)
  Leukotriene B_4 (LTB_4)
  Prostaglandin D_2 (PGD_2)

Exogenous
  N-formylated oligopeptides (ie, N-formylmethionyl or N-formylnorleucyl)

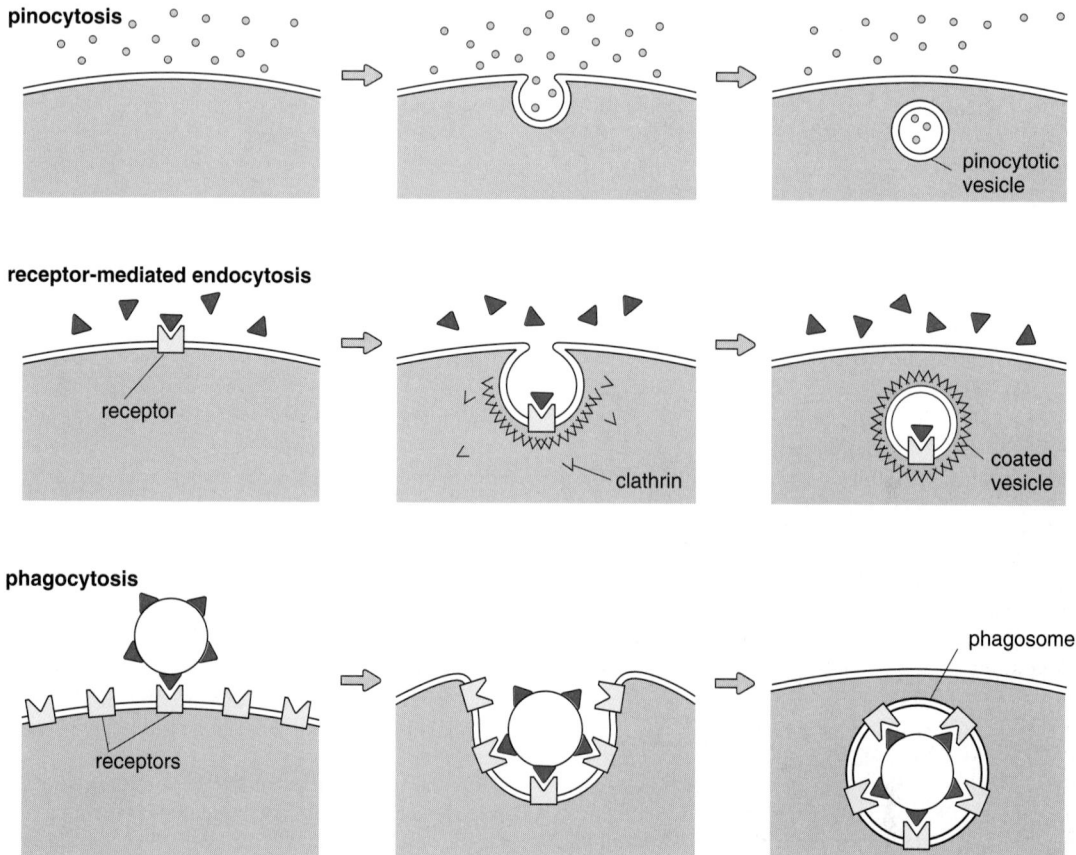

pinocytosis

pinocytotic vesicle

receptor-mediated endocytosis

receptor

clathrin

coated vesicle

phagocytosis

phagosome

receptors

Figure 2–6. Three major pathways for bringing extracellular materials into a cell. Pinocytosis ("cell drinking") occurs through formation of minute surface vesicles filled with unmodified extracellular fluid. Receptor-mediated endocytosis is triggered by the binding of a soluble ligand to one or more specific surface receptors; the resulting polymerization of clathrin protein on the cytoplasmic aspect of the plasma membrane leads to invagination of the receptor and formation of a coated pit. Phagocytosis occurs when multiple surface receptors sequentially engage the surface of a target particle, usually >100 nm in diameter. Pinocytotic and coated vesicles, like phagosomes, are lined by a single lipid bilayer derived from the plasma membrane.

group of proteins called **immunoglobulins** that are secreted by some cells of the lymphocyte lineage (see Chapters 3 and 7). Opsonization occurs because the phagocyte carries surface receptors for the opsonin protein: when such a protein coats a target particle, it allows receptor-mediated engulfment (Fig 2–7). The opsonizing effect of immunoglobulins, for example, is mediated through immunoglobulin receptors, called **Fc receptors,** on the phagocyte surface. Similarly, some components of the complement pathway act as very potent opsonins because the phagocytes express surface **complement receptors.**

Particles that have been engulfed by a neutrophil are initially contained within membrane-bounded vacuoles called **phagosomes.** Seconds after engulfment, storage granules in the neutrophil cytoplasm begin to fuse with each phagosome, emptying their contents into its lumen (Fig 2–8). This process is known as **degranulation.** The neutrophil granules contain an extensive array of enzymes and other substances that can kill and degrade bacteria or dissolve other phagocytized materials (see Table 2–6). Among the most abundant are a class of small (roughly 30 amino acids long) antimicrobial peptides called **defensins,** which kill by permeabilizing bacterial or fungal cell membranes and which constitute 30–50% of total granule protein. Other granule contents include the bactericidal enzyme **lysozyme,** numerous proteinases, and **lactoferrin**—a protein that inhibits bacterial growth by chelating iron. The cell also acidifies the phagosome by actively pumping hydrogen ions into its interior; this not only promotes hydrolysis of the target directly but also enhances the activities of many granular enzymes.

In addition, a family of potent **NADPH** (reduced form of nicotinamide-ademine dinucleotide phos-

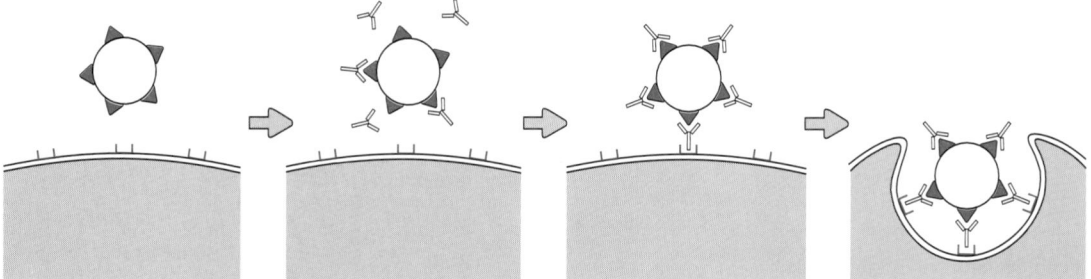

Figure 2–7. Opsonization. The opsonin protein (in this case, an immunoglobulin) binds to the surface of a particle, enabling the particle to be recognized by opsonin-specific receptors on the phagocyte surface.

phate)-**dependent oxidases** attached to the granule membranes project into the lumen of the phagocytic vacuole after degranulation. These oxidases act to convert molecular oxygen into highly reactive singlet oxygen, which spontaneously dismutates to form hydrogen peroxide (Table 2–8). In the presence of **myeloperoxidase** (which accounts for 5% of the dry weight of a neutrophil), this hydrogen peroxide combines with chloride ions to form hypochlorous acid (HOCl)—a potent oxidizing agent that is the active ingredient of household bleach. The hypochlorous acid is consumed almost instantaneously as it oxidizes amines, thiols, nucleic acids, proteins, and other biomolecules in the target particle, but a substantial portion reacts to form organic chloramines (R-NCl)—a less powerful but much longer-lived class of oxidizing agents.

Oxidative killing also occurs through a second pathway involving production of **nitric oxide (NO),** a soluble, highly labile, free radical gas. When activated, neutrophils express an enzyme called inducible nitric oxide synthase (iNOS) which can generate NO from the amino acid arginine and molecular oxygen (see Table 2–8). In the presence of other reactive oxygen species within the phagocytic vacuole, NO is con-verted to other products, such as peroxynitrite, which are highly toxic to bacteria, yeast, viruses, and other pathogens.

Together, these oxidative pathways provide some of the neutrophil's most important antimicrobial effects. Their vigorous action is manifested by a pronounced, transient increase in overall oxygen consumption by the neutrophil (called a **respiratory burst,** or **metabolic burst**) that occurs immediately after phagocytosis and can persist for as long as 3 hours.

The types of injuries that attract neutrophils into a tissue are nearly always accompanied by the local release of vasoactive mediators and other substances, which produces swelling, redness, heat, and pain at the involved site (see Chapter 12). These local effects, combined with an infiltration of neutrophils, constitute the pattern of host response known as **acute inflammation.** The first wave of invading neutrophils can be detected as early as 30 minutes after an acute injury; the cells generally accumulate to significant levels within 8–12 hours and continue to arrive in increasing numbers until the production of chemotactic signals subsides. Because neutrophils cannot replicate, and survive for only a few hours within tissues,

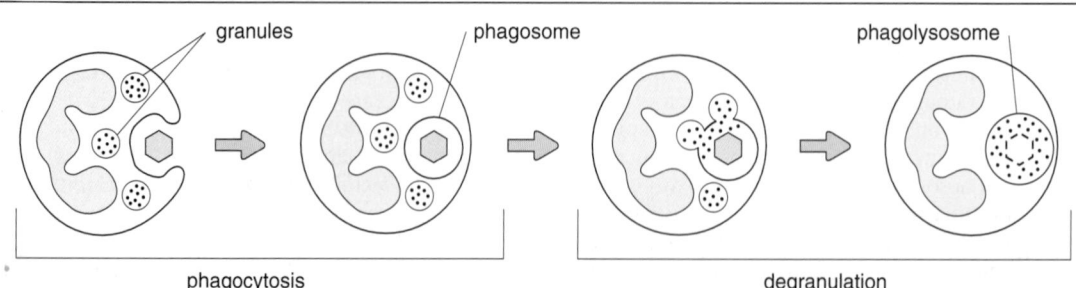

Figure 2–8. Engulfment and digestion of a target by a neutrophil. In the process of degranulation, multiple types of cytoplasmic granules may fuse with the phagosome, disgorging their contents into its lumen to inactivate and degrade the target particle.

Table 2–8. The major oxidative microbicidal pathways in neutrophils.

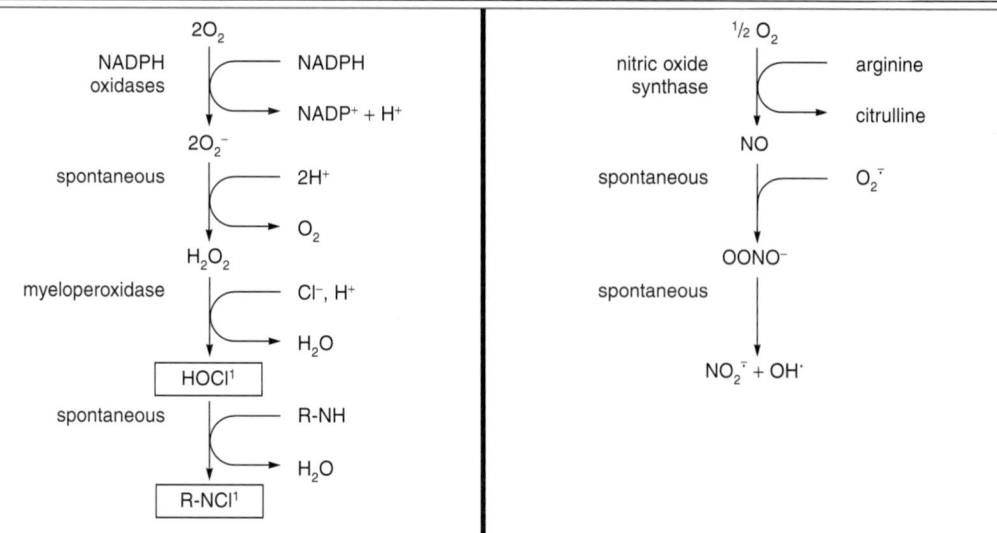

[1]Hypochlorous acid (HOCl) and organic chloramines (R-NCl) probably account for most of the target oxidation that takes place in vivo. The superoxide (O_2^-) and hydrogen peroxide (H_2O_2) intermediates in this pathway are also strong oxidizing agents but probably proceed along the pathway too quickly to play a major direct role in attacking target particles. "R-NH" denotes any organic primary or secondary amine.

many die at the site of inflammation and must be replaced by new cells from the circulation. In severe acute infections or other periods of high demand, the rate at which neutrophils are produced and released from storage in the bone marrow often increases dramatically, so that the blood neutrophil concentration rises several-fold. This greatly increases the number of cells available for delivery to the injured site. If marrow output is especially great, immature neutrophils that have unsegmented, rod-shaped nuclei (and hence are called **bands**) may also be released to the bloodstream. When the demand eventually wanes, the peripheral neutrophil concentration gradually returns to normal over a period of days or weeks.

If a localized response is prolonged or intense, enzymes released from dying neutrophils may liquefy nearby host cells and foreign material alike to form a viscous semifluid residue called **pus**—another hallmark of acute inflammation. Granule contents can also escape accidentally from living neutrophils during the course of phagocytosis, as degranulation often begins before a target particle has been completely engulfed (Fig 2–9). An extreme example of this occurs when neutrophils confront a target (such as a splinter) that is too large to engulf: in such a case, the cells attach themselves to the target and discharge granule contents (primarily from the specific granules) onto its surface, in a process called **extracellular degranulation.** Though beneficial in some cases, extracellular release of granule contents carries the risk of serious damage to host tissues, and plays a prominent role in the pathogenesis of several human diseases, including gout, some forms of glomerulonephritis, and autoimmune arthritis.

The neutrophilic phagocyte system has many advantageous properties as an agent of innate immunity. First, neutrophils are attracted by a limited number of stimuli that generally signal the presence of tissue injury no matter what its cause. This ensures that the cells can respond to many different types of injuries, including those that the host has never encountered before. Thus, acute trauma, foreign bodies, thermal or chemical burns, bacterial infections, and many other types of injuries each can provoke an intense neutrophil response. In addition, because large numbers of neutrophils are continually present in the blood, and because nearly all of them respond to the same set of chemotactic factors, vast numbers of the cells can be mobilized without delay. Moreover, neutrophils are highly effective at killing certain bacteria, and their ability to digest cellular debris and exogenous particulate matter provides an important first step in the healing process.

Nevertheless, a defense system based solely on neutrophils would have some very significant limitations. In particular, these cells are completely unable to recognize many types of potentially injurious agents, and so do not respond to them until tissue damage has occurred. For example, neutrophils cannot detect or eradicate most types of proteinaceous toxins or individual viral particles circulating in the blood, because these generally do not bind to any neutrophil surface receptor. When neutrophils are called into action, they have only a limited repertoire of possible responses, consisting mainly of phagocytosis and the intracellular or extracellular discharge of their granule contents. Finally, the neutrophil system by itself has almost no ability to modify its responses on

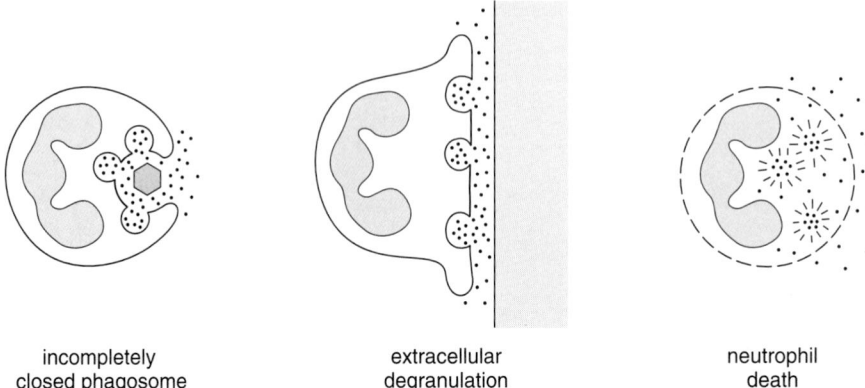

incompletely
closed phagosome

extracellular
degranulation

neutrophil
death

Figure 2–9. Some means by which the contents of neutrophil granules may be released into the extracellular milieu. Extracellular degranulation (also called "frustrated phagocytosis") occurs when the cell encounters a target that is too large to engulf. Neutrophil death, and the inadvertent release of granule contents from incompletely closed phagosomes, are common during intense or prolonged neutrophil reactions.

the basis of past exposure. Left on its own, this system of phagocytes would respond (or fail to respond) in the same stereotypical manner to a given pathogen no matter how many times it had encountered that same pathogen before.

Mononuclear Phagocytes: The Monocyte–Macrophage System

Nearly all tissues, organs, and serosal cavities harbor a population of resident phagocytes. Most contain only a diffuse scattering of individual phagocytic cells that remain inconspicuous under normal conditions and are very similar to one another in appearance and function. In some tissues, however, phagocytes are especially abundant or have distinctive morphologic features, and are known by specific names: examples include the Kupffer cells that line sinusoids of the liver (and account for nearly 10% of total liver mass), osteoclasts in bone, or microglial cells of the brain (Table 2–9). Regardless of their location or appearance, all of these tissue-associated phagocytes belong to a single lineage known as the **mononuclear phagocyte system** and are derived from a circulating white blood cell called the monocyte.

Monocytes are relatively large (12–20 μm in diameter) cells with kidney-shaped nuclei, loose nuclear chromatin, and fairly abundant cytoplasm that is well stocked with the types of organelles needed to synthesize secretory and membrane proteins (Fig 2–10). They also contain a substantial supply of cytoplasmic **lysosomes,** which contain most of the same enzymatic constituents found in neutrophil azurophilic granules; however, these are less numerous than the granules in neutrophils and are not readily seen under the light microscope. Monocytes are not very abundant in the peripheral circulation, ac-

counting for only 1–6% of all nucleated blood cells. They are produced in the bone marrow and are then released into the blood, where they circulate for only about a day before settling into a permanent site of residence in a tissue. Once settled in this manner, the cells are called tissue **macrophages,** or **histiocytes.** The criteria by which the cells select their tissue residence is presently unknown. Like other leukocytes, blood monocytes can be attracted into a site of injury or infection through a three-phase process of endothelial attachment that is essentially identical to that described for neutrophils and uses many of the same adhesion proteins and chemotactic factors (see earlier section). The specific chemokines recognized by monocytes and neutrophils differ, however, owing to the expression of distinct sets of chemokine receptors

Table 2–9. Cells of the monocyte–macrophage lineage.

Tissue	Cell Type Designation
Blood	Monocytes
Bone marrow	Monocytes and monocyte precursors (monoblasts, promonocytes)
Any solid tissue	Resident macrophages (histiocytes)
Skin	Langerhans' cells
Liver	Kupffer cells
Lung	Alveolar macrophages
Bone	Osteoclasts
Synovium	Type A synovial cells
Central nervous system	Microglia
Pleural cavity	Pleural macrophages
Peritoneal cavity	Peritoneal macrophages
Chronic inflammatory exudate	Exudate macrophages
Granuloma	Epithelioid cells, multinucleated giant cells

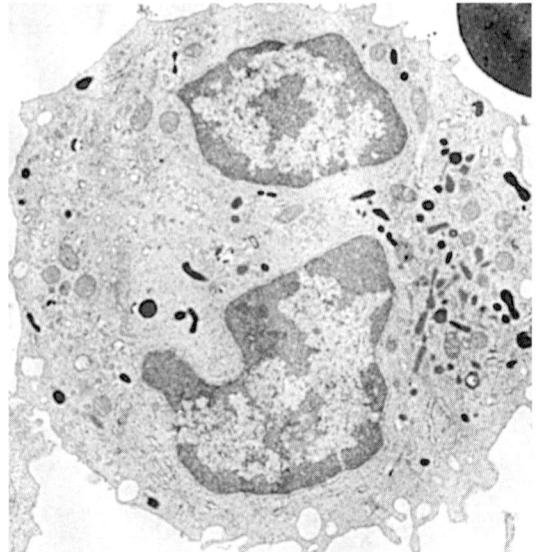

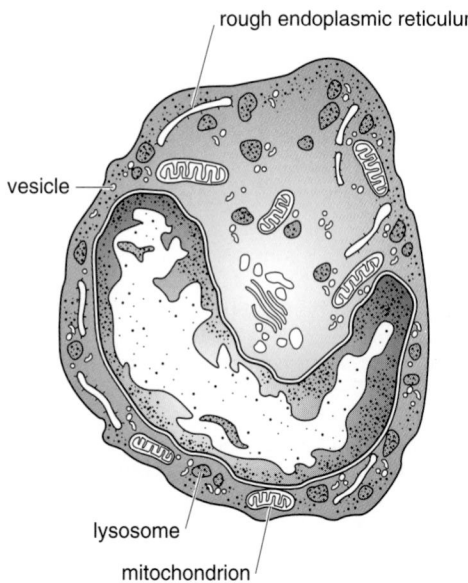

Figure 2–10. Electron micrograph of a human monocyte. Cytoplasmic granules (lysosomes) are present but are much less numerous than in neutrophils. However, the cell retains the abundant Golgi apparatus and rough endoplasmic reticulum needed to synthesize additional granules or secretory proteins as needed.

on each cell type; as a result, the particular combination of chemokines produced in a distressed tissue determines whether monocytes, neutrophils, or other leukocytes are attracted. It is not known whether these same factors also govern the entry and distribution of monocytes into normal tissues. Monocytes that colonize some tissues (such as the liver or brain) subse-

quently undergo changes in morphology or function, presumably in response to factors in the local microenvironment.

A tissue macrophage lives for approximately 2–4 months. During this time, some macrophages remain immobile, whereas others wander incessantly by amoeboid motion. In either case, the cell continually samples its surrounding environment by pinocytosis (see Fig 2–6) and through an extensive array of receptors on its surface (Table 2–10). Whenever it encounters certain stimuli, the cell undergoes a process known as **macrophage activation,** in which it rapidly increases its metabolic rate, motility, and phagocytic activity. Activated macrophages are somewhat larger than their inactive counterparts, owing mainly to an increase in cytoplasmic volume, and are much more efficient at killing bacteria and other pathogens. Many new proteins are synthesized on activation, including the inducible nitric oxide synthase, whose product (NO) has a major role in macrophage bactericidal function. The range of stimuli that can activate macrophages is very large: direct contact with certain microorganisms or inert particles, with bacterial LPS or host tissue breakdown products, or with protein components of the complement or blood coagulation systems can each lead to activation. Activation can also be induced by certain cytokines (notably one

Table 2–10. Ligands bound by macrophage surface receptors.

Opsonins
Complement components (C3 and C4 products)
Immunoglobulins (especially IgG; via Fc receptors)
Carbohydrates and carbohydrate-binding proteins (mannose-, fucose-, galactose-, and N-acetylglucosamine-containing oligosaccharides)

Chemotactic factors
N-formyl oligopeptides
Complement components (C5a)
Thrombin
Fibrin

Growth factors and cytokines
Colony-stimulating factors (GM-CSF, M-CSF)
Interleukins (IL-1, IL-3, IL-6, IL-10)
Interferons (IFNα, IFNβ, IFNγ)
Tumor necrosis factors (TNF)
Transforming growth factor β (TGFβ)

Hormones and other mediators
Insulin
Histamine
Epinephrine
Calcitonin
Parathyroid hormone
Somatomedins

Miscellaneous
Transferrin
Lactoferrin
Modified low-density lipoproteins
Fibronectin

Source: Modified and reproduced, with permission, from Klein J: *Immunology,* Blackwell Scientific, 1990.

known as interferon gamma, or **IFNγ**) that may be secreted by nearby lymphocytes (see Chapter 10).

Activated macrophages are avid phagocytes that engulf whatever foreign particles or cellular debris they encounter. They move somewhat less rapidly than neutrophils but have the advantage of being much longer-lived. They also are larger and hence can engulf larger targets, including entire senescent or damaged host cells. Like neutrophils, macrophages recognize some target particles directly by their surface properties. Some macrophage surface receptors have target specificities resembling those of the soluble proteins of innate immunity (see Table 2–1): for example, macrophages express a specific **mannose receptor,** an LPS receptor called **CD14** that is a membrane-bound version of soluble CD14, and a family of proteins, called **scavenger receptors,** that recognize carbohydrates or lipids in bacterial and yeast cell walls. In addition, macrophages also have receptors for complement components, immunoglobulins, and other opsonins, and a coating of such opsonins is essential for phagocytosis of many types of particles. Engulfment occurs through the "zippering" process described earlier (see Fig 2–6) and encloses the target particle in a phagosome; cytoplasmic lysosomes then fuse with the phagosome, disgorging their contents into its lumen.

In comparison with the action of neutrophils, macrophage phagocytosis tends to be a slower, less dramatic process: the metabolic burst that occurs after engulfment is less pronounced, and engulfed matter tends to be broken down gradually and relentlessly over time. This is in part a reflection of the limited number of lysosomes that are available in the macrophage at a given moment. Unlike neutrophils, however, macrophages retain all of the organelles needed to synthesize secretory proteins and so can produce new lysosomes as needed. Ultimately, the offending particles are usually completely annihilated. For example, red blood cells that leak from a damaged vessel to form a bruise, as well as any host cells that die by apoptosis (see Chapter 1), are soon engulfed by tissue macrophages and broken down into their component molecules. Most engulfed bacteria meet the same fate. Other materials may resist degradation but still remain sequestered within the macrophage and so are prevented from contacting the surrounding tissue. For example, large numbers of inhaled carbon particles often persist for years within macrophages in the lungs of cigarette smokers.

Activated macrophages not only function as phagocytes but also specifically secrete an enormous variety of biologically active substances into the surrounding tissues. Over 100 macrophage secretory products have been identified so far, a partial list of which is presented in Table 2–11. Certain of these can be secreted individually in response to specific stimuli, whereas others are released in combination with one another as part of a more generalized response.

Table 2–11. Secretory products of macrophages.

Enzymes
Lysozyme
Acid hydrolases (proteases, nucleases, glycosidases, phosphatases, lipases, etc)
Elastase
Collagenase
Plasminogen activator
Angiotensin-converting enzyme

Mediators
Interferons (IFNα, IFNβ)
Colony-stimulating factors (GM-CSF, M-CSF, G-CSF, and others)
Interleukins (IL-1, IL-6, IL-8, IL-10, IL-12)
Chemokines
Tumor necrosis factor α (TNFα)
Platelet-derived growth factor
Platelet-activating factor (PAF)
Transforming growth factor β (TGFβ)
Angiogenesis factors
Nitric oxide
Arachidonate derivatives (prostaglandins, leukotrienes)

Complement components
C1–C9
Properdin
Factors B, D, I, and H

Coagulation factors
Factors V, VII, IX, and X
Prothrombin
Thromboplastin

Reactive oxygen species
Hydrogen peroxide
Superoxide anion
Nitric oxide
Singlet oxygen
Hydroxyl radicals

Miscellaneous
Glutathione
Nucleotides (adenosine, thymidine, guanosine, etc)

Some products, such as lysozyme, complement components, and hydrogen peroxide, have antimicrobial activity. Others, such as elastases and collagenases, act to liquefy and remodel the extracellular matrix; this facilitates cellular migration and helps clear the way for the healing process. Macrophages also secrete numerous **cytokines** that influence the growth and activities of other cell types (Chapter 10). These include colony-stimulating factors (such as GM-CSF, which prolongs neutrophil survival in tissues by suppressing apoptosis), IL-6 (which induces the acute-phase response), fibroblast growth factors, prostaglandins, and chemokines that draw lymphocytes and other leukocytes into the vicinity. Interestingly, the NO secreted by activated macrophages not only has broad-spectrum antimicrobial activity but also acts as a messenger to regulate functions of other nearby cells; for example, NO triggers release of histamine and other vasoactive mediators from mast cells and platelets and so promotes the local vascular response to injury.

Most macrophages are thought to be terminally differentiated, though some appear capable of limited replication within tissues. Some of the factors secreted by activated macrophages attract other nearby macrophages and blood monocytes, but the relatively slow movement and small numbers of such cells limit the speed of their response. Generally, 7–10 days must pass before significant numbers of macrophages arrive at an injured site. In most cases, there is little or no accompanying increase in marrow production or blood concentration of these cells.

Eventually, large numbers of macrophages may congregate around targets that are large, numerous, or resistant to digestion. Such macrophage aggregates are called **granulomas** (Fig 2–11), and usually contain subpopulations of lymphocytes, fibroblasts, and other cell types. Macrophages in such lesions are often called **epithelioid cells** because they tend to interdigitate closely with one another through complex surface folds and microvilli, and so form a continuous sheet of cells that resembles an epithelium. This interdigitation serves to entrap material within the granuloma. Individual macrophages may also fuse to form large, **multinucleated giant cells** that are able to engulf correspondingly larger targets, such as splinters, multicellular parasites, or surgical suture material.

Viewed in isolation, macrophages are a significant factor in innate immunity but suffer from many of the same limitations that were described earlier for neutrophils. They are a fairly homogeneous group of phagocytic cells that recognize a fixed number of potential targets. They are, moreover, less numerous, slower to respond, and less effective than neutrophils at killing most bacteria. An additional facet of their biology, however, places macrophages among the most important components of the immune system: unlike neutrophils, macrophages are able to control the actions of lymphocytes—a far more abundant and versatile population of defensive cells, and the principal cells of acquired immunity. Macrophages affect

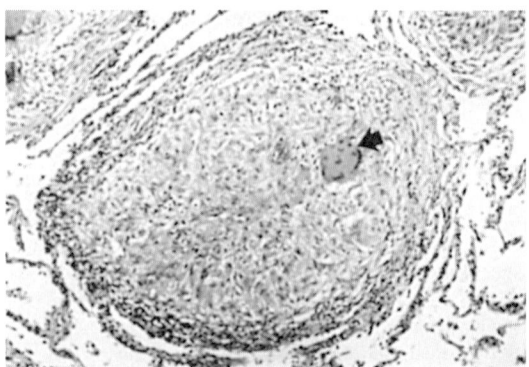

Figure 2–11. A granuloma—a distinctive pattern of macrophage reaction against foreign material. This photomicrograph shows a single roughly spherical granuloma, 1–2 mm in diameter, in the lung. It is composed almost entirely of epithelioid macrophages, with a thin, surrounding rim of fibroblasts and normal lung tissue. At one site, several individual macrophages have fused to form a multinucleated giant cell (arrow). In addition to macrophages, granulomas often contain other types of defensive cells (especially lymphocytes), fibroblasts, and collagen. (Courtesy of Martha Warnock)

lymphocyte responses in at least major two ways. First, activated macrophages secrete cytokines, such as TNF and IL-1, that control lymphocyte proliferation, differentiation, and effector function. Secondly, activated macrophages also are among the most important types of **antigen-presenting cells**—cells that process and display foreign substances in a form that can be recognized and responded to by lymphocytes. Through these two types of regulatory interactions with lymphocytes, macrophages play a crucial role in initiating and coordinating nearly all types of acquired immune responses. The mechanisms and consequences of these interactions will be explored in detail in subsequent chapters.

REFERENCES

INNATE IMMUNITY

Fearon DT, Locksley RM: The instructive role of innate immunity in the acquired immune response. *Science* 1996;**272**:50.

Nossal GJV: Life, death and the immune system. *Sci Am* 1993;**269**:52.

PHAGOCYTOSIS AND ENDOCYTOSIS

Gruenberg J, Howell KE: Membrane traffic in endocytosis: Insights from cell-free assays. *Annu Rev Cell Biol* 1989;**5**:453.

Kornfeld S, Mellman I: The biogenesis of lysosomes. *Annu Rev Cell Biol* 1989;**5**:483.

TARGET RECOGNITION AND ANTIMICROBIAL EFFECTOR MECHANISMS

Lehrer RI et al: Defensins: Antimicrobial and cytotoxic peptides of mammalian cells. *Annu Rev Immunol* 1993;**11**:105.

Nathan C: Natural resistance and nitric oxide. *Cell* 1995;**82**:873.

Roos D et al: Mutations in the X-linked and autosomal recessive forms of chronic granulomatous disease. *Blood* 1996;**87**:1663.

Rotrosen D, Gallin JI: Disorders of phagocyte function. *Annu Rev Immunol* 1987;**5**:127.

Weiss SJ: Tissue destruction by neutrophils. *New Engl J Med* 1989;**320**:365.

NEUTROPHILS AND MONOCYTE–MACROPHAGES

Borregaard N et al: Human neutrophil granules and secretory vesicles. *Eur J Hematol* 1993;**51:**187.

Cotter TG et al: Cell death in the myeloid lineage. *Immunol Rev* 1994;**142:**93.

Gallin JI et al (editors): *Inflammation: Basic Principles and Clinical Correlates,* 2nd ed. Raven Press, 1992.

ADHESION PROTEINS AND LEUKOCYTE–ENDOTHELIAL INTERACTIONS

Bevilacqua MP: Endothelial-leukocyte adhesion molecules. *Annu Rev Immunol* 1993;**11:**767.

Bokoch GM: Chemoattractant signaling and leukocyte activation. *Blood* 1995;**86:**1649.

Carlos TM, Harlan JM: Leukocyte-endothelial adhesion molecules. *Blood* 1994;**84:**2068.

Frenette PS, Wagner DD: Adhesion molecules—Part II: Blood vessels and blood cells. *New Engl J Med* 1996;**335:**43.

Kansas GS: Selectins and their ligands: Current concepts and controversies. *Blood* 1996;**88:**3259.

Lasky LA: Selectins: Interpreters of cell-specific carbohydrate information during inflammation. *Science* 1992;**258:**964.

Ruoslahti E: Integrins: *J Clin Invest* 1991;**87:**1.

Schall TI, Bacon KB: Chemokines, leukocyte trafficking, and inflammation. *Current Biol* 1994;**6:**865.

Springer TA: Traffic signals on endothelium for lymphocyte recirculation and leukocyte emigration. *Annu Rev Physiol* 1995;**57:**827.43

Lymphocytes & Lymphoid Tissues

3

Tristram G. Parslow, MD, PhD

The normal adult human body contains on the order of a trillion (10^{12}) lymphocytes, most of which appear virtually identical to one another when examined by conventional histologic techniques. The typical lymphocyte is a small, round, or club-shaped cell, 5–12 μm in diameter, with a roughly spherical nucleus, densely compacted nuclear chromatin, and cytoplasm so scanty as to be scarcely detectable under the light microscope. The cytoplasm contains scattered mitochondria and free ribosomes but lacks any distinctive organelles (Fig 3–1). Despite this uniform appearance, several very different types of lymphocytes can be distinguished on the basis of their functional properties and by the specific proteins they express. The most fundamental distinction is the division of these cells into two major lineages known as T (thymus-derived) cells and B (bone-marrow-derived) cells.

The relative proportions of T and B cells vary among tissues (Table 3–1); in peripheral blood, they account for about 75 and 10% of all lymphocytes, respectively. The remaining 15% of peripheral blood lymphocytes belong to a separate and rather enigmatic lineage known as natural killer (NK) cells, which differ from other lymphocytes in many significant respects and have some unusual properties that will be described later in this book (see Chapter 9). The present chapter focuses exclusively on T and B cells, which are the cells involved in most types of immune responses.

T- and B-lineage cells both arise from a subset of hematopoietic stem cells in the bone marrow or fetal liver that become committed to the lymphoid* pathway of development (Fig 3–2). There is considerable evidence for the existence of a committed marrow

---

* The word "lymphocyte" refers to cells at a specific stage in the T- or B-cell lineage. The term "lymphoid" is used to denote the entire lineages (encompassing cells at all developmental stages), or tissues in which cells from these lineages normally predominate.

progenitor, called the **lymphoid stem cell,** that serves as a common precursor for both T and B cells; however, such cells have not yet been purified or characterized definitively. The progeny of these putative stem cells follow divergent pathways to mature into either B or T lymphocytes. Human B-lymphocyte development takes place entirely within the bone marrow. T cells, on the other hand, develop from immature precursors that leave the marrow and travel through the bloodstream to the thymus, where they proliferate and differentiate into mature T lymphocytes.

The thymus and bone marrow are sometimes referred to as **primary lymphoid organs** because they provide unique microenvironments that are essential for **lymphopoiesis**—the initial production of lymphocytes from uncommitted progenitor cells. Together, the thymus and marrow produce approximately 10^9 mature lymphocytes each day, which are then released into the circulation. Lymphopoietic activity is controlled in part by soluble factors elaborated within these organs. For example, growth of early lymphoid progenitors requires at least two cytokines, called interleukin-3 **(IL-3)** and stem cell factor **(SCF),** found in both the thymic and marrow microenvironments. In addition, the thymus produces a number of hormones that selectively promote later stages of T-cell development. Lymphopoiesis also depends on direct contact of the lymphoid precursor cells with marrow and thymic stromal elements, with the extracellular matrix, and with one another. In general, lymphocytes are produced and released by the marrow and thymus at a more or less constant rate, irrespective of whether the cells are needed for an immune response at the moment. T lymphopoiesis in the thymus continues until about the time of puberty, at which time the organ normally involutes, but B cells continue to be produced by the marrow throughout life.

Mature lymphocytes that emerge from the thymus or bone marrow are in a quiescent, or **"resting,"** state: they are mitotically inactive (that is, they are in the G_0

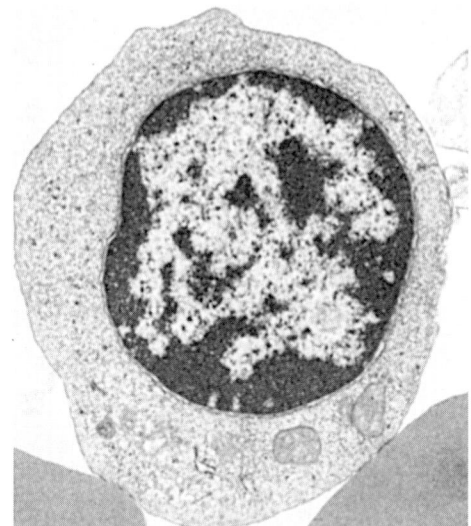

Figure 3–1. Electron micrograph of a normal human lymphocyte. This slightly tangential section exaggerates the amount of cytoplasm present: in most resting lymphocytes, the nucleus accounts for 90% of total cell volume. Note the dense nuclear chromatin and the bland cytoplasm, which lacks any obvious secretory organelles. (Courtesy of Imok Cha and Noel Weidner.)

phase of the cell cycle) and, although they are potentially capable of undergoing cell division and of carrying out immunologic functions, they have not yet been stimulated to do either. When dispersed into the bloodstream, these so-called "naive," or **"virgin,"** lymphocytes migrate efficiently into various **secondary** (or **peripheral**) **lymphoid organs,** such as the spleen, lymph nodes, or tonsils. The function of the secondary lymphoid organs is to maximize encounters between lymphocytes and foreign substances, and it is from these sites that most immune responses are launched.

Table 3–1. Proportions of lymphoid cell types in normal human tissues.

Tissue	Approximate % of [1]		
	T Cells	B Cells	NK Cells
Peripheral blood	70–80	10–15	10–15
Bone marrow	5–10	80–90	5–10
Thymus	99	<1	<1
Lymph node	70–80	20–30	<1
Spleen	30–40	50–60	1–5

[1] Includes cells at all recognizable stages of development in each lineage.

Most virgin lymphocytes have an inherently short life span and are programmed to die within a few days after leaving the marrow or thymus. If such a cell receives signals that indicate the presence of a specific foreign substance or pathogen, however, it may respond through a phenomenon known as **activation,** in the course of which it may undergo several successive rounds of cell division over a period of several days (Fig 3–3). Some of the resulting progeny cells then revert to the resting state to become **memory lymphocytes**—cells that resemble the virgin T or B lymphocyte from which they are derived but which can survive for many years. Such memory lymphocytes make up a large proportion of the cells in the immune system of an adult, and, like virgin lymphocytes, are constantly poised to undergo further cycles of activation and cell division. Thus, one consequence of activating a virgin lymphocyte is that some of its progeny become long-term constituents of the host immune system. The other progeny of an activated virgin lymphocyte differentiate into **effector cells,** which survive for only a few days but, during that time, carry out specific defensive activities against the foreign invader.

Lymphocyte proliferation can thus take place in two very different contexts. The first (lymphopoiesis) is confined to the thymus and marrow and results in the de novo production of short-lived, quiescent virgin lymphocytes that are then released into the periphery. This occurs autonomously at a rate dictated by the marrow and thymus themselves. The second form of replication takes place in peripheral tissues and occurs only when lymphocytes become activated as part of an immune response. This stimulus-dependent proliferation gives rise to long-lived memory cells and also to short-lived effector cells that actively carry out specific immune functions. The nature of these latter functions depends on the lymphocyte lineage from which the effector cells arose.

B CELLS

The defining feature of cells in the B-cell lineage is their ability to synthesize proteins called **immunoglobulins** (Fig 3–4). No other cell expresses these proteins. The immunoglobulins are an extremely diverse family of proteins, each made up of two related types of polypeptides called **heavy chains** and **light chains.** Each immunoglobulin binds specifically and with high affinity to its own particular small molecular ligand, which may be any of a vast number of chemical determinants found in proteins, carbohydrates, lipids, or other macromolecules. The molecular determinants bound by various immunoglobulin proteins can be referred to collectively as **antigens**—an important term that is considered more thoroughly in Chapter 5.

Mature B cells can express immunoglobulin in two

bone marrow

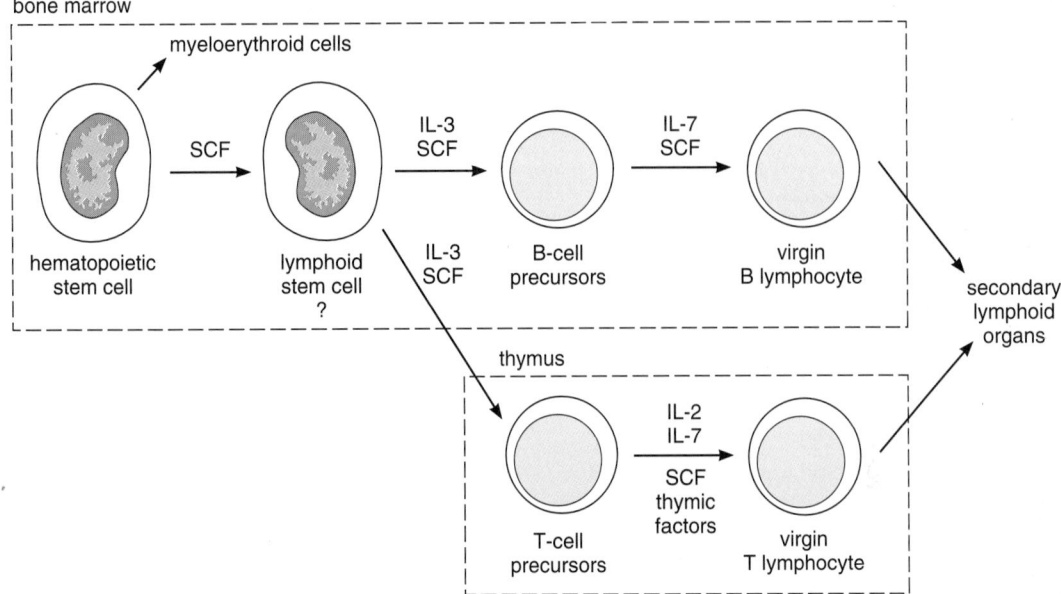

Figure 3–2. Schematic overview of lymphocyte development (lymphopoiesis). In this simplified diagram, most intermediate stages are omitted. The characteristics of cells that migrate to the thymus are unknown. A few of the regulatory molecules needed for proliferation at particular stages of development are indicated. SCF, stem cell factor; IL, interleukin.

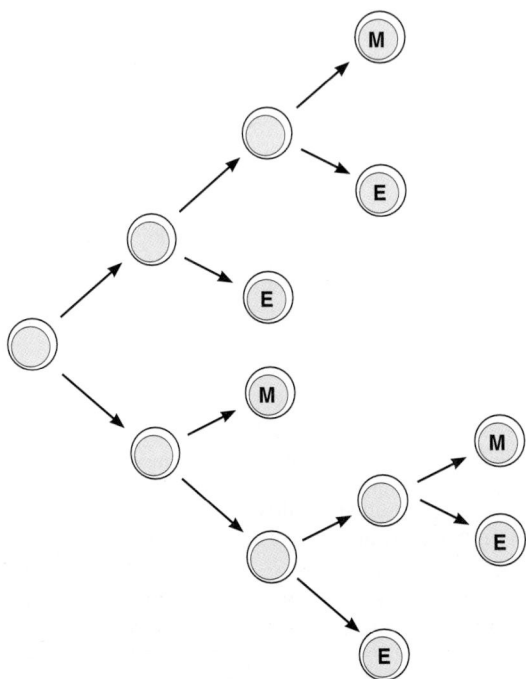

Figure 3–3. Lymphocyte activation leads to both cell division and differentiation. At each cell division, individual cells can cease dividing and differentiate into memory (M) or effector (E) cells. In this example, a single activated lymphocyte gives rise to four effector and three memory cells after four cycles of division.

different forms that each serve unique functions (Fig 3–5). In resting (virgin or memory) B lymphocytes, immunoglobulins are expressed only on the cell surface, where they serve as membrane-bound receptors for specific antigens. Each resting lymphocyte may express tens of thousands of membrane immunoglobulins on its surface. By contrast, the effector cells of the B lineage (called **plasma cells**) are uniquely specialized to secrete large amounts of immunoglobulin proteins into their surrounding milieu. Secreted immunoglobulins retain the ability to recognize and bind their specific ligands and are often referred to as **antibodies;** they normally circulate at a serum concentration of 7–26 g/L in an adult and so account for about 25% of total serum protein. Binding of an antibody to its target antigen can have a variety of effects that are beneficial to the host. For example, antibody binding may sequester and inactivate a toxic protein in the blood or may block receptors on a viral particle that would otherwise enable the virus to adhere to host cells. Many secreted immunoglobulins also are potent opsonins, in that they promote phagocytosis of bacteria or other targets to which they bind. The properties of immunoglobulins are discussed in much more detail in Chapter 7. For the present, it is enough to say that these binding proteins not only serve as surface receptors for foreign substances but also can be released to search out and bind their targets at a considerable distance from the cell.

When an activated B lymphocyte divides, some of its progeny become memory B cells, while the re-

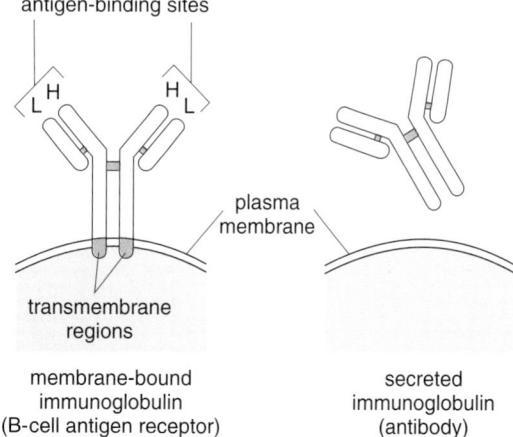

antigen-binding sites

plasma membrane

transmembrane regions

membrane-bound immunoglobulin (B-cell antigen receptor)

secreted immunoglobulin (antibody)

Figure 3–4. Membrane-bound and secreted forms of an immunoglobulin protein. This diagram depicts one of the many types of immunoglobulins, each of which is composed of paired light-chain (L) and heavy-chain (H) polypeptides. The amino termini of the L and H chains are juxtaposed to form the binding site for an antigen. A hydrophobic region (shaded) at the carboxy termini of the heavy chains anchors the membrane-bound protein onto the cell surface. When this region is absent, the immunoglobulin is secreted from the cell.

mainder differentiate into plasma cells. Plasma cells are oval or egg-shaped and have abundant cytoplasm and eccentrically placed round nuclei (Fig 3–6). Clumps of dark-staining chromatin are often distributed around the inner aspect of the nuclear membrane in plasma cells, giving the nuclei a characteristic "pinwheel" or "clock face" appearance under the light microscope. The protein-secretory organelles are well represented, including a large paranuclear Golgi apparatus and abundant rough endoplasmic reticulum. Immunoglobulins usually are not present on the surface of a plasma cell but are produced in copious

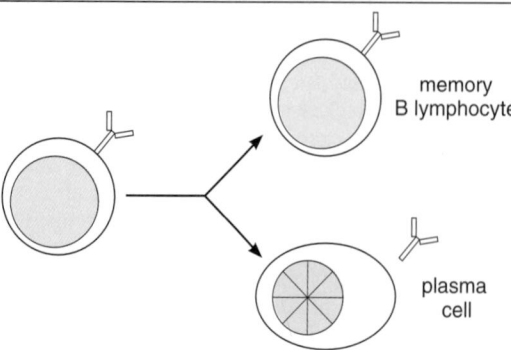

memory B lymphocyte

plasma cell

Figure 3–5. The progeny of an activated B lymphocyte can differentiate into either memory B lymphocytes or antibody-secreting plasma cells.

amounts in the cytoplasm and are then secreted into the extracellular space. Plasma cells have a relatively short life span (on the order of days to a few weeks) and are terminally differentiated. Unless new plasma cells are continually produced, the existing ones soon die out and immunoglobulins are no longer secreted. Thus, activation of B cells typically results in a transient wave of proliferation, followed by a burst of antibody secretion that increases and then subsides over several days or a few weeks.

The main function of B-lineage cells is to secrete antibodies into the blood and other body fluids and hence to make these fluids inhospitable to foreign invaders. They are the principal cell type involved in **humoral immunity**—that is, in protective effects that are mediated through tissue fluids. B cells also play two additional roles in the immune system. First, they can function as **antigen-presenting cells,** by processing and displaying foreign substances in a manner that can be recognized by T lymphocytes. Second, activated B cells can secrete certain **lymphokines** and other factors that influence the growth and activities of other immunologically important cells. These last two functions are discussed in more detail in later chapters.

T CELLS

T lymphocytes do not express immunoglobulins but, instead, detect the presence of foreign substances by way of surface proteins called **T-cell receptors.** These receptors form a heterogeneous class of membrane proteins, which, on most T cells, are made up of a pair of transmembrane polypeptides known as the α and β chains. T-cell receptors are closely related to immunoglobulins in evolution and share with them a number of structural and functional properties (see Chapters 7 and 9), including the ability to detect specific small molecular ligands called **antigens.** Unlike immunoglobulins, however, T-cell receptor proteins are never secreted, and, as a result, T cells lack the ability to strike their targets at long distance. Instead, they exert their protective effects either through direct contact with a target or by influencing the activity of other immune cells. Together with macrophages, T cells are the primary cell type involved in a category of immune responses called **cell-mediated immunity.**

Unlike B cells, T cells can detect foreign substances only in specific contexts. In particular, T lymphocytes will recognize a foreign protein only if it is first cleaved into small peptides, which are then displayed on the surface of a second host cell, called an **antigen-presenting cell.** Virtually all types of host cells can present antigens under some conditions, but certain cell types are specially adapted for this purpose and are particularly important in controlling T-cell activity. These specialized antigen-presenting

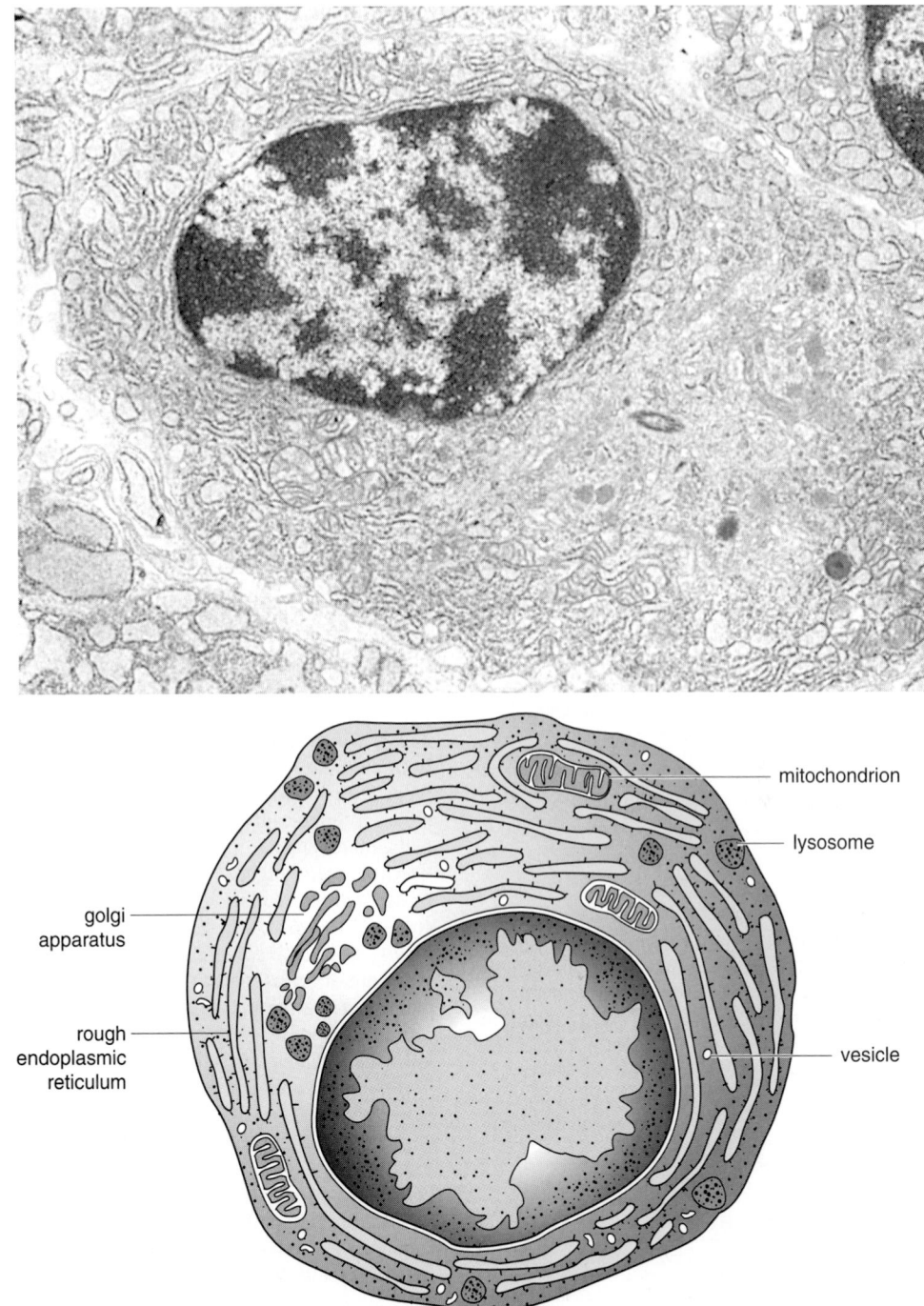

Figure 3–6. Electron micrograph *(top)* and diagram *(bottom)* of a plasma cell, the effector cell of the B-lymphoid lineage. The abundant rough endoplasmic reticulum and Golgi complex in the cytoplasm allow these cells to synthesize large amounts of immunoglobulin in a form that is then secreted from the cell. (Courtesy of DF Bainton.)

cells include macrophages and B lymphocytes, as well as other cell types that we will encounter later. Presentation depends in part on specific proteins, called **major histocompatibility complex (MHC)** proteins, on the surface of the presenting cells.

Foreign peptides are attached noncovalently onto the MHC proteins for display, and it is the combination of peptide and MHC protein that can be recognized by a T-cell receptor. Thus, T lymphocytes must directly touch the surfaces of other cells to detect antigens as well as to produce most of their immunologic effects.

Mature, functional T lymphocytes express a number of characteristic surface proteins in addition to T-cell receptors (Table 3–2). For example, surface T-cell receptors are always expressed in conjunction with five other transmembrane surface polypeptides that are known collectively as the **CD3 complex.** These CD3 proteins are physically associated with the T-cell receptors through noncovalent attachments; they serve to transmit signals from the receptors into the cytoplasm and must be present for the receptors to be transported onto the cell surface. Because the CD3 proteins are expressed almost exclusively by T-lineage cells and are easier to detect and much less structurally diverse than the receptors themselves, their presence is commonly used to identify T lymphocytes in extrathymic tissues. Surface expression of the receptor–CD3 complex, however, occurs relatively late in T-cell ontogeny. A different protein, called **CD2,** appears at an earlier stage of T-cell development in the thymus, continues to be displayed on the surfaces of virtually all T-lineage cells, and is almost never found on other cell types. CD2 therefore serves as a very

Table 3–2. Some important surface molecules on T lymphocytes.

Marker	Major Function or Significance
T-cell receptor	Antigen binding.
CD3 complex	Signal transduction from T-cell receptor; lineage-specific marker.
CD2, CD5, CD7	Lineage-specific markers.
CD4	Subset-specific marker (mainly on helper cells); interaction with class II MHC proteins.
CD8	Subset-specific marker (mainly on cytotoxic cells); interaction with class I MHC proteins.
CD28	Activation-specific marker; receives B7-mediated costimulation from APC.
CD40 ligand (CD40L)	Activation-specific marker; delivers contact-mediated help to B cells.
IL-2 receptor Class II MHC proteins Transferrin receptor CD25, CD29, CD54, CD69	Other activation-specific markers.
IL-1 receptor IL-6 receptor TNFα receptor	Other cytokine receptors.
Fc receptors	Immunoglobulin binding.
LFA-1, ICAM-1	Cell–cell adhesion molecules.

APC = antigen-presenting cell; IL = interleukin; TNF = tumor necrosis factor; LFA = leukocyte functional antigen; ICAM = intercellular adhesion molecule.

useful general marker for recognizing all cells in this lineage.

Nearly all mature T lymphocytes that are found in peripheral blood and secondary lymphoid organs are CD2+CD3+—that is, they each express CD2 and CD3 on their surface. The class of CD2+CD3+ T lymphocytes as a whole, however, is actually made up of distinct subpopulations that have very different immunologic functions and express their own distinctive surface markers. These subpopulations are often referred to as **T-cell subsets** (Table 3–3). The two most important T-cell subsets can be distinguished by two additional surface proteins known as CD4 and CD8. Mature, functional T lymphocytes almost always express only one of these two proteins, and this correlates with important differences in cell function (Fig 3–7). Most T lymphocytes that express surface **CD8** protein have **cytotoxic** activity—the ability to kill cells that have foreign macromolecules on their surfaces. Cytotoxic T lymphocytes (T_c **cells,** or **CTLs**) are extremely important in the defense against viral infections: for example, host cells that are infected by a virus can often be identified by the presence of viral peptides on their surfaces, and killing these cells is essential to eradicating the disease. In contrast, T lymphocytes that express **CD4** protein generally are not cytotoxic but instead function as **helper T cells (T_H cells),** which promote proliferation, maturation, and immunologic function of other cell types. For example, specific lymphokines secreted by helper T cells are very important in controlling the activities of B cells, macrophages, and cytotoxic T cells.

Altogether, roughly 70% of T cells in human blood or secondary lymphoid tissues are CD4+CD8– (also called CD4 cells), whereas 25% are CD4–CD8+ (or simply CD8 cells). Cells with either of these phenotypes are often referred to as **single-positive** lymphocytes and are the cells most commonly involved in immune responses. Approximately 4% of T cells outside the thymus are CD4–CD8– **double-negative** lymphocytes; nearly all of these express an alternative form of T-cell receptor composed of polypeptides called γ and δ (see Chapter 9). The remaining 1% of extrathymic T cells are **double-positive** CD4+CD8+ cells, whose function is unknown.

The correlation of CD4 or CD8 with T_H and T_C cell function, respectively, is strong but not absolute: a few CD8 cells have helper activity, and a few CD4 cells are cytotoxic. Expression of CD4 or CD8 actually correlates most closely with the type of MHC protein that a T cell can recognize, as will be described in Chapters 4 and 6. Nor are these the only functionally important ways in which T cells can differ from one another. Within the T_H-cell population, for example, additional subsets of cells can be distinguished that each secrete a characteristic group of cytokines when activated and so promote particular types of defensive reactions. This heterogeneity among T_H cells will be discussed in Chapter 9.

Table 3–3. Major T-cell subsets found in blood and peripheral tissues.

Surface Phenotype	Predominant Function	Proportion of Total Blood T Lympho-cytes	T-Cell Receptor Type
CD4⁺CD8⁻	Helper	70%	α/β
CD4⁻CD8⁺	Cytotoxic	25%	α/β, rarely γδ
CD4⁻CD8⁻	Cytotoxic	4%	γ/δ
CD4⁺CD8⁺	?	1%	α/β

Virgin and memory T lymphocytes ordinarily remain in the resting state, and in this state they do not exhibit significant helper or cytotoxic activity. When activated, however, these cells can undergo several rounds of mitotic division to produce multiple daughter cells. Some of these daughter cells return directly to the resting state as memory cells, but others become effector cells that actively express helper or cytotoxic activity. The daughter cells resemble their parents: activated CD4+ cells can produce only CD4+ daughter cells, whereas activated CD8+ cells yield only CD8+ progeny. The effector cells of the T lineage tend to have slightly more cytoplasm and looser chromatin than their resting counterparts but cannot

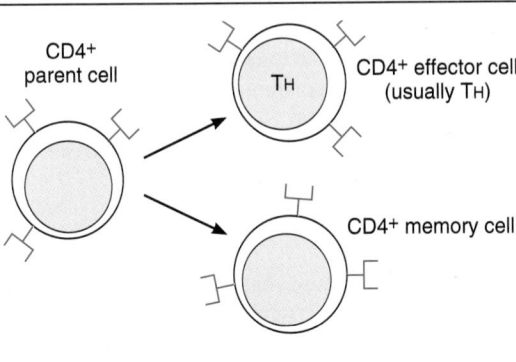

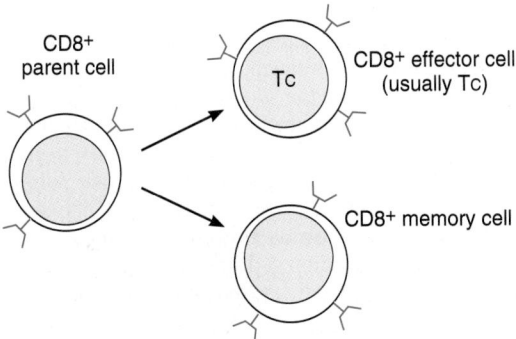

Figure 3–7. The progeny of activated T lymphocytes retain the surface phenotype (CD4+ or CD8+) of their parents.

reliably be distinguished from them under the light microscope. The effector cells, however, display several types of surface proteins (such as CD25, CD28, CD29, CD40L, transferrin receptors, and a group of MHC proteins known as class II MHC proteins) that are not found on resting T cells, and they also express increased amounts of some constitutive T-cell markers (such as CD2). When the activating stimuli are withdrawn, cytotoxic or helper activity gradually subsides over a period of several days as the effector cells either die or revert to the resting state.

AN OVERVIEW OF LYMPHOCYTE ACTIVATION

The term **"lymphocyte activation"** denotes an ordered series of events through which a resting lymphocyte is stimulated to divide and produce progeny, some of which become effector cells (Fig 3–8). The full response thus includes both the induction of cell proliferation (**mitogenesis**) and the expression of immunologic functions. Lymphocytes become activated when specific ligands bind to receptors on their surfaces. The ligands required are different for T cells and B cells (see following discussion), but the response itself is similar in many respects for all types of lymphocytes.

The earliest event known to take place when a T or B cell binds ligands that cause activation is a marked increase in activity of cytoplasmic **protein tyrosine kinases (PTKs)**—proteins that have the ability to catalyze the phosphorylation of tyrosine residues in other proteins. This increase occurs within seconds and reflects the functional activation of numerous different PTKs. Several important types of lymphocyte surface receptors (including membrane immunoglobulin and T-cell receptor proteins) are physically linked to specific cytoplasmic PTK proteins, which become active when the receptor binds its target ligand. As in many other receptor systems (see Chapter 1), the ligand-induced clustering of receptors on the B- or T-lymphocyte surface appears to be a key event in triggering PTK activation. The receptor-associated PTKs, in turn, may then activate other types of PTKs through phosphorylation, so that almost immediately a host of different PTKs are recruited into the response. By phosphorylating still other types of substrates, such as proteins that control cytoskeletal organization, expression of specific genes, and entry into the cell cycle, these newly activated PTKs appear to be either directly or indirectly responsible for triggering all subsequent events in lymphocyte activation. At present, however, the functions of most individual PTKs are uncertain.

One almost immediate effect of the PTK cascade is to activate the cytosolic enzyme **phospholipase C-γ1,** which then acts to hydrolyze a specific class of phospholipids, called phosphatidylinositides, that are

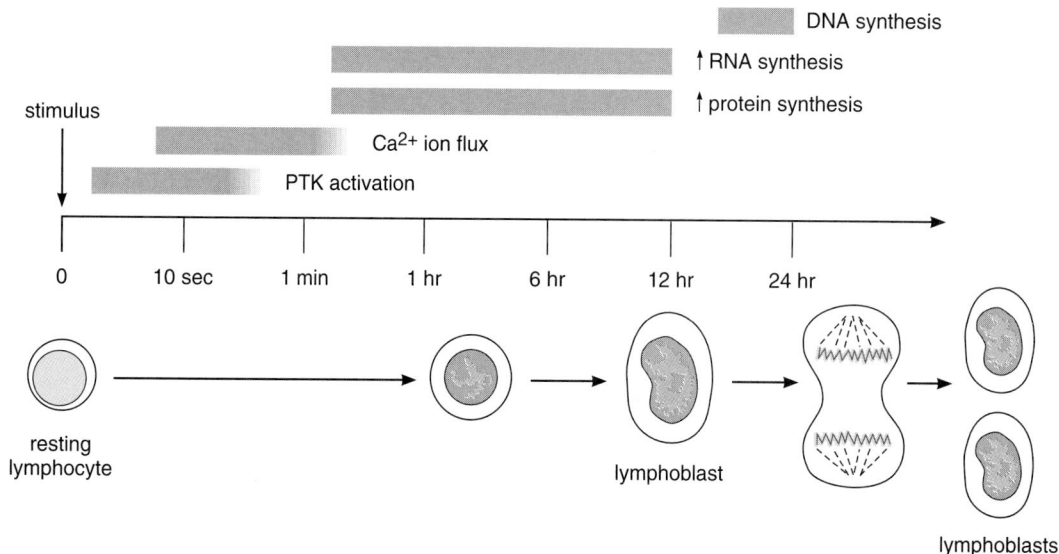

Figure 3–8. Major biochemical and morphologic events in lymphocyte activation. PTK, protein tyrosine kinase.

found in cellular membranes. The products of this hydrolysis include two small organic molecules, **diacylglycerol (DAG)** and **inositol 1,4,5-trisphosphate (IP3)**, which serve as second messengers to trigger additional changes in cellular physiology. DAG remains within the membrane of origin, where it binds and allosterically activates **protein kinase C**—a family of cytosolic enzymes that can phosphorylate other proteins at serine and threonine residues. IP$_3$ is released into the cytoplasm, binds to specific membrane receptors, and triggers a rapid, marked increase in the concentrations of **intracellular free calcium ions,** which flood into the cytosol from organellar storage pools, reaching maximal concentrations within 1 minute after contact with the activating stimulus. Like the PTK cascade, protein kinase C activation and these rapid calcium fluxes are thought to be critical for initiating the subsequent events in activation, though how they accomplish this is not yet known.

Within the first hour after stimulation, the rates of oxidative metabolism and of overall protein and RNA synthesis in the lymphocyte rise. The chromatin begins to decondense as previously silent genes are transcribed and the cell prepares to undergo mitosis. After 2–4 hours, specific proteins that are thought to regulate cell proliferation, such as the product of the protooncogene **c-myc,** become detectable in the nucleus. In parallel with these biochemical events, the morphology of the cell changes in a process known as **blast transformation:** its overall diameter increases to 15–30 μm as both its nucleus and cytoplasm enlarge; the nuclear chromatin becomes loose and pale-staining; and the cell acquires a prominent nucleolus (reflecting a high rate of RNA synthesis). Within 8–12 hours, the changes are sufficiently marked that the

cell can be recognized under the light microscope as a **lymphoblast**—a lymphocyte poised to begin mitosis. DNA synthesis takes place at around 18–24 hours after stimulation. The first cell division occurs 2–4 hours later and, depending on the conditions, can be repeated five or more times in succession, at intervals as brief as 6 hours. The effector cells produced as a result of each division mature completely within a few days and express the immune functions typical of their lineage for several days thereafter.

REQUIREMENTS FOR ACTIVATION OF B OR T LYMPHOCYTES

What are the stimuli that can lead to lymphocyte activation in vivo? Certainly, the most important are the innumerable foreign **antigens** that are recognized and bound by membrane immunoglobulins or T-cell receptor proteins. A few types of antigens are in themselves sufficient to activate B cells—these are usually highly polymeric proteins or polysaccharides that are able to interact simultaneously with many immunoglobulin proteins on the surface of a single cell. Such multivalent antigens act to **cross-link** the immunoglobulins to one another, so that eventually a great many immunoglobulins are gathered at one pole of the cell surface at the point of contact with antigen—a phenomenon known as **capping** (Fig 3–9A). This dense local aggregation of immunoglobulins, each of which is bound to antigen, transmits a very effective signal and is enough to trigger B-cell activation.

Activation can also be induced under artificial conditions by cross-linking other types of surface molecules (Table 3–4). Among the agents used for this pur-

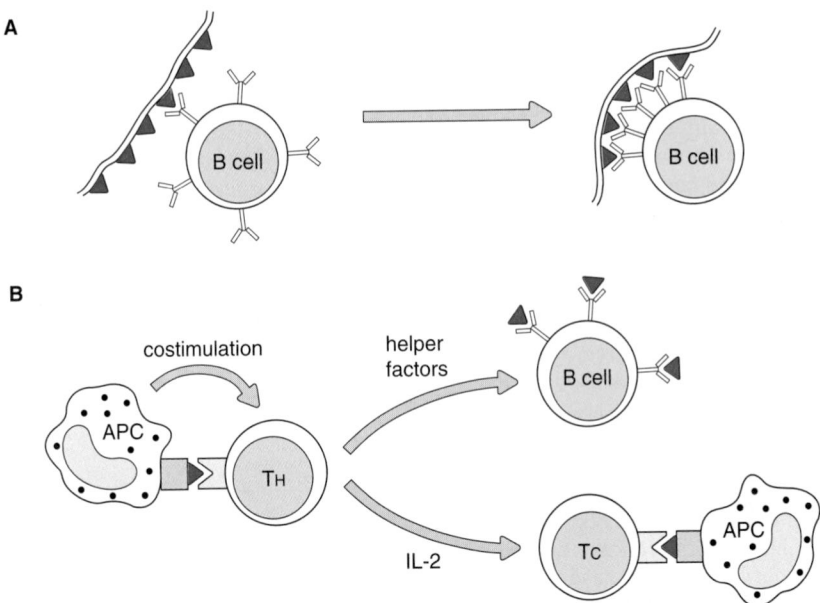

Figure 3–9. General requirements for lymphocyte activation. **A:** Some highly polymeric antigens that cross-link multiple antigen receptors are sufficient to activate B cells. **B:** Activation by a monomeric antigen requires additional stimuli supplied by another cell type. Costimulators from the antigen-presenting cell (APC) are necessary to activate a T_H cell, which in turn provides helper factors for B cells or interleukin-2 (IL-2) for T_C cells.

pose are certain lectins (sometimes called **mitogens**), which can activate T or B cells (or both) by cross-linking surface glycoproteins. Similar results can be obtained by using multivalent antibody complexes to cross-link some T-cell surface proteins (such as CD3) that are able to transmit signals to the cytoplasm. Alternatively, lymphocytes can be activated pharma-

Table 3–4. Mitogens and other conditions used to activate lymphocytes in vitro.

Mitogen or Condition	Specificity
Lectins	
Concanavalin A	T cells
Helix pomatia lectin	T cells
Phytohemagglutinin	T cells; few B cells
Pokeweed mitogen	T and B cells
Wheat germ agglutinin	T cells
Artificial cross-linking of specific surface proteins	
Immunoglobulins	B cells
T-cell surface markers (eg, CD3)	T cells
Pharmacologic agents	
Phorbol myristyl acetate plus calcium ionophore (eg, ionomycin)	T and B cells

cologically by treating them with agents that directly induce calcium fluxes and other important signaling events, thereby bypassing the surface receptors entirely. Such potent artificial activators are often used in clinical testing to study lymphocyte responses in vitro.

The majority of antigens encountered in nature, however, are not polymeric and so do not cross-link large numbers of receptors. Even when many copies of such an antigen bind individual immunoglobulins on a B cell, they generate only an incomplete signal, which fails to activate the cell. B cells can be activated by these more common antigens only if they are simultaneously stimulated by a nearby activated helper T lymphocyte. This stimulation may be delivered by lymphokines secreted from the T cell, but is transmitted most efficiently through direct contact of the B cell with T-cell surface proteins. In either case, the helper-cell-derived proteins (which will be referred to in this book as **helper factors**) interact with nonimmunoglobulin receptors on the B cell to generate a second signal. The combined effects of the helper factors and the bound antigen then act synergistically to cause B-cell activation.

In a similar manner, T-lymphocyte responses to most antigens also require two types of stimuli simultaneously. The first is provided by the antigen, which, if appropriately displayed by MHC proteins on an antigen-presenting cell, can be recognized and bound by T-cell receptors. When it binds an antigen–MHC complex, the T-cell receptor sends a signal to the cell interior, but this signal alone is usually not enough to cause activation. For helper T cells, full activation also requires contact with other specific ligands, known as **costimulators,*** that are expressed on the surface of the antigen-presenting cell. Activation of a cytotoxic T cell, on the other hand, generally requires **IL-2,** a cytokine secreted by activated helper T cells.

In summary, it is important to recognize that activation of a lymphocyte is controlled not only by antigen binding but also by interactions with other cells (Fig 3–9B): all T cells must cooperate with antigen-presenting cells, whereas B cells and cytotoxic cells depend on helper T lymphocytes. These interactions either require direct surface-to-surface contact or are mediated by cytokines that act only over extremely short distances. Owing to this interdependence among cell types, lymphocyte activation occurs most commonly and efficiently in the secondary lymphoid organs, where lymphocytes, antigens, and antigen-presenting cells encounter one another at close quarters.

LYMPHOID ORGANS

Lymphocytes are normally present in the blood at a concentration of approximately 2500 cells/mm³ and so account for roughly one third of all peripheral white blood cells. Each individual lymphocyte, however, spends most of its life within solid tissues, entering the circulation only periodically to migrate from one resting place to another. Indeed, at any given moment, no more than 1% of the total lymphocyte population can be found in the blood. Most of the remaining cells are contained in specialized lymphoid organs, such as the lymph nodes, thymus, tonsils, Peyer's patches, and white pulp of the spleen, where they carry out most of their functions.

Lymph Nodes & Lymphatic Circulation

Driven by the hydrostatic pressure within capillary lumens, water and low-molecular-weight solutes from the blood plasma continually leach out through blood vessel walls and into the lower pressure interstitial space. This slow leakage occurs in all solid organs and is the source of the nutrient-rich **interstitial fluid** that permeates every available niche in the tissues and

bathes each individual cell. Most of this fluid returns directly to the bloodstream through the walls of nearby venules, but a substantial amount (totaling approximately 120 mL/h in an adult at rest) does not. Instead, this portion of the interstitial fluid flows through the tissues at an almost imperceptible rate and is eventually collected in a branching network of flaccid, thin-walled channels known as primary lymphatic vessels. These vessels ramify throughout almost all organs of the body (except the brain, eyeballs, marrow cavities, cartilage, and placenta) but are often difficult to discern in tissue sections, since they collapse easily and are delimited only by a single delicate layer of lymphatic endothelial cells. Once the

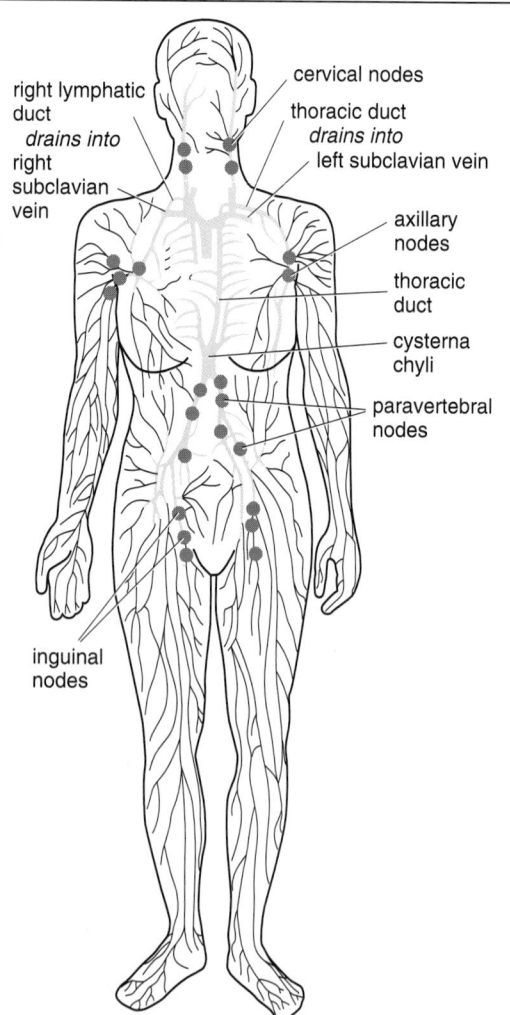

Figure 3–10. Lymphatic vascular system. Lymphatic vessels draining the right arm and right side of the head and neck converge to form the right lymphatic duct; the thoracic duct receives lymph from the remainder of the body. Only a few major collections of lymph nodes are depicted.

---

* Immunologists commonly use the prefix "co-" to indicate that a molecule intensifies or contributes to a particular function (and may even be essential for it) but cannot carry out that function by itself. Thus, any molecule that can activate T cells in the presence of antigen, but cannot do so alone, is a costimulator of T-cell activation. Examples of similar usage include the terms "coreceptor," "comitogen," and "coactivator."

fluid enters these vessels, it is known as **lymph.** Flowing slowly along the primary lymphatics, the lymph empties into progressively larger caliber lymphatic vessels, which ultimately converge and drain their contents into the right and left subclavian veins in the thorax (Fig 3–10). Thus, the lymphatic vasculature serves as a slow-flowing, low-pressure drainage system that collects a small proportion of the interstitial fluid from throughout the body and returns it to the bloodstream.

During its passage along the lymphatic vessels, the lymph flows through a series of bean-shaped organs called **lymph nodes,** which range from as little as 1 mm to about 25 mm in diameter. Nodes are distributed along the entire length of the lymphatic vasculature, tend to increase in size toward the venous end of the system, and often occur in chains or clusters that receive flow exclusively from a particular organ or region of the body (Fig 3–10). Especially prominent clusters of lymph nodes can be found in the neck and axillae (draining the head and arms), in the inguinal and paravertebral regions (draining the legs and pelvis), and in the root of the mesentery (draining the gut).

In its simplest form, a lymph node can be viewed as a localized dilatation of the lymphatic vessel, filled with dense aggregates of lymphocytes and macrophages that cling to a loose meshwork of connective tissue fibers called **reticulin** fibers. The reticulin mesh is produced by specialized fibroblasts known as reticular cells, small numbers of which are also present in the node. The node functions as a physical and biologic filter: as lymph fluid percolates through its internal lattice of cells, the macrophages and lymphocytes survey the fluid for any bacteria, viruses, or foreign macromolecules that may have been carried along with it from the tissues.

Larger nodes show an organized internal structure, which is schematized in Figure 3–11. The entire node is surrounded by a fibrous capsule. Lymph flows into the node along several **afferent lymphatic vessels** on one surface of the node and enters a narrow **subcapsular sinus** that is lined primarily by macrophages. The lymph then percolates sequentially through two more or less distinct regions of predominantly lymphoid tissue, called the **cortex** and the **medulla,** and finally exits through an **efferent lymphatic vessel** on the opposite side, at a region known as the hilus. Each node also receives a rich supply of blood that enters via an arteriole at the hilus, flows through a dense bed of capillaries and venules in the cortex and medulla, and then returns to the hilus to drain out through small veins.

The lymph node cortex usually contains several discrete spherical or ovoid cellular aggregates called **lymphoid follicles** (see Fig 3–11). These follicles are composed mainly of memory B lymphocytes, a smaller number of T cells (virtually all of which are helper cells), and a specialized type of supporting cell called the **follicular dendritic cell.** The latter cells are

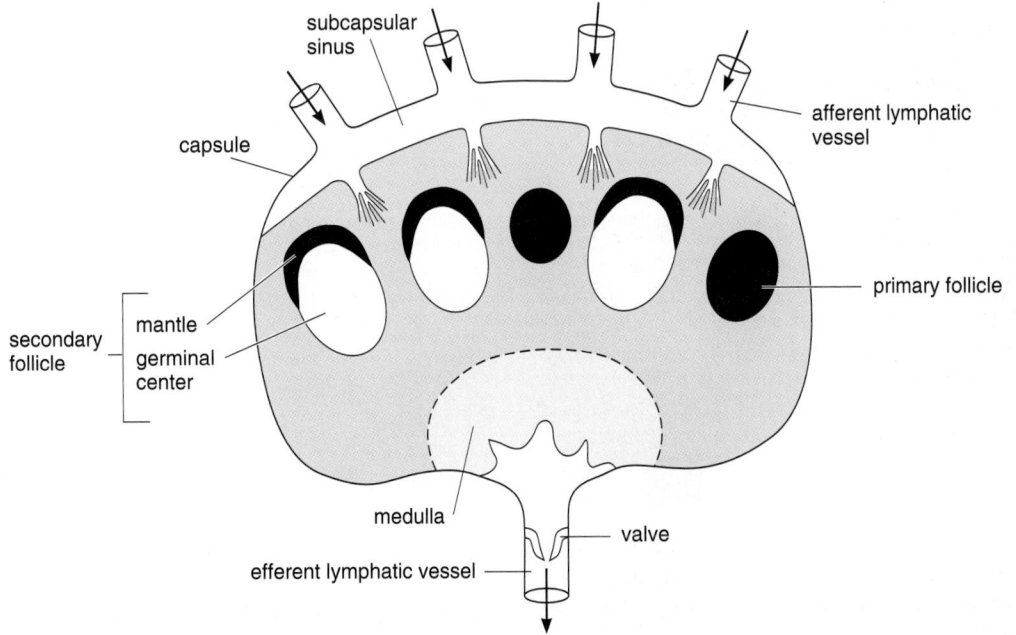

Figure 3–11. Idealized structure of a lymph node. Lymph enters via afferent vessels, passes through the cortex (shaded) and medulla, and exits via a single efferent vessel. Large lymphatic vessels often contain valves that prevent backward flow of the lymph.

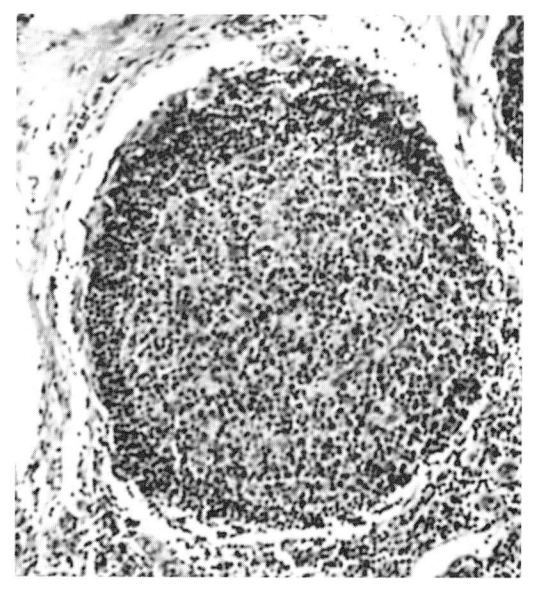

Figure 3–12. Structures of lymphoid follicles. **A:** A secondary follicle in the cortex of a lymph node, from a hematoxylin-eosin-stained section. Note the round, pale-staining germinal center and darker, overlying cap (mantle). Because follicles are often cut tangentially in standard tissue sections, the mantle is sometimes erroneously thought to completely encircle the germinal center. (Contributed by Brian Herndier.) **B:** At the top are photomicrographs of a primary *(left)* and a secondary *(right)* follicle from a hematoxylin-eosin-stained section of a lymph node. The diagrams below schematically depict the relationship between a follicular dendritic cell (white with shaded nucleus) and the surrounding lymphoid cells in a primary follicle *(left)* and a germinal center *(right)*. The relatively pale-staining properties of the germinal center result mainly from the abundant cytoplasm and large, pale-staining nuclei of the B-cell blasts it contains. (Contributed by Roger Warnke.)

A

primary

secondary

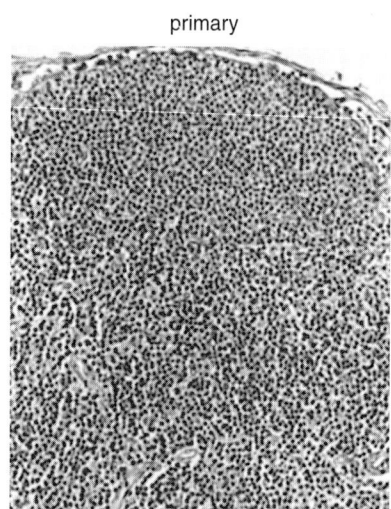

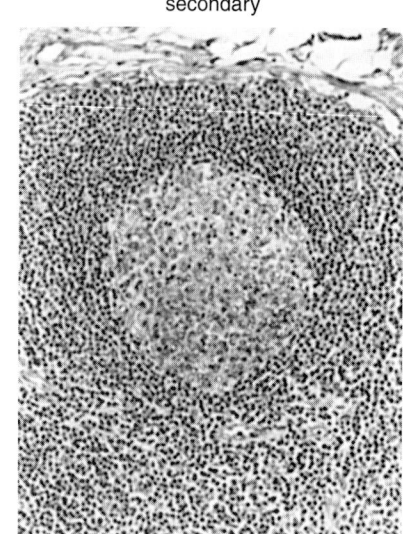

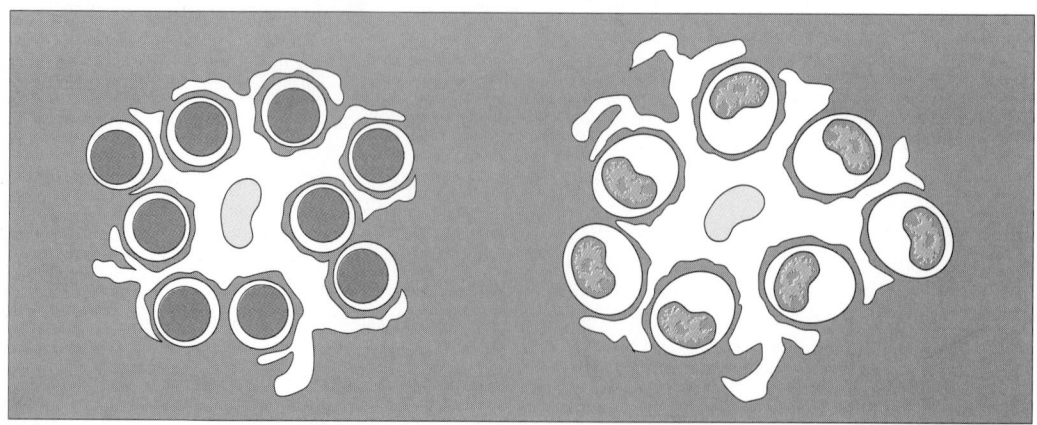

primary follicle

germinal center
of secondary follicle

B

so named because they are found only in lymphoid follicles and exhibit many long, delicate cytoplasmic processes that radiate out like tentacles to encircle each follicular lymphocyte. The origin and function of follicular dendritic cells are poorly understood, but they appear to be responsible for assembling memory B cells into follicles and regulating their subsequent activities.

Lymphoid follicles are labile structures that can disappear and re-form at different sites over time and can enlarge in response to infections or other immune challenges. They are of two types (Fig 3–12). **Primary follicles** contain predominantly mature, resting B cells; since these have dense nuclei and little cytoplasm, a primary follicle appears as a relatively dark-staining mass on conventional histologic preparations. **Secondary follicles,** on the other hand, appear as a pale-staining sphere known as the **germinal center,** with a cap (or **mantle**) of more darkly staining mature B lymphocytes overlying it on the afferent side of the node. The pale staining of the germinal center reflects the fact that, in this portion of the follicle, most of the lymphocytes are in various stages of activation and blast transformation and hence have more cytoplasm and looser chromatin than do resting lymphocytes. Numerous individual macrophages are also present in the germinal center, and occasional plasma cells may be seen.

Secondary follicles are not present at birth, and they form only after repeated exposure to substances that provoke an immune response. The presence of secondary follicles clearly denotes an ongoing B-cell immune response. Secondary follicles are thought to arise when a few B cells become activated in response to an antigen, migrate into a primary follicle, undergo blast transformation and begin to proliferate rapidly. Some of their progeny differentiate into plasma cells, which migrate from the follicle toward the medulla of the node; the antibodies that these cells secrete are carried away by the lymph flow and into the bloodstream. Proliferating B cells in a germinal center also undergo a process called **affinity maturation,** in which the B cells that respond most vigorously to the antigen are allowed to proliferate while others selectively die (see Chapter 8). The phagocytosed remains of B cells that have died in this process can be seen within the macrophages of a germinal center.

The regions of lymph node cortex lying outside the follicles are populated primarily by T cells, about two thirds of which are helper cells. T cells are especially abundant in the ill-demarcated region of cortex known as the **paracortex,** which lies between the lymphoid follicles and the medulla. Here, as in the T-cell-rich zones of all secondary lymphoid organs, the T cells are accompanied by a smaller population of supporting cells, called **interdigitating cells,** that have antigen-presenting activity. The **medulla** usually is less densely cellular than the cortex and often contains a scattering of plasma cells along with mature B and T lymphocytes and macrophages.

The lymph that flows into a node may carry with it microorganisms or other foreign matter from the tissues. When such a substance enters a lymph node, some of the lymphocytes and macrophages in the node may respond by activation. As a result, some of the resident lymphocytes begin to proliferate, inflammatory mediators are released locally, blood flow to the node increases markedly, and the normal, continual lymphocyte emigration from the node ceases entirely. If these responses are sufficiently pronounced, the node may become noticeably enlarged—a condition known as **lymphadenopathy.** Rapid enlargement of a lymph node can occur, for example, when an infection develops in the region it drains. Swelling usually decreases when the infection ends, although repeated bouts of swelling can lead to permanent enlargement and induration by scarring the interior of a node.

Spleen

The spleen (Fig 3–13) filters blood much as the lymph nodes filter lymph. Located just below the diaphragm on the left side of the abdomen, the spleen weighs approximately 150 g in an adult and is enclosed in a thin and rather fragile connective tissue capsule. Blood enters by way of the splenic artery at the hilum and passes into a branching network of progressively smaller arterioles that radiate throughout the organ. Each arteriole is encased in a cylindrical cuff of lymphoid tissue that consists mainly of mature T cells and is called the **periarteriolar lymphoid sheath.** Primary and secondary lymphoid follicles protrude at intervals from the sheath; these are identical to the follicles found in other lymphoid tissues and are composed mainly of B cells. The arterioles, sheaths, follicles, and a small amount of associated connective tissue are together called the splenic **white pulp,** which is visible as a delicate latticework on the cut surface of the organ. Blood flows from the arterioles into the **red pulp**—a spongy, blood-filled network of reticular cells and macrophage-lined vascular sinusoids that makes up the bulk of the spleen—and then exits by way of the splenic vein.

During the course of each day, approximately half the total blood volume passes through the spleen, where lymphocytes and macrophages survey it continually for evidence of infectious agents or other contaminants. The spleen thus serves as a critical line of defense against blood-borne pathogens. Splenic macrophages also have the important function of recognizing and eliminating any abnormal, damaged, or senescent red or white cells from the blood. Surgical removal of the spleen (most often performed because it has been lacerated by trauma) is usually well tolerated in an adult but causes a persistent rise in the percentage of malformed circulating erythrocytes and a

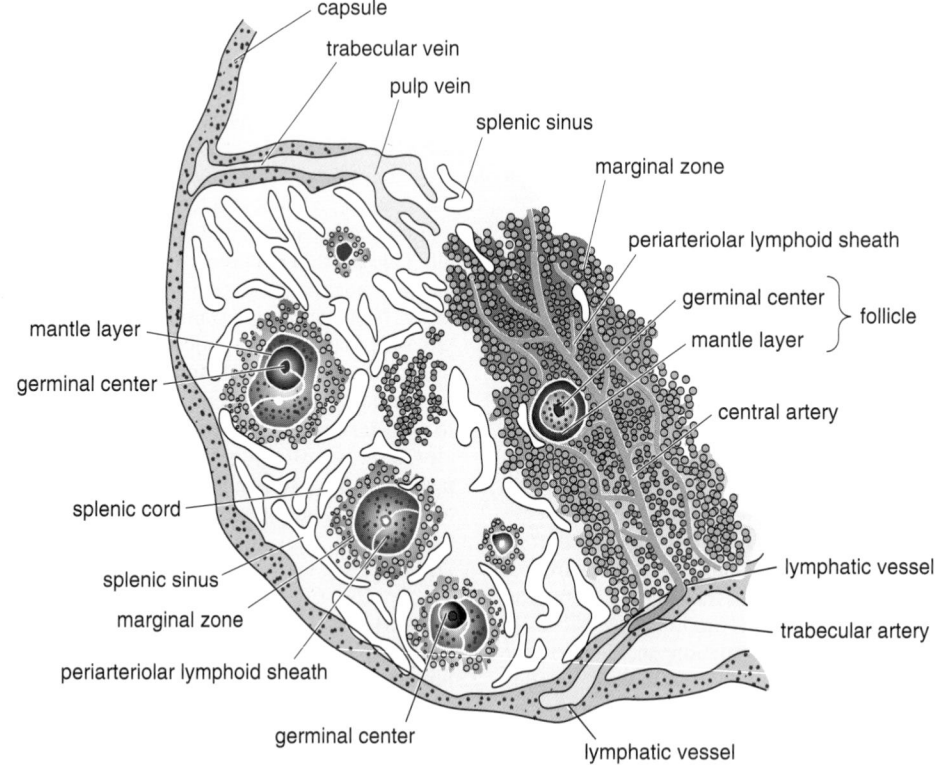

Figure 3–13. Microscopic anatomy of the spleen.

modestly increased risk of sepsis due to diplococci or other pyogenic bacteria.

Tonsils, Peyer's Patches, & Other Subepithelial Lymphoid Organs

Vast numbers of individual T and B lymphocytes, macrophages, and plasma cells lie just below the mucosal epithelia in many regions of the alimentary, genitourinary, and respiratory tracts. Especially dense populations of such cells can normally be found around bronchial lumens or in the lamina propria and submucosa of the large and small intestines, where they are well situated to detect any foreign substances that contact these body surfaces. In most areas, the cells form a diffuse, disorganized mass, punctuated only occasionally by isolated lymphoid follicles.

At other sites, the cells are organized into discrete, stable anatomic structures. For example, **tonsils** are nodular aggregates of macrophages and lymphoid tissue located immediately beneath the stratified squamous epithelium of the nasopharynx and soft palate. Tonsils lack a capsule and afferent lymphatic vessels but have many of the other constituents of a lymph node, including lymphoid follicles; their function is to detect and respond to pathogens in the respiratory and alimentary secretions. The overlying epithelium plunges downward into the substance of a tonsil to

form deep crypts whose contents are continually monitored by the tonsillar cells. Similar unencapsulated lymphoid nodules, called **Peyer's patches,** are present in the ileal submucosa of the small bowel, where they serve to detect substances that diffuse across the intestinal epithelium (Fig 3–14). Together, all of the organized and diffuse lymphoid tissues found in submucosal regions of the body can be viewed as a single functional unit, called the **mucosa-associated lymphoid tissue (MALT),** which will be discussed in Chapter 13. One important function of these tissues is to secrete antibodies across the mucosal surface as a defense against external pathogens.

The skin, too, is an important site of immune surveillance. Small populations of lymphocytes are constantly present in the dermis and epidermis, although they usually are inconspicuous and do not normally form lymphoid follicles. In addition, the epidermis contains a resident subpopulation of antigen-presenting cells, called **Langerhans' cells,** each of which sends out a network of dendritic branches that intertwine between epidermal epithelial cells over a relatively large area. These Langerhans' cells account for about 5% of all epidermal cells. When it encounters foreign substances, a Langerhans' cell secretes cytokines that attract additional lymphocytes from the nearby circulation and it also presents the foreign sub-

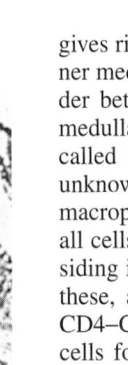

Figure 3–14. Microscopic anatomy of a Peyer's patch, a secondary lymphoid follicle beneath the mucosal epithelium of the small intestine. (Contributed by Linda Ferrell.)

stances on its surface to help initiate an immune response. Macrophages in the dermis play a similar role as antigen-presenting sentinels.

Thymus

Unlike the other lymphoid organs described earlier, the thymus is involved in lymphocyte production and maturation rather than in immune surveillance per se. It is the primary site at which T lymphocytes differentiate and become functionally competent. The organ itself arises during embryogenesis as two endodermal buds from the third pharyngeal pouches; these invade downward into the superior mediastinum and then fuse to form a solid, V-shaped epithelial mass. During the third month of gestation, this mass becomes colonized by primitive, marrow-derived lymphoid stem cells that are carried to it by way of the blood. It is not yet clear whether these migrating stem cells are already committed to T-cell differentiation or become committed only after entering the thymus. The epithelial component of the thymus is made up of sheets and islands of squamous cells that elaborate a variety of small peptide hormones, the best characterized of which are thymulin, thymopoietin, thymic humoral factor, and several forms of thymosin. These hormones have been proposed to play a role in attracting T-cell precursors from the blood and also to promote their subsequent maturation within the thymus. Once inside the organ, T cells pack themselves densely into the interstices between epithelial cells, stretching them apart until the epithelium comes to resemble a loose network of stellate cells that cling to one another via desmosomes. In this microenvironment, T cells proliferate briskly, giving the thymus one of the highest rates of cell division in the body.

The fully developed thymus is composed of two lobes, each comprising multiple lobules (Fig 3–15). Lymphocytes are packed more densely toward the periphery of each lobule than near its center, which

gives rise to the appearance of an outer cortex and inner medulla, although there is no sharp anatomic border between these two zones. In some areas of the medulla, the epithelium forms small keratized whorls, called **Hassall's corpuscles,** whose significance is unknown. Apart from the epithelial cells and a few macrophages and other supporting elements, virtually all cells in the thymus are T cells. T lymphocytes residing in the thymus are often called **thymocytes.** Of these, a minor proportion (approximately 10%) are CD4–CD8– cells. Unlike the rare double-negative T cells found outside the thymus, these are somewhat enlarged, have a high rate of mitotic activity, and are presumed to be primitive T-cell precursors. A second subpopulation (15% of thymic T cells) consists of single-positive thymocytes that express only CD4 or CD8 alone and are nearly indistinguishable from the mature T lymphocytes found elsewhere throughout the body. Such single-positive cells are most abundant in the thymic medulla and are thought to be fully mature virgin T lymphocytes that are preparing to leave the organ.

The vast majority of lymphoid cells in the thymus, however, are small T cells that express both CD4 and CD8 proteins together on their surfaces. These double-positive thymocytes account for roughly 75% of all thymic T cells. They are not immunologically functional and are thought to represent a transient intermediate stage in T-cell development. Amazingly, nearly all of these double-positive thymocytes (at least 99%) die without ever leaving the thymus: the thymic cortex is studded with individual dying thymocytes, and phagocytosed debris from the dead thymocytes can be seen within cortical macrophages and epithelial cells. Thus, the thymus is a site for both prolific replication and wholesale slaughter of T cells. As discussed in later chapters, the T-cell deaths that occur in the thymus are part of a rigorous **selection** process that is essential for creating a functioning immune system.

The developmental relationships among the various classes of thymocytes are outlined in Figure 3–16. Blood-borne lymphocyte progenitors enter the thymus and form a pool of replicating cells located mainly near the periphery of the cortex; it is not known whether this replicating pool is stable or must continually be replenished with new marrow precursors. The progeny of the replicating cells appear first as double-negative thymocytes and then progress to the double-positive stage in which they express T-cell receptors along with both CD4 and CD8 on their surfaces. Each individual thymocyte then selectively and permanently shuts off expression of either CD4 or CD8 (apparently choosing between these two markers at random), and so becomes a single-positive thymocyte. This differentiation process is plainly arduous, since fewer than 1% of the cells produced in the thymus are able to complete it. Although the factors that determine which thymocytes will survive are not entirely known, the selection process depends in part on

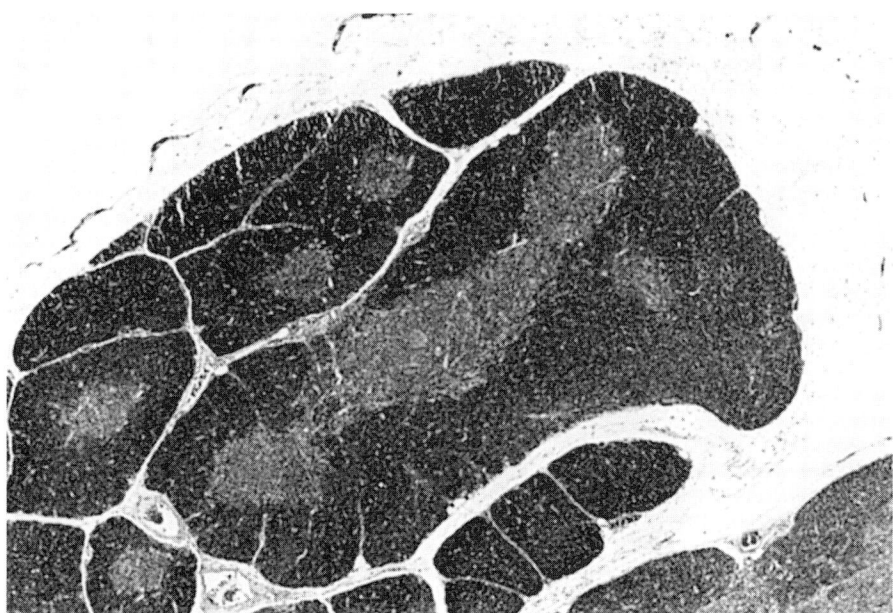

Figure 3–15. Microscopic anatomy of the thymus. This photomicrograph shows a portion of a thymic lobule from a hematoxylin-eosin-stained section, illustrating the dense outer cortex and pale inner medulla. (Contributed by Gordon Honda.)

specific interactions with thymic macrophages or epithelial cells, at least some of which are mediated through the T-cell receptor (see Chapter 9). The small percentage of single-positive cells that survive ultimately leave the thymus as mature T lymphocytes. There is a general tendency for the cells to migrate from the cortex toward the medulla as they differenti-

ate, though this may not be true of all thymocytes.

The thymus is relatively large and highly active at birth, weighing an average of 22 g. It continues to enlarge for several years, although at a lower rate than the rest of the body, and reaches its peak weight (around 35 g) at puberty. Thereafter, it begins to involute as the lymphoid components recede and are re-

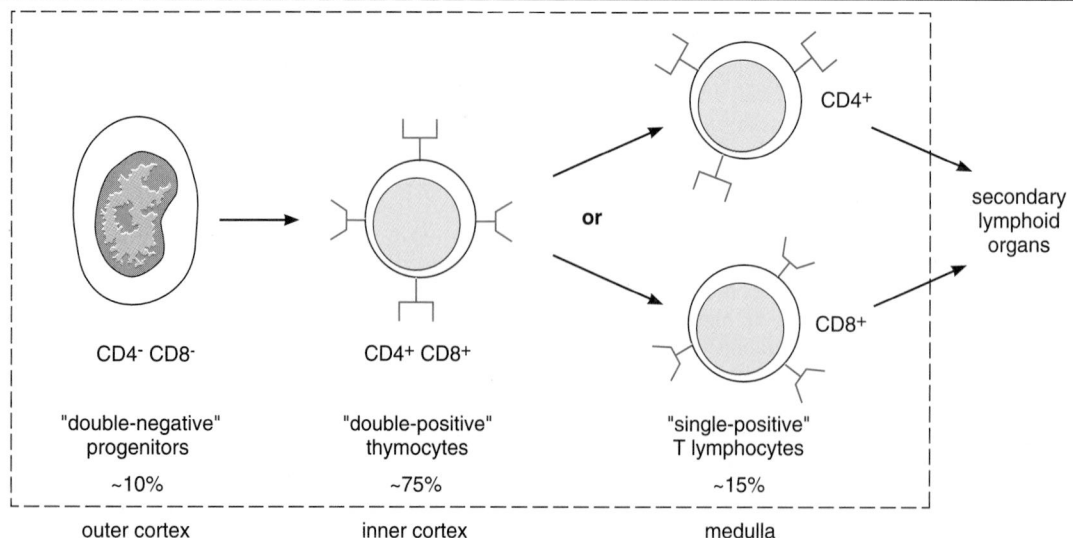

Figure 3–16. Model for intrathymic T-cell maturation. Developing thymocytes pass through three successive stages of differentiation as they migrate from the outer cortex to the medulla and then exit the thymus. Some identifiable intermediate stages have been omitted. The sequence depicted applies to most T cells that express α/β T-cell receptors. For details, see Chapter 9.

placed by fatty connective tissue. Little more than 6 g of thymic tissue (most of it epithelial) persists into adulthood. This normal regression probably signifies that the thymus produces enough virgin T lymphocytes early in life to seed the entire immune system and that it is then no longer necessary. Consistent with this view, removal of the thymus at any time after birth generally does not cause significant immunologic abnormalities. Complete congenital absence of the thymus, however, results in the absence of T lymphocytes and produces profound, life-threatening immunodeficiency.

LYMPHOCYTE CIRCULATION & HOMING

Lymphocytes are migratory cells; their distribution in the body reflects the rates at which they enter and depart particular sites, as well as their local replication. Individual lymphocytes in a lymph node, for example, linger there for an average of only 12 hours before detaching from the reticulin matrix and exiting through efferent lymphatics, swept along by the flowing lymph. These emigrating cells eventually are carried into the bloodstream, which disperses them throughout the body, but they generally remain in circulation for only a few minutes or hours before again taking up residence temporarily in another lymphoid organ (Fig 3–17). In a similar fashion, mature lymphocytes continually migrate in and out of all other secondary lymphoid tissues as well, changing locations on average once or twice each day, with roughly 1–2% of the total population in transit at any given moment. In most types of lymphoid organs, lymphocytes enter via blood vessels and exit through lymphatics, but in the spleen they enter and exit directly from the blood.

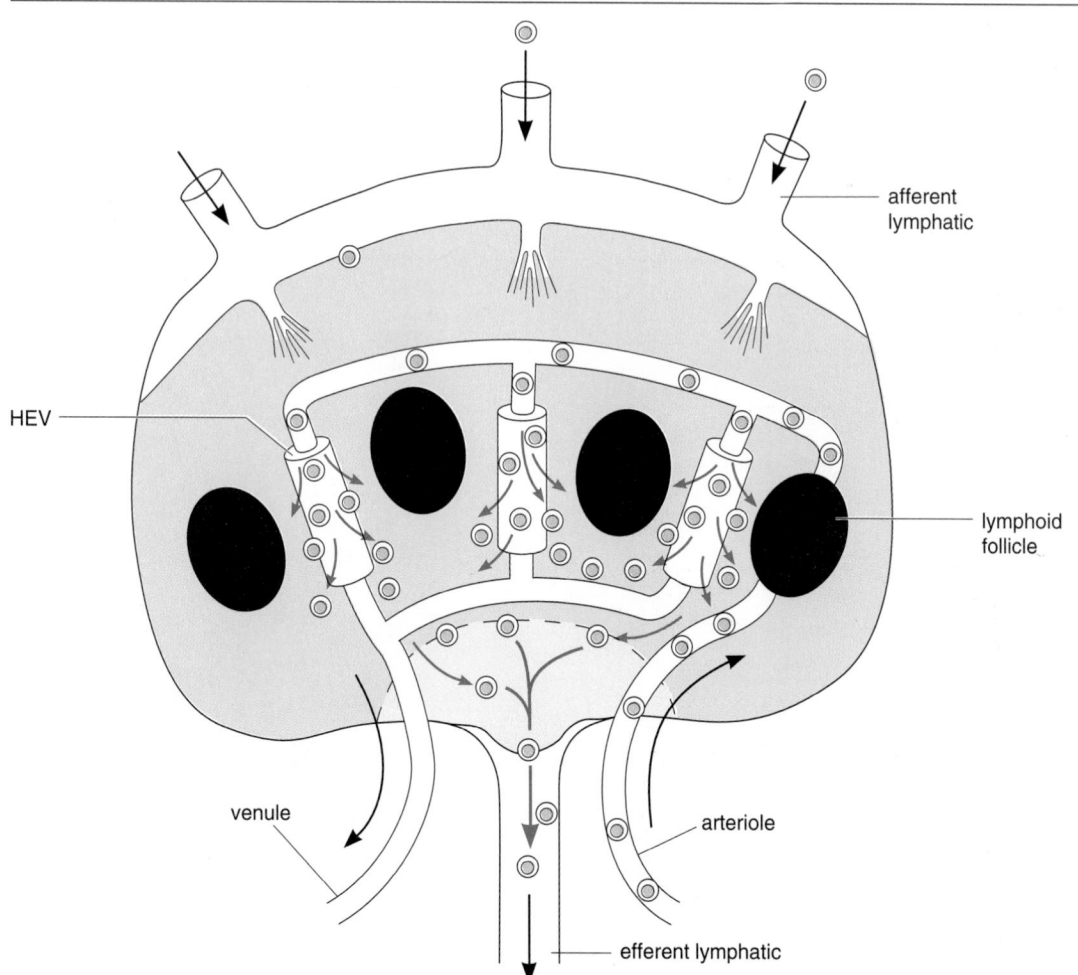

Figure 3–17. Schematic view of lymphocyte traffic through a lymph node. Some lymphocytes arrive from other nodes through the afferent lymphatic channels, but most enter from the blood by way of a high endothelial venule (HEV), migrate through the substance of the node and exit through afferent lymphatics. Average residence time in the node is approximately 12 hours. Note that the HEVs are located predominantly in the paracortex between lymphoid follicles.

These restless migrations serve several functions. First, as lymphocytes travel from organ to organ, they can survey the entire body for foci of infection or foreign antigens. This is especially important because, as we shall see in Chapter 4, only a small percentage of lymphocytes are able to respond to any given antigen—continually dispersing and reshuffling the population helps ensure that these rare, responsive lymphocytes will be present wherever in the body that antigen might appear. Second, such movements help maintain a balanced overall distribution of lymphocytes among tissues. In addition, because the microenvironments found in different tissues tend to favor specific aspects of lymphocyte development, migration through various sites can sequentially modulate and optimize a cell's growth and function. Finally, like a game of musical chairs, the shuttling process also places strong darwinian pressure on the population, as the migrating lymphocytes are forced to compete with one another for the limited space available in each tissue. Lymphocytes confront this competition from the earliest stages of their lives; for example, the bone marrow exports more new virgin B cells each day than can be accommodated in the periphery. Cells that compete least effectively for entry to the most favorable microenvironments tend to be weeded out over time, while the best adapted cells thrive.

Lymphocyte traffic among organs is not random.

Resting, virgin lymphocytes shuttle almost exclusively among the lymph nodes, Peyer's patches, tonsils, and spleen and have a roughly equal tendency to migrate into any of these tissues. In comparison, memory and effector cells can invade not only those sites but also the diffuse submucosal lymphoid tissues of the gut and lung, the pulmonary interstitium, and inflamed or infected sites in virtually any other organ. Moreover, once activated, individual effector and memory cells often show a very strong preference to return to the same type of tissue in which activation originally occurred. A memory cell originally activated in a lymphoid organ of the gut, for example, will tend to home preferentially to other gut-associated lymphoid tissues for the rest of its life.

These tissue-selective homing patterns result from interactions between surface molecules on lymphocytes and endothelial cells. Blood lymphocytes most commonly enter tissues by passing through the walls of specialized blood vessels known as **high endothelial venules (HEVs).** These vessels are a modified form of postcapillary venules, are found in all lymphoid organs, and can be recognized under the light microscopy by the cuboidal shape of the endothelial cells that line them (Fig 3–18). High endothelial cells in different target organs, such as lymph nodes or Peyer's patches, express particular surface glycoproteins, called **vascular addressins,** which are charac-

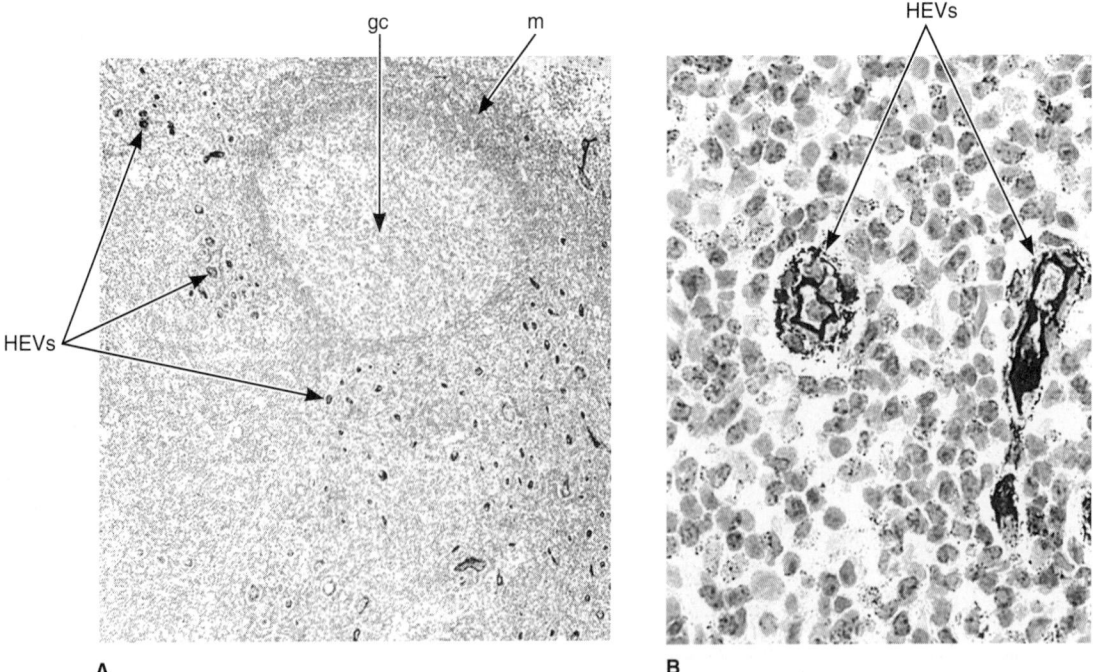

Figure 3–18. High endothelial venules (HEVs). **A:** Histologic section of a human lymph node, showing the distribution of HEVs, which are primarily found in the paracortex. gc, germinal center; m, mantle. **B:** High-power view showing the distinctive cuboidal shape of the high endothelial cells. The tissue in both photographs has been treated with reagents specific for the L-selectin ligand, which stain the high endothelial cell surfaces black. (Contributed by Michael Bell.)

teristic of that organ. Each type of addressin, in turn, is specifically recognized by one or more surface proteins, called **homing receptors,** on lymphocytes that home to that organ. Thus, when a circulating lymphocyte expresses a particular homing receptor, it will tend to bind HEV addressins found in the corresponding tissue or organ. Different types of lymphocytes are predisposed to express particular homing receptors, but the level of expression may increase or decrease markedly depending on whether the cell is activated, the nature of the activating antigen, and the microenvironment where activation occurred. Several of the receptor–addressin pairs that are known to mediate lymphocyte homing to lymph nodes, skin, the gastrointestinal tract, or sites of inflammation are listed in Table 3–5; addressins and receptors for other tissues are believed to exist but have not yet been identified. In particular, homing to lymph nodes can be initiated by contact between lymphocyte **L-selectin** and various endothelial surface glycoproteins, including **CD34.** Homing to gastrointestinal sites, on the other hand, depends on contact between a specific integrin on the lymphocyte and a glycoprotein ligand on the endothelium.

The process of lymphocyte binding and penetration of the vessel wall progresses in phases similar to those described earlier for the phagocytes (see Fig 2–5). The initial interaction of most nonintegrin-homing receptors with a vascular addressin is relatively weak and short-lived, so that the cell often continues to roll along the HEV wall under the force of the flowing blood. During this **primary adhesion** phase, which may last up to 20 seconds, the lymphocyte must receive signals that induce it to progress into the **secondary adhesion** phase, in which it rapidly translocates presynthesized integrin proteins (especially LFA-1) onto its surface, stops rolling, and becomes

firmly anchored to the endothelium. The signals that trigger this progression in lymphocytes have not yet been identified but may include HEV surface proteins, soluble factors diffusing from the tissues, or both.

After adhering to the HEV wall, a lymphocyte can then pass between high endothelial cells to enter the surrounding tissue. This process, called **diapedesis,** is usually completed within 10 minutes and depends on the continued expression of surface integrins that provide attachment to adjacent cells and to the extracellular matrix. The efficiency of lymphocyte recruitment can be very high; for example, about 25% of blood lymphocytes that enter a lymph node's vascular bed will invade across the HEVs. After exiting the bloodstream, each lymphocyte must then continue its migration within the lymphoid organ until it reaches an appropriate resting place, such as the paracortical region (for most T cells) or lymphoid follicles (for most B cells) of a lymph node. Each cell's movement into and through a lymphoid organ is probably controlled by chemotactic factors, including certain chemoattractant peptides, called chemokines, that will be discussed in Chapter 10. The pattern of localization can also change rapidly when cells contact antigen; for example, small numbers of T_H cells translocate from the paracortex into lymphoid follicles soon after they become activated, and this migration can play an essential part in triggering a B-cell response.

High endothelial venules are a constant feature of all secondary lymphoid organs (except the spleen) but may also appear transiently at any site in the body where an immune response is occurring. They arise by differentiation of preexisting capillaries in response to factors elaborated locally by activated immune cells. These vessels then serve as a portal

Table 3–5. Receptor–addressin interactions involved in lymphocyte homing.[1]

Lymphocyte-Homing Receptor	Vascular Addressin	Homing Specificity Conferred
L-selectin	CD34, glyCAM-1, others[2]	Virgin lymphocytes to lymph nodes.
L-selectin	MAdCAM	Virgin lymphocytes to Peyer's patches.
α_4/β_7 integrin	MAdCAM, VCAM-1	Virgin lymphocytes to Peyer's patches; memory–effector cells to lamina propria of GI tract.
CLA	E-selectin	Memory–effector cells to skin.
VLA-4	VCAM-1	Activated lymphoblasts and memory–effector cells to sites of inflammation.
CD44	Hyaluronate	Activated lymphoblasts to sites of inflammation.
PSGL-1	P-selectin	Unknown

Abbreviations: CLA = cutaneous lymphocyte antigens, a family of glycoproteins; PSGL = P-selectin glycoprotein ligand.
[1] Interactions involving the α_4/β_7 and VLA-4 integrins can support both the primary and secondary phases of adhesion (see Fig 2–5). All other molecular interactions listed here are sufficient for primary adhesion only. In most instances, secondary adhesion requires activation of surface integrins, particularly lymphocyte LFA-1, which binds ICAM-1 and ICAM-2 on the endothelial surface.
[2] L-selectin is thought to recognize a sulfated carbohydrate determinant based on sialyl Lewis-X, which is found on several distinct endothelial surface glycoproteins.

through which blood lymphocytes and other defensive cells can enter tissues to join in a response wherever they are needed. If the response is sufficiently intense and prolonged, the assembled lymphocytes, plasma cells, and antigen-presenting cells may arrange themselves spatially in a manner that resembles a permanent lymphoid organ, complete with secondary follicles. Such reactive, and usually temporary, encampments are sometimes referred to as **tertiary lymphoid organs.**

REFERENCES

ONTOGENY AND SUBTYPES
OF T- AND B-LYMPHOID CELLS

Ikuta K et al: Lymphocyte development from stem cells. *Ann Rev Immunol* 1992;**10:**759.

Kincade PW et al: Cells and molecules that regulate B lymphoiesis in bone marrow. *Ann Rev Immunol* 1989;**7:**111.

Adkins B et al: Early events in T-cell maturation. *Ann Rev Immunol* 1987;**5:**325.

Dorshkind K: Transcriptional control points during lymphopoiesis. *Cell* 1994;**79:**751.

Podack ER, Kupfer A: T cell effector functions: Mechanisms for delivery of cytotoxicity and help. *Ann Rev Cell Biol* 1991;**7:**479.

Robey E, Fowlkes BJ: Selective events in T cell development. *Ann Rev Immunol* 1994;**12:**675.

Ahmed R, Gray D: Immunological memory and protective immunity: Understanding their relation. *Science* 1996;**272:**54.

Sprent J, Tough DF: Lymphocyte life-span and memory. *Science* 1994;**265:**1395.

SECONDARY LYMPHOID ORGANS

Szakal AK et al: Microanatomy of lymphoid tissue during humoral immune responses: Structure function relationships. *Ann Rev Immunol* 1989;**7:**91.

Bohnsack JF, Brown EJ: The role of the spleen in resistance to infection. *Ann Rev Med* 1986;**37:**49.

Bos JD, Kapsenberg ML: The skin immune system: Its cellular constituents and their interactions. *Immunol Today* 1986;**7:**235.

MacLennan ICM: Germinal centers. *Ann Rev Immunol* 1994;**12:**117.

LYMPHOCYTE ACTIVATION

Clark EA, Lane PJL: Regulation of human B-cell activation and adhesion. *Ann Rev Immunol* 1991;**9:**97.

Janeway CA, Bottomly K: Signals and signs for lymphocyte responses. *Cell* 1994;**76:**275.

Parker DC: T cell-dependent B-cell activation. *Ann Rev Immunol* 1993;**11:**331.

Ullman K et al: Transmission of signals from T lymphocyte antigen receptor to the genes responsible for cell proliferation and immune function. *Ann Rev Immunol* 1990;**8:**421.

Weiss A, Littman DR: Signal transduction by lymphocyte antigen receptors. *Cell* 1994;**76:**263.

LYMPHOCYTE RECIRCULATION AND HOMING

Butcher EC, Picker LJ: Lymphocyte homing and homeostasis. *Science* 1996;**272:**60.

Rosen SD, Bertozzi CR: The selectins and their ligands. *Curr Opin Cell Biol* 1994;**6:**663.

Springer TA: Traffic signals for lymphocyte recirculation and leukocyte emigration: The multistep paradigm. *Cell* 1994;**76:**301.

The Immune Response

4

Tristram G. Parslow, MD, PhD

The immune system has at least three major functional properties that distinguish it from all of the body's other defenses. The first is its extreme **specificity**—the ability to recognize and distinguish among a vast number of different target molecules and to respond (or not respond) to each of these individually. Second, the immune system **discriminates between self and nonself,** so that it normally coexists peacefully with all of the innumerable proteins and other organic materials that make up the host but responds vigorously against foreign substances, including cells or tissues from other people. Third, the immune system has **memory,** that is, the ability to be molded by its experiences so that subsequent encounters with a particular foreign pathogen provoke more rapid and more vigorous responses than occurred at the initial encounter.

These properties of the immune system seemed impenetrable mysteries only a few decades ago, but in recent years they have begun to yield to research. A great deal is now understood about the mechanisms that give rise to immunologic specificity and memory, and the processes underlying self–nonself discrimination are beginning to be unraveled as well. What has emerged is the realization that the lymphocyte population in each person constitutes an extraordinarily interactive network of mobile cells that are almost as diverse as the foreign substances they respond to and that their diversity is the result of molecular genetic processes that may well be unique to these cells. Moreover, it is now recognized that each person's immune system is continually evolving in response to its environment and experience as the individual cells communicate and cooperate with one another to control their own proliferation, differentiation, and immunologic functions.

The interplay of molecular and cellular events that takes place during even the simplest immune response is dauntingly complex, and many aspects of immune system function are still incompletely understood. As a result, the subject can be especially bewildering and intimidating on first encounter. The goal of this chapter is therefore to present an introduction to the subject by describing the organization of lymphocyte populations and the essential elements of an immune response in a stepwise and simplified fashion. Each of these topics will then be addressed more rigorously and in much greater detail in subsequent chapters of this book.

CLONAL ORGANIZATION & DYNAMICS OF LYMPHOCYTE POPULATIONS

Virgin lymphocytes are continually released from the primary lymphoid organs into the periphery, each carrying surface receptors that enable it to bind substances called **antigens.** Antigen binding in B cells is mediated by surface immunoglobulin proteins, whereas in T cells it is mediated by T-cell receptors. The sequences of these two types of proteins are extremely diverse, so that as a group they can bind an enormous variety of antigens (see Chapters 7 and 9). Antigen binding, when accompanied by other stimuli, can lead to activation of a T or B cell. Virgin lymphocytes that fail to become activated die within a few days after entering the periphery, but those that become activated survive and proliferate, yielding daughter cells that may then undergo further cycles of activation and proliferation.

All of the progeny cells derived from any single virgin lymphocyte constitute a lymphocyte **clone.** Some members of each clone differentiate into effector cells, whereas the remainder are memory cells; however, apart from this, all cells within a clone are identical to one another in nearly all respects, reflecting their common ancestry. For example, B-cell clones contain only B cells, and each T-cell clone is made up entirely of either CD4+ or CD8+ cells.

A fundamental property of lymphocytes is that all

of the immunoglobulin or T-cell receptor proteins expressed by cells in a given clone are identical. Although each individual lymphocyte typically has thousands of such proteins on its surface, all of these have precisely the same amino acid sequence and are identical to those expressed by all other cells in the same clone. Since the sequence of an immunoglobulin or T-cell receptor protein determines which antigens it will bind, it follows that any single lymphocyte can recognize and respond to only a very small subset of the total universe of possible antigens. This same antigen specificity, moreover, is shared by all other cells in the clone (with the exception of occasional somatic mutants, discussed in Chapter 8). Thus, each lymphocyte or clone of lymphocytes has a uniquely restricted specificity for antigens—a phenomenon known as **clonal restriction.** The immune system as a whole is able to recognize many different antigens because it is made up of a vast number of different lymphocyte clones, each of which has very limited antigen specificity.

The antigen specificity of each virgin lymphocyte is determined through an essentially random genetic process during the early stages of its development and is permanently fixed by the time the cell enters the periphery (see Chapter 7). It has been estimated that the lymphopoietic system is able to produce lymphocytes with approximately 10^8 alternative antigen specificities. This range of possible specificities is known collectively as the **primary lymphocyte repertoire.** Roughly 10^9 virgin lymphocytes enter the periphery each day, so that at least a few with any given specificity are likely to be present at all times. Whenever any one of these encounters its specific antigen under conditions that favor activation, it can give rise to multiple daughter cells, some of which are long-lived memory cells. With each successive exposure to the same antigen, the antigen-specific clone expands further and so comes to represent an increasing proportion of the total lymphocyte population (Fig 4–1). In this manner, exposure to an antigen selectively promotes the growth of any clones that recognize it without affecting other cells in the population—a phenomenon known as **clonal selection.** On the other hand, if no further contact with an antigen occurs, the specific memory cells tend to die out, though this usually occurs over a period of years or decades. Thus, the lymphocyte population is continually evolving over time as individual clones expand or subside, depending on the specific antigens to which the host is exposed.

The antigen specificity of a given clone applies not only to its ability to recognize antigens but also to its effector functions. For example, cytotoxic effector T cells generally attack a target cell only if it bears the particular surface antigen recognized by their T-cell receptors; hence, the sequence of the T-cell receptor defines not only the antigen that can activate the T-cell clone but also the targets it will attack. Similarly, the antibodies secreted by a B-cell clone have exactly the same binding specificity as the surface immunoglobulins expressed on that clone. Clonal restriction thus ensures that the immune response mounted by a lymphocyte clone is directed with a high degree of specificity against the antigen that induced its activation. The speed and intensity of response to a given antigen is determined largely by clonal selection: the larger the specific clone, the more lymphocytes are available

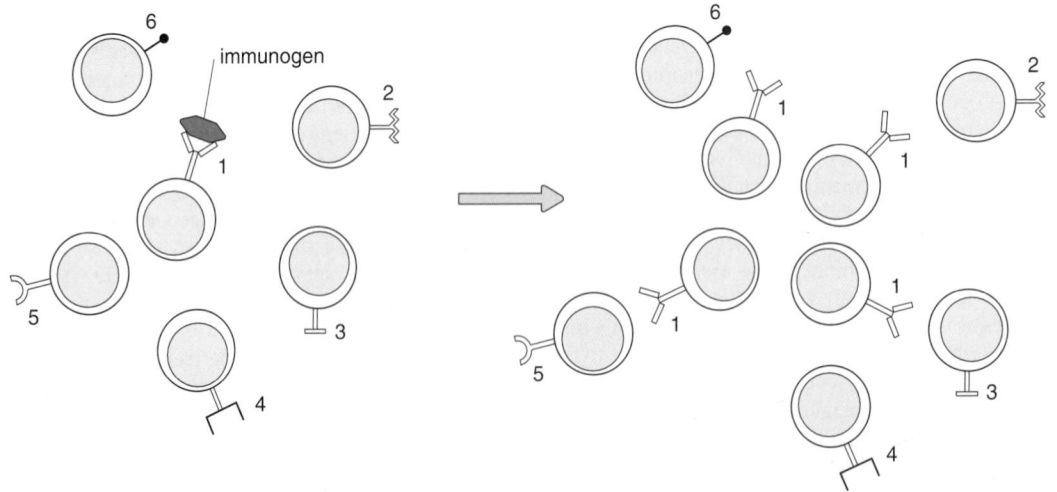

Figure 4–1. Clonal selection of lymphocytes by a specific immunogen. **Left:** The unimmunized lymphocyte population is composed of cells from many different clones, each with its own antigen specificity, indicated here by the distinctive shapes of the surface antigen receptors. **Right:** Contact with an immunogen leads to selective proliferation (positive selection) of any clone or clones that can recognize that specific immunogen.

that can recognize the antigen and can participate in the immune response.

The principles of clonal restriction and clonal selection were first postulated by Burnet, Jerne, Talmadge, and others in the 1950s and still rank among the most important conceptual insights in the history of immunology. Clonal restriction is the primary basis for the extreme specificity of immune responses: each clone of lymphocytes can respond only to the limited set of antigens recognized by its unique immunoglobulin or T-cell receptor proteins and, when activated, carries out effector functions that are specifically directed against that same antigen. Clonal selection, on the other hand, is principally responsible for the phenomenon of immunologic memory: exposure to an antigen sculpts and hones the lymphocyte population so that it can respond more quickly and more vigorously the next time the same antigen is encountered.

THE IMMUNE RESPONSE

Every **immune response** is a complex and intricately regulated sequence of events involving several cell types. It is triggered when an antigen enters the body and encounters a specialized class of cells called antigen-presenting cells (APCs). These APCs capture a minute amount of the antigen and display it in a form that can be recognized by antigen-specific helper T lymphocytes. The helper T cells become activated and, in turn, promote the activation of other classes of lymphocytes, such as B cells or cytotoxic T cells. The activated lymphocytes then proliferate and carry out their specific effector functions, which, in most cases, successfully inactivate or eliminate the antigen. At each stage in this process, the lymphocytes and APCs communicate with one another through direct contact or by secreting regulatory cytokines. They also may interact simultaneously with other cell types or with components of the complement, kinin, or fibrinolytic systems, resulting in phagocyte activation, blood clotting, or the initiation of wound healing. Immune responses may be either localized or systemic but are nearly always highly specific, focusing their full force against the antigen while causing little or no damage to normal host tissues. The responses are also precisely controlled and normally terminate soon after the inciting antigen is eliminated.

Figure 4–2 provides a schematic overview of the sequence of events that take place during a prototypical immune response. The following sections describe each step of this response in turn.

Immunogens & Antigens

Immunologists commonly use the term **antigen** when referring to the agent that triggers an immune response. Strictly speaking, however, this term actually refers to the ability of a molecule to be recognized by an immunoglobulin or T-cell receptor and hence to serve as the target of a response. For reasons that will be explained in Chapter 5, not all antigens are capable of inducing immune responses. Instead, a molecule or collection of molecules that can induce an immune response in a particular host is most properly referred to as an **immunogen.** Typical immunogens include pathogenic microorganisms (such as viruses, bacteria, or parasites), foreign tissue grafts, or otherwise innocuous environmental substances, such as the proteins in pollen, grasses, or food.

Proteins are, in general, the most potent immunogens. Other classes of molecules, such as lipids, carbohydrates, or nucleic acids, most commonly become the targets of immune responses when they are linked to an immunogenic protein (as in lipoproteins, glycoproteins, or nucleoprotein complexes). Many of the immunogens encountered in nature are actually composites of several different immunogenic substances. A single bacterium, for example, is made up of a multitude of proteins and other molecules that may each elicit a specific immune response. In the prototypic immune response depicted in Figure 4–2, the immunogen is a virus that, like most viruses, contains several immunogenic proteins.

ANTIGEN PROCESSING & PRESENTATION

Responses to most proteinaceous immunogens can begin only after the immunogen has been captured, processed, and presented by an APC (see Fig 4–2). The reason for this is that T cells only recognize immunogens that are bound to **major histocompatibility complex (MHC)** proteins on the surfaces of other cells (see Chapter 6). There are two different classes of MHC proteins, each of which is recognized by one of the two major subsets of T lymphocytes. **Class I MHC** proteins are expressed by virtually all somatic cell types and are used to present substances to **CD8** T cells, most of which are cytotoxic. Almost any cell can therefore present antigens to cytotoxic T cells and thus serve as the target of a cytotoxic response. **Class II MHC** proteins, on the other hand, are expressed only by macrophages and a few other cell types and are necessary for antigen presentation to **CD4** T cells—the subset that includes most helper cells. Since helper cell activation is necessary for virtually all immune responses, the class II-bearing APCs play a pivotal role in controlling such responses. In fact, unless otherwise stated, the term "antigen-presenting cell" usually refers only to these specialized cells that bear class II MHC proteins.

Exogenous immunogens can be captured in a variety of ways. The APC depicted in Figure 4–2 is a macrophage—a voracious phagocyte that can readily capture particulate immunogens. Other types of APCs

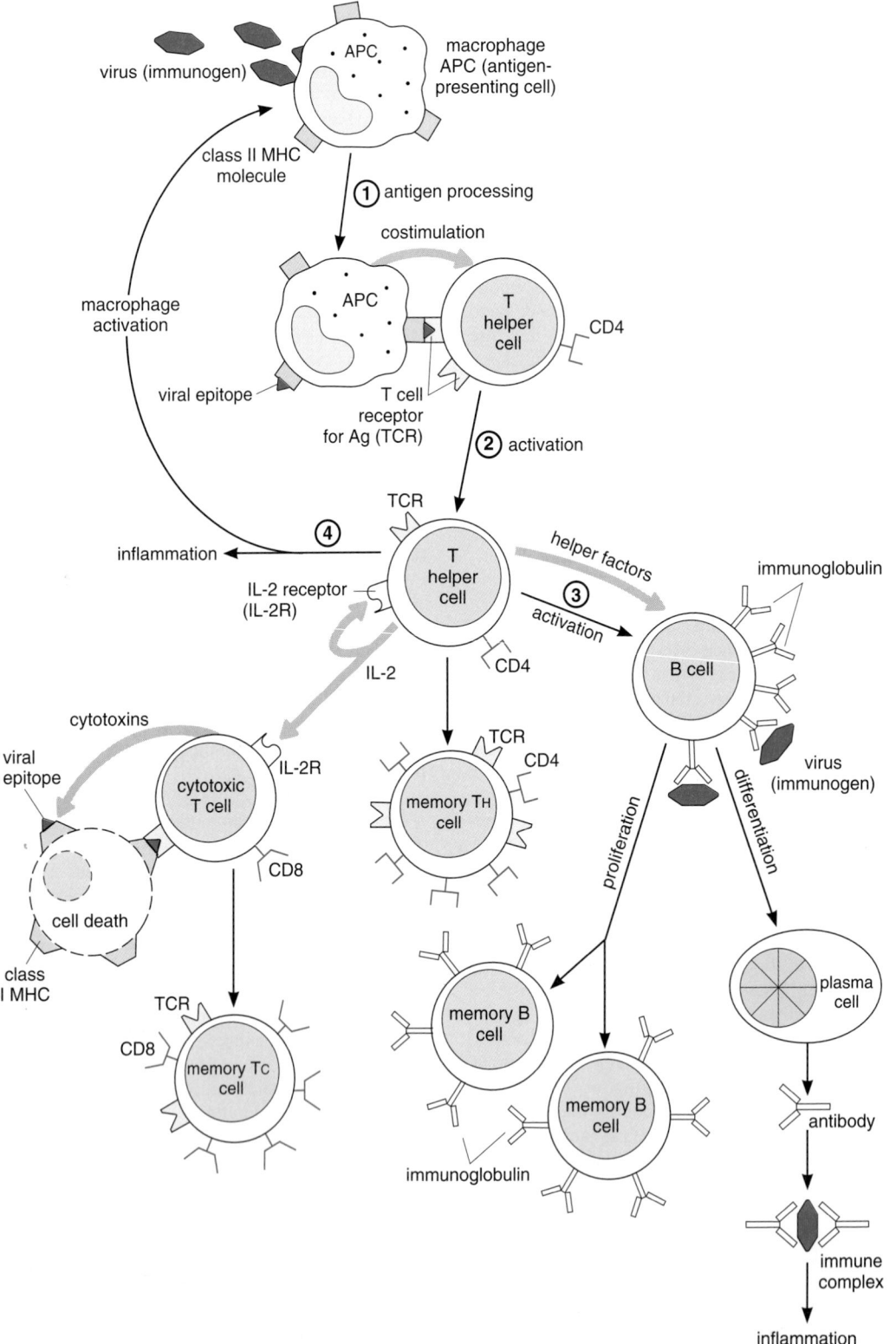

Figure 4–2. Sequence of events in a prototypical immune response (see text for details).

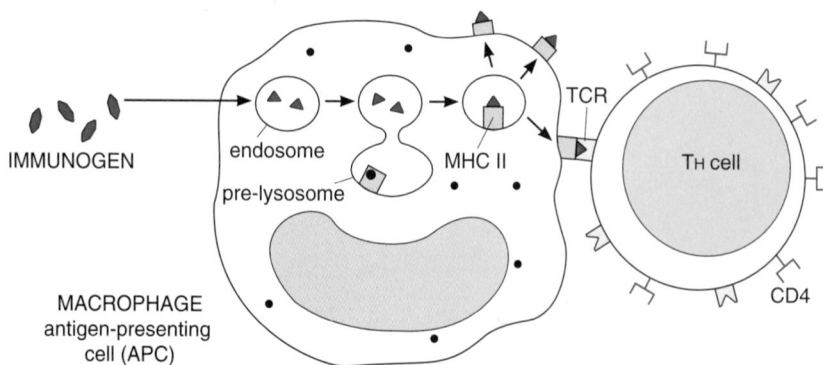

Figure 4–3. Capture, processing, and presentation of antigen by an APC. The immunogen is captured by phagocytosis, receptor-mediated endocytosis, or pinocytosis and is broken down into fragments. Some fragments (antigens) become associated with class II MHC proteins and are transported to the cell surface, where they can be recognized by CD4 T cells. TCR, T-cell receptor.

have less phagocytic capacity and tend to rely instead on receptor-mediated endocytosis or on pinocytosis (see Chapter 2)—pathways that are also used quite effectively by macrophages. By using these three pathways, APCs can capture a very broad range of different immunogenic substances, and most APCs exhibit little or no antigen specificity. Indeed, a given APC may present several different antigens simultaneously, one on each of its many surface MHC proteins. The capture mechanisms are relatively inefficient, however, so that relatively high local concentrations of an exogenous immunogen are required for optimal activity of most APCs.

Exogenous immunogens that are captured by an APC become enclosed within membrane-lined vesicles in its cytoplasm and, within these vesicles, undergo a series of alterations called **antigen processing** (Fig 4–3). The full range of chemical modifications that can occur during processing is not known; it probably depends on the chemical nature of the immunogen. Processing of most, if not all, proteinaceous immunogens appears to involve denaturation and partial proteolytic digestion, so that the immunogen is cleaved into short peptides. A limited number of the resulting peptides then associate noncovalently with class II MHC proteins and are transported to the APC surface, where they can be detected by helper T cells. This process is called **antigen presentation.** A CD4 helper T lymphocyte that comes into direct contact with an APC may become activated, but it will do so only if it expresses a T-cell receptor protein that can recognize and bind the particular peptide–MHC complex presented by the APC.

Activation of Helper T Lymphocytes

Helper T (T_H) cells are the principal orchestrators of the immune response because they are needed for activation of the two other lymphoid effector cell types: cytotoxic T (T_C) cells and antibody-secreting

plasma cells. T_H cell activation occurs early in an immune response (see Fig 4–2) and requires at least two signals. One signal is provided by binding of the T-cell antigen receptor to the antigenic peptide–MHC complex on the APC surface and is transmitted through the CD3 protein complex (see Chapter 9). The second, **costimulatory** signal also requires contact with the APC and is thought to result from binding of a separate signal-transmitting protein on the T-cell surface with a specific ligand on the APC. One interaction that is known to generate such a costimulatory signal is the binding of a T-cell surface protein designated **CD28** to any one of a small family of APC surface proteins designated **B7** (see Chapter 8). Other surface protein pairs may also mediate costimulation.

Together, the two signals induce the helper T cell to begin secreting a cytokine known as interleukin-2 **(IL-2)** and also to begin expressing specific high-affinity **IL-2 receptors** on its surface (Fig 4–4). IL-2 is a highly potent mitogenic factor for T lymphocytes and is essential for the proliferative response of activated T cells. The IL-2 protein has a very short half-life outside the cell and so acts only over extremely short distances. In fact, IL-2 is thought to exert its greatest effects on the cell from which it is secreted—a phenomenon known as an **autocrine effect.** Even if a T cell has received both activation signals from contact with an APC, it will not begin to proliferate in the absence of IL-2 activity or if its own surface IL-2 receptors are blocked. The IL-2 secreted by an activated T_H cell can also act on cells in the immediate vicinity, in a so-called **paracrine effect;** this is especially important for activating T_C cells, which generally do not produce enough IL-2 to stimulate their own proliferation (see below). In addition to IL-2, activated T_H cells secrete other cytokines that promote the growth, differentiation, and functions of B cells, macrophages, and other cell types (see Chapter 9).

The contact between an APC and an antigen-

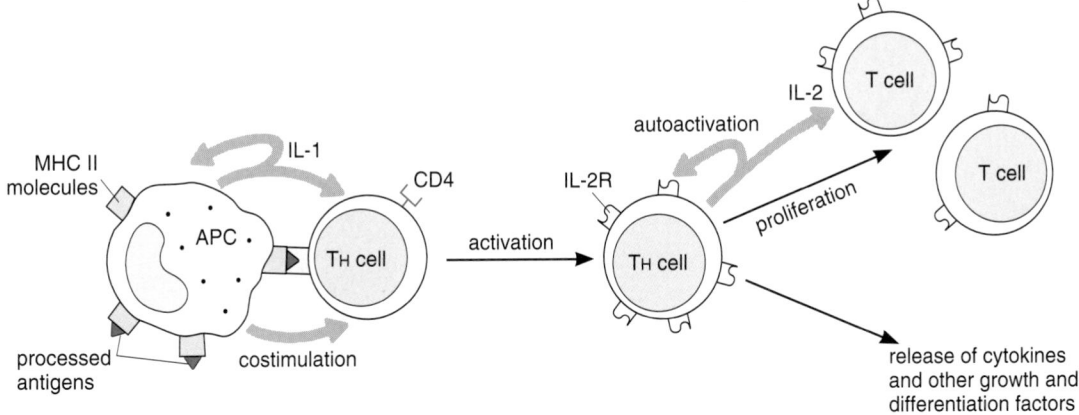

Figure 4–4. T_H-cell activation. The APC presents an antigenic peptide, bound to class II MHC, to the T_H cell and also provides a costimulatory signal. The two signals lead to activation of the T_H cell. The APC also releases IL-1, which acts on both the APC and the T_H cell to promote activation. Activation leads to IL-2 receptor expression and IL-2 secretion by the T_H cell, resulting in autocrine growth stimulation.

specific T_H cell also has effects on the APC. One of the most important is that the APC may begin to release a cytokine called interleukin-1 (**IL-1**). This cytokine appears to act primarily in an autocrine manner on the APC itself: it increases surface expression of class II MHC proteins and of various adhesion molecules and thereby strengthens binding of the T_H cell and enhances antigen presentation (see Fig 4–4). At the same time, IL-1 functions in a paracrine manner on the T_H cell to promote IL-2 secretion and IL-2 receptor expression, and thus it potentiates the T_H proliferative response. Macrophages produce relatively large amounts of IL-1 and smaller amounts of two additional cytokines—tumor necrosis factor (**TNF**) and interleukin 6 (**IL-6**)—that can mimic or synergize

with IL-1 activity (see Chapter 10). Other types of APCs produce the same cytokines, although in various proportions. The signal for their secretion appears to be transmitted to the APC at least in part by the class II MHC protein when it binds an appropriate T cell. Thus, T_H cell contact with an APC leads to bidirectional signaling events that enhance the immunologic functions of both cells.

Activation of B Cells & Cytotoxic T Cells

While the T_H cells are being activated as described earlier, some B cells may also have been engaging the immunogen through their antigen receptors, which are membrane-bound forms of the antibodies they will later secrete (see Chapters 7 and 8). Unlike T

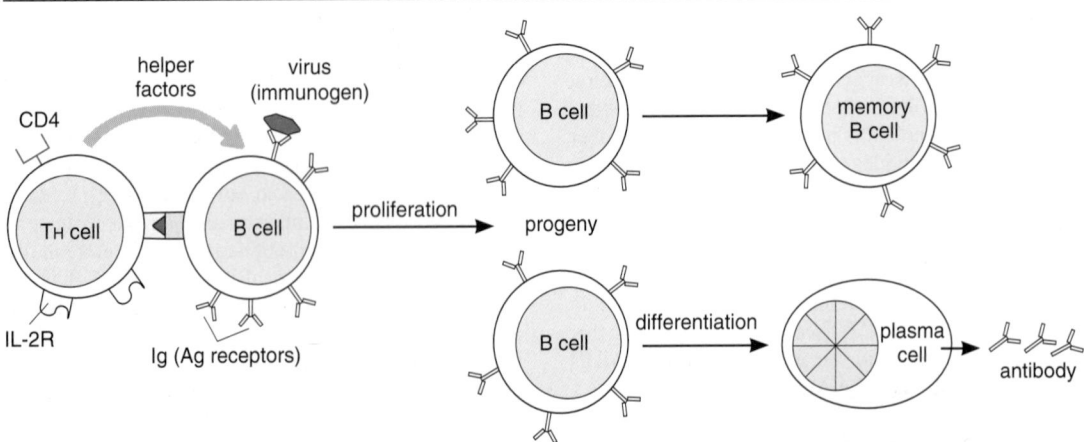

Figure 4–5. B-cell activation. Antigen binding to the surface immunoglobulins, coupled with soluble or contact-mediated helper factors from an activated T_H cell, lead to proliferation and differentiation. Cytokines involved in T_H-cell help include IL-2, IL-4, and IL-6. Contact-mediated help generally involves binding of CD40 on the B-cell surface to CD40 ligand (CD40L) on the activated T_H cell.

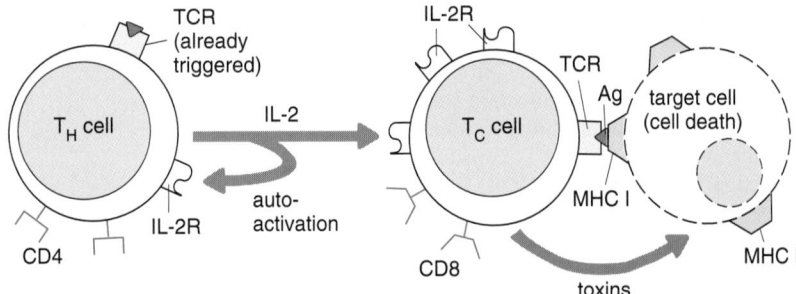

Figure 4–6. T_C-cell activation requires contact with a specific antigen complexed with a class I MHC molecule on the surface of a target cell. It also requires IL-2 from a nearby activated T_H cell. The activated T_C cell kills the target cell either by secreting cytotoxins (as shown) or by inducing it to commit suicide.

cells, B cells recognize an immunogen in its free, unprocessed form (see Fig 4–2). Specific antigen binding provides one type of signal that can lead to B-cell activation. A second type is provided by activated T_H cells, which express proteins that help activate the B cell by binding to nonimmunoglobulin receptors on its surface. These T_H-derived signals, which act on any B cell regardless of its antigen specificity, are known as **helper factors** (Fig 4–5). Some are cytokines that are secreted by activated T_H cells; these include IL-2 and two other interleukins—IL-4 and IL-6—each of which has a very short radius of action. Help is delivered even more efficiently, however, by cell–cell contact, which allows proteins on the T-cell surface to contact those on the B cell. The most effective form of contact-mediated help occurs when a protein called CD40 ligand (**CD40L),** which is expressed on T_H cells only after they become activated, binds to a protein called **CD40** on B cells. In fact, contact with an activated T_H cell may be sufficient to activate a resting B cell even though its surface immunoglobulins have not engaged an antigen; this is known as **bystander** B-cell activation. The combination of antigen binding and helper factors, however, yields the strongest mitogenic signals, so that over time antigen-specific clones quickly outgrow any activated bystanders. Some cells in the activated clone differentiate into plasma cells that secrete antibodies specific for the immunogen.

T_C lymphocytes function to eradicate cells that express foreign antigens on their surfaces, such as virus-infected host cells (Fig 4–6). Most T_C cells express CD8 rather than CD4 and hence recognize antigens in association with class I rather than class II MHC proteins. When a somatic cell is infected by a virus, some immunogenic viral proteins may undergo processing within the cell, and the resulting peptides may then appear as surface complexes with class I MHC molecules. These peptide–MHC complexes may then be recognized by the T-cell receptor of an antigen-specific clone, providing one of two signals necessary for T_C-cell activation. This first signal alone induces high-affinity IL-2 receptors on the T_C cell. The second

signal is furnished by IL-2 secreted from a nearby activated T_H lymphocyte. On receiving both signals, the activated T_C cell acquires cytotoxic activity, enabling it to kill the cell to which it is bound, as well as any other cells bearing the same peptide–MHC class I complexes. In some cases, killing occurs because the T_C releases specific toxins onto the target cell; in others, the T_C induces the target cell to commit suicide by apoptosis (see later discussion). The activated T_C cell also proliferates, giving rise to additional T_C cells with the same antigen specificity.

MECHANISMS OF ANTIGEN ELIMINATION

The ultimate function of the immune system is to seek out and destroy foreign substances in the body. Depending in part on the nature of the foreign substance, this can be accomplished in several ways. One, described in the preceding section, is the direct **cytotoxic** killing of antigen-bearing target cells by activated T_C cells (see Fig 4–6). Most other immunologic effector mechanisms require antibodies; the most important of these will now be described.

Toxin Neutralization

Antibodies specific for bacterial toxins or for the venom of insects or snakes bind these antigenic proteins and, in many cases, directly inactivate them by steric effects. In addition, formation of an antigen–antibody complex promotes the capture and phagocytosis of these toxins by macrophages and other phagocytes (see the section on opsonization, below). Because of their effectiveness, preformed antibodies against toxins or venom are often injected prophylactically or therapeutically as a means of protecting unimmunized individuals who have recently been, or are at risk of being, exposed to specific toxins.

Virus Neutralization

Antibodies specific for proteins on the surface of a virus may block the attachment of the virus to target cells, particularly if the antibodies bind at or close to the site of cell binding on the virus. This provides a means by which preexisting antibodies can protect against new viral infections. Once viral infection has become established, however, neutralization is often less important than the cytotoxic action of T_C cells for eradicating the infection.

Opsonization & Phagocyte Activation

Antibodies that coat bacteria or other particulate antigens can function as **opsonins** to promote phagocytosis. This occurs because macrophages and other phagocytes carry surface **Fc receptors** that facilitate engulfment of antibody-coated particles (see Chapters 2 and 7). Thus, just as macrophages control lymphocyte function through their role as APCs, B lymphocytes regulate macrophage function by directing these phagocytes to specific antigenic targets through the process of opsonization.

Immune responses also affect phagocyte functions in other ways. For example, IL-1 stimulates macrophages to express surface receptors for interferon gamma (**IFN-γ**) and other cytokines, released from activated T_H cells, that are potent macrophage activators. The resulting activation increases the phagocytic activity of the macrophage and may cause it to secrete numerous other cytokines and mediators (see Chapter 2). Activated lymphocytes also produce IL-2, IL-3, and IL-4, as well as colony-stimulating factors (see Chapter 10), which regulate macrophage growth and function.

Activation of Complement

Certain types of antibodies can activate the **complement pathway** when they are complexed with an antigen (see Chapters 7 and 11). If the antibody is bound to the surface of a cell, such as a bacterium, the cascade of complement enzyme reactions may lead to lysis of the cell, providing an important means of killing foreign invaders. Some products of the complement cascade also act as opsonins when bound to an antigen–antibody complex, whereas others are chemoattractive for neutrophils. Still others cause the release of inflammatory mediators such as histamine from mast cells and basophils (see Chapter 12).

Antibody-Dependent Cell-Mediated Cytotoxicity

One major class of antibodies, called IgG (see Chapter 7), binds to Fc receptors on the surfaces of natural killer (NK) cells and certain other cell types and enables them to carry out a form of antigen-specific cell killing called **antibody-dependent cell-mediated cytotoxicity (ADCC).** The IgG antibodies bound on the surface of the cell enable it to bind specifically to antigen-bearing target cells, which might be bacteria or multicellular parasites, and to kill the target cell with cytotoxins. The antibodies are said to "arm" the cells to perform ADCC, and they are ab-

solutely required for such killing; this fact distinguishes ADCC from T_C-mediated cytotoxicity, which occurs independently of antibodies.

INFLAMMATION

Although lymphocytes and APCs are the key cells in all immune responses, other types of cells may be recruited into the response. For example, cytokines or other products released by activated lymphocytes and macrophages may chemoattract neutrophils or eosinophils, stimulate proliferation of fibroblasts and endothelial cells, or cause mast cells and basophils to discharge other bioactive substances into the local tissues (see Chapter 12). These agents, as well as products of the complement cascade, may lead directly or indirectly to increased local vascular perfusion, capillary permeability, accumulation of extravascular fluid, and pain. In some instances, other enzymatic pathways such as the kinin, clotting, and fibrinolytic systems may also become activated (see Chapters 11 and 12).

The entire, integrated host reaction—encompassing the immune response along with all of its associated secondary phenomena—is called **inflammation.** Soluble factors that trigger the various secondary aspects of inflammation are known collectively as **inflammatory mediators** and are said to be **proinflammatory.** The cells involved (including lymphocytes, neutrophils, mast cells, and many others) are often referred to as **inflammatory cells.** Different features of inflammation predominate in different settings, giving rise to several distinct categories of inflammatory reactions (see Chapter 12). Most aspects of inflammation are potentially beneficial since they help to defend the host against toxins, pathogens, or other injurious substances. Excessive or inappropriate inflammatory reactions, however, can lead to discomfort, disability, and even death. For this reason, **antiinflammatory** drugs and other therapeutic measures that suppress inflammation play an important role in contemporary medical practice.

LOCALIZATION OF IMMUNE RESPONSES

The initial response to an immunogen depends partially on its route of entry into the body. Most immunogens enter via one of three routes. Those that enter through the bloodstream are most likely to be detected by macrophages and other APCs in the spleen, which then becomes the principal site of the immune response. By contrast, immunogens that enter the skin and subcutaneous connective tissues are usually detected by resident APCs, such as epidermal Langerhans cells or dermal macrophages, and, in addition, may be carried via the lymphatic circulation into regional lymph nodes; the immune response then begins both at the site of contact and in the affected nodes. Alternatively, an immunogen may enter the body by traversing mucosal surfaces of the respiratory or gastrointestinal tract; in this case, it immediately encounters the submucosal lymphoid tissues, which launch a response that is directed both locally and into the adjacent lumen from which the immunogen came (see Chapters 3 and 13).

Regardless of the site at which a response begins, there is always some trafficking of lymphocytes to other sites via the blood and lymphatic vessels, so that the entire immune system can eventually be recruited into the response if the immunogen is especially abundant, widely disseminated, or resistant to immune elimination. Some types of APCs are likewise capable of migrating through the blood or lymphatics (see Chapter 6), carrying immunogens along with them into distant lymphoid organs.

QUANTITATIVE & KINETIC ASPECTS OF IMMUNE RESPONSES

The quantitative aspects of immune function have been studied most extensively for B cells, since B-cell activity can easily be monitored by the concentrations of specific antibodies in the serum—an area of investigation known as **serology.** The general conclusions of such studies, however, are thought to be applicable to T-cell responses as well.

At any given moment, active T- and B-effector cells account for roughly 1% of the total lymphoid population in a normal host. These belong to many different clones (the exact number is unknown and no doubt varies widely), most of which are probably involved in ongoing, low-level immune responses against the many antigens encountered in everyday life. As a result, the serum of a normal, healthy adult contains innumerable different types of antibody molecules. Each is present in only minute amounts, but altogether they account for roughly 20% of total serum protein. Each of these circulating antibodies provides a low level of protection against its specific antigen.

When a person or animal is exposed to significant amounts of an antigen and mounts a B-cell response, the concentration of serum antibodies against that antigen generally rises. Serum from such an immunized individual is often called a **specific antiserum.** It is important to remember, however, that even in the serum of highly immunized individuals, antibodies against a given antigen make up only a small fraction of the total and antibodies with many other specificities are also present.

An individual's first encounter with a particular immunogen is called a **priming** event and leads to a relatively weak, short-lived response designated the **primary immune response.** This is divisible into several phases (Fig 4–7). The **lag,** or **latent, phase** is the time between the initial exposure to an immunogen and the detection of antibodies in the circulation, which averages about 1 week in humans. During this period, activation of T_H and B cells is taking place. The **exponential phase** is marked by a rapid increase in the quantity of circulating antibodies and reflects the increasing numbers of secretory plasma cells. After an interval during which the antibody level remains relatively constant because secretion and degradation are occurring at approximately equal rates (the **steadystate,** or **plateau, phase**), the antibody level gradually declines (**declining phase**) as synthesis of new antibody wanes. The decline indicates that new plasma cells are no longer being produced and that existing

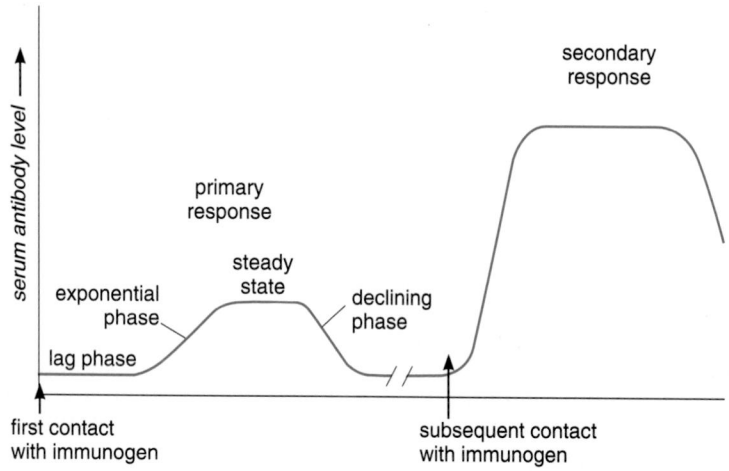

Figure 4–7. Primary and secondary immune responses (see text for details).

plasma cells are dying or ceasing antibody production; this generally signifies that the immunogen has been eradicated. Thus, the duration of a humoral immune response is limited primarily by the duration of the antigenic stimulus and by the relatively short life spans of the plasma cells involved in the response.

Subsequent encounters with the same immunogen lead to responses that are qualitatively similar to the primary response but manifest marked quantitative differences (see Fig 4–7). In such a **secondary,** or **anamnestic, immune response,** the lag period is shortened and antibody levels rise more rapidly to a much higher steady-state level, thereafter remaining in the serum at detectable levels for much longer periods. The large numbers of antigen-specific memory T and B cells generated during the primary response are responsible for the rapid kinetics and the greater intensity and duration of secondary responses.

PROGRAMMED CELL DEATH IN THE IMMUNE SYSTEM

Antigen-dependent proliferation of a lymphocyte clone is an example of **positive selection;** that is, the antigen promotes growth of the cells on which it acts. Under some conditions, however, contact with antigens or other stimuli results in **negative selection** of a responsive clone, meaning that cells in the clone selectively die. Negative selection of lymphocytes is a common event and is essential to the ability of the immune system to discriminate self from nonself. In particular, most virgin T or B cells whose antigen receptors recognize components found in normal host tissues are thought to be selectively killed before they leave the bone marrow or thymus, as a means of protecting the host against attack by these potentially **autoreactive** (ie, self-reactive) cells. This may account for the observation that at least 99% of developing thymocytes die within the thymus (see Chapter 3). Thus, the clonal composition of the immune system is shaped not only by positive clonal selection but also by the active elimination of potentially deleterious clones.

Lymphocytes frequently die after being instructed to commit suicide by signals in their environment. These signals often include events such as antigen binding to surface immunoglobulins or TCRs which, under other circumstances, would lead to clonal proliferation. When delivered in particular combinations or at certain vulnerable stages in a cell's life, however, these signals instead induce death by **apoptosis** (see Chapter 1). Because death in these cells is preceded by biochemical changes indistinguishable from those of activation, it is often termed **activation-induced cell death (AICD).** AICD triggered by contact with self-antigens is an important mechanism for eliminating autoreactive B- and T-lymphoid cells (see

Chapters 8 and 9), and occurs commonly among normal thymocytes, bone marrow progenitors, and germinal center B cells.

Another signaling pathway that is especially important for killing of and by lymphocytes involves a surface transmembrane protein called **Fas** (MW 45,000; also called APO-1 or **CD95**), which is expressed constitutively by many normal or neoplastic cell types as well as on activated B and T lymphocytes. The extracellular portion of Fas serves as a receptor for a different surface protein—a homotrimer of polypeptides called Fas ligand **(FasL),** found on many activated T cells and certain other cell types. When cells expressing these two proteins contact one another, binding of FasL causes Fas to trimerize and this, in turn, induces apoptosis in the Fas-bearing cell. The signaling pathway involved is incompletely understood, but depends on an 80-amino-acid "death domain" in the cytoplasmic portion of Fas. Cytotoxic T lymphocytes exploit this as one mechanism for killing: activated T_C cells express FasL, which enables them to induce apoptosis in target cells that express Fas. But lymphocytes themselves can also be killed in this way. For example, after prolonged or repeated activation, helper T cells express both Fas and FasL, and so may kill either themselves or one another; this is thought to be one mechanism for limiting the intensity of an immune response. The same mechanism might also act to eradicate autoreactive T_H cells that encounter abundant self-antigens in peripheral tissues— and indeed, mutations in Fas are responsible for certain rare autoimmune diseases. Fas-mediated killing may also account in part for the phenomenon of **immune privilege**—the observation that foreign tissues transplanted to certain sites in the body are much less prone to immunologic attack than they would be at other sites. Cells in two of the best studied privileged sites (the testes and anterior chamber of the eye) have been found to express FasL constitutively; this tends to induce apoptosis of any lymphocytes that become activated (and hence express Fas) within these tissues, and so suppresses any local immune responses.

The importance of negative selection is also illustrated by **follicular lymphoma,** the most common form of B-cell cancer in humans (see Chapters 7 and 46). A major factor in the genesis of this disease is **Bcl-2**—a normal cellular protein that acts to inhibit apoptosis in some lymphocytes and other cell types (see Chapter 1). Follicular lymphoma arises when a clone of B cells expresses abnormally high levels of Bcl-2 protein and so becomes resistant to killing; as a result, these cells accumulate in abnormally large numbers and eventually evolve into a cancer. This implies that a high, controlled rate of programmed lymphocyte death normally benefits the host by restricting the growth of individual clones and of the lymphoid population as a whole, providing a counterforce against the stimuli that might otherwise drive excessive lymphocyte proliferation.

REFERENCES

Abbas AK: Die and let live: Eliminating dangerous lymphocytes. *Cell* 1996;**84:**655.

Brodsky FM, Guagliardi LE: The cell biology of antigen processing and presentation. *Ann Rev Immunol* 1991;**9:**707.

Burnet FM: A modification of Jerne's theory of antibody production using the concept of clonal selection. *Aust J Sci* 1957;**20:**67.

Cohen JJ et al: Apoptosis and programmed cell death in immunity. *Ann Rev Immunol* 1992;**10:**267.

Gray D: Immunological memory. *Ann Rev Immunol* 1993;**11:**49.

Green DR et al: Activation-induced apoptosis in lymphoid systems. *Semin Immunol* 1992;**4:**379.

Parker DC: T cell-dependent B-cell activation. *Ann Rev Immunol* 1993;**11:**331.

Podack ER, Kupfer A: T cell effector functions: Mechanisms for delivery of cytotoxicity and help. *Ann Rev Cell Biol* 1991;**7:**479.

Streilein JW: Unraveling immune privilege. *Science* 1995;**270:**1158.

Vitetta ES et al: Cellular interactions in the humoral immune response. *Adv Immunol* 1989;**45:**1.

von Boehmer H, Kisielow P: Self–nonself discrimination by T cells. *Science* 1990;**248:**1369.

5 Immunogens, Antigens, & Vaccines

Tristram G. Parslow, MD, PhD

Any substance that is capable of inducing an immune response is called an **immunogen** and is said to be **immunogenic.** The response may involve exclusively the humoral or the cellular limb of the immune system but most commonly involves both. As a rule, immune responses are carried out only by those B- and T-cell clones whose surface immunoglobulin or T-cell receptor (TCR) proteins recognize the immunogen. Substances that are recognized by a particular immunoglobulin or TCR, and so can serve as the target of an immune response, are called **antigens** and are said to be **antigenic.** Thus, all immunogens are also antigens (Fig 5–1).

Most of the immunogens encountered in nature, including essentially all microbial pathogens, are complex assemblages made up of several different types of molecules, not all of which are antigenic. For example, the response to an enveloped virus is usually directed against proteins of the viral particle but not against the lipids that make up much of the viral envelope. Even when a single pure protein serves as an immunogen, the response is usually directed against only a few discrete clusters of amino acid residues within the larger polypeptide. The specific set of chemical features that is recognized by a given antibody or TCR is called an **epitope** (or, in older terminology, an **antigenic determinant**). In other words, an epitope is the specific site to which a particular immunoglobulin or TCR binds. It follows that every immunogen must contain one or more epitopes that enable it to serve as an antigen. Not all antigens or epitopes are immunogenic, however; in other words, not every chemical substance that can be bound by an immunoglobulin or TCR is, by itself, capable of inducing an immune response. This chapter explores the properties that enable a substance to serve as the stimulus for, or the target of, an immunologic attack.

IMMUNOGENS

The ability to evoke an immune response, and the nature and intensity of this response, depend not only on the physicochemical properties of the immunogen itself but also on other factors, such as the characteristics of the organism being immunized, the route of contact, and the sensitivity of the methods used to detect the response. The factors that influence immunogenicity are complex, but several important generalizations can be made.

Properties of the Immunogen

Large proteins are, as a rule, the most potent immunogens. Polysaccharides, short polypeptides, and some synthetic organic polymers (eg, polyvinyl pyrrolidone) can also be immunogenic under certain circumstances. At least one simple lipid—an unusual fatty acid, called mycolic acid, present in mycobacteria—is known to be immunogenic. Most mammalian cellular lipids, as well as nucleic acids, are not immunogenic, but antibodies that react with them can be elicited by immunization with nucleoprotein or lipoprotein complexes; this is probably the mechanism of origin of the anti-DNA antibodies found in the serum of many patients with autoimmune diseases (see Chapter 33). Thus, nucleic acids and most lipids are examples of molecules that are antigenic but not immunogenic.

Immunogenicity is influenced by molecular size. The most potent immunogens are proteins with molecular weights greater than 100,000. Extremely small molecules, such as amino acids, monosaccharides, and most other species smaller than MW 10,000, usually are not immunogenic. A few substances with molecular weights below 1000 can induce immune responses but in most cases will do so only when bound to a larger, host-derived macromolecule such as a protein; this is the mechanism by which many people become allergic to metals (such as nickel) or to certain drugs.

Immunogenicity is also a function of chemical complexity. This principle is most clearly illustrated by synthetic polypeptides. Homopolymers of a single amino acid are poor immunogens regardless of size, whereas copolymers of two or—even better—three amino acids are often quite active. Aromatic amino

74

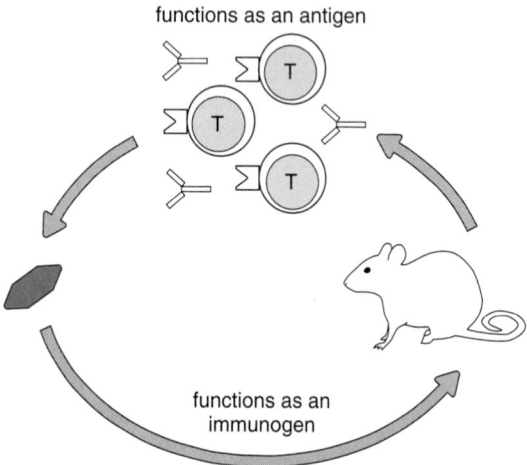

functions as an antigen

functions as an
immunogen

Figure 5–1. Immunogens and antigens. An immunogen induces an immune response; antigens serve as the target of the response.

acids contribute more to immunogenicity than do nonaromatic residues; thus, simple random polypeptides that contain tyrosine are better immunogens than are comparable polypeptides without tyrosine, and immunogenicity of such polymers is directly proportional to their tyrosine contents. Attachment of tyrosine chains to the weakly immunogenic protein gelatin (which contains few aromatic amino acids) markedly enhances its immunogenicity.

Most important, however, is foreignness: the immune system normally discriminates between self and nonself, so that only molecules that are foreign to the host are immunogenic. Thus, albumin isolated from the serum of a rabbit and injected back into the same or another rabbit will not yield an immune response—every rabbit is **tolerant** to this endogenous protein. Yet the same protein, if injected into other vertebrate species, is likely to evoke substantial antibody responses, depending on the dose of antigen and the route and frequency of injection. The mechanisms that enable an animal to discriminate self from nonself are not yet fully understood, but some of the known processes that contribute to this discrimination are considered in Chapters 8 and 9.

Genetic Constitution of the Host Animal

The ability to respond to a particular immunogen is genetically predetermined. For example, pure polysaccharides are immunogenic when injected into mice or humans but not when injected into guinea pigs or rabbits. Much information about the genetics of immune responsiveness has accrued from studies using inbred strains of animals. For example, some strains of guinea pig produce a vigorous antibody response against the simple polypeptide poly-L-lysine, whereas other strains give no detectable response; crossbreeding studies among these strains indicate that the abil-

ity to respond to poly-L-lysine is inherited as an autosomal-dominant trait. Many analogous phenomena have been described in humans. Selective responsiveness of this type reflects a number of hereditary factors, the best understood of which include the particular collection (repertoire) of different immunoglobulins and TCR proteins that an individual is able to produce (Chapters 7–9), and the ability of antigen-presenting cells (APCs) to present specific types of molecules to T lymphocytes (Chapter 6). Individuals whose APCs cannot present a substance or whose lymphocytes cannot recognize it will not respond to this substance as an immunogen.

Mode of Contact

Whether or not a substance will evoke an immune response also depends on the dosage and the route by which it enters the body. A quantity of substance that has no effect when injected intravenously may evoke a copious antibody response when injected subcutaneously. Route of contact also can influence the qualitative nature of a response; for example, an immunogen that contacts the intestinal mucosa typically evokes the production of a different type of antibody than would be produced if it entered through the bloodstream, and this can affect subsequent events in the immune response (see Chapter 7). The threshold dose required for a response under particular conditions varies among immunogens. In general, once the threshold dose is exceeded, increasing doses lead to increasing, though less than proportionate, responses. Excessive doses, however, may not only fail to induce a response but may instead establish a state of specific unresponsiveness, or tolerance, to subsequent exposures to that substance—a phenomenon that is sometimes referred to as **high-zone tolerance.**

Both the intensity and the character of the response to an immunogen can be altered if it is administered in combination with other immunogens. This is because an ongoing response to one substance can affect local cytokine concentrations as well as the type and activation state of local immune cells, and these may, in turn, favor or disfavor particular types of responses to other immunogens. Certain substances, called **adjuvants** and **immunomodulators,** are especially effective at enhancing or modifying the responses to many different immunogens when administered along with them, and have been exploited therapeutically for this purpose in the development of vaccines (see later section).

B-CELL ANTIGENS & B-CELL EPITOPES

Large molecules are the strongest immunogens and usually are correspondingly strong antigens. Any given antibody or TCR, however, will recognize and bind to only a limited portion of such a molecule, and

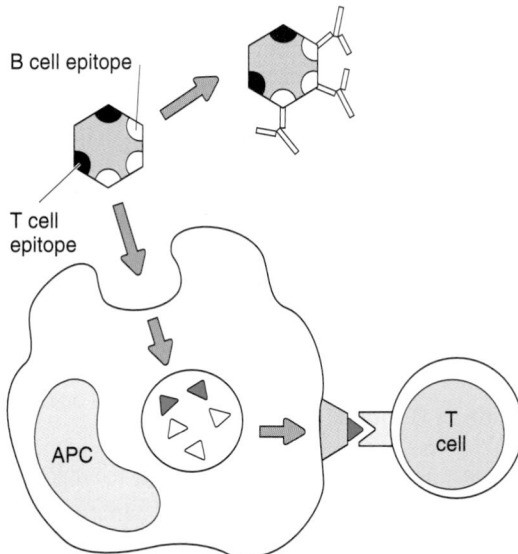

Figure 5–2. Most large antigens contain multiple epitopes. B-cell epitopes (white) are regions that can be bound by immunoglobulin proteins. T-cell epitopes (black) are recognized by T lymphocytes only after being processed and presented in association with an MHC protein on the surface on an antigen-presenting cell (APC).

specific. Conversely, when the alanines were situated near the backbone and the tyrosines and glutamates were exposed, tyrosine- and glutamate-specific antibodies were obtained. In each instance, the most exposed residues made up the predominant epitopes of the antigen. Similarly, antibodies raised against branched polysaccharide antigens preferentially recognize the terminal sugar residues of each branch.

A more detailed appreciation of this relationship has emerged from studying x-ray crystallograms that show the precise, three-dimensional structures of protein antigens and of individual antibodies bound to them. Globular proteins tend to fold into compact masses with the majority of their constituent amino acids (particularly those with hydrophobic side chains) buried in the interior, leaving a minority of residues (including most of those that have polar side chains) on the surface, exposed to the surrounding environment. Because the overall folding pattern is fairly rigid, the exposed residues occupy more-or-less fixed locations with respect to one another, which together define the contoured, water-accessible surface of the protein. A given antibody typically binds to a specific subset of residues that are clustered together on this surface. The epitope for such an antibody, then, is best thought of as a particular array of chem-

this binding site is called an epitope, or antigenic determinant. A single antigenic molecule may contain several distinct epitopes, and most large antigens do (Fig 5–2). For any given antigen in a particular individual, the regions that are recognized by immunoglobulins (called **B-cell epitopes**) are usually different from those that are recognized by TCRs (called **T-cell epitopes**). The concept of T-cell epitopes is somewhat complicated in that T cells only recognize their epitopes in association with MHC molecules on cell surfaces. In contrast, epitope recognition by an antibody is a relatively straightforward bimolecular interaction that occurs in solution and so is correspondingly easier to study experimentally and to understand. We therefore begin by focusing on B-cell antigens and epitopes.

Size and Locations of B-Cell Epitopes

Antibody responses against native, folded proteins are almost always directed against residues on the protein surface, since it is these residues that are exposed and accessible for binding. An early demonstration of this principle came from immunizing animals with synthetic polypeptides that constituted an invariant backbone decorated with numerous side branches composed of alanine, tyrosine, and glutamate (Fig 5–3). When the branches were synthesized so that all alanines were clustered at the outer termini, with tyrosine and glutamate nearer the backbone, most of the antibodies produced were alanine-

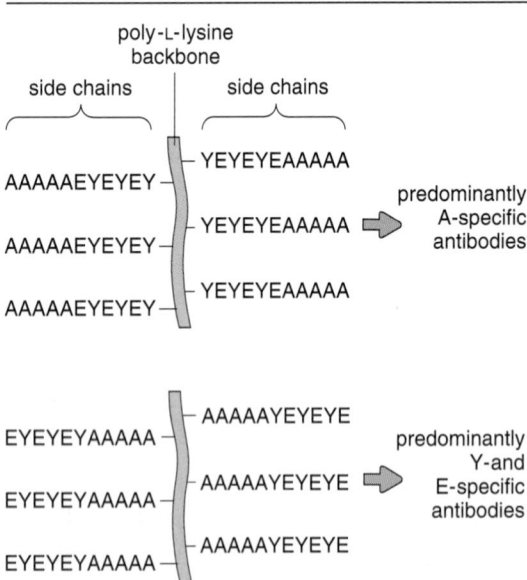

Figure 5–3. The most exposed residues on an antigen are most likely to function as B-cell epitopes. In this schematic representation of an experiment by Sela and colleagues (*Science* 1969;**166**:1365), animals were immunized with synthetic polypeptides consisting of a poly-L-lysine backbone with side chains composed of alanine (A), tyrosine (Y), and glutamate (E) residues. The residues that were located at the most exposed termini of the side chains served as the preferred (immunodominant) B-cell epitopes.

ical features arranged in a specific spatial contour on the accessible surface of the antigen.

The antigen-binding site on any single immunoglobulin molecule has a fixed size (Chapter 7), and this, in turn, dictates the maximum spatial dimensions of its epitope. Studies using homopolymers of sugars or amino acids, either alone or conjugated to immunogenic proteins, indicate that a single epitope can encompass as few as three to six amino acid or sugar residues. On the other hand, x-ray crystallograms of individual antibodies bound to native, globular proteins have revealed contacts involving as many as 20 amino acid residues on the antigen simultaneously. Thus, a reasonable rule of thumb may be that B-cell epitopes generally comprise about 3–20 amino acid residues on the antigen. A typical epitope extends over a total area of up to about 700 Å² on the antigen surface, which means that a single epitope might occupy roughly 10% of the total surface of a small protein such as human lysozyme (130 amino acids, MW 14,700).

The number of separate epitopes on an antigenic molecule generally is proportional to its size and chemical complexity. One way to estimate how many B-cell epitopes are present on a given antigen is to determine the number of antibody molecules that can bind to each molecule of antigen under saturating conditions. Using this approach, it has been estimated, for example, that hen egg albumin (MW 42,000) has about five B-cell epitopes, whereas thyroglobulin (MW 700,000) has about 40. This approach provides only minimal estimates, however, since epitopes can overlap one another, so that not all possible epitopes on a molecule can be occupied by bound antibodies simultaneously. Moreover, these numbers are somewhat misleading, since different regions of an antigen can be used preferentially as epitopes by different individuals or different animal species, or even by a single individual at different times. In fact, the weight of evidence currently suggests that virtually any region on the exposed surface of a folded protein has the potential to serve as a B-cell epitope.

These observations can be of use in predicting the locations of B-cell epitopes on a folded protein whose sequence is known but whose precise structure is not: since polar residues are situated on the surface much more frequently than nonpolar residues, the regions of highest average polarity within a polypeptide sequence have the highest likelihood of being targets for antibody binding.

Conformational and Linear Epitopes

In many instances, all of the amino acid or sugar residues that form a given epitope are positioned sequentially in the linear sequence of a protein or polysaccharide antigen. Because these residues are covalently linked to one another and cannot move far apart, epitopes of this type are not affected by heat denaturation or other treatments that alter the three-dimensional structure of a protein. Such epitopes are called **linear** (or **sequential**) **epitopes** (Fig 5–4).

Other B-cell epitopes, by contrast, form only when the critical residues are brought together in space through folding of the polypeptide or polysaccharide chain into its normal three-dimensional conformation. Epitopes of this type are called **conformational epitopes,** and, by definition, are lost if the antigen is denatured and fails to refold properly. Many conformational epitopes are made up of residues located at two or more discontinuous sites along the linear sequence of an antigen, as depicted in Figure 5–4. This is not always the case, however. For example, repeating polymers of the tripeptide tyrosine-alanine-glutamine form α helices in solution and can evoke specific antibodies. Individual tripeptides with this sequence, by contrast, do not have an ordered conformation and will not bind to antibodies prepared against the helical polymer, even though they can be recognized by specific antibodies prepared in other ways. Thus, the α-helical form of this simple, continuous peptide sequence can function as a conformational epitope.

Antibodies that recognize conformational epitopes are often used to study changes that occur in the three-dimensional structures of proteins during physiologic processes such as ligand binding. Such conformational shifts may eliminate certain epitopes on a protein while causing new ones to form. For example, antibodies have been described that can discriminate between the oxygenated and nonoxygenated forms of hemoglobin by detecting small differences in alignment of the globin subunits. There are many other examples of such conformation-specific antibody binding.

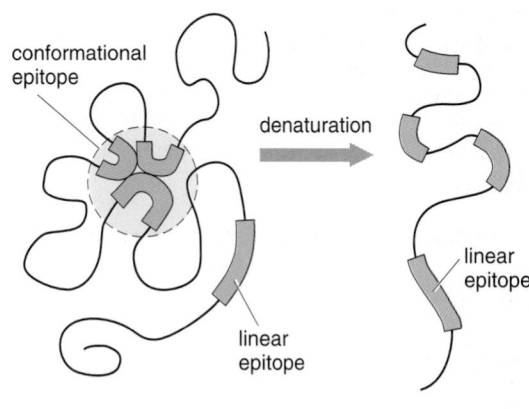

Figure 5–4. Conformational and linear epitopes in a polypeptide antigen. After denaturation, the conformational epitope can no longer be recognized by antibodies, but the linear epitope is unaffected.

THE PHYSICOCHEMICAL BASIS OF ANTIGEN–ANTIBODY BINDING

Much of our understanding of antigen–antibody interactions comes from studies of small molecules that are not immunogenic but that can be bound by antibodies of appropriate specificity. Molecules with these characteristics were first uncovered in the early 20th century by the pioneering experiments of Karl Landsteiner, who was studying the immunologic properties of certain small aromatic amines (Fig 5–5). These compounds in free form cannot induce antibody responses. Landsteiner found, however, that when they were coupled covalently to immunogenic proteins that were then injected into animals, the resulting immune responses included antibodies that were capable of binding the free aromatic amine. This demonstrated that a nonimmunogenic molecule could become the target of an antibody response when attached to an immunogenic protein. Landsteiner named substances that had this property **haptens,** from the Greek word *haptien* ("to fasten"). The proteins or other immunogens onto which haptens are fastened for such experiments are called **carriers.** We now know that most small, nonimmunogenic compounds behave as haptens if coupled to an appropriate carrier. This has practical importance, since it provides a simple way of obtaining antibodies directed against virtually any small molecule, regardless of its inherent immunogenicity. Even antibodies that are specific for particular metal ions have been obtained in this manner.

Just as importantly, the discovery that antibodies could be raised against small, chemically defined haptens provided an experimental system that could be used to determine precisely which chemical features of an epitope are responsible for its interaction with antibodies. At the time haptens were discovered, protein biochemistry was in its infancy, but organic chemists had become quite adept at synthesizing small molecules with defined structures. Taking this approach, Landsteiner and others were able to demonstrate that antibodies raised against a particular hapten would also bind other, chemically similar molecules.

In general, the more structurally similar a compound was to the original hapten, the more likely it was to bind the antihapten antibody (Table 5–1). Through studies of these simple model epitopes, it soon became clear that an antibody not only recognizes specific chemical features (such as polarity, hydrophobicity, or ionic charge) of its epitope but also recognizes the overall shape of the epitope and the locations of these chemical features in three-dimensional space.

This then led to the more general realization that antibodies bind to their epitopes because the two molecules are **complementary** to each other: the antigen-binding residues in an antibody protein form a contoured surface that molds closely onto that of its epitope, so that epitope and antibody fit together in a "lock-and-key" relationship (Fig 5–6). This complementarity refers not only to the shapes of the two binding surfaces (with peaks in one fitting into valleys in the other) but also to their chemical features: individual amino acids from the antigen and antibody are positioned so as to allow the formation of salt bridges (that is, bonding between positively and negatively charged residues), hydrogen bonds, van der Waals contacts, and localized hydrophobic interactions between the two surfaces. These multiple, discrete, noncovalent linkages are the basis for bonding between an antibody and its epitope, and the sum of the individual strengths of these linkages determines the overall bonding energy. The more perfectly an epitope matches the chemical and spatial contours of an antibody, the more tightly it is bound. This complemen-

Table 5–1. Effect of variations in epitope structure on the strength of binding by antihapten antibodies.[1]

	ortho	meta	para
R = sulfonate	+	+++	±
R = arsonate	–	+	–
R = carboxylate	–	±	–

[1] In this typical experiment, an antiserum raised against the hapten *m*-aminobenzene sulfonate (R = sulfonate, in the *meta* position) was tested for its ability to bind this or various structurally related compounds. Binding affinity was graded from absent (–) to very strong (+++). Sulfonate and arsonate are both tetrahedral and negatively charged, but arsonate is the bulkier of the two owing to the larger size of the arsenic atom as well as the presence of additional hydrogen atoms. Carboxylate is also negatively charged but is planar rather than tetrahedral. (Based on data from Landsteiner K, van der Scheer J: On cross reactions of immune sera to azoproteins. *J Exp Med* 1936;**63**:325.)

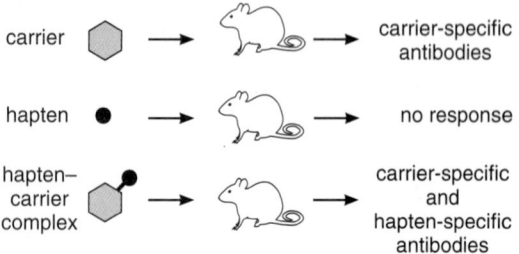

Figure 5–5. Haptens are substances that are antigenic but not immunogenic.

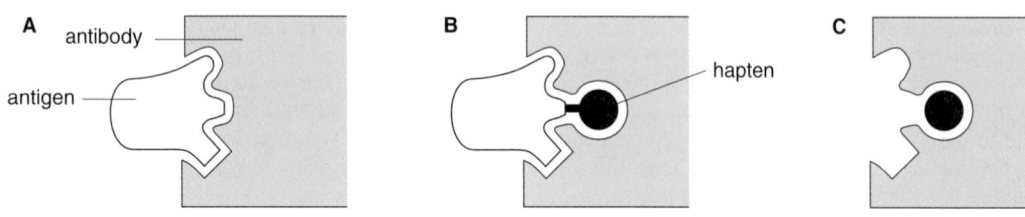

Figure 5–6. Schematic illustration of the complementarity between a B-cell epitope and the antigen-binding site on an antibody protein. Antibodies raised against **A:** an antigen or **B:** a hapten–carrier complex are fully complementary to their cognate epitopes. **C:** An antibody whose epitope includes a hapten will also bind the isolated hapten, although it usually has lower affinity for the free hapten than for the hapten–carrier complex. Note that binding of the hapten interferes with binding of the hapten–carrier complex; this fact is often used as a basis for demonstrating low-affinity hapten binding by hapten-specific antibodies.

tarity between immunoglobulins and their epitopes is an extremely important concept to understand, since it is the mechanism by which the humoral immune system recognizes and distinguishes among antigenic molecules.

Quantitative Aspects of Antigen–Antibody Interactions

A hapten alone rarely constitutes the entire epitope for an antihapten antibody. More typically, the hapten serves as only one of the residues that contribute to the epitope, together with amino acid residues from the carrier, and for this reason the antibody usually binds less strongly to free hapten than to the hapten–carrier complex (see Fig 5–6). Changes in chemical structure of the hapten tend to distort its complementarity with the antibody, weakening or eliminating individual chemical contacts and so further weakening the interaction overall. In similar fashion, mutation of an amino acid residue that forms part of a protein epitope may weaken or eliminate antibody binding, depending on how much that residue contributed quantitatively to the binding and to what extent the new amino acid can substitute for it. Systematic studies of this phenomenon show that not all chemical linkages contribute equally; in general, salt bridges and hydrogen bonds are individually more critical than van der Waals or hydrophobic interactions, and in some cases the loss of even one salt bridge or hydrogen bond can abolish antigen–antibody binding.

B-cell responses to most antigens involve many structurally different antibody molecules, which may each recognize separate epitopes or different groups of residues within any single epitopic region. Because different chemical contacts are involved in each case, some antibodies bind very strongly, and others more weakly, to the same antigen. Similarly, a given antibody may be capable of binding not only one antigen but also other molecules containing regions that happen to resemble its epitope. The binding of an antibody to an antigen other than the one that induced its formation is called a **cross-reaction.** Cross-reacting antigens generally have some, but not all, of the features responsible for the strong binding of an antibody to its original (or **cognate**) antigen. Though the antigen-binding sites on most antibodies are somewhat flexible and can compensate for minor variations in epitope structure, antibodies generally have a lower affinity for a cross-reacting antigen than for their cognate antigen.

The term **affinity** is used to describe the strength of interaction between two molecules that interact in a simple one-to-one fashion. One measure of affinity is the relative rates at which such molecules tend to associate and disassociate from each other, which can be depicted as:

$$[AB] \underset{k_2}{\overset{k_1}{\rightleftharpoons}} [A] + [B]$$

where k_1 and k_2 are the rate constants for dissociation and association, respectively. This relationship can be described most simply by a single value, called the **dissociation constant (K_d),** defined as the ratio of concentrations of the unbound and bound molecules at equilibrium:

$$K_d = \frac{[A]\,[B]}{[AB]}$$

so that small K_d values indicate strong, high-affinity interactions. In the case of antigen–antibody binding, K_d values in the range of 10^{-7} to 10^{-10} molar (M) are typical for high-affinity interactions with cognate antigens. Cross-reactions and low-affinity cognate interactions may be characterized by K_d values as high as 10^{-4} to 10^{-6} M; weaker interactions often are not detectable and may not be physiologically significant.

T-CELL ANTIGENS, T-CELL EPITOPES, & IMMUNOGENICITY

Epitope recognition by a TCR occurs through complementary interactions that are, in most respects, identical to those described earlier. Unlike an antibody, however, a TCR does not bind free antigens appreciably and instead recognizes its epitope as part of a complex with MHC proteins on the surface of an APC. Both the epitope and the MHC molecule contribute to the complementarity required for effective TCR binding (see Chapter 6) and so determine the affinity of the interaction. Before being presented by an APC, most proteinaceous antigens must undergo processing, in the course of which the antigen is degraded into peptides that then can serve as T-cell epitopes. Because they recognize only processed antigens, T cells show no preference for epitopes that lie on the surfaces (as opposed to the interior) of globular proteins and rarely recognize specific conformational features of the native antigen. Moreover, APCs often present only a few of the many possible peptides that can be obtained from an antigen (see Chapter 6), which strictly limits the number that can function as T-cell epitopes. Nevertheless, some large proteins have been found to contain as many as 50 separate T-cell epitopes, and T cells show the same exquisite specificity as antibodies in recognizing their cognate antigens.

Studies with small, well-defined antigens have shown that humoral and cell-mediated immune responses can be directed against different regions of a single molecule. For example, the human hormone glucagon, which is only 29 amino acids long, contains separate B-cell and T-cell epitopic regions: when mice are immunized with human glucagon, they produce antibodies only against the amino-terminal part of the molecule, whereas their T cells respond only to the carboxy-terminal portion. Similarly, the small organoarsenate molecule L-tyrosine-p-azobenzenearsonate (ABA-Tyr), with a molecular weight of only 409, induces cellular immunity but little or no antibody production in a variety of animal species. When animals are immunized with a hapten covalently attached to ABA-Tyr, they respond with hapten-specific antibodies and ABA-Tyr-specific T cells.

T-cell epitopes not only serve as the targets for cytotoxic T-cell responses but are essential for nearly all B-cell responses as well. This is because T-cell epitopes are needed to activate helper T lymphocytes, which, in turn, are required for B-cell responses against nearly all antigens. Thus, as a rule, a molecule must contain at least one T-cell epitope to be immunogenic. Molecules that contain only B-cell epitopes (such as haptens, or the amino-terminal portion of human glucagon) may serve very well as targets for antibody responses but are unable to induce such responses themselves.

Immunodominance

Individual residues within a single epitope that contribute disproportionately to interactions with an antibody or TCR are said to be **immunodominant** residues. This might be said, for example, of a residue that forms a salt bridge with the antibody or TCR.

When an antibody recognizes a sequence at the end of a polymer, the terminal residue of this polymer is almost invariably the most critical for binding and, hence, is immunodominant, whereas the other residues generally exhibit decreasing degrees of immunodominance with increasing distance from the terminus. The same term can also be applied to a particular epitope within a large antigen that contains numerous epitopes; in a given individual, and under a given set of circumstances, only one or a few of these may serve as the primary target of an immune response. In a B-cell response, for example, one epitope might evoke antibodies in larger quantities and with higher binding affinities than do the other available epitopes and so would be said to be the immunodominant epitope.

Thymus-Independent Antigens

A few types of molecules have been reported to induce antibody responses without the apparent participation of T lymphocytes. Most such **thymus-independent antigens** are polymers composed of many repeating chemical units, and may activate B lymphocytes directly by cross-linking specific B-cell surface receptors (Chapter 3). Certain lectins, some polymeric proteins, and many polysaccharides have been reported to be thymus-independent antigens. Careful analysis of the responses to such antigens indicates, however, that many, though not all, do require some degree of T-cell help, albeit significantly less than that required by conventional **thymus-dependent antigens.** It may therefore be more accurate to view them as thymus-efficient, rather than thymus-independent.

One striking property of the responses to thymus-independent antigens is that no apparent **memory** is engendered; even after repeated exposures, the antibody responses are quantitatively modest, occur after a relatively long lag period, and in all other respects resemble primary humoral responses. (In particular, the antibodies produced are nearly all of the IgM class; see Chapter 7). This implies that clonal expansion of antigen-specific helper T cells is required for many of the characteristic features of secondary antibody responses, and that an immunogen must contain at least one T-cell epitope in order to induce functional immunologic memory.

VACCINES

A **vaccine** is a nonpathogenic immunogen that, when inoculated into a host, induces protective immunity against a specific pathogen. Vaccines rank among the most important contributions of science to human health, and the development of the first vaccines against smallpox (by Edward Jenner, in 1798) and rabies (by Louis Pasteur, in 1880) are landmarks in the history of immunology. Effective vaccination programs have drastically reduced the incidence of

Table 5–2. Representative vaccines for human use.[1]

Vaccine	Type	Administration
Smallpox	Nonpathogen (vaccinia virus)	Subcutaneous
Polio—Salk	Killed	Oral
Polio—Sabin	Live, attenuated	Oral
MMR: Measles	Live, attenuated	Subcutaneous
Mumps	Live, attenuated	Subcutaneous
Rubella	Live, attenuated	Subcutaneous
DTP: Diphtheria	Toxoid	Intramuscular
Tetanus	Toxoid	Intramuscular
Pertussis	Killed	Intramuscular
Haemophilus influenzae B	Glycoconjugate	Intramuscular
Hepatitis A virus	Killed	Intramuscular
Hepatitis B virus	Subunit	Intramuscular

[1] Properties of some vaccine preparations as approved for use in the US; alternative forms of some are also available. Smallpox vaccine is no longer in general use, as the disease has been eradicated worldwide. MMR and DTP are combination vaccines, each directed against three pathogens as shown.

many infectious diseases that once were common, and in the case of smallpox eradicated the disease. To be effective, a vaccine must induce long-standing immunity that acts at the appropriate body sites and against the appropriate microbial antigens to prevent disease in all persons at risk; to be practical, it must also be safe, inexpensive, and easy to store and administer. Vaccines currently in use, some of which are listed in Table 5–2, generally satisfy these criteria. But useful vaccines have yet to be developed against many major infectious diseases, including malaria and AIDS, and for this reason, as well as the need to improve existing preparations, vaccinology remains a very active area of research.

Some useful vaccines consist of live, naturally occurring microbes that share important antigens with a pathogen but are not pathogenic themselves. For example, **vaccinia** (cowpox) virus, a relative of the smallpox virus, causes an inapparent, self-limiting infection in normal people while inducing immunity against smallpox as well as against itself. Similarly, the nonpathogenic mycobacterium called **Bacillus Calmette-Guérin (BCG)** can be used as a live vaccine against *Mycobacterium tuberculosis.* An advantage of these agents is that, being infectious, they can be transmitted from vaccinees to others in the population; a drawback is that they may cause serious disease in persons with defective immune systems (see Chapter 20).

Other vaccines are prepared from potentially pathogenic bacteria or viruses that have either been **killed** (with heat or chemical treatments) or are **attenuated** (that is, have lost the ability to produce disease in humans). Because of the way in which their antigens are

presented to T cells (see Chapter 6), killed vaccines induce humoral but not cell-mediated immunity, whereas attentuated vaccines induce both types of immunity and so are generally much more potent and efficacious than killed vaccines. This is the main reason why the original, killed-virus polio vaccine developed by Jonas Salk has since been superseded by the Sabin vaccine, which uses live, attenuated poliovirus. The usual method of attenuating a virus is to grow it for prolonged periods in cells from a species other than its usual host; over time, the virus accumulates mutations that favor growth under the new conditions but which often reduce its growth and virulence in the original host. This approach was first developed by Pasteur, who attentuated the canine rabies virus by adapting it to growth in rabbits. In many cases, the exact mutations responsible for attenuation are not known. One problem with attenuated vaccines is that, very rarely, further mutations allow the virus to revert to a pathogenic form. For example, approximately one case of polio occurs among every million vaccinees receiving the Sabin virus. A newer approach to attenuation is to employ recombinant DNA techniques to introduce large gene deletions and other mutations that may be less prone to reversion.

Certain vaccines are made of purified macromolecules rather than entire microorganisms. For example, the tetanus and diphtheria vaccines contain only inactive forms of the soluble bacterial toxins responsible for these diseases; these **toxoid** vaccines induce antitoxin antibodies but no immunity against the bacteria themselves. **Subunit vaccines,** such as the hepatitis B vaccine, consist of only a single immunogenic protein from the pathogen of interest, usually produced in laboratory bacteria, yeast, or cultured cells using recombinant DNA techniques. Several effective **glycoconjugate vaccines** against *Haemophilus influenzae* type B have been produced by linking polysaccharide B-cell epitopes from the capsule of this organism onto immunogenic carriers such as tetanus toxoid; similar vaccines against pneumococci and some meningococci are also under development. A related approach is to attach short (usually <20 amino acid), chemically synthesized peptides that correspond to known epitopes from an infectious organism onto a carrier to create **peptide vaccines.** These strategies are based on the concept that isolated carbohydrate or polypeptide epitopes can act as haptens to induce antibodies, which may then recognize the same epitopes in the native pathogen, though usually with lower affinity. For this approach to succeed, however, the vaccine must incorporate both B- and T-cell epitopes, since B-cell epitopes alone induce little or no immunologic memory. Moreover, T-cell epitopes must be carefully chosen to ensure that they can be recognized, presented, and responded to by all members of the populations at risk.

One very new strategy for immunization is the use of **DNA vaccines.** These are based on the discovery that when DNA encoding a chosen microbial protein is injected intramuscularly, host cells at the site of injection take up these artificial genes and express the foreign protein for several weeks. Depending on the protein expressed, this can induce specific humoral or cellular immunity, or both. DNA vaccines appear to offer many advantages of safety and convenience and have yielded promising results in animals, but their clinical usefulness has not yet been proven. Fundamental questions also remain concerning their mechanism of action; for example, it is not known whether immunization results from DNA expression in the muscle cells themselves or in lymphocytes and APCs present at the injection site.

ADJUVANTS

The response to an immunogen can often be enhanced if it is administered as a mixture with substances called **adjuvants.** Adjuvants function in one or more of the following ways: (1) by prolonging retention of the immunogen, (2) by increasing the effective size of the immunogen, and so promoting phagocytosis and presentation by macrophages, (3) by stimulating the influx of macrophages or other immune cell types to the injection site, or (4) by promoting local cytokine production and other immunologic activities of such immune cells.

A number of adjuvants have been used in experimental animals, the most potent being **complete Freund's adjuvant (CFA),** a water-in-oil emulsion containing killed mycobacteria. CFA appears to work by providing a depot for the immunogen and by stimulating macrophages and certain lymphocytes, but its very strong inflammatory effects preclude its use in humans. The only adjuvants approved for clinical use in the US are **aluminum salts**—fine particles of aluminum phosphate or hydroxide onto which the immunogen is adsorbed. These widely used adjuvants increase the stability and effective particle size of an immunogen and also promote release of certain cytokines, such as interleukin-1. Unfortunately, aluminum adjuvants only stimulate humoral immunity, do not work with all antigens, and cannot be frozen or freeze-dried. Several other types of adjuvants are being explored for human use, most of which contain either mycobacterial cell walls or specific glycosylated protein fragments, called **muramyl di-** or **tripeptides,** derived from such walls, usually emulsified with oils, phospholipids, or other surfactants as a complex mixture. Another promising approach may be to incorporate specific **immunomodulators** into vaccines in order to promote particular types of immune responses. For example, **interleukin-12** influences helper T-cell development in such a way as to promote cell-mediated, as opposed to humoral, immune reactions (see Chapter 9); its inclusion in a vaccine preparation might selectively promote a protective cytotoxic response against the target pathogen.

REFERENCES

Benjamin DC et al: The antigenic structure of proteins: A reappraisal. *Ann Rev Immunol* 1984;**2**:67.

Good MF et al: The T cell response to the malaria circumsporozoite protein: An immunological approach to vaccine development. *Ann Rev Immunol* 1988;**6:**663.

Goodman JW, Sercarz EE: The complexity of structures involved in T cell activation. *Ann Rev Immunol* 1983;**1:**465.

Goodman JW: Modelling determinants for recognition by B cells and T cells. *Prog Allergy* 1989;**56:**1.

Landsteiner K: *The Specificity of Serological Reactions.* Harvard University Press, 1945.

Livingston AM, Fathman CG: The structure of T cell epitopes. *Ann Rev Immunol* 1987;**5:**477.

Milch DR: Synthetic T and B cell recognition sites: Implications for vaccine development. *Adv Immunol* 1989;**45:**195.

Rabinovich NR et al: Vaccine technologies: View to the future. *Science* 1994;**265:**1401.

Reichlin M: Amino acid substitution and the antigenicity of globular proteins. *Adv Immunol* 1975;**20:**71.

Sela M: Antigenicity: Some molecular aspects. *Science* 1969;**166:**1365.

Zanetti ME et al: The immunology of new generation vaccines. *Immunol Today* 1987;**8:**18.

Antigen Presentation & the Major Histocompatibility Complex

6

Frances M. Brodsky, DPhil

The cells and humoral factors of the innate immune system have, for the most part, evolved to recognize distinctive carbohydrate or lipid markers found on many types of pathogens but not in the normal host (see Chapter 2). The acquired immune system, by contrast, mainly targets peptide antigens derived from foreign proteins. This focus on peptides reflects the antigen specificity of T lymphocytes, whose antigen receptors (TCRs) only recognize the complexes formed by peptides bound to **major histocompatibility complex (MHC) proteins** on the surfaces of host cells. The use of a peptide-based recognition system has important advantages: since the structural diversity of peptides is much greater than that of carbohydrates or lipids, the acquired immune system is able to detect and discriminate among a much broader range of immunogens, which allows for much greater specificity in its responses. In addition, peptide-specific responses can be directed against virally encoded proteins that are synthesized by infected host cells even though they lack any unusual carbohydrate or lipid modifications.

As part of this focus on peptide antigens, the immune systems of humans and other mammals have evolved mechanisms for sampling the many proteins in their environments and cleaving them into peptides (a sequence of events called **antigen processing**) and then making those peptides accessible for recognition by T cells (**antigen presentation**). These are early, indispensable steps in nearly all acquired immune responses, and so are critical to the immune system's ability to detect and respond to antigenic challenges. In this chapter, we examine in detail the cellular and molecular basis of antigen processing and presentation, emphasizing the ways in which these processes influence whether and how lymphocytes react to a potential immunogen. Against this backdrop, we also explore the important role these processes play in determining resistance or susceptibility to disease and their unique importance in the context of organ transplantation.

ORIGINS OF ANTIGENIC PEPTIDES

To function as T-cell antigens, proteins must first be processed into peptides that can associate with host cell MHC molecules. Depending on the source of the antigen, processing can occur through either of two major pathways, and the pathway that is used has decisive consequences for any subsequent immune response (Table 6–1).

The Endocytic (Class II) Pathway

Many antigenic peptides are derived from proteins that have been captured and taken into a cell from its external environment. These include proteins that were part of a microorganism or other large particle engulfed through phagocytosis; smaller particles or individual proteins that bound to the cell surface and were then captured through receptor-mediated endocytosis; or free, soluble proteins in the extracellular fluid that were imbibed nonspecifically during pinocytosis (see Fig 2–6). Proteins captured through any of these routes are taken into the cell in membranous endosomal vesicles, where they are then gradually broken down by exposure to an acidic pH and to cellular proteolytic enzymes. Although the bulk of each protein is ultimately destroyed, many short peptides are produced as intermediates in this process, their lengths and sequences varying in accordance with the sequence of the original protein, the cleavage specificities of the proteinases acting on it, its folded conformation and accessibility to cleavage, and many other factors. Through a mechanism that will be described later, some of these peptides are spared from further degradation, and are instead transported back to the cell surface for presentation to T cells. This is sometimes termed the "exogenous" pathway of antigen processing because it acts mainly on proteins from outside the presenting cell.

Peptides generated by the endocytic pathway vary widely in sequence and in length. Importantly, this pathway delivers peptides to **MHC class II** mole-

Table 6–1. The Antigen-Processing Pathways.

	Endocytic Pathway	Cytosolic Pathway
Major antigen sources	Endocytosed extracellular proteins (host and foreign) Membrane proteins (host and foreign)	Cytosolic proteins of host or intracellular pathogens (viral, bacterial, parasitic) Signal peptides (host and foreign)
Processing machinery	Lysosomal enzymes	Proteasomes (including LMPs)
Cell types where active	Professional APCs	All nucleated cells
Site of antigen–MHC binding	Endocytic vesicles, prelysosomes	Rough endoplasmic reticulum
MHC utilized	Class II	Class I
Presents to	CD4 (helper) T cells	CD8 (cytotoxic) T cells

cules, which are expressed by macrophages and other "professional" antigen-presenting cells (APCs) that present antigens to CD4+ T lymphocytes, most of which are helper cells. The endocytic pathway therefore supplies the antigenic peptides used by specialized APCs to activate helper T cells.

The Cytosolic (Class I) Pathway

Antigenic proteins can also be derived from pathogens that live inside infected host cells. This category includes not only viruses, which rely on the protein synthetic machinery of the host, but also some intracellular bacteria (such as *Chlamydia, Shigella, Rickettsia,* and *Listeria*) and intracellular parasites (such as *Toxoplasma*), which synthesize their own proteins. Antigens from such intracellular pathogens are processed through a sequence of events involved in normal protein turnover. In this case, protein cleavage occurs in the cytosol within large, multisubunit enzyme assemblages called **proteasomes,** which ordinarily carry out the routine function of degrading host cytosolic proteins that have been damaged, improperly folded, or otherwise targeted for destruction or rapid turnover. Two distinct size classes of proteosomes (20S and 26S) have been described, and both are implicated in antigen processing. Each proteasome is made up of 15–20 different proteolytic subunits and has multiple substrate specificities. As a result, they can degrade a broad range of cytosolic proteins, including not only normal cellular constituents but also proteins from intracellular pathogens.

In the process of cleaving these substrates, the proteasomes liberate a myriad of short peptides into the cytosol. Selected peptides from this pool are then actively pumped into the lumen of the rough endoplasmic reticulum (RER) through channels created by a pair of proteins called the transporters of antigenic peptides: **TAP-1** and **TAP-2.** Each of the TAP subunits is an integral RER membrane protein that has seven transmembrane regions and an adenosine triphosphate (ATP)-hydrolyzing domain on its cytoplasmic surface; the TAPs therefore belong to the family of structurally related membrane channel proteins called ATP-binding cassette (ABC) transporters—a family that also includes P-glycoprotein (which pumps drugs and other small molecules out of cells, conferring drug resistance in some human cancers) and the cystic fibrosis transmembrane conductance regulator (an ion channel whose mutation causes cystic fibrosis). TAP-1 and TAP-2 together form a heterodimeric channel that selectively pumps a wide assortment of peptides of 8–12 residues (or occasionally longer) from the cytosol into the RER lumen in an ATP-dependent manner. As described later on, some of these peptides then associate with **MHC class I** proteins and are delivered to the cell surface for presentation to CD8+ T lymphocytes. All components of this cytosolic pathway, including class I MHC proteins, are expressed by nearly every nucleated human cell type, ensuring that any cell that becomes infected can present antigens to cytotoxic T cells. This, in turn, leads to killing of the infected cell, which helps to limit spread of the pathogen it contained.

Though the endocytic and cytosolic degradative pathways are largely separate, some pathogens are processed through both. For example, the contents of endocytic vesicles are occasionally released into the cytosol (perhaps by lysis of the vesicle membrane) in a phenomenon called **macropinocytosis,** which transfers potential antigens from the endocytic to the cytosolic pathway. Conversely, virally encoded proteins that integrate into cellular membranes (such as the surface glycoproteins of enveloped viruses) are targeted to endocytic vesicle membranes and consigned to the endocytic pathway, as are membrane proteins of the host cells. Interestingly, the signal peptides that target membrane proteins to the RER, and which are proteolytically removed during protein synthesis, often survive in the RER lumen and bind class I MHC proteins, whereas the remainder of the same polypeptide enters the endocytic pathway and is presented by class II MHC. Despite these exceptions, however, most immunogenic proteins primarily follow one pathway or the other. That is why, for example, live virus vaccines (which are processed through the cytosolic pathway) stimulate cytotoxic immune responses much more effectively than killed virus or subunit vaccines (which must be processed through the endocytic pathway).

STRUCTURE, FUNCTION, & GENETICS OF MHC PROTEINS

Before describing how antigenic peptides become bound to MHC proteins, we must first consider the proteins themselves. The human MHC proteins were first discovered in the 1950s, when it was recognized that many people, especially those who had received multiple blood transfusions or had been pregnant several times, had antibodies in their serum that reacted against a new class of surface glycoproteins on leukocytes from other members of the population. The membrane proteins recognized by these antibodies were termed **human leukocyte antigens (HLA)**—a term that is still used as a synonym for the human MHC proteins. It was soon realized that these same HLA molecules could also be targets of cellular immunity: when leukocytes from two unrelated individuals are incubated together, T cells from each nearly always react strongly (by activation and proliferation) against HLA proteins expressed by the other. Similarly, HLA proteins are usually the main targets of the cellular immune reactions that cause rejection of solid tissues transplanted between unrelated individuals. In these artificial settings, the HLA proteins behave as immunogenic markers that distinguish each person's cells from most others in the population and are the major barrier to **histocompatibility**—the ability of tissue transplants from one person to be accepted by another, rather than rejected immunologically. Despite their clinical importance, however, these properties of the MHC proteins are simply byproducts of their normal function of presenting antigenic peptides to T cells.

The Structures of Classical MHC Proteins and Their Peptide-Binding Sites

Most peptide antigens are presented as complexes with the **"classical"** MHC proteins: class I, which presents antigens to CD8+ (usually cytotoxic) T cells, and class II, which presents to CD4+ (usually helper) T cells. Class I and class II proteins are encoded by separate genes but are closely related in evolution and structurally similar in many respects. Each is expressed on the cell surface as a heterodimer composed of two noncovalently linked polypeptide chains (Fig 6–1). A class II molecule is formed by polypeptides called α and β, which are similar in size and are both anchored in the surface membrane at their carboxy termini. The extracellular regions of the class II α and β chains each fold to form a pair of globular domains, designated α_1 and α_2, or β_1 and β_2, respectively. Each class I molecule, by contrast, consists of a structurally distinct α chain associated with a second, shorter polypeptide called β_2-**microglobulin.** The class I α chain is organized in three folded domains (α_1, α_2, and α_3) and has a carboxy-terminal membrane anchor. The smaller β_2-microglobulin, with one folded domain, is linked to the membrane only indirectly through its association with the α chain; this association is critical for stabilizing the class I molecule and for facilitating its transport to the cell surface.

Each MHC molecule can bind one antigenic peptide. Binding occurs at a site formed by the two domains that are situated farthest from the cell surface and, hence, are most accessible to other cells. The **peptide-binding site** in a class I protein is formed by the α_1 and α_2 domains; that in a class II protein is formed by the α_1 and β_1 domains. In either case, sequences from the two adjacent domains combine to create an eight-stranded β-pleated sheet that serves as the floor of the binding site, above which are positioned two α helices, oriented adjacent and roughly parallel to each other, so that they form two walls with a groove between them (Fig 6–2).

Peptides bind inside the groove of an MHC protein in an extended conformation. The structure of the groove determines the types of peptides that can bind (Fig 6–3). For example, the groove in a class I molecule is constricted at both ends, and so can only accommodate peptides that are 8–10 amino acids long. The ends of the class II binding cleft are more open, which enables these proteins to bind the somewhat longer and irregular peptides (8–12 amino acids) generated by the endocytic processing pathway.

The specificity of binding in both class I and class II proteins is further determined by the amino acid residues that make up the β-sheet floor and α-helical walls of the peptide-binding groove: these create minute pockets with unique spatial and chemical features that can bind complementary features in a peptide, such as a particular amino acid side chain at a particular position. The characteristics of these pockets, which reflect the sequence of the MHC protein, determine whether a given peptide can be bound. The constraints are fairly liberal, however, so that any single MHC protein can accommodate peptides with a wide variety of different sequences. The important point is that peptide binding by a given MHC protein is somewhat selective but much less specific than antigen binding by a TCR or an immunoglobulin protein. Since a single cell may express on the order of 10^6 class I proteins on its surface, each cell has the potential to present many alternative peptides simultaneously.

MHC Polymorphism

The MHC genes have evolved by successive duplications so that each person inherits multiple class I and class II genes (Fig 6–4). There are three separate genes, designated **HLA-A, -B,** and **-C,** that each code for classical MHC class I α chains. Similarly, there are three classical MHC class II gene loci, known as

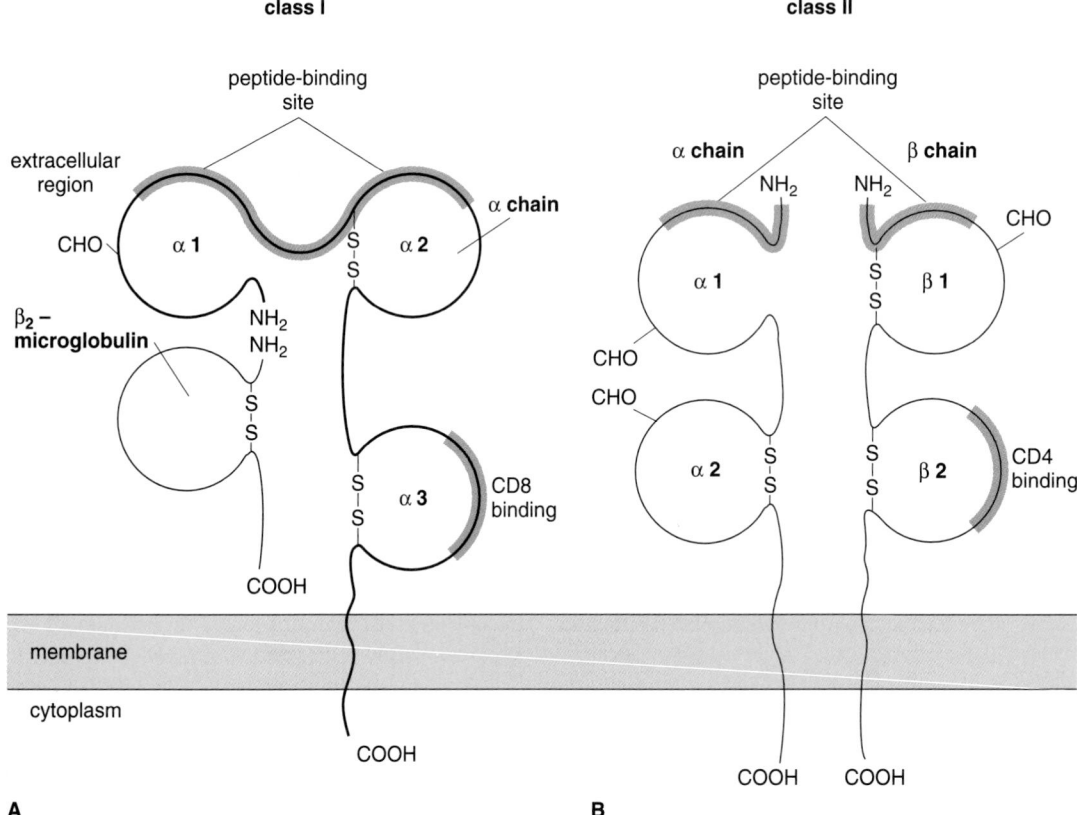

Figure 6–1. Schematic representations of MHC class I and class II proteins. **A:** The class I molecule consists of a MW 44,000 polymorphic transmembrane polypeptide (α chain) noncovalently associated with a MW 12,000 nonpolymorphic polypeptide (β_2-microglobulin) that is not anchored in the membrane. The three extracellular domains of the α chain are designated α_1, α_2, and α_3. The binding site for antigenic peptides is formed by the cleft between the α_1 and α_2 domains; CD8 contacts a portion of the α_3 domain. **B:** The class II molecule consists of a MW 34,000 α chain noncovalently associated with a MW 29,000 β chain, both of which are polymorphic. Antigenic peptides bind a cleft formed by the α_1 and β_2 domains; CD4 contacts sequences in the β_2 domain. Locations shown for the peptide-, CD4-, and CD8-binding sites are approximations only.

HLA-DP, -DQ, and **-DR,** each of which includes genes for one α and at least one β polypeptide. A person normally inherits two copies of each gene locus (one from each parent), and so carries a total of six class I and six class II loci. Moreover, multiple different **alleles** of each locus exist in the human population—that is, there are many alternative versions of each MHC gene that yield proteins with slightly distinct sequences (Table 6–2). For example, there are at least 67 known HLA-A alleles, 149 HLA-B alleles, and 179 HLA-DR-β alleles. Diversity of this type is called allelic **polymorphism,** and the MHC genes are the most polymorphic genetic system known.

Almost all of the polymorphism among MHC alleles involves amino acid residues located in and around the peptide-binding groove. As a result, each allelic form has its own unique peptide-binding properties. Because many allelic forms are common in the population, a typical person is likely to inherit two differ-

ent alleles of many of the MHC loci. This is advantageous to the individual, since it increases the range of different antigenic peptides that can be presented to T cells. MHC polymorphism also benefits humanity at large, since it increases the likelihood that at least some individuals will be able to present antigens from any new pathogen that might be encountered, thus helping to ensure survival of the population as a whole.

The HLA Gene Complex

All of the classical MHC gene loci previously described reside together in the HLA gene complex (see Fig 6–4), which spans 3.5×10^6 bp on the short arm of chromosome 6. The three class I α loci (HLA-A, -B, and -C) are together on one side of this region, and the three class II loci (HLA-DP, -DQ, and -DR, each with its α and β genes) occupy the other. The particular combination of alleles found at these six loci on

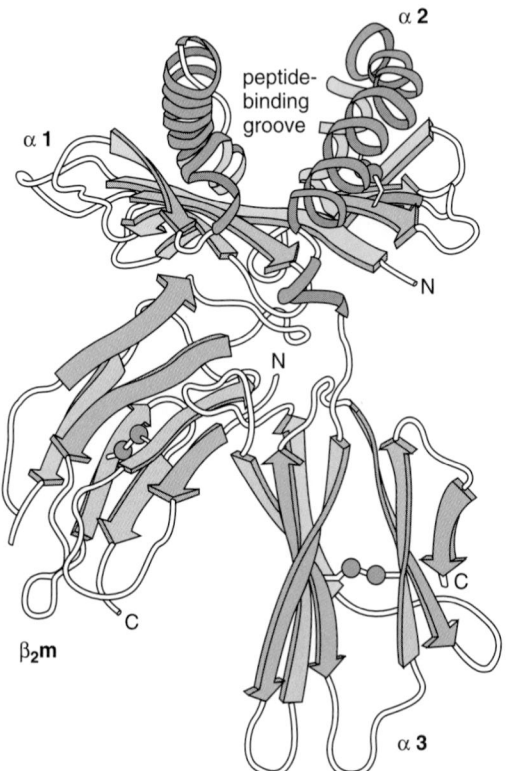

Figure 6–2. Diagrammatic structure of a class I MHC molecule (side view). In this ribbon diagram of the polypeptide backbone, the protein is oriented as in Figure 6–1, but only the extracellular region is depicted. The peptide-binding site is a groove (or cleft) formed by eight strands of β-pleated sheet and a pair of α helices from the α_1 and α_2 domains. The β sheet forms the floor and the two α helices form the walls of the cleft. β strands are depicted as broad arrows and α helices as narrow coils. (Modified and reproduced, with permission, from Bjorkman PJ et al: Structure of the human class I histocompatibility antigen HLA-A2. *Nature* 1987;**329:**506.)

any single chromosome (and which are therefore inherited together) is called a **haplotype.**

MHC genes are expressed **codominantly,** which means, for example, that all six class I alleles (three on each copy of chromosome 6) are expressed together on the surface of every nucleated cell. HLA-C, however, is generally expressed at a lower level than HLA-A and HLA-B. All of these class I α chains pair with β_2-microglobulin, which is the product of a single, nonpolymorphic gene located on chromosome 15. The class II loci are also expressed codominantly but are only active in the subset of cells that express class II (as well as class I). HLA-DR tends to be expressed at higher levels than HLA-DP or HLA-DQ. The α and β genes of each class II locus pair preferentially with each other, so that cross-locus pairings do not contribute significantly to HLA diversity.

Also encoded in the HLA complex are several other proteins that contribute to antigen processing or presentation. These include the genes for **TAP-1** and **TAP-2,** which transport peptides into the RER as part of the endogenous pathway, and are encoded in the class II region. Although some allelic variability of the human TAP proteins has been observed (see Table 6–2), this is thought to have little effect on their peptide-transporting function; by contrast, TAP genes in rats are more polymorphic and strongly influence the repertoire of endogenous peptides that can be processed. Two other genes in the class II region encode low-molecular-weight proteins **(LMPs)** that also participate in the endogenous pathway. The LMPs are subunits of proteasomes and appear to modify proteasome cleavage patterns so as to enhance production of peptides that can bind MHC class I molecules. The HLA locus also includes genes for certain **nonclassical MHC proteins,** which are structurally similar to class I or class II but have different roles in immunity. One of these, HLA-G, is encoded in the class I region and forms a dimer with β_2-microglobulin that acts to control immune responses at the fetal–maternal interface. Another, called **HLA-DM,** is a heterodimer of α and β chains that localizes to endocytic vesicle membranes and helps promote loading of peptides processed through the endocytic pathway onto MHC class II proteins, as is described later on.

The HLA complex can thus be regarded as a cluster of tightly linked genes, many of which are evolutionarily related, and most of which contribute to antigen processing or presentation. A few genes in this region, however, do not share these attributes. The latter include genes for the cytokines tumor necrosis factor α and β (see Chapter 10); for complement factors C2, C4, B, and F (see Chapter 11); for two heat shock proteins; and for the steroidogenic enzyme 21-β-hydroxylase. The significance of the latter associations, if any, is unknown.

ASSEMBLY & PRESENTATION OF PEPTIDE–MHC COMPLEXES

Like other integral membrane proteins, class I and class II MHC proteins are synthesized in association with the RER. The individual chains translocate across the RER membrane as they are produced, so that when synthesis is complete the majority of each protein projects into the RER lumen, with its carboxy terminus remaining embedded in the membrane (see Fig 6–1). The class I and class II biosynthetic pathways then diverge immediately, as the subunits begin to assemble in the lumen of the RER (Fig 6–5).

MHC Class I. Each newly formed class I α chain associates with β_2-microglobulin and binds antigenic peptide during its assembly in the RER. The chaper-

class I

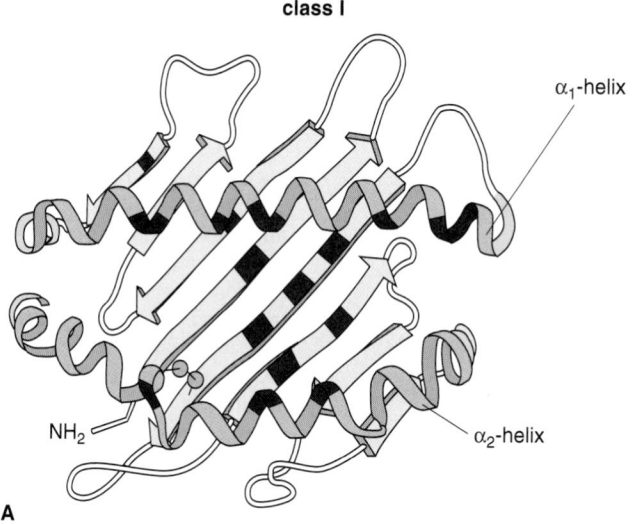

α₁-helix

NH₂

α₂-helix

A

class II

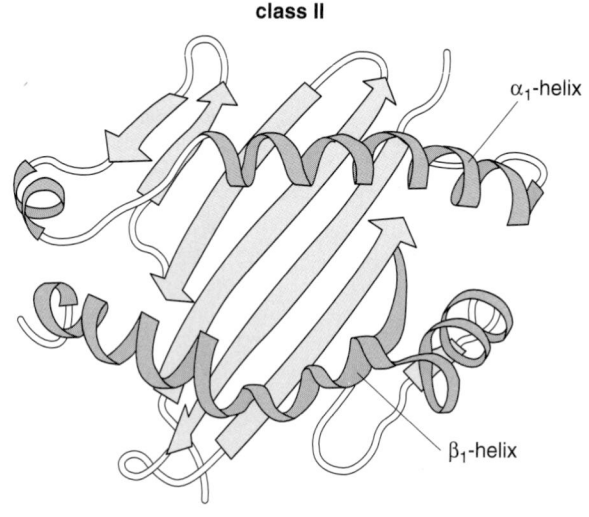

α₁-helix

β₁-helix

B

Figure 6–3. Peptide-binding sites of MHC class I and class II molecules. Each binding site has a floor composed of eight β strands and two α-helical walls. **A:** In the class I molecules, β sheets appear as broad arrows, α helices as narrow coils, and residues that are highly polymorphic among alleles are shown in black. The helices at either end of the class I binding site are closely apposed, so that peptides of only eight to nine residues can be bound. **B:** The class II groove, by comparison, has relatively open ends, which enable it to accommodate somewhat longer peptides. (Modified and reproduced, with permission, from Bjorkman PJ et al: Structure of the human class I histocompatibility antigen HLA-A2. *Nature* 1987;**329:**506, with additional data supplied by Peter Parham; and from Brown JH et al: Three-dimensional structure of the human class II histocompatibility antigen HLA-DR1. *Nature* 1993;**364:**33.)

one proteins calnexin and calreticulin help to mediate the initial folding and association of the α-chain/β₂-microglobulin heterodimer, which then physically associates with TAP transporter complexes in the membrane. The TAP proteins deliver cytosolically processed peptides to the peptide-binding site, inducing an additional conformational change that stabilizes the peptide–MHC complex. Although the TAP proteins preferentially import peptides 8–12 residues long, most peptides bound to class I proteins are only eight to nine residues long, suggesting that some exopeptidase trimming may occur within the RER. The peptide–MHC complex is then transported through the cytoplasm along the usual route of vesicular transport, passing sequentially through the Golgi apparatus and *trans*-Golgi network (where the single carbohydrate side chain is attached to the α chain in the RER and modified to a complex carbohydrate) before

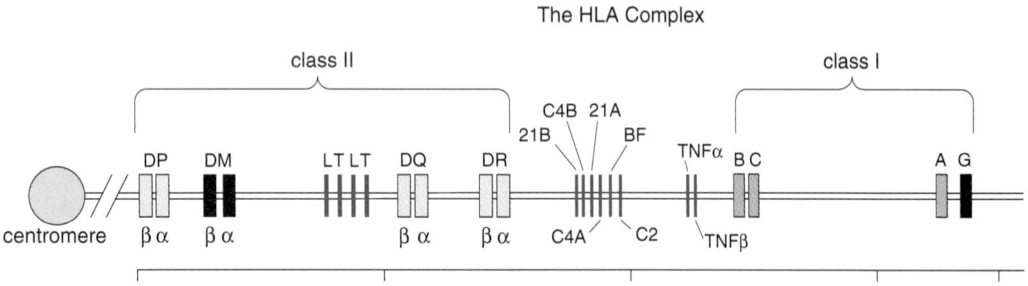

The HLA Complex

Figure 6–4. Organization of the HLA gene complex on the short arm of human chromosome 6. Regions encoding the class I and class II MHC proteins are indicated by braces. A cluster of four genes within the class II region encodes TAP (T) and LMP (L) proteins, which are peptide transport proteins and proteasome components, respectively, required for processing cytosolic antigens (see text). Of the several genes for nonclassical MHC molecules encoded in the HLA locus, only those for HLA-G (G) and HLA-DM (DM) are shown. The region between the class I and class II loci (sometimes called the class III locus) contains genes for tumor necrosis factors α and β (TNFα and TNFβ); steroid 21-β-hydroxylase (21A and 21B); and complement factors C2, C4, B, and F. Scale is approximate.

emerging on the cell surface (see Fig 6–5). Class I proteins that fail to bind peptides are unstable and are degraded within the cell.

MHC Class II. Class II α and β chains associate with each other soon after synthesis in the RER, where they, like class I proteins, are exposed to the

Table 6–2. Number of alleles in the human MHC (HLA region).[1]

Locus	Known Alleles
Class I	
Classical	
HLA-A	67
HLA-B	149
HLA-C	39
Nonclassical	
HLA-G	6
Class II	
Classical	
HLA-DRα[2]	2
HLA-DRβ	179
HLA-DQα	18
HLA-DQβ	29
HLA-DPα	8
HLA-DPβ	69
Accessory Molecules[3]	
HLA-DMα	4
HLA-DMβ	5
TAP-1	5
TAP-2	4

Abbreviations: HLA = human leukocyte antigen; TAP = transporter of antigenic peptides; LMP = low-molecular-weight protein.
[1] These are the number of alleles officially assigned by the WHO Nomenclature Committee for Factors of the HLA System, as of January 1996. Provided by Steven G. E. Marsh.
[2] The class II genes designated α or β encode the α or β subunits, respectively.
[3] Allelic variation of the LMP genes in humans has not yet been fully characterized.

pool of cytosolically processed peptides. The class II molecules, however, do not bind these peptides, because they associate instead with a third polypeptide, called the **invariant chain,** which blocks the class II peptide-binding site (see Fig 6–5). The invariant chain received its name because it has no polymorphic variants in the human population, though it is expressed in four different forms as a result of alternative splicing and alternative translational initiation sites. The major form of the polypeptide spans the RER membrane and has an amino-terminal domain that projects into the cytoplasm; it assembles to form a trimer that can bind three class II α/β heterodimers simultaneously. In addition to blocking peptide binding, the bound invariant chain functions as a chaperone that promotes stable folding of the class II proteins. It also alters the intracellular trafficking so that, after passing through the *trans*-Golgi network (where carbohydrate side chains on the α, β, and invariant chains are modified) vesicles containing the class II protein complex are routed into the endocytic pathway. The signals that trigger this change in trafficking are provided mainly by the cytoplasmic portion of the invariant chain, though lumenal sequences may also play a role. It is not clear whether the class II-containing vesicles enter the endocytic pathway directly from the *trans*-Golgi network or instead are first delivered to the cell surface for endocytosis, or both. Whatever the route, this is a critical event, since it directs the class II proteins toward an encounter with endocytosed peptides from the extracellular environment.

As vesicles bearing the class II/invariant chain complexes mature into **prelysosomes,** cellular proteinases (including cathepsins B, D, and S) in the vesicle lumen progressively cleave the invariant chain to produce a shorter, residual peptide called **CLIP.** The CLIP peptide is then catalytically removed by the

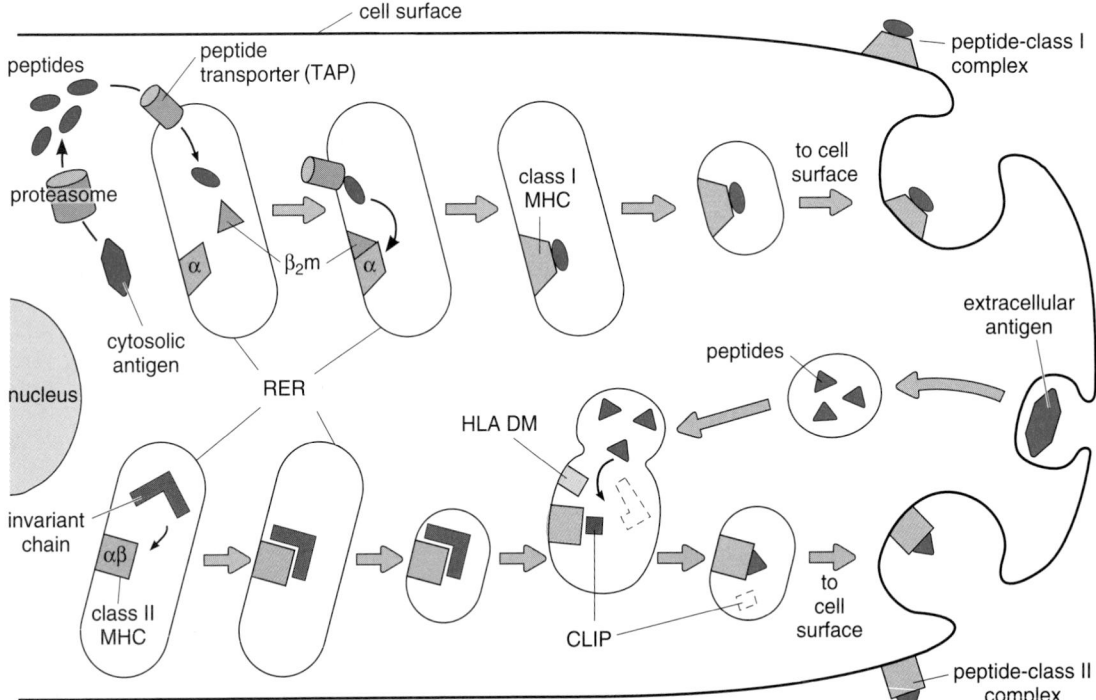

Figure 6–5. Pathways of assembly and transport for antigen–MHC complexes containing class I *(top)* and class II *(bottom)* HLA molecules. MHC polypeptides of both classes are initially expressed in the rough endoplasmic reticulum (RER) lumen. Peptides from cytosolic antigens processed by proteasomes are actively pumped into the RER by TAP transporters; they bind class I α chain and $β_2$-microglobulin in the RER lumen and are then transported to the cell surface. Class II proteins associate with the invariant chain in the RER and so are prevented from binding cytosolically processed peptides. Class II proteins are instead translocated to an endosomal compartment (either directly or by way of the cell surface), where the invariant chain is degraded to the CLIP peptide and then removed entirely to be replaced by peptides from the endocytic pathway. Peptide loading onto class II is assisted by the nonclassical MHC molecule HLA-DM.

HLA-DM molecule, which is exclusively localized to the class II-rich prelysosomal compartment. Removal of CLIP exposes the peptide-binding groove and allows endocytically processed peptides to bind the class II molecule. Peptide binding stabilizes the MHC proteins and allows the peptide/class II complex to be transported to the cell surface (see Fig 6–5).

Thus, class I and class II MHC molecules travel different routes within the cell and acquire antigenic peptides in different cellular compartments. The effect is to segregate these two groups of molecules, so that class I proteins selectively present peptides derived from proteins synthesized within the cell, whereas class II proteins present peptides from the extracellular environment. MHC proteins of both classes that fail to bind peptides are unstable and are rapidly degraded within the cell, ensuring that most MHC molecules are displayed on the cell surface as peptide–MHC complexes.

Control of the Antigen-Processing and Presentation Pathways

Though antigen processing and presentation occur constitutively, their efficiencies can be enhanced in

times of need. For example, levels of expression of class I molecules, TAP transporters, and LMP subunits all increase in response to interferon-gamma (IFNγ), a cytokine produced by macrophages, helper T lymphocytes, and other cell types during immune responses. IFNγ also can induce the expression of class II molecules on a variety of cell types (including endothelial cells, fibroblasts, and epithelial cells) that normally do not express them, temporarily enabling these cells to present antigens to helper T cells. On the other hand, some infectious pathogens actively subvert these processes: for example, herpes simplex viruses have been found to produce proteins that bind and inactivate the TAP transporters, enabling these viruses to block the endogenous pathway in an infected cell and so evade detection by the immune system.

PEPTIDE–MHC RECOGNITION BY T CELLS

TCRs recognize peptide–MHC complexes by binding simultaneously to specific residues both in the peptide and in the highly polymorphic region of the MHC molecule in and around the peptide-binding groove. As a result, individual TCRs are capable of discriminating not only among peptides but also among different allelic forms of a given MHC protein.

A T cell's ability to distinguish among peptide–MHC complexes is further enhanced by the CD4 or CD8 proteins on its surface. These two coreceptor molecules each specifically recognize one of the nonpolymorphic, immunoglobulin-like domains found in MHC proteins: CD4 binds the β_2 domain in all MHC class II polypeptides, whereas CD8 binds the α_3 domain of MHC class I. Recognition by CD4 or CD8 increases the overall avidity of the interaction and delivers a strong activation signal to the T cell (see Chapter 9). As a consequence, CD8+ T cells generally recognize peptides bound to class I MHC proteins and are said to be **class I-restricted,** whereas CD4+ T cells recognize peptides complexed with MHC class II and are said to be **class II-restricted.** This is an important factor in determining the type of immune response induced by a particular antigen. Cytosolic (class I-associated) antigens are mainly recognized by CD8+ cytotoxic T cells, which can kill the infected cells that present them. On the other hand, peptides from the endocytic pathway, associated with class II molecules, are mainly presented to CD4+ helper T cells, and these, in turn, may help to initiate a B-cell antibody response against the extracellular antigen.

Positive & Negative T-Cell Selection

The antigen-processing machinery operates continually within all normal cells, even in the absence of infection. Malfolded or otherwise unstable cellular proteins from the cytosol are constantly being cleaved into peptides that are then processed through the cytosolic pathway. Consequently, every nucleated human cell normally presents a great many host-derived ("self") peptides as MHC class I complexes on its surface. Similarly, class II-bearing cells routinely endocytose and present self peptides from proteins in the extracellular fluid and from their own surface membranes. When an infection occurs, peptides from the pathogen comingle with those from the host in the endogenous or exogenous pools (or both) and are presented along with them on the cell surface. Even during an intense infection, foreign peptides rarely account for more than a small fraction of all surface complexes. In short, the antigen presentation pathways do not distinguish between foreign and self peptides.

If self antigens are processed and presented at all times, why do they not trigger immune reactions? The answer lies mainly in an important—but incompletely understood—process of **negative selection** that operates on T cells as they develop in the thymus. Through negative selection, any T cells whose TCRs can bind to a self peptide/MHC complex are either killed or functionally inactivated before they are released to the periphery. This thymic censorship functions to eliminate **autoreactive** (ie, self-reactive) T cells that might otherwise attack normal host tissues.

A different selective process in the thymus, called **positive selection,** acts to ensure that mature T cells recognize only peptides that are bound to MHC proteins. This process selectively favors the growth of T cells whose TCRs recognize epitopes that include at least some residues from the MHC molecule—particularly those that flank the peptide-binding groove. Because this region of the MHC is highly polymorphic in the population, one consequence of this selection is that any individual's T cells respond primarily to peptides bound to a specific MHC allele expressed by that individual, that is, to "self" MHC. T cells that are not positively selected in this way fail to survive in the thymus.

The mechanisms of positive and negative selection during thymic T-cell development are considered in more detail in Chapter 9. For the present, it is enough to say that they are critical to the adaptive immune system's ability to discriminate self from nonself. Positive selection ensures that an individual's T cells respond only to peptides complexed with self MHC proteins. Negative selection ensures that any T cells capable of recognizing MHC complexes that contain a self peptide are eliminated or inactivated before they can attack host tissues.

Alloreactivity & Transplant Rejection

When cells or tissues are transplanted between individuals who express different alleles at one or more MHC loci, the recipient's T cells encounter the donor's MHC molecules, which carry different polymorphic residues and also present a very different set of self peptides derived from the donor's proteins. Responding to features in both the MHC and the peptides as nonself, a high proportion of the recipient's T cells (as much as 30%) are strongly activated. This so-called **alloreaction** (*allo-* means "other") is a major cause of transplant rejection. Avoiding it requires finding donors whose MHC alleles match those of the recipient as closely as possible, but the extensive polymorphism of these alleles makes matching difficult except between related individuals. Determining an individual's MHC alleles is called **HLA typing,** or histocompatibility typing. Ideally, if data from several family members are available to provide information about heredity, complete haplotypes can be determined. Although HLA typing has in the past relied on the use of antibodies to detect specific alleles, this has now been almost entirely supplanted by methods based on DNA sequence analysis of the HLA genes, which are far more accurate in determining allelic variation (see Chapter 17).

ANTIGEN-PRESENTING CELLS

Unless otherwise stated, the term "antigen-presenting cell" (APC) refers to cells that constitutively express class II MHC molecules, and so can present antigens to helper T cells. (These are sometimes also called "professional" APCs.) There are three major classes of cells that function as APCs (macrophages, dendritic cells, and B cells), and each has unique properties that make it important for particular aspects of the immune response.

Macrophages

Most types of macrophages express class II proteins, and their levels of class II expression increase when they become activated (see Chapter 2). Macrophages are widely distributed in lymphoid and nonlymphoid tissues and, because of their prodigious phagocytic capacity, are especially important for presenting antigens from particulate immunogens such as bacteria. Their many broad-specificity receptors enable macrophages to capture a wide range of pathogens, and so to play a prominent role in primary immune responses (ie, to pathogens that have not been encountered before), but their affinity for most ligands is low, so that most unopsonized immunogens must occur at relatively high concentrations to be presented efficiently by these cells. In addition, however, macrophages are highly efficient at capturing antibody-coated antigens using their surface Fc receptors, and so continue to play an important role in processing antigens during secondary immune responses.

Dendritic Cells

Cells in this category are known by a variety of names depending on their location in the body but are all thought to represent different forms of a single cell type derived from a marrow precursor. All have in common an unusual, spidery shape imparted by their many long cytoplasmic processes, called dendrites. Dendritic cells are found as a diffuse, minor resident population in all surface epithelia and many solid organs but can also migrate through the blood and lymph. Members of this group include epidermal **Langerhans' cells,** the "veiled" cells of lymph, **blood dendritic cells** (which make up less than 0.1% of all nucleated blood cells), and the **interdigitating cells** that are found throughout the T-cell zones of lymphoid organs. (Follicular dendritic cells, which are discussed later on, are not included in this group, though they have a similar morphology.)

Dendritic cells have little or no phagocytic capacity but express abundant class II protein and are highly efficient at capturing and presenting antigens. They appear to be particularly effective at initiating primary immune responses. As sentinels in the skin and epithelia, dendritic cells are ideally situated to intercept antigens that contact the body surfaces. Being motile, they also are important for transporting antigens through the body in search of T cells with appropriate antigen specificity. For example, within minutes after an immunogen is applied to the skin, Langerhans' cells carrying processed antigen on their surfaces begin to migrate from the site into dermal lymphatics, which carry them to the T-cell zones of regional lymph nodes, where they can present the antigens to T cells and help initiate an immune response.

Despite the unfortunate similarity in names and morphology, follicular dendritic cells (FDCs) are not related to the dendritic cells described previously and are not considered to be APCs. FDCs are found only in primary and secondary lymphoid follicles and may, in fact, be responsible for assembling such follicles (see Chapter 3). Their origin remains obscure, but they do not appear to be descendants of any marrow precursor. FDCs are not appreciably phagocytic and do not express class II MHC protein. They do, however, express abundant surface Fc receptors, which make them very efficient at capturing antigen–antibody complexes, thus helping to potentiate secondary immune responses (see Chapter 8). Once displayed on the FDC surface, antigens may persist for weeks or even months, suggesting a possible role for these cells in maintaining immunologic memory.

B Lymphocytes

Although B cells lack significant phagocytic activity, they are able to capture, process, and present some antigens to helper T cells. They are especially effective in presenting the antigens that bind specifically to their surface immunoglobulins. B cells with appropriate specificity are usually very scarce the first time an antigen is encountered but become increasingly significant as APCs with each subsequent exposure. Antigen presentation by B cells and its importance for humoral immunity are considered in detail in Chapter 8.

Specialized Forms of Antigen Presentation

As noted earlier, cytokines (especially IFNγ) released at sites of ongoing immune reactions can induce class II MHC expression in epithelial and mesenchymal cells, enabling these cells to function temporarily as APCs. In addition, epithelial cells and some other cell types are able to present certain nonpeptide antigens to T cells (see Chapter 13). These are presented as complexes with a family of nonclassical MHC molecules, called the **CD1** proteins, which are encoded outside the HLA gene locus. The CD1 proteins structurally resemble conventional class I molecules, except that the CD1 antigen-binding groove is narrower and deeper, enabling it to accommodate nonpeptide antigens such as the mycobacterially derived lipid, mycolic acid.

MHC AND DISEASE

The allelic forms of class I and class II MHC molecules that are expressed by any one individual dictate the repertoire of peptides that can be presented. Due to the relatively small number of proteins in a typical pathogen and the peptide-binding constraints imposed by a given set of MHC alleles, usually only a few epitopes from any one pathogen can be presented effectively to an individual's T cells. These few epitopes therefore dominate the cellular response to that pathogen and are called the dominant T-cell epitopes with respect to that individual (see Chapter 5). This genetically determined capacity to react immunologically against a particular immunogen is called **immune responsiveness.** Historically, the phenomenon was first observed in mice, where it became evident that inbred strains differed in their ability to mount an antibody response against particular synthetic peptide antigens; this was attributed to "immune response" genes, which were ultimately shown to be class II MHC alleles.

Because immune responses directed against some features of a pathogen are likely to be more effective than others at preventing or limiting infection, it might be expected that different individuals would show differences in their ability to resist infectious diseases and that these differences would be genetically correlated with the presence of particular MHC alleles. This expectation has been confirmed repeatedly in animals but has been harder to demonstrate in humans, in part because the population is highly outbred, and in part because disease development is influenced by numerous other genetic and environmental factors in addition to the MHC. Nevertheless, a few recent studies in humans indicate a role for MHC alleles in susceptibility to infectious diseases. For example, in Gambia, where malaria is highly prevalent, it has been observed that three specific HLA alleles are statistically less common among children dying of this disease than in the Gambian population at large. These alleles are, conversely, more frequent among children who develop a low-level, less virulent infection, suggesting that these alleles may confer the ability to mount a more effective immune response.

Studies on MHC-binding epitopes from human immunodeficiency virus (HIV) proteins have also revealed the importance of the interplay between host and pathogen in modulating immune responsiveness. The HLA-B8 allele is known to present a peptide derived from a region of the HIV Gag protein where mutations do not interfere with Gag function; therefore, the virus easily escapes a T-cell response directed against this epitope. The antigenic peptide presented by the HLA-B27 allele, however, is derived from a region of HIV protein that is less tolerant of mutation; as a result, the cytotoxic T-cell responses generated by individuals expressing HLA-B27 have a more sustained antiviral effect in vitro. It has not yet been determined whether this particular difference in immune responsiveness is associated with a more effective antiviral immune response or a better clinical outcome

overall. Nevertheless, such observations support a role for HLA alleles in natural disease resistance in humans and suggest their importance for designing effective vaccination strategies.

Another statistical link between MHC alleles and human disease has been observed in the case of **autoimmune disorders**—that is, disorders that are thought to involve an inappropriate immune attack against self tissues (see Chapter 32). As indicated in Table 6–3, several autoimmune disorders have been found to occur significantly more frequently among persons who carry particular HLA alleles than among those who do not. For example, in the US Caucasian population, inheritance of the HLA-B27 allele is associated with an 80-fold increased risk of developing ankylosing spondylitis, a degenerative inflammatory disease of the spine whose cause is unknown. One possible interpretation of this finding is that the HLA-B27 allele confers susceptibility to an as-yet-unidentified infectious agent that is directly responsible for the disease. Another possibility is that HLA-B27 presents peptides derived from a normal component of vertebral tissue, which resemble peptides from such an agent and so become the target of an immunologic cross-reaction in infected individuals. Still another hypothesis is that no external agent is required, but that HLA-B27 inappropriately presents self antigens from vertebral tissues in such a way that it becomes the target of an immune attack, due to a failure of T-cell negative selection. Although investigations of these and other possible etiologies are continuing, it is important to emphasize that no HLA allele is associated with disease in 100% of cases. Hence, the effect of MHC proteins is likely to be only one among several genetic and environmental factors that determine susceptibility to autoimmune disease.

Table 6–3. Some MHC-associated disorders in the US Caucasian population.

Disorder	Relative HLA Allele	Risk[1]
Ankylosing spondylitis	B27	80
Juvenile rheumatoid arthritis	Dw14	47
	Dw4	26
Reiter's syndrome	B27	40
Insulin-dependent diabetes mellitus	DQw8	32
Acute anterior uveitis	B27	8
Sjögren's syndrome	DR3	6
Graves' disease	DR3	4
Systemic lupus erythematosus	DR2	3

[1] Chance that a person who is heterozygous for the indicated allele will develop the disease, expressed as a multiple of the risk in the population that does not carry this allele.

REFERENCES

Bjorkman P, Parham P: Structure, function, and diversity of class I major histocompatibility complex molecules. *Ann Rev Biochem* 1990;59:253.

Cresswell P: Assembly, transport, and function of MHC class II molecules. *Ann Rev Immunol* 1994;**12:**259.

Germain RN, Margulies DH: The biochemistry and cell biology of antigen processing and presentation. *Ann Rev Immunol* 1993;**11:**403.

Hansen TH et al: The major histocompatibility complex. In: *Fundamental Immunology,* WE Paul (editor), Raven Press, 1993, p. 577.

Hill AVS et al: Common West African HLA antigens are associated with protection from severe malaria. *Nature* 1991;**352:**595.

Howard J: Supply and transport of peptides presented by class I MHC molecules. *Curr Opin Immunol* 1995;**7:**69.

Madden DR: The three-dimensional structure of peptide-MHC complexes. *Ann Rev Immunol* 1995;**13:**587.

Nepom GT, Erlich H: MHC class II molecules and autoimmunity. *Ann Rev Immunol* 1991;**9:**493.

Phillips RE et al: Human immunodeficiency virus genetic variation that can escape cytotoxic T cell recognition. *Nature* 1991;**354:**453.

Sanderson F et al: Accumulation of HLA-DM, a regulator of antigen presentation, in MHC class II compartments. *Science* 1994;**266:**1566.

Schmidt CM, Orr HT: Maternal/fetal interactions: The role of the MHC class I molecule HLA-G. *Crit Rev Immunol* 1993;**13:**207.

Sloan VS et al: Mediation by HLA-DM of dissociation of peptides from HLA-DR. *Nature* 1995;**375:**802.

Steinman RM: The dendritic cell system and its role in immunogenicity. *Ann Rev Immunol* 1991;**9:**271.

Stroynowski I, Forman J: Novel molecules related to MHC antigens. *Curr Opin Immunol* 1995;**7:**97.

Immunoglobulins & Immunoglobulin Genes

7

Tristram G. Parslow, MD, PhD

Immunoglobulin proteins are the critical ingredients at every stage of a humoral immune response. When expressed on the surfaces of resting B lymphocytes, they serve as receptors that can detect and distinguish among the vast array of potential antigens present in the environment. On binding their cognate antigens, surface immunoglobulins can initiate a cascade of molecular signaling events that may culminate in B-cell activation, clonal proliferation, and the generation of plasma cells. The immunoglobulins that are secreted as a result then function as **antibodies,** traveling through the tissue fluids to seek out and bind to the specific antigens that triggered their production.

The two hallmarks of immunoglobulins as antigen-binding proteins are the **specificity** of each for a particular epitope target and their **diversity** as a group. In addition to antigen binding, however, immunoglobulins also possess **secondary biologic activities** that are critical for host defense. These include, for example, the ability to function as opsonins, to activate the complement cascade, or to cross the placental barrier. Immunoglobulin proteins are heterogeneous with respect to these latter activities, which are determined by structural features independent of those that dictate antigen specificity. In this chapter, we first consider how the structures of immunoglobulins account for their specificity, diversity, and secondary biologic activities. We then examine the remarkable genetic mechanisms that give rise to these proteins.

IMMUNOGLOBULIN PROTEINS

Organization & Diversity of Immunoglobulin Proteins

The immunoglobulins are an enormous family of related, but nonidentical glycoproteins. It has been estimated that each person is capable of producing at least 10^8 different antibody molecules, each with its own distinct properties. Though carbohydrate may account for up to one fifth of an antibody's mass, almost all of its significant biologic attributes are determined by its polypeptide components. Antibodies are bifunctional molecules in that they bind specifically to antigens and also initiate a variety of secondary phenomena—such as complement activation, opsonization, or signal transduction—that are unrelated to their antigen-binding specificity. As we shall see, these two independent aspects of immunoglobulin function reside in separate regions of each protein.

The sheer diversity of immunoglobulins was for a long time a major barrier to understanding their structures. A serum specimen from any normal person contains a tremendous number of different antibody molecules, each of which is present in only minute amounts and (owing to its unique structure) has its own distinctive set of physical properties, such as molecular weight and isoelectric point. When a serum specimen is fractionated by electrophoresis, for example, most immunoglobulins are found to migrate as a broad band (called the **gamma-globulin** fraction) that reflects the presence of innumerable different proteins, each with slightly different electrophoretic properties. This extreme diversity made it virtually impossible to isolate sufficient amounts of any single antibody protein from a normal donor to permit a thorough biochemical analysis.

A series of key discoveries beginning in the 1950s finally opened up the field of immunoglobulin protein chemistry. The first was the finding that enzymes and reducing agents could be used to digest or dissociate immunoglobulins into smaller components. This revealed that diversity was largely confined to specific regions of the immunoglobulin molecules; other regions were much more uniform and could be isolated in pure form that made them accessible for structural analysis. A second breakthrough came with the realization that patients who had certain types of B-lym-

95

phoid cancers (such as **multiple myeloma**) contained in their blood and urine large amounts of a single, homogeneous type of immunoglobulin protein secreted by a single malignant B-cell clone. Purification of such **myeloma proteins** made it possible to study individual antibodies and permitted (by 1969) the determination of the first complete amino acid sequence of an immunoglobulin. The development, in 1975, of laboratory methods for immortalizing individual clones of antibody-secreting cells gave birth to **monoclonal antibody** technology (see later section) and made it possible to obtain homogeneous antibodies of virtually any specificity in unlimited quantities. At about the same time, the isolation and analysis of immunoglobulin genes revolutionized the study of this protein family by making it relatively easy to isolate, modify, and even design immunoglobulin proteins of all types. Information gleaned from all these approaches forms the basis for our current, detailed understanding of immunoglobulin protein structure.

The Four-Chain Basic Unit. Every immunoglobulin molecule is made up of two different types of polypeptides. The larger, **heavy (H) chains** are roughly twice as large as the smaller, **light (L) chains.**

Every immunoglobulin contains equal numbers of heavy- and light-chain polypeptides and can be represented by the general formula $(H_2L_2)n$. The chains are held together by noncovalent forces and also by covalent interchain disulfide bridges to form a bilaterally symmetrical structure as depicted in Figure 7–1. All normal immunoglobulins conform to this basic structure, although some, as we shall see, are composed of more than one of these four-chain units.

The heavy and light polypeptide chains are both composed of folded globular **domains,** each of which is 100 to 110 amino acids long and contains a single intrachain disulfide bond (see Fig 7–1). Though the amino acid sequences of the individual domains vary, they fold into very similar three-dimensional conformations (a roughly cylindrical assembly of β strands known as the **immunoglobulin barrel**), owing in part to the fairly constant location of the intrachain disulfide. Light chains always contain two of these domains, whereas heavy chains contain either four or five.

All of the light chains and all of the heavy chains in any single immunoglobulin protein are identical. When compared among different immunoglobulins,

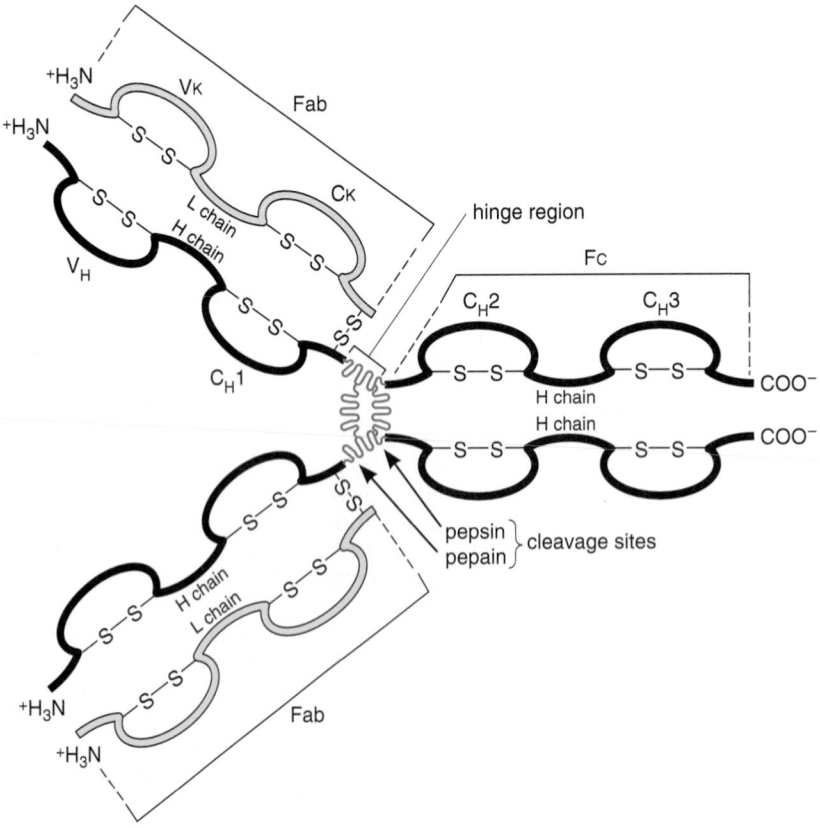

Figure 7–1. Schematic model of an IgG1 (κ) human antibody molecule showing the basic four-chain structure and domains (V_H, C_H1, etc). Sites of enzymatic cleavage by pepsin and papain are shown.

however, the sequences of these chains vary widely. In both heavy and light chains, this variability is most pronounced in the *N*-terminal domain, whereas the sequences of the other domains remain relatively constant. For this reason, the *N*-terminal domain in a heavy- or light-chain polypeptide is called the **variable region,** abbreviated V_H or V_L, respectively. The other domains are collectively termed the **constant region,** abbreviated C_H or C_L. Light-chain polypeptides contain only a single C_L domain, but heavy chain C_H regions comprise three or more domains that are numbered sequentially (C_H1, C_H2, etc.) beginning with the domain closest to V_H.

Within an immunoglobulin unit, the heavy and light chains are aligned in parallel as shown in Figure 7–1. Each V_H domain is always positioned directly beside a V_L domain, and this pair of domains together forms a single **antigen-binding site.** Each basic four-chain unit thus contains two separate but identical antigen-binding sites and so is said to be **divalent** with respect to antigen binding. The antigen specificity of a given protein is determined by the combined sequences of its V_H and V_L domains and for this reason varies widely among immunoglobulins. Each C_H1 domain interacts closely with the C_L domain, and in most types of immunoglobulins the two are linked covalently by one or more disulfide bridges. Each of the remaining C_H domains is aligned with its counterpart on the opposite heavy chain and may be linked to it by disulfide bonds. Overall, the protein has a T- or Y-shaped configuration when viewed schematically. The region at the base of each arm in the T or Y, located between the C_H1 and C_H2 domains, is called the **hinge region;** in most immunoglobulins, it has a loose secondary structure that makes it flexible, enabling the two arms to move relatively freely with respect to each other.

Enzymatic Digestion Products of Immunoglobulins. Immunoglobulins are rather resistant to proteolytic digestion but are most susceptible to cleavage near the hinge region (see Fig 7–1), which usually lies adjacent to the site of interchain disulfides linking the two heavy chains together. The enzyme **papain** happens to cleave this region on the *N*-terminal side of the inter-heavy-chain disulfides, and so splits an immunoglobulin into three fragments of roughly similar size. Two of these are identical to each other, consisting of an entire light chain along with the V_H and C_H1 domains of one heavy chain; these fragments thus contain the antigen-binding sites of the protein, and so are called **Fab fragments** (ie, antigen-binding fragments). Each Fab fragment is **monovalent** with respect to antigen-binding activity. The third fragment comprises the carboxy-terminal portions of both heavy chains held together by disulfides. The structure of this third fragment is identical for many different immunoglobulin molecules, so that fragments of this type can often be crystallized even if they are derived from a heterogeneous antibody population. Hence, this third fragment is designated the crystallizable or **Fc fragment.** Most of the secondary biologic properties of immunoglobulins (such as the ability to activate complement) are determined by sequences in the Fc region of the protein. This is also the region that is recognized by the **Fc receptors** found on many types of cells.

A somewhat different pattern of cleavage occurs with the enzyme pepsin, which cleaves on the carboxy-terminal side of the inter-heavy-chain disulfides. This yields a single large fragment called an **F(ab)′2** fragment, which roughly corresponds to two disulfide-linked Fab fragments and has divalent antigen-binding activity. The Fc region, on the other hand, is extensively degraded by pepsin, and usually does not survive as an intact fragment.

Characterization of these proteolytic fragments in the 1960s was an important step toward understanding antibody structure, as it provided the first evidence that the antigen-binding and secondary functions of antibodies reside in separate regions of the protein. Such fragments are still used today when it is necessary to dissociate different aspects of antibody function for diagnostic or research purposes.

Classification of Immunoglobulins & Their Constituent Chains

Immunoglobulins are composed of heavy and light chains. The *N*-terminal domain (V region) in both types of chains is highly variable and mediates antigen binding. The remaining portion (C region) of each chain, by comparison, is far less variable. Nevertheless, every normal person produces several alternative forms of heavy and light chains that each have distinctly different C-region amino acid sequences (Table 7–1). These alternative forms of the immunoglobulin chains can be distinguished from one another by their physical properties (such as molecular weight) or serologically by using antibodies (usually obtained from animals that have been immunized with human Fc fragments) that recognize specific features in the various human C regions. Although these normal variations in sequence of the C_L region have no effect on immunoglobulin function, those in the C_H region significantly affect the secondary biologic properties of immunoglobulins.

Light-Chain Types and Subtypes. All light chains have protein molecular weights of approximately 23,000 but can be classified into two distinct **types,** called **kappa** (κ) and **lambda** (λ), on the basis of their C_L-region sequences. There are no known functional differences between these two types, and each can associate with any of the various classes of heavy chains. Nevertheless, expression of two distinct light-chain types is common among mammals. Indeed, the amino acid sequence similarities between human and mouse kappa chains are much greater than those between the kappa and lambda chains within each species—indicating that the primordial kappa

Table 7–1. Properties of human immunoglobulin chains and related polypeptides.

Chain	H Chains					L Chains		Secretory Component	J Chain
	γ	α	μ	δ	ε	κ	λ	SC	J
Classes in which chain occurs	IgG	IgA	IgM	IgD	IgE	All classes	All classes	IgA	IgA, IgM
Subclasses or subtypes	1,2,3,4	1,2	—	—	—	—	1,2,3,4,5,6	—	—
Molecular weight (approximate)	50,000[1]	55,000	70,000	62,000	70,000	23,000	23,000	70,000	15,000
V region subgroups	V_{HI}–V_{HIV}					$V_{\kappa I}$–$V_{\kappa IV}$	$V_{\lambda I}$–$V_{\lambda IV}$		
Carbohydrate (average percentage)	4	10	15	18	18	0	0	16	8
Number of oligosaccharides (average)	1	2 or 3	5	?	5	0	0	?	1

[1] 60,000 for γ3.

and lambda genes separated from one another during evolution prior to the divergence of these mammalian species.

The C regions of all κ light chains produced by an individual are essentially identical. In contrast, a single person may express as many as six slightly different forms of the λ C region. These various **subtypes** of λ differ from one another only slightly in C-region amino acid sequences and are functionally identical, though each is encoded by a separate chromosomal locus.

A given immunoglobulin molecule always contains exclusively κ or one of the λ chains, never a mixture. Similarly, any given B-lineage cell produces only one type of light chain. When the entire population of serum immunoglobulins (or of B-lineage cells) in an individual is considered, the proportion of kappa to lambda chains that are produced varies from species to species; in humans, the ratio is about 2:1.

Heavy-Chain Classes and Subclasses. Humans express five different classes (or isotypes) of immunoglobulin heavy chains, which differ considerably in their C_H-region sequences and in their physical and biologic properties. All of the heavy chains in any given immunoglobulin are identical. The five classes of heavy chains are designated μ, δ, λ, α, and ε, and immunoglobulins that contain these heavy chains are designated the IgM, IgD, IgG, IgA, and IgE classes, respectively. The γ and α classes are further divided into subclasses (γ1, γ2, γ3, γ4, α1, and α2) based on relatively minor differences in C_H sequence and function; the corresponding immunoglobulin subclasses are denoted IgG1, IgG2, etc. Heavy chains representing the various subclasses within a class are much more similar to one another than to the other classes. Normal individuals express all nine classes and subclasses, because each is encoded by a separate genetic locus and is inherited independently.

The heavy-chain polypeptides range in molecular

weight from about 50,000 to 70,000. The μ and ε chains are made up of five globular domains apiece (one V_H and four C_H), whereas γ, α, and δ chains each contain only four domains (one V_H and three C_H). The δ chain has an intermediate molecular weight attributable to an enlarged hinge region. The γ3 chain also has a large hinge that consists of about 60 amino acid residues; of these, 14 are cysteines, which accounts for the large number of inter-heavy-chain disulfide bonds in IgG3 (see section on IgG). In some mammalian species, the charge characteristics of the various IgG subclasses differ sufficiently to permit their separation by electrophoretic techniques, but this is not true of humans.

Composition of Immunoglobulin Classes and Subclasses. The class of the H chain determines the class of the immunoglobulin. Thus, there are five classes of immunoglobulins: IgG, IgA, IgM, IgD, and IgE. A given molecule in any of these classes may contain either κ or λ light chains. For example, two γ chains (of any of the four subclasses), combined with either two κ or two λ L chains, constitute an IgG molecule—the most abundant class of immunoglobulins in sera from adults. Similarly, two μ chains together with two L chains form an IgM monomer unit of the type found on the surfaces of many B cells. The secreted form of IgM, however, is a pentameric macroglobulin, which consists of five of these basic four-chain units along with an additional polypeptide called J chain (Fig 7–2). Each IgM pentamer contains 10 identical antigen-binding sites and so has polyvalent binding activity. IgA accounts for only about 10–15% of serum immunoglobulin but is the predominant class of antibody found in body secretions. The membrane-bound form of IgA is a single four-chain unit, but the secreted form can polymerize to form assemblages comprising two to five of these basic units along with J chain and (in secreted IgA) yet another polypeptide called secretory component (see Fig

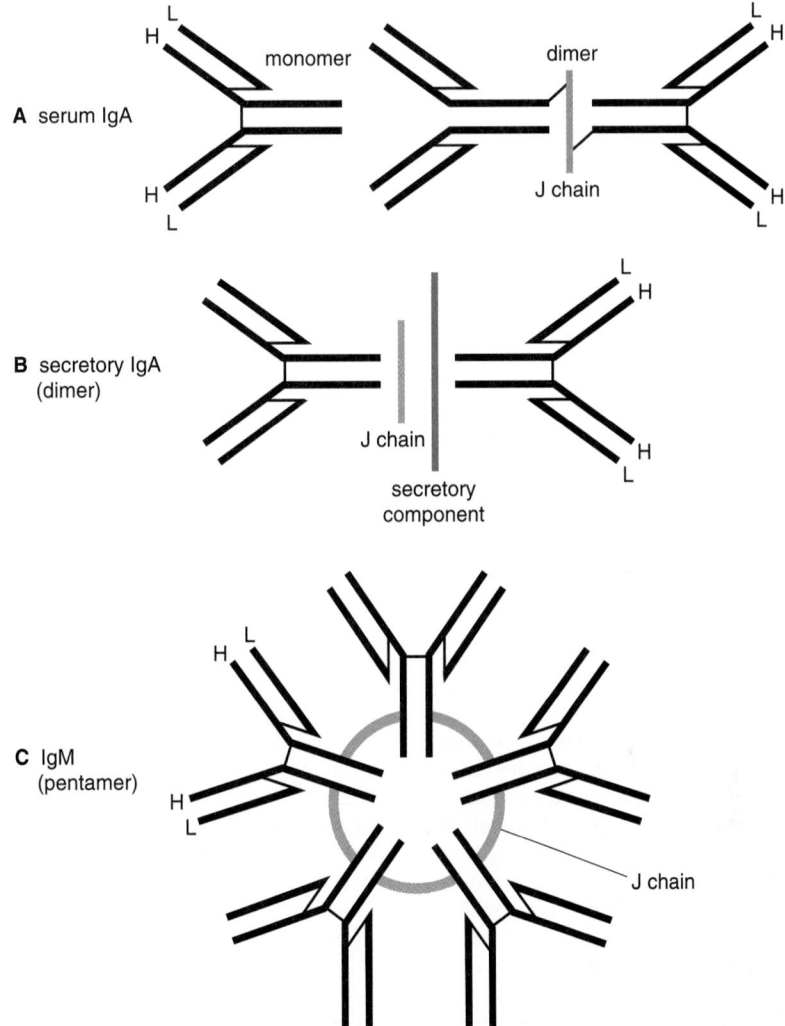

A serum IgA — monomer, dimer, J chain

B secretory IgA (dimer) — J chain, secretory component

C IgM (pentamer) — J chain

Figure 7–2. Highly schematic illustration of polymeric human immunoglobulins. Polypeptide chains are represented by thick lines; disulfide bonds linking different polypeptide chains are represented by thin lines.

7–2). The properties of the individual chains are summarized in Table 7–1, and those of the immunoglobulin classes are compared in Table 7–2.

One noteworthy structural difference among the immunoglobulin classes or subclasses lies in the number and arrangement of interchain disulfide bridges within each four-chain unit (Fig 7–3). In IgA2, for example, the L chains are covalently linked to each other rather than to the H chains, so that L–H binding is entirely due to noncovalent forces. In other subclasses, the L–H bond may be situated either close to the junction of the V_H and C_H1 domains (as in IgG2 or IgA1) or, alternatively, near the junction between C_H1 and C_H2 (as in IgG1).

Membrane and Secreted Immunoglobulins. Immunoglobulins of all classes can exist in either membrane-bound or secreted forms. The membrane forms always exist as individual four-chain units and have on their heavy chains an additional carboxy-terminal sequence of approximately 40 amino acid residues. This sequence consists of a highly acidic region of 12–14 residues, followed by a strikingly hydrophobic sequence of about 26 residues. The hydrophobic portion is the transmembrane component, which anchors the heavy chain (and, hence, the entire four-chain unit) into the cell membrane. It is similar in hydrophobicity and length to known transmembrane segments of other proteins and probably forms a single membrane-spanning α helix. The acidic portion of the membrane segment shows little amino acid sequence conservation among heavy-chain classes, but the hydrophobic sequences tend to be quite similar.

Table 7–2. Properties of human immunoglobulins.

	IgG	IgA	IgM	IgD	IgE
H-chain class	γ	α	μ	δ	ε
H-chain subclasses	$\gamma1, \gamma2, \gamma3, \gamma4$	$\alpha1, \alpha2$			
L-chain type	κ and λ	κ and λ	κ and λ	κ and λ	κ and λ
Molecular formula	$\gamma_2 L_2$	$\alpha_2 L_2{}^1$ or $(\alpha_2 L_2)_2 SC^2 J^3$	$(\alpha_2 L_2)_5 J^3$	$\delta_2 L_2$	$\varepsilon_2 L_2$
Sedimentation coefficient (S)	6–7	7	19	7–8	8
Molecular weight (approximate)	150,000	160,000[1] or 400,000[4]	900,000	180,000	190,000
Electrophoretic mobility (average)	γ	Fast γ to β	Fast γ to β	Fast γ	Fast γ
Complement fixation (classic)	+	0	++++	0	0
Serum concentration (approximate; mg/dL)	1000	200	120	3	0.05
Serum half-life (days)	23	6	5	3	2
Placental transfer	+	0	0	0	0
Mast cell or basophil degranulation	?	0	0	0	++++
Bacterial lysis	+	+	+++	?	?
Antiviral activity	+	+++	+	?	?

[1] For monomeric serum IgA.
[2] Secretory component.
[3] J chain.
[4] For secretory IgA.

This probably reflects the requirement that membrane-bound heavy chains of all classes must associate with the same pair of integral membrane proteins, called Ig-α and Ig-β, in order to transduce signals into the cell (see Chapter 8). The direct anchoring of immunoglobulins into surface membranes occurs only in B-lineage cells and should not be confused with the indirect association that results when soluble antibodies bind to Fc receptors found on many cell types.

Secreted immunoglobulins lack the terminal transmembrane segment as a result of alternative RNA splicing (see later discussion). In its place, the secreted forms of μ and α (but not of the other classes) contain short terminal sequences, called **tail pieces,** that mediate polymerization of four-chain units and also serve as contact sites for the J chain.

Allotypic (Allelic) Forms of Heavy and Light Chains. The heavy-chain classes and subclasses and the light-chain types and subtypes are each encoded by separate genetic loci, so that all are normally present in a single haploid genome. Some of these individual loci, however, exist in more than one form within the population; the alternative forms (alleles) generally differ from one another by only one or, at most, a few amino acid substitutions. Such minor alternative forms at a given immunoglobulin locus are called allotypes. In humans, allotypes have been found for γ, α, and ε H chains and for κ L chains. Thus far, allotypic forms of λ L chains or of μ and δ H chains have not been observed.

Allotypic variation has no effect on immunoglobulin function and is primarily of interest because the variant C-region sequences can be immunogenic in some circumstances. For example, mothers may become immunized during the course of pregnancy against paternal allotypic determinants expressed on fetal immunoglobulins. Alternatively, immunization may result from blood transfusions. In addition, patients with rheumatoid arthritis can develop **"rheumatoid factors"**—antibodies that are directed against normal IgG—which occasionally recognize allotypic determinants.

J Chain and Secretory Component. As noted above, the secreted forms of IgM and IgA generally exist as polymers of the basic four-chain unit that include a single additional polypeptide called J chain. J chain is a small (MW 15,000) acidic protein that is structurally unrelated to heavy and light chains but is synthesized by all plasma cells that secrete polymeric immunoglobulins. In these polymeric assemblies, J chain is disulfide-bonded to the penultimate cysteine residue in the tail segment of the α or μ chains. Its function seems to be to facilitate proper polymerization, though whether or not it is required for polymerization remains controversial.

Secretory component is a single glycopeptide with a peptide molecular weight of approximately 70,000 and a high carbohydrate content. It is associated only with IgA and is found almost exclusively in body secretions. Its amino acid sequence is invariant and shows no appreciable resemblance to J chain or to any of the immunoglobulin polypeptides. Secretory component can exist either in free form or bound to IgA molecules; the latter interaction is usually noncovalent, but disulfide bonds have been implicated in a small proportion of human IgA. Free secretory com-

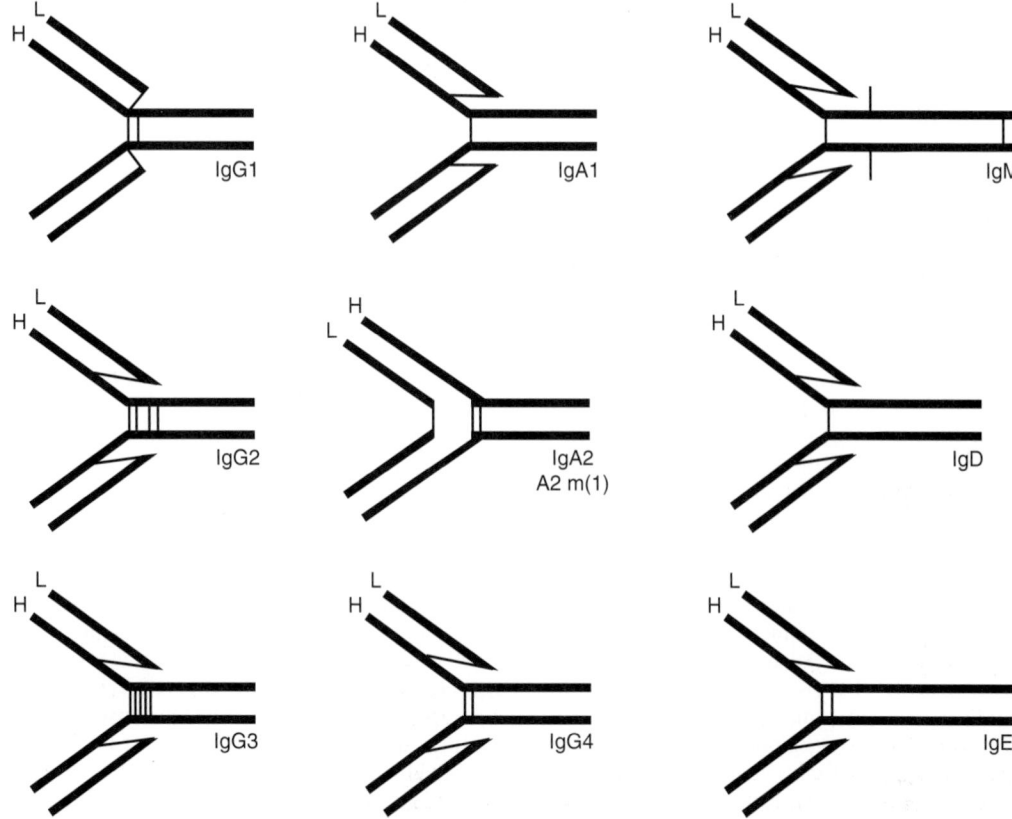

Figure 7–3. Distribution of interchain disulfide bonds in various human immunoglobulin classes and subclasses. H chains are represented by long thick lines and L chains by short thick lines. Disulfide bonds are represented by thin lines. The number of inter-heavy-chain disulfide bonds in IgG3 may be as large as 14.

ponent can even be observed in secretions from individuals who lack measurable IgA in their serum or secretions.

Secretory component is not synthesized by lymphocytes but rather by mucosal epithelial cells that overlie Peyer's patches and other submucosal lymphoid tissues (see Chapter 13). Such epithelial cells take up IgA that is secreted from the lymphoid cells beneath them, link it with secretory component, and transport the resulting complex across the epithelial barrier into secretions. Linkage with secretory component is presumed to facilitate the transepithelial passage of IgA.

Biologic Activities of Immunoglobulins

As previously noted, immunoglobulins are bifunctional molecules that bind antigens and, in addition, initiate other biologic processes that are independent of antibody specificity. These two kinds of activities are each localized to a particular part of the protein: antigen binding to the combined V_H and V_L domains, and the other activities to the C_H domains (particularly those of the Fc segment). The latter activities,

some of which are summarized in Table 7–2, are considered in this section.

Immunoglobulin G. Immunoglobulin G (IgG) accounts for approximately 75% of the total serum immunoglobulin in normal adults and is the most abundant antibody produced during secondary humoral immune responses in the blood. Within the IgG class, the relative concentrations of the four subclasses are approximately as follows: IgG1, 60–70%; IgG2, 14–20%; IgG3, 4–8%; and IgG4, 2–6% (Table 7–3). These values vary somewhat among individuals; it appears that the propensity to produce IgG antibodies of one subclass or another is at least partly an inherited trait.

Table 7–3. Properties of human IgG subclasses.

	IgG1	IgG2	IgG3	IgG4
Abundance (% of total IgG)	70	20	6	4
Half-life in serum (days)	23	23	7	23
Placental passage	+++	+	+++	+++
Complement fixation	+	+	+++	—
Binding to Fc receptors	+++	+	+++	—

IgG is the only class of immunoglobulin that can cross the placenta in humans, and it is responsible for protection of the newborn during the first months of life (see Chapter 43). The subclasses are not equivalent in this respect, IgG2 being transferred less efficiently than the others, but the biologic significance of this inequality, if any, is unknown.

Antigen-bound IgG is also capable of fixing (that is, binding and activating) serum complement, and once again the subclasses do so with unequal efficiency (IgG3 > IgG1 > IgG2). IgG4 is completely unable to fix complement by the classic pathway, which requires binding of a protein called C1q, but it may be active in the alternative pathway (see Chapter 11). The C1q binding site on the other IgG proteins appears to reside in the C_H2 domain.

Macrophages and certain other cell types express surface receptors that bind the Fc regions of IgG molecules. These interact principally with C_H2 domains and bind IgG1 and IgG3 with much higher affinity than the other subclasses. The properties of these receptors are considered in a later section.

Immunoglobulin A. Immunoglobulin A (IgA) is the predominant immunoglobulin produced by B cells in Peyer's patches, tonsils, and other submucosal lymphoid tissues. Thus, although it accounts for only 10–15% of serum immunoglobulin, it is by far the most abundant antibody class found in saliva, tears, intestinal mucus, bronchial secretions, milk, prostatic fluid, and other secretions. On B-cell surfaces, IgA exists as a monomer (MW 160,000) comprising only one four-chain unit. In the blood or in secretions, it multimerizes to form disulfide-linked polymers of up to five such units that are associated with one molecule each of J chain and (in secretions) secretory component. The predominant secreted forms of IgA are dimers and trimers (see Fig 7–2). The two subclasses, IgA1 and IgA2, are expressed at a 5:1 ratio in the blood and have similar properties. High-affinity Fc receptors specific for IgA have been observed but are not well characterized.

Immunoglobulin M. Immunoglobulin M (IgM) constitutes approximately 10% of normal serum immunoglobulins and is normally secreted as a J-chain-containing pentamer with a molecular mass of approximately 900 kD. IgM antibody predominates in early primary immune responses to most antigens, though it tends to become less abundant subsequently. IgM (often accompanied by IgD) is the most common immunoglobulin expressed on the surfaces of B cells, particularly virgin B lymphocytes. IgM is also the most efficient complement-fixing immunoglobulin: a single molecule of antigen-bound IgM suffices to initiate the complement cascade. Fc receptors specific for IgM exist but have not been well characterized.

Immunoglobulin D. The immunoglobulin D (IgD) molecule is a monomeric four-chain unit with a molecular mass of approximately 180 kD. Though IgD is commonly found on the surfaces of B lympho-cytes that also bear surface IgM, it is rarely secreted in significant amounts, and only traces of it are normally found in the blood. In cells that coexpress IgD and IgM, both classes of heavy chains are produced by alternative splicing of a single RNA (see later discussion) and have identical antigen specificity. The IgD on these cells can bind antigen and transmit signals to the cell interior, with consequences that appear identical to those produced by IgM. When such B cells become activated, surface IgD expression ceases.

The physiologic function of IgD is unknown. It is relatively labile to degradation by heat or proteolytic enzymes. There are isolated reports of IgD with antibody activity toward insulin, penicillin, milk proteins, diphtheria toxoid, nuclear components, or thyroid antigens. Its presence on many mature virgin lymphocytes has suggested an as-yet-unproven role in B-cell differentiation or tolerance.

Immunoglobulin E. Though it normally represents only a minute fraction (0.004%) of all serum antibodies, immunoglobulin E (IgE) is extremely important from the clinical standpoint because of its central involvement in **allergic disorders.** Two specialized types of inflammatory cells that are involved in allergic responses—the **mast cell** and the **basophil**—carry a unique, high-affinity Fc receptor that is specific for IgE antibodies. Thus, despite the very low concentration of IgE (roughly 10^{-7} M) in blood and tissue fluids, the surfaces of these cells are constantly decorated with IgE antibodies, adsorbed from the blood, that serve as antigen receptors. When its passively bound IgE molecules contact an antigen, the mast cell or basophil releases inflammatory mediator substances that produce many of the acute manifestations of allergic disease (see Chapters 12 and 27). Elevated levels of serum IgE may also signify infection by **helminths** or certain other types of multicellular **parasites** (Chapter 51). Like IgG and IgD, IgE exists only in monomeric form. Fc receptors appear to recognize primarily the C_H3 domain of the ε chain.

Immunoglobulin Variable Regions

The V regions, which coincide with the *N*-terminal domains of light and heavy chains, mediate antigen binding and are by far the most heterogeneous portions of these proteins. Indeed, no two human myeloma proteins from different patients have ever been found to have identical V-region sequences. Some clear patterns can be discerned, however. V_H regions show significantly more resemblance to one another than to V_L regions, whereas V_κ and V_λ sequences each have characteristic features that distinguish them from each other and from V_H. Thus, V_H, V_κ, and V_λ sequences can be recognized as separate groups that each associate with their own characteristic constant regions. There is never any mixing: a given V_H sequence, for example, may be found on heavy chains of any class (μ, δ, γ, α, or ε), but is never found on a light chain.

Framework and Hypervariable Regions. Variable regions within any single group are not uniformly variable across their entire 110-amino-acid spans. Instead, they consist of relatively invariant stretches (called **framework regions**) of 15–30 amino acids, separated by shorter regions of extreme variability (called **hypervariable regions**) that are each 9–12 amino acids long. V_H and V_L regions each contain three hypervariable regions, whose approximate locations are depicted in Figure 7–4. Antigen binding is mediated by noncovalent interactions that primarily involve amino acids in the hypervariable regions of each chain; hence, the sequences of these regions are the primary determinants of antigen specificity. Hypervariable regions are also called **complementarity-determining regions (CDRs),** and within each chain are designated CDR1, CDR2, and CDR3, beginning with the one nearest the amino ter-

minus. CDR3 is usually the longest and most variable of the three, as specialized genetic mechanisms act to increase sequence diversity in this region (see later section).

V-Region Subgroups. When sequences of many variable regions from any one type of chain (V_H, V_κ, or V_λ) are compared, they are found to form subgroups that are more similar to one another than to the remaining V regions in the group. For example, human V_κ regions have been classified into four subgroups, and similar subgroups exist for the V_H and V_λ regions. The subgroups differ from one another principally in the length and position of amino acid insertions and deletions within their framework regions.

Idiotypes. The term idiotype refers to the unique V-region amino acid sequences of the homogeneous immunoglobulin molecules produced by a single B-cell clone. Thus, there are as many idiotypes as there are B-cell clones (perhaps about 10^8 in an adult).

The concept of idiotype (which means "self-type") was first derived from experiments in which inbred animals were inoculated with purified antibody proteins that had been raised against a particular antigen in genetically identical animals. The inoculated animals mounted an antibody response against the injected immunoglobulin, implying that some sequences within it were recognized as foreign, but these antibodies would not react with other immunoglobulins from the same strain of animal. The antiserum produced in such a response was called an **anti-idiotype** antiserum. It was soon observed that the reaction between an antihapten antibody and its corresponding anti-idiotypic antiserum could, in some cases, be inhibited by the hapten, indicating that the idiotypic determinants were close to or within the antigen-binding site. It is now known that anti-idiotype antibodies specifically recognize sequences in the hypervariable regions of the target antibody, which are unique to that antibody and determine its antigen specificity. Thus, in current usage, the term idiotype refers to the global characteristics of the antigen-binding site in a given immunoglobulin, which are determined by the hypervariable sequences of its particular V_H and V_L domains.

The Three-Dimensional Structure of Immunoglobulins

The complete three-dimensional structures of many immunoglobulin molecules have been deduced from x-ray crystallographic studies. Such studies provided conclusive evidence that all of the individual globular domains in heavy and light chains share a common folded structure, despite the considerable differences in their amino acid sequences. Each domain is folded into a rigid, roughly cylindrical scaffold made up of seven to nine strands of antiparallel β sheets that are aligned like the staves of a barrel (Fig 7–5). In V_H and V_L domains, the three hypervariable sequences each

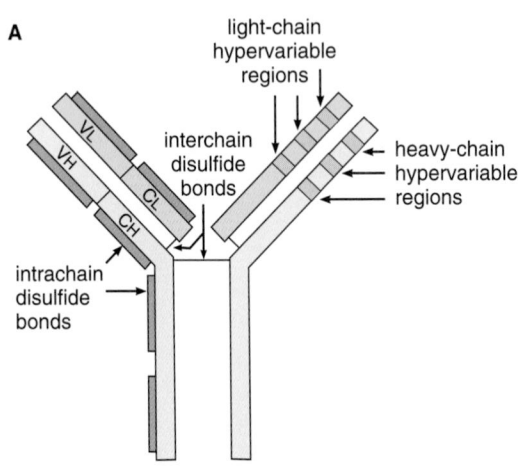

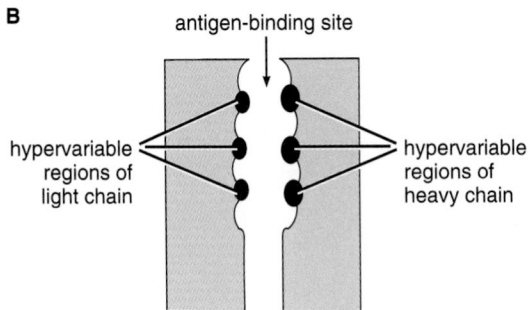

Figure 7–4. ***A:*** Schematic depiction of an IgG molecule showing the approximate locations of the hypervariable regions (also called complementarity-determining regions [CDRs]) in the heavy and light chains. Each CDR is roughly 9–12 residues long and is centered on residues 30–33, 56, or 94–98 of the polypeptide chain. ***B:*** Schematic depiction of how the three CDRs in each heavy- and light-chain pair form an antigen-binding site.

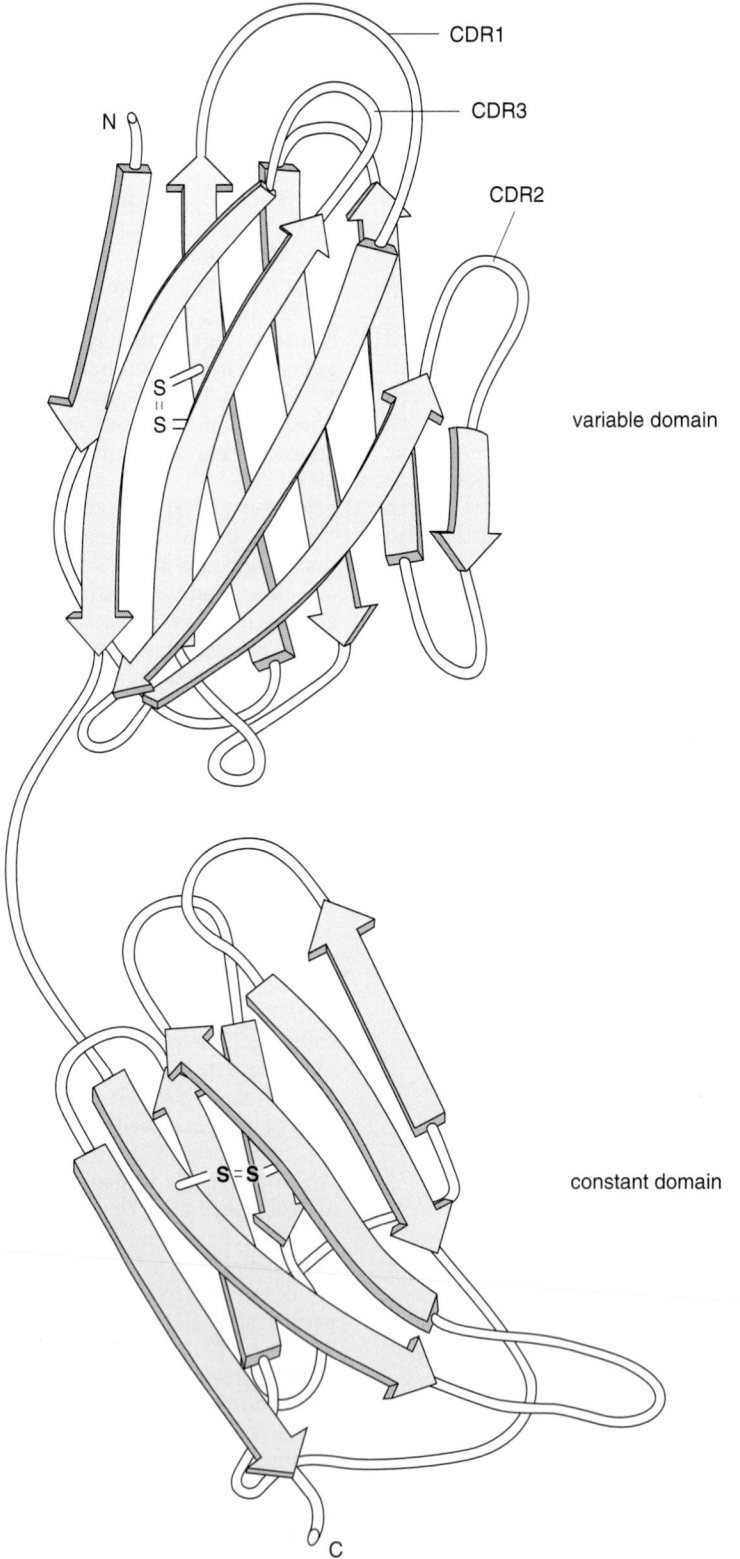

Figure 7–5. Three-dimensional structure of a light chain. In this ribbon diagram tracing the polypeptide backbone, β strands are shown as wide ribbons, other regions as narrow strings. Each of the two globular domains consists of a barrel-shaped assembly of seven to nine antiparallel β strands. The three hypervariable regions (CDR1, CDR2, and CDR3) are flexible loops that project outward from the amino-terminal end of the V_L domain.

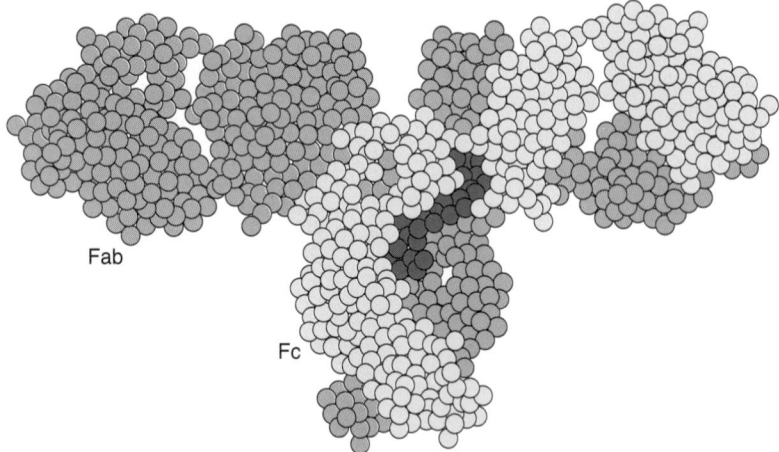

Figure 7–6. Three-dimensional structure of an immunoglobulin molecule. (Reproduced, with permission, from Silverton EW, Navia MA, Davies DR: Three-dimensional structure of an intact human immunoglobulin. *Proc Natl Acad Sci USA* 1977;**74**:5140.)

occupy a position between individual β strands and form relatively flexible loops that project outward from one "rim" of the barrel to participate in antigen binding. A single antigen-binding site is formed by the apposition of six hypervariable loops: three from V_H and three from V_L.

Complete crystallographic structures have also been obtained for antibodies or Fab fragments complexed with their target antigens or with haptens. These structures confirm the expectation that antigen-binding is mainly carried out by residues in the hypervariable regions (especially CDR3) but demonstrate that nearby residues in the framework regions can also participate in binding. In general, haptens tend to bind by nestling into small (10–15 Å) crevices in the antigen-binding site, whereas macromolecular antigens interact over larger regions on the surface of the site. For example, 16 separate residues in lysozyme were found to interact with nearly 20 residues spread over a 20 × 30 Å surface formed by the six CDR loops of one antilysozyme Fab fragment.

Structural studies also reveal the strong tendency of immunoglobulin domains to adhere to one another laterally through noncovalent (especially hydrophobic) interactions (Fig 7–6). Thus, pairs of heavy and light chains are held together side by side not only by disulfide bonds but also by extensive noncovalent interactions between the C_H1 and C_L domains. Similarly, the heavy chains within each four-chain unit adhere to one another in part through strong hydrophobic contacts between C_H3 domains. These interdomain interactions are mediated by hydrophobic residues that occupy one lateral face of the barrel and that tend to be relatively conserved among all immunoglobulin domains.

The Immunoglobulin Supergene Family

The repetitive domain structure of immunoglobulin polypeptides reflects the manner in which their genes evolved. It is thought that the common ancestor of all immunoglobulin proteins was a small primordial gene that encoded a single copy of the barrel-like polypeptide domain. In light of the tendency of modern immunoglobulin domains to adhere to one another noncovalently, it could be speculated that the protein product of this gene originally served to mediate some useful protein–protein interaction in—or, perhaps, cell–cell interactions among—the ancestral cells that expressed it. Over evolutionary time, this single progenitor gene appears to have been reduplicated many times at the DNA level, so that additional copies were produced at both nearby and distant chromosomal locations. The sequences of individual copies then diverged as a result of random mutations and natural selection. Every modern immunoglobulin light chain can thus be viewed as a tandemly duplicated descendant of the primordial domain, whereas heavy chains each represent four or five tandem variants of this domain.

The descendants of this hypothetical primordial domain can be found not only in immunoglobulins but also in many other types of proteins (Table 7–4). Although their sequences have diverged greatly, the single or multiple immunoglobulin-like domains in each of these proteins can be recognized by their size and three-dimensional shape, by the characteristic position of the intrachain disulfide bond, and by a few other conserved features. In recognition of their common ancestry, these proteins (or their corresponding genes) are known collectively as the **immunoglobulin gene superfamily.** Most, but not all, are integral

Table 7–4. The immunoglobulin gene superfamily.

Immunoglobulin heavy and light chains

T-cell receptor α, β, γ, and δ chains

CD3 complex γ, δ, and ε chains

MHC proteins: class I α and β_2-microglobulin, and class II α and β

T-cell differentiation antigens CD2, CD4, CD7, and CD8

B-cell signal transducers Ig-α and Ig-β

Costimulatory surface proteins (B7.1 and B7.2) and their receptor (CD28)

Fc receptor α chains: FcαRI, FcεRI, FcεRII (CD23), FcγRI (CD64), FcγRII (CD32), and FcγRIII (CD16)

Complement receptors: CR1 (CD35) and CR2 (CD21)

Adhesion proteins: VCAM-1 (CD106), ICAM-1 (CD54), ICAM-2 (CD102), LFA-3 (CD58), and NCAM

Other CD proteins: eg, CD1, CD5, CD19, CD22, CD31, CD33, CD48, and CD56

Cytokine receptors for IL-1, IL-6 family, M-CSF, G-CSF, stem cell factor (SCF), and platelet-derived growth factor (PDGF)

Poly-Ig receptor

Thy-1

Carcinoembryonic antigen

Myelin protein Po

Abbreviations: VCAM-1, vascular cell adhesion molecule type 1; ICAM-1 and -2, intercellular adhesion molecule types 1 and 2; LFA-3, leukocyte functional antigen type 3; NCAM, neural cell adhesion molecule.

membrane proteins. In any given member of this family, the immunoglobulin-like domains may be found in association with other unrelated types of domains that confer specialized activities, such as transmembrane signalling. Superfamily members are found at widely scattered chromosomal locations, are expressed in diverse cell types, and subserve many different functions, but in each case the immunoglobulin-like sequences appear to retain their ancestral function of interacting with other immunoglobulin-like domains in the same or other proteins.

ANTIBODY TECHNOLOGIES

The diversity and specificity of antibodies make them potentially invaluable reagents for diagnostics and research. Early serologists discovered, for example, that **antiserum** from an animal immunized against a particular microbe could be used to detect that microbe in blood or tissue specimens to diagnose infections. Even today, antisera raised in this way against snake venom proteins are widely used to treat snake bites, and antisera against human T cells have been used to suppress rejection of transplanted tissues. But this approach has serious limitations: even when a well-defined immunogen is used, the antiserum obtained is a complex mixture of structurally diverse antibodies recognizing multiple epitopes on

the immunogen, and its composition fluctuates unpredictably over the life of the animal. Moreover, the supply of antiserum from any single animal is limited, and there is no way of ensuring that antiserum obtained from a different animal would have identical properties.

To harness the full potential of antibodies, it was necessary to devise a way of obtaining abundant, pure preparations of homogeneous immunoglobulin directed against any desired antigen. This was first accomplished in 1975 by Kohler and Milstein, who discovered that fusing a normal B cell with an immortal, malignant plasma cell could give rise to a hybrid cell line that proliferated indefinitely while secreting the immunoglobulin encoded by the parental B cell. An immortal, antibody-producing clone of hybrids obtained in this way is called a **hybridoma,** and the antibody it produces is termed a **monoclonal antibody.** The production of hybridomas (Fig 7–7) is now routine and typically uses one of several mouse plasma cell lines developed for this purpose that do not express immunoglobulins of their own, so that any hybrids they form secrete only antibodies derived from the B-cell parent. First, a mouse is immunized with the target antigen in order to maximize the number of cognate B cells, and a single-cell suspension of its splenic cells is then combined with plasma cells in the presence of an agent that induces cell fusion. The mixture is next treated with a combination of antibiotics that selectively kill the parental plasma cells but not B cells or hybrids. Because any unfused B cells have a short life span in culture, the only proliferating cells that remain after a few weeks are hybrids, whose nuclei contain a mixture of chromosomes from both parents in varying proportions. These can then be grown as individual clones and screened to identify those that secrete antibody with the desired properties, which can then be produced in large quantities by propagating the hybridoma in culture or in animals.

Monoclonal antibodies have revolutionized the study of immunology and cell biology and have found numerous applications in diagnosis (see Chapter 14). They are also being explored as tools for clinical imaging and therapy, especially in cancer. For example, certain radioactively labeled monoclonal antibodies that recognize tumor surface antigens can, if injected into the bloodstream, home to the tumor and reveal its location by radioactive emission. Similarly, monoclonal antibodies coupled to toxins such as ricin or diphtheria toxin (forming a so-called **immunotoxin**) have shown some promise as antitumor chemotherapeutic agents capable of targeting toxin activity specifically to tumor cells. Unfortunately, the use of mouse monoclonal antibodies in humans is often limited by their immunogenicity, and it can be technically difficult to obtain the immunized human B cells needed to produce useful human hybridomas. One possible solution is to isolate the heavy- and light-chain genes encoding a murine antibody of in-

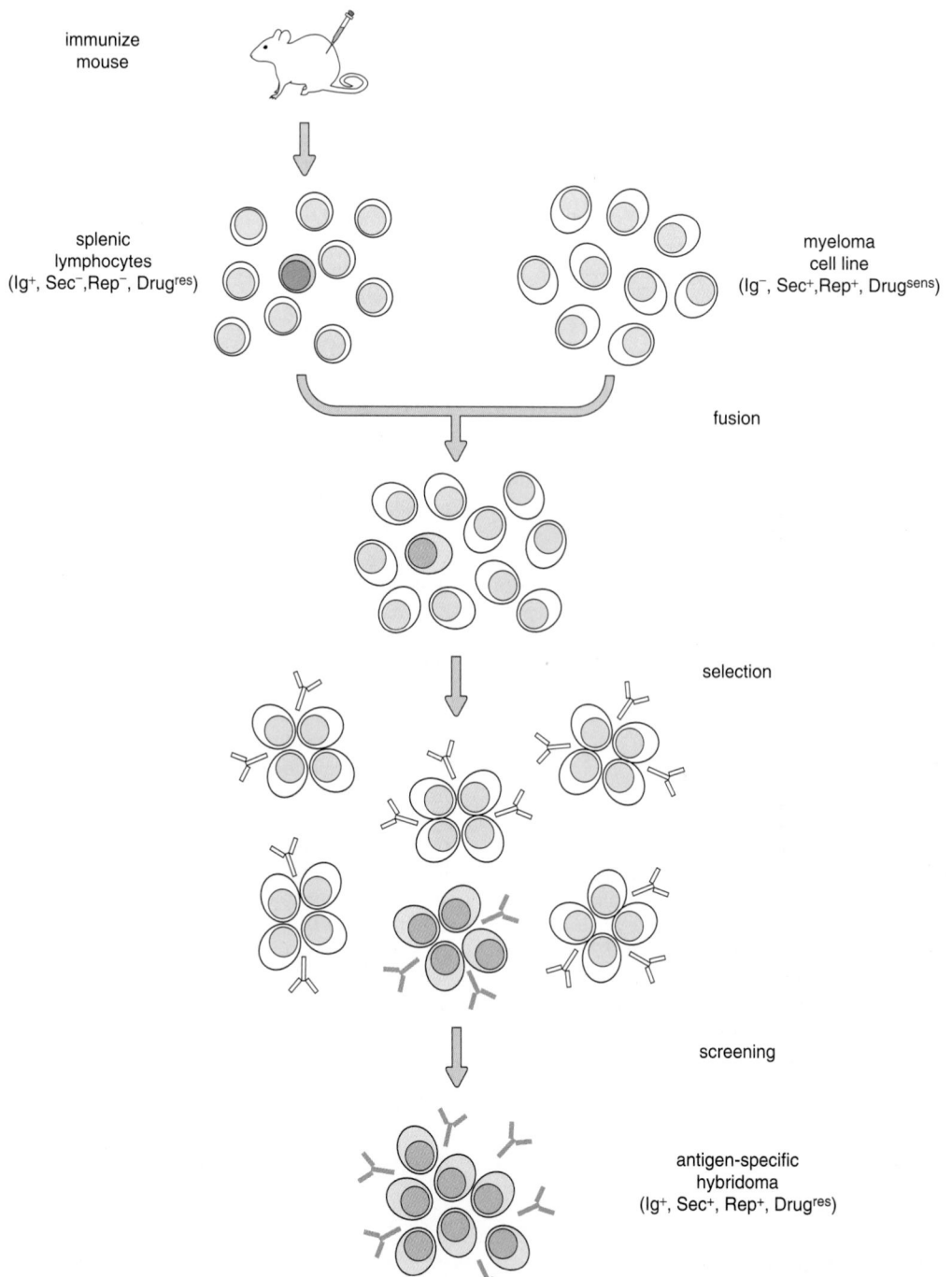

immunize
mouse

splenic
lymphocytes
(Ig^+, Sec^-, Rep^-, $Drug^{res}$)

myeloma
cell line
(Ig^-, Sec^+, Rep^+, $Drug^{sens}$)

fusion

selection

screening

antigen-specific
hybridoma
(Ig^+, Sec^+, Rep^+, $Drug^{res}$)

Figure 7–7. Preparation of an antigen-specific mouse hybridoma. A mouse is immunized with the antigen of interest, and its splenocytes are isolated as a source of B cells, a few of which (in dark blue) express surface immunoglobulin (Ig) specific for the antigen. The B cells express Ig but do not secrete it and cannot replicate in cell culture (ie, they are Ig^+, Sec^-, Rep^-). The splenocytes are fused with a myeloma cell line that replicates actively in culture and has an intact secretory apparatus but does not express endogenous Ig (ie, it is Ig^-, Sec^+, Rep^+). The myeloma cells also carry a mutation ($Drug^{sens}$) that makes them vulnerable to killing by a drug or other conditions to which the normal B cells are resistant ($Drug^{res}$). The B cells and myeloma cells are fused in vitro to produce hybrid cells carrying chromosomes from both parental cells together in a single nucleus. The mixed population that results from this fusion also includes a few unfused parental cells of each type. The population is exposed to the drug for two weeks or more, which kills any unfused myeloma cells ($Drug^{sens}$). Unfused B cells (Rep^-) also die during this time, so that the only proliferating cells that remain are hybrids with features of both parents (Rep^+, $Drug^{res}$). These are then grown as individual clones and screened to identify those that secrete antibody with the desired specificity. The antigen-specific hybridomas identified in this way can be grown indefinitely in culture or as ascites tumors and produce a limitless supply of the desired monoclonal antibody.

terest, use recombinant DNA techniques to alter their C-region sequences to encode proteins that more closely resemble a human antibody, and then reintroduce this **humanized** antibody gene into a plasma cell for expression.

Antibody diversity can also be exploited for less obvious purposes. For example, certain V regions have been found to have enzymatic activity, in that they can catalyze specific organic chemical reactions. As is true of other enzymes, such **catalytic antibodies** generally have affinity for a transition state intermediate along the reaction pathway, and deliberate immunization with a transition-state analog offers one approach to obtaining monoclonal antibodies that promote a particular reaction. But catalytic antibodies also occur spontaneously; among the anti-DNA antibodies produced by patients with autoimmune disorders, for example, one can identify rare antibodies that catalyze cleavage of the DNA strand! Though the study of catalytic antibodies is in its infancy, the range of reactions they can catalyze is already surprisingly broad, and it appears likely they will find many industrial and research applications.

Fc RECEPTORS

Many cell types are able to bind circulating antibodies or antigen–antibody complexes using surface **Fc receptors.** The physiologic function of these receptors varies among cell types. Receptors specific for each of the heavy-chain classes are thought to exist, but only those for γ and ε have been characterized at the molecular level. Three types of Fcγ receptors and two types of Fcε receptors can be distinguished based on their binding affinities, which differ from one another by one or two orders of magnitude (Table 7–5). Moreover, humans express up to three structurally different forms of a given Fcγ receptor, each encoded by a separate gene on chromosome 1, and each with a characteristic tissue distribution and biologic activity. Some of these receptors consist only of a single ligand-binding (α) polypeptide, but others are complexes containing an α subunit along with the CD3-γ or -ζ chains (or both). These are the same CD3-γ and -ζ polypeptides that form part of the antigen-receptor complex in T cells (see Chapters 3 and 9), and they serve an identical function in transducing signals from the Fc receptors into the cell interior. FcεRI also includes CD3-γ, as well as a unique signal-transducing β chain.

Only the high-affinity receptors of each type (FcγRI and FcεRI) are able to bind monomeric immunoglobulins to a significant degree at the concentrations normally found in the blood. Cells that express these high-affinity Fc receptors can therefore adsorb circulating antibodies onto their surfaces, where they may function as antigen receptors. For example, binding of unliganded IgG molecules onto FcγRI receptors on macrophages or natural killer cells serves to "arm" these cells to carry out **antibody-dependent cellular cytotoxicity (ADCC)** (Chapter 4). On the other hand, antigen binding to FcεRI-associated IgE on the surface of a basophil or mast cell can stimulate these cells to degranulate, producing symptoms of **allergy** (see Chapter 12). There is some evidence that people who inherit particular sequence variants of the FcεRI β-chain gene are predisposed to developing allergies, though this finding remains controversial.

Cells that carry only the low-affinity Fc receptors (FcγRII, FcγRIII, and FcεRII) cannot adsorb appreciable amounts of free antibody but instead bind their cognate immunoglobulin only in antigen–antibody complexes, where its effective concentration is increased. Binding of such multivalent complexes also serves to cross-link the Fc receptors and transmit signals into the cell. Interactions of this type are responsible for facilitating phagocytosis through the phenomenon of **opsonization** (Chapter 2) and are also important for triggering chemotaxis and degranulation in neutrophils and other phagocytes. In addition, low-affinity Fc receptors on B-lymphoid cells enable these cells to sense the presence of antigen–antibody

Table 7–5. Properties of human Fc receptors.

	Associated Markers[1]	Affinity (Kd)	Relative Subclass Preference	Cell Type Distribution
IgG receptors				
FcγRI	CD64	10^{-8}M	IgG1 = IgG3 > IgG4	Monocytes, macrophages.
FcγRII	CD32	10^{-7}M	IgG1 = IgG3 > IgG2	Monocytes, macrophages, neutrophils, eosinophils, B lymphocytes.
FcγRIII	CD16	10^{-6}M	IgG1 = IgG3	Macrophages, neutrophils, eosinophils, NK cells.
IgE receptors				
FcεRI	—	10^{-9}M	—	Mast cells, basophils.
FcεRII	CD23	10^{-7}M	—	Eosinophils, monocytes, macrophages, platelets, some T and B cells.

Abbreviation: NK, natural killer (see Chapter 9).
[1] CD designations generally apply only to the ligand-binding (α) chains of these receptors.

complexes, providing an important feedback-signalling pathway that limits further antibody production in the late stages of an immune response (see Chapter 8).

IMMUNOGLOBULIN GENES

Immunoglobulin Genes Are Formed Through DNA Rearrangement in B Cells

To contend with the almost unlimited variety of antigens that it may encounter, the human immune system is able to produce an estimated 10^8 different antibody molecules, each with a unique specificity for antigen. How can so many different antibody proteins be encoded in the genes of every human being? The antigen specificity of an antibody is determined by amino acid sequences within its paired heavy- and light-chain variable domains, which together form the antigen-binding site. To produce antibodies with many different specificities, the immune system must have the genetic capability to produce a very large number of different variable domain sequences. The sequence of the constant region, on the other hand, is generally the same for all heavy or light chains of a given immunoglobulin class and has no effect on antigen specificity. In fact, the entire family of immunoglobulin proteins consists of a relatively small number of different constant region domains linked in various combinations with an almost unlimited assortment of variable region sequences. In 1965, Dreyer and Bennett first recognized that these interchangeable combinations of protein domains must be the result of an active reshuffling of gene fragments that took place within the B-cell chromosomes. This was a revolutionary insight, because it implied that a cell could efficiently manipulate its chromosomes to change the structure of genes that it had inherited. And yet this proved to be only a part of the story: nearly a decade later, Susumu Tonegawa made the astonishing discovery that the inherited chromosomes contain no immunoglobulin genes at all, but only the building blocks from which these genes can be assembled. Since that time, studies by many investigators have revealed in detail the extraordinary process through which a B-cell precursor assembles an immunoglobulin gene.

As with most human genes, the information that codes for an immunoglobulin protein is dispersed along the DNA strand in multiple coding segments (**exons**) that are separated by regions of noncoding DNA (**introns**); after the gene is transcribed into RNA, introns are removed from the transcript and the exons are joined together by RNA splicing. Unlike nearly all other genes, however, the immunoglobulin DNA sequences that are found in germ cells or other nonlymphoid cell types do not exist as intact, functional genes. This is because the exons that code for variable domains are normally broken up along the chromosome into still smaller gene segments; these segments each lack some of the features needed for proper RNA splicing and so cannot function individually as exons. Before a developing B cell can begin to synthesize immunoglobulin, it must first fuse two or three of these gene segments together to assemble a complete variable region exon. This fusion of gene segments is achieved through a highly specialized process that requires cutting, rearrangement, and rejoining of the chromosomal DNA strands. Only developing lymphocytes possess the enzymatic machinery that is needed to carry out this process of immunoglobulin gene rearrangement.

Light-Chain Genes. The kappa light-chain genes are simplest and are therefore considered first. All of the genetic information needed to produce kappa chains lies within a single locus on chromosome 2 (Fig 7–8). The constant domain of the protein (amino acid residues 109–214) is encoded by an exon called C_κ, and only one copy of this exon is found on the chromosome. The sequence encoding any given variable domain, however, is contained in two separate gene segments called the variable (V_κ) and joining (J_κ) segments. The V_κ segment encodes approximately the first 95 amino acids of the variable domain; the shorter J_κ segment codes for the remaining 13 (amino acids 96–108). In contrast to the single C_κ exon, multiple V_κ and J_κ segments are present, each with a somewhat different DNA sequence. The five J_κ segments are clustered together near the C_κ exon, whereas approximately

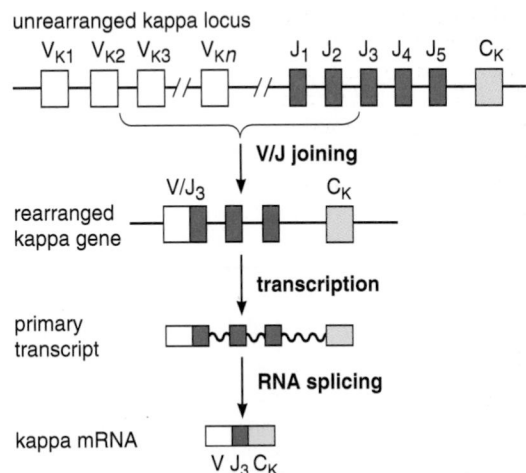

Figure 7–8. Assembly and expression of the κ light-chain locus. A DNA rearrangement event fuses one V segment (in this example, $V_{\kappa2}$) to one J segment ($J_{\kappa3}$) to form a single exon. The V/J exon is then transcribed together with the unique C_κ exon, and the transcript is spliced to form mature κ mRNA. Note that any unrearranged J segments on the primary transcript are removed as part of the intron during RNA splicing.

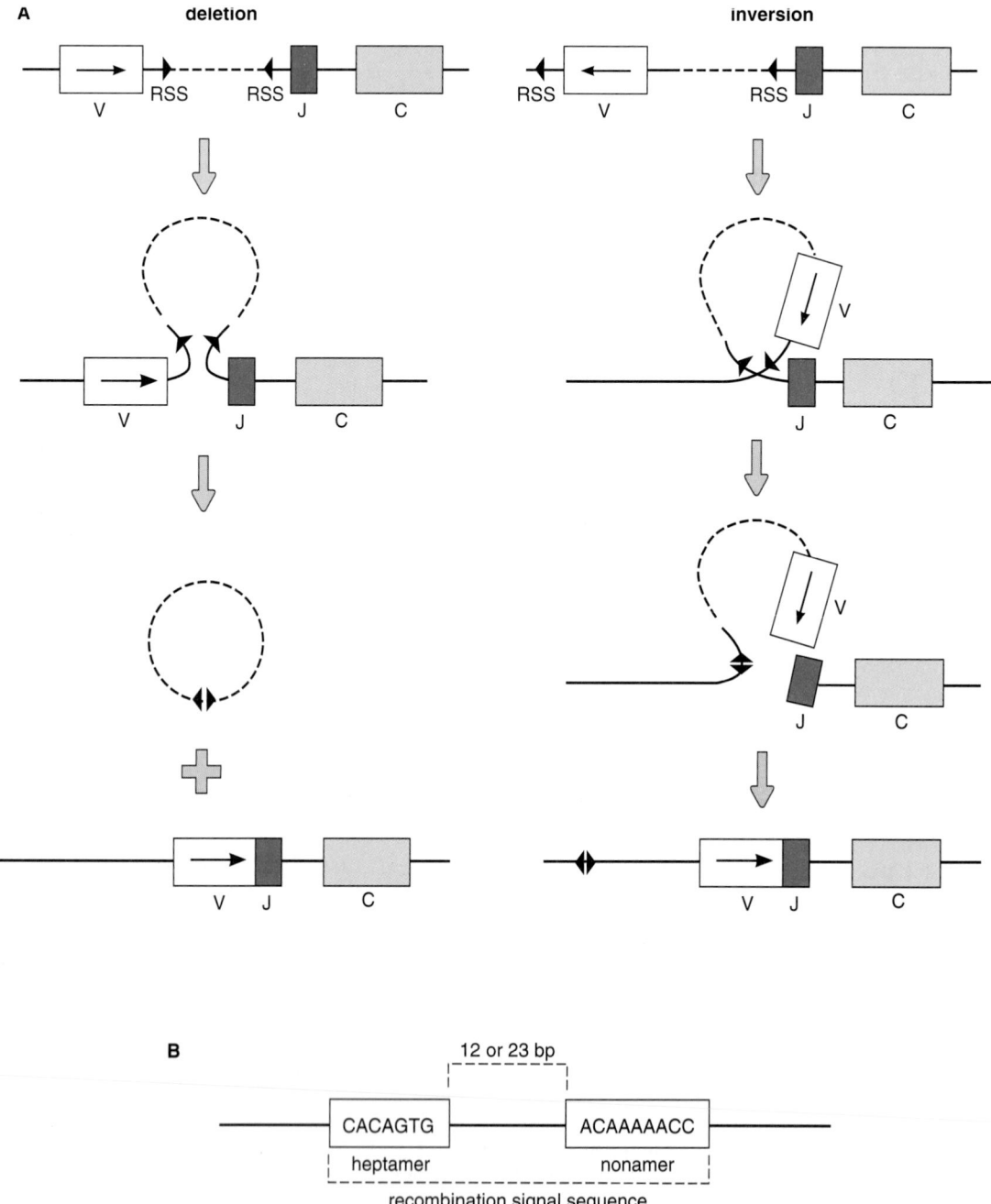

Figure 7–9. Mechanism of immunoglobulin κ gene rearrangement. *A:* Site-specific cleavage and religation of the chromosomal DNA is guided by a pair of recombination signal sequences (RSS) flanking V and J gene segments. The chromosome segment undergoes either deletion *(left)* or inversion *(right),* depending on the original orientation of the V segment with respect to the J and C segments. If deletion occurs, the DNA that originally separated V and J is released as a covalently closed circle and subsequently is degraded. *B:* The RSS, consisting of a pair of short DNA sequences (heptamer and nonamer) separated by either 12 or 23 base pairs (bp) of DNA, marks all sites of recombinase action in both heavy- and light-chain genes.

30–35 different V_κ segments lie scattered over a region that spans roughly 1 million base pairs (bp) of DNA (less than 1% of the length of chromosome 2). This wide separation between V_κ and J_κ segments is found in the DNA of all nonlymphoid cells. When an immature hematopoietic cell becomes committed to the B-lymphocyte lineage, however, it selects one V_κ and one J_κ segment and fuses these together. This process of **V/J joining** is accomplished by highly precise enzymatic manipulation of specific sites in the chromosomal DNA. In some instances, this involves precise deletion of all the DNA that normally separates the V_κ and J_κ segments; in others, the two segments are brought together by inverting a portion of the chromosomal strand with no overall loss of DNA (Fig 7–9). The result in either case is that the V_κ and J_κ segments become permanently and covalently joined to one another, side by side on the rearranged chromosome, to form a single continuous exon. Transcription can then begin at one end of the V_κ segment, and pass through both the fused V_κ/J_κ exon and the nearby C_κ exon. When transcribed together, these two exons contain all of the information needed to synthesize a particular kappa protein.

The organization of the kappa genes thus accounts for the unusual properties of this light-chain protein family. As there is only one C_κ exon, all kappa proteins must have identical constant region sequences. On the other hand, because the cell can choose from among many alternative V_κ and J_κ segments, and can join these together in various combinations, a large number of different variable domain sequences can result. For example, 30 V_κ and 5 J_κ segments could in theory give rise to ($30 \times 5 =$) 150 different variable domains. This reshuffling process, known as **combinatorial joining,** is the most important source of light-chain protein diversity.

Lambda light chains arise from a similar gene complex on chromosome 22. Joining of V_λ and J_λ segments occurs in a manner identical to that of the kappa segments. A given chromosome 22, however, may contain up to six slightly different copies of the C_λ exon (corresponding to various subtypes of lambda protein), each with a nearby J_λ segment. A V_λ segment (of which there are approximately 100) may fuse to any of these alternative J_λ segments, and the resulting

V_λ/J_λ exon can then be transcribed together with the adjacent C_λ exon. The B cell selects only one of the available J_λ segments for V/J joining, and in so doing determines which C_λ subtype will be expressed (Fig 7–10).

Heavy-Chain Genes. All immunoglobulin heavy chains are derived from a single region spanning 685,000 bp on chromosome 14 (Fig 7–11). Each heavy-chain constant region is encoded by a cluster of several short exons. The μ constant region, for example, is divided among five exons known collectively as the C_μ sequence. Constant region (C_H) sequences for each of the nine heavy-chain isotypes are arrayed in tandem along the chromosome in the following order: C_μ, C_δ, $C_{\gamma3}$, $C_{\gamma1}$, $C_{\alpha1}$, $C_\gamma2$, $C_\gamma4$, C_ε, $C_\alpha2$; only a single copy of each is present. The six J_H segments and approximately 65 V_H segments are arranged in a manner analogous to those of the kappa gene. In contrast to the light-chain genes, however, a third type of gene segment, called the diversity (D_H) segment, must also be used in forming a heavy-chain variable region. Several of these D_H segments (the exact number is unknown), each coding for two or three amino acids, lie between the J_H and V_H segments on the unrearranged chromosome. In assembling the heavy-chain gene, a B cell must complete two DNA rearrangement events, first bringing together one D_H and one J_H segment, and subsequently linking these to a V_H segment—a sequence termed **V/D/J joining.**

Use of the D_H segment greatly increases the amount of heavy-chain diversity that can be produced. For example, 65 V_H, 10 D_H, and 6 J_H segments could give rise to ($65 \times 10 \times 6 =$) 3900 different heavy-chain variable domains, and these, when combined with 150 kappa-chain variable domains, could form (150 × 3900 =) nearly *600,000* different antigen-binding sites! Even using a relatively small number of gene segments, then, the immune system can generate enormous antibody diversity through combinational joining.

Additional diversity of immunoglobulin variable regions arises because the V/(D)/J (that is, either V/J or V/D/J) rearrangement process is somewhat imprecise, so that the site at which one segment fuses with another can vary by a few nucleotides. As a result, the DNA coding sequence that remains at the junction be-

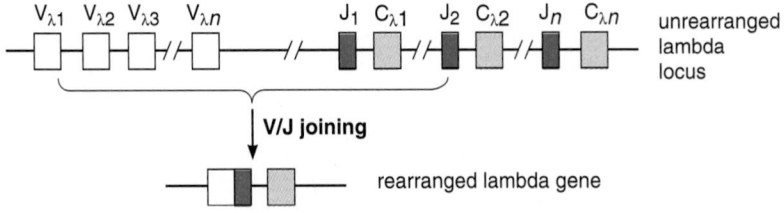

Figure 7–10. Assembly of a λ light-chain gene. An individual λ locus contains up to six alternative C_λ exons, each with a nearby J_λ segment. In this example, DNA rearrangement fuses $V_{\lambda1}$ with $J_{\lambda2}$; the resulting gene produces light chains that contain $C_{\lambda2}$.

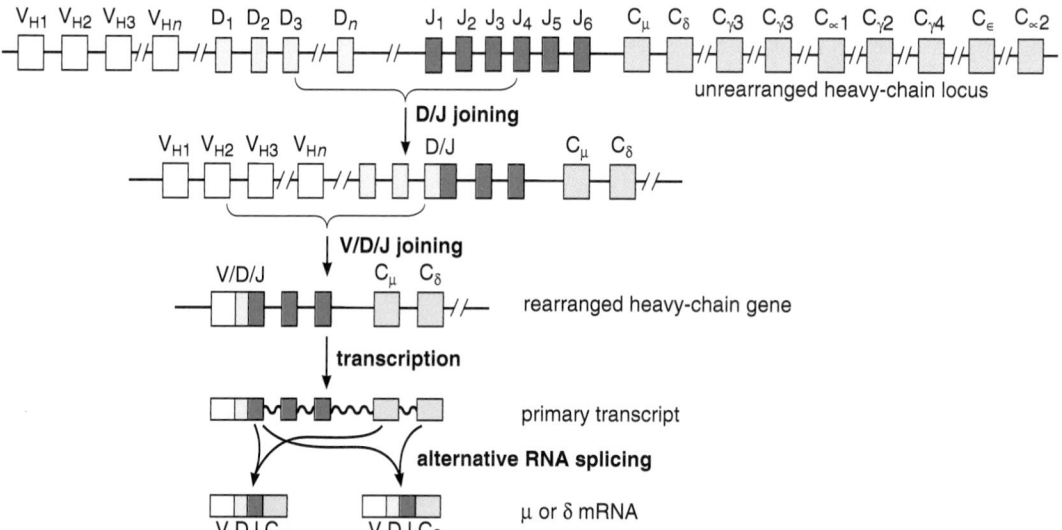

Figure 7–11. Rearrangement and expression of the heavy-chain locus. Unlike the light-chain genes, assembly of a heavy-chain V region exon requires two sequential DNA rearrangement events involving three different types of gene segments. The D_H and J_H segments are joined first and are then fused to a V_H segment. Nine alternative C-region sequences are present; of these, however, only C_μ and C_δ are initially transcribed. The primary transcript can be spliced in either of two ways to generate mRNAs that encode μ or δ heavy chains with identical V domains. This diagram is highly schematic: each C_H sequence is actually composed of multiple exons whose aggregate length is more than three times longer than that of the V/D/J exon.

tween any two segments can also vary. Moreover, during assembly of a heavy-chain gene (but not of light-chain genes), a few nucleotides of random sequence (called **N regions**) are often inserted at the points of joining between the V, D, and J segments; these insertions are carried out by **terminal deoxynucleotidyl transferase (TdT),** a nuclear enzyme that is expressed in immature lymphocytes. The variations in gene sequence that result from **imprecise joining** or from the insertion of N regions contribute substantially to overall antibody diversity. Moreover, these processes affect the sequences within each V/(D)/J exon that code for the **third hypervariable region (CDR3)** of the heavy- or light-chain variable domain; hence, the diversity they engender has a disproportionately strong effect on antigen specificity. At the same time, however, these processes greatly increase the risk that two segments may be joined in an improper translational reading frame, resulting in a nonfunctional gene. In practice, such unsuccessful rearrangements occur frequently and generally cannot be reversed or repaired; they represent a cost paid by the immune system in exchange for greater potential gene diversity.

In general, only the C_H region located immediately downstream of the V/D/J exon can be expressed. Because the V/D/J exon is originally assembled at a site adjacent to the C_μ locus, the gene always produces μ heavy chains when it is first rearranged. For this reason, virgin B lymphocytes always express IgM

on their surfaces. Expression of one of the other C_H regions can occur only after a cell becomes activated in the periphery, as is described in Chapter 8. One important exception to this rule is the C_δ sequence, which lies very near the C_μ region and is often transcribed along with the V/D/J and C_μ exons. This produces RNA that can be spliced to yield either μ or δ mRNA (see Fig 7–11) and so enables the cell simultaneously to express IgM and IgD antibodies that have identical variable domain sequences. Such coexpression of IgM and IgD on the surface membrane is a common phenotype of mature B lymphocytes.

The Molecular Basis of V/(D)/J Rearrangement

Active gene rearrangements of the type that produce V/(D)/J joining were first thought to be a unique property of the immunoglobulin genes. Subsequently, however, it was found that the genes encoding T-cell antigen receptors (TCRs) also are assembled from germline V, D, J, and C segments through a virtually identical series of DNA rearrangements (see Chapter 9). Among the similarities, for example, the rearrangement sites in both immunoglobulin and TCR genes always coincide with so-called **recombination signal sequences** (see Fig 7–9B)—a pair of short DNA sequences (7 and 9 bp long, respectively) that are located immediately adjacent to each unrearranged V, D, or J segment. It is now thought that rearrangement of both the immunoglobulin and TCR gene families is carried out by the same molecular machinery: a presumably complex system of enzymes and other proteins known collectively as the **V/(D)/J recombinase.** This term must be used loosely, however, as only a few of the proteins that carry out these rearrangements have been identified so far. The most important are two nuclear proteins called **RAG-1** and **RAG-2** (the products of recombination activating genes 1 and 2, respectively), which are expressed only in immature B- and T-lineage cells. Acting together, though perhaps with the help of other unknown cellular proteins, RAG-1 and RAG-2 have the ability to recognize and cleave DNA specifically at recombination signal sequences, suggesting that they are critical ingredients in these early steps of recombination. It appears likely that at least some of the later steps, such as religating the various gene segments together, are carried out by cellular enzymes that are also involved in more common types of DNA repair that occur in all cells.

V/(D)/J recombinase activity appears to be unique to B and T lymphoid cells: no other cell type has yet been proven to manipulate its chromosomes in this way. Moreover, recombinase activity is present only during the early phases of lymphoid development that take place within the lymphopoietic organs. By the time a virgin B cell emerges from the marrow, it has rearranged both its heavy- and light-chain genes and has forever lost the ability to perform further V/(D)/J rearrangements. The orderly manner in which the recombinase carries out its task defines the stages of B-cell ontogeny, as will be discussed in the following chapter.

Immunoglobulin Gene Rearrangements & B-Cell Malignancy

Apart from their role in generating antibody diversity, immunoglobulin gene rearrangements are gaining increasing importance in clinical diagnosis and research. Rearrangement of these genes can be detected in biopsies or blood specimens by using a technique known as the Southern blot, and their presence provides a highly sensitive and specific means of diagnosing lymphoid cancers (see Chapter 18). Perhaps more importantly, errors in immunoglobulin gene rearrangement are now thought to contribute to the genesis of several major types of leukemia and lymphoma. For example, the cells of **Burkitt's lymphoma,** a B-lymphocytic malignancy, usually contain a specific chromosomal abnormality called **t(8,14),** in which a portion of chromosome 8 has been translocated onto chromosome 14 (Fig 7–12). In this translocation, breakage of chromosome 14 occurs within the immunoglobulin heavy-chain locus, whereas the breakpoint on chromosome 8 coincides with a cellular protooncogene known as **c-*myc*,** which encodes the transcription factor c-Myc (see Chapter 1). As a result, the c-*myc* gene is moved to a position directly adjacent to the heavy-chain gene. It is thought

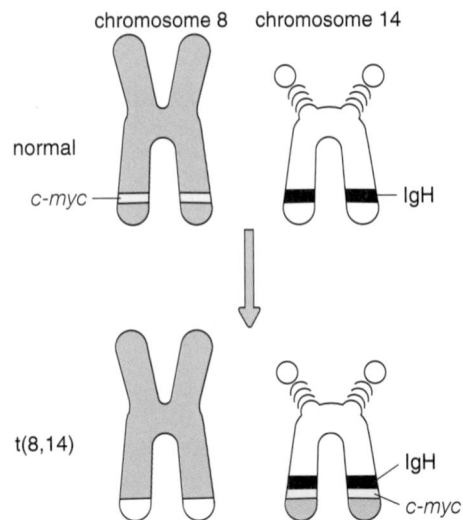

Figure 7–12. The t(8,14) chromosomal anomaly of Burkitt's lymphoma. A reciprocal translocation of genetic material exchanges the distal ends of the long arms of chromosomes 8 and 14. This transposes the c-*myc* protooncogene from chromosome 8 into the active immunoglobulin heavy-chain locus on chromosome 14 and contributes to the development of a malignancy.

that this proximity to the transcriptionally active heavy-chain locus alters the expression of the protooncogene, and that this, along with other damage to c-*myc* that can occur during translocation, contributes to malignant transformation. Less commonly, Burkitt's lymphoma may lack t(8,14) and instead exhibit a closely related anomaly in which the c-*myc* locus is translocated into the kappa or lambda light-chain gene on chromosomes 2 or 22, producing the same effects.

A similar type of chromosomal anomaly, designated **t(14,18),** is observed in at least 90% of cases of **follicular lymphoma**—the most common human B-cell malignancy. In this translocation, the gene on chromosome 18 that encodes the cytoplasmic membrane protein **Bcl-2** is moved to a position immediately adjacent to the heavy-chain locus on chromosome 14. B-cells carrying the t(14,18) anomaly express unusually high levels of structurally normal Bcl-2 protein and hence are resistant to being killed by many of the physiologic processes that normally induce apoptosis (Chapter 1). As a result, they tend to accumulate in great numbers and evolve into a malignancy (Chapter 46). In both t(14,18) and the Burkitt's anomalies, the chromosomal breakpoint in affected immunoglobulin loci occurs directly beside a J segment, which strongly implies that each of these translocations results in part from an error in immunoglobulin gene rearrangement.

REFERENCES

EARLY STUDIES OF IMMUNOGLOBULIN PROTEIN CHEMISTRY

Hilschmann N, Craig LC: Amino acid sequence studies with Bence Jones protein. *Proc Natl Acad Sci USA* 1965; **53**:1403.

Porter RR: Structural studies of immunoglobulins. *Science* 1973;**180**:713.

Wu TT, Kabat EA: An analysis of the variable regions of Bence Jones proteins and myeloma light chains and their implications for antibody complementarity. *J Exp Med* 1970;**132**:211.

IMMUNOGLOBULIN CHAINS & RELATED POLYPEPTIDES

Kehry M et al: The immunoglobulin μ chains of membrane-bound and secreted IgM molecules differ in their C-terminal segments. *Cell* 1980;**21**:393.

Koshland ME: The coming of age of the immunoglobulin J chain. *Ann Rev Immunol* 1985;**3**:425.

Natvig JB, Kunkel HG: Immunoglobulins: Classes, subclasses, genetic variants, and idiotypes. *Adv Immunol* 1973;**16**:1.

BIOLOGICAL PROPERTIES OF IMMUNOGLOBULINS

Blattner FR, Tucker PW: The molecular biology of immunoglobulin D. *Nature* 1984;**307**:417.

Spiegelberg HL: Biological activities of immunoglobulins of different classes and subclasses. *Adv Immunol* 1974;**19**:259.

ANTIBODY STRUCTURE

Alzari PN et al: Three-dimensional structure of antibodies. *Ann Rev Immunol* 1988;**6**:555.

Amit AG et al: Three-dimensional structure of an antigen–antibody complex at 2.8 Å resolution. *Science* 1986;**233**:747.

Colman PM: Structure of antibody–antigen complexes: Implications for immune recognition. *Adv Immunol* 1988;**43**:99.

Davie JM et al: Structural correlates of idiotypes. *Ann Rev Immunol* 1986;**4**:147.

Davies DR, Padlan EA: Antibody–antigen complexes. *Ann Rev Biochem* 1990;**59**:439.

ANTIBODY TECHNOLOGIES

Morrison SL: In vitro antibodies: Strategies for production and application. *Ann Rev Immunol* 1992;**10**:239.

Kohler G, Milstein C: Continuous cultures of fused cells secreting antibody of predefined specificity. *Nature* 1975;**256**:495.

Lerner RA et al: At the crossroads of chemistry and immunology: Catalytic antibodies. *Science* 1991;**252**:659.

Schultz PG, Lerner RA: From molecular diversity to catalysis: Lessons from the immune system. *Science* 1995; **269**:1835.

IMMUNOGLOBULIN SUPERGENE FAMILY

Hunkapiller T, Hood L: Diversity of the immunoglobulin gene superfamily. *Adv Immunol* 1989;**44**:1.

Williams AF, Barclay AN: The immunoglobulin superfamily—domains for cell surface recognition. *Ann Rev Immunol* 1988;**6**:381.

Fc RECEPTORS

Ravetch JV, Kinet J-P: Fc Receptors. *Ann Rev Immunol* 1991;**9**:457.

Ravetch JV: Fc receptors: Rubor redux. *Cell* 1994;**78**:553.

IMMUNOGLOBULIN GENE ORGANIZATION & REARRANGEMENTS

Dreyer WJ, Bennett JC: The molecular basis of antibody formations: A paradox. *Proc Natl Acad Sci USA* 1965;**54**:864.

Honjo T et al (editors): *Immunoglobulin Genes*. Academic Press, 1989.

Rowen L et al: The complete 685-kilobase DNA sequence of the human β T cell receptor locus. *Science* 1996; **272**:1755.

Tonegawa S: Somatic generation of antibody diversity. *Nature* 1983;**302**:575.

V(D)J RECOMBINASE

Akira SJ et al: Two pairs of recombination signals are sufficient to cause immunoglobulin V-(D)-J joining. *Science* 1987;**238**:1134.

Gellert M: Molecular analysis of V(D)J recombination. *Ann Rev Genetics* 1992;**26**:425.

Lewis SM: The mechanism of V(D)J joining: Lessons from molecular, immunological, and comparative analyses. *Adv Immunol* 1994;**56**:27.

Schatz D et al: V(D)J recombination: Molecular biology and regulation. *Ann Rev Immunol* 1992;**10**:359.

OTHER SOURCES OF ANTIBODY DIVERSITY

French DL et al: The role of somatic hypermutation in the generation of antibody diversity. *Science* 1989;**244**:1152.

Komori T et al: Lack of N regions in antigen receptor variable region genes of TdT-deficient lymphocytes. *Science* 1993;**261**:1171.

Max EE et al: Variation in the crossover point of kappa immunoglobulin gene V-J recombination: Evidence from a cryptic gene. *Cell* 1980;**21**:793.

CHROMOSOMAL TRANSLOCATIONS IN LYMPHOID NEOPLASIA

Croce CM, Nowell PC: Molecular basis of human B cell neoplasia. *Blood* 1985;**65**:1.

Korsmeyer SJ: Chromosomal translocations in lymphoid malignancies reveal novel proto-oncogenes. *Ann Rev Immunol* 1992;**10**:785.

B-Cell Development & the Humoral Immune Response

8

Anthony L. DeFranco, PhD

The clonal selection theory, formulated by Burnet in the 1950s to explain the specificity of immune responses, postulates that each of the cells that make antibodies—the B lymphocytes—makes only antibodies of a single specificity and, moreover, that antigen selectively induces the expansion of those cells that can make antibody against it. This theory was soon expanded to account for the fact that the immune system normally makes antibodies to foreign entities but not to self-components. In subsequent years, a great deal has been learned about B lymphocytes and how they participate in immune responses. The tenets of the clonal selection theory have been upheld, and the molecular mechanisms by which it occurs are now largely understood. In this chapter, we consider the mechanisms by which B lymphocytes develop from precursors and how these mechanisms ensure that each B cell makes a unique antibody molecule. This, in turn, forms the basis for clonal selection. We then consider how antigen induces an immune response from the appropriate B cells and the role of helper T cells in this process, as well as the mechanisms by which B-cell responses are diversified to give different classes of immunoglobulin (IgM, IgG, etc) and to maximize the affinities of the antibodies produced. Finally, we review what is known about the mechanisms that act to prevent B-cell immune responses directed against self.

B-LYMPHOCYTE ONTOGENY

THE GENERATION OF B LYMPHOCYTES

Development of B cells from hematopoietic stem cells occurs in the bone marrow. In humans, approximately 10^9 B cells are generated each day. Their development proceeds through a series of distinct stages that are accompanied, and in many cases defined, by the DNA rearrangements that assemble their immunoglobulin genes. These rearrangements occur in a strict developmental sequence (Fig 8–1). The first rearrangements take place in a population of mitotically active bone marrow cells, sometimes referred to as **pro-B cells,** which are the most primitive recognizable cells in the B lineage. These cells express the surface proteins CD10 and CD19, as well as the nuclear proteins terminal deoxynucleotidyl transferase (TdT), RAG-1, and RAG-2 (Fig 8–2). These latter proteins play important roles in V/D/J recombination as described in Chapter 7.

The first rearrangement that occurs in a pro-B cell is the joining of D_H and J_H segments in the heavy-chain genes. This occurs on both copies of chromosome 14 in virtually all developing B cells. The cell then joins a V_H segment to the fused D_H/J_H segment on one of its two chromosomes. If this first attempt yields a functional gene in which the V and J regions are linked in such a way that they can be translated in the same reading frame of the genetic code and hence produce a functional protein, the cell (for reasons that will be discussed presently) carries out no further rearrangements of its other heavy-chain locus. If, on the other hand, the first rearrangement fails, a second attempt at V/D/J assembly is made using the other chromosome 14. Because of the error-prone nature of V/D/J joining, about 50% of pro-B cells fail at both tries to produce a functional heavy-chain gene; unable to proceed further through the maturation pathway, these cells simply die in the marrow.

Successful V/D/J rearrangement on either chromosome allows the cell immediately to begin synthesizing heavy-chain proteins. The heavy chains produced at this stage are all of the μ isotype and have a short hydrophobic region at their carboxy termini that causes them to integrate into cellular membranes.

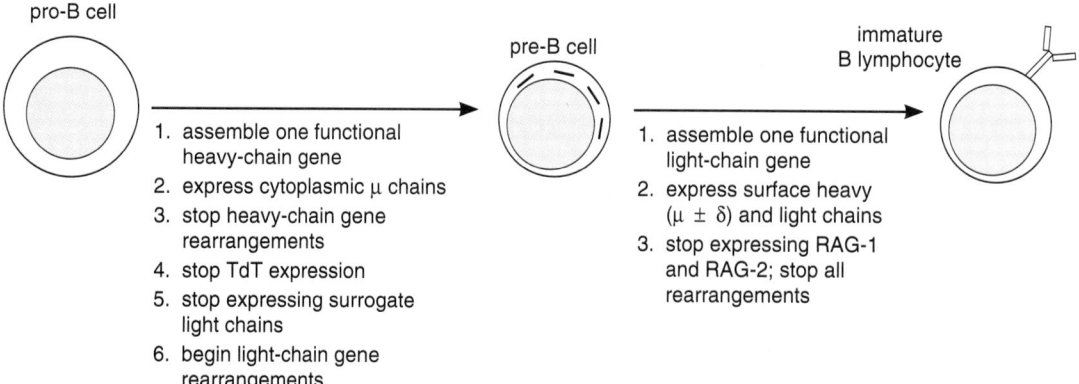

Figure 8–1. Major genetic events in early B-cell ontogeny. Listed are the sequences of events that occur in progressing from each stage of development to the next. Note that the ability to perform V/(D)/J rearrangements is lost by the time the cell becomes an immature B lymphocyte.

This membrane-associated form of μ protein is called **μm.** Heavy chains ordinarily cannot be transported to the cell surface unless they are complexed with light chains. Pro-B cells express two proteins, known as **surrogate light chains,** that can bind to heavy chains, take the place of light chains, and be displayed transiently on the surface membranes of these immature cells. The surrogate light chains are not true immunoglobulin proteins; they are expressed only in primitive B-cell precursors, are derived from genes that do not undergo somatic rearrangement, and have no role in immune responses per se. Nevertheless, they are essential for regulating early B-cell development. When the $μ_m$ and surrogate light-chain proteins reach the cell surface, they are believed to transmit a signal back into the cell, perhaps after contacting some unknown ligand. In effect, this signal notifies the cell that it has produced a functional heavy-chain protein. In response, the cell permanently halts any further rearrangements of its heavy-chain genes and stops expressing TdT. At about the same time, the cell gains the ability to rearrange its light-chain genes. This shift from heavy-chain to light-chain rearrangements does not appear to be due to changes in the recombinase machinery itself, but rather to changes in accessibility of the various immunoglobulin loci on the chromosomes, and is probably mediated by many of the same proteins that control transcription of these genes. Once the developing B cell expresses $μ_m$, it also ceases to synthesize new surrogate light chains, so that the temporary signaling complex soon disappears from the cell surface. The $μ_m$ chain now lacking a light-chain partner is trapped in the endoplasmic reticulum at this stage. These events mark the transition into the next phase of ontogeny, known as pre-B cell stage (see Fig 8–1).

Pre-B cells are defined as cells that do not yet express immunoglobulin light chains but contain $μ_m$ heavy chains intracellularly (Figs 8–1 and 8–2). They

are found almost exclusively in the bone marrow and represent a transient phase in B-cell development that lasts for about two days. Interestingly, generation of pre-B cells is deficient in a fairly common hereditary immunodeficiency disease known as **X-linked agammaglobulinemia,** or Bruton's agammaglobulinemia. The defect in this disorder is in the gene encoding an intracellular protein tyrosine kinase, called **Btk.** Although the exact role of Btk in B-cell development is not understood, its absence leads to decreased maturation of pro-B cells to pre-B cells and also to a reduction in subsequent steps in B-cell development. As a result, there are very few B cells in these patients and they make little or no antibody.

On entering the pre-B-cell phase, the B-cell precursors divide several times in response to interleukin 7 (IL-7) produced locally by bone marrow stromal cells. Pre-B cells then cease dividing and do not resume mitosis until they have become fully mature and encounter antigen in the periphery. The most important event taking place in pre-B cells is the rearrangement of light-chain genes, which begins only after heavy-chain rearrangements have ceased. Because TdT is no longer expressed, no N-region nucleotides are inserted as the light-chain genes rearrange. V/J joining is attempted on each chromosome 2 or 22 in succession, until a functional κ or λ gene is produced. As soon as either type of light-chain protein appears, it associates with the existing $μ_m$ heavy chains, and the resulting four-chain units are transported to the cell surface as membrane IgM. At that moment, the cell enters the B-lymphocyte stage of development and ordinarily loses the ability to perform additional V/J rearrangements because RAG-1 and RAG-2 expression ceases. It seems likely that the signal to shut off the recombinase is sent by the IgM molecules themselves when they first reach the cell surface.

The successful assembly of a single heavy- or light-

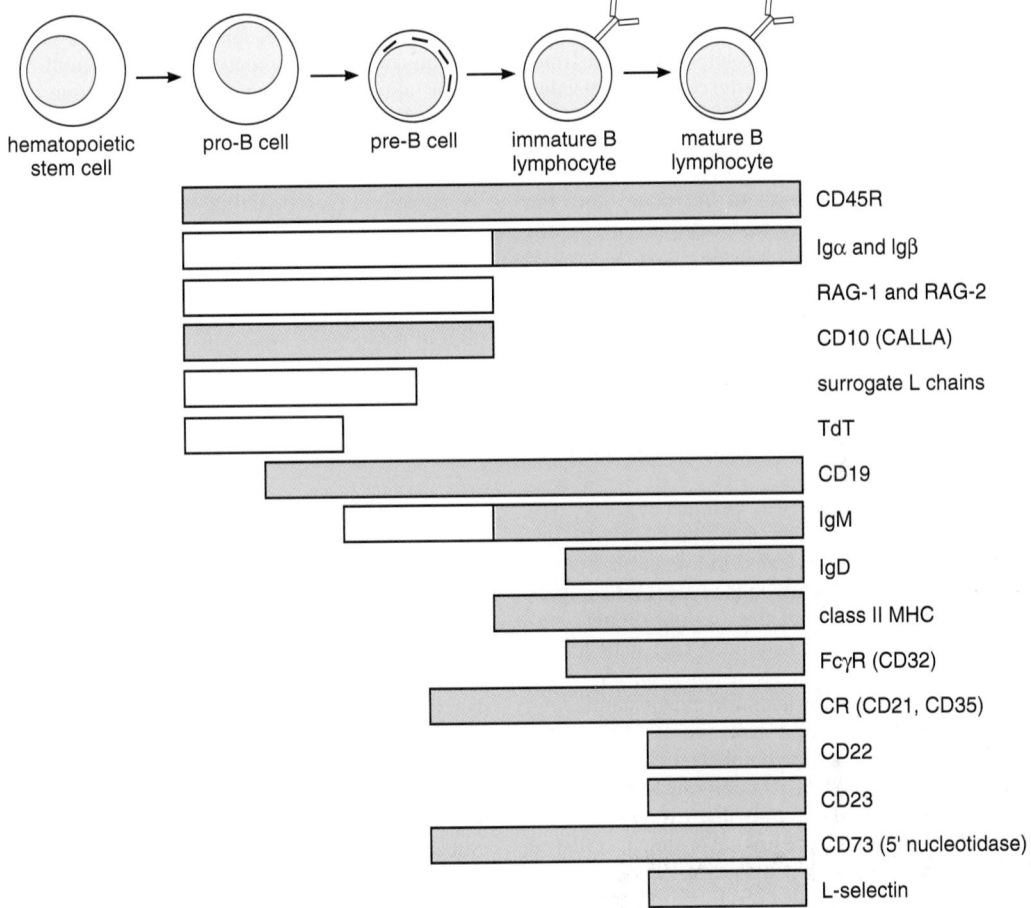

Figure 8–2. Expression of selected marker proteins at various stages of B-cell development. Open bars indicate that a protein is expressed only within the cytoplasm of a cell; filled bars indicate surface expression. CR = complement receptors.

chain gene prevents all other genes of that type from undergoing rearrangement in the same cell. Consequently, only one heavy-chain and one light-chain gene can give rise to protein in any individual B lymphocyte—a phenomenon termed **allelic and isotypic exclusion.** If the lymphocyte subsequently divides in the periphery, chromosomes bearing the active rearranged genes are passed on to its progeny, and the daughter cells continue to express these genes without performing further V/J or V/D/J rearrangements. For this reason, all of the immunoglobulin molecules produced by a given B lymphocyte and its progeny have identical antigen specificity and light-chain type (κ or λ). This is the molecular basis of the phenomenon known as **clonal restriction** (Chapter 4). The diversity of antibody molecules produced by the immune system as a whole reflects the fact that innumerable B-cell precursors each rearrange their genes independently and in different combinations, resulting in a large assortment of clones that each possess a unique specificity for antigen.

MATURATION & RELEASE OF VIRGIN B LYMPHOCYTES

The moment it begins to express surface IgM, a cell is considered to have become a B lymphocyte. Nevertheless, it is not yet ready to exit the bone marrow or to participate in immune responses. Instead, such **immature B lymphocytes** remain in the marrow for another one to three days before maturing further and exiting the bone marrow. During this time, the cells acquire additional surface molecules that distinguish them as **mature B lymphocytes** (see Fig 8–2). One such marker is surface **IgD,** which, as noted in Chapter 7, is produced by alternative splicing of some of the RNA transcripts arising from the rearranged heavy-chain gene. The IgM and IgD on any individual lymphocyte both incorporate the same light chains and have identical antigen specificity. Other surface markers that appear on mature B lymphocytes include complement receptors (CR1 and CR2, the latter also known as CD21); a membrane-anchored enzyme called **5'-nucleotidase (CD73),** whose function is unknown; the lectin-like oligosaccharide-binding protein **CD23;** and the adhesion proteins **leukocyte functional antigen-1 (LFA-1), intercellular adhesion molecule-1 (ICAM-1),** and **CD22.** Individual cells also begin to express surface-homing receptors, such as **L-selectin,** which targets them to lymph nodes or other peripheral sites. At about the same time, the cells acquire **class II major histocompatibility complex (MHC)** proteins, which enable them to present antigens to helper T cells, and they also begin surface expression of **CD40**—a protein involved in receiving T-cell help (see later discussion). With the acquisition of these various accessory molecules, the mature lymphocytes become competent for immunologic function. They are then released from the bone marrow to disseminate through the bloodstream and colonize secondary lymphoid organs.

The developmental pathway outlined earlier is typical of the B-cell population as a whole but does not apply strictly to all of its cells. Individual B-lineage cells may differ significantly in the types and amounts of surface markers they express or the sequence in which these markers are acquired. This may reflect the existence of functionally distinct subsets of B cells. Indeed, there is considerable circumstantial evidence for the existence of distinct subsets. At present, however, only two types of B cells are clearly recognizable: the "conventional" B cells and a small, enigmatic subpopulation of B cells that express on their surface CD5—a protein of unknown function that is also expressed on most T lymphocytes. These **CD5 B cells** are long-lived cells that are found principally in the peritoneal cavity and appear to be derived from precursor cells that are present in infant but not adult bone marrow. As these B cells arise soon after birth, they are the major source of antibody production in young individuals. The heavy-chain gene rearrangements of these B cells principally involve a few V_H genes near the D_H and J_H gene segments and often lack N regions. Thus, these B cells have a less diverse antibody repertoire than do the B cells that dominate mature individuals. No unique immunologic function has yet been assigned to CD5 B cells, although they may be especially important for T-cell-independent antibody responses such as those directed at antigens of bacterial cell walls (see next section). Curiously, CD5 B cells are disproportionately more likely than other B cells to produce autoreactive immunoglobulins (that is, antibodies that recognize determinants in host tissues). Remarkably, the malignant cells in nearly all cases of human B-cell **chronic lymphocytic leukemia** carry the CD5 marker, suggesting that this malignancy arises from the CD5 B cell subpopulation.

Production of virgin B lymphocytes occurs continually in the bone marrow and independently of exogenous antigens. The marrow of an adult releases approximately 1 billion virgin B cells into the circulation each day regardless of the immunologic history of the individual. The vast repertoire of variable regions expressed by these cells is also unaffected by prior antigen exposure, being determined by the more-or-less random joining of V, D, and J gene segments into various combinations. As a result, no more than about 1 in 100,000 newly minted B cells is capable of recognizing any individual epitope. Moreover, although they can home efficiently into lymphoid tissues or sites of ongoing inflammation, virgin B cells are mitotically and immunologically inert and have very limited life spans. Nearly all die within a few days unless they are roused from their quiescent state. Only those that become activated survive.

THE HUMORAL IMMUNE RESPONSE

THE B-CELL ANTIGEN RECEPTOR

The production of large amounts of specific antibody in response to antigenic challenge depends on the ability of the immune system to activate only those rare B cells capable of producing antibody that can react with the antigen. These cells are induced to proliferate rapidly to expand their numbers. Subsequently, these cells either differentiate into antibody-secreting plasma cells or become memory B cells, which are long-lived cells that produce an antibody response later on reexposure to the antigen. This process is referred to as **clonal selection,** because a small number of B cells are selected, based on their antigen specificity, and then divide and give rise to a clone of progeny, all of which produce the same or nearly the same antibody as the founder cell.

Clonal selection requires each B cell to recognize the antigen that binds to the antibody secreted by that cell. This is accomplished by differential RNA splicing yielding the expression of two forms of immunoglobulin heavy chains—a secreted form and a membrane form, the latter containing a hydrophobic transmembrane domain and a very short cytoplasmic tail. All heavy-chain isotypes can give rise to both secreted and membrane forms. The membrane form combines with immunoglobulin light chains to make membrane immunoglobulin. Interestingly, membrane immunoglobulin is retained in the endoplasmic reticulum unless it can associate with two additional proteins expressed exclusively in cells of the B-cell lineage. These proteins, called **Ig-α** and **Ig-β,** associate with membrane immunoglobulin to form the **B-cell antigen receptor (BCR),** which can transit to the cell surface (Fig 8–3A). Ig-α and Ig-β are transmembrane glycoproteins, each of which has a moderately large

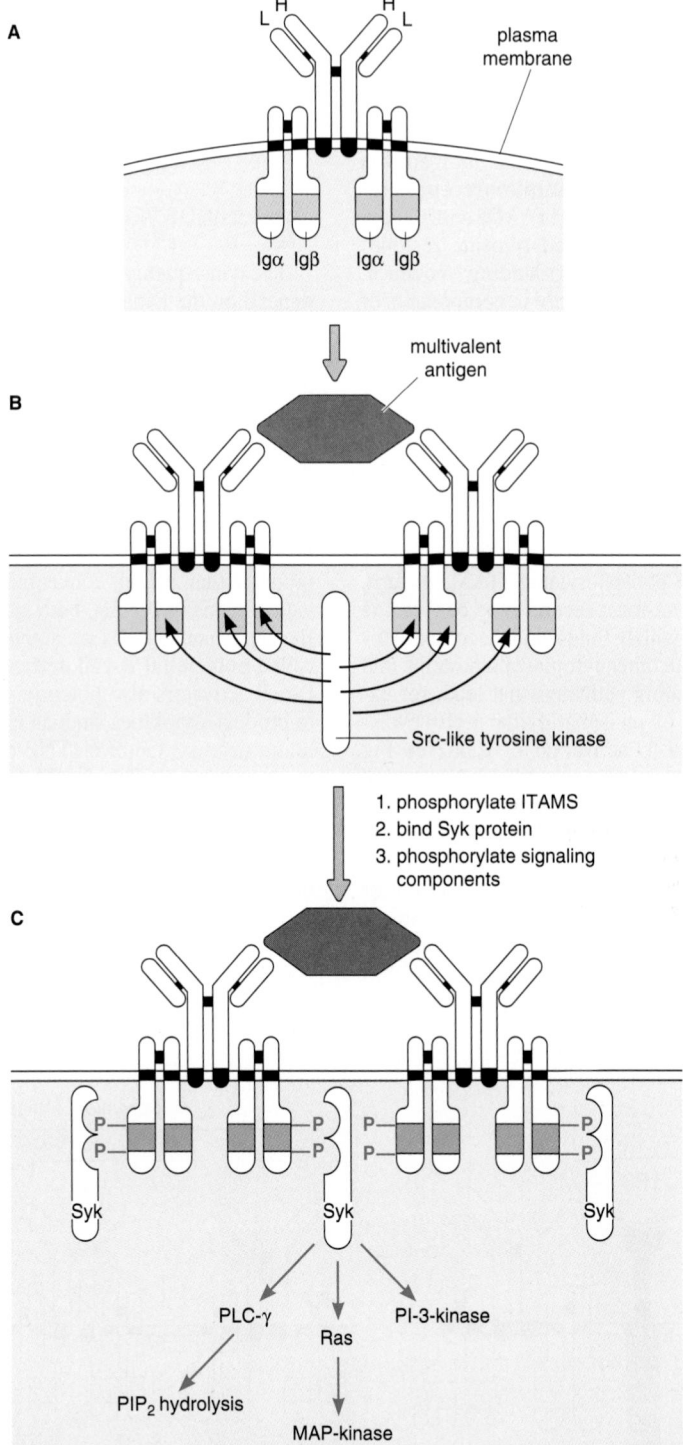

Figure 8–3. Signaling through the B-cell antigen receptor (BCR). **A:** Antigen receptor transmembrane-signaling complex on mature B cells. Ig-α and Ig-β are disulfide-linked to each other but associate with membrane immunoglobulins noncovalently through their transmembrane and extracellular domains. The number of Ig-α/Ig-β heterodimers per membrane immunoglobulin unit is not known but is believed to be two, as shown, for reasons of symmetry. Both Ig-α and Ig-β cytoplasmic domains contain copies of the immunoreceptor tyrosine-based activation motif (ITAM). The consensus sequence for the ITAM is YxxL/IxxxxxxxYxxL/I, where Y = tyrosine; L/I = leucine or isoleucine; and x = any amino acid. In the resting state, the ITAM tyrosines (Y) of Ig-α and Ig-β are largely unphosphorylated. **B:** On cross-linking with multivalent antigen, a Src-family tyrosine kinase phosphorylates ITAM tyrosines. **C:** Doubly phosphorylated ITAMs serve as binding sites for a second type of tyrosine kinase, called Syk. Once bound, Syk becomes phosphorylated on tyrosines and its activity is increased. Syk is thought to be largely responsible for phosphorylating downstream signaling targets, such as activators of Ras, phosphatidylinositol-3-kinase (PI-3-kinase), and phospholipase C-γ (PLC-γ), which hydrolyzes inositol-containing phospholipids (eg, PIP$_2$).

cytoplasmic domain. These cytoplasmic domains each include a short region important for transmitting into the cell a signal indicating that antigen has bound. This region is called an **immunoreceptor tyrosine-based activation motif (ITAM),** and its key features are two precisely spaced tyrosine residues within a partially conserved surrounding sequence. ITAM sequences are found not only in components of the BCR, but also in the T-cell antigen receptor complexes and in various Fc receptors, and in each case are thought to induce transmembrane signaling in a fundamentally similar way. In B cells, cross-linking of two or more BCRs by a bivalent or multivalent antigen brings together several Ig-α and Ig-β cytoplasmic domains with their ITAMs. This clustering leads to phosphorylation of the ITAM tyrosines by protein tyrosine kinases belonging to the Src-family (see Chapter 1). The phosphorylated ITAM, in turn, becomes a binding site for a second type of tyrosine kinase, called **Syk,** which binds and becomes activated to phosphorylate other cytoplasmic proteins that activate various signaling pathways that lead, for example to hydrolysis of phosphatidylinositol 4,5-bisphosphate (PIP_2) and to activation of Ras (see Fig 8–3). The subsequent events are poorly understood at this time, although a number of transcription factors ultimately become activated, which leads to the expression of specific genes that contribute to cellular activation. In any case, it is the ability of bivalent or multivalent antigen to bring together multiple antigen receptors and their attached ITAMs that initiates the signaling events that inform a B cell it has encountered antigen.

T-CELL-INDEPENDENT ANTIGENS

The consequences of antigen contact with the BCR depend on the nature of the antigen and on other signals received by the B cell at that time. Generally, antigen contact alone is insufficient to activate B cells, as most protein antigens require antigen-specific T-cell help to generate an antibody response. Some antigens do not require the presence of helper T cells, however, and are called **T-independent antigens.** These antigens typically fall into either of two categories, with different mechanistic properties (Fig 8–4). The first group, called **TI-1 antigens,** have the property that at high concentrations they induce activation of many B cells, both specific and nonspecific. Because many B cells are activated, these antigens are called **polyclonal B-cell activators.** Often polyclonal B-cell activators also potently stimulate macrophages to produce cytokines such as interleukin-1 (IL-1) and tumor necrosis factor α (TNF-α), which augment immune responses. Typical TI-1 antigens are bacterial cell wall components, and their recognition by cells of the immune system appears to be an evolved feature of innate immunity. For example, the TI-1 antigen **lipopolysaccharide,** from gram-negative bacterial cell walls, can induce immunologic defense reactions in a number of invertebrate as well as vertebrate or-

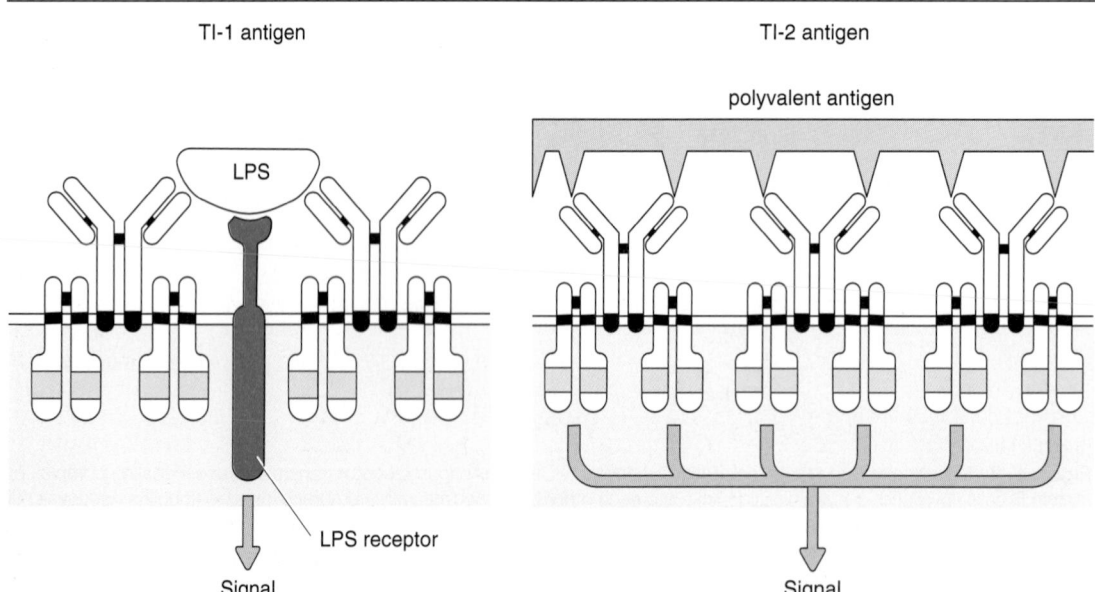

Figure 8–4. B-cell activation by T-independent antigens. TI-1 antigens *(left)* activate B cells by signaling primarily through nonimmunoglobulin receptors, although specific surface antibodies can enhance signalling by concentrating the antigen on the cell surface. A hypothetical receptor for lipopolysaccharide (LPS) is shown. TI-2 antigens *(right)* are highly repetitive structures and therefore can activate B cells by specifically binding and cross-linking numerous surface immunoglobulins.

ganisms. Interestingly, at low concentrations TI-1 antigens often do elicit an antigen-specific antibody response. It has been postulated that this occurs because BCRs that specifically recognize the TI-1 antigen can concentrate it onto the surfaces of specific B cells, where it can then stimulate other types of receptors more efficiently and trigger activation.

In contrast, **TI-2 antigens** do not have polyclonal B-cell activator properties, nor do they activate macrophages. These antigens are generally highly repetitive polymeric antigens such as polysaccharides from bacterial cell walls, or polymeric protein structures such as bacterial flagella. It has been postulated that their B-cell-activating properties derive from their ability to cross-link numerous BCR molecules and induce either intense, or especially prolonged, intracellular-signaling reactions (see Fig 8–4). Antibody responses to TI-2 antigens, although they do not require helper T cells, do appear to require low levels of cytokines, such as might be generated by a nearby immune response.

T-CELL HELP
& ACCESSORY SIGNALS

Most protein antigens only induce antibody production in the presence of CD4+ helper T cells. Typically, T-cell help can be provided in two forms: by soluble cytokines (especially IL-4 and IL-5), or by a cell–cell contact-dependent signal (Fig 8–5). Contact-mediated help results from specific interactions between membrane proteins on the T_H- and B-cell surfaces. The most important interaction of this type occurs between the B-cell protein **CD40** and a protein called **CD40 ligand** (or **CD40L**), which appears on T_H cells only after they become activated. In some circumstances, the CD40L signal in combination with the cytokines IL-4 and IL-5 can fully activate B cells even in the absence of antigen. In other circumstances, however, CD40L stimulation in the absence of antigen contact leads to death of the B cell via apoptosis. In general, however, the combination of antigen binding and CD40L acts synergistically to trigger B-cell activation. Binding of CD40 to CD40L is an extremely important mechanism of delivering T-cell help in vivo. An inherited defect in CD40L causes a form of congenital immunodeficiency known as **hyper-IgM syndrome,** in which humoral immunity is impaired due to a deficiency of T-cell help. In these patients, the antibody response to many antigens is markedly abnormal, and no IgG, IgA, or IgE is produced. IgM levels, on the other hand, are abnormally high, possibly as a secondary effect of recurrent infections. This IgM response may be due to T-independent antigen stimulation or possibly to residual T-cell-dependent antibody responses in the absence of CD40L.

In B cells that coexpress surface IgM and IgD, both

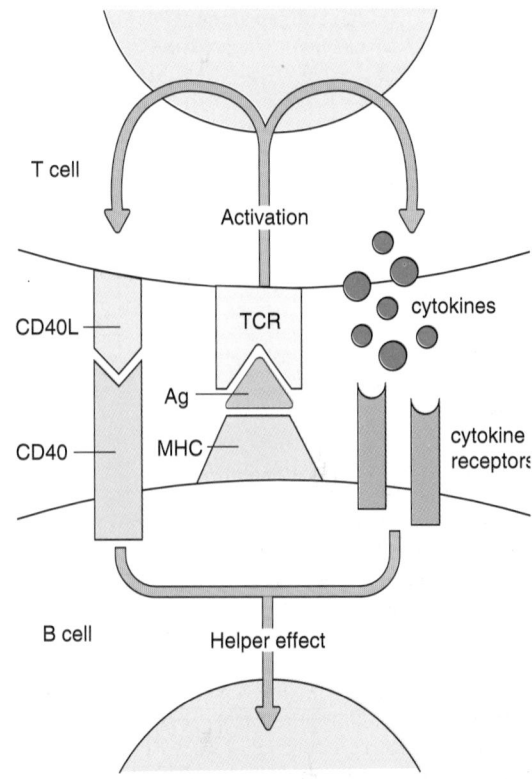

Figure 8–5. B-cell activation by a helper T cell. Antigen-specific B cells are stimulated by antigen contact with the BCR. They also take up the antigen (Ag) for digestion into peptides that combine with class II major histocompatibility complex (MHC) molecules and then go to the cell surface to be presented to antigen-specific helper T cells. T-cell-receptor (TCR)-based recognition of the antigen leads to T-cell activation, which stabilizes the association between the T and B cells and induces T-cell synthesis of CD40L and cytokines, which provide coactivating signals for the B cell.

are capable of antigen binding and signal transduction, and they produce identical effects. Certain accessory molecules on the B cell (such as CD22, complement receptors, and class II MHC proteins) can also send signals that augment activation when they bind their cognate ligands. Antigens that have complement fragments bound to them can simultaneously bind the BCR and CR2 complement receptor, bringing them together in the plasma membrane; this bridging greatly promotes B-cell activation (Fig 8–6B). In contrast, activation is suppressed by the binding of antigen–antibody complexes (especially those containing IgG) to B-cell surface **Fc receptors**—this provides a negative feedback mechanism that may be important for terminating B-cell responses once saturating amounts of antibody have been produced. The mechanism of this suppression appears to involve the clustering of the Fc receptors together with the engaged BCRs, interfering in some way with the ITAM-based signaling mechanisms (see Fig 8–6C). Thus,

A antigen alone

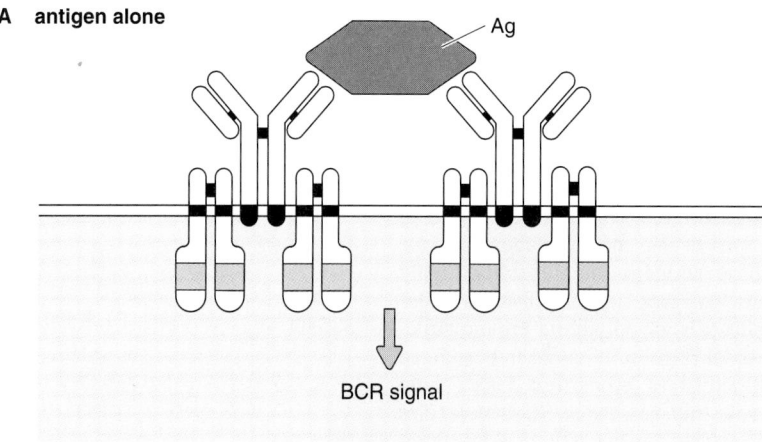

B antigen + complement
(C3d)

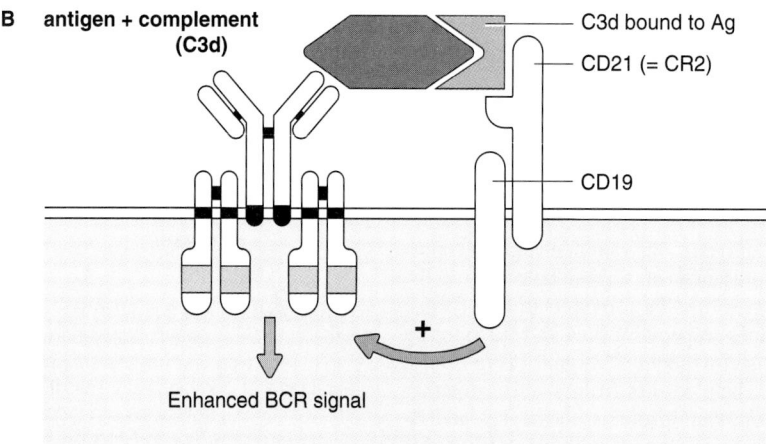

C antigen – antibody
complex

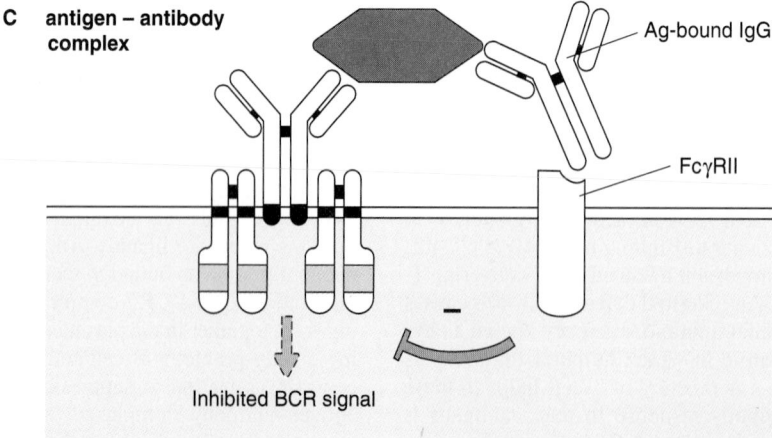

Figure 8–6. Recognition of complex ligands by B cells. **A:** Immunoglobulin cross-linking by antigen can transmit a signal through the BCR alone. **B:** Signaling is enhanced when the antigen is complexed with other immunologically relevant ligands such as the C3d fragment of complement (see Chapter 11), which engages a separate receptor called complement receptor 2 (CR2) that synergizes with the BCR. **C:** Signaling may be inhibited if the antigen is complexed with an antibody (ie, the antigen exists as an antigen–antibody complex) because the antibody engages a surface Fc receptor (in this case, FcγRII), which antagonizes signaling by the BCR.

the B cell can recognize complex antigenic ligands in which the antigen has either complement components or antibodies bound to it, as distinct from simple antigens, and can modulate its response appropriately.

Another surface protein that may modulate lymphocyte activation is **CD45,** a membrane-spanning glycoprotein whose cytoplasmic domain has **protein tyrosine phosphatase** activity (ie, the ability to dephosphorylate phosphotyrosines of other proteins). CD45 is found on all hematopoietic cells, but its molecular mass varies considerably among cell types owing to differences in the size of the extracellular domain that result from alternative mRNA splicing. B lymphocytes express the largest (220 kd) isoform of CD45, designated **CD45R.** Although its precise role is unknown, CD45 paradoxically stimulates BCR or TCR signaling. It appears to do this by removing an inhibitory tyrosine phosphorylation of the Src-family tyrosine kinases, which initiate signal transduction by phosphorylating ITAMs in antigen-clustered receptors.

B LYMPHOCYTES AS ANTIGEN-PRESENTING CELLS

The activation of B cells in response to T-cell-dependent antigens usually requires direct contact between the antigen-stimulated B cell and an antigen-activated T_H cell. T cells are constantly binding to other cells to determine whether they have ligands (specific antigenic peptide bound to an MHC molecule) for the TCR of that T cell. This interaction is short-lived, however, if the T cell fails to detect the appropriate ligand. On the other hand, if a T cell encounters antigen presented by the bound cell, this greatly strengthens the interaction between the two cells. In the case of T_H cells, the resulting interaction can last for many hours and allow for efficient delivery of cytokines and contact-dependent signals involving CD40L. For efficient activation of B cells to occur, the B cell must present antigen to T_H cells to induce such a stable interaction. B cells are inefficient at taking up antigens by phagocytosis or pinocytosis but are extremely efficient at taking up antigen via the BCR. This is because the immunoglobulin acts as a high-affinity receptor, enabling the B cell to capture its cognate antigen at concentrations several orders of magnitude lower than those needed to engage the low-affinity, broad-specificity receptors on other types of antigen-presenting cells. The bound antigen is taken into the B cell by receptor-mediated (in this case, immunoglobulin-mediated) endocytosis. It is then processed by proteases in late endosomes or lysosomes. The resulting antigenic peptides can combine with newly synthesized class II MHC molecules, which are specially routed to endocytic compartments. Class II MHC molecules are constitutively synthesized by B cells, but their synthesis is upregu-

lated by various activation stimuli, including specific antigen, IL-4, and polyclonal B-cell activators. The resulting class II MHC–peptide complexes are then displayed on the B-cell surface, where they may be recognized by T cells that have the appropriate antigen- and MHC-specificities (Fig 8–7). Note that, if the antigen is a complex protein, the B cell may produce and display from it many different processed peptides that can serve as T-cell epitopes; these may or may not correspond to the B-cell epitope originally recognized by the immunoglobulin. If this sequence of events leads to helper T-cell activation, the presenting B cell is also likely to become activated, since it not only is receiving signals from the bound antigen but also is already in direct contact with the helper cell (see Fig 8–6). Activated B cells express surface **B7.1** and **B7.2** proteins, which are T-cell costimulators that are important for activating naive T cells. In the absence of costimulation, B-cell presentation of antigen to naive T cells leads to their inactivation. In contrast, a T_H cell that has recently been activated by antigen presented by other cells expressing B7.1 or

A   antigen uptake by B cell

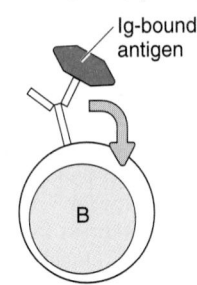

1. internalization
2. processing to peptides
3. binding of peptides to class II MHC
4. Express peptide–MHC II complex on cell surface

B   antigen presentation to T_H cell

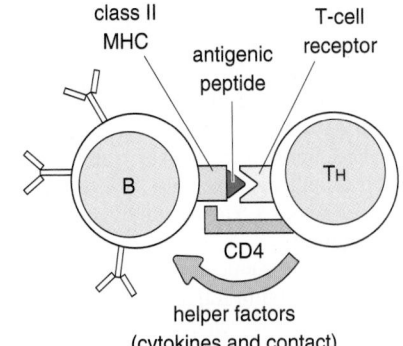

Figure 8–7. Antigen presentation by a B lymphocyte to a CD4+ T lymphocyte. **A:** The antigen-specific B cell can bind antigen via membrane immunoglobulin (Ig), **B:** internalize the antigen and present it to helper T cells. Presentation does not require, but is likely to result in, activation of the B cell.

B7.2 can provide help to a B cell even if it does not express the costimulatory molecules. Activated B cells may also secrete IL-6 and TNFα, which (like IL-1) increase the efficiency of T_H-cell activation.

In addition to antigen uptake, the BCR stimulates the ability of a B cell to present antigen to T cells via its signaling function. BCR signaling induces increased expression of class II MHC molecules, induces expression of B7.1 and B7.2, and enhances cell–cell adhesion by increasing the binding affinity of the adhesion molecule LFA-1. These features of BCR function serve to promote antigen-specific antibody responses by favoring interactions between antigen-specific T_H cells and antigen-stimulated B cells.

Although they offer unique advantages, B cells also have important limitations as antigen-presenting cells. They are not present in large numbers at most sites in the body, and, because they have little phagocytic capacity, they are unable to process many types of particulate antigens. Most importantly, in an unimmunized person, B cells specific for any given antigen are exceedingly rare. Consequently, other types of antigen-presenting cells, such as dendritic cells or macrophages, usually play the dominant role in initiating primary humoral responses. B cells then become increasingly important in this capacity at each subsequent encounter with antigen.

IMMUNOGLOBULIN SECRETION

When a B cell becomes activated and divides, its daughter cells do not regain the capacity for V/(D)/J rearrangement, but rather continue to express the rearranged genes they inherited from their clonal forebears. Some undergo further differentiation to become **plasma cells,** which secrete large amounts of immunoglobulin derived from the same genes. Many of the cells that commit to becoming plasma cells migrate to the bone marrow in order to do so. As a result, the marrow contains the great majority of the body's plasma cells and is the main source of circulating antibodies, especially during secondary immune responses. Plasma cells cannot replicate, and survive for only a few days before undergoing programmed cell death; hence, humoral responses wane quickly after an antigenic challenge subsides. At its peak, however, a plasma cell may secrete thousands of antibody molecules per minute.

The shift from producing membrane-bound to secreted immunoglobulin reflects a subtle change in the structure of the heavy-chain mRNA. The short hydrophobic tail that anchors a heavy-chain protein onto the cell membrane is encoded by the final two exons of every C_H region; when a B cell differentiates into a plasma cell, it produces an alternative form of heavy-chain mRNA that lacks these final exons and so encodes a heavy-chain protein that can be secreted from the cell (see Fig 3–4). In the case of μ heavy chains,

this slightly truncated mRNA is designated μs. B cells that coexpress surface IgM and IgD almost always secrete only IgM (in pentameric form, complexed with J chains); IgD is rarely secreted.

MEMORY B LYMPHOCYTES

Most cells within a proliferating clone that do not differentiate into plasma cells instead revert to the resting state to become memory B lymphocytes. Many of these memory cells ultimately take up residence within lymphoid follicles, where they survive for years; if subsequently activated, they undergo further cycles of replication to produce still more memory and plasma cells. In general, the progeny at each stage continue to express the same immunoglobulin genes as their parents. Two specialized types of genetic processes, however, occur at high frequency whenever memory B cells proliferate in the periphery. These processes—known as class switching and somatic hypermutation—further diversify the immunoglobulin genes expressed by some of the replicating cells and can permanently alter the characteristics of the B-cell clone. In the following sections, we consider each of these phenomena in turn.

THE HEAVY-CHAIN CLASS SWITCH

As a B-cell clone proliferates, individual daughter cells often appear that express a heavy-chain class (such as γ or α) that differs from that of the founder (Fig 8–8A). This phenomenon is called **class switching,** or isotype switching. It results from a specialized type of DNA rearrangement in the expressed heavy-chain gene, whereby a new C_H region is moved to a position adjacent to the existing V/D/J exon by deleting all intervening C_H sequences on the chromosome (see Fig 8–8B). Although class switching bears some resemblance to V/(D)/J joining, the two processes are believed to occur through entirely different enzymatic pathways. In particular, switching occurs in mature B cells that no longer express RAG-1 and RAG-2 and hence cannot carry out V/(D)/J joining. In addition, switching takes place at distinct chromosomal sites (called **switch regions**) that are located within the introns upstream of the first C_H exon of each heavy-chain gene. As switching occurs within introns, it does not change the structure of the V/D/J exon and therefore does not affect antigen specificity. Because class switching occurs by deleting one or more heavy-chain isotype genes, it is normally irreversible.

Through the process of class switching, a pre-assembled V/D/J exon that was originally linked to C_μ can become associated with any of the other heavy-chain constant region sequences. By this means, the effector function of an antibody can be changed with-

A

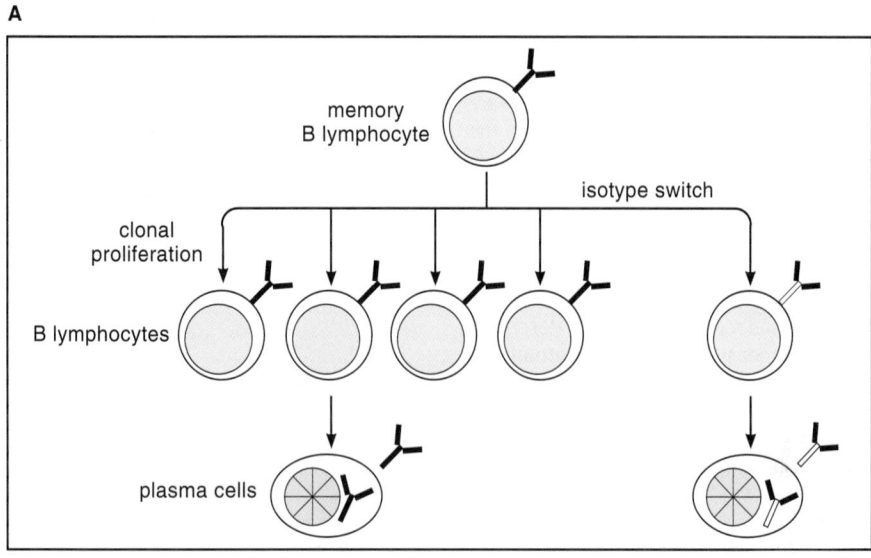

B

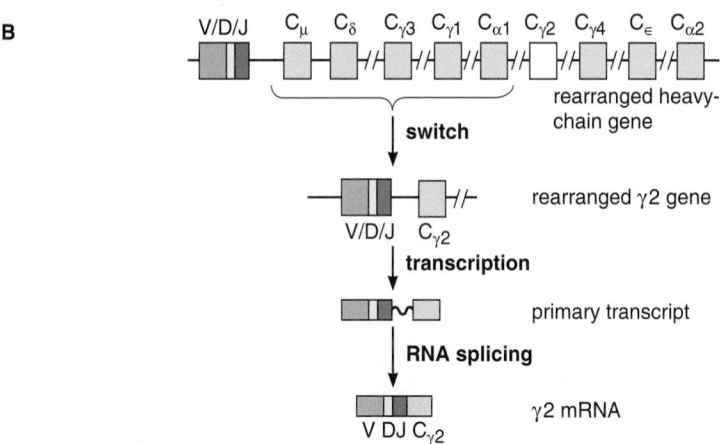

Figure 8–8. Heavy-chain class switch. **A:** During clonal proliferation of an activated memory B cell, some daughter cells may arise that express a different heavy-chain isotype and pass this trait on to their progeny. **B:** Class switching takes place when a fully assembled heavy-chain locus undergoes an additional DNA rearrangement event that places a new C_H sequence adjacent to the V/D/J exon. This occurs by deletion of the intervening C_H exons and is carried out by an enzymatic pathway distinct from that of V/D/J rearrangement. In the example shown, the gene switches to the $C_{\gamma 2}$ isotype.

out altering its specificity for antigen. The choice of a new C_H isotype is strongly influenced by cytokines and other factors acting on the B cell. For example, the microenvironment found in Peyer's patches favors switching to $C_{\alpha 1}$, resulting in the production of IgA. This appears to be due to the action of a cytokine called transforming growth factor beta (TGFβ). Similarly, exposure of the activated B cell to IL-4 promotes switching to C_ε. In the mouse, IL-4, TGF-β, and interferon gamma (IFNγ) each promote class switching to different IgG subtypes. In the human, less is known about the control of switching, although IFNγ and IL-4 are known to promote switching to IgG1 and IgG4, respectively. If a cell that has switched continues to divide, its progeny (both mem-

ory and plasma cells) also express the new heavy-chain isotype. As a rule, subclones expressing non-μ isotypes become increasingly prevalent during a T-cell-dependent antibody response, and their isotype distribution increasingly reflects the peripheral tissue in which the proliferation has occurred: memory cells in subepithelial regions most commonly express IgA, whereas IgM- and IgG-expressing memory cells are predominant elsewhere.

SOMATIC HYPERMUTATION

Fully assembled V/J and V/D/J exons in B cells undergo point mutation at an unusually high rate during the course of an immune response. The mechanism of this phenomenon, termed **somatic hypermutation,** is unknown but appears quite specific, as adjacent regions on the chromosome (including the C_H exon) are not affected. As the mutations are introduced into the variable region exon at random, they can have the effect of either increasing or decreasing affinity of the resulting immunoglobulin for its target antigen. Individual cells that express higher affinity mutants are selected from this pool of cells by virtue of their high affinity for antigen. This occurs by a complicated process in the germinal center, which is described later. This selection process is thought to account for a phenomenon known as **affinity maturation:** the observation that antibodies produced later in an immune response tend to have higher affinity for the target antigen than those produced earlier.

LYMPHOID FOLLICLES & GERMINAL CENTERS

The initial encounter between B cells and antigen most commonly occurs within a lymphoid organ, such as a lymph node or submucosal lymphoid tissue, since that is where most B cells normally reside. An antigen may be transported into the lymphoid organ by a dendritic cell (see Chapter 6), which can then present it directly to cognate T_H cells. Alternatively, free antigen may enter by way of the blood or lymphatic channels to be captured and presented by resident macrophages or other antigen-presenting cells. In either case, antigen presentation and T_H-cell activation take place within the T-cell-rich zone of the organ, such as in the paracortex of a lymph node. Numerous B cells pass through the T-cell zones at all times, either flowing with the lymph or entering from the bloodstream through high endothelial venules, and this B-cell traffic tends to increase when local T cells become activated. If one of these B cells can recognize the antigen through its BCR and also receives appropriate T-cell help, including CD40L contact, it becomes activated and migrates from the T-cell zone into a nearby lymphoid follicle (Fig 8–9A).

In the absence of an ongoing immune response, a lymphoid follicle consists mainly of a polyclonal collection of resting B lymphocytes, each enveloped within the spidery cytoplasmic processes of specialized supportive cells called **follicular dendritic cells (FDCs).** The FDCs, which are unrelated to other types of dendritic cells despite the unfortunate similarities in name and morphology, appear to be responsible for organizing the follicle and controlling many of its activities. Unlike dendritic cells, FDCs are not derived from a bone marrow precursor cell, and they do not ordinarily present antigens to T cells. FDCs express abundant surface Fc receptors, however, and are therefore very efficient at capturing antigen-antibody complexes; in the presence of preformed antibodies,

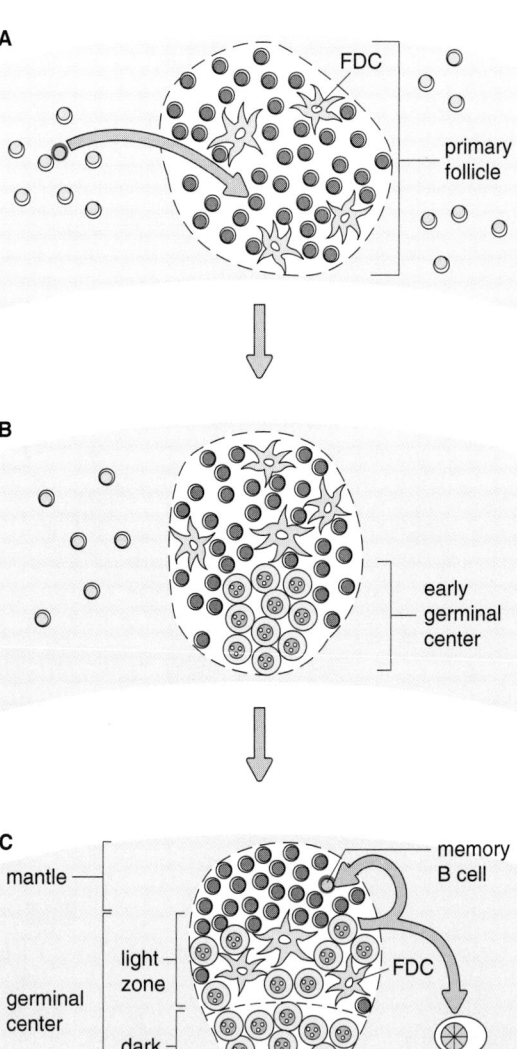

Figure 8–9. Dynamics of a lymphoid follicle during a humoral response. **A:** An antigen-specific B cell (in dark blue) contacts antigen and receives help from an activated T_H cell in the T-cell-rich zone of a lymphoid organ (in this case, the paracortex of a lymph node). It migrates into an adjacent primary lymphoid follicle and undergoes blast transformation. FDC = follicular dendritic cell. **B:** After three to seven days, clonal progeny of the B cell (in dark blue) appear as an early germinal center, which displaces the FDCs and resting polyclonal B cells of the original follicle toward the afferent surface of the node. **C:** After one to four weeks, the germinal center has matured to form a dark zone, populated mainly by proliferating blasts, and an apical light zone, where nonproliferating progeny of these blasts contact FDCs. Cells that survive selection in the light zone emerge as memory cells or plasma cells. The newly formed memory B cells, as well as those from the original primary follicle, make up the follicular mantle overlying the germinal center. Photographs of germinal centers exhibiting these features can be seen in Figures 3–12 and 3–14.

this enables FDCs to trap unprocessed antigens within follicles, where they may persist for weeks or even months on the FDC surface.

It is currently believed that any activated B cell that migrates into a follicle dies by apoptosis within a few days unless it is able to capture an antigen from the FDC surface using its surface immunoglobulin, process the antigen, present it to local T_H cells, and receive effective T-cell help in return. The rare B cell that succeeds in this process undergoes blast transformation and begins to proliferate very rapidly, with a generation time as short as six hours. Its clonal progeny become visible within three days to a week as a **germinal center**—a roughly spherical group of blast cells that tend to push aside the surrounding FDCs and resting lymphocytes of the original follicle (see Fig 8–9B). Each germinal center results from the clonal expansion of only one or a few activated B-cell founders. Over time, the germinal center enlarges and becomes polarized into two morphologically distinct zones (see Fig 8–9C). The **dark zone** (which, in a lymph node, tends to be located near the efferent side of the follicle—that is, near the medulla) is composed of rapidly proliferating B cells called **centroblasts.** It is during the proliferation of centroblasts in the dark zone that hypermutation takes place within the V/D/J and V/J exons of the rearranged immunoglobulin genes.

As individual centroblasts cease dividing, they move into the adjacent **light zone,** where they acquire the name **centrocytes** and come into contact with FDCs that bear unprocessed antigens. The light zone is believed to be a region of intense selective pressure where numerous centrocytes compete to bind a limited amount of cognate antigen on the surface of the FDCs. Centrocytes whose BCR binds antigen survive, whereas those that fail to bind die by apoptosis. This is thought to be the basis for selecting cells that produce high-affinity immunoglobulins: in a competitive situation, surface immunoglobulins of higher affinity are thought to compete for antigen more effectively than those of lower affinity. Cells with higher affinity immunoglobulins not only are stimulated more strongly through their BCRs, but also compete more effectively in internalizing antigen and presenting it to

local T_H cells, and hence receive more effective help, as described earlier. Together, these selective processes likely account for the antibody affinity maturation that occurs as a humoral response proceeds.

Centrocytes that survive the selection process emerge from the germinal center as either plasma cells or memory B cells. The plasma cells generally exit the follicle, either remaining in the lymphoid organ or migrating to the bone marrow. Memory cells often move into the follicular mantle, joining the original polyclonal population of memory B cells that remain in the follicle after the immune response subsides and the germinal center regresses. The T_H-cell surface molecule CD40L appears to play a role in inducing centrocytes to develop into memory cells rather than into plasma cells. Interestingly, patients with the X-linked hyper-IgM syndrome, in which CD40L is defective, fail to develop germinal centers at all.

PRIMARY & SECONDARY HUMORAL RESPONSES

Of necessity, the properties of a primary humoral immune response (that is, the antibody response that occurs the first time an individual encounters a given antigen) reflect the properties of virgin lymphocytes. Because B cells with the appropriate specificity are rare in unimmunized hosts, most of the antigen must be processed by macrophages or dendritic cells and presented to antigen-specific helper T cells, which are also correspondingly rare. These antigen-activated T_H cells multiply and then must contact and promote the activation of antigen-specific B cells, which must in turn proliferate and differentiate into plasma cells in sufficient numbers to be effective. The initially low frequencies of antigen-specific T cells and B cells and the necessity of their expansion account for the lag time (typically 5–10 days) required to reach peak serum antibody concentrations in a primary response, and for the relatively low concentrations achieved (Table 8–1). The antibodies initially produced are predominantly IgM—the type secreted by most direct progeny of virgin B cells—and have, on average, low

Table 8–1. Comparison of primary and secondary humoral immune responses.

	Primary response	Secondary response
Antigen presentation	Mainly by non-B cells	B lymphocytes increasingly important
Antigen concentration needed to induce response	Relatively high	Relatively low

Antibody response
  Lag phase
  Peak concentration
  Class(es)
	
	5–10 days
	Relatively low
	Mostly IgM
		
		2–5 days
		Relatively high
		Other classes (IgG, IgA, etc) often predominate, in tissue-specific manner

Average antigen affinity	Relatively low	Relatively high

antigen affinities. The pentameric structure of IgM helps compensate for this low intrinsic affinity by providing multiple binding sites so that antigens with multiple copies of individual epitopes can be bound with a higher avidity.

Subsequent responses, by contrast, are increasingly dominated by antigen-specific memory cells, whose sheer numbers enhance both the speed and intensity of the response (see Table 8–1). In a highly immunized lymph node, as many as one in a few hundred B cells may be specific for the target antigen. Memory B cells may serve as the principal antigen-presenting cells in secondary responses, and so enable helper T cells to become activated at very low concentrations of antigen. In the process, the B cells themselves are ideally positioned for activation, as they are stimulated strongly both by antigen induction of BCR signaling and by direct contact with the helper cells (see Fig 8–7). The responding B cells are more likely to express high-affinity antibodies, following selection in the germinal center during either the initial response or the secondary response. Although some plasma cells still produce IgM in a secondary response, a substantial number of plasma cells arise from class-switched B-cell subclones and instead secrete IgG, IgA, or IgE. These latter isotypes therefore tend to predominate in secondary responses, depending on the site at which the response occurs: secondary responses in the peripheral lymph nodes are predominantly IgG, whereas those at mucosal surfaces are mainly IgA.

B-CELL TOLERANCE

The random assembly of V, D, and J segments during lymphopoiesis inevitably produces some B-cell clones whose immunoglobulins recognize self-determinants on normal host cells or tissues. Because such autoreactive immunoglobulins are potentially deleterious to the host, stringent measures are needed to ensure that they are not secreted. In most cases, these measures operate successfully; the immune system remains specifically **tolerant** toward the many self-determinants to which it is continually exposed. In contrast, in some people antibodies to certain self-components are made and lead to tissue or organ damage. These diseases are referred to as autoimmune diseases because the immune system has lost tolerance to certain self-components.

There are two main ways in which B cells that make autoreactive immunoglobulins are silenced. The first applies to the situation in which an immature B cell contacts antigen in the bone marrow shortly after it begins expressing surface immunoglobulins. This results in maturational arrest; the cell fails to mature further and does not exit the marrow. Instead, the cell

reactivates expression of the RAG-1 and RAG-2 recombinase proteins, so that it is able to resume rearranging its light-chain genes. Like 60–70% of all human B lymphocytes, many autoreactive B cells initially express κ light chains; in those cells, the reactivated recombinase is able to carry out a special type of DNA rearrangement in which a V_κ or J_κ segment in the active κ-gene locus becomes fused to a site downstream of the C_κ segment which is called the **κ-deleting element** (Fig 8–10). As a result of this rearrangement, the C_κ segment and other important regions are deleted, the gene is permanently inactivated, and the cell can then attempt to assemble a new κ or λ gene on one of its other chromosomes. This process has been called **receptor editing.** If the original κ chain contributed to recognition of self-antigen, then replacing it with a new light chain may eliminate autoreactivity. In that case, it is believed that the cell can resume maturation, shut off its recombinase activity, and eventually be released from the marrow. If receptor editing fails, then the autoreactive B cell remains arrested in the undifferentiated state and eventually dies.

The receptor-editing mechanism applies only to immature B cells, and so would be effective only for eliminating cells that recognize self-antigens found in the bone marrow, such as serum proteins and ubiqui-

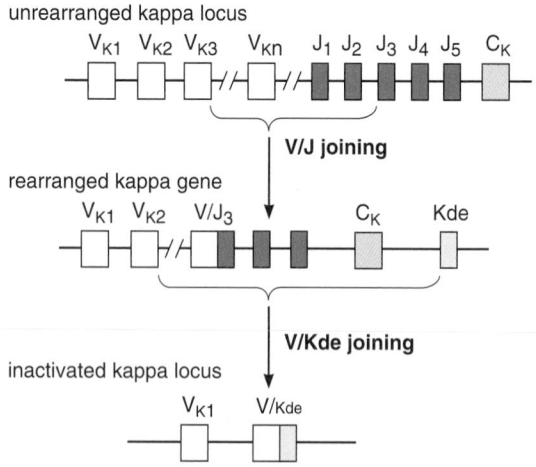

Figure 8–10. Rearrangements that remove a functionally rearranged κ light-chain gene. In immature B cells that contact self-antigen, maturation is arrested and RAG-1 and RAG-2 are reexpressed. Among the reactions that can be performed by the V/D/J recombinase is a rearrangement between either an unrearranged V_κ gene (as shown) or a sequence in the intron between J_κ and C_κ with a sequence 24 kb downstream of the C_κ gene called the κ-deleting element (Kde). This deletes the intervening DNA, including C_κ, and results in a nonfunctional gene. This reaction may occur as part of receptor editing, whereby a self-reactive immature B cell attempts to change light chain and thereby its antigen specificity.

tous cell surface or extracellular matrix proteins. Many other self-antigens, however, are found only outside the marrow, and for these antigens a different mechanism is needed to ensure B-cell tolerance. This mechanism acts only on mature B cells in peripheral tissues and relies on the fact that B-cell activation by most protein antigens requires the participation of helper T cells. When a mature B cell contacts antigen in the absence of appropriate T-cell help, the B cell either dies or loses its ability to carry out an immune response. The fate of the B cell depends on the physical nature of the antigen involved. In the case of membrane-bound or particulate antigens, the self-reactive B cell generally dies—a phenomenon referred to as **clonal deletion.** Soluble protein antigens, which presumably generate weaker signals through the BCR of

a self-reactive B cell, do not cause cell death but instead make the cell unresponsive to activating stimuli—a phenomenon called **clonal anergy.** Anergic B cells can become activated under some circumstances, so clonal anergy is thought to be a less absolute mechanism for enforcing tolerance to self. Anergic B cells, however, cannot compete effectively with nonanergic B cells for survival and proliferation in the body; as a result, the anergic cells probably die within a few days, so that clonal anergy and clonal deletion differ only in the short term. It remains to be determined precisely what roles clonal anergy and clonal deletion each play in maintaining self-tolerance and how these mechanisms come to be circumvented in autoimmune disease.

REFERENCES

B-CELL DEVELOPMENT

Hayakawa K, Hardy RR: Normal, autoimmune, and malignant CD5+ B cells: The Ly-1 B lineage. *Ann Rev Immunol* 1988;**6:**197.

Kincade PW et al: Cells and molecules that regulate B lymphopoiesis in bone marrow. *Ann Rev Immunol* 1989;**7:**111.

Kitamura D et al: A B cell-deficient mouse by targeted disruption of the membrane exon of the immunoglobulin µ chain gene. *Nature* 1991;**350:**423.

Li Y-S et al: The regulated expression of B lineage associated genes during B cell differentiation in bone marrow and fetal liver. *J Exp Med* 1993;**178:**951.

Rolink A, Melchers F: Molecular and cellular origins of B lymphocyte diversity. *Cell* 1991;**66:**1081.

Vetrie D et al: The gene involved in X-linked agammaglobulinemia is a member of the src-family of protein-tyrosine kinases. *Nature* 1993;**361:**226.

B-CELL SURFACE RECEPTORS & SIGNALING

Immunology Today, September 1994 (entire issue): B-cell signaling.

DeFranco AL: Transmembrane signaling by antigen receptors of B and T lymphocytes. *Curr Opin Cell Biol* 1995;**7:**163.

Reth M: Antigen receptors on B lymphocytes. *Ann Rev Immunol* 1992;**10:**97.

Venkitaraman A et al: The B-cell antigen receptor of the five immunoglobulin gene classes. *Nature* 1991;**352:**777.

Zola H: The surface antigens of human B lymphocytes. *Immunol Today* 1987;**8:**308.

B-CELL ACTIVATION

Arpin C et al: Generation of memory B cells and plasma cells in vitro. *Science* 1995;**268:**720.

Aruffo A et al: The CD40 ligand, gp39, is defective in activated T cells from patients with X-linked hyper-IgM syndrome. *Cell* 1993;**72:**291.

Banchereau J et al: The CD40 antigen and its ligand. *Ann Rev Immunol* 1994;**12:**881.

Clark EA, Lane PJL: Regulation of human B-cell activation and adhesion. *Ann Rev Immunol* 1991;**9:**97.

Clark EA, Ledbetter JA: How B and T cells talk to each other. *Nature* 1994;**367:**425.

Liu Y-J et al: Mechanism of antigen-driven selection in germinal centres. *Nature* 1989;**342:**929.

MacLennan ICM: Germinal centers. *Ann Rev Immunol* 1994;**12:**117.

Mond JJ et al: T cell-independent antigens type 2. *Ann Rev Immunol* 1995;**13:**655.

Parker DC: T cell-dependent B-cell activation. *Ann Rev Immunol* 1993;**11:**331.

Vitetta ES et al: Cellular interactions in the humoral immune response. *Adv Immunol* 1989;**45:**1.

HEAVY-CHAIN CLASS SWITCHING & IMMUNOGLOBULIN SECRETION

Cebra JJ et al: C_H isotype "switching" during normal B-lymphocyte development. *Ann Rev Immunol* 1984;**2:**493.

Early P et al: Two mRNAs can be produced from a single immunoglobulin µ gene by alternative RNA processing pathways. *Cell* 1979;**20:**313.

Finkelman FD et al: Lymphokine control of in vivo immunoglobulin isotype selection. *Ann Rev Immunol* 1990;**8:**303.

Harriman W et al: Immunoglobulin class-switch recombinations. *Ann Rev Immunol* 1993;**11:**385.

B-CELL TOLERANCE

Cyster JG et al: Competition for follicular niches excludes self-reactive cells from the recirculating B-cell repertoire. *Nature* 1994;**371:**389.

Goodnow CC et al: The need for central and peripheral tolerance in the B repertoire. *Science* 1990;**248:**1373.

Goodnow CC: Transgenic mice and analysis of B cell tolerance. *Ann Rev Immunol* 1992;**10:**489.

Schwartz RH: Acquisition of immunological self-tolerance. *Cell* 1989;**57:**1073.

Tiegs SL et al: Receptor editing in self-reactive bone marrow B cells. *J Exp Med* 1993;**177:**1009.

9

T Lymphocytes & Natural Killer Cells

John B. Imboden, MD

The success of virtually all immune responses depends on the remarkable ability of thymus-derived (T) lymphocytes to recognize and discriminate among a wide range of different foreign antigens. As is the case with B lymphocytes, the enormous diversity of the T-cell repertoire stems from the ability of developing T cells to rearrange and modify the genes that encode their antigen receptors. An appreciation of the structure and function of the T-cell antigen receptor is essential for understanding T-cell development and the complexities of the responses of mature T cells to antigen.

T-CELL ANTIGEN RECEPTOR

STRUCTURE OF THE T-CELL ANTIGEN RECEPTOR

T lymphocytes do not "see" soluble antigens but rather recognize antigen in the form of peptide fragments that are bound to class I and class II molecules of the major histocompatibility (MHC) locus. The T-cell receptor for antigen (TCR) is a complex of at least eight polypeptide chains (Fig 9–1). Two of these (the α and β chains) form a disulfide-linked dimer that recognizes antigenic peptides bound to MHC molecules and, therefore, is the actual ligand-binding structure within the TCR. The amino-terminal regions of the α and β chains are polymorphic, so that within the entire T-cell population there are a large number of different TCR α/β dimers, each capable of recognizing a particular combination of antigenic peptide and MHC. The TCRs on individual T cells generally contain only a single type of α/β dimer and, therefore, individual T cells respond only to a specific combination of antigen and MHC.

The α/β dimer is associated with a complex of proteins designated CD3. The CD3 chains are not polymorphic and range in size from 16 to 28 kd. They are involved in signal transduction and thus allow the TCR to convert the recognition of antigen–MHC into intracellular signals for activation. Compared with TCR α and β, whose intracellular regions are only several amino acids in length, the CD3 chains have large cytoplasmic domains, ranging from 45 to 55 amino acids for CD3 ε, δ, and γ to 113 amino acids for CD3ζ.

TCR α & β GENES AND THE GENERATION OF TCR DIVERSITY

To generate the diversity of TCRs required to recognize a wide spectrum of antigenic determinants, the TCR α and β genes use a strategy of recombination similar to that of the immunoglobulin genes (see Chapter 7). The germline TCR β-gene locus contains 20 to 30 V (variable), 2 D (diversity), and 13 J (joining) gene segments (Fig 9–2). When the TCR β gene rearranges early in T-cell ontogeny, one of the V_β segments is linked to one of the D_β regions and to one of the J_β segments to form a complete exon. After transcription, RNA processing combines the V/D/J exon with a C_β (constant) region to form a TCR β-messenger RNA that encodes a functional protein. The potential diversity generated by this combinatorial joining is equal to the product of the number of possible V segments × the number of D segments × the number of J segments. Similarly, in the TCR α locus, there are approximately 100 V segments and 50 J segments (but no D segments). To form a functional TCR α-chain gene, a V_α segment joins to a J_α segment. As in immunoglobulin genes, diversity is further enhanced by imprecise joining and by the insertion of non-germline-encoded nucleotides (N regions) between

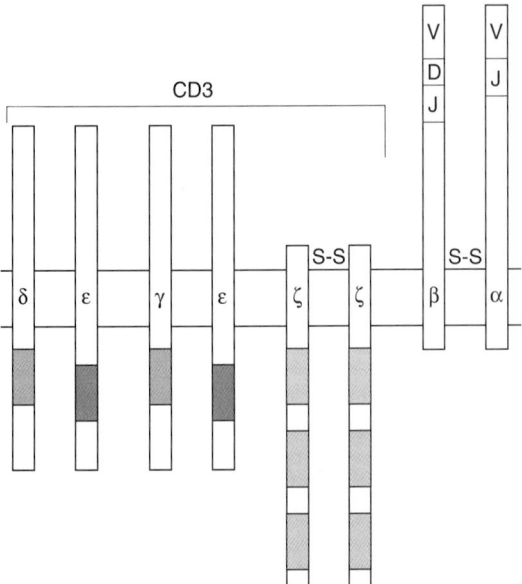

Figure 9–1. The T-cell antigen receptor (TCR). The TCR is a complex of eight transmembrane proteins. The α and β chains form a disulfide-linked (S–S) dimer that is responsible for the recognition of antigenic peptides bound to class I and class II MHC molecules. The amino-terminal regions of the α and β chains, which are formed through rearrangements of V, D, and J segments, are highly polymorphic. The α/β dimer is noncovalently associated with the CD3 complex, which converts the recognition of antigen into transmembrane signals. The CD3 polypeptides are not polymorphic and have larger cytoplasmic domains than TCR α and β. The CD3 complex consists of three sets of dimers. There are two CD3ε chains, one paired with CD3γ and the other with CD3δ. The ζ chain exists either as a disulfide-linked ζ/ζ homodimer (as shown here) or as a heterodimer with either η (an alternatively spliced form of ζ) or the γ chain. The functional importance of this variation in the ζ dimer is not understood. The cytoplasmic domains of CD3 chains contain one or more immune receptor tyrosine-based activation motifs (ITAMs), depicted here as shaded boxes.

segments during the rearrangement process. These mechanisms each enhance the diversity of sequences at the junctions between V_α and J_α and between the V_β, D_β, and J_β segments (junctional diversity). N-region insertion is carried out by the enzyme terminal deoxynucleotidyltransferase (TdT), which is expressed in the nuclei of immature T cells at the stage when V/(D)/J recombination occurs. Unlike immunoglobulin genes, TCR genes do not undergo somatic hypermutation.

TCR RECOGNITION OF ANTIGEN

For T cells to respond to an antigen, the antigen must be processed into peptides, which in turn bind to the groove on the "top" of class I and class II MHC molecules. The resulting complex of peptide and MHC molecule forms the ligand for the TCR. It is likely, but not yet formally proven, that contacts with both the peptide and the MHC molecule are critical for TCR binding. It is important to emphasize a further constraint on TCR recognition: the T-cell system is heavily biased toward recognizing peptides bound to self-MHC molecules. This restriction to self-MHC molecules results from a process of positive selection in the thymus that selectively favors the growth of developing T cells whose TCRs have the potential to recognize peptides presented by self-MHC, as will be described later on.

INTERACTION OF THE TCR WITH SUPERANTIGENS

Superantigens are a class of bacterial toxins and retroviral proteins that have the remarkable ability to bind both MHC class II molecules and the TCR β chain. In so doing, they act as a "clamp" between the TCR and class II molecule, providing signals to the T cells. It is important to grasp the differences between

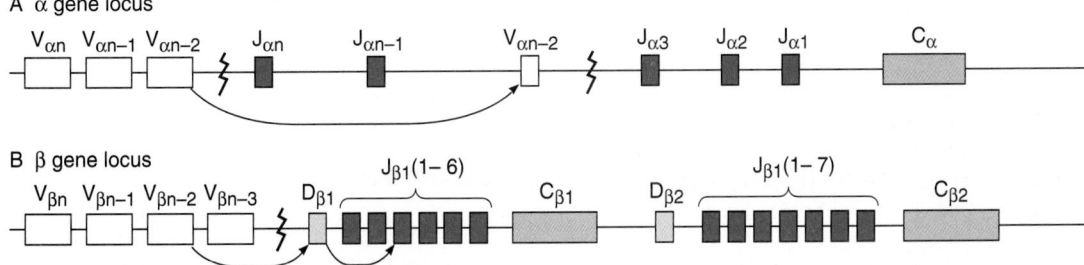

Figure 9–2. Rearrangement of the TCR α and β genes. The TCR α-gene locus contains multiple V and J segments, only several of which are shown here. Similarly, the TCR β-gene locus contains multiple V, D, and J segments. During T-cell ontogeny, the TCR genes rearrange (arrows), so that one of the V_α segments pairs with the J_α segment and a V_β segment pairs with a D_β and J_β segment. The two C (constant) segments in the β gene are very similar, and differential use of $C_{\beta1}$ and $C_{\beta2}$ does not contribute to TCR diversity.

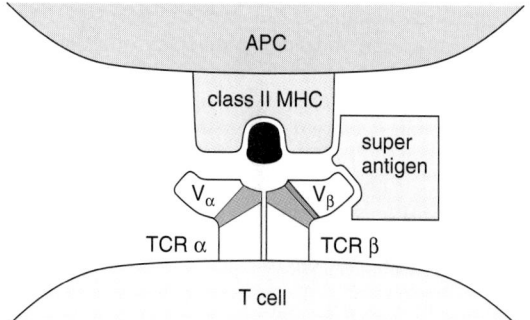

Figure 9–3. Model of the interactions between the TCR, class II MHC molecule, and a superantigen. The superantigen interacts with the MHC molecule outside the peptide groove and binds only to the V_β segment of the TCR.

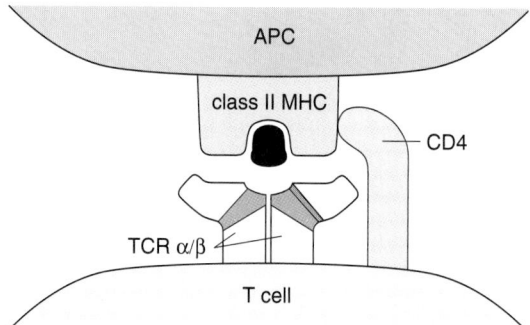

Figure 9–4. CD4 coreceptor. CD4 binds class II MHC molecules at a membrane-proximal region not directly involved in peptide binding. In the model depicted here, the coreceptor binds the same MHC molecule that engages the TCR. CD8 plays a similar coreceptor role on T cells that recognize antigen in association with class I MHC molecules. CD8 binds a nonpolymorphic region on MHC class I molecules. Be-cause the cytoplasmic domains of CD4 and CD8 interact with Lck, the coreceptors can bring this Src-like protein tyrosine kinase into proximity with the TCR.

classical antigenic peptides and superantigens. Superantigens are not processed, and interact with the MHC molecule outside of the peptide-binding groove. On the T-cell side, superantigens bind to V_β segments only, without regard to the D_β and J_β regions or to any part of the TCR α chain (Fig 9–3). Superantigens differ in the V_β sequences that they can bind, with any given superantigen binding only those encoded by one or a few V_β gene segments. Activation of T cells by individual superantigens, therefore, is selective for T cells whose TCRs express particular V_β segments.

Because superantigens only recognize the V_β segment and not the other components of the TCR α/β dimer, a superantigen has the capability of activating between 1–10% of peripheral T cells (this is orders of magnitude more than a conventional antigen). Exposure to a superantigen, therefore, can lead to massive T-cell activation, and the ensuing release of large amounts of lymphokines accounts for many of the manifestations of acute exposure to bacterial toxins that have superantigen capabilities. This likely explains the clinical features of **toxic shock syndrome,** which can be induced by *Staphylococcus aureus* toxin TSST-1, a superantigen that activates human T cells expressing $V_{\beta2}$. In the acute phase of toxic shock syndrome there is a marked, and selective, expansion of T cells that bear $V_{\beta2}$: in one case, 70% of peripheral T cells were $V_{\beta2}^+$ in the acute phase of the disease. Under other conditions, however, the activation induced by a superantigen leads to apoptosis of the activated cells, so that eventually T cells expressing the cognate V_β segment are selectively depleted from the population.

CD4 & CD8 CORECEPTORS

The expression of CD4 and CD8 divides mature T cells into two mutually exclusive subsets: those that recognize antigen in the context of class II MHC molecules (CD4+ cells) and those that recognize antigen bound to class I molecules (CD8+ cells). CD4 binds to a membrane-proximal region of MHC class II molecules that is not directly involved in peptide binding; CD8, on the other hand, binds to a corresponding region on MHC class I molecules (see Fig 6–1). It is possible, therefore, that CD4 or CD8 interacts with the same MHC molecule as the TCR during T-cell activation (Fig 9–4). There is considerable evidence to support this notion and to suggest that CD4 and CD8 are in close proximity to the TCR, functioning as coreceptors. Both CD4 and CD8 carry large cytoplasmic signaling domains that have intrinsic protein tyrosine kinase (PTK) activity, and the signals transmitted by those domains on contact with an MHC molecule create synergy with signals emanating from the TCR (see later discussion).

T-CELL ONTOGENY

STAGES OF THYMOCYTE DEVELOPMENT

T cells develop from bone-marrow-derived progenitor cells that undergo maturation in the thymus (Fig 9–5). Early in development, thymocytes express several cell surface molecules, such as CD2, that are characteristic of the T-cell lineage, but they lack many others, including CD4 and CD8, and thus are known as **double-negative thymocytes.** Rearrangement of

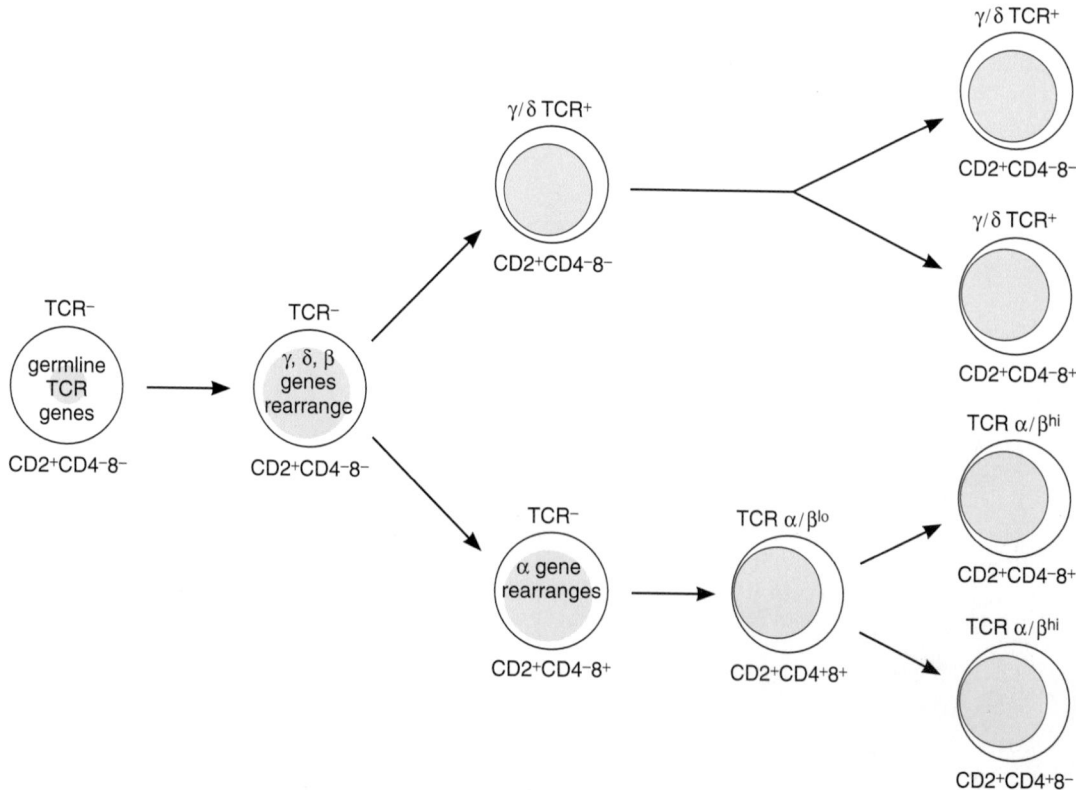

Figure 9–5. Stages in thymocyte development. Progenitor cells migrate from the bone marrow to the thymus. At the earliest stages of development, thymocytes express several T-cell surface molecules, such as CD2, but still have germline configurations of their TCR genes. Thymocytes destined to become α/β T cells pass through a critical CD4+CD8+ phase during which positive and negative selection occur.

the TCR genes begins in the double-negative stage. Cells that are destined to become α/β T cells rearrange the TCR β gene first, then the α gene. If rearrangements lead to the formation of functional TCR α and β proteins that can form a dimer, then the α/β dimer and CD3 molecules are coexpressed at low levels on the cell surface. At this point in development, the thymocytes express both CD4 and CD8 and are called **double-positive thymocytes.** As thymocytes mature into T cells, the level of TCR expression increases and the cells lose expression of either CD4 or CD8, becoming **single-positive.** At this stage, thymocytes have acquired the phenotype of mature peripheral T cells and soon exit the thymus.

POSITIVE & NEGATIVE SELECTION OF THYMOCYTES

The generation of TCRs is a largely stochastic process and can produce T cells with antigen specificities that are undesirable. For this reason, enormous selective pressures are exerted within the thymus in order to allow survival of only those mature T cells whose TCRs are restricted by self-MHC molecules and are not autoreactive. The great majority of thymocytes fail this process: at least 99% of developing T cells die within the thymus. Two distinct types of selection have been observed, both of which occur at the stage when thymocytes are CD4+CD8+ (double-positive) and express low levels of TCR on the cell surface. **Positive selection** promotes the survival of thymocytes whose TCRs have the capability of recognizing antigens bound to self-MHC molecules. **Negative selection** leads to the deletion of thymocytes whose TCRs recognize peptides derived from self-proteins.

Thymocytes are programmed to die by apoptosis unless they are rescued on the basis of the ability of their TCRs to recognize antigen in association with self-MHC molecules. A remarkable feature of this positive selection is that it leads to the selection of TCRs with specificity for foreign antigens bound to self-MHC yet occurs in the absence of the foreign antigen. Positive selection takes place in the thymic cortex, where developing thymocytes encounter epithelial cells that express both class I and class II MHC molecules loaded with self-peptides (Fig 9–6).

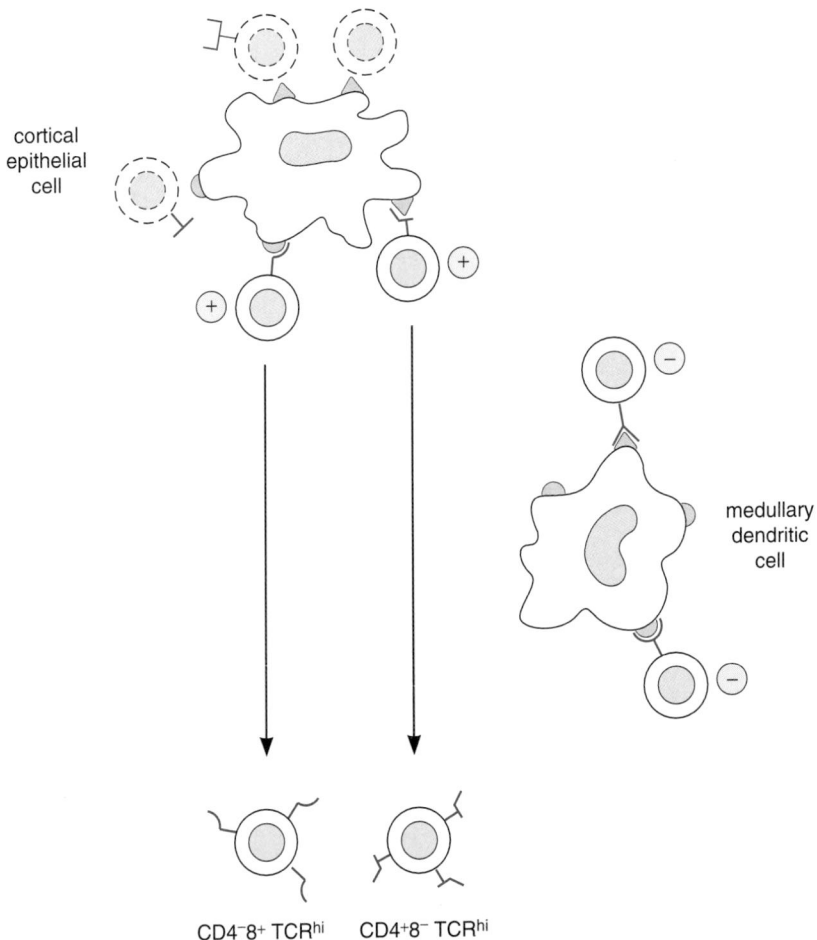

CD4⁻8⁺ TCRʰⁱ   CD4⁺8⁻ TCRʰⁱ

Figure 9–6. Positive and negative selection of thymocytes. CD4⁺CD8⁺TCRˡᵒ thymocytes encounter self-peptides bound to class I (▲) and class II (▲) MHC molecules on epithelial cells in the thymic cortex and on macrophages and dendritic cells in the medulla. Thymocytes whose TCRs are unable to recognize antigens in association with self-MHC die of neglect (dotted outlines). Thymocytes that recognize the combination of self-peptide and self-MHC with low affinity receive a survival signal that allows their positive selection (+). Thymocytes whose TCRs recognize self-peptides and self-MHC with high affinity are deleted (negative selection) (–). The net result of thymic selection is the survival of T cells whose TCRs are restricted by self-MHC molecules but are not autoreactive. Positive selection occurs largely as a result of interactions with cortical epithelial cells, and negative selection largely stems from interactions with medullary macrophages and dendritic cells.

The molecular basis for positive selection remains uncertain, but clearly involves signaling through the TCR. It appears that TCR binding to self-peptide–MHC complexes in the thymic cortex transmits a survival signal to the thymocyte, resulting in its positive selection. Thymocytes whose TCRs are unable at all to recognize self-peptide–MHC do not receive a survival signal, fail positive selection, and die. Failure of positive selection accounts for the great majority of intrathymic death.

Negative selection, which eliminates potentially autoreactive T cells, appears to occur primarily in the thymic medulla, where CD4⁺CD8⁺ thymocytes migrate from the cortex. There, thymocytes encounter self-peptides presented in association with class I and class II MHC molecules on bone-marrow-derived dendritic cells and macrophages (see Fig 9–6). If a thymocyte recognizes these self-peptides with high affinity, it undergoes apoptosis. Thus, at this stage in T-cell development and in this context, recognition of antigen delivers signals that result in cell death rather than activation. Cells that do not receive this cell death signal mature and are exported from the thymus.

One recent hypothesis, called the **avidity model** of T-cell selection, proposes that, to a large extent, positive and negative selection represent qualitatively different responses to different intensities of signaling through the TCR (Fig 9–7). The overall strength of signaling in a T cell is proportional to TCR oc-

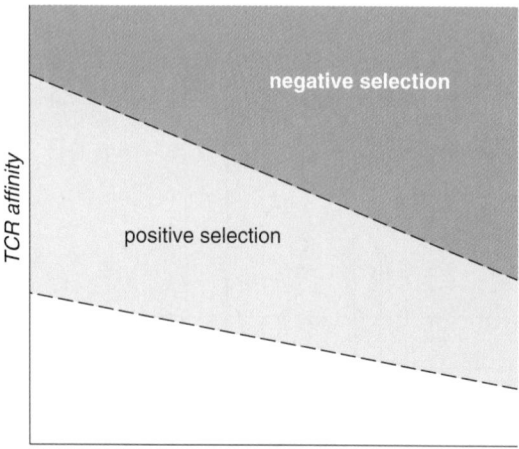

Figure 9–7. The avidity model of T-cell selection in the thymus. Overall TCR signal intensity is the product of both the density and binding affinities of peptide–MHC complexes on the thymic epithelial cell surface. Intermediate levels of signaling promote cell survival; excessive signaling yields cell death. The units depicted are arbitrary and the thresholds unknown.

cupancy, which in turn reflects both the number of TCRs engaged and their affinity for binding the antigen–MHC complex. Below a certain level of TCR occupancy, no effective signal is transmitted. According to the avidity model, a moderate level of occupancy provides a positive signal that allows thymocyte growth and maturation, whereas excessive occupancy (above a certain, undefined threshold) causes cell death by apoptosis. Thymocytes whose receptors bind strongly to self-peptide–MHC complexes in the medulla would thus be eliminated (negative selection), whereas those that give weak but perceptible binding to the same complexes in the cortex would be positively selected. We do not yet know, in biochemical terms, exactly what constitutes the critical difference between the survival signal delivered by low-avidity TCR binding and the apoptotic signal triggered by high-avidity interactions. Nevertheless, the avidity model offers a plausible schema by which TCR–MHC interactions could guide both positive and negative thymic selection, and considerable evidence is accruing to support it.

For negative selection to eliminate all potentially autoreactive T cells, one might imagine that thymic medullary dendritic cells and macrophages would need to present all potential antigenic self-peptides, including those derived from proteins expressed in a highly tissue-specific fashion. To what extent this occurs is not yet clear; the array of peptides presented in the thymus is an area of ongoing investigation. It is known, however, that negative selection is not 100%

effective and that some potentially autoreactive T cells do escape. These autoreactive cells are then either deleted in peripheral tissues or are rendered anergic (unresponsive to antigen). Alternatively, such cells may never encounter antigen simply because the antigens are normally sequestered from the immune system. In certain pathologic states, however, one or more of these mechanisms for peripheral tolerance fails, leading to autoimmunity.

T-CELL ACTIVATION

When a T cell encounters an antigen-presenting cell (APC), the specificity of its TCR determines the outcome. Only if the TCR recognizes its particular antigen–MHC combination does activation occur. The recognition of appropriately presented antigen activates T cells to proliferate, differentiate, and perform their effector functions. Activation of helper T cells leads to the production of lymphokines that promote cellular and humoral immune responses, whereas activation of cytotoxic T cells results in killing of the antigen-bearing cells. Each of these T-cell responses depends on the ability of the TCR to generate intracellular signals for activation.

SIGNAL TRANSDUCTION BY THE TCR

Key to the ability of the TCR to deliver intracellular signals is its interactions with PTKs. In unstimulated T cells, **Fyn,** a member of the Src family of PTKs, associates with the cytoplasmic domains of CD3 chains (Fig 9–8). A second Src-like PTK, called **Lck,** binds to the cytoplasmic domains of CD4 and CD8 and thus can be brought into proximity with the TCR through the interactions of these coreceptors with the MHC. Stimulation of the TCR by antigen–MHC triggers the phosphorylation of tyrosine residues in the cytoplasmic domains of the CD3 chains of the receptor complex. According to a widely accepted model of TCR signaling, Lck and Fyn are responsible for these initial phosphorylation events.

The antigen-induced tyrosine phosphorylation sites lie within particular amino acid sequences, designated immune receptor tyrosine-based activation motifs **(ITAMs),** found in the cytoplasmic domains of CD3 molecules. ITAMs are also present in the signaling chains of the B-cell antigen receptor and of certain Fc receptors. When tyrosine-phosphorylated, the CD3 ITAMs form a recognition unit for another PTK, called **ZAP-70,** and thus recruit ZAP-70 to the TCR complex. ZAP-70, either alone or together with the Src-like PTKs, appears largely responsible for the phosphorylation of a number of intracellular proteins.

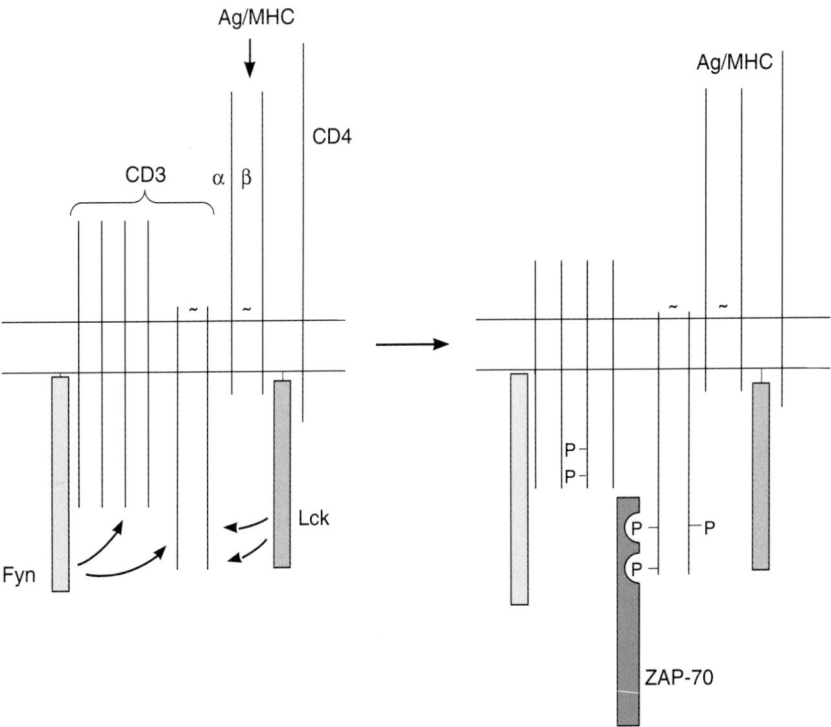

Figure 9–8. Model for the interactions of the T-cell antigen receptor with protein tyrosine kinases. In resting T cells, the CD3 components of the TCR are associated with the protein tyrosine kinase Fyn, and the CD4 coreceptor is associated with Lck. On stimulation of the TCR, the CD3 chains are tyrosine phosphorylated on ITAMs, probably through the action of Fyn or Lck. The tyrosine phosphorylated ITAMs in turn recruit a third protein tyrosine kinase, ZAP-70, to the receptor.

The recent recognition that mutations in ZAP-70 result in immunodeficiency in humans underscores the importance of ZAP-70 in TCR signaling.

Key signaling pathways activated by the TCR-associated PTKs include the Ras pathway, which activates a cascade of serine–threonine kinases, and the phospholipase C pathway (Fig 9–9). TCR stimulation leads to the tyrosine phosphorylation and activation of phospholipase $C\gamma$-1 (PLCγ-1), which hydrolyzes phosphatidylinositol bis-phosphate (PIP$_2$), a membrane phospholipid. The ensuing breakdown of PIP$_2$ generates two second messengers: diacylglycerol and inositol 1,4,5-tris-phosphate (IP$_3$). Diacylglycerol activates the protein kinase C family of serine–threonine protein kinases. IP$_3$ releases Ca^{2+} from internal stores into the cytoplasm, causing an increase in the concentration of cytoplasmic free calcium ([Ca^{2+}]$_i$). Elevations in [Ca^{2+}]$_i$, activated protein kinase C, and the Ras pathway appear to be important mediators for many of the T-cell responses, including the induction of lymphokine gene transcription and the triggering of cytolytic activity. One consequence of the increase in [Ca^{2+}]$_i$ is the activation of calcineurin, a Ca^{2+}-dependent serine phosphatase that plays a key role in activating the interleukin-2 (IL-2) gene. Calcineurin is the target of **cyclosporin** and FK506, two immunosuppressive drugs that block TCR-mediated production of IL-2. These drugs are widely used after clinical transplantation to prevent graft rejection.

CD45: A TYROSINE PHOSPHATASE REQUIRED FOR TCR SIGNALING

CD45 is a large (180–220 kd) transmembrane cell surface molecule that is expressed by all leukocytes, including all T lymphocytes. The cytoplasmic domain of CD45 has tyrosine phosphatase activity. Variants and mutants of T-cell lines that lack CD45 have been isolated in vitro. Remarkably, these CD45-negative T cells cannot respond to antigen, even though they express normal levels of the TCR. The block is at the very early steps of TCR signaling, indicating that CD45 is required for the functional coupling of the TCR and its PTKs. At first glance a positive role for a tyrosine phosphatase in TCR signaling seems counterintuitive. It appears, however, that the CD45 phosphatase removes tyrosine phosphorylations that inhibit the activation of Src-like PTKs. Phosphorylation of a tyrosine residue found in the carboxy terminal tails of Src-like PTKs inactivates these kinases (Fig 9–10). By removing this inhibitory phosphorylation, CD45 allows these PTKs to be activated during antigen recognition.

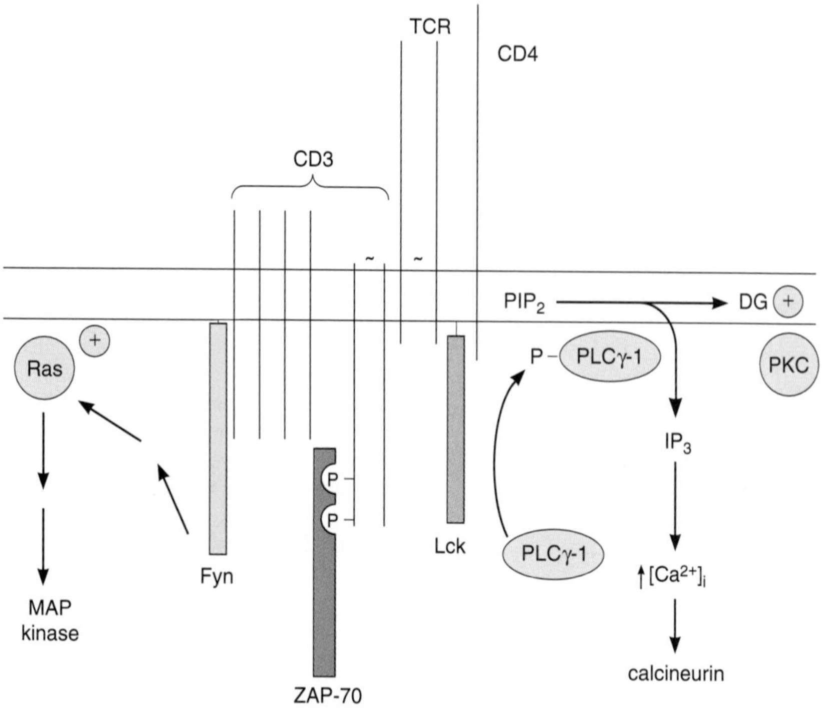

Figure 9–9. Activation of the signaling pathways by the TCR. The TCR-activated protein tyrosine kinases phosphorylate a variety of intracellular molecules, including phospholipase Cγ-1 (PLCγ-1) and upstream regulators of Ras. Tyrosine phosphorylation (P) activates PLCγ-1 which then hydrolyzes its substrate, the membrane phospholipid phosphatidylinositol bis-phosphate (PIP$_2$), releasing diacylglycerol (DG) and inositol trisphosphate (IP$_3$). DG activates protein kinase C (PKC), a family of serine–threonine kinases, and IP$_3$ triggers an increase in the concentration of cytoplasmic free Ca^{2+}.

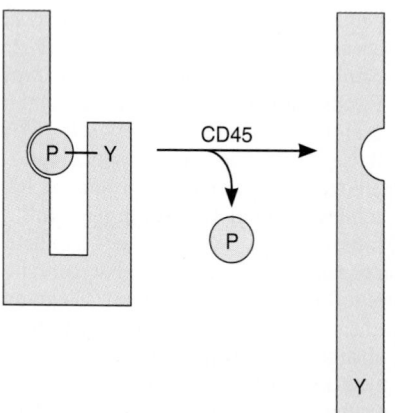

Figure 9–10. Regulation of Src-like protein tyrosine kinases by CD45. Src-like protein kinases, such as Lck and Fyn, can be phosphorylated (P) on a carboxy-terminal tyrosine (Y) by a kinase designated Csk. Phosphorylation at this site induces a conformational change in Src kinases that renders them catalytically inactive. The CD45 phosphatase removes the phosphate from this regulatory tyrosine and restores activity. An inability to activate Lck and Fyn likely explains the impaired TCR signaling observed in T cells that lack CD45.

COSTIMULATION BY CD28

Despite their complexity, the signals delivered by the TCR are not sufficient to fully activate T cells. Rather, T-cell activation requires the delivery of both the TCR signals and a second set of signals generated by costimulatory molecules. In the absence of the proper costimulus, stimulation of the TCR alone can induce a T cell to enter a state in which it remains viable but is refractory to stimulation by antigen. This state, which is known as **anergy,** can be long-lived, persisting for weeks to months in vitro.

The best characterized (and probably the most important) costimulatory molecule is **CD28,** a 44-kd glycoprotein that is expressed as a homodimer on the surfaces of virtually all CD4$^+$ T cells and approximately 50% of CD8$^+$ T cells. CD28 binds two distinct cell surface molecules, **B7.1** and **B7.2,** found on macrophages, dendritic cells, and activated B cells. The combination of TCR stimulation and the interaction of CD28 with its B7 ligands fully activates T cells and results in substantially greater lymphokine production than can be induced by TCR signals alone (Fig 9–11). This enhanced lymphokine production reflects the ability of CD28 signals to promote lymphokine gene transcription and to increase the stability of lymphokine messenger RNAs. The signaling

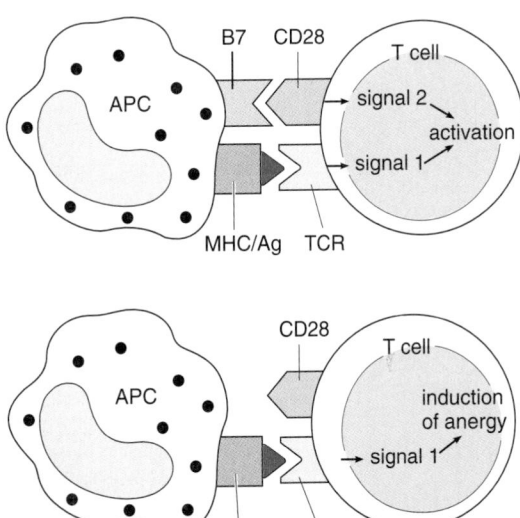

Figure 9–11. The role of CD28 in T-cell activation. Activation of T cells is thought to require TCR-derived signals (signal 1) and a costimulus (signal 2). The major costimulatory molecule, CD28, binds to two cell surface molecules, B7.1 and B7.2, on antigen-presenting cells. The combination of TCR signals and CD28 signals results in a substantial increase in lymphokine production over that seen with TCR stimulation alone. In the absence of the costimulus, the unopposed TCR signals can cause the T cell to enter a state of unresponsiveness known as anergy.

pathways involved in costimulation by CD28 have not been defined.

Because T-cell activation requires both the TCR signals and a costimulus, costimulatory molecules such as CD28 may provide a means of manipulating the immune response to specific antigens. Indeed, in vivo blockade of B7.1 and B7.2 (which prevents CD28 from binding) results in prolongation of allograft survival in experimental animals and reverses autoimmunity in mouse models, raising the possibility that disrupting the CD28/B7 interaction may prove to be a powerful means of suppressing undesirable immune responses. The CD28 costimulus can also be exploited to enhance responses. For example, the immune response to many types of tumors, which generally lack B7.1 and B7.2, is not adequate to prevent tumor growth following implantation in mice. In certain experimental models, however, an effective antitumor immune response is initiated in animals immunized with tumor cells that have been genetically altered so that they express B7.1.

INTERACTION OF T CELLS WITH APCs: THE ROLE OF ADHESION MOLECULES

It is likely that the initial interaction between a T cell and an APC is not mediated by the TCR. This is because the affinity of a TCR for its ligand (antigen–MHC) is generally not sufficient to mediate stable binding to another cell, particularly if relatively small numbers of MHC molecules are complexed with the appropriate peptide. T cells, however, express a number of adhesion molecules, such as leukocyte functional antigen-1 (LFA-1, also called CD11a/CD18) and CD2, that bind ligands on the surface of APCs and thus promote cell–cell contact. The binding of these adhesion molecules to their ligands probably initiates the interaction between the T cell and the APC, allowing the T cell to "survey" the surface of the APC for the appropriate combination of antigenic peptide and MHC molecule. If the TCR recognizes its antigen, then TCR-mediated signals stabilize the interaction between the T cell and the APC, at least in part by modifying LFA-1 so as to increase its affinity for its ligand on the APC. In addition to facilitating the association between T cell and APC, LFA-1 and CD2 also transmit intracellular signals that promote TCR-mediated activation.

T-CELL-MEDIATED IMMUNE RESPONSES

The frequency of occurrence of T cells whose TCRs recognize antigenic peptides derived from any particular pathogen or immunogen is low—on the order of 1 in 1000 or less. An important component of any T-cell immune response is a rapid expansion in the numbers of antigen-specific T cells. This expansion is mediated largely by IL-2 produced by helper T cells. Because high-affinity receptors for IL-2 are induced on antigen recognition and are not expressed by resting T cells, only activated T cells respond to IL-2. IL-2, therefore, induces a relatively selective expansion of those T cells capable of responding to the inciting pathogen. Polyclonal expansions of 1000-fold can be achieved within 10 days through this mechanism. Moreover, as is discussed later on, the effector function of naive T cells is limited but can evolve dramatically following initial activation. The immune response, therefore, entails qualitative as well as quantitative changes in the responding T cells.

The mechanisms that act to terminate a T-cell immune response are incompletely understood. The great majority of the newly expanded T cells die, probably as a result of apoptosis. One candidate for an important negative regulator is **CTLA-4,** a T-cell surface molecule whose expression is induced by activation. CTLA-4 shares considerable sequence similarities with CD28, and, like CD28, binds B7.1 and B7.2. Unlike CD28, however, CTLA-4 appears to inhibit, rather than promote T-cell responses. Mice genetically engineered to lack CTLA-4 die with massive polyclonal proliferation of T lymphoblasts, indicating that CTLA-4 plays a critical role in maintaining T-lymphocyte homeostasis.

The T-cell population is heterogenous with respect to both functional capabilities and cell surface phenotypes. Broadly speaking, T cells are divided into helper cells, which promote cell-mediated and antibody responses, and cytotoxic cells, which kill antigen-bearing target cells. Helper T cells usually express CD4, and cytotoxic T cells generally are CD8$^+$. It should be emphasized, however, that expression of CD4 and CD8 really correlates with MHC restriction. Thus, some CD4$^+$ T cells have cytolytic activity, and certain CD8$^+$ T cells function as helper cells.

HELPER T CELLS: THE T$_H$1 & T$_H$2 SUBSETS

Helper T cells provide signals that augment cell-mediated immune responses and that are necessary for B cells to differentiate into antibody-producing cells. When activated, helper T cells produce soluble lymphokines that can regulate the activities of T cells, B cells, monocyte-macrophages, and other cells of the immune system. T-cell help for B-cell differentiation also occurs through direct contact between the two cell types, which results in direct stimulation of receptors on the B cells and also exposes the B cell to high local concentrations of T$_H$-derived lymphokines.

The lymphokine repertoire of virgin helper T cells is very limited; on their initial encounter with antigen, helper T cells produce IL-2 but little in the way of other lymphokines. When activated, however, virgin T$_H$ cells give rise to effector T cells that can produce a considerable array of different lymphokines. Most of these mature T$_H$ effector cells belong to one of two distinct subsets, designated T$_H$1 and T$_H$2 cells, that are distinguished by the particular lymphokines they produce (Table 9–1). Their divergent patterns of lymphokine expression, in turn, allow each of these T$_H$ subsets to promote distinct types of immune reactions that are best suited to eliminating particular types of microorganisms.

T$_H$1 cells produce IL-2, interferon-gamma (IFNγ), and tumor necrosis factor beta (TNFβ, also called lymphotoxin alpha). Broadly speaking, these lymphokines promote defensive reactions that are mediated by macrophages and other phagocytes, and so involve intracellular killing of pathogens. IFNγ, for example, potently activates macrophages by inducing nitric oxide synthase and other metabolic enzymes that increase microbicidal activity. At the same time, IFNγ acts on activated B cells to induce immunoglobulin class switching to IgG1—an isotype that binds strongly to all three classes of macrophage Fcγ receptors and so functions as an extremely potent opsonin. The overall effect is to potentiate both engulfment and killing by phagocytes.

T$_H$2 cells, by contrast, do not make IL-2, IFNγ, or TNFβ but instead secrete IL-4, IL-5, IL-6, IL-10, and

Table 9–1. Lymphokine expression by T$_H$1 and T$_H$2 cells.

TH Subtype	Cytokines Secreted	Major Immunologic Effects[1]
T$_H$1	IFNγ	Activate macrophages.
		Promote B-cell proliferation and class switching to IgG1.
	IL-2	Promotion activation of antigen-specific T$_H$ and T$_C$ cells.
	TNFβ	Activate macrophages and neutrophils.
		Promote B-cell growth and immunoglobulin production.
T$_H$2	IL-4	Chemoattract lymphocytes, mast cells, and basophils.
		Enhance growth of mast cells and eosinophils.
		Promote B-cell proliferation and class switching to IgE and IgG4.
		Inhibit T$_H$1-cell differentiation.
		Inhibit cytokine production by macrophages.
	IL-5	Enhance growth and development of eosinophils.
	IL-6	Promote B-cell growth and immunoglobulin production.
	IL-10	Inhibit production of cytokines (including IFNγ) by T$_H$1 cells, macrophages, and other APCs.
		Inhibit T$_H$1-cell differentiation.
		Promote B-cell growth and immunoglobulin production.
	IL-13	Same as IL-4.

Abbreviations: IFNγ = interferon gamma, IL = interleukin, TNFβ = tumor necrosis factor beta, APC = antigen-presenting cell.
[1] Only a few pertinent effects of these cytokines are listed here; a more complete discussion can be found in Chapter 10. Each of the processes listed is enhanced by the cytokine unless otherwise stated.

IL-13. These T$_H$2-derived cytokines act together to chemoattract B cells, mast cells, basophils, and eosinophils and then to promote the growth and differentiation of those cell types at the site of an immune response. In addition, IL-4 promotes B-cell class switching to IgE—the isotype bound uniquely by Fcε receptors on mast cells and eosinophils, and which enables those cells to recognize and respond to antigens. By these means, T$_H$2 cells cause an influx of mast cells and eosinophils and help focus their attack on an antigen. This type of defense reaction is particularly effective against large, multicellular parasites such as helminths, which can often be killed extracellularly by eosinophils but are too large to be engulfed by macrophages. Indeed, macrophages play little role in T$_H$2-mediated immune reactions, in part, because IL-10 acts to inhibit IFNγ production and because IL-4 selectively favors production of two immunoglobulin isotypes (IgE and IgG4) that are not recognized by macrophage Fc receptors.

T_H1 and T_H2 cells appear to derive from common precursor T cells and have the capacity to differentiate into either T_H subtype. Such differentiation probably involves an intermediary stage, designated the **T_H0 cell,** which is defined by its ability to secrete both IFNγ and IL-4 (Fig 9–12). The subsequent pathway that each T_H0 cell follows is determined by the cytokines present in its milieu. IL-12 causes antigen-primed virgin T_H cells to differentiate into T_H1 cells, whereas IL-4 drives differentiation into T_H2 cells. Activated macrophages are known to secrete IL-12: this promotes local development of T_H1 cells, which, in turn, would amplify the macrophage response. The source of IL-4 during the initial phase of an immune response (before the appearance of T_H0 and T_H2 cells) is uncertain, but attention recently has focused on a relatively minor T-cell subset that, in mice, expresses a cell surface molecule called natural killer 1.1 (NK1.1) and produces IL-4 on primary stimulation. Later in the response, IL-4 released by activated mast cells would enhance T_H2 differentiation and further amplify the mast cell reaction. If either IL-4 or IL-12 predominates over a prolonged period, individual T_H cell clones may become permanently biased toward the corresponding developmental pathway. Moreover, the two subtypes reciprocally inhibit each other: T_H1-derived IFNγ inhibits the development of T_H2 cells, and T_H2-derived IL-4 interferes with T_H1 cell development. Indeed, one important function of T_H2

cells may be to suppress T_H1 production so as to limit the tissue damage that can accompany an overly vigorous T_H1-mediated response.

As a result of these positive and negative feedback effects, an immune response can become strongly polarized toward either T_H1 or T_H2 production over time, so that one subtype or the other comes to dominate. Immune responses that are chronic, such as those to parasitic infections, are especially prone to such polarization. This can be highly advantageous if it yields the optimal response against a pathogen. A well-characterized example of a T_H1-dominated response is the brisk cell-mediated reaction of most mouse strains against the protozoan *Leishmania major.* This intracellular pathogen invades macrophages, stimulating them to produce IL-12 and thus promoting T_H1 development. The T_H1 lymphokines, in turn, activate the macrophages to kill the parasites and clear the infection. For reasons that are not well understood, certain mouse strains develop a T_H2-dominated response to *L major;* this leads to a vigorous antibody response but no macrophage response. In these strains, the parasite evades killing, disseminates widely, and eventually kills the host. A similar dichotomy can be seen in humans infected with *Mycobacterium leprae*—the causative agent of **leprosy.** *M leprae* produces two patterns of disease that correlate with the T_H response of the host. Patients with a T_H1-dominated response develop the less ag-

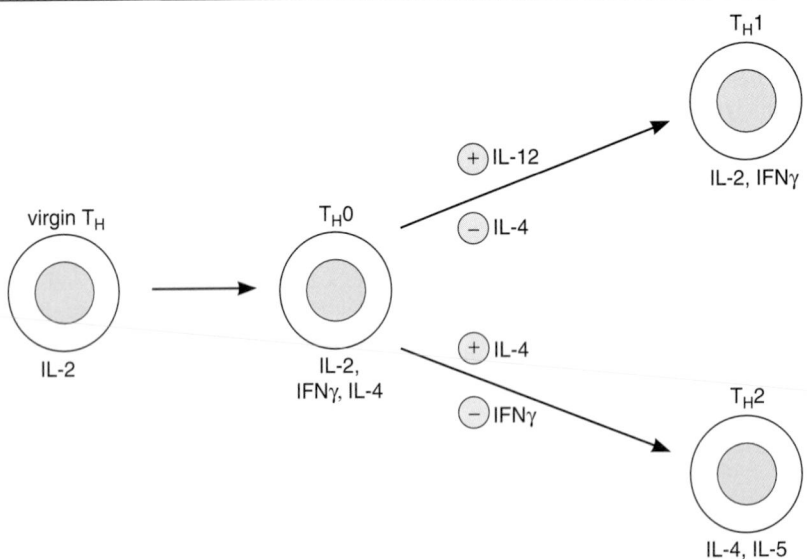

Figure 9–12. Differentiation of helper T cells into T_H1 and T_H2 cells. Virgin T_H cells produce IL-2 and little in the way of other cytokines on initial activation. Repeated stimulation in the presence of IL-12, a macrophage-derived cytokine, causes T_H cells to differentiate into T_H1 cells, which produce IL-2 and IFNγ and are particularly effective in enhancing immune responses that involve macrophages and other phagocytes. Stimulation in the presence of IL-4, on the other hand, promotes the development of T_H2 cells, which produce IL-4 and other cytokines that promote mast cell- and eosinophil-mediated responses. The differentiation into either T_H subtype probably involves a common intermediary, designated T_H0, which produces IL-2, IFNγ, and IL-4. T_H1 and T_H2 cells have the ability to mutually downregulate the development of the other: the T_H1 product IFNγ impairs the generation of T_H2 cells, and the T_H2 cytokine IL-4 inhibits the development of T_H1 cells.

gressive, tuberculoid form of the disease, in which the infectious agent is contained by a brisk macrophage response at multiple foci in the body. Those with a T_H2-dominated response, on the other hand, develop the disseminated, lepromatous form of leprosy.

The divergent effects of T_H1 and T_H2 cells are also seen in their association with deleterious immune reactions in humans. In particular, **autoimmune disorders** associated with the destruction of host tissues, as occurs in diabetes mellitus, multiple sclerosis, or inflammatory bowel disease, predominantly involve T_H1 responses. By contrast, **allergic disorders** (such as seasonal rhinitis, asthma, and contact dermatitis) in which IgE, mast cells, and eosinophils play a prominent role are dominated by T_H2 cells. It is not yet clear to what extent the development of such disorders might reflect an inborn predisposition toward T_H1 or T_H2 responses. Nevertheless, it may someday be possible to treat or prevent these disorders by selectively influencing the development or functions of individual T_H subtypes. Similar approaches might also be used to promote desirable immune responses. For example, IL-12 administered at the time of vaccination has been found to enhance protective T_H1 reactions against certain pathogens in animals.

CYTOLYTIC T CELLS

Cytolytic T lymphocytes (CTLs) respond to antigen recognition by killing the antigen-bearing cell. These cells are usually CD8$^+$ and recognize antigen in the context of MHC class I molecules. CTLs play a prominent role in the host defense against viral infections. Proteins from viral pathogens enter the endogenous pathway for antigen presentation, resulting in the expression of MHC class I molecules bearing viral peptides. CTLs also are involved in the response to certain intracellular bacterial pathogens, including *Listeria* and mycobacteria. CTLs are important in allograft rejection and may play a role in immune surveillance against malignancy.

Killing by Cytotoxic Granules

CTLs arise from virgin T precursors that have limited killing capability. Differentiation into cytolytic cells results from the combination of antigen recognition and exposure to IL-2. In addition to triggering proliferation, IL-2 increases the expression of cytoplasmic granules involved in the killing of target cells (Fig 9–13). The CTL granules contain **perforin** (also known as cytolysin) and **granzymes,** a family of re-

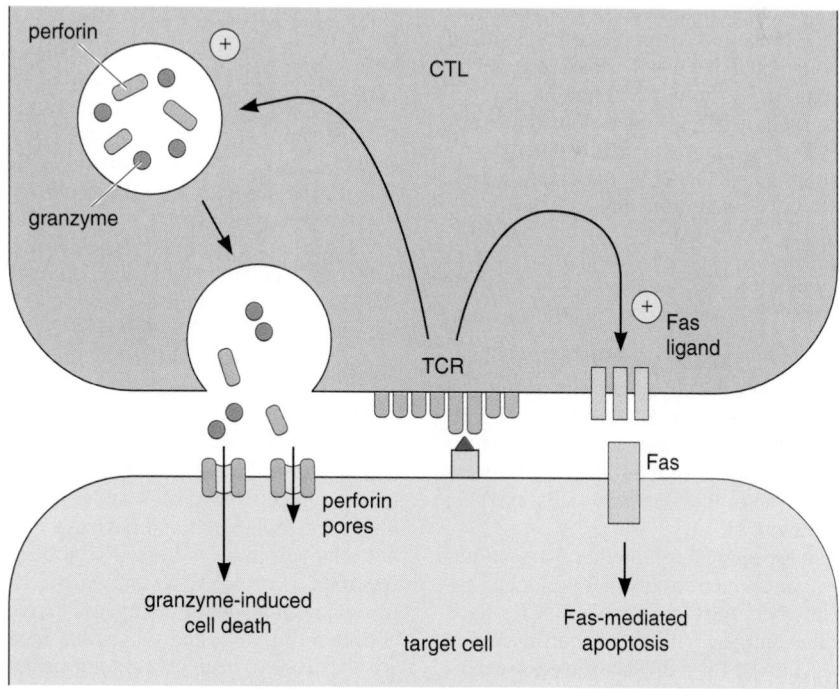

Figure 9–13. Mechanisms of target cell killing by cytolytic T cells. Antigen recognition by cytolytic T cells triggers the exocytosis of granules, leading to the release of perforins, which form pores in the target cell membrane and permit the entry of granzymes into the target cell. Granzymes trigger target cell death through as yet undefined pathways that lead to cell membrane disintegration and to apoptosis. Cytolytic T cells also can kill targets through the Fas ligand–Fas pathway. TCR stimulation induces the expression of Fas ligand on the cytolytic T cell. If the target cell expresses Fas, its engagement by Fas ligand transduces a signal that triggers apoptosis in the target cell.

lated serine proteases. During target cell recognition, the contents of these granules are directionally released toward the target. The perforin molecules, which are evolutionarily related to complement component C9, form 10- to 20-nm pores in the plasma membrane of the target. These perforin pores are not sufficient to kill nucleated target cells, which have the ability to repair membranes and thereby avoid osmotic lysis. Rather, the pores appear to function as a means of delivering granzymes into the target, and it is the granzymes that induce death of the target by triggering apoptosis. One important step in this process is carried out by granzyme B, which proteolytically cleaves and activates ICE-like proteases (caspases) in the target cell, which are components of the apoptotic pathway (see Chapter 1).

Killing by the Fas Ligand–Fas Pathway

The release of cytolytic granules is not the only means by which CTLs can kill antigen-bearing cells. Antigen recognition stimulates CTLs to express Fas ligand, a member of the tumor necrosis factor (TNF) family. The interaction of Fas ligand with Fas (a cell surface molecule related to TNF receptors) induces apoptosis in the Fas-expressing cell (see Chapter 4). The Fas death pathway is also used by CD4$^+$ T$_H$1 cells, which do not express cytolytic granules.

T cells can be activated to express Fas, and activated T cells can become susceptible to Fas-induced apoptosis. Fas-mediated death of T cells, triggered by Fas ligand-expressing T cells, is important for immune regulation. Humans and mice with mutations that interfere with Fas expression or function develop a clinical disorder characterized by massive accumulation of T cells and by autoimmunity.

MEMORY T CELLS

A remarkable feature of the adaptive immune system is its memory; a second challenge with an antigen results in a prompter and more effective immune response than does the initial exposure to the same antigen. T-cell memory reflects antigen-induced differentiation of naive T cells into memory cells and can involve T$_H$ cells and CTLs.

One important aspect of T-cell memory is quantitative; exposure to an antigen results in a prolonged increase in the numbers of T cells whose TCRs have specificity for that antigen. Unlike the short-lived virgin T cells, which exist for a matter of weeks, memory T cells are either long-lived or capable of self-renewal and persist for years. Indeed, antigen-specific memory CTLs have been detected in humans as long as 30 years after vaccination. On rechallenge, therefore, there can be up to 100 times more T cells available to respond to the antigen in question.

There are also important qualitative distinctions between memory T cells and virgin T cells. Memory T$_H$ cells, for example, proliferate sooner and express a broader array of lymphokines after contact with an antigen and are more effective helpers. Memory and virgin T cells also differ in their surface phenotypes, most notably in their expression of CD45 isoforms. Alternative splicing of CD45 mRNA gives rise to a number of different isoforms of CD45 that differ in the size and composition of their extracellular domains. Virgin T cells express 205- to 220-kd isoforms designated CD45RA, whereas memory T cells express a 180-kd isoform called CD45RO. Memory T cells also express higher levels of adhesion molecules on their surfaces; this enables them to adhere more tightly to APCs, and may account for their ability to respond to lower concentrations of antigens. In addition, memory and virgin T lymphocytes express different types of surface homing receptors and so follow different patterns of trafficking to and within tissues (see Chapter 3).

γ/δ T CELLS

A small subset (<5%) of mature T cells does not express a TCR α/β dimer. These cells have a second form of the TCR, composed of a CD3 complex together with a dimer of polypeptides designated γ and δ. The TCRγ and δ genes are highly homologous to the TCRα and β genes and, as is the case with α and β, functional gene products are formed by the rearrangements of germline V and J segments (in the case of γ) or V, D, and J segments (TCRδ). Indeed, the TCRδ gene lies within the TCRα locus.

Interestingly, the first T cells to mature during fetal development are γ/δ T cells. The development of these early γ/δ T cells is highly regulated. They appear in successive waves, with each wave characterized by the use of particular Vγ segments. The γ/δ T cells that mature in the postnatal thymus use different Vγ segments.

The physiologic roles of γ/δ T cells remain uncertain. These cells are either CD4$^-$CD8$^-$ or CD4$^-$CD8$^+$ and appear to be the predominant T-cell type in certain epithelial tissues, such as the skin. γ/δ T cells can produce lymphokines and have cytolytic capabilities, but relatively little is known regarding their antigen specificities or MHC restriction. Certain γ/δ T cells recognize nonpeptide antigens derived from mycobacteria in vitro, and substantial increases in these γ/δ T cells have been observed in patients with tuberculosis and other mycobacterial infections. One subclass of γ/δ T cells in the epidermis appears to react to unknown distress signals expressed by damaged epidermal keratinocytes; when activated, these T cells secrete keratinocyte growth factor—a cytokine that may facilitate wound healing.

NATURAL KILLER CELLS

Natural killer (NK) cells are large granular lymphocytes that, like CTLs, use cytoplasmic granules containing perforins and granzymes to kill target cells. NK cells were defined initially by their ability to lyse certain tumor cell lines and virally infected cells in vitro. NK cell activity against these in vitro targets is spontaneous; it is readily apparent in individuals who have not been previously exposed to the target cell antigens (hence the term "natural killing"). A detectable CTL response, in contrast, requires prior sensitization.

NK cells constitute a discrete lymphoid lineage distinct from T lymphocytes. Unlike T cells, NK cells do not productively rearrange their TCR genes and do not express a cell surface TCR/CD3 complex. Most NK cells express CD16 (a low-affinity Fc receptor that binds IgG in immune complexes) and CD56, whereas these molecules are not found on most T cells. Thus, analysis of CD3, CD16, and CD56 serves to distinguish NK cells (always CD3$^-$ and usually CD16$^+$CD56$^+$) from T cells (always CD3$^+$ and usually CD16$^-$CD56$^-$).

DEVELOPMENT & TISSUE DISTRIBUTION OF NK CELLS

Like T and B lymphocytes, NK cells derive from a bone marrow precursor, but, apart from this, little is known about their ontogeny. The requirements for development of the NK cell lineage are clearly distinct from those of T cells and B cells. For example, children with severe combined immunodeficiency may lack T cells and B cells but have normal NK cells. Conversely, a few individuals have been identified in whom NK cells are absent but T and B lymphocyte development is normal. The development of NK cells does not require a thymus.

NK cells make up about 15% of peripheral blood lymphocytes and 3–4% of splenic lymphocytes. Appreciable numbers of NK cells are also found in the lung interstitium, the intestinal mucosa, and the liver. Unlike T cells, they are rare in the thymus and lymph nodes and are not usually found in the thoracic duct lymph.

NATURAL KILLING

The cell surface molecules that NK cells use to recognize and respond to targets have not been well defined and remain an area of intense investigation. In marked contrast to killing by CTLs, whose ability to recognize targets depends on antigen presentation by MHC class I molecules, natural killing is inhibited by MHC class I molecules and is enhanced by their absence. In teleologic terms, sensing diminished or aberrant class I expression could be useful in the detection of virally infected cells and malignant cells. These observations have led to the hypothesis that NK cells express two types of receptors: one set that triggers cytolytic activity, and a second that binds MHC class I molecules and inhibits killing.

Ly-49 INHIBITORY RECEPTORS

Little is known about the identity of stimulatory NK cell receptors or the nature of their ligands on target cells. There has been, however, considerable progress in understanding the inhibition of natural killing. The first inhibitory molecule to be identified was Ly-49A, a cell surface molecule found on subsets of mouse NK cells. Ly-49A interacts with certain MHC class I molecules and, as a result, prevents the NK cell from killing its target. Disruption of the Ly-49A/MHC interaction (by the addition of monoclonal antibodies to either component) enables NK cells to lyse formerly resistant targets. Conversely, expression of a class I molecule known to be a ligand for Ly-49A renders formerly susceptible targets resistant. The Ly-49A inhibitory signals, therefore, are dominant over stimulatory signals. Ly-49A is a member of a family of closely related molecules, raising the possibilities that individual NK cells express multiple family members with distinct abilities to recognize particular class I molecules. Differential expression of members of the Ly-49 family may define NK cell subsets with differing spectra of susceptible targets.

KILLER CELL INHIBITORY RECEPTORS

The human homologues of the Ly-49 family have not yet been found. Remarkably, studies of human NK cells have led to the identification of a completely separate set of NK cell inhibitory molecules: the killer cell inhibitory receptor (KIR) family. Like the Ly-49 molecules, KIR molecules interact with MHC class I molecules and, as a result of this interaction, inhibit natural killing. Individual KIR molecules (there appear to be at least 10 members of the family) differ in the particular class I molecules they recognize. Differential expression of KIR molecules may generate subsets of NK cells with differing abilities to kill targets.

Despite their functional similarities, the Ly-49 and KIR families have radically different structures. Ly-49 molecules are type II integral membrane proteins (meaning that their amino termini are intracellular) and are expressed as disulfide-linked dimers. KIR molecules are members of the immunoglobulin supergene family and are expressed as monomers, oriented with their amino termini extracellularly. The existence of two very different families of NK cell molecules that can bind class I MHC molecules and inhibit natural killing is perplexing. One possibility is that there are important, yet subtle and so far unappreciated, differences in the functions of the Ly-49 and KIR molecules. Alternatively, since Ly-49 molecules have thus far not been identified in humans and KIR molecules have not been found in rodents, these two families may represent a remarkable example of convergent evolution, in which very different structures have been used to obtain the same, essential function.

ANTIBODY-DEPENDENT CELL-MEDIATED CYTOTOXICITY

In addition to their ability to mediate natural killing, NK cells can kill antibody-coated cells. This antibody-dependent cell-mediated cytotoxicity (ADCC) requires the binding of the Fc portion of the antibody to the NK cell surface Fc receptor, CD16, which in turn activates the cytolytic apparatus of the NK cell. Like natural killing, ADCC is inhibited by ligation of Ly-49 molecules on rodent NK cells and KIR molecules on human NK cells.

CYTOKINE PRODUCTION BY NK CELLS

Activated NK cells produce cytokines such as IFNγ, TNFα, and granulocyte-macrophage colony-stimulating factor, and thus have immunoregulatory abilities. By producing IFNγ, for example, NK cells can augment cell-mediated immune responses by activating macrophages and by skewing the differentiation of T_H cells away from T_H2 cells and toward the T_H1 subtype. NK cell-derived cytokines also modulate hematopoiesis and enhance the production of granulocytes and macrophages.

ROLES OF NK CELLS IN HOST DEFENSE

Although the ability of NK cells to kill tumor cells in vitro has been a focus of research interest, the major physiologic roles of NK cells appear to be in the early host defense against microbial agents. In humans, recurrent viral infections, particularly with varicella-zoster virus, cytomegalovirus virus, and Epstein-Barr virus, dominate the clinical manifestations of a selective deficiency in NK cells. This experiment of nature suggests a major role of NK cells in viral immunity, a conclusion that is further supported by animal studies. The latter also implicate NK cells in early host defenses against certain bacterial and parasitic infections. NK cells, therefore, help protect against a range of infectious agents, particularly early in the course of infections before the T-cell and B-cell responses have developed. NK cells may thus function as a bridge between the innate and the acquired immune systems, acting as a front line of defense while producing cytokines to promote the development of a specific immune response.

REFERENCES

THE TCR, T-CELL ONTOGENY, & T-CELL ACTIVATION

Appleby MW et al: Defective T cell receptor signaling in mice lacking the thymic isoform of p59*fyn*. *Cell* 1992;**70**:741.

Bluestone JA: New perspectives of CD28-B7-mediated T cell costimulation. *Immunity* 1995;**2**:555.

Chan AC et al: ZAP-70: A 70 kd protein tyrosine kinase that associates with the TCR ζ chain. *Cell* 1992; **71**:649.

Davis MM, Bjorkman PJ: T-cell antigen receptor genes and T-cell recognition. *Nature* 1988;**334**:395.

Green JM et al: Absence of B7-dependent responses in CD28-deficient mice. *Immunity* 1994;**1**:501.

Harding FA et al: CD28-mediated signalling co-stimulates murine T cells and prevents induction of anergy in T-cell clones. *Nature* 1992;**356**:607.

Janeway CA: The T cell receptor as a multicomponent signaling machine: CD4/CD8 coreceptors and CD45 in T cell activation. *Ann Rev Immunol* 1992;**10**:645.

Janeway CA: Thymic selection: Two pathways to life and two death. *Immunity* 1994;**1**:3.

Jenkins MK et al: CD28 delivers a costimulatory signal involved in antigen-specific IL-2 production by human T cells. *J Immunol* 1991;**147**:2461.

Kappler JW et al: T cell tolerance by clonal deletion in the thymus. *Cell* 1987;**49**:273.

Marrack P, Kappler J: The staphylococcal enterotoxins and their relatives. *Science* 1990;**248**:705.

Nossal GJV: Negative selection of lymphocytes. *Cell* 1994;**76**:229.

Schreiber SL, Crabtree GR: The mechanism of action of cyclosporin and FK506. *Immunol Today* 1992;**13**:136.

Rudd CE et al: The CD4 receptor is complexed in detergent lysates to a protein tyroine kinase (pp58) from human T lymphocytes. *Proc Natl Acad Sci USA* 1988;**85**:5190.

Veillette A et al: The CD4 and CD8 T cell surface molecules are associated with the internal membrane tyrosine protein kinase p56*lck*. *Cell* 1988;**55**:301.

von Boehmer H. Positive selection of lymphocytes. *Cell* 1994;**76**:219.

Weiss A, Littman DR: Signal transduction by lymphocyte receptors. *Cell* 1994;**76**:263.

T-CELL SUBSETS & EFFECTOR FUNCTION

Havran WL, Allison JP: The immunobiology of T cells with invariant $\gamma\delta$ antigen receptors. *Ann Rev Immunol* 1991;**9:**679.

Henkart PA: Lymphocyte-mediated cytotoxicity: Two pathways and multiple effector molecules. *Immunity* 1994;**1:**343.

Kojima H et al: Two distinct pathways of specific killing revealed by perforin mutant cytotoxic T lymphocytes. *Immunity* 1994;**1:**357.

Mosmann TR, Coffman RL: T_H1 and T_H2 cells: Different patterns of lymphokine secretion lead to different functional properties. *Ann Rev Immunol* 1989;**7:**145.

Paul WE, Seder RA: Lymphocyte responses and cytokines. *Cell* 1994;**76:**241.

Sprent J: T and B memory cells. *Cell* 1994;**76:**315.

Watanabe-Fukunaga R et al: Lymphoproliferation disorder in mice explained by defects in Fas antigen that mediates apoptosis. *Nature* 1992;**356:**314.

NK CELLS

Trinchieri G: Biology of natural killer cells. *Adv Immunol* 1989;**47:**187.

Yokoyama W. Natural killer cells: Right-side-up and upside-down NK-cell receptors. *Curr Biol* 1995;**5:**982.

10

Cytokines

Joost J. Oppenheim, MD, & Francis W. Ruscetti, PhD

Many critical interactions among cells of the immune system are controlled by soluble mediators called **cytokines.** Over the past three decades, much has been learned about the molecular nature and biologic effects of these important regulatory molecules. The cytokines are a diverse group of intercellular-signaling proteins that regulate not only local and systemic immune and inflammatory responses but also wound healing, hematopoiesis, and many other biologic processes.

Over 100 structurally dissimilar and genetically unrelated cytokines have been identified to date. Most are peptides or glycoproteins with molecular weights (MW) of between 6000 and 60,000. They are extremely potent compounds that act at concentrations of 10^{-9}–10^{-15} M by binding to specific surface receptors on target cells. Unlike endocrine hormones, they are not produced by specialized glands but, rather, by a variety of different tissues and individual cells. Cytokines produced by lymphocytes are also known as **lymphokines,** whereas those produced by monocytes or macrophages are called **monokines.** Only a few cytokines—such as transforming growth factor β (TGFβ), erythropoietin (EPO), stem cell factor (SCF), and monocyte colony-stimulating factor (MCSF)—are normally present in detectable amounts in the blood and are able to influence distant target cells. Most other cytokines act only locally over extremely short distances, in either a **paracrine** manner (ie, on adjacent cells) or an **autocrine** manner (ie, on the producing cell itself).

Each cytokine is secreted by particular cell types in response to a variety of stimuli and produces a characteristic constellation of effects on the growth, motility, differentiation, or function of its target cells. A given cytokine may be secreted individually or as part of a coordinated response along with other, unrelated cytokines. Many are functionally redundant—meaning that their activities overlap extensively. Furthermore, one cytokine may induce the secretion of other cytokines or mediators, thus producing a cascade of biologic effects.

This chapter focuses primarily on the participation of cytokines and their receptors in immune and inflammatory responses. Cytokine nomenclature has little to do with structural relationships among molecules: some of them have been termed interleukins (IL) and been assigned a number in sequence (Table 10–1), but many others retain their descriptive and frequently misleading historical names (Table 10–2). We first consider the IL-1, IL-2, IL-4, IL-6, tumor necrosis factor (TNF), and interferon (IFN) cytokine families, and then briefly review the cytokines that regulate growth, differentiation, and function of leukocytes. Cytokines that function primarily on other tissue types are not covered.

Because of their redundancy and complex interactions, it can be quite perilous to extrapolate from in vitro studies of a cytokine to assess its role in the intact organism. An additional source of information, however, has become available in recent years with the development of gene knockout technology: the use of homologous DNA recombination to disrupt specific chromosomal genes and thereby create mice (called **knockout mice**) with homozygous congenital deficiencies in any protein of interest. This technology has been applied to numerous cytokines and cytokine receptors and has provided important new insights into their biologic roles, as summarized later on. In addition, cytokines can now be produced in large quantities by using recombinant DNA techniques, and a number are being tested as potential therapeutic agents; we briefly summarize the resultant clinical experience to date. For more detailed information readers are referred to cited texts, monographs, and reviews.

INTERLEUKIN-1 & TUMOR NECROSIS FACTOR

Interleukin-1 (IL-1) and tumor necrosis factor (TNF) are structurally unrelated cytokines that bind to different cellular receptors, yet their spectra of bio-

Table 10–1. Major properties of human interleukins.

Interleukins	Principal Cell Source	Principal Effects
IL-1α and β	Macrophages, other APCs, other somatic cells.	Costimulation of APCs and T cells. B-cell growth and Ig production. Acute-phase response of liver. Phagocyte activation. Inflammation and fever. Hematopoiesis.
IL-2	Activated T_H2 cells, T_C cells, NK cells.	Proliferation of activated T cells. NK and T_C cell functions. B-cell proliferation and IgG2 expression.
IL-3	T lymphocytes.	Growth of early hematopoietic progenitors.
IL-4	T_H2 cells, mast cells.	B-cell proliferation, IgE expression, and class II MHC-expression. T_H2- and T_C-cell proliferation and functions. Eosinophil and mast cell growth and function. Inhibition of monokine production.
IL-5	T_H2 cells, mast cells	Eosinophil growth and function.
IL-6	Activated T_H2 cells, APCs, other somatic cells.	Synergistic effects with IL-1 or TNF. Induces fever. Acute-phase response of liver. B-cell growth and Ig production.
IL-7	Thymic and marrow stromal cells.	T and B lymphopoiesis. T_C-cell functions.
IL-8	Macrophages, other somatic cells.	Chemoattractant for neutrophils and T cells. Angiogenic.
IL-9	Cultured T cells.	Some hematopoietic and thymopoietic effects.
IL-10	Activated T_H2, CD8 T, and B lymphocytes, macrophages.	Inhibition of cytokine production by T_H1 cells, NK cells, and APCs. Promotion of B-cell proliferation and antibody responses. Suppression of cellular immunity.
IL-11	Stromal cells.	Synergistic effects on hematopoiesis and thrombopoiesis.
IL-12	B cells, macrophages.	Proliferation and function of activated T_C and NK cells. IFNγ production. Promotes T_H1-cell induction; suppresses T_H2-cell functions. Promotion of cell-mediated immune responses.
IL-13	T_H2 cells.	Mimics IL-4 effects.
IL-14	T cells, B cells, tumor cells.	Proliferation of activated B cells.
IL-15	Epithelial cells, monocytes. Nonlymphocytic cells.	Mimics IL-2 effects.
IL-16	CD8+ > CD4+ lymphocytes.	Chemoattracts CD4+ cells (T cells, eosinophils and monocytes.) Comitogenic for CD4+ T cells.

Abbreviations: IL = interleukin; Ig = immunoglobulin; APC = antigen-presenting cell; NK = natural killer; IFN = interferon.

logic effects overlap considerably (Table 10–3). Their importance in immune responses stems largely from their ability to enhance the activation of helper T (T_H) lymphocytes by antigen-presenting cells (APCs). IL-1 and TNF are each secreted by APCs on contact with an antigen- and major histocompatibility complex (MHC)-specific T_H cell, and provide costimulatory signals that promote T-cell activation (see Chapter 4). By inducing the expression of various adhesion molecules, IFNγ receptors, and class II MHC proteins on the surface of an APC, IL-1 and TNF increase the efficiency with which an APC can bind and activate T_H cells. In addition, IL-1 and TNF act in a paracrine

fashion on the T_H cell, augmenting IL-2 secretion, expression of surface receptors for IL-2 and IFNγ, and other subsequent events leading to clonal proliferation. Through their ability to potentiate T_H-cell activation, IL-1 and TNF can promote both humoral and cellular immune responses. Furthermore, these cytokines act synergistically with one another and also with IL-6 to produce markedly augmented effects.

IL-1 and TNF also act directly on many other types of immune and inflammatory cells (see Table 10–3). For example, they can directly promote the growth and differentiation of B cells, particularly during the transition from pre-B cells into mature B lymphocytes

Table 10–2. Major properties of human noninterleukin immunoregulatory cytokines.

	Principal Cell Source	Principal Effects[1]
TNFα	Activated macrophages, other somatic cells.	IL-1-like effects. Vascular thrombosis and tumor necrosis.
TNFβ	Activated T$_H$1 cells.	IL-1-like and TNF-like effects. Development of peripheral lymphoid organs.
IFNα and β	Macrophages; neutrophils, other somatic cells.	Antiviral effects. Induction of class I MHC on all somatic cells. Activation of macrophages, NK cells, and "bystander" CD8+ T cells.
IFNγ	Activated T$_H$1 and NK cells.	Induction of class I MHC on all somatic cells. Induction of class II MHC on APCs and somatic cells. Activation of macrophages, neutrophils, and NK cells. Promotion of cell-mediated immunity (inhibits T$_H$2 cells). Induction of high endothelial venules. Antiviral effects.
TGFβ	Activated T lymphocytes, platelets, macro-phages, other somatic cells.	Anti-inflammatory (suppression of cytokine production and class II MHC expression). Antiproliferative for myelomonocytic cells and lymphocytes. Promotion of B-cell expression of IgA. Promotion of fibroblast proliferation and wound healing.

Abbreviations: TNF = tumor necrosis factor; IFN = interferon; IL = interleukin; MHC = major histocompatibility complex; NK = natural killer; APC = antigen-presenting cell; TGF = transforming growth factor; Ig = immunoglobulin.
[1] All of the listed processes are enhanced unless otherwise indicated.

and from lymphocytes into plasma cells. They also can activate neutrophils and macrophages, stimulate hematopoiesis, and induce expression of numerous other cytokines and inflammatory mediators. Moreover, both IL-1 and TNF produce a broad range of effects on nonhematopoietic cell types (see Table 10–3).

THE INTERLEUKIN-1 FAMILY

IL-1 is produced by virtually all nucleated cell types, including all members of the monocyte–macrophage lineage, B lymphocytes, natural killer (NK) cells, T-lymphocyte clones, keratinocytes, dendritic cells, astrocytes, fibroblasts, neutrophils, endothelial cells, and smooth muscle cells. Like all other species examined to date, humans express two distinct molecular forms of IL-1, called **IL-1α** and **IL-1β.** These are peptides, 159 and 153 amino acids long, respectively, that are encoded by separate genes and share only 26% amino acid sequence similarity. Nevertheless, the potency and biologic activities of IL-1α and IL-1β are virtually identical, and they bind with about the same affinity to the same cell surface receptors. Many cell types express both IL-1 genes, but their relative levels of expression can vary widely. For example, human monocytes produce predominantly IL-1β, whereas keratinocytes produce mainly IL-1α. The biologic significance of this disparity is unknown. A number of cell types can also express a third gene that codes for a protein known as **IL-1 receptor antagonist (IL-1RA),** which is biologically inactive but competes for binding of IL-1 receptors and so is a competitive inhibitor of IL-1α and IL-1β.

IL-1α and IL-1β are initially synthesized as propeptides (MW 31,000) that are then processed enzymatically, either at or beyond the outer cell membrane, to yield the mature cytokines (MW 17,000). The IL-1α propeptide is biologically active, but the IL-1β precursor is not. Precursor IL-1β is selectively cleaved by the IL-1β-converting enzyme (**ICE,** or caspase-1), which enables the resultant mature form of IL-1β to exit the cell. Although IL-1 acts as a soluble extracellular protein, biologically active IL-1α (but not IL-1β) has also been detected on the surfaces of cells and may thus participate in interactions that require cell-to-cell contact.

We briefly review the production of IL-1 as a model for cytokine production in general. A few tissues express IL-1 constitutively; for example, the skin contains significant amounts of IL-1, as do amniotic fluid, sweat, and urine. In contrast, macrophages and most other cell types produce IL-1 only in response to external stimuli, such as bacterial lipopolysaccharide (**LPS**); urate or silicate particles; or **adjuvants,** such as aluminum hydroxide and muramyl dipeptide (see Chapter 5). It is thought that, during the process of antigen presentation, IL-1 production by the presenting cell is initially triggered by contact with the T cell and may then be increased further in response to TNF, colony-stimulating factor (CSF), or IL-2 released from the T cell when it becomes activated. Prostaglandins, a class of small molecules that are important mediators of inflammation (Chapter 12), can also regulate IL-1 expression; for example, IL-1 production by macrophages is enhanced by leukotrienes but is suppressed by products of the cyclooxygenase pathway, such as prostaglandin E$_2$. Increased circulating levels of IL-1 are also observed during the luteal phase of the menstrual cycle and during strenuous exercise.

Table 10–3. Target cells and actions of IL-1 or TNF.

Target Cells or Tissues	Effects	IL-1	TNF
T lymphocytes	Costimulate T-cell activation.	+	+
	Induce IL-2 and IFNγ receptors.	+	+
	Induce lymphokine production.	+	+
B lymphocytes	Promote proliferation.	+	+
	Enhance immunoglobulin expression.	+	+
Monocytes and macrophages	Chemoattract.	−	±
	Activate cytotoxic state.	+	+
	Induce production of prostaglandins, IL-1, IL-6, GM-CSF, and chemokines.	+	+
Neutrophils	Activate to produce cytokines.	+	+
Endothelial and vascular smooth muscle cells	Increase adhesiveness for leukocytes (ICAM-1).	+	+
	Induce procoagulant activity, cytokine production, and class I MHC.	+	+
	Induce mitogenesis and angiogenesis.	+	+
Hematopoietic cells	Inhibit some precursor growth and differentiation.	−	+
	Stimulate precursor cells.	+	−
Hepatocytes	Induce some acute-phase proteins.	+	+
	Decrease cytochrome P-450.	+	+
	Increase plasma Cu; decrease plasma Fe and Zn.	+	+
Neuroendocrine cells	Stimulate glucocorticoid secretion.	+	+
	Induce fever.	+	+
	Induce somnolence and anorexia.	+	+
Osteoblasts	Decrease alkaline phosphatase.	+	+
Osteoclasts	Increase bone resorption and collagenase.	+	+
Chondrocytes	Increase cartilage turnover.	+	+
Fibroblasts and synovial cells	Induce collagenase, chemokines, other cytokines.	+	+
Adipocytes	Decrease lipoprotein lipase.	+	+
	Increase lipolysis.	+	+
Epithelial cells	Induce proliferation.	+	ND[1]
	Increase type IV collagen secretion.	+	ND
Pancreatic β cells	Modulate insulin secretion.	+	−
Dendritic cells	Enhance ability to activate T cells.	+	ND
Tumor cells	Cytostatic and cytolytic effects.	+	+

Abbreviation: IL = interleukin; IFN = interferon; GM-CSF = granulocyte–macrophage colony-stimulating factor; ICAM = intercellular adhesion molecule; MHC = major histocompatibility complex.
[1] ND, no data available.

IL-1 RECEPTORS & SIGNAL TRANSDUCTION

IL-1α and IL-1β bind high-affinity receptors (Kd = 10^{-10} M) which are present on most nucleated cell types. The numbers of receptors range from 50 or fewer on T lymphocytes to several thousand on fibroblasts. Two distinct receptors have been characterized, both of which are transmembrane glycoproteins that bind IL-1α and IL-1β equally. These IL-1 receptors share only 28% sequence similarity but have comparable three-dimensional structures with three extracellular immunoglobulin-like domains. The type-I receptor (**IL-1RI**) is 517 amino acids long, has a 217-amino-acid cytoplasmic tail, and transmits signals intracellularly when it binds IL-1; it is responsible for signaling in all IL-1 responsive cells. The type

II receptor (**IL-1RII**), by contrast, has only a 29-amino-acid cytoplasmic tail and cannot transduce signals. The extracellular domain of IL-1RII is released in soluble form at sites of local inflammation and into the serum during times of systemic inflammation. This soluble IL-1RII is produced in relatively large amounts, binds IL-1β much more strongly than it binds IL-1α or IL-1RA, and functions as an endogenous inhibitor of IL-1β at inflammatory sites and has therefore been called an IL-1 decoy.

Receptors for IL-1 are expressed constitutively on responsive cells, but their levels of expression can be modulated by a variety of agents. For example, IL-4, IL-13, and corticosteroids each increase the expression of IL-1RII and thus suppress IL-1 responsiveness. Conversely, granulocyte–monocyte colony-stimulating factor (GM-CSF) and granulocyte colony-stimulating factor (G-CSF) induce IL-1RI and enhance IL-1 responsiveness, whereas TGFβ suppresses IL-1 effects by decreasing IL-1RI expression. In contrast, T-cell activation is accompanied by increased surface expression of both types of IL-1 receptors.

The mechanism of signal transduction by IL-1 is still controversial. After IL-1 binds, the receptor–cytokine complex is immediately internalized and subsequently degraded, and it must then be replaced by newly synthesized receptors. IL-1 binding to only 5–10% of the IL-1RI molecules on a cell (ie, occupancy of fewer than 50–200 receptors/cell) appears sufficient to trigger cellular responses. The earliest events observed after binding include phosphorylation of serine and threonine residues on a number of cytoplasmic proteins. Some of the phosphorylated proteins directly or indirectly activate specific transcription factors such as NFκB, which in turn bind to chromosomal DNA containing IL-1 responsive genes, leading to activation or suppression of those genes.

TUMOR NECROSIS FACTOR

Human TNF exists in two distinct forms called TNFα and lymphotoxin-α (**LTα**, also known as TNFβ). TNFα was first described as an activity in the serum of LPS-treated animals that was capable of inducing hemorrhagic necrosis of certain tumors. It was later discovered independently as **cachectin,** a circulating mediator of the wasting syndrome associated with certain parasitic diseases. TNFα is produced predominantly by activated macrophages and less so by other cell types. LTα is primarily a product of activated T lymphocytes. TNFα and LTα both bind to the same receptors on target cells and consequently also have overlapping biologic activities, which also overlap with those of IL-1 (see Table 10–3). The activities of TNFα and LTα are not identical, however, because LTα also binds to a cell surface molecule known as **LTβ,** the gene for which is expressed by T and B cells and to a limited degree by myelomonocytic cells. The LTα/LTβ complex stimulates an unrelated receptor, thus accounting for the unique properties of LTα, such as promoting the development of lymphoid organs.

The degree of similarity between TNFα and LTα is only 28% at the amino acid level. They are encoded by two separate genes that are both located within the MHC complex on chromosome 6; hence, they are sometimes referred to as class III MHC proteins, although they have no structural resemblance to class I or class II MHC molecules. Both are synthesized as propeptides and are processed intracellularly to yield the mature forms, which are 157 and 171 amino acids long, respectively. An active membrane-bound form of TNFα exists that can mediate tumor cell killing through cell contact.

TNF RECEPTORS & SIGNAL TRANSDUCTION

Two types of high-affinity receptors for TNFα and TNFβ have been identified. The 75,000 (type II) receptor binds TNFα and TNFβ with about 10-fold higher affinity ($K_d = 5 \times 10^{-11}$ M) than does the MW 55,000 (type I) receptor. Each TNF receptor has a large extracellular binding domain, a hydrophobic transmembrane region, and an intracellular signal-transducing tail. TNFα and LTα bind to these receptors as trimers, with each trimer binding simultaneously to two or three of either type I or type II receptors. This ligand-mediated cross-linking of the receptors is thought to initiate signal transduction, resulting in a cascade of protein phosphorylation and gene activation similar to that produced by IL-1. The two types of TNF receptor are thought to elicit distinct responses: the type I receptor reportedly promotes cytotoxic activity and endotoxin shock, whereas the type II receptor promotes T-lymphocyte proliferation.

Like the IL-1 receptors, TNF receptors are internalized after ligand binding and are modulated by a variety of regulatory factors. For example, IL-2 increases expression of both types of TNF receptors, whereas IFNγ selectively induces type II. Activated cells shed cell-surface TNF receptors, which can bind TNF and may antagonize TNF activity during inflammatory responses.

NONIMMUNOLOGICAL INFLAMMATORY EFFECTS OF IL-1α OR IL-1β & TNFα

TNFα appears primarily responsible for a laboratory phenomenon known as the localized **hemorrhagic Shwartzman reaction,** in which two successive injections of bacterial LPS given 24 hours apart into the same local tissue site produce localized coagulation, hemorrhage, and tissue necrosis. This occurs because LPS-induced secretion of TNFα by macrophages can stimulate endothelial cells to produce prostaglandins, IL-6, and a protein called procoagulant factor (or tissue factor III), which can initiate the clotting cascade. These local coagulation and inflammatory effects block the blood supply and may account for the ability of TNFα to cause infarcts and hemorrhagic necrosis of tumors—the property that led to its initial discovery. There is also a systemic form of the Shwartzman reaction, in which two doses of LPS given intravenously induce **disseminated intravascular coagulation (DIC)**—widespread thrombosis that obstructs capillaries, depletes the supply of coagulation factors, and may lead to hemorrhages, shock, and death. This systemic reaction is thought to mimic certain effects of severe bacterial sepsis and is mediated, at least in part, by TNFα. Repeated

Table 10–4. Plasma proteins of the acute-phase response.[1]

Inducible by IL-1, IL-6, or TNF
Complement factors C3, C9, and B
Mannose-binding protein
Serum amyloid proteins A and P
C-reactive protein
Haptoglobin
α_1-Acid glycoprotein

Regulated only by IL-6
Albumin
Prealbumin
Fibrinogen
Fibronectin
Cysteine proteinase inhibitor
α_1-Antichymotrypsin
Ceruloplasmin
Angiotensin

Abbreviations: IL = interleukin; TNF = tumor necrosis factor.
[1] Hepatocyte synthesis and plasma concentration of each of the listed proteins are increased during the acute-phase response, except those of albumin and prealbumin, which are decreased.

injections of IL-1 can also yield local Shwartzman reactions, and low doses of IL-1 act synergistically with TNFα to mimic the fatal systemic effects of **septic shock.** TNFα and IL-1 are among the most important inducers of the **acute-phase response,** in which hepatocytes produce increased amounts of certain plasma proteins that are thought to be of value in nonspecific host defense against infections (Table 10–4). Their effect in this regard is exceeded by that of IL-6 (see following discussion).

Both IL-1 and TNFα can activate endothelial cells and thus promote neutrophil margination and migration into an inflamed site. They induce the production of endothelial growth factors and have angiogenic activity. Acting alone or synergistically, they can induce a number of effects that are mediated through the hypothalamus: they are **endogenous pyrogens** (ie, they induce **fever**) and stimulate the secretion of corticotropin-releasing factor, which stimulates the release of adrenocorticotropic hormone (ACTH) from the pituitary and in turn induces the production of glucocorticoids by the adrenals. This activation of the hypothalamic–pituitary–adrenal axis has anti-inflammatory effects, since glucocorticoids suppress the production of both IL-1 and TNFα.

Both IL-1 and TNFα stimulate alkaline phosphatase activity in osteoblasts, bone resorption by osteoclasts, cartilage turnover by chondrocytes, and proliferation by fibroblasts and synovial cells. Increased levels of IL-1 and TNFα are found in inflammatory joint fluids and may contribute to the fibrosis and thickening of arthritic joints. The administration of TNF antagonists can ameliorate the symptoms and signs of rheumatoid arthritis.

IL-1 synergizes with colony-stimulating factors (CSFs, see later discussion) to stimulate proliferation and differentiation of early hematopoietic progenitors in the bone marrow. In addition, IL-1 induces bone marrow stromal cells to produce a number of the hematopoietic CSFs, as well as receptors for G-CSF and SCF. TNFα also actively induces CSF production by bone marrow stromal cells and macrophages but suppresses rather than promotes stem cell proliferation. Both TNF and IL-1 enhance the production and release of neutrophils from the marrow. IL-1 and, to a lesser extent, TNFα can protect against the marrow-suppressive effects of radiation if given a day prior to exposure.

Overall, the considerable functional redundancy of IL-1 and TNFα is probably protective in that it provides alternative pathways for mobilizing host reactions to emergencies. Moreover, IL-1 and TNFα regulate each other, and their ability to synergize enables them to achieve maximal effects at suboptimal concentrations. This is economical, results in enormous amplification of host reactions, and increases the efficiency of the host defense system. Despite this redundancy, however, the considerable differences in the phenotypes of various IL-1 and TNF ligand and receptor knockout mice indicate that each of these cytokines does have unique pathophysiologic roles. (Table 10–5).

IL-1, TNF, & THEIR INHIBITORS AS THERAPEUTIC AGENTS

Both IL-1 and TNFα have been investigated as possible therapeutic agents, with emphasis on their immunostimulatory and antineoplastic activities. Neither has yet proven useful in practice, however, largely because of their numerous side effects. The pharmacologic properties of TNFα and IL-1 at high concentrations are similar, although TNFα causes more vascular occlusion, tumor necrosis, and capillary leakage, whereas IL-1 (owing to its more potent hematopoietic effects) provides greater protection against lethal doses of radiation and against bone marrow suppression caused by cancer chemotherapeutic agents.

Antagonists of IL-1 and TNFα are of considerable therapeutic interest as a means of ameliorating chronic inflammatory diseases. IL-1 and TNFα activities can potentially be inhibited by factors that affect their synthesis, release, receptor binding, or signal transduction. Potent nonspecific antagonism to both these cytokines is exhibited by TGFβ and by corticosteroids. In addition to reducing IL-1 production, TGFβ inhibits IL-1RI expression and induces the production of IL-1RA—it is a "triple threat!" Corticosteroids not only reduce the production of IL-1 and TNFα, but also increase expression of IL-1RII, which can further inhibit IL-1 effects. Inhibitors of the lipoxygenase pathway likewise reduce the amount of IL-1 released, whereas leukotrienes appear to increase it (see Chapter 12). β-Melanocyte-stimulating factor has been reported to inhibit IL-1 activity through an unknown mechanism.

Table 10–5. Phenotypic characteristics of proinflammatory cytokine knockout mice.

Targeted Gene	Phenotypic Abnormalities
IL-1β	Reduced IL-6 production and acute-phase responses to turpentine but normal IL-1α levels. Resistance to collagen-induced arthritis.
ICE (caspase-1)	Reduced production of IL-1β and partially of IL-1α. Resistance to LPS lethality.
TNF-R p55	Lower LPS lethality and decreased serum IL-6 levels. Lower resistance to intracellular bacteria.
TNF-R p75	Lower LPS lethality.
TNFα	Lower LPS lethality and reduced resistance to bacterial infection.
LTα (TNFβ)	Failure of lymph node development, absent Peyer's patches, and splenic hypoplasia.
CD40 ligand	No immunoglobulin response to T-dependent antigens. Human gene defect results in hyper-IgM syndrome with neutropenia and intracellular bacterial infections.
Fas ligand	Failure of apoptosis of old T cells and CTL target cells. Mice with gld gene defect develop autoimmunity.
Fas antigen	lpr/lpr mice develop lymphoid hyperplasia and autoimmunity. Humans with gene defect develop autoimmune lymphoproliferative syndrome (ALPS).
IL-6	LPS increases serum TNF, but lower fever response. Reduced acute-phase protein response to turpentine.
IL-6R (gp130)	Embryonic lethal with cardiac hypoplasia.
LIF	Failure of blastocyst implantation.
CNTF	Loss of motor neurons and muscle atrophy.
TGFβ-1	Early death from wasting and polyinflammatory state.
TGFβ-2 or 3	Embryonic lethal.
IL-8R	Deficient neutrophil inflammatory response and reduced antibacterial resistance.
MIP-1α	Reduced mononuclear cell response to influenza virus and reduced post-coxsackie viral myocarditis.

Abbreviations: IL = interleukin; ICE = interleukin-converting enzyme; LPS = lipopolysaccharide; LT = lymphotoxin; LIF = leukocyte inhibitory factor; CNTF = ciliary neurotrophic factor; TGF = transforming growth factor; MIP = macrophage inflammatory protein; CTL = cytotoxic T lymphocyte.

IL-1RA can competitively inhibit IL-1 binding to its receptor; however, it must be present in substantial (at least 100-fold) molar excess over IL-1 to compete effectively. Moreover, IL-1RA is unable to prevent activation of helper T cells by APCs, presumably because alternative pathways of costimulation are available. The shed extracytoplasmic domain of IL-1RII can selectively bind and inhibit IL-1β and probably plays a significant antagonistic role in vivo. Interestingly, certain poxviruses have also been found to encode soluble homologues of the receptors for IL-1 (type II), TNFα and IFNγ that are secreted by infected cells and suppress antiviral immune responses.

THE TNF RECEPTOR SUPERFAMILY

The type-I (p55) and type-II (p75) TNF receptors belong to a larger family of structurally related membrane proteins, called the TNF receptor superfamily (TNFR-SF), which also includes Fas, the nerve growth factor (NGF) receptor, a TNFR-related protein (TNFR-RP, the receptor for the LTα/LTβ complex), CD27, CD30, and CD40 (Table 10–6). The receptors in this superfamily each contain three or four copies of a cysteine-rich repeat of about 40 amino acids in their extracellular domains. These repeats contain four or six conserved cysteine residues in a characteristic pattern that is distinct from cysteine-rich repeats in other molecules. Some of these receptors bind more than one ligand and, unlike most other cytokines, the ligands bind as dimers or trimers. The mode of signal transduction by the TNFR-SF is being elucidated. The cytoplasmic portions of the family members have little homology with one another or with any other receptors.

All members of the TNFR-SF transmit signals that stimulate T or B cells (or both). Indeed, one member—CD40—serves as the principal receptor on B cells for contact-mediated help provided by T$_H$ cells, which express the CD40 ligand protein (see Chapter 9). Recent reports indicate that CD40 is also expressed on APCs and participates in T-cell costimulation. Another member is Fas, which, in conjunction with its ligand (FasL), transmits signals that trigger apoptosis in various settings, including target-cell killing by cytotoxic T lymphocytes (CTLs; see Chapters 4 and 9). Resting human B lymphocytes express the NGF receptor and secrete NGF, which appears to function as an autocrine growth factor that is essential for survival of memory (ie, class-switched), but not virgin, B cells. CD27 is expressed on activated T cells but also by Ig-producing B cells and NK cells. The CD27 ligand (also known as CD70) is expressed on monocytes and some T and B cells and is thought to participate in IL-2 independent T-cell stimulation and CTL development. CD30 is reported to be expressed by the Reed-Sternberg cells of Hodgkin's disease, as well as B- and T-cell lymphomas and other tumors, and to a greater extent by T$_H$2 than by T$_H$0 and T$_H$1 lymphocytes. The CD30 ligand is a costimulator of T cells.

Table 10–6. TNF receptor superfamily members and their ligands.

Ligand	Receptor	Major Effects
TNFα	TNFR-I (p75)	Cytotoxicity and lymphocyte proliferation.
	TNFR-II (p55)	Apoptosis and septic shock.
Lymphotoxin α/β complex	TNFR-RP	Development of lymph nodes and Peyer's patches.
Nerve growth factor (NGF)	NGFR (low-affinity)	Promotes neuronal survival and differentiation.
		Autocrine growth factor for memory B cells.
Fas ligand (FasL)	Fas	Apoptosis.
CD40 ligand (CD40L)	CD40	Promotes B-cell growth, survival, differentiation, and Ig class-switching.
CD27 ligand (CD27L = CD70)	CD27	Costimulates T-cell activation.
CD30 ligand (CD30L)	CD30	Costimulates T-cell activation.

Abbreviations: TNF = tumor necrosis factor; TNFR = TNF receptor; TNFR-RP = TNFR-related protein; Ig = immunoglobulin.

INTERLEUKIN-2

Interleukin-2 (IL-2) is an autocrine and paracrine growth factor that is secreted by activated T lymphocytes and is essential for clonal T-cell proliferation. It was first discovered in 1976 by virtue of its ability to enhance mitogenesis of human T lymphocytes and to support continuous growth of normal T cells in culture. The discovery of IL-2 (then called **T-cell growth factor**) was a major advance in immunology, because it made it possible for the first time to propagate and study individual clones of normal T cells that maintained their immunologic properties. Its essential role in T-cell proliferation, together with its effects on cytokine production and on the functional properties of B cells, macrophages, and NK cells, places IL-2 among the most critical immunoregulatory cytokines.

The IL-2 molecule is a MW 15,400 polypeptide, 133 amino acids long, that is encoded by a single gene on human chromosome 4. It can be glycosylated to various degrees to produce higher molecular weight species, although the glycosylated side chains are not necessary for function. Its amino acid sequence bears no similarity to that of any other known cytokine, but x-ray crystallographic analysis indicates that it has a three-dimensional structure resembling those of IL-4 and GM-CSF. IL-2 is a globular protein composed of two α helices that are arranged to form hydrophobic planar faces around a very hydrophobic core. This configuration is maintained in part by the single intrachain disulfide bond, which is essential for biologic activity.

Resting T lymphocytes do not synthesize or secrete IL-2 protein but can be induced to do both by the appropriate combinations of antigen and costimulatory factors (see Chapter 4) or by exposure to polyclonal mitogens (see Chapter 3). Studies of isolated T-cell subtypes indicate that antigen-induced IL-2 production occurs mainly in CD4 T_H cells. CD8 lymphocytes and some NK cells, however, also can be induced to secrete IL-2 under certain conditions. When normal human lymphocytes are exposed to a T-cell mitogen, IL-2 mRNA expression becomes detectable after four hours, reaches peak concentration at 12 hours, and thereafter declines rapidly. The abrupt disappearance of the mRNA reflects not only the cessation of IL-2 gene transcription but also the instability of IL-2 mRNA, which has a half-life of less than 30 minutes. Synthesis and release of IL-2 protein follow a similar time course, resulting in a transient burst of secretion that quickly subsides. Because IL-2 has a very short half-life in the circulation, it acts only on the cell that secreted it or on cells in the immediate vicinity.

IL-2 RECEPTORS
& SIGNAL TRANSDUCTION

The high-affinity IL-2 receptor **(IL-2R)** is not expressed on resting T cells but is induced to maximal levels within two or three days after the cells become activated. Expression then declines to undetectable levels by 6–10 days after activation. The decline in receptor expression occurs regardless of whether IL-2 is present, indicating that it is autonomously regulated. This ensures that, within a few days after activation, the T cell will become refractory to IL-2, so that clonal proliferation will cease. If such a cell is then reactivated, IL-2R reappears on the cell surface, and IL-2-dependent proliferation resumes until the receptors again disappear four to seven days later. The transient nature of IL-2R expression helps to maintain the cyclical, self-limiting pattern of normal T-cell growth in vivo. In contrast, T cells that have been transformed by **human T-cell leukemia virus type I (HTLV-I),** the agent of **adult T-cell leukemia** syndrome, constitutively express IL-2R. Some HTLV-1-infected cells also produce **IL-15,** a cytokine normally expressed by nonlymphoid cells, which can bind the IL-2R and produces many of the same effects as IL-2 itself; this suggests that autocrine growth stimulation plays a role in T-cell transformation by HTLV-1.

The high-affinity IL-2 receptor consists of a complex of three distinct integral membrane polypeptides, designated α, β, and γ. The IL-2R α chain (also called Tac, CD25, or p55) binds IL-2 with low affinity (K_d 1.4×10^{-8} M), but does not signal. Surprisingly, IL-2Rα knockout mice have markedly enlarged peripheral lymphoid organs, suggesting that the α chain is needed for normal T-cell homeostasis (Table 10–7). The other components of the IL-2R, the IL-2R β-chain (p75), and the IL-2R γ-chain (p64), are members of the hematopoietin receptor superfamily (see following discussion) and are both signal transducers. Both proteins bind other cytokines in addition to IL-2 (Fig 10–1). The IL-2R β-chain binds IL-2 with intermediate affinity (K_d 1.2×10^{-7} M), whereas the γ-chain (p64) by itself does not bind IL-2. Receptor complexes consisting of α/γ or β/γ heterodimers bind IL-2 with an affinity of about 10^{-9} M. The higher-affinity α/β/γ heterotrimer has an equilibrium K_d of 1.3×10^{-11} M and a dissociation half-life of 50 minutes. Both β/γ dimers and heterotrimers are able to mediate IL-2-induced signal transduction. IL-15 can also signal through β/γ dimers but is a more effective stimulant when it binds a heterotrimer consisting of the IL-2R β and γ chains plus a unique IL-15Rα chain.

Several distinct cytoplasmic regions of the IL-2 β chains can be involved in IL-2-mediated cellular sig-

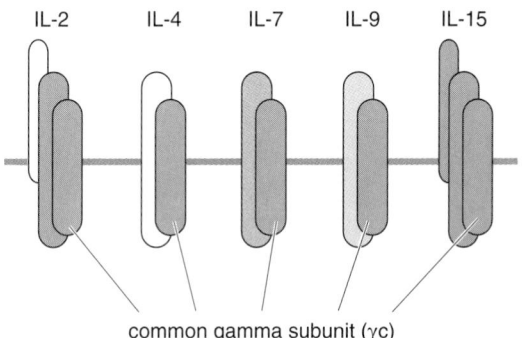

Figure 10–1. The IL-2 γ-chain family.

naling. A serine-rich region is critical for induction of c-Myc and cell proliferation, whereas an acidic region is required for physical association with the Src-like protein tyrosine kinase (PTK) Lck, for activation of the Ras pathway through binding of Shc, and for induction of Fos and Jun (see Chapter 1). In addition, the Janus kinase (Jak) family member Jak1 binds to the β chain. The IL-2R γ chain binds Jak-3 and has an SH2-like homology domain that may be involved in binding to phosphotyrosine residues on other signaling proteins (see Chapter 1). The IL-2R γ chain is also a functional component of the IL-4R, IL-7R, IL-9R, IL-13R, and IL-15 receptor complexes (see Fig 10–1). Recently, mutations in the IL-2R γ chain have been shown to cause **X-linked severe combined immunodeficiency (X-SCID)** in humans because they abolish responsiveness to all these interleukins (Table 10–7). X-SCID is a lethal disease characterized by absent or greatly reduced T cells and severely depressed cell-mediated and humoral immunity.

EFFECTS OF IL-2 ON T LYMPHOCYTES

When exposed to appropriate activating stimuli, resting CD4 T lymphocytes begin to express both IL-2 and surface IL-2R and shortly thereafter begin to proliferate. Interference with either the IL-2 or its receptor (eg, by treatment with specific antibodies) blocks the proliferative response. CD8 T cells are generally unable to produce adequate amounts of IL-2 and so require exogenous IL-2 from helper cells in order to proliferate. Because of its effect on lymphocyte proliferation, IL-2 can be used to establish proliferating clones of normal human CD4 or CD8 T cells in vitro, provided the cells are also continually exposed to mitogens or other activating stimuli that serve to maintain IL-2 receptor expression. The addition of IL-2 to activated normal human lymphocytes promotes several other cellular functions as well as proliferation. For example, IL-2-stimulated T cells

Table 10–7. Phenotypic deficiencies of immunoregulatory cytokine knockout mice.

Targeted Gene	Phenotypic Abnormalities
IL-2	Lethal gastrointestinal ulcerations, inflammatory bowel disease. Lymphoid hypertrophy in survivors.
IL-2Rα	Older mice develop massive enlargement of lymphoid organs and autoimmunity.
IL-2Rβ	Hyperactivation of T-cell autoimmunity.
IL-2Rγ	Greatly reduced lymphoid numbers including NK cells (defective in human X-SCID).
IL-7	Failure of thymic and peripheral lymphocyte development.
IL-7R	Greatly underdeveloped thymic and lymphoid tissues.
IFNγ	Susceptibility to bacterial and large virus infections. No deficiency in T_H1 responses. Deactivated macrophages.
IFNα/βR	Reduced antiviral resistance.
IFNγR	Reduced LPS lethality and cytokine production. Lower resistance to bacterial infection.
IL-4	Reduced IgG1 and IgE levels. Reduced T_H2 cytokine production.
IL-10	Chronic enterocolitis secondary to elevated levels of proinflammatory cytokines; growth defects.

Abbreviations: IFN = interferon; IL = interleukin; Ig = immunoglobulin; LPS = lipopolysaccharide; NK = natural killer; X-SCID = X-linked severe combined immunodeficiency.

exhibit enhanced cytotoxicity and produce lymphokines, such as IFNγ, TNFβ, and TGFβ; B-cell growth factors, such as IL-4 and IL-6; and hematopoietic growth factors, such as IL-3, IL-5, and GM-CSF. Surprisingly, T-cell development in mice with a disrupted IL-2 gene appears normal. Paradoxically, however, after six to eight weeks, increased numbers of T cells are found in the periphery, many of which are activated. This leads to a lethal syndrome characterized by enlarged lymphoid organs, T-cell infiltration of marrow and gut, and severe colitis. It has been observed that activation-induced T-cell apoptosis is deficient in these IL-2 knockout mice, and their lymphoproliferative abnormality may reflect this deficiency.

IL-2 EFFECTS ON NON-T CELLS

NK cells are unique among lymphoid cells in that they constitutively express IL-2R and thus are IL-2-responsive even in a resting state. Because they express only the β and γ chains, unstimulated NK cells bind IL-2 with relatively low affinity and proliferate only in response to correspondingly higher IL-2 concentrations. Once stimulated by IL-2, however, NK cells begin to express the IL-2R α chain and so acquire high-affinity receptors. IL-2-stimulated NK cells have enhanced cytolytic activity and secrete numerous cytokines, including several (IFNγ, GM-CSF, and TNFα) that are potent activators of macrophages. IL-2 also induces **lymphokine-activated killer (LAK)** activity, which is predominantly due to NK cells.

Activated or transformed B lymphocytes express high-affinity IL-2R at approximately 30% the density found on activated T cells. IL-2 enhances proliferation and antibody secretion by normal B cells, although at concentrations two to threefold higher than are required to obtain T-cell responses. It also influences the heavy-chain class switch, biasing B cells toward expression of IgG2 antibodies.

Human monocytes and macrophages constitutively express low levels of IL-2R β chain but inducibly express high-affinity receptors containing all three chains on exposure to IL-2, IFNγ, or other activating agents. Continued exposure of an activated macrophage to higher concentrations of IL-2 enhances its microbicidal and cytotoxic activities and promotes secretion of hydrogen peroxide, TNFα, and IL-6. Higher concentrations of IL-2 can activate neutrophils as well.

IL-2 AS A THERAPEUTIC AGENT

Administration of IL-2 to normal or immunodeficient mice has been shown to enhance immune responses, particularly those mediated by cytotoxic T lymphocytes or NK cells. Its potential use in humans, unfortunately, is limited by severe toxic side effects that occur at pharmacologic IL-2 dosages. One of the most important of these is the "vascular leak syndrome," characterized by the accumulation of edema fluid in the pleural cavities, peritoneum, and other extravascular spaces; this may result from the ability of IL-2 to induce other cytokines that activate endothelial cells. IL-2 treatment can also lead to elevated serum cortisol levels, with consequent immunosuppressive effects. High-dose IL-2 has been tested as an immunostimulatory agent in the treatment of a variety of cancers and has produced partial remissions in about 20% of patients with renal cell carcinoma or metastatic melanoma. IL-2 has also been tested at low doses as a treatment for the T-cell anergy that occurs in patients with lepromatous leprosy; although some clinical benefit was observed, the anergy persisted, and the beneficial effects have been attributable to activation of macrophages and NK cells.

INTERLEUKIN-6 (IL-6) & RELATED CYTOKINES

IL-6 is a cytokine with multiple biologic activities on a variety of cells (Table 10–8). Its major activities include synergizing with IL-1 and TNF to costimulate T cells; inducing the **acute-phase response** in liver cells (see Table 10–4) and the hypothalamic fever center; enhancing B-cell replication, differentiation, and immunoglobulin production; promoting hematopoiesis and thrombopoiesis; and supporting growth of transformed hepatocyte and myeloma cell lines in tissue culture.

The gene for IL-6 is located on human chromosome 7. The reported MW of IL-6 ranges between 22,000 and 30,000, owing to variations in the degree of glycosylation and phosphorylation of a single polypeptide. IL-6 can be produced by many cell types, including activated T and B lymphocytes, monocytes, endothelial cells, epithelial cells, and fibroblasts. Its expression is induced by a variety of stimuli, including TNF, IL-1, platelet-derived growth factor, and agents that activate T and B lymphocytes and macrophages.

THE IL-6 RECEPTOR FAMILY

High-affinity binding sites for IL-6, with a K_d of 10^{-10} to 10^{-12} M are expressed by a variety of cell types, including macrophages and myelomonocytic cell lines, hepatocytes, resting T cells, activated or Epstein-Barr virus-infected B cells, and plasma cell lines. Target cells express from 10^2 to 10^4 IL-6 receptors. The receptor consists of two glycoprotein chains. The MW 80,000 IL-6Rα chain lacks a cytoplasmic

Table 10–8. The human IL-6 family of cytokines.

	IL-6	IL-11	LIF	OSM	CNTF	CT-1
Prominent cell sources	Activated T$_{H2}$ cells. Macrophages. Endothelial fibroblasts	Stromal cells.	T cells. Macrophages. Fibroblasts.	Macrophages. T cells.	Glial cells.	Embryonic stem cells. Heart and skeletal muscle. Fibroblasts.
Unique effects	T-cell costimulator. Coinduces cachexia. Induces glucocorticoids, bone resorption, and keratinocyte growth.	Thrombopoietic.	Inhibits leukemic cell growth. Inhibits melanoma growth.	Promotes smooth muscle and fibroblast growth.	Enhances survival of ciliary neurons.	Cardiac myocyte hypertrophy.
Shared effects[1]	Acute-phase response.	+	+	+	+	+
	B-cell and plasma cell growth, Ig production.	+	—	—	—	—
	Hematopoiesis.	+	+	+	—	?
	Leukemic cell growth.	?	↓	↓	—	↓
	Neurotrophic activity.	?	+	+	+	+
	Endothelial cell growth.	?	+	+	—	?

[1] Ability to induce or enhance the indicated processes.
↓ = inhibits.

domain and binds IL-6 with low affinity; the resulting complex of IL-6Rα and IL-6 is then bound with high affinity by the MW 130,000 IL-6Rβ chain, which transduces a signal into the cytoplasm.

Over the past decade, the IL-6Rβ chain has been found to form part of the receptors for five additional structurally unrelated cytokines: interleukin-11 (**IL-11**), leukocyte inhibitory factor (**LIF**), oncostatin M (**OSM**), ciliary neurotrophic factor (**CNTF**), and cardiotrophin-1 (**CT-1**). Each of these cytokines has its own specific receptor containing one or more unique chains that mediates ligand binding. The IL-6Rβ chain (gp130) functions as a common signal-transducing subunit in each of these receptors, which may account for the reported overlap in the biologic activities of these structurally dissimilar cytokines (Table 10–8).

ACTIVITIES OF THE IL-6 CYTOKINE FAMILY

IL-6 acts as a costimulant that synergistically augments the mitogenic effects of IL-1 and TNF on helper T cells. This effect is in part (but not entirely) due to its ability to increase IL-2R expression. IL-6 is also very effective in enhancing TNF- or IL-1-in-duced cachexia and glucocorticoid synthesis and is able independently to stimulate osteoclast activity and keratinocyte growth. It does not induce the production of any other known cytokines and has relatively little direct effect on immune cells at physiologic concentrations. This suggests that its main immunologic function is to potentiate the effects of other cytokines.

IL-6 is the most important inducer of the hepatic acute-phase response (see Table 10–4), although IL-11, CT-1, LIF, and OSM share this activity, as do IL-1 and TNF. IL-6 knockout mice, however, are phenotypically normal except for a lowered acute-phase and fever response, and increased production of TNF (Table 10–5). The capacities of IL-6 to stimulate the growth of lymphoid cell lines and to promote immunoglobulin synthesis are shared by IL-11. Since malignant plasma cells of multiple myeloma both produce and respond to IL-6, it may act as an autocrine growth factor for these cells. IL-11 has stimulatory effects on hematopoiesis, as do IL-6 and LIF. Mutation of the LIF gene inhibits blastocyst implantation. The leukemic cell inhibitory and myelocytopoietic activities of LIF are also exhibited by OSM and IL-6. OSM was initially discovered as an inhibitor of melanoma cell growth. CNTF promotes survival of ciliary neurons by preventing apoptosis.

Most effects of CNTF are neuron-specific, because expression of its receptor appears to be largely confined to neural tissues. CNTF knockout mice lose their motor neurons. IL-6 and LIF also have some trophic effects on neural cells. The recently discovered CT-1 is a more potent stimulant of cardiac myocytes than other members of the IL-6 family. Knockout of the IL-6R β gene, which blocks the activities of all the IL-6 family members, is lethal for the embryos and causes developmental abnormalities, including cardiac hypoplasia.

INTERFERONS

In 1957, it was discovered that cells exposed to inactivated viruses produce at least one soluble factor that can "interfere" with viral replication when applied to newly infected cells. The factor was named **interferon (IFN).** It has since been shown that the interferons consist of a large family of secretory proteins that not only share antiviral activity but also have the ability to inhibit proliferation of vertebrate cells and to modulate immune responses. Interferons do not exert their antiviral effects by acting on viral particles but rather by inducing an antiviral state within the host cell that makes it inhospitable to viral replication. This, as well as the antiproliferative and immunomodulatory effects of interferons, reflects their ability to regulate specific gene expression and metabolic activity in their target cells. Many different types of proteins can induce an antiviral state in vertebrate cells and therefore are, by definition, interferons. Their molecular and biologic properties differ so widely that it is useful to classify the interferons into distinct types.

THE ANTIVIRAL INTERFERONS
(IFNα, IFNβ, & IFNω)

Most cell types can synthesize type I IFNs and will do so in response to infection by viruses, bacteria or protozoa, or when exposed to certain cytokines (Fig 10–2). These IFNs can also be induced artificially by treating cells with double-stranded RNA molecules, which presumably mimic the genomes of certain RNA viruses. One inducer of type I IFN that is used frequently is **poly(I:C)**—a heteroduplex of polyinosinate and polycytidinate RNA chains. Type I IFNs are not normally found in tissues or serum but appear rapidly during viral infections.

There are three major forms of type I IFN, called IFNα, IFNβ, and IFNω. **IFNα** is the primary IFN produced by **leukocytes** and consists of glycosylated proteins (MW 16,000–27,500) encoded by a family of at least 18 closely related genes, of which 14 are functional. The amino acid sequences of these various IFNα proteins are approximately 73% identical to one another. **Fibroblasts** and most other nonleukocytic cells primarily express **IFNβ,** a protein that is only about 30% identical to IFNα. Small amounts of IFNβ are also expressed by leukocytes. There are six **IFNω** genes, of which only one is functional; it resembles the IFNγ genes and is primarily expressed by leukocytes.

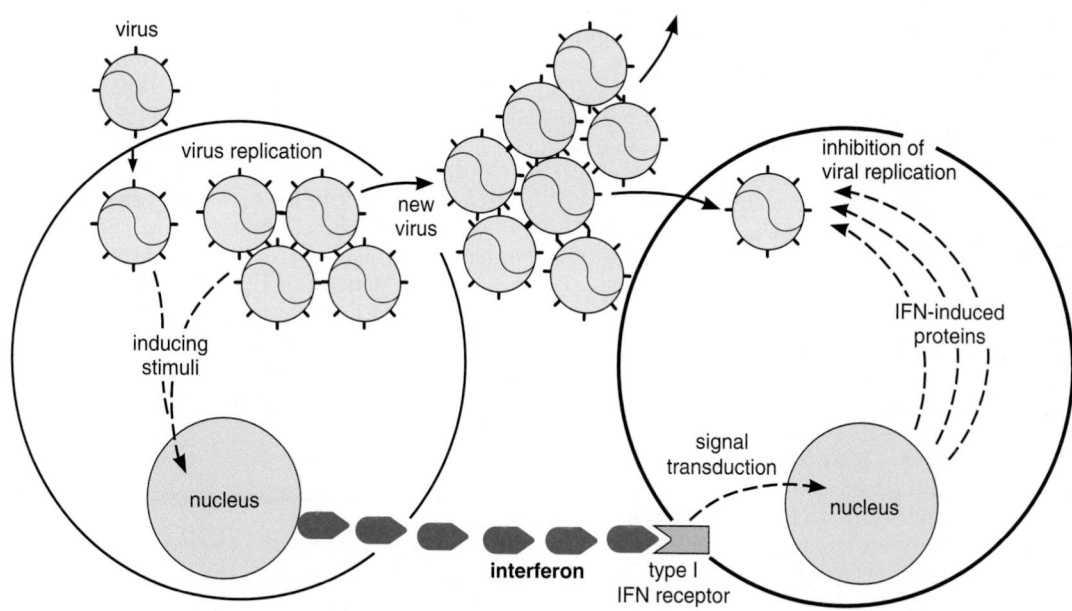

Figure 10–2. Schematic representation of the induction and activity of a type I interferon.

All three forms of type I IFN bind to a single multi-chain receptor, which is expressed on nearly all cell types. The molecular characteristics of the receptor are not fully known. Binding of type I IFN to this receptor induces or increases expression of at least 30 different gene products in the target cell (see Fig 10–2). Among the proteins whose expression is increased are the **class I MHC** molecules, which function to present endogenous antigens to CD8 T cells. Induction of class I MHC enhances the ability of virally infected cells to present viral antigens and so to be killed by cytotoxic T cells. Other IFN-inducible proteins include a specific protein kinase and **2′-5′ oligoadenylate (2-5A) synthetase,** both of which require the presence of double-stranded RNA for activity. When activated, this protein kinase phosphorylates a component of the cellular translational machinery (called eukaryotic initiation factor 2), and thereby inhibits protein synthesis. The 2-5A synthetase produces short chains of adenylate residues joined by 2′-5′ phosphodiester bonds; these bind and activate a cellular endoribonuclease that specifically degrades single-stranded RNA. These enzymes, together with other IFN-inducible proteins, combine to yield a relatively nonspecific inhibition of gene expression that provides a potent defense against viruses.

In addition to inhibiting viral replication, type I IFNs can modulate specific cellular functions. They are able to arrest the growth of (but generally do not kill) many types of cells in culture, including transformed cell lines. They also may either inhibit or promote cellular differentiation, depending on the cell type and the timing and dosage of IFN.

Interestingly, type I IFN also has some capacity to activate T lymphocytes; indeed, it is the only cytokine thus far shown to be sufficient to induce T-cell proliferation. The effect is greatest on CD8+ memory T cells and is antigen-independent. It is not yet known whether IFN activates these cells directly or by inducing other cytokines. Although each affected cell undergoes, on average, only a single round of cell division, the polyclonal nature of the response can lead to significant expansion of the CD8+ population overall. Type I IFN may therefore contribute to the striking "bystander" activation of CD8+ T cells that typically accompanies viral infections.

IMMUNE INTERFERON (IFNγ)

IFNγ (also called type II IFN or **immune IFN**) arises from a single gene and differs in virtually all respects from the type I IFNs. There is only a single active form of IFNγ protein—a homodimer of MW 18,000 polypeptides that can be glycosylated to various degrees. The receptor to which it binds is likewise unrelated to the receptor for type I IFN. Although IFNγ has some antiviral activity (which led to its discovery and is the source of its name), it is less active in this regard than the type I IFNs. Moreover, IFNγ expression is not inducible by infection or by double-stranded RNA. It is therefore best regarded as a distinct **immunoregulatory** cytokine.

IFNγ is a lymphokine that is secreted by nearly all CD8 T cells, by some CD4 T cells (particularly by the T_H1 and, to a lesser extent, the T_H0 subsets, but not by the T_H2 subset [see Chapter 9]), and by NK cells. Each of these cell types secretes IFNγ only when activated, usually as part of an immune response and especially in response to IL-2 and IL-12. IFNγ production is inhibited by IL-4, IL-10, TGFβ, glucocorticoids, cyclosporin A, and FK506.

Nearly all cell types express heterodimeric receptors for IFNγ and respond to this cytokine by increasing the surface expression of class I MHC proteins. As a result, virtually any cell in the vicinity of an IFNγ-secreting lymphocyte becomes more efficient at presenting endogenous antigens and hence a better target for cytotoxic killing if it harbors an intracellular pathogen. Unlike the type I IFNs, IFNγ also increases the expression of class II MHC proteins on class II-bearing-cells and so promotes antigen presentation to CD4 T lymphocytes as well. It also induces do novo expression of class II MHC proteins on venular endothelial cells and on some other epithelial and connective tissue cells that do not otherwise express them, thus recruiting these cell types to function as APCs at sites of intense immune reactions.

IFNγ is also a potent activator of macrophages. Exposure to IFNγ greatly enhances the microbicidal (and, to a lesser degree, cytotoxic) activity of murine macrophages and induces them to secrete monokines such as IL-1, IL-6, IL-8, and TNFα. It also activates neutrophils, NK cells, and vascular endothelial cells. IFNγ synergistically enhances the cytotoxic effects of TNF. In the presence of IFNγ, venular endothelial cells become more adhesive for neutrophils (see Chapter 2) and may differentiate to form high endothelial venules, which attract lymphocytes from the circulation (see Chapter 3).

Although IFNγ tends to promote the differentiation of B cells and CD8 T cells into immunologically active effector cells, IFNγ does not promote lymphocyte proliferation. IFNγ enhances the activity of T_H1 cells and therefore augments macrophage reactions, but it inhibits the proliferation of T_H2 cells and thus tends to suppress mast cell and eosinophil responses. IFNγ not only decreases the production IL-4 by T_H2 cells but also potently inhibits the effects of IL-4 on B cells, promoting IgG1 production but preventing immunoglobulin class switching to IgE.

INTERLEUKIN-4 & INTERLEUKIN-13

Interleukin-4 (IL-4) is an MW 15,000–20,000 glycoprotein secreted by activated CD4 T cells of the T_H2

subset and by mast cells. It was initially identified as a helper factor for B-cell proliferation and was therefore called B-cell growth factor-I (**BCGF-I**). It is mitogenic for activated B cells, although its effect is usually less pronounced than that of IL-2 and always requires other activating stimuli. IL-4 was also previously called B-cell stimulatory factor-I (**BSF-I**) because of its ability to induce class II MHC expression on resting B cells. IL-4 is a major regulator of the heavy-chain class switch, since it promotes switching to IgG4 and IgE. It also induces expression of the low-affinity Fcε receptor (CD23). Thus, IL-4 acts on B cells at many stages.

IL-4 also promotes the induction of T_H2 cells, which control (among other things) the proliferation and activities of eosinophils and mast cells. The indirect effect of IL-4 on these cells, coupled with its direct effect on IgE production, suggests a central role in **allergic diseases.** In contrast, IL-4 suppresses the induction and function of T_H1 cells, which control many facets of cellular immunity, suggesting that IL-4 may have clinical utility in the treatment of T-cell-mediated autoimmunity and graft-versus-host disease.

In addition to the preceding effects, IL-4 promotes cytotoxic T-cell activity, enhances IL-3-mediated mast cell growth, acts synergistically with CSFs to enhance the growth of various hematopoietic cells, and induces the vascular cell adhesion molecule (VCAM)-1 on endothelial cells. IL-4 also has multiple effects on macrophages: it can activate macrophage cytocidal functions and increase macrophage expression of class II MHC proteins. It suppresses the synthesis of proinflammatory cytokines, however, such as IL-1, IL-6, IL-8, and TNFα, by activated monocytes. Despite all the aforementioned effects, IL-4 knockout mice exhibit only deficiencies in the production of IgE and T_H2 cytokines (Table 10–7).

A newly characterized lymphokine, **IL-13,** was recently found to have many properties overlapping those of IL-4. It is a T-cell product that enhances the production of IgE and suppresses the production of monokines. The receptors for IL-13 and IL-4 share the IL-2 γ and IL-4 β chains but use distinct binding (α) chains.

INTERLEUKIN-5

Interleukin-5 (IL-5) is a disulfide-linked homodimeric glycoprotein with a MW of 40,000–50,000. It was originally described as a growth factor for murine B cells and eosinophils but does not have significant stimulatory activity on human B cells. CD4+ T_H2 cells are the major source of this cytokine. The IL-5 receptor shares a common β chain with the receptors for IL-3 and GM-CSF but also includes an α chain that

specifically binds IL-5 and is restricted to eosinophils and basophils in humans. The major function of IL-5 in humans is to stimulate the production of **eosinophils.** IL-5 not only increases the numbers of eosinophils but also has been reported to increase their function. In vivo studies have clearly demonstrated that IL-5 is the major cytokine regulating eosinophilia during helminth infections and allergic diseases. Human IL-5 also enhances the activities of basophils by priming them to release mediators, such as histamine and leukotrienes, in response to other signals.

INTERLEUKIN-7

Interleukin-7 (IL-7) is an MW 25,000 glycoprotein secreted by thymus, spleen, and bone marrow stromal cells that functions as a growth factor for both T- and B-cell precursors. The heterodimeric receptor for IL-7 contains a specific binding chain and the shared IL-2Rγ signal transducer. IL-7R is expressed on B- and T-cell progenitors and mature T cells as well as on macrophages and monocytes. IL-7 enhances β-integrin-mediated adhesion of thymocytes to matrix proteins. Together with SCF, it provides a powerful mitogenic stimulus to thymocytes and pre-B cells. IL-7 provides the signal that promotes rearrangement of T-cell receptor genes during fetal thymocyte development. It induces IL-2R expression, but most of its proliferative effect occurs independently of IL-2. Mature human peripheral blood T lymphocytes do not respond significantly to IL-7 unless costimulated or previously activated. IL-7 administration results in pronounced leukocytosis in normal mice and hastens recovery of leukocytes in mice made leukopenic by sublethal irradiation or cytotoxic agents; the majority of its pharmacologic in vivo effect is on B-lineage cells, with a more modest increase observed in T lymphocytes.

IL-7 enhances the function of mature, activated lymphocytic cells, particularly those with cytotoxic activity. It can also induce LAK activity, but to a substantially lesser degree than IL-2. At higher concentrations, IL-7 also increases macrophage cytotoxic activity and induces cytokine secretion by monocytes. On the other hand, the major defect in IL-7 knockout mice is lymphoid hypoplasia due to failure of T- and B-lymphocyte development (Table 10–7).

INTERLEUKIN-9

Interleukin-9 (IL-9) is a heavily glycosylated polypeptide lymphokine with an apparent MW of 30,000–40,000. It is secreted by IL-2-activated T cells and has growth-promoting effects on mast cells in vitro. IL-9 can costimulate T cells together with IL-2 or IL-4 and may potentially stimulate hematopoietic progenitors. Its physiologic role has not been firmly established.

INTERLEUKIN-10

Interleukin-10 (IL-10) is an 18,000-MW protein that is produced late in the activation process by T_H2 cells, CD8 T cells, monocytes, keratinocytes, and activated B cells. It was originally called **cytokine synthesis inhibitory factor** because of its ability to inhibit cytokine production by activated T lymphocytes. For example, IL-10 inhibits the production of cytokines, such as IL-2 and IFNγ by T_H1 cells, and therefore tips the regulatory balance in favor of T_H2 responses. IL-10 inhibits cytokine production by NK cells and macrophages. IL-10 further deactivates macrophages by suppressing their production of reactive oxygen intermediates, nitric oxide, and adhesion proteins. Indeed, the suppression T_H1 activity appears to be due to an indirect effect resulting from suppression of class II MHC expression and consequent impairment of the accessory cell functions of macrophages and dendritic cells. On the other hand, IL-10 also has a direct comitogenic effect on mast cells, T cells, and B cells and promotes B-cell antibody production. A viral analogue of IL-10 is encoded by the *bcrf*-1 gene in the Epstein-Barr virus (EBV). The production of this virokine enables EBV to subvert the host immune response both by suppressing cellular immune responses and by promoting proliferation of its B-cell hosts. The virokine lacks the T-cell stimulating effects of authentic IL-10.

INTERLEUKIN 12

Interleukin-12 (IL-12) is a structurally unique heterodimer composed of two distinct disulfide-linked subunits (MW 35,000 and 40,000). It was originally called cytotoxic lymphocyte maturation factor (CLMF) or NK cell stimulatory factor (NKSF). IL-12 is produced predominantly on activation by B cells and macrophages. Production of IL-12 by activated macrophages is suppressed by IL-4 and IL-10. It promotes the proliferation of activated T lymphocytes and NK cells, enhances the lytic activity of NK and LAK cells, and is the most potent inducer of IFNγ production by resting or activated T and NK cells. In addition, it selectively induces the differentiation of T_H0 into T_H1 lymphocytes, but suppresses T_H2-

dependent functions, such as the production of IL-4, IL-10, and IgE antibodies. The latter capabilities are being exploited for vaccine development, in the hope that including IL-12 in vaccine preparations can selectively promote T_H1 immune responses. IL-12 also induces the production of GM-CSF, TNF, IL-6, and, to a small extent, IL-2. It synergizes with IL-2 in promoting cytotoxic T-cell responses. As such, IL-12 may hold promise as an immunopotentiating antitumor agent.

INTERLEUKIN-14

Interleukin-14 (IL-14) is a 50–60-kd glycosylated cytokine otherwise known as the high-molecular-weight B-cell growth factor. IL-14 is produced only by follicular dendritic cells and T cells, and IL-14 receptors are found only in cells of the B-cell lineage. IL-14 is mitogenic for activated B cells but inhibits antibody production. Thus, IL-14 participates mainly in secondary humoral immune responses.

INTERLEUKIN-15

Many of the biologic properties of IL-15 were discussed earlier in relationship to IL-2, with which it has much in common, including the ability to induce proliferation of activated T cells, generate specific cytotoxic T cells, and activate LAK cells. Unlike IL-2, IL-15 is widely expressed in placenta, skeletal muscle, kidney, lung, liver, heart, and bone marrow stroma. It is produced most abundantly by epithelial cells and monocytes, but not by T lymphocytes. It functions as a signal from nonlymphoid cells for generating T-cell-dependent immune responses.

INTERLEUKIN-16

Interleukin-16 (IL-16), which was previously known as lymphocyte chemoattractant factor (LCF), is produced by stimulated T lymphocytes and induces the directional migration of CD4+ T cells, eosinophils, and monocytes. LCF also upregulates IL-2Rα and MHC class II expression on T cells. The chemoattractant effect of LCF is blocked by anti-CD4 Fab fragments, suggesting that CD4 or CD4-related molecules are required for the effects of LCF on target cells. The physiologic role of IL-16 remains to be established.

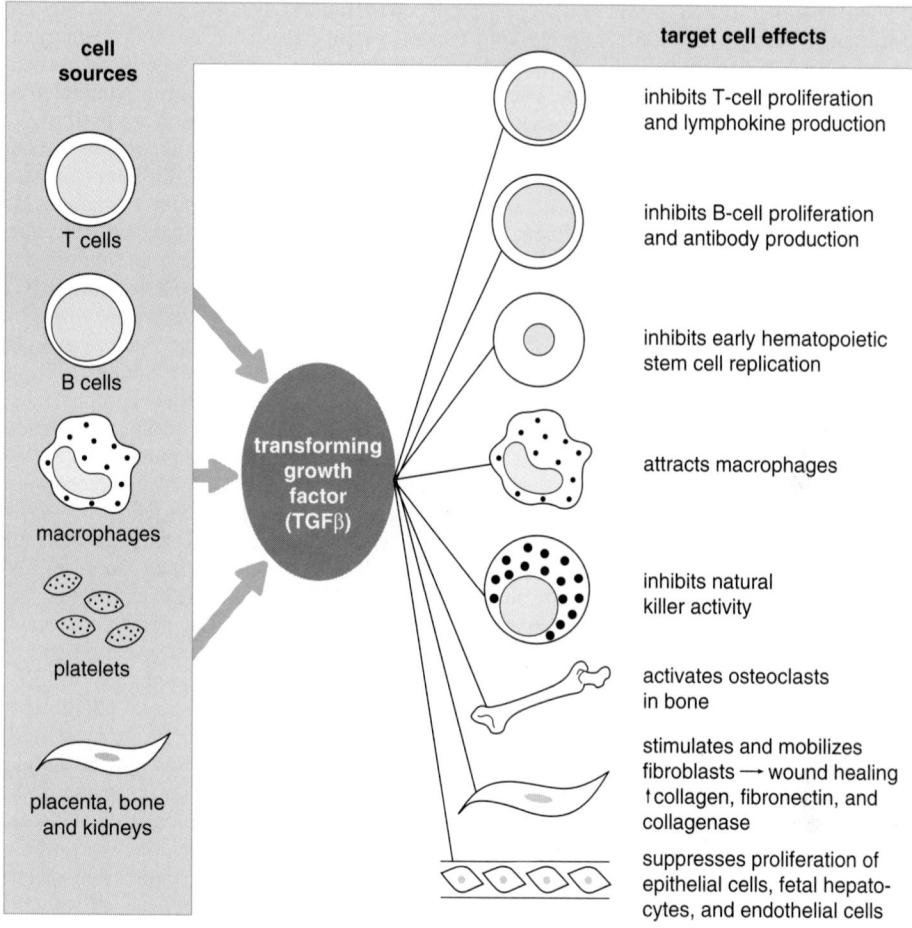

cell
sources

T cells

B cells

macrophages

platelets

placenta, bone
and kidneys

transforming
growth
factor
(TGFβ)

target cell effects

inhibits T-cell proliferation
and lymphokine production

inhibits B-cell proliferation
and antibody production

inhibits early hematopoietic
stem cell replication

attracts macrophages

inhibits natural
killer activity

activates osteoclasts
in bone

stimulates and mobilizes
fibroblasts ⟶ wound healing
↑collagen, fibronectin, and
collagenase

suppresses proliferation of
epithelial cells, fetal hepatocytes, and endothelial cells

Figure 10–3. Cell sources and effects of TGFβ.

TRANSFORMING GROWTH FACTOR β

Transforming growth factor β (TGFβ) was initially discovered as a growth factor for fibroblasts that promoted wound healing. It also has considerable antiproliferative activity, however, and acts as a negative regulator of immunity and hematopoiesis. TGFβ is produced by many cell types, including activated macrophages and T lymphocytes. Humans express at least three forms of TGFβ, called TGFβ-1, -2, and -3 (Fig 10–3). These are the products of separate genes, but they all bind to five types of high-affinity cell surface receptors. Type I and II receptors transduce signals, whereas the function of type III, IV, and V receptors is not yet clear. TGFβ receptors are expressed in widely different numbers by many cell types. The results of mouse knockout experiments indicate that

all three forms of TGFβ are essential for development and confirm an important immunoregulatory role for TGFβ-1 (see Table 10–5).

TGFβ has antiproliferative effects on a wide variety of cell types, including macrophages, endothelial cells, and T and B lymphocytes. It also suppresses the production of most lymphokines and monokines and reduces the cellular expression of class II MHC proteins and of IL-1 receptors. TGFβ at 10^{-10} to 10^{-12} M blocks the proliferative effects of IL-2 on T and B cells and of IL-1 on thymocytes. In addition, TGFβ inhibits T-cell-dependent polyclonal antibody production, mixed-leukocyte reactions, and the in vitro generation of cytotoxic T cells. It also inhibits the induction of NK cell activities and of LAK cells by IL-2. Thus, TGFβ is unique in that it can act as a negative-feedback regulator that dampens immunologically mediated reactions.

TGFβ also has some activities that tend to potentiate inflammation. It is chemoattractive for neutrophils and monocytes, and it stimulates monocyte expression of adhesion proteins. In humans, TGFβ promotes switching of B cells to the IgA antibody class. These effects may account for the observation that injection of TGFβ directly into inflamed joints exacerbates the inflammation. On the other hand, systemic administration of TGFβ1 has anti-inflammatory effects and TGFβ1 knockout mice develop a lethal polyinflammatory state due to overproduction of proinflammatory cytokines.

INTERLEUKIN-8 & THE CHEMOKINE FAMILY OF CYTOKINES

Over the past 10 years, a new family of cytokines has been characterized whose members have **chemoattractant** activity for leukocytes and fibroblasts (Table 10–9). These chemoattractant cytokines, called **chemokines,** range in molecular weight from 8000 to 16,000, share 20–50% amino acid sequence similarity with one another, bind to structurally related **7-transmembrane receptors,** and are active at concentrations of 10^{-8}–10^{-11} M. Chemokines act predominantly to influence the functions, rather than the growth, of target cells. In particular, they appear to play a crucial role in attracting specific types of cells into sites of tissue injury and inflammation.

Chemokines are produced by a variety of cell types (most notably by activated monocyte–macrophages and endothelial cells), are chemoattractive for various combinations of cell types, and exhibit considerable redundancy (see Table 10–9). No uniform system of nomenclature has yet been adopted for these proteins, and they carry names that focus on a variety of attributes. One, **IL-8,** is an interleukin. Nearly all chemokines contain two intramolecular disulfide bonds formed by two pairs of conserved cysteine residues and can be classified into two subfamilies according to the sequences of the cysteine pair nearest the amino terminus. In the **C-X-C (or α) chemokines,** which are encoded by a cluster of genes on chromosome 4, these cysteines are separated by one amino acid, whereas in the **C-C (or β) chemokines,** whose genes are clustered on chromosome 17, the two cysteines are adjacent. Most α chemokines attract neutrophils, whereas all β chemokines attract monocytes and T lymphocytes and some also attract eosinophils, basophils, and NK cells. A newly identified chemokine, called lymphotactin, preferentially attracts T cells and is the sole representative of the **C chemokines,** which contain only a single disulfide bond.

Nine chemokine receptors have been identified to date (see Table 10–9). All belong to the rhodopsin-like receptor family, members of which are single polypeptides that have seven transmembrane regions. This extremely diverse family also includes the leukocyte receptors for *N*-formylmethionyl peptides and for complement factor C5a (both of which have chemoattractant activity), as well as beta-adrenergic receptors and the odorant receptors of nasal epithelium. Four receptors bind α chemokines: one (CXCR1) binds IL-8 and GCP-2; the second (CXCR2) binds IL-8 and at least four other α-subfamily members; a third (CXCR3) binds IP10 and Mig, and the fourth (CXCR4, also called fusin) binds SDF. Similarly, the five known receptors for β chemokines (CCR1–5) can each bind multiple ligands. This promiscuity at the receptor level probably accounts for the overlapping activities of the chemokines. At least two of the chemokine receptors (CXCR4 and CCR5) also function as highly effective coreceptors that allow the type-1 **human immunodeficiency virus (HIV-1)** to enter and infect CD4+ T cells and macrophages, respectively; this may account for the finding that chemokines that bind CCR5 can interfere with HIV-1 replication in vitro and that some persons who remain uninfected despite repeated exposure to HIV-1 have elevated levels of these chemokines in their blood or inherited defects in CCR5. In addition, the Duffy blood group antigen on erythrocytes (which also serves as the receptor for the malarial parasite, *Plasmodium vivax*) binds many α and β chemokines and is thought to act as a nonfunctional sink that limits free cytokine diffusion in the bloodstream.

Agents that induce the expression of chemokines include a battery of macrophage activators (including LPS), polyclonal mitogens and antigens that activate T cells, and inducers of platelet aggregation. In addition, a number of proinflammatory cytokines, such as IL-1, IL-2, IFNγ, TNF, and platelet-derived growth factor (PDGF), potently induce various chemokines. The chemokines have limited ability to induce one another but can in some cases induce other mediators.

As a group, the chemokines appear capable of selectively attracting all types of leukocytes to an inflamed site. They appear to do so in part by inducing binding activity and surface expression of leukocyte integrins, which promote binding to endothelium and subsequent tissue invasion. In this way, for example, IL-8 enhances endothelial binding by neutrophils, and MIP-1α does the same for T cells. Chemokine secretion by endothelial cells also appears to promote leukocyte migration across vessel walls, and gradients of chemokines may guide their migrations through tissue. All known chemokines bind tightly to glycosaminoglycans, such as those found in the extracellular matrix and on endothelial surfaces, suggesting a mechanism whereby secreted chemokines might accumulate regionally and direct cells along specific routes. At high concentrations, chemokines also can activate cellular effector functions: for example, degranulation and the metabolic burst are triggered in

Table 10–9. Properties of selected human chemokines.

Chemokine	Chemoattracted Cells	CXCR 1	CXCR 2	CXCR 3	CXCR 4	CCR 1	CCR 2B	CCR 3	CCR 4	CCR 5	DAg	Other Major Activities
C-X-C (α) Subfamily												
IL-8	N, T, Mc, NK, Ec, Bs, Es, K, Ms	■	■								■	Stimulates neutrophil degranulation, adhesion, and microbicidal effects. Angiogenic.
GRO-α	N, T, Mc, F		■								■	Neutrophil degranulation. Mitogenic for fibroblasts and melanoma cells.
GRO-β, ENA78, and GCP-2	N		■									Activate neutrophils.
NAP-2	N	▨										Activates neutrophils.
PF-4	N, Ec, F											Antiangiogenic.
Mig	T, Ec, F			■								Antiangiogenic and antitumor effects.
IP-10	T, NK, Ec, M			■								Antiangiogenic and antitumor effects.
SDF	N, T, B, M				■							B-cell and cardiac development. Competitively inhibits T-cell entry by HIV-1.
C-C (β) Subfamily												
MIP-1α	M, T, NK, BS, Es, Ms, Dc, B					■		■	■	■		Activates T cells and β-integrin adhesion. Suppresses myeloid colony formation.
MIP-1β	M, T, NK, Dc									■		Activates T cells and β-integrin adhesion.
MCP-1	M, T, NK, Bs, Ms, Dc					▨	■		▨		■	Activates macrophages. Degranulates basophils.
MCP-2	M, T, Es, Ms					■						Activates macrophages. Degranulates basophils.
MCP-3	M, T, Bs, Es, Dc, N					■						Activates macrophages. Degranulates basophils.
RANTES	M, T, NK, Bs, Es, Ms, Dc					■		■	■	■		Activates T cells and β-integrin adhesion. Degranulates basophils. Antitumor effects.
I-309	M							■				Activates macrophages.
Eotaxin	M, T, Es, N							■				Eosinophil chemoattraction.

Abbreviations: IL = interleukin; GRO = growth-related peptide; ENA = epithelial-derived neutrophil attractant; GCP = granulocyte chemotactic protein; NAP = neutrophil-activating peptide; PF = platelet factor; Mig = monokine induced by interferon gamma; IP = interferon γ-inducible protein; SDF = stromal-derived factor; HIV = human immunodeficiency virus; MIP = macrophage inflammatory protein; MCP = monocyte chemoattractant protein; RANTES = regulated on activation, normal T expressed and secreted; N = neutrophil; T = T cell; B = B cell; NK = natural killer cell; Ec = endothelial cell; F = fibroblast; M = monocyte; Mc = melanoma cell; Bs = basophil; Ms = mast cell; Es = eosinophil; Dc = dendritic cell; K = keratinocyte.
[1] Not all receptor specificities are known. Solid color and crosshatching denote strong and weak binding, respectively.
Abbreviations: CXCR = C-X-C (α) subfamily receptor; CCR = C-C (β) subfamily receptor; DAg = Duffy blood-group antigen.

neutrophils by IL-8, in monocytes by MCP-1, and in eosinophils by RANTES or MIP-1α.

IL-8 and other α chemokines have been found in the blood of patients with inflammatory reactions and severe trauma and can readily be detected at inflammatory sites, as in the synovial fluid of patients with rheumatoid arthritis, in psoriatic skin, and in the circulation of patients in septic shock. Thus, α chemokines are implicated as a major participant in acute inflammatory reactions, though they are not, in general, pyrogenic and do not induce the acute-phase proteins. Local injections of some of the β chemokines can induce primarily lymphocytic or macrophage infiltrates in tissue, suggesting a role in chronic inflammation, whereas others attract eosinophils and stimulate basophil degranulation with histamine release, and so might play a role in allergy and in parasitic infections. Mice with disrupted genes for the IL-8 receptor homologue are more susceptible to bacterial infections, whereas MIP-1α knockout mice mount a diminished mononuclear cell response to influenza infection and allow greater replication of the influenza virus.

HEMATOPOIETIC COLONY-STIMULATING FACTORS

Colony-stimulating factors are cytokines that stimulate individual pluripotent stem cells or their committed progeny (found mainly in the bone marrow in adults) to produce large numbers of erythrocytes, platelets, neutrophils, monocytes, eosinophils, and basophils (see Chapter 1). Each CSF acts on progenitor cells with particular developmental capabilities and is named according to the predominant cell types whose production it supports in stem cell cultures in vitro (Table 10–10). Thus, granulocyte–monocyte CSF stimulates production of neutrophils and monocytes; granulocyte CSF (**G-CSF**) yields neutrophils; monocyte CSF (**M-CSF**) yields monocytes; erythropoietin (**EPO**) stimulates production of erythrocytes; and thrombopoietin (TPO) stimulates production of platelets. Interleukin-3 (**IL-3**), also known as multi-CSF, stimulates myeloerythroid progenitor cells to produce mature myeloid, megakaryocytic, and erythroid progeny. Primitive hematopoietic stem cells do not proliferate in response to any single cytokine, but their growth is promoted by combinations of factors that include one from each of the following three groups: (1) either stem cell factor (SCF) or Flt3 ligand; (2) IL-1, IL-6, IL-11, IL-12, TPO, or G-CSF; and (3) IL-3, IL-4, or GM-CSF. These synergistic effects are direct (being observed in single-cell assays). Synergy can be due to either induction of cycling in resting cells or enhanced proliferative rate (or both). In addition to maintaining homeostasis under normal conditions, these cytokines marshall bone marrow responses to environmental stresses, such as infection or trauma. In vivo administration of CSFs can also yield effects that extend beyond their in vitro activities, presumably because CSFs can induce other cytokines or their receptors, and directly influence the functions of some mature leukocytes.

The various CSFs are unrelated to one another structurally and bind to distinct cell surface receptors. Nevertheless, many have overlapping functions and induce quite similar biologic effects. This is particularly true of CSFs that influence granulocyte and macrophage production (see Table 10–10). The bio-

Table 10–10. Human hematopoietic growth factors.

	Predominant Cell Source	Cells Whose Production Is Enhanced
SCF	Fibroblasts, hepatocytes, endothelial cells, epithelial cells, stromal cells.	All hematopoietic cell types, gonadal cells, melanocytes, mast cells.
Flt 3	Stromal cells.	All hematopoietic cell types.
IL-3	T lymphocytes.	Neutrophils, monocytes, eosinophils, erythrocytes, basophils.
IL-5	T lymphocytes.	Eosinophils.
IL-11	Stromal cells, fibroblasts.	All primitive hematopoietic progenitors, platelets.
GM-CSF	T lymphocytes, monocytes, fibroblasts, endothelial cells.	Neutrophils, monocytes, eosinophils, dendritic cells.
G-CSF	Monocytes, fibroblasts.	Neutrophils.
M-CSF	Monocytes, lymphocytes, fibroblasts, endothelial cells, epithelial cells.	Monocytes, placental trophoblast cells.
EPO	Kidney cells.	Erythrocytes.
TPO	Kidney, liver.	Platelets.

Abbreviations: SCF = stem cell factor; IL = interleukin; GM-CSF = granulocyte–macrophage colony-stimulating factor; G-CSF = granulocyte colony-stimulating factor; M-CSF = macrophage colony-stimulating factor; EPO = erythropoietin; TPO = thrombopoietin.

logic significance of this redundancy is not clear. Some cytokines (eg, IL-1, IL-6, and IL-11) have little or no independent effect on hematopoiesis but act synergistically with others that do. Stem cell factor (SCF) is the most potent of these synergistic CSFs: it interacts with many other cytokines to promote growth of myeloerythroid and lymphoid stem cells and hence increase the production of all blood cells.

Hematopoiesis is controlled by at least 30 known cytokines. Most of these cytokines have overlapping functions but some have unique functions as revealed by studies in knockout mice (Table 10–11). Some of these—such as SCF, M-CSF, and EPO—are constitutively produced and present at all times in the plasma, whereas others are produced in response to specific stimuli. For example, IL-3, IL-5, and CM-CSF are expressed by T cells only when these cells become activated. Similarly, fibroblasts and endothelial cells secrete G-CSF and GM-CSF only when stimulated by IL-1, TNFα, or other products of activated macrophages.

Many aspects of hematopoiesis and its control are incompletely understood. At any given moment, the

Table 10–11. Phenotypic deficiencies of hematopoietic cytokine knockout mice.

Targeted Gene	Phenotypic Abnormalities
G-CSF	Defective myelopoiesis and neutropenia. Susceptible to *Listeria* infections.
GM-CSF	Accumulation of pulmonary surfactants and pulmonary fibrosis. No hematopoietic defects.
cMPL (thrombo-poietin receptor)	Thrombocytopenia.
SCF (c-*kit* ligand)	Steel locus mutation in this gene result in altered coat color, anemia, and defective gonadal development.
SCF-receptor (c-*kit* (w) mutant genes)	Maldevelopment of melanocyte, germ cell and hematopoietic lineages. Piebaldism: dominant hypopigmented spotting.
CSF-1 (M-CSF)	Reduced bone resorption and osteope-trosis in mice. Hypoactive macrophages.
FLR-2	Defective hematopoiesis.

Abbreviations: G-CSF = granulocyte colony-stimulating factor; GM-CSF = granulocyte–macrophage colony-stimulating factor; cMPL = cellular counterpart of viral myeloproliferative leukemia gene; SCF = stem cell factor; CSF = colony-stimulating factor; M-CSF = macrophage colony-stimulating factor.

majority of pluripotent stem cells are thought to be in a resting, nonmitotic state (ie, in the G_0 phase of the cell cycle). Their entry into the mitotic cycle can be induced by SCF, IL-11, IL-6, and IL-1. Other factors, such as TGFβ, IFNγ, MIP-1α, and TNFα, cause cycling stem cells to revert to the resting state. It is not clear how the progeny of stem cells become committed to a particular cell lineage or how CSFs might influence this process. Most evidence is compatible with the view that commitment occurs randomly, but that committed cells subsequently survive only if the appropriate CSFs are present (see Chapter 1). According to this model, IL-3 is required to support the growth of the most primitive progenitors; GM-CSF supports early multilineage precursors; and EPO, G-CSF, M-CSF, IL-5, or IL-7 is required for survival of cells committed to specific lineages.

Several of the CSFs profoundly affect cells that participate in immunity and inflammation. Macrophages produced in the presence of GM-CSF alone have better APC activity and, when activated, have greater cytotoxic activity than those produced by M-CSF. In contrast, M-CSF-treated macrophages are less functionally active, in part because M-CSF reduces MHC protein expression and stimulates production of IL-1RA. GM-CSF is essential for the generation of dendritic cells from their marrow-derived precursor forms, and the local release of this cytokine by activated macrophages, T cells, and keratinocytes in the course of an immune response is thought to stimulate circulating dendritic cell progenitors to differentiate into functional APCs. GM-CSF also potentiates the activity of mature dendritic cells.

Many CSFs are currently being tested for possible clinical use. GM-CSF and G-CSF may prove to be of value in preventing the therapy-induced granulocytopenia that is the major cause of death among cancer patients undergoing chemotherapy or radiation therapy. Both of these cytokines may also have protective activity against bacterial septicemia. A combination of SCF and IL-11 shows promise for preventing thrombocytopenia in several therapeutic settings. In comparison with many of the other pluripotent cytokines, G-CSF, EPO, and TPO, which have more restricted activities, produce relatively few toxic side effects and are more useful clinically.

CYTOKINE RECEPTOR FAMILIES

The characterization of many cytokine receptors and their corresponding genes has revealed that most belong to larger multigene families (Table 10–12). The members of each family share distinctive structural features and are thought to be evolutionarily related. For example, the receptors for IL-1, M-CSF, SCF, G-CSF, and IL-6 each contain an immunoglobulin-like domain in their extracellular regions and thus belong to the **immunoglobulin gene superfamily** (see Chapter 7). Distinctive characteristics of the TNF and IL-6 receptor families have been described in previous sections.

Many of the remaining cytokines belong to the **hematopoietin receptor family.** This family includes the receptors for IL-2, IL-3, IL-4, IL-5, IL-6, IL-7, IL-9, GM-CSF, G-CSF, EPO, LIF, growth hormone, and prolactin. Members of this receptor family can be recognized by a distinctive set of four spaced cysteines in their extracellular domains as well as by a conserved sequence motif (Trp-Ser-X-Trp-Ser) located near the external membrane surface. As a rule, receptor dimerization is required for signal transduction by receptors of this family. The dimers can be either homodimers, as in the IL-4 receptors, or more complex heterodimers, as in the IL-6 receptor and some of the other members of this family.

The divisions among families are not mutually exclusive, and some receptors can be assigned to multiple families. For example, the IL-6 receptor belongs to both the hematopoietin receptor and immunoglobulin superfamilies and also is the prototype of the IL-6 receptor family.

One important result of cytokine signaling is the transcriptional activation of specific target genes, which is rapid and may require new protein synthesis. Many cytokines achieve this effect through the Jak-

Table 10–12. Cytokine receptor families.

	Distinguishing Features	Ligands of Member Receptors
Hematopoietin	Trp-Ser-X-Trp-Ser motif; four extracellular Cys residues.	IL-2, IL-3, IL-4, IL-5, IL-6 family, IL-7, IL-9, GM-CSF, G-CSF, EPO, growth hormone, prolactin.
Immunoglobulin superfamily	Ig-like extracellular domain.	IL-1, IL-6, M-CSF, G-CSF, SCF.
TNF family	Four Cys-rich extracellular regions.	TNFα, CD27L, CD30L, CD40L, Fas antigen, LT α/β complex, NGF.
IL-3 family	Common β subunit.	IL-3, IL-5, GM-CSF.
IL-6 family	Common β subunit.	IL-6, IL-11, LIF, OSM, CNTF, CT-1.
IL-8 family	Rhodopsin-like proteins with seven transmembrane domains.	IL-8, GRO, RANTES, NAP-2, GCP-2, MCP-1, 2, 3, MIP-1 α and β, and others.
Tyrosine kinase family	Intrinsic Tyr kinase activity in cytoplasmic domain.	M-CSF, SCF, platelet-derived growth factor, fibroblast growth factor.
TGFβ family	Intrinsic Thr/Ser kinase activity in cytoplasmic domain.	TGFβ, inhibins, activins, Mullerian inhibiting substance, bone morphogenetic protein.
IFN family	Type 1 (for IFNα, β, and ω), type II (for IFNγ).	IFNα, β, ω, and γ, IL-10.

Abbreviations: TNF = tumor necrosis factor; IL = interleukin; TGF = transforming growth factor; IFN = interferon; GM-CSF = granulocyte–macrophage colony-stimulating factor; G-CSF = granulocyte colony-stimulating factor; M-CSF = macrophage colony-stimulating factor; SCF = stem cell factor; LIF = leukocyte inhibitory factor; OSM = oncostatin M; CNTF = ciliary neurotrophic factor; CT-1 = cardiotrophin-1; GRO = growth-related peptide; RANTES = regulated on activation, normal T expressed and secreted; NAP = neutrophil-activating peptide; GCP = granulocyte chemotactic protein; MCP = monocyte chemotactic protein; MIP = macrophage inflammatory protein.

Stat signaling pathway (see Chapter 1) using various combination of Jaks and Stats (Table 10–13). It remains to be determined how the activation of particular members of the Jak-Stat families leads to specificity of cytokine-mediated signaling.

Table 10–13. Activated Jak kinases and Stat signal transducers used by cytokines.

Receptor	Activated Jaks	Activated Stats[1]
IFNα/β	Jak1, Tyk2	Stat1, Stat2, Stat3
IFNγ	Jak1, Jak2	Stat1, Stat3
IL-2, IL-7, IL-9, IL-15	Jak1, Jak3	Stat3, Stat5
IL-3, IL-5, GM-CSF	Jak2	Stat1, Stat3
IL-4, IL-13	Jak1, Jak3	Stat6
IL-6 family	Jak1, Jak2, Tyk2	Stat1, Stat2, Stat3
IL-10	Unknown	Stat1, Stat3
IL-12	Jak2, Tyk2	Stat3, Stat4
G-CSF	Jak2	Stat1
CSF-1	Jak1	Stat1, Stat3
SCF	Jak2	Stat1, Stat3
TPO	Jak2, Tyk2	Stat1, Stat3, Stat5
EPO	Jak2	Stat5

Abbreviations: IFN = interferon; IL = interleukin; GM-CSF = granulocyte–macrophage colony-stimulating factor; G-CSF = granulocyte colony-stimulating factor; TGF = transforming growth factor; CSF = colony-stimulating factor; SCF = stem cell factor; TPO = thrombopoietin; EPO = erythropoietin; Stat = signal transducers and activators of transcription.
[1] The ligands shown have been selected (from more than 20 ligands that activate Stats) to emphasize the relative selectivity of Stat activation.

VIROKINES & VIRORECEPTORS

It has recently become clear that some viruses encode cytokine-like proteins or receptor homologues that probably play important roles in viral life cycles. For example, Epstein-Barr virus produces an IL-10-like activity, denoted vIL-10. Since IL-10 stimulates the proliferation and differentiation of B cells, the natural reservoir of EBV, vIL-10 has an augmenting effect on viral replication and B-cell transformation. Similarly, a new T-cell cytokine, IL-17, which is highly similar to a protein encoded by the T-cell transforming virus herpes saimiri, has been identified. IL-17 may have a role in normal T-cell activation or proliferation and thereby increase viral replication. Other viruses, such as the poxviruses, encode cytokine-binding proteins whose structures sometimes resemble those of the corresponding cellular receptors, such as IL-1RII, TNFR, and IFNγR, and that are able to bind and inhibit the active cytokines in vivo. In addition, herpes viruses such as cytomegalovirus encode soluble receptors for chemokines such as IL-8 or MIP-1α. It has been proposed that all of these so-called virokines, or viroreceptors, may be descendants of cellular proteins whose genes were usurped by the viruses to enable them to interfere with host defenses.

OVERVIEW & PROSPECTS

The cytokines as a group serve as crucial intercellular-signaling molecules that are responsible for the multidirectional communication among immune and inflammatory cells engaged in host defense, repair, and restoration of homeostasis, as well as among other somatic cells in the connective tissues, skin, nervous system, and other organs.

Cytokines regulate one another's production and activities through competition, synergism, and mutual induction, resulting in a complex network of cytokine cascades and regulatory circuits with positive and negative feedback effects. In addition, other types of biologic mediators, such as corticosteroids and prostaglandins, have agonistic or antagonistic effects on cytokine activities. The biologic responses to cytokines can also be regulated through effects on the specific cytokine receptors expressed by responsive cells, and these receptors may provide a useful therapeutic target for modulating cytokine activity.

Owing to the complexity of cytokine interactions, the therapeutic use of these agents is still in its infancy. Nevertheless, some disease states have already been shown to respond to IFN or to IL-2. Specific agonists and antagonists of the cytokines and their receptors can be expected to play an important role in future therapy of inflammatory, infectious, autoimmune, and neoplastic diseases.

REFERENCES

GENERAL

Callard RG, Gearing A (editors): *The Cytokine Fact Book.* Academic Press, 1994.

Durum SK, Oppenheim JJ: Proinflammatory cytokines and immunity. In *Fundamental Immunology,* 3rd ed. Paul WE (editor). Raven Press Ltd, 1993.

Howard M et al: T cell derived cytokines and their receptors. In *Fundamental Immunology,* 3rd ed. Paul WE (editor). Raven Press Ltd, 1993.

Nicola NA (editor): *Guidebook to Cytokines and Their Receptors.* Oxford Univ Press, 1994.

Oppenheim JJ et al (editors): *Clinical Applications of Cytokines.* Oxford Univ Press, 1993.

Thompson A (editor): *Cytokine Handbook,* 2nd ed., Academic Press, 1994.

INTERLEUKIN-1

Colotta F et al: The type II decoy receptors: A novel regulatory pathway for IL-1. *Immunol Today* 1994;**15:**562.

Dinarello CA: IL-1 and IL-1 antagonism. *Blood* 1991; **77:**1627.

Fantuzzi G, Dinarello CA: The inflammatory response in IL-1β-deficient mice: Comparison with other cytokines-related knockout mice. *J Leuk Biol* 1996;**59:**489.

Neta R, Oppenheim JJ: IL 1: Can we exploit Jekyll and subjugate Hyde. *Biol Ther Cancer Updates* 1992;**2:**1.

Neta R et al: Relationship of TNF to interleukins. In *Tumor Necrosis Factor: Structure, Function, and Mechanism of Action.* Vilcek J, Aggarwal B (editors). Marcel Dekker, 1992.

TUMOR NECROSIS FACTOR FAMILY

Aggarwal B, Vilcek J (editors): *Tumor Necrosis Factor: Structure, Function, and Mechanism of Action.* Marcel Dekker, 1992, pp 1–624.

Beutler B (editor): *Tumor Necrosis Factors: The Molecules and Their Emerging Role in Medicine.* Raven Press, 1992.

Beutler B, Van Huffel C: Unraveling function in the TNF ligand receptor. *Science* 1994;**264:**667.

Nagata S, Golstein P: The FAS death factor. *Science* 1995;**27:**1449.

Old LJ: Tumor necrosis factor (TNF). *Science* 1985; **230:**630.

Torcia M et al: Nerve growth factor is an autocrine survival factor for memory B lymphocytes. *Cell* 1996;**85:**345.

IL-6 FAMILY

Ip NY et al: CNTF and LIF act on neuronal cells via shared signaling pathways that involve the IL-6 signal transducing component gp130. *Cell* 1992;**69:**1121.

Metcalf D: Leukemia inhibitory factor—A puzzling polyfunctional regulator. *Growth Factors* 1992;**7:**169.

Paul SR, Schendel P: The cloning and biological characterization of recombinant human interleukin 11. *Int J Cell Cloning* 1992;**10:**135.

Pennica D et al: Cardiotrophin-1: Biological activities and binding to the LIP receptor/gp130 signaling complex. *J Biol Chem* 1995;**270:**10:915.

Taga T, Kishimoto T: Cytokine receptors and signal transduction. *FASEB J* 1992;**6:**3387.

Wallance P et al: In vivo properties of oncostatin M. *Ann NY Acad Sci* 1995;**762:**42.

INTERFERONS

Diaz MO et al: Nomenclature of the human interferon genes. *J Interferon Res* 1993;**13:**61.

Farrar MA, Schreiber RD: The molecular cell biology of interferon-γ and its receptor. *Ann Rev Immunol* 1993;**11:**571.

Halloran PF. Interferon-γ, prototype of the proinflammatory cytokines—importance in activation, suppression, and maintenance of the immune response. *Transplant Proc* 1993;**25:**Suppl 1:10.

Sen GC, Lengyel P: The interferon system. A bird's eye view of its biochemistry. *J Biol Chem* 1992;**267:**5017.

Tough DF et al: Induction of bystander T cell proliferation by viruses and type I interferon in vivo. *Science* 1996;**272:**1947.

van den Broek MF et al: Immune defense in mice lacking Type I and/or Type II interferon receptors. *Immunol Rev* 1995;**148:**5.

Williams BRG: Signal transduction and transcriptional regulation of interferon α stimulated genes. *J Interferon Res* 1991;**11:**207.

Williams JG et al: Interferon-γ: A key immunoregulatory lymphokine. *J Surg Res* 1993;**54:**79.

Young HA, Hardy KJ: Role of interferon gamma in immune cell regulation. *J Leuk Biol* 1995;**58:**373.

IMMUNOREGULATORY CYTOKINES (IL-2, IL-4, IL-5, IL-10, IFNγ, ETC)

Giri J et al: Utilization of the beta and gamma chains of the IL-2 receptor by the novel cytokine IL-15. *EMBO J* 1994;**13:**2822.

Leonard W et al: The molecular basis of X-linked severe combined immunodeficiency: The role of the interleukin-2 receptor γ chain as a common γ chain, γc. *Immunol Rev* 1994;**138:**61.

Minami Y et al: The IL-2 receptor complex: Its structure, function, and target genes. *Ann Rev Immunol* 1993; **11:**245.

Moore KW et al: IL 10. *Ann Rev Immunol* 1993;**11:** 165.

Mosmann TR, Moore KW: The role of IL 10 in cross-regulation of T_{H1} and T_{H2} responses. *Immunol Today* 1991;**12:**A49.

Muller G et al: Gene targeting in immunology. In: *Immunological Review*, No 148, Goran Moller (editor). Munksgaard Copenhagen, Stockholm, 1995.

Schwartz RH: Costimulation of T lymphocytes: Role of CD28 in interleukin-2 production and immunotherapy. *Cell* 1992;**71:**1065.

Smith KA: Low dose IL-2 immunotherapy. *Blood* 1993;**81:**1414.

INTERLEUKIN-4, -5, & -7

Komschlies K et al: Diverse immunological and hematologic effect of IL-7: Implications for clinical application. *J Leuk Biol* 1995;**58:**623.

Paul WE: Interleukin 4: A prototypic immunoregulatory lymphokine. *Blood* 1991;**77:**1859.

Sanderson CJ: Interleukin 5, eosinophils, and disease. *Blood* 1992;**79:**3101.

HEMATOPOIETIC CYTOKINES

Gearing A et al: Elevated levels of GM-CSF and IL 1 in the serum, peritoneal, and pleural cavities of GM-CSF transgenic mice. *J Exp Med* 1992;**175:**877.

Metcalf D: Hematopoietic regulation, redundancy or subtlety. *Blood* 1993;**82:**3515.

Moore MAS et al: Cytokine networks involved in hemopoietic stem cell proliferation and differentiation. In: *Molecular Control of Hemopoiesis* CIBA Symposium. 1990;**148:**43.

Muller-Sieburg CE, Deryugina E: The stromal cells' guide to the stem cell universe. *Stem Cells* 1995;**13:**447.

Lord B, Dexter TM: Growth factor in hematopoiesis. In *Bailliere's Clinical Hematology.* Tindall, 1992.

Ogawa M: Differentiation and proliferation of hematopoietic stem cells. *Blood* 1993;**81:**2844.

Verfaillie CM: Can human hematopoietic stem cells be cultured ex vivo? *Stem Cells* 1994;**12:**466.

Zsebo KM et al: Radioprotection of mice by recombinant rat stem cell factor. *Proc Natl Acad Sci USA* 1992;**89:**9464.

CHEMOKINES & INTERLEUKIN-16

Alkhatib G et al: CC CKR5: MIP-1α, MIP-1β receptor as a fusion cofactor for macrophage-tropic HIV. *Science* 1996;**272:**1955.

Baggiolini M et al: IL-8 and related chemotactic cytokines—CXC and CC chemokines. *Adv Immunol* 1994;**55.**

Ben-Baruch A et al: Signals and receptors involved in recruitment of inflammatory cells. *J Biol Chem* 1995;**270:**11703.

Canter DM et al: The lymphocyte chemoattractant factor. *J Lab Clin Med* 1995; 125.

Furie MB, Randolph G: Chemokines and tissue injury. *Am J Pathol* 1995;**146:**1287.

Oppenheim JJ et al: Properties of the novel proinflammatory supergene intercrine cytokine family. *Ann Rev Immunol* 1991;**9:**617.

GROWTH FACTORS

Kingsley D: The TGF-β superfamily: New members, new receptors, and new genetic tests of function in different organisms. *Genes Dev* 1994;**8:**133.

Massague J et al: The TGF-β family and its composite receptors. *Trends Cell Biol* 1994;**4:**172.

Shull NM et al: Targeted disruption of mouse TGFβ1 gene results in multifocal inflammatory disease. *Nature* 1992;**359:**693.

Wahl SM: Transforming growth factor beta: The good, the bad, and the ugly. *J Exp Med* 1994;**180:**1587.

CYTOKINE RECEPTORS

Honda M et al: Human soluble IL-6 receptor: Its detection and enhanced release by HIV infection. *J Immunol* 1992;**148:**2175.

Layton MJ et al: A major binding protein for LIF in normal mouse serum: Identification as a soluble form of the cellular receptor. *Proc Natl Acad Sci USA* 1992;**89:**8616.

Lee J et al: Characterization of two high affinity human IL-8 receptors. *J Biol Chem* 1992;**267:**M283.

Massague J: Receptors for the TGFβ family. *Cell* 1992;**69:**1067.

Miyajima A et al: Common subunits of cytokine receptors and the functional redundancy of cytokines. *TIBS* 1992;**17:**378.

VIROKINES & VIRORECEPTORS

Spriggs MK: Cytokine and cytokine receptor genes "captured" by viruses. *Curr Opin Immun* 1994;**6:**526.

Smith GL: Virus strategies of evasion of the host response to infection. *Trends Microbiol* 1994;**2:**81.

McFadden G: DNA viruses that affect cytokine networks. In *Human Cytokines: Their Role in Disease and Therapy.* Aggarwal B, Puri K (editors). Blackwell Science, 1995.

Ruby JR et al: CD40 ligand has potent antiviral activity. *Nature Medicine* 1995;**1:**437.

Complement & Kinin

11

Michael M. Frank, MD

Complement activation, kinin generation, blood coagulation, and fibrinolysis are physiologic processes that occur through sequential cascade-like activation of enzymes normally present in their inactive forms in plasma. Although they are four distinct systems and perform different functions, they interact with one another and with various cell membrane proteins. The first two—complement and kinin—are the subjects of this chapter because of their involvement in immunologic effector responses.

THE COMPLEMENT SYSTEM

Complement is a collective term used to designate a group of plasma and cell membrane proteins that play a key role in the host defense process. Table 11–1 lists the major proteins, their molecular weights, and their serum concentrations.

FUNCTIONS OF COMPLEMENT

This complex system, which now numbers more than 25 proteins, acts in at least three major ways. The first and best known function of the system is to cause **lysis** of cells, bacteria, and enveloped viruses. The second is to mediate the process of **opsonization,** in which foreign cells, bacteria, viruses, fungi, and so forth, are prepared for phagocytosis. This process involves the coating of the foreign particle with specific complement protein fragments that can be recognized by receptors for these fragments on phagocytic cells (see Chapter 2).

The third function of the complement proteins is the generation of peptide fragments that regulate features of the inflammatory and immune responses. These proteins play a role in vasodilatation at the site of inflammation, in adherence of phagocytes to blood

Table 11–1. Molecular weights and serum concentrations of complement components.

	Molecular Weight	Serum Concentration (μg/mL)
Classic pathway component		
C1q	410,000	70
C1r	85,000	34
C1s	85,000	31
C2	102,000	25
C3	190,000	1200
C4	206,000	600
C5	190,000	85
C6	128,000	60
C7	120,000	55
C8	150,000	55
C9	71,000	60
Alternative pathway component		
Properdin	53,000	25
Factor B	90,000	225
Factor D	25,000	1
Inhibitors		
C1 Inhibitor	105,000	275
Factor I	88,000	34
Regulatory proteins		
C4-binding protein	560,000	8
Factor H	150,000	500
S protein (vitronectin)	80,000	500

vessel endothelium, in egress of the phagocytes from the vessel, in directed migration of phagocytic cells into areas of inflammation, and, ultimately, in clearing infectious agents from the body.

PATHWAYS OF COMPLEMENT ACTIVATION

Most of the early-acting proteins of the complement cascade are present in the circulation in an inactive form. The proteins undergo sequential **activation** to ultimately cause their biologic effects.

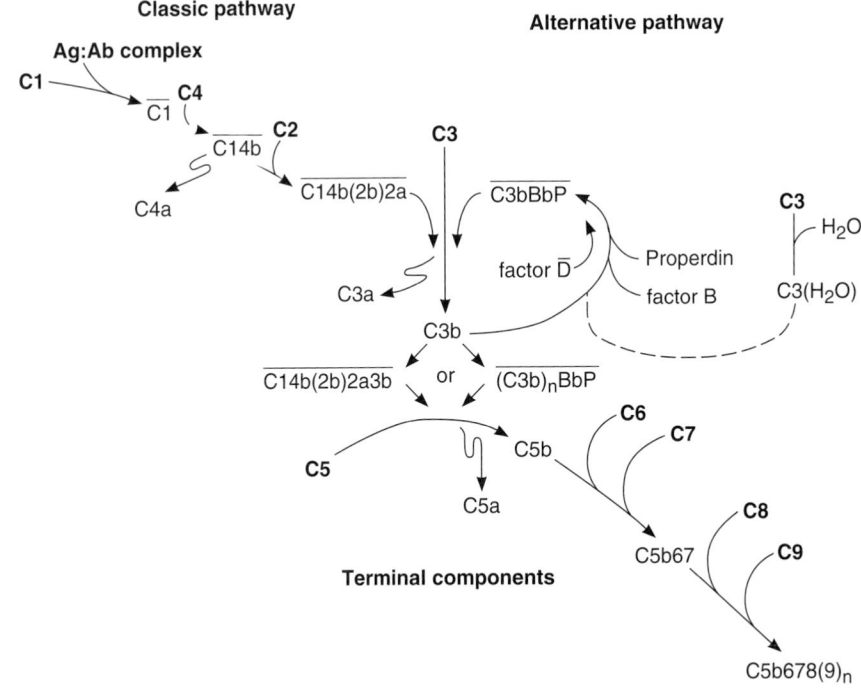

Figure 11–1. The complement cascade.

Two major pathways of complement activation operate in plasma. A general scheme of the system is shown in Figure 11–1. The first complement activation pathway to be discovered is termed the **classic complement pathway.** Under normal physiologic conditions, activation of this pathway is initiated by antigen–antibody complexes. The second pathway, known as the **alternative complement pathway,** was discovered more recently, although phylogenetically it probably is the older activation pathway. It does not have an absolute requirement for antibody for activation. Both pathways function through the interaction of proteins termed **components,** or **factors.** Both proceed by means of sequential activation and assembly of a series of components, leading to the formation of a complex enzyme capable of binding and cleaving a key component, C3, which is common to both pathways. Thereafter, the two pathways proceed together through binding of the terminal components to form a membrane attack complex, which ultimately causes cell lysis.

NOMENCLATURE

The proteins of the classic pathway and the terminal components are designated by numbers following the letter C. Proteins of the alternative pathway are generally given letter designations, as are other proteins that have major regulatory effects on the system.

The proteins of each pathway interact in a precise sequence. When a protein is missing, as occurs in some of the genetic deficiencies, the sequence is interrupted at that point. The early steps in the activation process are associated with the assembly of complement cleavage fragments to form enzymes that bind the next proteins in the sequence to continue the reaction cascade. These enzymes are designated with a bar placed over the symbol of the component to indicate active enzymatic activity.

THE CLASSIC COMPLEMENT PATHWAY

Initiation

The sequence of events that take place in the classic complement cascade is depicted in Figure 11–2. In most cases, the classic pathway is initiated by binding of antibody to an antigen. A single molecule of immunoglobulin M (IgM) on an antigenic surface, or two molecules of IgG of appropriate subclass bound side by side, can bind and activate the first component of the pathway, **C1.** C1 is a macromolecular complex composed of three different proteins (C1q, C1r, and C1s) held together by calcium ions. Each C1 complex is composed of one C1q, two C1r, and two C1s chains. The enzymatic potential of the complex resides in the C1r and C1s chains, each of which is an MW 85,000 proenzymatic form of a serine protease.

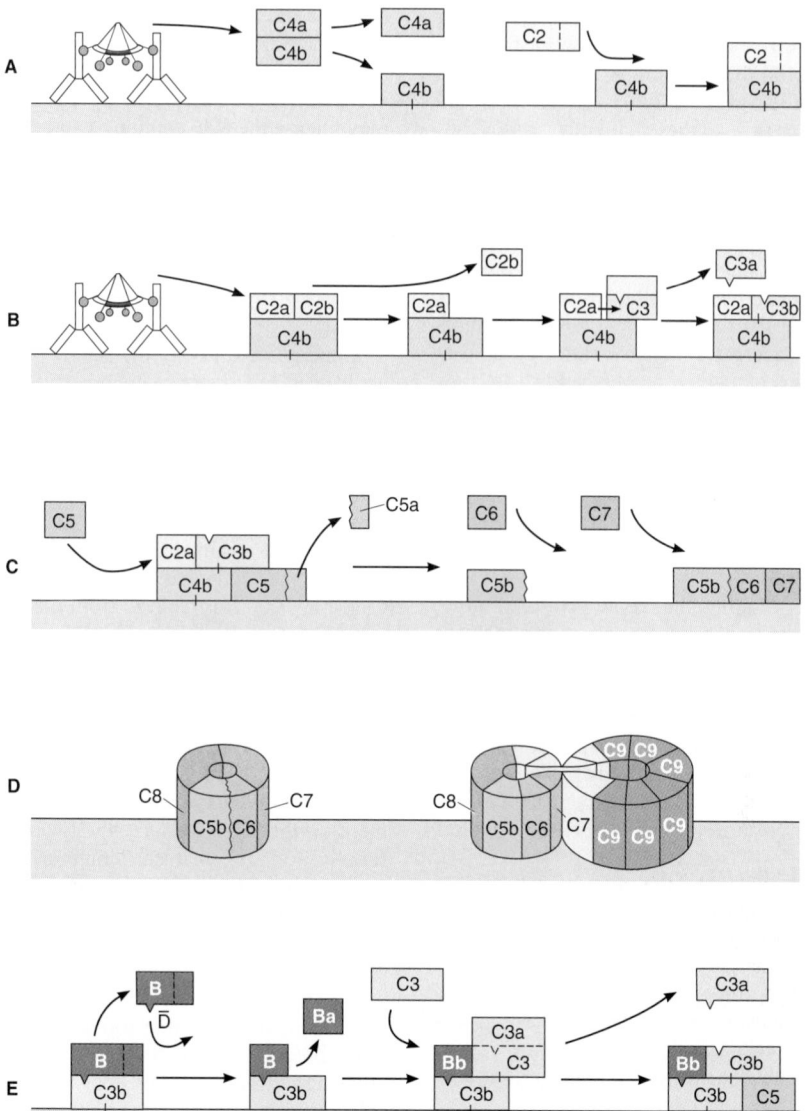

Figure 11–2. Diagram of the complement cascade. **A:** The classic complement pathway. A doublet of IgG antibody molecules on a surface can bind and activate C1, a three-part molecule composed of C1q, C1r, and C1s. C1q has a core and six radiating arms, each of which ends in a pod. The pod recognizes and binds to the Fc fragment of the IgG. On activation the C1 binds and cleaves C4. The small fragment, C4a, is released. The large fragment, C4b, binds to the target to continue the cascade. In the presence of magnesium ion, C2 recognizes and binds to C4b. **B:** Once C2 is bound to C4b, it can be cleaved by C1. A small fragment, C2b, is released, and the large fragment, C2a, remains bound to the C4b. This newly formed complex of two protein fragments can now bind and cleave C3. This molecule is, in turn, cleaved into two fragments: C3a and C3b. The small fragment, C3a, is released, and the large fragment, C3b, can bind covalently to a suitable acceptor. C3b molecules that bind directly to the C4b continue the cascade. **C:** The complex formed of C2a, C4b, and C3b can bind and cleave C5. A small fragment of C5, C5a, is released. The large fragment, C5b, does not bind covalently. It is stabilized by binding to C6. Here for clarity the C4b2a3b complex is no longer shown, although it is still present on the surface. When C7 binds, the complex of C5b, C6 and C7 becomes hydrophobic. It is partially lipid-soluble and can insert into the lipid of the cell membrane bilayer. **D:** When the C5b67 binds C8, a small channel is formed in the cell membrane. Multiple molecules of C9 can bind and markedly enlarge the channel. The channel has a hydrophobic outer surface and a hydrophilic central channel that allows passage of water and ions. **E:** The alternative complement pathway. In the presence of magnesium ion, C3b on a surface can bind factor B, just as C4b can bind C2. Factor D, a fluid-phase factor, can cleave bound factor B into two fragments, Ba and Bb. Ba is released. The C3bBb complex can now bind an additional molecule of C3 and cleave it, just as C4b2a can bind and cleave C3. C3a is released, and the new complex of C3bBbC3b, usually written (C3b)2Bb, can bind C5 to continue the cascade.

Antibody binding is mediated by the much larger (MW 410,000) C1q portion of the complex, which binds the Fc portion of immunoglobulins. C1q can bind to IgM, IgG1, IgG2, or IgG3. It does not bind IgG4, IgE, IgA, or IgD, so these antibody classes cannot activate the classic pathway.

C1q is itself composed of six identical subunits, each containing one copy each of three different polypeptide chains. Portions of these three chains closely resemble collagen and coil around one another to form a triple-helical collagen-like arm that is highly flexible. In the C1q complex, the six subunits are arranged to create a globular central core from which the six arms radiate outward (see Fig 11–2). At the end of each arm is a pod-like hand that is formed by the carboxy termini of all three chains, and that mediates binding to the C_{H2} domains in immunoglobulins of appropriate subclasses. The binding specificity of C1q has been exploited in creating clinical assays (called **C1q binding assays**) to detect immune complexes in serum.

If the antibody-binding sites (epitopes) on a target antigen are too low in density for proper arrangement of antibody molecules, C1 binding does not occur. This is seen with erythrocytes coated with anti-Rh0 (D) antibody as a result of maternal–fetal **Rh incompatibility.** Although complement-activating subclasses of IgG are formed against such erythrocytes, complement is not usually activated and has no role in their destruction because the necessary IgG doublets do not form.

Binding of C1 to antibody results in activation of the proteolytic enzyme activities of C1r and, subsequently, C1s. Each of these polypeptides becomes activated upon cleavage into two fragments, the shorter of which has protease activity. It is believed that the function of the activated C1r enzyme, $\overline{C1r}$, is to cleave C1s, which then develops enzymatic activity. $\overline{C1s}$ then cleaves the next component of the pathway, C4 (see Figs 11–1 and 11–2A).

C4 & C2

C4 is a three-chain molecule. The largest of the three chains, the α chain, is cleaved at a single site by $\overline{C1s}$, with the release of a small peptide, C4a. The larger peptide, consisting of most of the α chain together with the β and γ chains of C4, binds to the target cell to continue the complement cascade. Binding involves the formation of a covalent amide or ester bond between the target cell and the α chain of C4 (see the discussion of chemistry under the section on C3). In the presence of magnesium ion, C4b on a target cell is capable of interacting with and binding the next component in the series, a single-chain molecule of MW 102,000, termed C2. C2 binds to C4b and, in the presence of $\overline{C1s}$, is cleaved. The larger cleavage fragment of C2 (C2a), which contains the enzymatic site, remains in complex with C4b to continue the complement cascade (see Fig 11–2B). The complex of C4b

and C2a develops a new capacity: the ability to bind and cleave the next component in the series, C3. For this reason it is termed the **classic pathway C3 convertase.** The peptide complex C4b2a is unstable and may release the C2a peptide as an enzymatically inactive fragment; however, target-bound C4b can accept another C2 and, in the presence of active C1, regenerate a convertase capable of continuing the complement cascade. These early steps in the classic pathway are under tight regulation, as discussed later.

C3

The C3 convertase of the classic pathway binds and activates C3, a glycoprotein present at a concentration of about 1.2 g/L of plasma. C3 consists of two disulfide-linked chains, termed α and β (MW 110,000 and 75,000, respectively). Two amino acids in the C3 α chain are linked by a thiolester bond that lies buried in a hydrophobic pocket of the protein and twists the α chain into a strained configuration (see Fig 11–4). When C3 is activated by the convertase, a peptide C3a (MW 9000) is cleaved from the α chain. As a result, the internal thiolester on the remaining C3b fragment becomes exposed to the surrounding medium. This highly reactive thiolester has a half-life of roughly 30–60 ms and, during this time, reacts to form a covalent bond with any suitable acceptor in its vicinity.

If C3b bonds covalently to the adjacent C4b fragment on the target surface, the two (along with C2a) form a complex that can continue the complement cascade (see Fig 11–2B). In addition, the presence of bound C3b strongly **opsonizes** the target particle, increasing its phagocytosis by cells that carry **C3b receptors** (CR1; see section on C3 Receptors). C3b also has a strong tendency to interact with nearby IgG molecules, and the dimer formed by C3b and IgG is a more potent opsonin than is C3b alone. If, on the other hand, the thiolester does not encounter a suitable acceptor, it reacts with water to form the conformationally altered inactive species **C3(H2O)**; this rapid inactivation helps to ensure that the reactive form of C3b is destroyed and does not produce unwanted activation.

THE CLASSIC PATHWAY C5 CONVERTASE

The complex on a target surface consisting of C4b, C2a, and C3b ($\overline{C4b2a3b}$) has a newly expressed enzymatic activity: it can coordinate with and cleave C5, and so is called the **classic pathway C5 convertase.** Again, two fragments, C5a and C5b, are formed, with C5a being the smaller. The larger fragment (C5b) remains noncovalently associated with the $\overline{C4b2a3b}$ complex and is available to interact with later components. It is C5b that initiates the segment of the complement cascade that leads to membrane attack.

In summary, the early steps of the complement cascade lead to the generation of a series of enzymatically active peptides and peptide complexes. As each complex is formed, it has a different specificity from the preceding complex, and interacts with the next protein in the complement cascade. Each enzyme interacts with multiple molecules of the next substrate protein in the cascade of reactions either until it decays, as occurs with the C3 and C5 convertases, or until it is inhibited by regulatory proteins present on cells or in plasma. Thus, there is a potential for considerable biologic amplification: a limited number of antigen–antibody complexes lead to the activation of large numbers of complement molecules.

Nonimmunologic Classic Pathway Activators

It is of interest that a number of nonimmunologic activators of the classic pathway exist. Certain bacteria (eg, certain *Escherichia coli* and *Salmonella* strains of low virulence) and viruses (eg, parainfluenza virus, human immunodeficiency virus) interact with C1q directly, causing C1 activation and, in turn, classic pathway activation in the absence of antibody. Such an interaction in most cases aids the natural defense process of the host. Other structures, such as the surface of urate crystals, myelin basic protein, denatured DNA, bacterial endotoxin, and polyanions (such as heparin) also may activate the classic pathway directly. Such activation by urate crystals is thought to contribute to the inflammation and pain associated with gout.

THE ALTERNATIVE COMPLEMENT PATHWAY

C3 not only serves as a pivotal component of the classic pathway but also is the key component of the **alternative complement pathway.** This pathway provides yet another means of activating the complement cascade in the absence of bound antibodies. As described earlier, C3 can undergo hydrolysis of its thiolester bond to form a conformationally altered species called $C3(H_2O)$. Spontaneous decay of C3 to $C3(H_2O)$ is thought to occur continually but at a very low rate in the blood. In the presence of magnesium ions, $C3(H_2O)$ can bind another circulating protein called **factor B,** which is similar in many respects to C2; in fact, factor B and C2 are encoded by adjacent genes on chromosome 6 and may well have arisen through duplication of a single gene. The complex of $C3(H_2O)$ and factor B can be acted on by a third blood protein, **factor D,** which is a C1-like serine proteinase. As a result, factor B is cleaved, and the remaining complex acquires C3 convertase activity. This initial complex can then cleave additional C3 proteins to produce highly reactive C3b.

This spontaneous sequence of reactions ensures that minute amounts of C3b are constantly being produced in the blood. Under normal circumstances, these fragments are rapidly inactivated by cleavage; stringent control mechanisms (see later discussion) operate to limit the extent of the reaction and so prevent massive complement activation and damage to host cells. If these reactions happen to occur near a foreign particle, however, some C3b fragments may become covalently bound to its surface (see Fig 11–2E). C3b is capable of binding factor B, which can then be acted on by factor D, forming a complex (C3bBb) called the **alternative pathway C3 convertase.** The C3 convertase, in turn, can bind and cleave an additional molecule of C3 to form a larger complex (denoted C3bBbC3b) that has **C5 convertase** activity. The latter complex then efficiently triggers subsequent steps in the complement cascade and so promotes an attack on the particle to which it is bound.

The alternative pathway C3 convertase (C3bBb) is extremely unstable and would ordinarily dissociate rapidly. In the blood, however, a protein called **properdin** binds to this convertase and stabilizes it, thus slowing its decay and allowing it to continue the complement cascade.

For many years, investigators have used a protein derived from cobra venom (**cobra venom factor**) to activate complement in the laboratory. Recent studies have shown that this protein is related to cobra C3 and is a physiologic analogue of C3b in this reptile. Cobra venom factor, when added to human plasma, functions just like human C3b to activate the alternative pathway. As described later on, endogenous C3b is under tight regulatory control by other plasma proteins. By contrast, cobra venom factor is not inhibited by these regulators and therefore can induce massive complement activation.

THE LATE COMPONENTS C5–9 & THE MEMBRANE ATTACK COMPLEX

The late phase of the complement cascade (see Fig 11–2C) begins when C5 is bound and then cleaved by either the alternative or classic pathway convertase into C5a and C5b. C5a is released and produces biologic effects, which are described in a later section. C5b continues the lytic sequence; however, it does not form a covalent bond with the surface of its target. C5b is rapidly inactivated unless it is stabilized by binding to the next component in the cascade, C6. The C5b6 complex can bind C7, the third protein involved in membrane attack. The C5b67 complex is strongly hydrophobic and interacts with nearby membrane lipids. It is capable of inserting into the lipid bilayer of cell membranes. In that location, one C5b67 complex can accept one molecule of C8 and multiple molecules of C9, ultimately forming a cylindrical transmembrane channel, C5b678(9)n, which has been termed the **membrane attack complex (MAC)** (Fig 11–3). This structure has a hydrophobic outer surface,

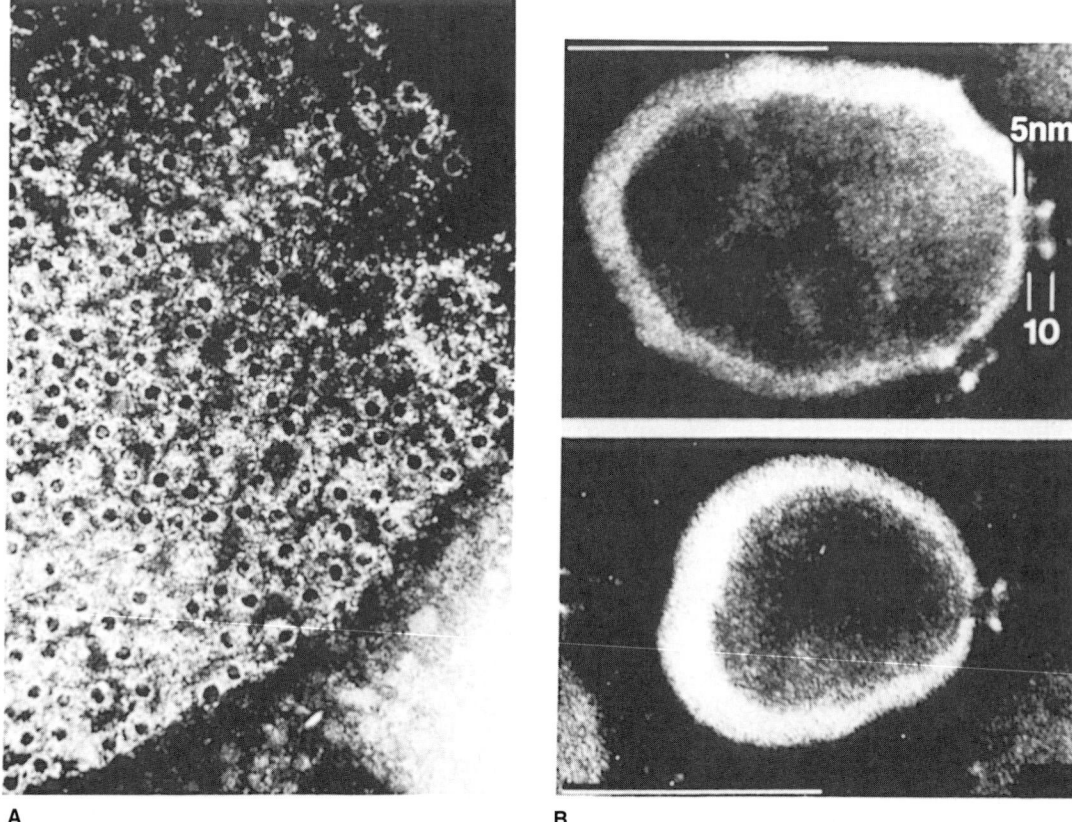

Figure 11–3. Lysis of cells by C5b-9, the membrane attack complex (MAC). **A:** Surface of cells lysed by antibody and complement. Note the surface lesions. (Micrograph courtesy of R. Dourmashkin.) **B:** Two views of the purified lesions allowed to attach to lipid micelles. The hollow cylinder formed by the C5b-9 has allowed the electron-dense dye to enter the lipid droplet. (Photograph courtesy of S. Bhakdi.)

which associates with the membrane lipid of the bilayer, and a hydrophilic core through which small ions and water can pass. The ionic environment of the extracellular fluid then communicates with that inside the cell, so that once this complex is inserted into the membrane, the cell cannot maintain its osmotic and chemical equilibrium. Water enters the cell because of the high internal oncotic pressure, and the cell swells and bursts. The assembly of C5b–C8 appears to form a small membrane channel that is increasingly enlarged and stabilized by the binding of multiple molecules of C9. One such channel penetrating the erythrocyte membrane is sufficient to destroy the cell. Cells with more complex metabolic machinery can, to some extent, internalize and destroy complement complexes that form on the cell surface or shed them as vesicles from the cell surface, thereby providing some protection against complement attack.

CONTROL MECHANISMS

The complement system has evolved to aid in the host defense process by directly damaging invading organisms and by producing tissue inflammation. Strict regulatory control of this system is of critical importance to prevent complement-mediated destruction of the individual's own tissues. When complement is involved in causing disease, it usually is functioning normally but is misdirected, that is, damaging to the host tissues. Many control proteins have evolved to defend against such attack.

The C1 Inhibitor

The first of these, **C1 inhibitor (C1INH),** recognizes activated $\overline{\text{C1r}}$ and $\overline{\text{C1s}}$ and destroys their activity. This glycoprotein (MW 105,000) not only inhibits $\overline{\text{C1r}}$ and $\overline{\text{C1s}}$, but also acts as an inhibitor of activated Hageman factor (see section on Proteins of the Kinin Cascade) and of all the enzyme systems activated by Hageman factor fragments. Thus, C1INH regulates enzymes formed during activation of the kinin-generating system, the clotting system, the fibrinolytic system, and the complement cascade. In each of these systems, C1INH binds physically to the active site of the enzyme to destroy its activity and in the process is consumed. Interestingly, during C1 inactivation the

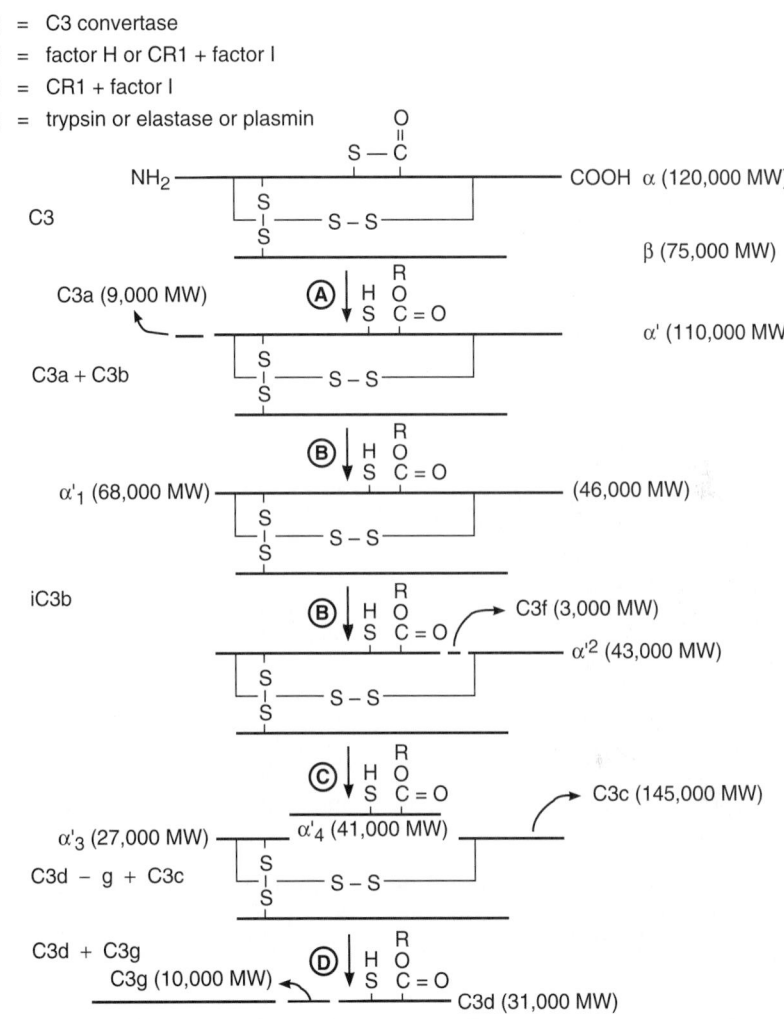

(A) = C3 convertase
(B) = factor H or CR1 + factor I
(C) = CR1 + factor I
(D) = trypsin or elastase or plasmin

Figure 11–4. The C3 degradation pathway. The a and b chains of C3 are shown. Activation of C3 with the formation of C3a and C3b by the C3 convertases is shown (step A). C3b is degraded to iC3b by the action of factor H or CR1 plus factor I (step B). Two forms of iC3b have been described, differing in loss of a 3-kDa fragment. In the presence of CR1 and factor I, C3c is released and C3dg remains target-bound (step C). C3dg can be further degraded to C3d by proteolytic enzymes (step D). Specific cellular receptors exist for each of these fragments.

C1 is dissociated, with the C1INH binding to each of the C1r and C1s enzymatic sites and freeing C1q of its subunits. Since C1INH is consumed when acting as an inhibitor, the synthetic product of two active genes is necessary to provide the relatively high plasma concentration of the protein gene product required for effective inhibitor activity. A relative deficiency occurs in patients with **hereditary angioedema,** who have a defect in one of the two genes responsible for formation of C1INH. These patients have one half to one third the normal level of C1INH and have frequent attacks of angioedema—painless swelling of deep cutaneous tissues—whose cause is still uncertain. It may arise from activation of the kinin-generating system or from activation of the complement system,

with generation of peptides that cause vascular leakage.

C4-binding Protein, Factor I & Factor H

C4-binding protein **(C4bp)** and a second protein, factor I, are responsible for regulation of C4b. C4bp binds to C4b and facilitates its cleavage by the proteolytic enzyme **factor I.** On target surfaces, C4bp is not required for C4b cleavage by factor I, but its presence may accelerate the cleavage process.

Factor I also acts proteolytically to inactivate C3b and $C3(H_2O)$ (Fig 11–4). This activity requires a cofactor termed **factor H.** Factor H acts as an obligate cofactor in the fluid phase and as an accelerator of C3 cleavage on cell surfaces (see Fig 11–4). In the presence of factors H and I, the C3b or C3(H$_2$O) α chain is cleaved at two sites to form a partially degraded molecule, **iC3b.** This molecule, although inactive in continuing the complement cascade, is active as an opsonin and is discussed further later on. Under the appropriate conditions, as discussed later, factor I can cleave iC3b further to form a molecule termed C3dg, which also interacts with specific receptors that recognize this C3 degradation peptide.

Vitronectin (S Protein)

Yet another control protein, **S protein** (also called **vitronectin**), interacts with the C5b67 complex as it forms in the fluid phase and binds to its membrane-binding site to prevent the binding of C5b67 to biologic membranes. Following binding of S protein to fluid-phase C5b67, binding of C8 and C9 to the fluid-phase complex can proceed, but the complex does not insert into lipid membranes and does not lyse cells.

Protected Site Concept

In the control of complement attack against host tissue, it would be beneficial if complement proteins such as C3b were rapidly degraded when bound to host cells but not degraded when bound to the surface of a microorganism. A process for accomplishing this goal has evolved. When deposited on a microorganism, C3b is often in a "protected site," which is protected from the action of the control proteins factors H and I. The C3b persists to activate the alternative pathway and destroy the organism. In contrast, on host cells C3b interacts with factors H and I and is degraded. The biochemical basis for this protection of C3b on an organism surface is not yet completely understood but appears to relate to the presence of charged carbohydrates such as sialic acid on mammalian cells, which may facilitate the binding of factor H.

GENETIC CONSIDERATIONS

Most of the genes encoding proteins of the classic and alternative pathways have been cloned, and their amino acid sequences have been determined. Moreover, the activation peptides have been studied in some detail. Allotypic variants of many of the proteins have been found that show genetic polymorphisms, as demonstrated by differences in surface charge. Almost all of the variants of complement proteins show autosomal-codominant inheritance at a single locus. The genes for C4, C2, and factor B are located within the major histocompatibility locus on the short arm of chromosome 6 in humans and are termed class III histocompatibility genes. The significance of the intimate colocalization of histocompatibility genes and complement genes is unknown at present.

Interestingly, there are two C4 loci on chromosome 6; thus, there are four C4 genes: two on each chromosome 6. The two loci code for proteins termed C4A and C4B, which differ in functional activity. Individuals with at least one null allele at one of the C4 loci are thought to be prone to the development of autoimmune disease. Genes for many of the regulatory proteins that interact with C4 and C3 are grouped as a supergene family on chromosome 1 (Table 11–2). This family is now known to encode factor H, C4-binding protein, decay-accelerating factor, CR1, and CR2. The gene products of this family each have one or more 60-amino-acid domains or short consensus repeats (SCRs) that may repeat multiple times in the molecule. They presumably originated from a common gene precursor. See Chapter 25 for a discussion of inherited complement component deficiencies with associated syndromes.

Mannose Binding Protein

Although not considered one of the complement sequence proteins, **mannose-binding protein (MBP)** must be considered at this time (see also Chapter 2). Inherited defects in this protein have been found particularly in children with frequent infections and opsonic defects. The protein has a tail segment that structurally resembles C1q and a head region that binds to mannose residues present on the surface of many microbes. It tends to form a trimer. The bound protein can activate the classical complement pathway much as bound antibody and C1 activate the pathway, ultimately opsonizing the organism. Point mutations in MBP have been shown to cause partial or complete loss of opsonic activity. Studies of the protein may prove very important in evaluation of individuals, particularly young children, with frequent infection.

BIOLOGIC CONSEQUENCES OF COMPLEMENT ACTIVATION IN INFLAMMATION

In general, the larger fragments formed during complement component cleavage tend to continue the complement cascade, whereas the smaller fragments mediate aspects of inflammation. For example, the cleavage of C3 and C5 generates C3a and C5a fragments, which consist of the first 77 and 74 amino acids of the C3 and C5 α chains, respectively. Cleavage of C4 generates C4a, a MW 77,000 amino acid fragment from the α chain of C4. All of these small activation peptides have **anaphylatoxic** activity: they cause smooth muscle contraction and degranulation of mast cells and basophils, with consequent release of histamine and other vasoactive substances that induce capillary leakage. **C5a** is the most potent of these anaphylatoxins.

C5a and C3a also have important immunoregulatory effects on T-cell function, either stimulating (C5a) or inhibiting (C3a) aspects of cell-mediated immunity.

Table 11–2. Regulators of complement activation encoded on chromosome 1.[1]

Name	Ligand	Distribution	Structure	Biochemical acceleration of decay of convertase	Cofactor for cleavage of C3b or C4b
Membrane cofactor protein (MCP; CD46)	C3b/C4b	On most cell surfaces including trophoblast and sperm	Single chain ≈68 kd 4 SCRs	–	+
CR1 (CD35)	C3b/C4b	Erythrocytes, phagocytes, most B lymphocytes, some T lymphocytes, follicular dendritic cells, glomerular podocytes	Single chain 190 kd (multiple forms) 30 SCRs	+	+
CR2 (CD21)	C3d, C3dg	Most B lymphocytes, some T lymphocytes, follicular dendritic cells, some epithelial cells	Single chain 145 kd 15 SCRs	–	+
DAF (CD55)	C3b/C4b	On most cell surfaces, all peripheral blood cells, trophoblast, and sperm	Single chain 70 kd 4 SCRs	+	–
C4-binding protein (C4bp)	C4b	Plasma	520 kd 7 α chains, 1 β chain Each α 7 SCRs Each β 3 SCRs	+	+
Factor H	C3b	Plasma	Single chain 160 kd 20 SCRs	+	+

Abbreviations: SCR = short consensus repeat; DAF = decay accelerating factor.
[1] A number of these proteins have multiple allelic forms differing in molecular weight.

C5a has profound effects on phagocytic cells. By interacting with specific cell membrane C5a receptors, it is strongly chemotactic for neutrophils and mononuclear phagocytes, inducing their migration along a concentration gradient toward the site of generation. It increases neutrophil adhesiveness and causes neutrophil aggregation. In addition, it dramatically stimulates neutrophil oxidative metabolism and the production of toxic oxygen species, and it triggers lysosomal enzyme release from a variety of phagocytic cells. Cellophane membranes used in **renal dialysis** machines and membrane oxygenators may activate the alternative pathway with C5a generation. This, in turn, may lead to neutrophil aggregation, embolization of the aggregates to the lungs, and pulmonary distress. It is suspected that C5a generation plays an important deleterious role in the development of **adult respiratory distress syndrome.**

The life span of these biologically potent peptides, C3a and C5a, is limited by a serum carboxy-peptidase that cleaves off the terminal arginine from the peptides, in most cases markedly reducing their activity.

COMPLEMENT RECEPTORS & RELATED MEMBRANE PROTEINS

C1q Receptors

The surfaces of many cell types bear complement receptors. Receptors for the **C1q** component of C1 have been identified on neutrophils and monocytes, the majority of B lymphocytes, and a small population of lymphocytes lacking both B- and T-cell markers. Binding via this receptor has been shown to activate cells for a variety of cellular functions, including phagocytosis and oxidative metabolism. C1q can also augment the cytotoxicity of human peripheral blood lymphocytes to antibody-sensitized chicken erythrocytes and supports antibody-independent cytolytic activity by certain lymphoblastoid cell lines. The C1q receptor does not interact with C1q in intact C1 but interacts once the C1 has been dissociated by the C1 inhibitor.

C3 Receptors

The best studied receptors are those that recognize C3 fragments (see Table 11–2). Importantly, these receptors do not recognize native circulating C3 and are not blocked by the normal plasma protein. Receptors exist for C3b, iC3b, C3d, and C3dg. These receptors have characteristic cellular distributions, with the C3b receptor (termed **CR1**) being prominent on erythrocytes, granulocytes, mononuclear phagocytes, B lymphocytes, and 25% of T cells in humans. In contrast, the C3bi receptor (**CR3**) is present only on phagocytic cells. The C3d receptor (**CR2**) is present on lymphoblastoid cells, B lymphocytes, and a proportion of T cells. These receptors bind the various C3 fragments as indicated. If the C3 is bound to an antigen or target particle, the antigen or target binds via the C3 ligand to the surface of cells with the receptor. For phagocytic cells, binding of the target to the phagocyte surface can augment the ingestion process (see Chapter 2).

Thus, CR1 and CR3 are both important in the process of phagocytosis. They also serve several other functions, however. They both act as cofactors for the further degradation of C3 fragments by the serum enzyme factor I. In each case, a C3 fragment bound to the receptor can be cleaved by factor I to the decay fragment C3dg. This fragment is not formed in the absence of complement receptors. CR3 is a member of the **integrin** protein family and plays a major role in cell adherence (see Chapter 1); phagocytes from CR3-deficient patients have marked abnormalities in adherence and ingestion. Another integrin, p150/95, binds C3b and C3dg and has recently been identified as **CR4**. Recently, a number of children with deficiency of all of the CR3-related proteins have been identified. They present with a history of delayed separation of the umbilical cord at birth and frequent soft-tissue and cutaneous infections by a variety of organisms, especially staphylococci and *Pseudomonas aeruginosa*. Neutrophils lacking these receptors do not marginate normally, and affected children have a marked leukocytosis.

CR2 (also designated **CD21**) is a receptor for the C3d and C3dg fragments of C3. It is present on B lymphocytes, some T cells, and nasal epithelial cells.

Regulatory Molecules

Several other cellular membrane proteins act not as receptors but rather to control untoward complement activation. **Decay-accelerating factor (DAF)** is a single-chain membrane protein (MW 70,000) that is a potent accelerator of C3 convertase decay, but, unlike CR1 and CR3, it has no factor I cofactor activity (see Table 11–2). Functionally, the protein acts to limit membrane damage if, by chance, complement is activated at the cell surface. CD46, also called membrane cofactor protein (MCP), facilitates degradation of C3b and C4b (see Table 11–2). **C8-binding protein,** also known as **homologous restriction factor (HRF),** acts to prevent successful completion and membrane insertion of the MAC. This membrane protein therefore acts to prevent cell lysis at yet another step in the complement cascade. It is called homologous restriction protein because it recognizes C8 and C9 of the same species far better than it recognizes late components of other species. Human homologous restriction protein on cells prevents the action of human C8 and C9 on those cells far better than it prevents the action of C8 and C9 from other species. Any potential advantage of this function is completely obscure.

CD59 is yet another regulatory protein that prevents assembly of the complete C5b–9 complex on target cells and so prevents complement-mediated lysis. Interestingly, DAF, HRF, and CD59 are each bound to the cell surface by a **phosphoinositide glycosidic linkage** rather than by a transmembrane domain within the amino acid backbone of the protein. This phosphoinositide linkage is reported to give the protein far greater lateral mobility within the cell membrane, increasing its ability to intercept damage-causing complement complexes. In patients with **paroxysmal nocturnal hemoglobinuria,** phosphoinositide-linked proteins are incorrectly assembled or inserted into cellular membranes of hematologic cells due to a specific enzyme defect, rendering these cells exquisitely sensitive to complement-mediated lysis.

Mimicry of Complement Proteins

Given the stability of the complement proteins and receptors in evolution and their importance in host defense, it is not surprising that microbes have evolved mechanisms for inhibiting activity of the proteins or using them for their own ends. In general, pathogenic organisms have mechanisms for decreasing the effectiveness of complement peptides. These range from the presence of capsules surrounding the outer membrane that prevent the interaction of complement peptides with phagocyte complement receptors, to the synthesis of proteins that aid degradation of complement peptides. Organisms have also subverted the complement peptides to their own ends. For example, Epstein-Barr virus (EBV) produces a surface protein that mimics the C3 fragment C3d, thereby gaining entry to B cells by binding to CR2 (CD21), the B-cell C3d receptor. Measles virus enters cells by binding to CD46, the membrane cofactor protein.

THE KININ CASCADE

The kinin-generating system is a second important mediator-forming system in blood. Here there is one major final product, **bradykinin,** a nonapeptide with potent ability to cause increased vascular permeability, vasodilatation, hypotension, pain, contraction of many types of smooth muscle, and activation of phospholipase A_2 with attendant activation of cellular arachidonic acid metabolism. Bradykinin effects are in most cases mediated by interaction with one of two

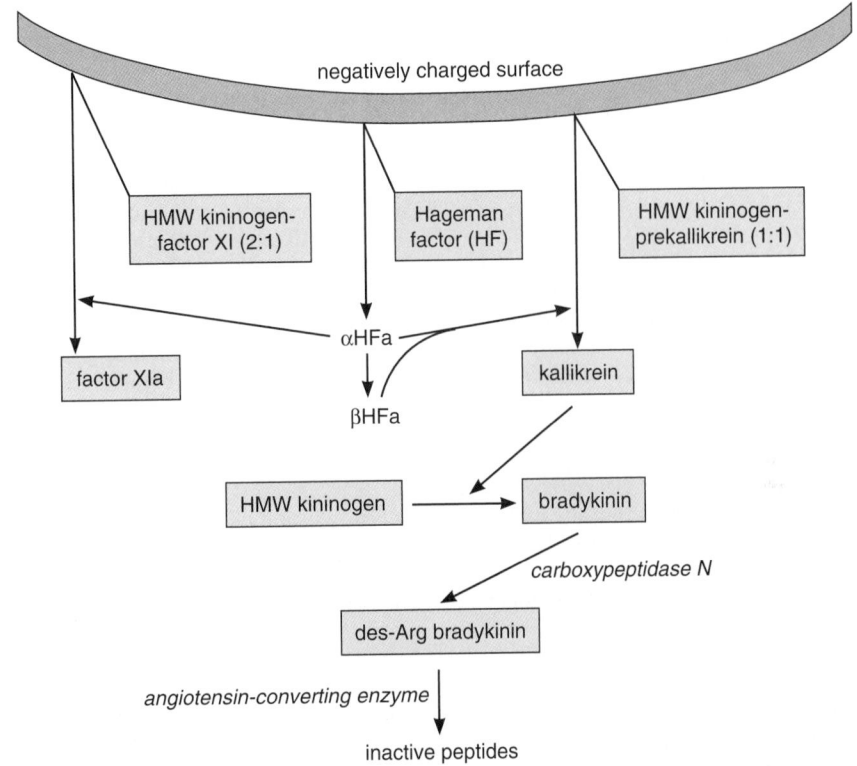

Figure 11–5. The kinin-generating pathway. Emphasized is the fact that complexes of high-molecular-weight (HMW) kininogen with both factor XI and prekallikrein associate on a surface with Hageman factor. The Hageman factor is activated and in turn is responsible for the activation of factor XI and prekallikrein. Active kallikrein cleaves high-molecular-weight kininogen to release bradykinin.

types of bradykinin receptors—B-1 and B-2—present on the membrane of many cell types, including vessel endothelial cells, smooth muscle, nerve cells, and synovial lining cells. Specific bradykinin receptor antagonists are now available, and a wide range of physiologic effects of bradykinin are being established. Often interaction with bradykinin causes the release of a variety of cytokins, altering cellular function. Recent studies have suggested an important role for bradykinin in blood pressure homeostasis and aspects of renal function, including glomerular filtration rate and renal plasma flow.

PROTEINS OF THE KININ CASCADE

Four plasma proteins make up the bradykinin-generating system: **Hageman factor, clotting factor XI, prekallikrein,** and **high-molecular-weight kininogen** (Fig 11–5). Factor XI circulates as a complex with high-molecular-weight kininogen in a molar ratio of 2:1. Prekallikrein also circulates in a complex with high-molecular-weight kininogen in a molar ratio of 1:1. In contrast, Hageman factor circulates as an uncomplexed single-chain plasma protein.

STEPS IN KININ ACTIVATION

On interaction with a negatively charged surface such as is supplied experimentally by glass or naturally by many biologically active materials like the lipid A of gram-negative bacterial endotoxin, Hageman factor is cleaved and activated. The cleaved Hageman factor (αHFa) has proteolytic activity and can cleave additional molecules of Hageman factor to generate more αHFa. Cleavage of the single chain of Hageman factor (MW 80,000) yields heavy and light chains (MW 50,000 and 28,000, respectively) that remain linked by disulfide bonds. The active enzymatic site of Hageman factor resides in its light chain. Cleavage is also catalyzed by other proteolytic enzymes, particularly kallikrein. αHFa can interact with the complex of factor XI and high-molecular-weight kininogen to activate factor XI to factor XIa. This, in turn, can activate the intrinsic coagulation cascade. αHFa can also interact with the high-molecular-weight kininogen–prekallikrein complex to cleave the single-chain prekallikrein into a two-chain molecule (kallikrein), with the chains associated via a disulfide linkage. The cleaved molecule has proteolytic enzymatic activity associated with the lower molecular weight chain. To facilitate these cleavages of both factor XI and prekallikrein, high-molecular-weight kininogen complexes are bound to the surface, presumably near the Hageman factor.

AMPLIFICATION & REGULATION OF KININ GENERATION

Active kallikrein is capable of further cleaving αHFa, with loss of the heavy chain but not the light chain. The resulting molecule, βHFa, remains capable of activating the high-molecular-weight kininogen–prekallikrein complex, but it does not remain surface-bound and does not interact efficiently with the high-molecular-weight kininogen–factor XI complex. Prekallikrein is also a single-chain glycoprotein that is converted to an active form by cleavage within a disulfide bridge, resulting in a two-chain molecule with the chains linked by disulfide bonds. The enzymatic site resides in the light chain, and the surface-binding site in the heavy chain. Active kallikrein can cleave high-molecular-weight kininogen at several sites to release bradykinin from the kininogen. Bradykinin has a short half-life, since it is rapidly attacked by carboxypeptidase N, which removes the C-terminal arginine to form the molecule termed des-Arg bradykinin. des-Arg bradykinin no longer has the smooth muscle-contracting activity of bradykinin and cannot induce capillary plasma leakage when injected into skin, but it retains some vascular effects. des-Arg bradykinin is, in turn, cleaved by angiotensin-converting enzyme to form low-molecular-weight peptides that lack biologic activity.

PLASMA INHIBITORS OF KININ GENERATION

The inhibitors of this mediator-generating system include C1 inhibitor, α_2-macroglobulin, and α_1-proteinase inhibitor. C1 inhibitor and α_2-macroglobulin are the principal inhibitors of active kallikrein, with C1 inhibitor contributing most to inhibitory activity. C1 inhibitor and α_1-proteinase inhibitor are the major inhibitors of factor XIa, and C1 inhibitor is the principal inhibitor of active Hageman factor.

LOW-MOLECULAR-WEIGHT KININOGEN & TISSUE KALLIKREINS

A low-molecular-weight kininogen also exists in plasma. This protein has an identical heavy chain to that of high-molecular-weight kininogen. Low-molecular-weight kininogen can act as a source of bradykinin, but it is not easily cleaved by kallikrein. Tissue kallikreins—low-molecular-weight kallikreins found in multiple tissues—that can cleave low-molecular-weight kininogen to lysylbradykinin (bradykinin with an additional linked lysine). Presumably, lysylbradykinin undergoes the same degradation pathway as does bradykinin.

FUNCTIONS OF KININS IN DISEASE

The physiologic role of the kinin-generating system is uncertain, and in only a few cases do we understand its role in disease. Free bradykinin and lysylbradykinin have been found in nasal secretions during **rhinitis** and viral nasal inflammation, and it is reasonable to believe that both blood and tissue kallikreins contribute to its presence. It is believed that kinins, via their ability to cause smooth muscle contraction and capillary leakage, contribute to **asthma,** but this is by no means proven. Kinin generation has been found following antigen challenge of human lung fragments passively sensitized with specific IgE antibody, but the exact pathways involved in its generation are still uncertain. It has also been suggested that release of tissue kallikreins and activation of the kinin system is responsible for the severe pain of **pancreatitis** and plays a role in the synovitis of rheumatoid arthritis. The kinin-generating system has been reported to be involved in edema formation in **hereditary angioedema,** because kinins are present in fluid from suction-induced blisters over angioedema areas and because levels of circulating prekallikrein fall during attacks of this disease. Nevertheless, the kinin-forming system has not yet been conclusively proved to be responsible for the attacks of edema in hereditary angioedema.

REFERENCES

GENERAL
Borsos T: *The Molecular Basis of Complement Action.* Appleton-Century-Crofts, 1970.
Frank MM: The complement system. In: *Samter's Immunologic Diseases,* 5th ed. Frank MM et al (editors). Little Brown, 1995, pp. 331–353.

CLASSIC PATHWAY
Cooper NR: The classical complement pathway: Activation and regulation of the first complement component. *Adv Immunol* 1985;**37**:151.
Kerr MA: The second component of human complement. *Methods Enzymol* 1981;**80**:54.

Tack BF: The β-Cys-τ-Glu thioester bond in human C3, C4, and α$_2$-macroglobulin. *Springer Semin Immunopathol* 1983;**6**:259.

Ziccardi RJ: The first component of human complement (C1): Activation and control. *Springer Semin Immunopathol* 1983;**6**:213.

ALTERNATIVE PATHWAY

Pangburn MK, Muller-Eberhard HJ: The alternative pathway of complement. *Springer Semin Immunopathol* 1984;**7**:163.

MEMBRANE ATTACK COMPLEX

Mayer MM et al: Membrane damage by complement. *Crit Rev Immunol* 1981;**2**:133.

Nicholson-Weller A, Halperin JA: Membrane signaling by complement S56–9: The membrane attack complex. *Immunol Res* 1993;**12**:244.

CONTROL MECHANISMS

Frank MM et al: Hereditary angioedema: The clinical syndrome and its management. *Ann Intern Med* 1976;**84**:580.

Ochs HD et al: Regulation of antibody responses: The role of complement and adhesion molecules. *Clin Immunol Immunopathol* 1993;**67**:533.

Zahedi K et al: Structure and regulation of the C1 inhibitor gene. *Behring Inst Mitt* 1993;**93**:115.

GENETIC CONSIDERATIONS

Campbell RD et al: Complement system genes and the structures they encode. *Prog Immunol* 1992;**5**:25.

Perlmutter DH, Colton HR: Complement molecular genetics. In: *Inflammation: Basic Principles and Clinical Correlates,* 2nd ed. Gallin JE et al (editors). Raven Press, 1992, p. 81.

MANNOSE-BINDING PROTEIN

Sommerfield JA et al: Mannose binding protein gene mutations associated with unusual and severe infections in adults. *Lancet* 1995;**345**:886.

Thompson C: Research News: Protein proves to be a key link in innate immunity. *Science* 1995;**269**:301.

BIOLOGIC EFFECTS

Gerard C, Gerard NP: C5a anaphylatoxin and its seven transmembrane segment receptor. *Ann Rev Immunol* 1994;**12**:775.

Goldstein IM: Complement: Biologically active products. In: *Inflammation: Basic Principles and Clinical Correlates,* 2nd ed. Gallin JE et al (editors). Raven Press, 1992, p. 63.

Hugli TE: Biochemistry and biology of anaphylatoxins. *Complement* 1986;**3**:111.

Reid KBM et al: Complement system proteins which interact with C3b or C4b. *Immunol Today* 1986;**7**:230.

CELL MEMBRANE RECEPTORS & REGULATORY MOLECULES

Brown EJ: Complement receptors, adhesion, and phagocytosis. *Infect Agents Dis* 1992;**1**:63.

Fearon DT, Carter RH: The CD19/CR2/TAPA-1 complex of B lymphocytes: Linking natural to acquired immunity. *Ann Rev Immunol* 1995;**13**:127.

Morgan BP, Meri S: Membrane proteins that protect against complement lysis. *Springer Semin Immunopathol* 1994;**15**:369.

Schifferli JA et al: The role of complement and its receptor in the elimination of immune complexes. *N Engl J Med* 1986;**315**:488.

Zalman LS et al: Deficiency of the homologous restriction factor in paroxysmal nocturnal hemoglobinuria. *J Exp Med* 1987;**165**:689.

MOLECULAR MIMICRY

Fishelson Z: Complement related proteins in pathogenic organisms. *Springer Semin Immunopathol* 1994;**15**:345.

KININS

Colman RW: Contact systems in infectious disease. *Rev Infect Dis* 1989;**4**(suppl):689.

Kozin F, Cochrane CH: The contact activation system of plasma: Biochemistry and pathophysiology. In: *Inflammation: Basic Principles and Clinical Correlates,* 2nd ed. Gallin JI et al (editors). Raven Press, 1992, pp. 103–122.

Proud D, Kaplan AP: Kinin formation: Mechanisms and role in inflammatory disorders. *Ann Rev Immunol* 1988;**6**:49.

Wetsel RA: Structure, function, and cellular expressions of complement anaphylatoxin receptors. *Curr Opin Immunol* 1995;**7**:48.

12

Inflammation

Abba I. Terr, MD

The immune response is not limited to interactions of lymphocytes and antigen-presenting cells. In vivo it often is accompanied by additional physiologic manifestations that may involve other cell types, extracellular proteins, or even other organ systems. For example, when an immunogen is injected into the skin, the resulting immune response is frequently accompanied by redness (**erythema), warmth,** and **swelling** at the injection site. These signs reflect changes in blood vessels of the surrounding tissues: arterioles dilate so that local vascular perfusion is increased (producing erythema and warmth), and post-capillary venules become abnormally permeable, allowing vascular fluid to leak into the affected tissues to cause swelling (**edema).** In addition, various types of nucleated blood cells may migrate into the affected site to join in the response, becoming visible under the microscope as a **cellular infiltrate.** When a response occurs at or near a mucosal surface, glandular epithelial cells may dramatically increase their production of mucus or other secretions. If a response is intense and protracted, fibroblasts and endothelial cells at the site may proliferate and form a permanent scar. Additionally, some immune responses are accompanied by local or disseminated blood-clotting and coagulation, by activation of the serum complement or kinin cascades, or by systemic manifestations such as fever.

This multifaceted host reaction that results from and accompanies the "pure" immune response in vivo is termed **inflammation,** or the **inflammatory response.** There are several distinct inflammatory pathways, each of which proceeds via a cascade of biologic events. Many of the individual steps in the inflammatory cascade are controlled by cytokines or other soluble regulatory molecules known as **inflammatory mediators.** A given mediator may not only produce effects directly but may also stimulate production of other mediators that control different aspects of the response. At the same time, other sec-

ondary events may be triggered by antigen–antibody complexes or by products of the activated complement cascade. Thus, each step in the process has the capability to induce subsequent steps, giving rise to an integrated response. The particular pathways and constellation of events that occur during an inflammatory response depend on many factors, including the nature of the inciting stimulus, its portal of entry, and the characteristics of the host. Not all inflammation is immunologically mediated. For example, some foreign substances can directly activate neutrophils and evoke neutrophil-mediated **acute inflammation** without the participation of lymphocytes (see Chapter 2). Even these reactions, however, may be controlled and modulated by the immune system in an immunized host through the opsonizing effect of antibodies.

An inflammatory response can be either beneficial or detrimental to the host. Increases in local vascular perfusion, for example, may have the beneficial effect of enhancing delivery of neutrophils, lymphocytes, and other circulating defensive cells to the site of an immune response. Similarly, leakage of protein-rich edema fluid into the site may help to dilute or inactivate a harmful immunogen, while increased glandular secretion helps flush foreign irritants off an epithelial surface. Localized clotting and coagulation may act to limit dissemination of an antigen through the circulation, and scarring is an integral component of the healing process. Inflammation is detrimental, on the other hand, when it temporarily or permanently injures host tissues and interferes with their normal functions. The terms **allergy** and **hypersensitivity** are used to describe the harmful effects of immunologically mediated inflammatory reactions that are directed against innocuous foreign substances such as dust, pollen, foods, or drugs. The pathogenic consequences of **autoimmune diseases** occur in part because of immunologically mediated inflammation directed against host tissues.

Table 12–1. Inflammatory cells.

Circulating	Tissue-Resident
Lymphocytes	Mast cells
Neutrophils	Macrophages
Eosinophils	
Basophils	
Platelets	

This chapter describes immunologically mediated inflammatory reactions, that is, those mediated either by antigen-specific lymphocytes or by preformed antibodies. The types of accessory cells and mediator substances that participate in these reactions are considered first, and then the characteristics of the reactions themselves are discussed. There are several distinct types of immunologic inflammatory reactions, each of which occurs through a specific mechanism and produces a characteristic pattern of associated phenomena. From a clinical standpoint, it is extremely important to recognize and understand these reaction patterns, since they offer insight into the pathologic processes at work in a given patient and provide clues that can guide the choice of appropriate therapy.

INFLAMMATORY CELLS

Any cell that participates in inflammatory reactions can be called an **inflammatory cell.** The term is thus applicable to many different cell types (Table 12–1). Some are long-term residents of normal tissues; others are circulating cells that enter tissues only in the course of an inflammatory response. Three types of inflammatory cells—neutrophils, macrophages, and lymphocytes—are the principal effector cells of most acute inflammatory or immune reactions and have been considered at length in earlier chapters. This section focuses on the properties of the other inflamma-

tory cell types. Most of these cells express surface receptors for complement components, for the Fc portions of antibody molecules (Table 12–2), and for various cytokines. As a result, their activities tend to be controlled directly or indirectly by ongoing immune responses or by activation of the complement cascade.

Eosinophils

Eosinophils are bone marrow-derived granulocytes whose clinical significance derives from their strong association with **allergic reactions** and with **helminthic parasite infections.** An eosinophil in blood or tissue can be recognized by its bilobed nucleus and by the characteristic eosinophilic granules in its cytoplasm. Human eosinophils are slightly larger than neutrophils, being 12–17 μm in diameter, but they contain substantially fewer specific granules (approximately 200 per cell). Eosinophil granules are spherical or oblong and 0.5 μm in diameter; they can be seen under the electron microscope to contain an electron-dense crystalloid core surrounded by a less dense amorphous matrix (Fig 12–1). The major contents of these granules include an **eosinophil peroxidase** (which is biochemically distinct from the myeloperoxidase of neutrophils but mediates the same reaction; see Chapter 2) and other enzymes that can generate toxic oxygen metabolites, a cytotoxic lysophosphatase called **Charcot-Leyden crystal protein,** and at least three other abundant basic proteins. One of the latter, called the **major basic protein,** has a strong affinity for acidic dyes such as eosin and is responsible for the intense red staining of the granules.

Circulating eosinophils normally make up about 1–3% of peripheral white blood cells. These circulating cells, however, represent only a very small proportion of the total eosinophil population: it is estimated that, for every circulating eosinophil, there are approximately 200 mature eosinophils in the bone marrow and 500 in connective tissues throughout the body. Eosinophil production in the bone marrow is

Table 12–2. Inflammatory cell immunoglobulin Fc receptors.[1]

Receptor[2]	Present on:					
	Neutrophils	Monocytes	Mast Cells	Basophils	Eosinophils	Platelets
IgM	–	–	–	–	–	–
IgG						
IgG1	+	+	–	?	+	+
IgG2	+	+	–	–	?	+
IgG3	+	+	–	–	?	+
IgG4	+	+	–	–	?	+
IgA	+	+	–	–	?	–
IgD	–	–	–	–	+	–
IgE	–	+	+	+	+	+
(FcεRI)	–	–	+	+	–	–
(FcεRII)	–	+	?	?	+	+

[1] Symbols: +, receptor present; –, receptor absent; ?, presence unknown.
[2] Immunoglobulin isotype for which the cell has a receptor.

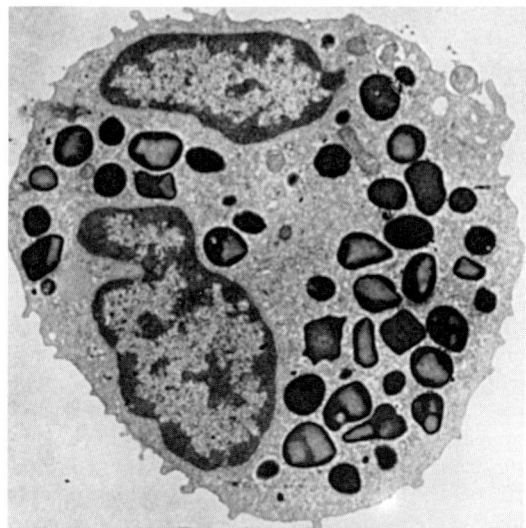

Figure 12–1. Electron micrograph of a mature human eosinophil. The numerous cytoplasmic granules stain darkly owing to the presence of peroxidase and contain characteristic central electron-dense crystalline cores with a surrounding amorphous matrix. The nucleus typically has two lobes. The cell is 15 μm in diameter. (Courtesy of Dorothy F Bainton.)

dependent not only on granulocyte–macrophage colony-stimulating factor (GM-CSF) and interleukin-3 (IL-3), which promote differentiation of all types of granulocytes, but also on **IL-5,** which functions as a specific eosinophil growth factor (see Chapter 10). The life span of an eosinophil is relatively short: it has a marrow maturation time of 2–6 days, a circulating half-life of 6–12 hours, and a connective tissue residence time of only a few days. Increased concentrations of eosinophils **(eosinophilia)** in the blood can occur in several clinical settings but are most commonly encountered in allergic or parasitic diseases; the increase is thought to be mediated by IL-5. Eosinophilia of solid tissues also can occur in these disorders, as a result of chemokines and other mediators released locally by mast cells, macrophages, lymphocytes, and other cells. Intracellular and protozoan parasites do not evoke eosinophilic responses (see Chapter 51).

Eosinophils bear surface immunoglobulin E (IgE) receptors, but these are of the low-affinity **(FcεRII)** type and so are largely unoccupied when the serum IgE concentration is within the normal range. Approximately 10–30% of eosinophils from normal individuals also have low-affinity **(FcγRIII)** or intermediate-affinity **(FcγRII)** IgG receptors (see Table 12–2). In addition, 40–50% display receptors for complement components. These various receptor types enable an eosinophil to recognize and bind to particulate antigens that are coated with IgE, IgG, or complement derivatives, much as a neutrophil or macrophage rec-

ognizes an opsonized particle. Binding, in turn, leads to eosinophil activation, which is characterized by (1) an increase in the number of surface Fc and complement receptors and certain other surface markers, (2) enhanced oxidative metabolism, (3) de novo synthesis and release of the arachidonate derivative leukotriene C_4 (LTC$_4$; see later discussion) and certain other proinflammatory mediators, and (4) increased cytotoxic activity. Activation can also be induced or enhanced by contact with activated endothelial cells, by T-cell-derived lymphokines (GM-CSF, IL-3, and IL-5), or by monokines such as IL-1 and tumor necrosis factor alpha (TNFα).

Activated eosinophils can phagocytose many types of particles in vitro (including bacteria, fungi, mycoplasmas, inert particles, and antigen–antibody complexes), but the evidence that they play a significant role as phagocytes in vivo remains inconclusive. Instead, they appear to act primarily by attaching themselves tightly onto an antibody-coated or complement-coated particle and discharging their granule contents onto its surface through **extracellular degranulation.** This occurs, for example, when eosinophils aggregate around a large tissue parasite, such as *Trichinella, Schistosoma,* or *Fasciola.* The cationic granular proteins may attach themselves to the negatively charged surfaces of these parasites to exert their cytotoxic effects. For example, eosinophil peroxidase tends to attach itself in this manner and so concentrates production of toxic oxygen metabolites onto the target surface. Eosinophils also bind and attack large deposits of antigen–antibody complexes in the tissues (see later discussion). Granular contents released during particularly intense responses can damage host tissues. For example, major basic protein is toxic to respiratory epithelium and is found in elevated concentrations in the sputum and airway secretions of people with asthma. Hexagonal, bipyramidal crystals of granule proteins, called **Charcot-Leyden crystals,** are also found in the sputum of asthmatics; they provide a useful clinical marker for eosinophil-mediated airway reactions.

Mast Cells

Mast cells are marrow-derived, tissue-resident cells that are essential for **IgE-mediated** inflammatory reactions (Table 12–3). Human mast cells are relatively large (10–15 μm in diameter) and heterogeneous in shape but generally are round, oval, or spindle-shaped, and they bear numerous surface projections (Fig 12–2). They possess a single round or oval eccentrically located nucleus. Their most distinctive feature under the light microscope is the presence in each cell of 50–200 densely packed granules that appear to fill the cytoplasm and that exhibit a distinctive purplish **(metachromatic)** coloration in hematoxylin-stained tissue preparations. Each granule is membrane-bounded and 0.1–0.4 μm in diameter; the granules contain relatively large amounts of **histamine,**

Table 12–3. Properties of human mast cells and basophils.

	Mast Cells	Basophils
Cell diameter	10–15 µm	5–7 µm
Nucleus	Bilobed or multi-lobed	Round or oval; eccentric
Cell surface contour	Smooth with occasional short, broad projections	Numerous narrow projections
Predominant localization	Connective tissues	Blood
Life span	Weeks or months	Days
Terminally differentiated	No	Yes
Major granule contents	Histamine, chondroitin sulfate, neutral proteinases, heparin, TNFα	Histamine, chondroitin sulfate, neutral proteinases, major basic protein, Charcot-Leyden protein
Mediators that are synthesized and released after degranulation	TNFα, PAF, LTC$_4$, PGD$_2$, IL-4	LTC$_4$

Abbreviations: TNF = tumor necrosis factor; PAF = platelet-activating factor; LTC$_4$ = leukotriene C$_4$; PGD$_2$ = prostaglandin D$_2$.

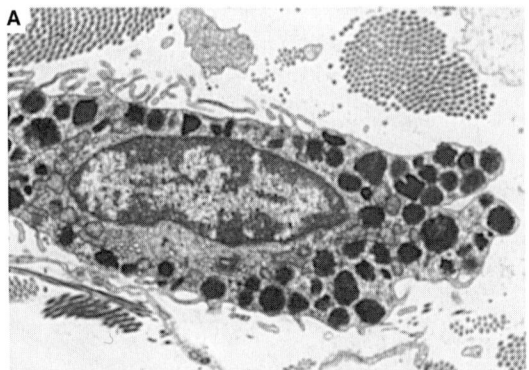

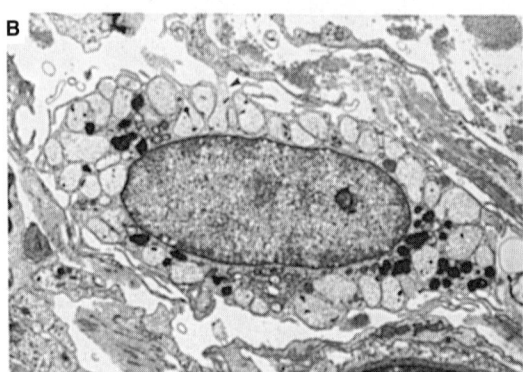

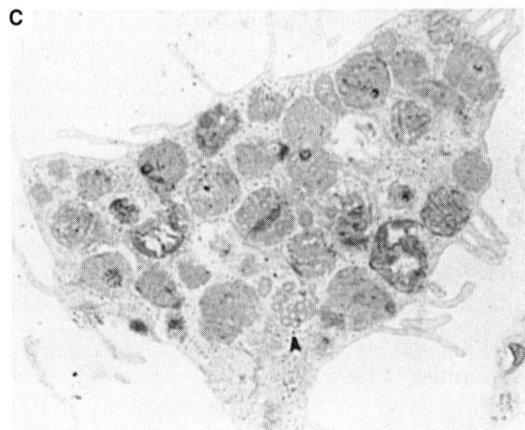

Figure 12–2. Electron micrographs of skin mast cells. *A:* An unstimulated mast cell. (Courtesy of Marc M Friedman.) *B:* A mast cell activated 5 minutes earlier with ragweed antigen. Note the swollen, lucent appearance of the secretory granules. (Courtesy of Marc M Friedman.) *C:* Cytoplasm of an unstimulated mast cell, showing the diverse appearances of the granules, which may contain crystalline, whorled, or granular material. (Courtesy of Karen Oetkon.) Each cell is 10–15 µm in diameter.

heparin, TNFα, and other preformed inflammatory mediators that are described later in this chapter. They also contain superoxide dismutase, peroxidase, and numerous acid hydrolases (such as β-hexosaminidase, β-glucuronidase, and arylsulfatase) that may act to degrade the extracellular matrix. Under the electron microscope, the granules may be seen to contain amorphous electron-dense granular zones as well as highly ordered crystalline arrays (see Fig 12–2).

Mast cells express on their surfaces large numbers of high-affinity Fc receptors for IgE (**FcεRI**). As a result, the surface of each cell is coated with lymphocyte-derived IgE molecules that have been adsorbed from the circulation and serve as receptors for specific antigens. Mast cells are scattered in connective tissues throughout the body but are found in especially large numbers beneath surface tissues such as the skin (which contains 10^4 mast cells/mm^3), lung alveoli (10^6 mast cells/g of tissue), gastrointestinal mucosa, and nasal mucous membranes. They are thus strategically positioned to detect inhaled or ingested antigens. When its surface IgE molecules bind antigens, a mast cell promptly undergoes activation, characterized by granule enlargement, solubilization of the crystalline structures within the granules, and then **degranulation** with release of granule contents into the surrounding tissues. Some of the substances within the granules increase local vascular permeability, smooth muscle contraction, and epithelial mucus secretion, whereas others act as chemotactic factors to attract other inflammatory cells. These regulatory factors are sometimes referred to as **mast cell mediators.** Some of the granular proteinases and other enzymes may have nonspecific effects on an antigen, but otherwise

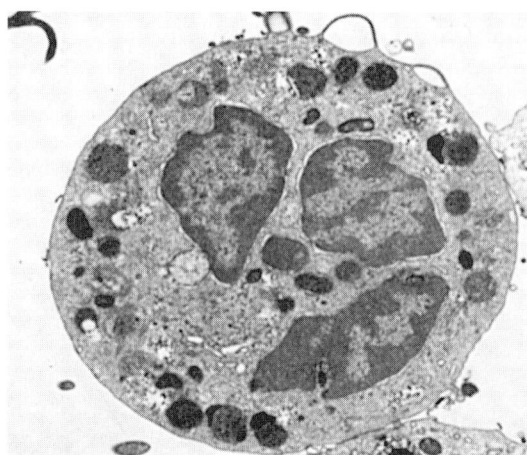

Figure 12–3. Electron micrograph of a peripheral blood basophil. The nucleus is multilobed, and the cytoplasmic surface is smooth with occasional short blunt folds or uropods. The cell is 5–7 μm in diameter. (Courtesy of Marc M Friedman.)

mast cells do not appear to carry out any other significant direct effector activities such as phagocytosis.

Histochemical and biochemical analyses indicate that mast cells at various body sites differ in the relative amounts of two neutral proteinases in their cytoplasmic granules. The two proteinases, called tryptase and chymase, together make up 25–70% of granule protein by weight; their physiologic substrates are undetermined. Most mast cells in the lungs and gastrointestinal mucosa contain only tryptase, whereas the majority in the skin and gastrointestinal submucosa contain both tryptase and chymase. This difference appears to be reversible and depends on factors in the local microenvironment; its functional significance is unknown.

Basophils

Basophils are circulating marrow-derived cells that have many of the same properties as tissue mast cells, although they represent an independent cell lineage. At 5–7 μm in diameter, they are the smallest cells of the granulocyte series and account for no more than 1% of nucleated cells in the marrow or peripheral blood. Like mast cells, basophils bear high-affinity Fc receptors for IgE (approximately 270,000 FcεRI receptors are present on each cell) and contain histamine-rich cytoplasmic granules. These two attributes distinguish mast cells and basophils from all other human cell types. Basophils, however, differ from mast cells morphologically and biochemically in several respects (Fig 12–3; Table 12–3).

Small to moderate numbers of basophils accumulate in tissues in a variety of inflammatory conditions involving the skin (such as late-phase cutaneous allergic

responses, cutaneous basophil hypersensitivity reactions, and lesions of bullous pemphigoid), the small intestine (Crohn's disease), the kidneys (allergic interstitial nephritis, renal allograft rejection), nasal mucosa (allergic rhinitis), and eyes (allergic conjunctivitis). In view of these associations and the many similarities between basophils and mast cells, it is generally presumed that basophils participate in IgE-mediated reactions in a manner analogous to that of mast cells. Nevertheless, the importance of basophils in immunity and hypersensitivity has yet to be proven.

Platelets

Platelets are anucleate cytoplasmic fragments derived from bone marrow megakaryocytes and are the smallest circulating blood cells (2 μm in diameter). They have a 10-day life span in the circulation. Their primary function is in blood-clotting, but they also store and can release mediator substances that have important proinflammatory effects. During clot formation, platelets undergo an **activation** response that causes them to aggregate with one another and also to discharge the contents of the three types of storage granules in their cytoplasm (called dense bodies, α granules, and lysosomal granules, respectively) to the exterior. The released products may include various arachidonate metabolites (prostaglandin G_2 [PGG_2], PGH_2, and thromboxane A_2 [TXA_2]; see later discussion), growth factors, and bioactive amines, as well as neutral and acid hydrolases. Occlusion of a blood vessel by platelet aggregates has the useful effects of entrapping leukocytes and preventing the spread of antigen through the circulation. Platelets express surface Fc receptors for IgG and also low-affinity **(FcεRII)** receptors for IgE. The latter receptor allows platelets to bind and secrete cytotoxic products (probably hydrogen peroxide or other oxygen metabolites) onto IgE-coated tissue parasites but without inducing platelet aggregation or degranulation. Antigen binding through the platelet FcεRII also induces production of **platelet-activating factor (PAF),** a potent inflammatory mediator (see later discussion).

Endothelial Cells

Although not usually classified as inflammatory cells themselves, endothelial cells can participate actively in immune responses by promoting immigration and modulating the responses of circulating inflammatory cells. When endothelial cells are exposed to cytokines (such as IL-1, TNF, or gamma interferon [IFNγ]) or other products released at the site of an ongoing immune response, they may become activated and acquire increased adhesiveness for monocytes, neutrophils, and other circulating cells. Such increased adhesiveness is important in attracting leukocytes into the involved tissue (see Chapter 2). Activated endothelial cells sometimes express class II major histocompatibility complex (MHC) proteins (and so may function as antigen-presenting cells) and

Table 12–4. Some major inflammatory mediators.[1]

Vasoactive and smooth muscle-constricting mediators
Histamine
Arachidonate metabolites (PGD_2, LTC_4, LTD_4, TXE_4)
PAF
Adenosine

Chemotactic factors
Chemokines
PAF
Complement components, especially C5a
Arachidonate metabolites (LTB_4)

Enzymatic mediators
Tryptase, others

Proteoglycan mediators
Heparin

Abbreviations: PGD_2 = prostaglandin D_2; LT = leukotrienes; TXE_4 = thromboxane E_4; PAF = platelet-activating factor.
[1] The limited selection represented here omits many proinflammatory cytokines (see Chapter 10) and other mediators.

can also secrete the cytokines IL-1 and GM-CSF, which modulate immune responses.

MEDIATORS OF INFLAMMATION

Inflammatory mediators are host-derived compounds that are secreted by activated cells and serve to trigger or enhance specific aspects of inflammation. Such compounds are said to be **proinflammatory;** meaning that they promote inflammation. Many of the **cytokines** act as inflammatory mediators, as detailed in Chapter 10. This section describes some of the other major mediators (Table 12–4), classifying them somewhat arbitrarily into four groups: (1) those with vasoactive and smooth muscle-constricting properties, (2) those that attract other cells and are termed chemotactic factors, (3) enzymes, and (4) proteoglycans. These categories are not mutually exclusive, and several mediators can be assigned to more than one group.

1. VASOACTIVE & SMOOTH MUSCLE-CONSTRICTING MEDIATORS

Histamine

Histamine (Fig 12–4) is an inflammatory mediator that is found preformed in the granules of mast cells and basophils. It is synthesized within these granules by the action of histidine decarboxylase on the amino acid histidine and may make up as much as 10% of granule contents by weight. Histamine is bound through ionic linkages to proteoglycans and proteins within the granules and is bound particularly tightly to mast cell heparin; however, it dissociates from these ligands when released to the extracellular space by degranulation. Histamine exerts its physiologic effects by interacting with any of three different target cell receptors, designated H1, H2, and H3. The receptors are

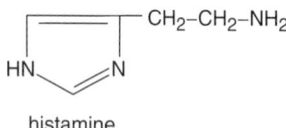

histamine

Figure 12–4. Chemical structure of histamine.

expressed in a tissue-specific manner and each produces characteristic effects (Table 12–5). Major effects mediated by the **H1 receptor** include contraction of bronchial, intestinal, and uterine smooth muscles and augmentation of vascular permeability in postcapillary venules. **Antihistamine** drugs used to treat allergies act by selectively blocking H1 receptor binding. In contrast, binding of **H2 receptors** augments gastric acid and airway mucus secretion and can be inhibited by such compounds as cimetidine and ranitidine, which are useful for treating peptic ulcer disease. **H3 receptor** binding principally affects histamine synthesis and release.

Arachidonic Acid Metabolites

The prostaglandins and leukotrienes are metabolites produced by enzymatic cyclooxygenation and lipoxygenation, respectively, of arachidonic acid (Fig 12–5). They constitute two major families of inflammatory mediators, whose members exhibit diverse vasoactive, smooth muscle-constricting, and chemotactic properties. Many **nonsteroidal anti-inflammatory drugs,** such as **aspirin,** act primarily by blocking the synthesis of prostaglandins. Inhibitors of leukotrienes that are sufficiently selective for clinical use have recently been developed and shown in clinical trials to be effective in treating asthma.

Arachidonic acid is a 20-carbon fatty acid containing four double bonds (Fig 12–6). It can be liberated from membrane phospholipids either through the sequential action of phospholipase C and diacylglycerol lipase, or by the direct action of phospholipase

Table 12–5. Histamine receptors.

Receptor	Histamine Actions
H1	Increased postcapillary venular permeability Smooth muscle contraction Pulmonary vasoconstriction Increased cGMP levels in cells Enhanced mucus secretion Leukocyte chemokinesis Prostaglandin production in lungs
H2	Enhanced gastric acid secretion Enhanced mucus secretion Increased cAMP levels in cells Leukocyte chemokinesis Activation of suppressor T cells
H3	Histamine release inhibition Histamine synthesis inhibition

Abbreviations: cGMP = cyclic guanosine monophosphate; cAMP = cyclic adenosine monophosphate.

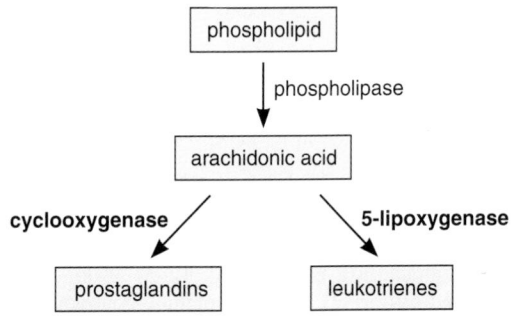

Figure 12–5. Major pathways of arachidonic acid formation and metabolism.

A_2, on membrane phospholipids. Once liberated, arachidonic acid can be metabolized by either the cyclooxygenase or lipoxygenase pathway. Each of these pathways can give rise to many alternative products (see Fig 12–6), each with its own spectrum of effects, and any of these metabolites may be produced by many different cell types in response to various stimuli. A complete discussion of the arachidonate metabolites is beyond the scope of this text, which instead considers only a few representative mediators of this class that are involved in inflammation.

A. Cyclooxygenase Products: The main product of the cyclooxygenase pathway in connective tissue mast cells is **prostaglandin D2** (PGD_2). This mediator promotes local vascular dilatation and vascular permeability (although to a lesser extent than does histamine) and also is a chemoattractant for neutrophils. PGD_2 is thought to have a role, along with histamine, in mediating **wheal-and-flare** reactions in IgE-mediated allergic responses and may be responsible for the systemic flushing and hypotensive episodes that occur in patients with systemic mastocytosis. Basophils do not generate cyclooxygenase products.

B. Lipoxygenase Products: The four principal products of the **lipoxygenase** pathway are the leukotrienes: LTB_4, LTC_4, LTD_4, and LTE_4 (see Fig 12–6). These are the principal arachidonate metabolites released by mucosal mast cells. LTB_4 is a potent chemoattractant (see later discussion). LTC_4, LTD_4, and LTE_4 collectively make up what was once termed "slow-reacting substance of anaphylaxis": they induce smooth muscle contraction, bronchoconstriction, and mucus secretion in the airways and the wheal-and-flare reaction in the skin. When injected intravenously, the last two compounds can cause hypotension and cardiac dysrhythmias. The leukotrienes are several hundred-fold more potent on a molar basis than is histamine and are therefore believed to have an important role in the genesis of allergic disorders.

Platelet-Activating Factor

PAF is a lipophilic organic mediator (Fig 12–7) that is released from activated mast cells and platelets and can also be produced by other activated cell types. It was originally named because of its ability to activate platelets, but it has since been found to have many other proinflammatory effects, including the ability to cause activation and degranulation of neutrophils and eosinophils, to activate complement, and to induce synthesis of prostaglandins and LTC_4. By stimulating the production of collagenases and other metalloproteinases that degrade the extracellular matrix, PAF is thought to promote cartilage destruction in inflammatory arthritis. It is also the most potent eosinophil chemoattractant known. When injected into the skin, PAF causes a wheal-and-flare response and leukocyte infiltration. When inhaled, it causes acute bronchoconstriction, an eosinophilic infiltrate, and a state of nonspecific bronchial hyperreactivity that may persist for days or weeks following a single administration. Injected intravenously, it can cause widespread activation of neutrophils, platelets, and basophils, as well as profound hypotension.

The bioactive form of PAF, depicted in Figure 12–7, consists of a glycerol backbone linked to three substituents: (1) a long-chain alcohol, usually of 16–18 carbons; (2) an acetyl group; and (3) a phosphorylcholine moiety. Platelets and other cells normally store an inactive form of PAF that contains arachidonate at position 2; when a cell becomes activated, the arachidonate is excised by phospholipase A_2 and replaced by acetate to produce the active compound. Once outside the cell, PAF is rapidly degraded by plasma- and cell-associated hydrolases, which remove the acetyl group. Some inhibitors of PAF are currently being tested for therapeutic use, but none is yet available clinically.

Adenosine

The nucleoside adenosine (Fig 12–8) is liberated from degranulating mast cells and can then bind to surface adenosine receptors on many cell types. Its effects include bronchoconstriction and the induction of fluid secretion from intestinal epithelial cells. Blood adenosine concentrations may rise during acute asthmatic episodes.

2. CHEMOTACTIC MEDIATORS

Among the most important chemotactic mediators are the peptides that make up the **chemokine** family of cytokines, which are considered in detail in Chapter 10. Certain complement components, notably **C5a**, are also potent chemoattractants (see Chapter 11). In addition, several nonpeptide inflammatory mediators have been found to have significant chemoattractant activity. These include PAF and LTB_4 (see previous discussion), which, together with C5a, are potent neutrophil chemoattractants that are active at concentrations as low as 10^{-10} M. PAF also has strong chemoattractant effects on eosinophils.

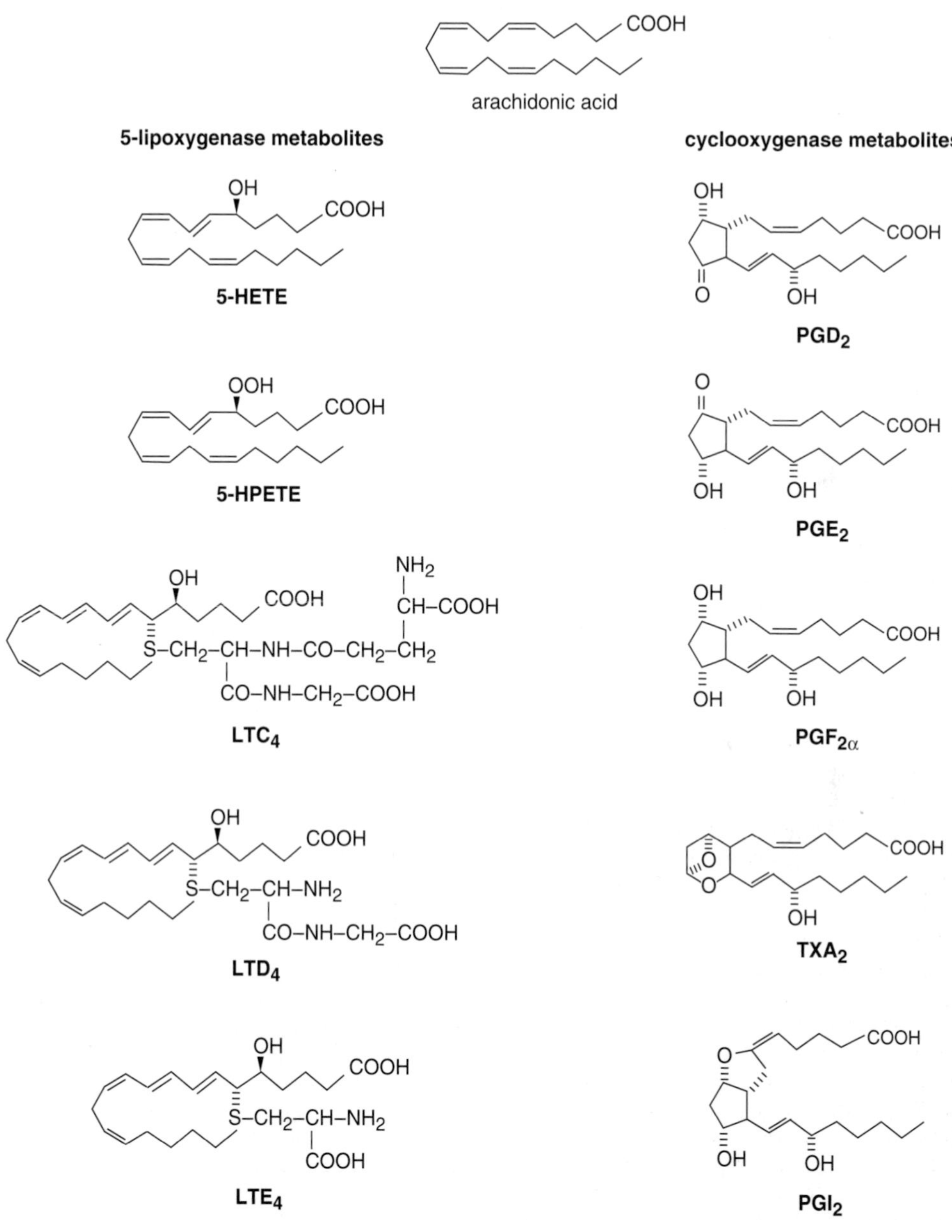

Figure 12–6. Chemical structures of arachidonic acid and of some principal 5-lipoxygenase and cyclooxygenase metabolites. Each of the compounds depicted is a physiologically active inflammatory mediator. *Abbreviations:* 5-HETE = 5-hydroxyeicotetraraenoic acid; 5-HPETE = 5-hydroperoxyeicotetraraenoic acid; LT = leukotrienes; PG = prostaglandins; TX = thromboxane.

3. ENZYMATIC MEDIATORS

A panoply of enzymes can be found in the storage granules of inflammatory cells and can be released to the exterior on degranulation. In addition to their effects on antigens and host tissues, a few of these can act to initiate the complement, clotting, or kinin cascade. For example, mast cell tryptase can cleave complement factor C3 to generate C3a, and it also acts on many clotting proteins. Other mast cell proteinases can proteolytically activate kallikrein or kininogen (see Chapter 11).

4. PROTEOGLYCANS

Mast cell and basophil granules are rich in protein–polysaccharide complexes called proteoglycans, which form much of the structural matrix of these granules and also serve as binding sites for heparin

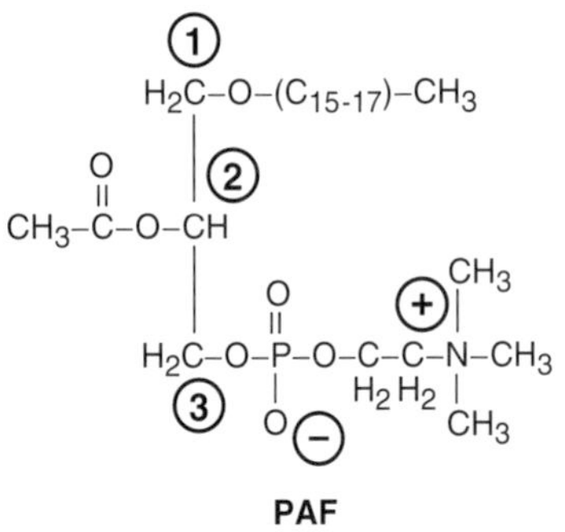

PAF

Figure 12–7. Chemical structure of the secreted, bioactive form of platelet-activating factor (PAF).

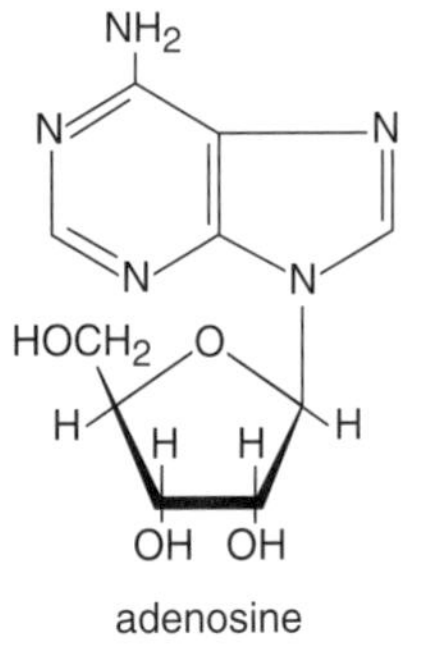

adenosine

Figure 12–8. Chemical structure of adenosine.

and other mediators. These may be the primary functions of the chondroitin sulfate that is present in such granules. Other proteoglycans, however, also have intrinsic regulatory activity. For example, the major granular proteoglycan in human mast cells is heparin (MW 60,000), which has anticoagulant activity and also is capable of modulating tryptase activity (see previous discussion). Each human mast cell contains about 5 pg of heparin.

TYPES OF IMMUNOLOGICALLY MEDIATED INFLAMMATORY RESPONSES

Much of what is now known about inflammatory reactions in humans was derived from use of the **skin test**—a procedure in which a small amount of a purified antigen is injected beneath the skin and the response to the injection is then observed. Skin testing is widely used in clinical practice to assess whether patients are hypersensitive to particular antigens. It is also very useful experimentally for studying the mechanisms of immune reactions: for example, biopsies of test sites can be performed to examine the cellular infiltrates induced by an antigen, and fluids extracted from the sites can be assayed for inflammatory mediators.

More than a century of experience with skin testing in humans has revealed at least four distinct patterns of immunologically mediated inflammatory reactions (Table 12–6). Under the somewhat artificial conditions of the skin test, a single pure antigen may induce exclusively one type of reaction in a given patient. By contrast, responses against the more complex, multicomponent antigens encountered in nature often include two or more of these patterns simultaneously. Thus, these reaction patterns are not mutually exclusive but, rather, serve to highlight the major integrated pathways by which humans respond to foreign substances.

Cell-Mediated Immunity

Cell-mediated immunity (CMI) is the term applied to defensive reactions that are mediated primarily by activated T lymphocytes and macrophages. Reactions of this type are very common. They occur through the sequence of events outlined in Chapter 4, in which contact with antigen leads to activation, proliferation, and differentiation of T cells that have the appropriate specificities. Owing to the time required for these events to take place and for significant numbers of cells to be recruited into the response, CMI reactions develop rather slowly. Even in a highly immunized host, CMI responses exhibit a relatively long lag phase and do not achieve their maximal intensity until approximately 36 hours after exposure to the antigen. Consequently, CMI responses are also called **delayed-type hypersensitivity (DTH)** reactions.

The evolution of a DTH reaction is schematized in Figure 12–9. The reaction is initiated by activation of an antigen-specific T_H cell, which then releases numerous immunoregulatory and proinflammatory lymphokines and other substances into the surrounding tissues. These compounds, together with bioactive substances released by the antigen-presenting cell, promote clonal expansion of the responsive T_H cell and serve to attract additional inflammatory cells from the circulation. The chemoattracted cells may include antigen-specific and nonspecific T or B lymphocytes, as well as monocytes, neutrophils, eosinophils, and basophils. Some of the cytokines promote differentiation and activation of macrophages and so enhance the phagocytic, bactericidal, and antigen-presenting functions of these cells. These activated macrophages, in turn, secrete other cytokines including IL-12, which promotes differentiation of the T_H cells toward a T_H1 phenotype, so that eventually the effects of T_H1-derived cytokines come to predominate (see Chapter 9). Local blood vessels are induced to dilate, which further enhances immigration of cells from the bloodstream. The coagulation–kinin systems also become activated, so that fibrin is formed and deposited at the

Table 12–6. Classes of immunologically mediated inflammation.

Type of Inflammation	Skin Test Terminology	Time to Maximal Reaction (hours)	Predominant Cellular Infiltrate	Principal Mediators	Principal Mechanism Inducing the Inflammatory Response
Cell-mediated (CMI)	Delayed (DTH)	36	Lymphocytes, macrophages	Lymphokines	Lymphokines released from activated T_H1 cells induce primarily macrophage and T-cell responses.
Immune complex-mediated	Late	8	Neutrophils	Complement factor C5a	Immune complexes fix complement, inducing neutrophil reaction.
IgE-mediated Immediate phase	Immediate	0.25	Eosinophils	Histamine, leukotrienes	Antigen binding to surface IgE leads to mast cell degranulation, with release of stored mediators.
Late phase	Late	6	Eosinophils, neutrophils	PAF, TNFα, PGD_2, IL-4, leukotrienes	Mediators synthesized and released by mast cells after degranulation.
Cutaneous basophil hypersensitivity	Delayed	36	Basophils	Unknown	Unknown

Abbreviations: CMI = cell-mediated immunity; DTH = delayed-type hypersensitivity; PAF = platelet-activating factor; TNF = tumor necrosis factor; PGD_2 = prostaglandin D_2; IL-4 = interleukin-4; IgE = immunoglobulin E.

site. Fibrin deposition is probably important in confining the inflammatory reaction to a discrete location and imparts a firm consistency **(induration)** that is characteristic of tissues undergoing DTH reactions.

Viewed under the light microscope, the site of an ongoing DTH reaction can be seen to contain a tissue infiltrate composed mainly of lymphocytes and macrophages, along with variable numbers of plasma cells and other inflammatory cells. This is sometimes referred to as a **chronic inflammatory infiltrate** to indicate the relatively long time (several days or more) needed for its development and to distinguish it from acute inflammatory infiltrates, which are composed primarily of neutrophils (see Chapter 2).

Certain types of antigens induce CMI with an especially pronounced macrophage response, leading to the formation of granulomas (see Chapter 2). Such **granulomatous inflammation** is therefore a subtype of CMI. It develops most commonly in response to particulate antigens that are large, insoluble, and resistant to elimination. These include foreign bodies (such as suture material; silica; talc; or mineral oil); fungi; metazoan parasites; or mycobacteria, such as *Mycobacterium tuberculosis* or *M leprae.*

CMI reactions are encountered in many clinical settings, including numerous infectious diseases and certain types of vaccination sites, or following contact of many different types of chemicals with the skin or mucous membranes. CMI is also a major mechanism of allograft rejection and graft-versus-host disease and plays a role in some autoimmune disorders and in tumor immunity. Cytotoxic T-cell reactions against

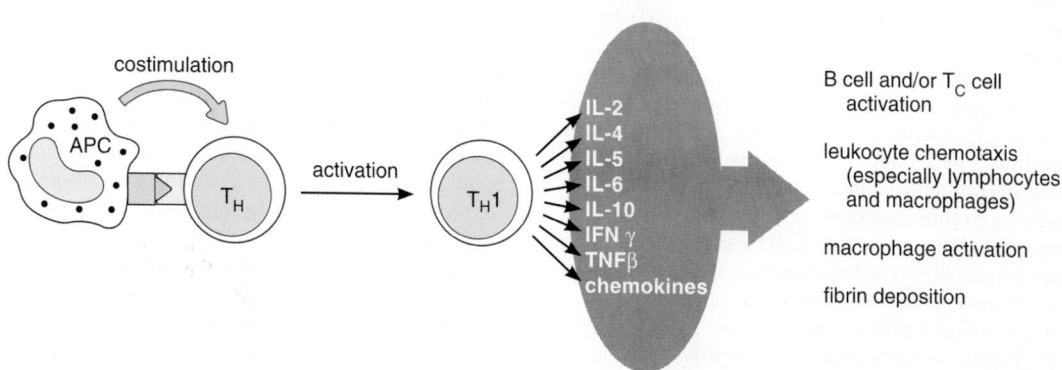

Figure 12–9. Schematic depiction of the immunologic events that give rise to a cell-mediated inflammatory response.

virus-infected host cells are another example of this type of response. Indeed, immunity to infection by any type of intracellular pathogen is mediated by CMI; the types of organisms that provoke this type of immunity include viruses; fungi; protozoa; helminthic parasites; and some bacteria, such as *Chlamydia.*

Hypersensitivity diseases mediated by DTH are discussed in Chapter 30. The most common disease in this category is **allergic contact dermatitis.** In this disease, the sensitizing agents are usually haptens that form antigenic complexes when they bind to host proteins in the skin and are then processed and presented by Langerhans' cells. Examples of common substances that act in this manner are pentadecyl catechol (the active immunogen in the oil of **poison ivy**) and **nickel** found in jewelry.

Despite their potential protective effects, prolonged or intense CMI reactions can lead to permanent injury to host tissues. Perhaps for this reason, active feedback inhibition mechanisms exist that limit the intensity of CMI reactions. The mechanisms involved in this inhibition are unknown but appear to be antigenically nonspecific. Thus, persons with severe or widespread diseases that induce CMI are sometimes found to have reduced or absent cellular immunity to various unrelated antigens. This state of generalized, nonspecific depression of cellular immunity is called **anergy.** It is usually defined clinically as the absence of DTH skin test reactivity to commonly encountered antigens or loss of a previously positive DTH skin test. Anergy may occur in individuals with extensive granulomatous disorders such as miliary tuberculosis, severe coccidioidomycosis, lepromatous leprosy, or sarcoidosis. It also occurs in Hodgkin's disease. A temporary loss of CMI can occur during the acute phase of certain viral infections such as measles. Not surprisingly, CMI is also impaired in the various congenital forms of cellular immunodeficiency and in the acquired immune deficiency syndrome (AIDS).

Immune Complex-Mediated Inflammation

Immune complex-mediated inflammation refers to the inflammatory responses that occur when an antibody binds to antigen and activates the complement cascade. Reactions of this type do not require the active participation of the lymphocytes that originally generated the antibody. Thus, they can occur relatively rapidly in an immunized host who has preformed circulating antibodies of the appropriate specificity (see Table 12–6). There are two classic types of immune complex-mediated reactions—the localized **Arthus reaction,** and systemic **serum sickness**—but their underlying mechanisms are similar. Each occurs through the sequence of immune complex formation and deposition, complement activation, and cellular infiltration.

A. Immune-Complex Formation: The classic complement pathway is activated when antibody molecules of an appropriate class bind to an antigen in a spatial conformation that allows subsequent binding of complement component C1 (see Chapter 11). For this to occur, the chemical nature of the antigen is generally less important than the number and types of antibody molecules it binds. IgM antibodies, or IgG antibodies of any subclass except IgG4, can activate the classic pathway, whereas IgA, IgE, and IgD cannot. As few as one IgM or two IgG molecules can suffice to activate (or "fix") complement when bound to the surface of a particulate antigen, such as a bacterium or a virus-infected host cell.

By contrast, soluble molecular antigens generally fix complement only after they have been incorporated into larger, multimeric **antigen–antibody complexes.** Such complexes (also called **immune complexes**) form because each immunoglobulin four-chain unit contains two independent and identical antigen-binding sites and can therefore bind to two antigen molecules simultaneously. Thus, when soluble antigen and antibody molecules are present in an appropriate molar ratio, they can cross-link one another to form a multimolecular lattice, as depicted in Figure 12–10. Because they contain numerous antibody molecules, immune complexes are often highly efficient at activating complement.

B. Complex Deposition: The physical properties of immune complexes are strongly influenced by the molar ratios of the molecules they contain (see Chapter 14). Complexes formed with a substantial excess of either antigen or antibody are small and relatively soluble, whereas those formed at near-stoichiometric equivalence are larger and have a tendency to precipitate out of solution (the so-called **precipitin reaction**). Large, insoluble complexes of the latter type can form in the circulation when a large amount of antigen is introduced into the bloodstream of an immunized person. The complexes then tend to be deposited in tissues throughout the body, particularly in the internal elastic lamina of arteries and in perivascular regions. They also tend to become trapped as the serum is filtered through renal glomeruli, and so they accumulate within the basement membranes of glomerular capillaries. Thus, massive systemic antigen exposure can lead to the widespread deposition of complement-fixing immune complexes. This is the pathogenic mechanism of **serum sickness.**

Alternatively, high concentrations of antigen–antibody complexes can form at a discrete site where antigen is present in a solid tissue. This can occur, for example, when an antigen is injected into the dermis of an immunized person. The resulting complexes precipitate as focal deposits in the blood vessels and fix complement, producing a localized inflammatory response that is called the **Arthus reaction.**

C. Complement Activation and Cellular Infiltration: The principal inflammatory factor derived from the complement cascade appears to be C5a, which is a powerful chemoattractant for neutrophils. When immune complexes in and around a

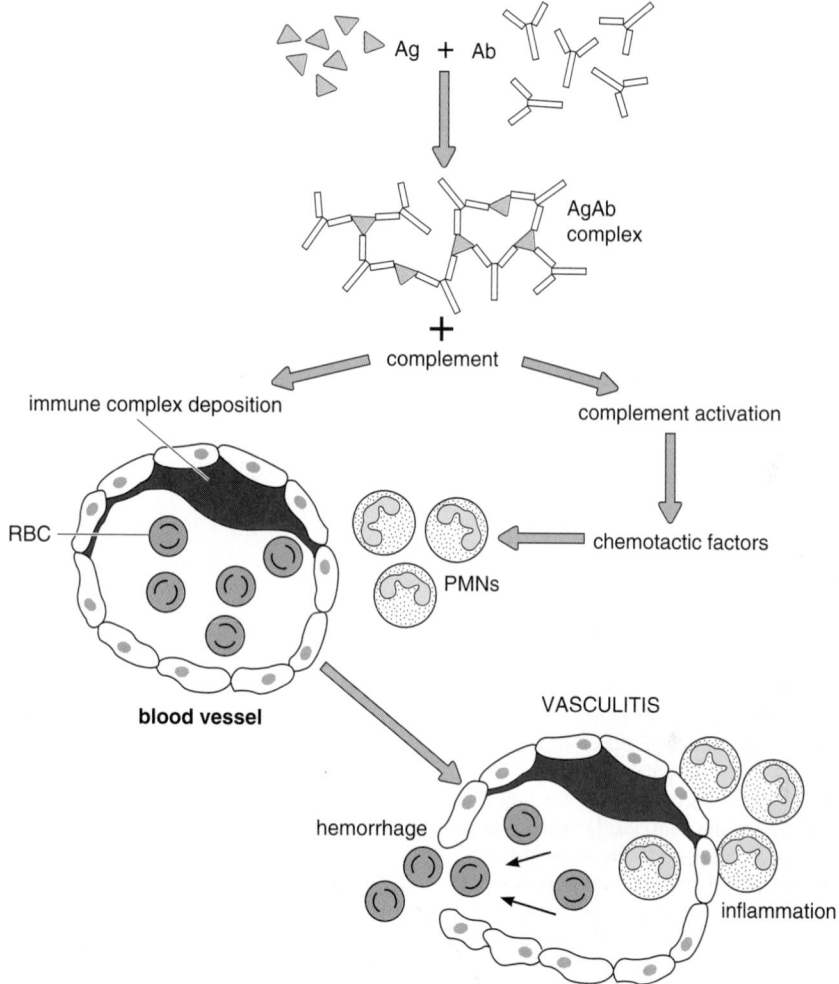

Figure 12–10. Schematic depiction of the immunologic events in immune complex-mediated inflammation. Ag = antigen; Ab = antibody; RBC = red blood cell; PMN = polymorphonuclear leukocyte.

blood vessel wall fix complement, C5a is released and stimulates neutrophilic infiltration (ie, acute inflammation) of the vessel. The resulting **vasculitis** has several components (see Fig 12–10). Neutrophils release lysosomal enzymes and toxic oxygen metabolites while phagocytosing the immune complexes, and these cause destruction of the vessel wall with associated microhemorrhages into the tissues. Endothelial cells swell and proliferate, platelets aggregate in the lumen, and fibrin is deposited in and around the vessel owing to activation of the coagulation cascade. Later in the progression of the injury, macrophages and lymphocytes also infiltrate the area, although the precise factors that attract them have not been determined. One possibility, suggested by recent research, is that antigen–antibody complexes deposited in a tissue can be recognized directly by local mast cells or other resident cells that express low-affinity Fc receptors and so might provoke the secretion of

chemokines or other mediators that attract inflammatory cells.

Clinical Manifestations

As is true of all other types of inflammation, immune complex-mediated reactions can be beneficial, detrimental, or both. This type of inflammation often occurs in concert with other antibody-mediated phenomena (such as opsonization) during normal immune responses. In addition, it is the primary mechanism underlying several types of hypersensitivity. The Arthus reaction, for example, can frequently be observed at inoculation sites in persons who receive subcutaneous antigen injections as a treatment for allergy, and it also occurs occasionally as a response to insect bites or injected medications. These reactions are generally limited to mild edema and cellular infiltration, with little or no vascular destruction. More severe Arthus reactions also occur in two autoimmune disorders—autoimmune thyroiditis and Goodpasture's syndrome—in which the action of antithyroglobulin antibodies and antiglomerular basement membrane antibodies, respectively, can lead to destruction of the involved tissues.

Serum sickness is a systemic vasculitis of variable severity that is characterized clinically by fever, lymphadenopathy, arthralgias, and dermatitis. It once occurred commonly in persons receiving intravenous injections of large quantities of foreign immune serum—a widely used treatment for various infectious or toxic diseases prior to the antibiotic era. Today, it occurs occasionally among transplant patients who receive heterologous serum as a source of antilymphocyte or antithymocyte antibodies to suppress transplant rejection. Serum sickness also can occur as an allergic reaction to penicillin or other drugs or during the prodromal phase of some viral infections, most notably viral hepatitis.

A chronic form of serum sickness can be induced in animals by repeated intravenous infusions of antigen. Depending on the specific animal, antigen, and dosage regimen used, this can result in widespread vasculitis, glomerulonephritis, pulmonary alveolitis, or other lesions. This has been proposed as an experimental model for the immunopathogenesis of the human disorders systemic lupus erythematosus, rheumatoid arthritis, polyarteritis nodosa, and other diseases of unknown etiology that are characterized by the presence of circulating immune complexes and by vasculitis. The serum sickness model, however, does not fully mimic the pathologic and clinical manifestations of these disorders, and the antigens responsible for vasculitis in the human diseases remain unknown.

The presence of circulating immune complexes does not always indicate disease. In fact, small quantities of immune complexes can be found in the serum of normal persons. The antigens responsible for these complexes are not all known, although at least some are antigens from ingested foods. The remainder may be other environmental antigens or autoantigens. Most such complexes are promptly eliminated through phagocytosis by splenic macrophages and other cells, whose surface Fc and complement receptors enable them to bind the IgG and C3 proteins present in these complexes. Immune complex disease thus appears to require (1) large amounts of antigen; (2) generation of immune complexes large enough to activate complement; and (3) in some cases, impaired function of the phagocyte system, possibly because of abnormalities in the Fc or complement receptors.

IgE-Mediated Inflammation

IgE-mediated inflammation occurs when antigen binds to the IgE antibodies that occupy the FcεRI receptor on mast cells. Within minutes, this binding causes the mast cell to degranulate, releasing certain preformed mediators. Subsequently, the degranulated cell begins to synthesize and release additional mediators de novo. The result is a two-phase response: an

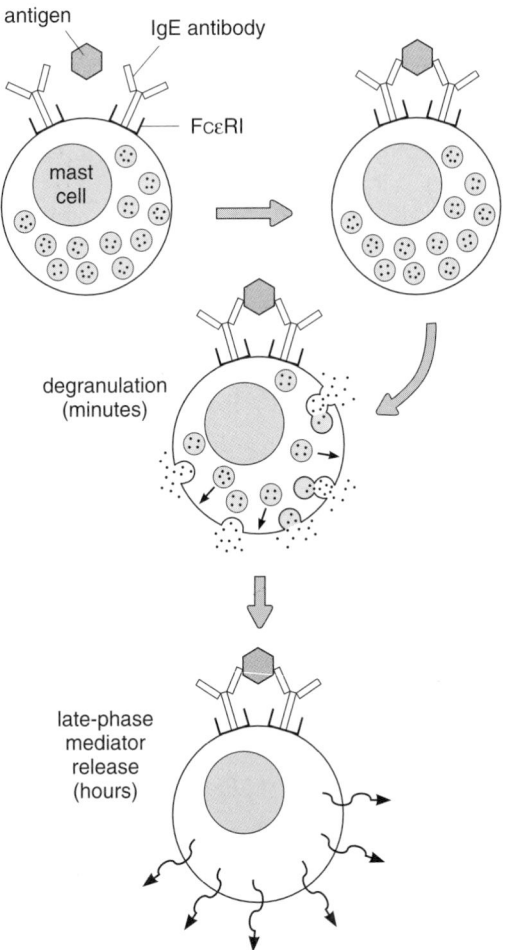

Figure 12–11. Schematic depiction of the immunologic events in an IgE-mediated inflammatory response.

initial immediate effect on blood vessels, smooth muscle, and glandular secretion, followed a few hours later by cellular infiltration of the involved site. This type of inflammatory reaction is commonly referred to as **immediate hypersensitivity.**

As just mentioned, IgE antibodies bind to mast cells via the numerous high-affinity Fcε receptors on the surface of each cell. The binding is noncovalent and reversible, so that the bound antibodies are in constant equilibrium with the pool of circulating IgE. As a result, each mast cell can bind many different antigens. The events that occur on binding are depicted in Figure 12–11. The response is initiated when a multivalent antigen binds and cross-links two or more IgE antibodies occupying FcεRI receptors. This cross-linking transmits a signal that activates the mast cell, resulting in activation of protein tyrosine kinases and increases in intracellular free calcium levels. These signaling events are complete within 2–3 minutes after antigen binding. Soon thereafter, cytoplasmic granules fuse with one another and with the surface membrane, discharging their contents to the exterior. Basophils are the only other cell type that express FcεRI receptors, but it is not known whether they contribute significantly to immediate hypersensitivity reactions.

The **immediate phase** of the inflammatory response is due mainly to preformed mediators (especially **histamine**) that are stored in the mast cell granules, and also to certain rapidly synthesized arachidonate derivatives. It reaches maximal intensity within about 15 minutes after antigen contact. This phase is characterized grossly by erythema, localized edema in the form of a wheal, and **pruritus** (itching), all of which can be attributed to histamine. Microscopic examination at this stage reveals only vasodilation and edema. The granule contents, however, also induce local expression of the vascular addressin VCAM-1 (see Chapter 2), as well as secretion of RANTES and other chemokines (see Chapter 10), which promote subsequent recruitment of inflammatory cells to the site. Manifestations of the **late phase** are due in part to presynthesized TNFα and in part to other mediators (principally PAF, IL-4, and various arachidonate metabolites) whose synthesis begins after the mast cell degranulates. The effects of these mediators become apparent about 6 hours after antigen contact and are marked by an infiltrate of eosinophils and neutrophils. Clinical features of the late phase include erythema, induration, warmth, pruritus, and a burning sensation at the affected site. Fibrin deposition probably occurs transiently, but there is no evidence of significant immunoglobulin or complement deposition. Mast cell-derived IL-4 promotes the pro-

duction of T_H2 cells (see Chapter 9). TNFα not only functions in the short term as a leukocyte chemoattractant but also can stimulate local angiogenesis, fibroblast proliferation, and scar formation during prolonged hypersensitivity reactions.

IgE-mediated inflammation is the mechanism underlying **atopic allergy** (such as hay fever, asthma, and atopic dermatitis), systemic **anaphylactic reactions,** and allergic **urticaria** (hives). It is also at least partially responsible for immunity to helminthic parasites. It may normally play a facilitative role as a first line of immunologic defense, since it causes rapid vasodilation and thus facilitates the entry of circulating soluble factors and cells to the site of antigen contact. Many serious sequelae of allergic disease can be ascribed to the actions of the chemoattracted leukocytes rather than to the mast cells themselves.

Cutaneous Basophil Hypersensitivity

The physiologic significance of cutaneous basophil hypersensitivity (previously called Jones-Mote hypersensitivity) is presently unknown. It is elicited by protein antigens that, when injected into the skin, produce a localized area of swelling that develops over the same time course as a DTH reaction but which is softer than a typical DTH lesion and is pruritic. Viewed under the microscope, the lesions reveal a prominent infiltrate of basophils but no granulomas or other features of DTH. Lesions of this type appear to be antibody-mediated, but their mechanism of formation is uncertain. Basophilic infiltrates are sometimes seen in renal allografts, suggesting that the process may be one component of transplant rejection.

REFERENCES

Barnett EV: Circulating immune complexes: Their biologic and clinical significance. *J Allergy Clin Immunol* 1986;**78**:1089.

Beer DJ, Rocklin RE: Histamine modulation of lymphocyte biology: Membrane receptors, signal transmission, and functions. *Crit Rev Immunol* 1987;**7**:55.

Braquet P, Rola-Pleszczynski M: Platelet-activating factor and cellular immune responses. *Immunol Today* 1987;**8**:345.

Dahlen B, Dahlen SE: Leukotrienes as mediators of airway obstruction and inflammation in asthma. *Clin Exp Allergy* 1994;**25**(suppl)2:50.

Erffmeyer JE: Serum sickness. *Ann Allergy* 1986;**56**:105.

Galli SJ: New concepts about the mast cell. *N Engl J Med* 1993;**328**:257.

Kinet JP: The high-affinity receptor for IgE. *Curr Opin Immunol* 1989;**2**:499.

Parker CW: Lipid mediators produced through the lipoxygenase pathway. *Ann Rev Immunol* 1987;**5**:65.

Samuelsson B et al: Leukotrienes and lipoxins: Structures, biosynthesis, and biological effects. *Science* 1987;**237**:1171.

Serafin WE, Austen KF: Current concepts: Mediation of immediate hypersensitivity reactions. *N Engl J Med* 1987;**317**:30.

Spencer DA: An update on PAF. *Clin Exp Allergy* 1992;**23**:521.

Stevens RL, Austen KF: Recent advances in the cellular and molecular biology of mast cells. *Immunol Today* 1989;**10**:381.

Valent P, Bettelheim P: The human basophil. *Crit Rev Oncol Hematol* 1990;**10**:327.

Wardlaw AJ et al: Eosinophils: Biology and role in disease. *Adv Immunol* 1995;**60**:151.

Weller PF: The immunobiology of eosinophils. *N Engl J Med* 1991;**324**:1110.

13

The Mucosal Immune System

Warren Strober, MD, & Ivan J. Fuss, MD

The mucosal immune system is composed of the lymphoid tissues that are associated with the mucosal surfaces of the gastrointestinal, respiratory, and urogenital tracts. It has evolved within an antigenic environment quite distinct from that existing in the interior of the body and is thus characterized by a number of features that differentiate it from the systemic lymphoid system. These consist of a mucosa-related immunoglobulin, IgA; a complement of T cells with mucosa-specific regulatory properties or effector capabilities; and a mucosa-oriented cell-homing system that allows lymphocytes initially activated in the mucosal follicles to migrate selectively to the diffuse mucosal lymphoid tissues underlying the epithelium. This last feature leads to the partial segregation of mucosal cells from systemic cells and thus qualifies the mucosal immune system as a somewhat separate immunologic entity.

The primary function of the mucosal immune system is to provide for host defense at mucosal surfaces. In this role, it operates in concert with several nonimmunologic protective factors, including: (1) resident bacterial flora that inhibit the growth of potential pathogens; (2) mucosal motor activity (peristalsis and ciliary function) that maintains the flow of lumenal constituents and thus reduces the interaction of potential pathogens with epithelial cells; (3) substances such as gastric acid and intestinal bile salts that create a mucosal microenvironment unfavorable to the growth of pathogens; (4) mucous secretions that create a barrier (glycocalyx) between potential pathogens and the epithelial surfaces; and, finally, (5) substances, such as lactoferrin, lactoperoxidase, and lysozyme, that have inhibitory effects on one or another specific microorganism. Optimal host defense at the mucosal surface depends on both intact mucosal immune responses and nonimmunologic protective functions. Thus, antibiotic therapy that eliminates normal flora may result in infection by an organism that ordinarily cannot gain a foothold at the mucosal surface, despite the existence of an intact immune system. Conversely, mucosal infections are common in congenital and acquired immunodeficiency states even in the presence of normal nonimmunologic protective factors.

A second but equally important function of the mucosal immune system is to prevent the entry of mucosal antigens into the circulation and thus to protect the systemic immune system from inappropriate antigenic exposure. This occurs both at the mucosal surface, by preventing the entry of potentially antigenic materials, and in the circulation, by providing for the clearance of mucosal antigens via a specific transport system. In addition, the mucosal immune system contains regulatory T cells that act to inhibit systemic immune responses to antigens that breach the mucosal barrier. This latter aspect of mucosal immune function may be important in the development of autoimmune processes and could conceivably be manipulated to treat a variety of autoimmune diseases.

ANATOMY

The mucosal system can be divided morphologically and functionally into two major parts: (1) the organized lymphoid tissues consisting of mucosal follicles (also called gut-associated lymphoid tissue [GALT] or bronchus-associated lymphoid tissues [BALT]) and (2) a diffuse lymphoid tissue compartment consisting of widely distributed cells located in the mucosal lamina propria (see Fig 13–1 and Chapter 3). The organized tissues are "afferent" lymphoid areas and are sites of antigen entry and induction of immune responses, whereas the diffuse tissues are "efferent" lymphoid areas and are sites where antigens interact with differentiated cells and cause the secretion of antibodies by B cells or induce helper or cytotoxic activities of T cells. The two parts of the mucosal immune system are linked by a mucosal homing

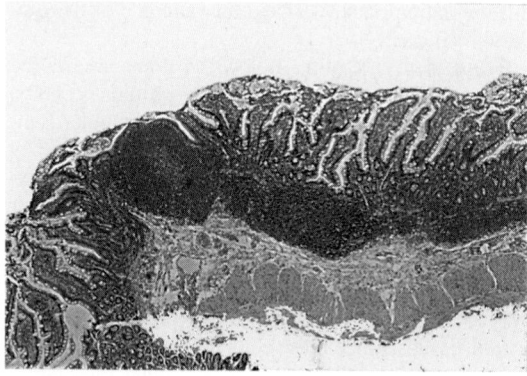

Figure 13–1. Histologic section of primate ileum showing a large lymphoid aggregate (Peyer's patch) and diffuse lymphoid tissue in the lamina propria. B- and T-lymphoid cells contact antigen and are induced to differentiate in the Peyer's patches; they then migrate to the lamina propria, where they perform their effector functions. Antigens enter the Peyer's patches through specialized cells (M cells) in the overlying epithelium.

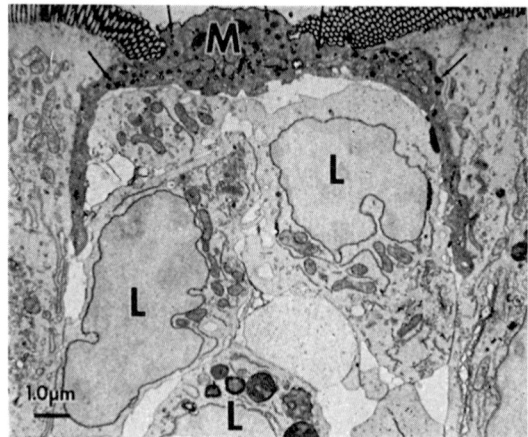

Figure 13–2. Transmission electron micrograph of a mouse M cell (M). Antigens pinocytosed from the mucosal lumen are transported without digestion to the underlying tissue, which includes lymphocytes (L) and dendritic cells. Arrows indicate pinocytotic vesicles in the M-cell cytoplasm.

mechanism, so that activated cells from the lymphoid follicles travel to the diffuse lymphoid areas where they can best interact with their cognate antigens. Both the organized and diffuse immune cell populations are exquisitely antigen-dependent in that their numbers are remarkably reduced in germ-free states and are expanded under conditions of antigen overload. The normal state is more or less midway between these extremes and is characterized by sufficient antigen stimulation to expand the mucosal population to a size that far exceeds that of the spleen and lymph nodes combined; on this basis, the mucosal immune system is quantitatively the predominant part of the overall lymphoid system.

MUCOSAL LYMPHOID AGGREGATES

The mucosal lymphoid aggregates are morphologically different from those of the systemic lymphoid system in that they receive antigen via the epithelium rather than through the lymphatic or blood circulation. This necessitates a distinct morphology that contains a number of unique elements.

M Cells. M cells are flattened epithelial cells with poorly developed brush borders and a thin overlying glycocalyx; they are distinguished from absorptive epithelial cells by their ability to pinocytose materials in the overlying mucosal lumen and to transport the latter in an undegraded form to the follicle proper (Fig 13–2). A wide range of substances are taken up by M cells, including soluble proteins, inert particulates, and various microorganisms. Although for the most part this uptake appears to be nonspecific, some degree of selectivity must exist, since otherwise trans-

port function would be overwhelmed by bacteria from the normal intestinal flora. One theoretic mechanism of exclusion involves secreted IgA antibodies that coat bacteria in the normal flora and retard their uptake.

Following transport via M cells, particulates and other substances accumulate in the follicular dome areas or interfollicular areas, where they are taken up by dendritic cells or phagocytic cells. In addition, some materials migrate to other lymphoid organs. M cells have been shown to bear major histocompatibility complex (MHC) class II proteins; nevertheless, it is doubtful that they act as antigen-presenting cells.

Dome Cells. The area just below the epithelium in the lymphoid follicle (the so-called dome area) contains a dense band of dendritic cells that are well positioned to take up antigens emerging from the M cells (Fig 13–3). Recent work has shown that these MHC class II-expressing cells take up ingested protein antigen and then present it to T cells to elicit T-cell proliferation and cytokine production. This implies that the lack of response to orally administered antigens (discussed in greater detail later on) is not due to lack of antigen-presenting cells in the mucosal follicles. There is some evidence that, following antigen uptake, dendritic cells move from the dome area to the interfollicular areas where they become functionally mature and interact with T cells.

Follicular T Cells. T cells are scattered through the dome area and other areas of the follicle, including the germinal centers; however, they are most dense in the interfollicular areas, where they frequently bear activation markers such as the IL-2Rα chain. Whereas CD4 T cells are widely distributed throughout the mucosal follicle, CD8 T cells are found exclusively in the interfollicular areas (see Fig 13–3).

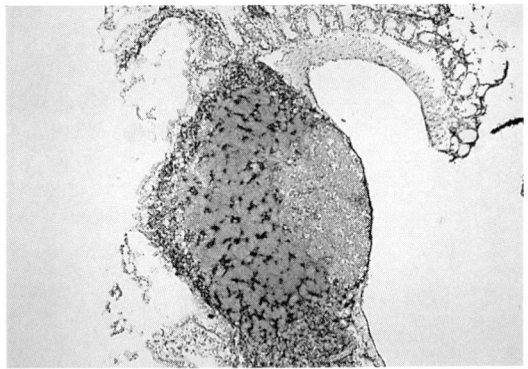

A

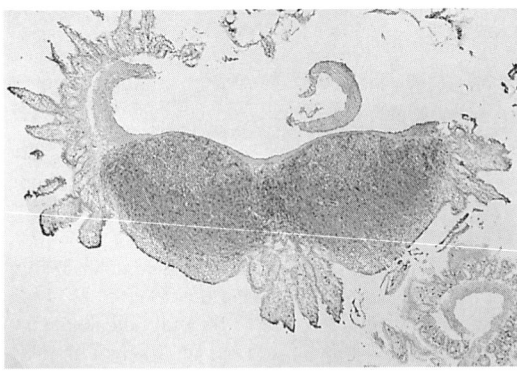

B

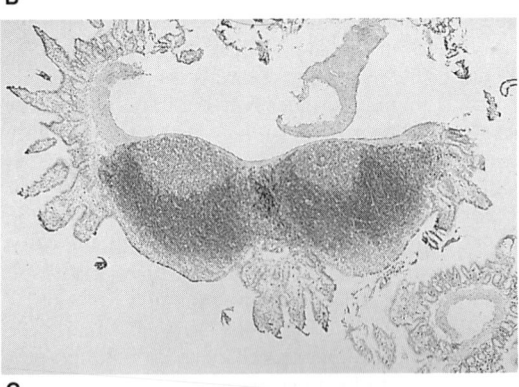

C

Figure 13–3. Histologic sections of mouse Peyer's patches, stained with antibodies (brown) that distinguish specific cell types in the patch. ***A:*** Antibody specific for dendritic cells (anti-CD11c), showing the layer of these cells immediately beneath the epithelium. ***B:*** Anti-CD4 antibody, showing CD4+ T cells. ***C:*** Anti-CD8 antibody, showing CD8+ T cells.

T cells in mucosal follicles produce a variety of both T_H1- and T_H2-type cytokines, depending on the conditions of immunization. In recent studies it was shown that T_H1-type responses predominate when protein antigen is administered orally in the absence of adjuvants, whereas T_H2-type responses occur when such antigen is given along with certain adjuvants such as cholera toxin. As noted later on, these different T-cell

differentiation patterns shape the outcome of the mucosal response.

Follicular B Cells. Below the dome area is the follicular area, which contains the germinal centers. The latter are generally similar to those in other lymphoid tissues except for the fact that the B cells they contain differentiate primarily into surface IgA-expressing (sIgA+) B cells. Thus, whereas the outer zones contain sIgM+/sIgD+ B cells intermixed with numerous T cells, the inner zones contain sIgA+ B cells and relatively few sIgG+ B cells. Interestingly, very few if any IgA plasma cells are present in the follicular tissues, since these cells develop only after additional differentiation in the draining mesenteric lymph nodes and in the lamina propria.

DIFFUSE MUCOSAL LYMPHOID TISSUE

The diffuse lymphoid tissues of the mucosal immune system consist of cell populations present in two separate compartments: the **intraepithelial lymphocyte (IEL) compartment** and the **lamina propria lymphocyte (LPL) compartment** (Fig 13–4).

Intraepithelial Lymphocytes

The IEL population, as the name implies, comprises cells lying above the lamina propria and basement membrane, among the epithelial cells. There is about one IEL for every four to six epithelial cells, so that this population is surprisingly large. The IELs are a phenotypically and morphologically distinct population that differs from cell populations in lamina propria or other lymphoid organs. For instance, most IELs are CD8 T cells (90% in mice; 50–80% in humans), many of which are granulated and some of which express FcεRI, a receptor typically found on mast cells. Perhaps more strikingly, a significant subpopulation bears the γδ T-cell receptor (TCR) rather than the αβ TCR (20–80% in mice; 5–10% in humans).

The origin of IELs also sets them apart from other cell populations. Studies of thymectomized mice indicate that many of these cells (including both αβ- and γδ-bearing IELs) are not of thymic origin and are instead composed of bone marrow cells that undergo development and selection in association with the intestinal epithelium. The significance of this extrathymic development is not clear, but one possibility is that it ensures that TCR specificities in the IEL are biased toward antigens encountered in the mucosal environment.

The function of IELs is not fully understood. What is clear is that they are mature, differentiated T cells that, on stimulation via the TCR, proliferate poorly yet produce ample amounts of various cytokines. In addition, they display the capacity to mediate cytotoxic function and this, along with the fact that they are CD8 T cells, suggests that they act in vivo as

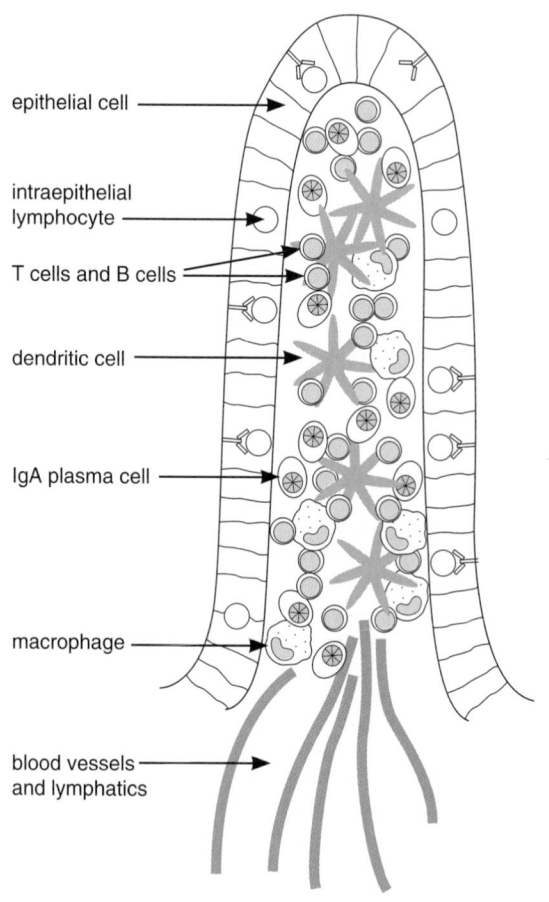

epithelial cell

intraepithelial lymphocyte

T cells and B cells

dendritic cell

IgA plasma cell

macrophage

blood vessels and lymphatics

Figure 13–4. Diagrammatic representation of cells in an intestinal villus. Intraepithelial lymphocytes (IELs) are present above the basement membrane and between epithelial cells. The lamina propria lies beneath the basement membrane, and contains a mixture of B cells, T cells, macrophages, dendritic cells, and other cell types.

cytolytic effector cells. It should be noted that this functional characterization applies to both the $\alpha\beta$ and $\gamma\delta$ TCR-bearing T-cell subpopulations, and it is likely that these subpopulations differ from one another more in their range of antigen specificities than in their overall function. One unifying hypothesis of IEL function, based on the above-mentioned considerations, is that IELs respond to a restricted set of "stress" proteins expressed on or released by epithelial cells in response to bound microorganisms; this leads, in turn, to elimination of the epithelial cells along with the bound organism. Thus, IELs may undercut the ability of pathogens to colonize the mucosa by reacting against the cellular substrate necessary for such colonization, rather than against the organisms themselves.

Lamina Propria Cells

The lamina propria contains a complex array of cells, including T cells, B cells, macrophages, dendritic cells, and mast cells. This population is dynamic in that its size depends to a great extent on the antigenic environment of the organism: animals in germ-free environments have relatively few lamina propria cells, whereas those in highly infected environments have expanded populations of such cells.

The lamina propria T-cell population is composed mainly of CD4 cells (60–70%) expressing the $\alpha\beta$ TCR (>95%), as in the peripheral blood; however, these cells differ from peripheral blood cells in that most (95%) display CD45RO, a marker associated with memory cells. In addition, they contain increased numbers of highly activated cells expressing MHC class II molecules and the IL-2Rα chain. Finally, recent studies have shown that lamina propria T cells also differ from peripheral blood T cells by the fact that they respond poorly to proliferative stimuli when stimulated via the TCR/CD3 receptor alone and thus appear to be partially anergic; on the other hand, they retain considerable ability to respond via the CD2 receptor, probably when the latter is costimulated via the TCR/CD3 receptor. When lamina propria cells are stimulated via the CD2 receptor (or costimulated via the CD2 and TCR/CD3 receptor) they produce large amounts of lymphokines, particularly IFNγ. Overall, lamina propria T cells appear to mount relatively poor proliferative responses but produce large amounts of cytokines; they therefore can be defined as highly differentiated effector T cells.

Lamina propria B cells are similar to lamina propria T cells in that these cells are also highly differentiated, existing mostly as plasma cells. In addition, most of these B cells express IgA and, in humans, produce IgA2 rather than IgA1 as one moves distally along the gastrointestinal tract. IgG and IgM plasma cells are also present but are relatively infrequent compared with B-cell populations in other lymphoid organs. The percentage of the total B-cell population, however, expressing IgG and IgM increases during inflammation; this may reflect proliferation of ordinarily inapparent sIgM+ B cells that are present in the lamina propria at all times.

Antigen-Presenting Cells. The chief "professional" antigen-presenting cells in the lamina propria are probably dendritic cells. These are found in the Peyer's patches, as well as in the diffuse mucosal tissues lying below the lamina propria. Macrophages are also abundant in the diffuse mucosal areas but appear to function primarily as phagocytes rather than as antigen-presenting cells. In this regard, lamina propria macrophages usually bear markers associated with cell activation and are thus likely to be a population of activated cells oriented toward intracellular degradative function.

Another cell type associated with the lamina propria that has antigen-presenting cell capability is the

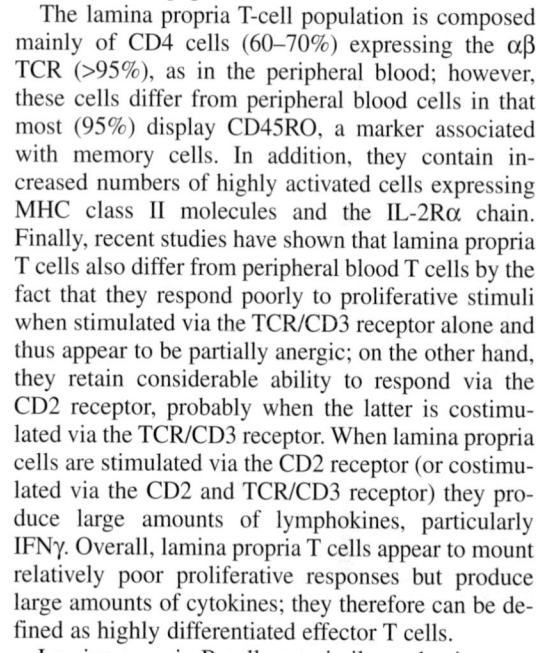

intestinal epithelial cell. These cells can express MHC class II antigens, particularly during inflammatory responses when exposed to IFNγ. Epithelial cells have been shown to function as antigen-presenting cells in vitro but probably do so only in relation to IEL in vivo since they probably have relatively little contact with lamina propria T cells. Recently, it has been shown that CD1d, an MHC class I-like molecule, is expressed on epithelial cells and may act as a restriction element for antigens presented by epithelial cells. CD1d may also facilitate interaction between epithelial cells and CD8 on IELs, since it is known that epithelial cells interact preferentially with CD8 T cells.

Lamina Propria Natural Killer and Lymphokine-Activated Killer Cells. Cells bearing natural killer (NK) markers (CD16, CD56) are sparse in the human lamina propria, and NK activity is difficult to demonstrate in human lamina propria cell populations unless procedures to enrich them are used. On the other hand, primate and rodent lamina propria cell populations manifest more robust NK activity, which would suggest that the lack of NK activity in human lamina propria is due in part to the fact that human habitats and habits are not conducive to the development of mucosal NK cells, even though the potential for such development does exist. This view is supported by the fact that cells with lymphokine-activated killer (LAK) function, by contrast, are relatively easily demonstrated among the human lamina propria cell populations.

Lamina Propria Mast Cells. Mucosal areas are rich in mast cell precursors, which rapidly differentiate into mature mast cells when they are appropriately stimulated. Through their release of mediators, mast cells constitute an important mechanism by which inflammatory cells are chemoattracted to mucosal tissues and participate in local host defense.

In humans, mast cells in mucosal tissue produce relatively small amounts of histamine and tryptic proteinase on activation, whereas those in connective tissue produce relatively large amounts of histamine as well as both tryptic and chymotryptic proteinases. Differential mast cell development in these two tissues may depend on the types of cells and cytokines present in their local environments. In this regard, mast cell precursors differentiate into "mucosal" mast cells under the influence of T-cell-derived lymphokines such as IL-3, whereas "connective-tissue" mast cells require other factors such as stem cell factor. This may account for the rapid appearance of mast cells in mucosal tissues infected with nematode parasites, since presumably the parasites can stimulate mucosal T cells to secrete lymphokines that cause differentiation of mast cell precursors into mucosal mast cells. Thus, the significance of the mucosal mast cell type to the mucosal immune system (and to the body as a whole) may lie in its unique capacity to expand rapidly in number under the influence of a T-cell-derived signal.

IMMUNOGLOBULIN A

STRUCTURE & FUNCTION OF IgA

As noted earlier, one of the distinguishing features of the mucosal immune system is that humoral responses induced in mucosal follicles result predominantly in the production of IgA antibodies. Not unexpectedly, this is tied to the fact that IgA exhibits a number of properties that allow it to function efficiently in the mucosal environment. The biochemical structure, genetics, and synthesis of IgA are discussed in Chapter 7; we will concentrate here on IgA function.

IgA is quantitatively the most abundant of the immunoglobulins, having a synthetic rate exceeding that of all other immunoglobulins combined when secretory as well as circulating IgA is taken into account. In humans, IgA is encoded by two separate genetic loci within the immunoglobulin heavy-chain region, downstream of the γ and ε heavy-chain loci. The first IgA gene encodes IgA1, which is the predominant circulating IgA (about 80% of the total circulating IgA) as well as a major component of IgA in mucosal secretions of the proximal gastrointestinal tract. The second IgA gene encodes IgA2, the IgA that is particularly abundant in secretions, especially those of the distal gastrointestinal tract, and that accounts for about 60% of total secretory IgA. Whereas circulating IgA1 generally occurs as a monomer, both mucosal IgA1 and IgA2 generally occur as a dimer (or a multimer), which allows both forms to bind to secretory component on the surface of epithelial cells (Fig 13–5). These secretory forms of IgA are capable of being transported to the mucosal surface via a specific transport mechanism, as discussed in greater detail later on.

IgA1 and IgA2 heavy chains differ by only 15–20 amino acids scattered through their respective constant region domains; these differences, however, are strategic and lead to molecules with somewhat disparate properties. One difference is that IgA1, unlike IgA2, has a long proline-rich hinge region that both confers considerable flexibility to the antigen-binding sites and renders the molecule susceptible to cleavage by proteinases secreted by a number of bacteria. This latter property limits the efficacy of IgA1 on the mucosal surface where proteinase-producing bacteria often reside. Another distinction is that IgA1 and IgA2 differ with respect to the amount and composition of carbohydrate side chains they contain. In particular, IgA1 has more available penultimate galactose and *N*-acetyl galactose residues and thus is able to bind to the asialoglycoprotein receptor present on hepatocytes. On the other hand, IgA2 displays more truncated oligosaccharides with exposed mannose residues, thus allowing IgA2 to bind to certain organ-

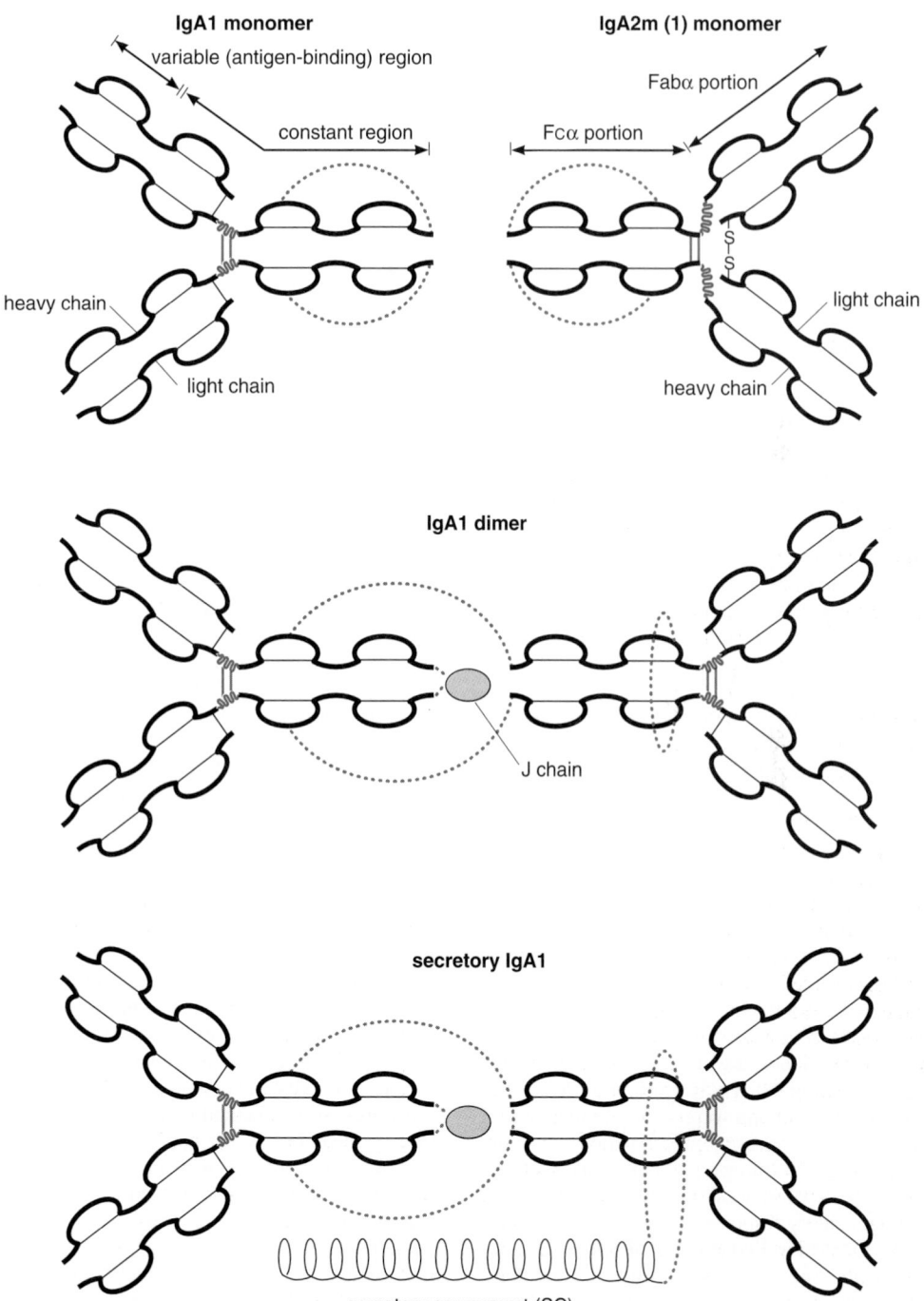

Figure 13–5. Diagrammatic representation of IgA structural forms. Shaded areas indicate immunoglobulin domains. Beads indicate disulfide bonds. In the actual IgA dimer and secretory IgA molecule, the J chain and secretory component protein are intertwined with Cα heavy chains.

isms and thus to prevent their colonization of the mucosal surface. Finally, the two classes of IgA differ with respect to allotypy: IgA2, but not IgA1, has two allotypic forms, designated A2M(2) and A2M(1).

IgA exhibits four properties that facilitate its function at mucosal surfaces.

IgA Polymerization and Interaction with Secretory Component. The IgA heavy chain, in common with the IgM heavy chain, has an extra C-terminal domain (tail segment) containing cysteine residues (see Fig 13–5). This domain permits IgA to interact with a bivalent (or multivalent) molecule, also produced by B cells, known as J chain, and thus to form IgA dimers (or trimers). IgA polymerization is important to IgA function because polymerized IgA (pIgA) has an increased capacity to bind and agglutinate antigens. In addition, dimeric (or trimeric) IgA (but not monomeric IgA) has the ability to interact with secretory component (SC), a 95-kd protein produced by epithelial cells (see Fig 13–5). The latter acts as a transport receptor for IgA and becomes part of the secreted IgA molecule (secretory IgA).

Resistance to Proteolysis. Interaction of the IgA molecule with SC to form secretory IgA renders the IgA molecule less susceptible to proteolytic digestion in the proteinase-rich environment of the intestine. This results from the fact that proteinases cannot find target sites on the IgA/SC complex owing to the latter's greater rigidity and increased carbohydrate display (as compared with uncomplexed IgA or other immunoglobulins). In addition, IgA contains a glycosylated, proline-rich hinge region that is generally more resistant to intestinal proteinases than is that of IgG.

Anti-Inflammatory Properties of IgA. The Fc region of IgA, unlike that of IgM or IgG, does not react with components of either the classic or alternative complement pathway, except possibly when the IgA is highly polymerized or is in the form of an immune complex, and even in the latter instance it does not bind C3b and therefore does not recruit inflammatory cells and mediators. In addition, the binding of IgA to neutrophils and other phagocytic cells via the Fc domain results in inhibition of phagocytic and lytic functions in these cells. Finally, the Fc/SC end of IgA is hydrophilic and mucophilic; thus, binding of IgA to a microorganism retards the latter's attachment to epithelial cells by enmeshing it in the mucous layer. Taken together, the Fc or Fc/SC properties of IgA allows this immunoglobulin to prevent colonization of pathogens without inducing inflammation. This, of course, is a highly useful property in an area of the body replete with substances that have the potential to induce inflammatory responses.

Proinflammatory Properties of IgA. The earlier consideration notwithstanding, IgA can and does mediate certain proinflammatory effects under certain circumstances. Thus, IgA bound to phagocytes via the Fc receptor does generate increased phagocytic function when the IgA is cross-linked at the cell surface by antigen. In this context, there is some evidence that IgA can mediate antibody-dependent cell-mediated cytotoxicity via binding to the Fc receptor. Moreover, IgA interacts via its Fc region with lactoferrin and lactoperoxidase and thereby enhances the function of these nonspecific host defense elements.

TRANSPORT OF IgA

As noted earlier, the capacity of dimeric IgA to bind to SC enhances its capacity to function in the intestinal lumen. More importantly, however, such binding is the key initial step in the IgA transport mechanism that allows the mucosal immune system to deliver IgA to mucosal sites (Fig 13–6). The sequence of events occurring during IgA transport involves, first, the binding of polymeric IgA to SC expressed on the basolateral surface of the epithelial cell or hepatocyte (via a covalent interaction); this is followed by endocytosis of IgA/SC into vesicles, movement of those vesicles to the apical surface of the cell and, finally, release of IgA/SC complexes into the mucosal lumen. This final step is accompanied by proteolytic cleavage of the SC receptor molecule, so that a portion of this receptor, too, is incorporated into secreted IgA. Interestingly, the cellular synthesis and translocation of SC is independent of the presence of IgA, and the amount of SC synthesized usually exceeds the amount necessary for transport; this leads to the secretion of free (unbound) SC.

IgA transport mediated by SC occurs in the epithelium of the digestive tract, the salivary glands, the bronchial mucosa, and lactating mammary glands. In addition, it occurs in the uterine epithelium, where it is regulated by the effects of estrogen on SC synthesis by uterine epithelial cells. Finally, IgA transport mediated by SC also occurs in the liver, where it results in secretion of IgA into the bile. In rodents, SC is present on hepatocytes and on biliary epithelial cells, and thus SC-mediated hepatic transport is a robust process leading to rapid clearance of circulating IgA. This is underscored by the fact that in rats (but not in humans) biliary obstruction leads to increased IgA levels. In humans, SC is present on biliary epithelial cells but not on hepatocytes, so that SC-mediated transport is a relatively minor process. This is not to say, however, that hepatic uptake of IgA in humans is negligible, since it now appears that SC-mediated transport is supplemented in this species by an uptake process mediated by the asialoglycoprotein receptor present on hepatocytes, which binds IgA1 and galactose and N-acetyl galactose on carbohydrate side chains. This uptake mechanism differs from SC-mediated transport in that it acts selectively on monomeric IgA1 rather than dimeric IgA2 and results in intracellular degradation of IgA rather than transport into the bile.

Although the function of SC-mediated transport at mucosal surfaces is primarily the delivery of IgA to the lumen, such transport in the liver (as well as uptake mediated by the asialoglycoprotein receptor) has the additional (and perhaps more important) role of clearing the circulation of material that has penetrated the mucosal barrier and that has the potential of evoking untoward immune responses. IgA immunoglobulin

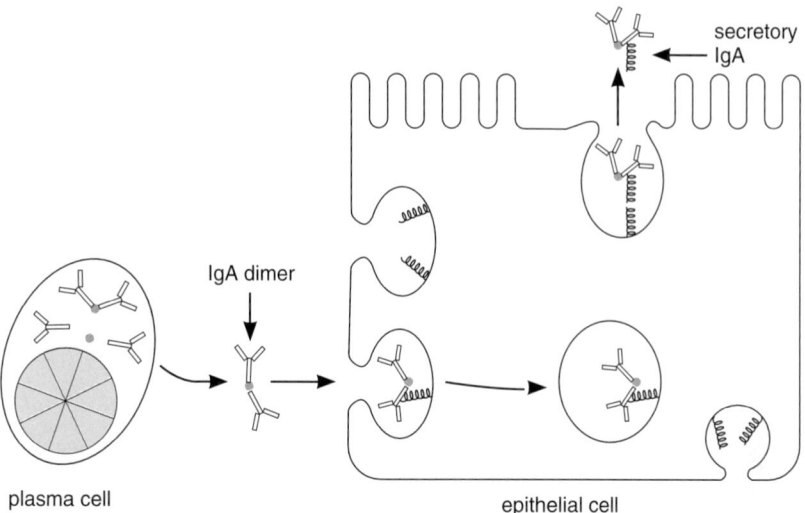

Figure 13–6. Secretory component (SC)-mediated transport of IgA across an epithelial cell. Transport depends on binding of dimeric IgA to SC, followed by uptake into vesicles and ultimate delivery of intact IgA to the mucosal lumen in association with a part of the SC protein (secretory IgA).

is particularly suited to this task because, as the immunoglobulin that has been induced at mucosal sites it is the immunoglobulin whose receptors are specific for mucosal antigens.

IMMUNE EXCLUSION

Macromolecules in the mucosal environment are capable of transepithelial transport into the circulation in an intact form. As indicated earlier, this could lead to stimulation of the systemic immune system by antigens capable of evoking unnecessary or harmful immune responses, including those that lead to auto-immunity. This potentiality, however, is countered by **immune exclusion**—the process by which IgA provides a barrier to macromolecular absorption. Immune exclusion involves the binding of antigens at the mucosal surface by IgA, which leads to their entrapment in the mucous layer, where the antigen becomes subject to degradation by intestinal proteinases. This process operates in tandem with the aforementioned hepatic clearance mechanism, with immune exclusion preventing entry of antigens, and hepatic clearance cleansing the system of antigens that have entered. That IgA is necessary to both processes is shown by the fact that individuals with selective IgA deficiency (ie, those who have low IgA levels and normal IgM and IgG levels) show increased absorption of macromolecules and high levels of circulating immune complexes following ingestion of antigens. Finally, immune exclusion and hepatic clearance have the effect of restricting immune responses against mucosal antigens to the mucosal lymphoid system and thus to the unique mucosal regulation of such responses, as discussed later on.

SECRETORY VERSUS CIRCULATING IgA

In recent years, in vivo and in vitro studies of IgA synthesis and catabolism have provided insights into the source of IgA present in various body compartments. The results of these studies show that, in humans, most circulating IgA is produced in the bone marrow and is in the form of IgA1 monomers, whereas secretory IgA is produced mainly at mucosal sites (either as IgA1 or IgA2 dimers or polymers). Polymeric IgA (whether IgA1 or IgA2) is more rapidly catabolized than monomeric IgA, because polymeric IgA is subject to additional catabolic mechanisms such as SC-mediated transport and asialoglycoprotein receptor-mediated uptake. In rats and rabbits, polymeric IgA accounts for about half of the circulating IgA, although most IgA delivered into the circulation is polymeric. This is explained by the fact that, as alluded to earlier, SC-mediated transport in the liver is a quantitatively important process in those species, and thus, polymeric IgA is more rapidly cleared than monomeric IgA.

The separate origins of mucosal and circulating IgA in humans have led some investigators to suggest that the IgA system in humans is bipartite, that is, it is composed of two relatively independent synthetic centers that are separately regulated. An alternative view, more in keeping with the concept that the bone marrow is not an inductive site for IgA B cells, is that

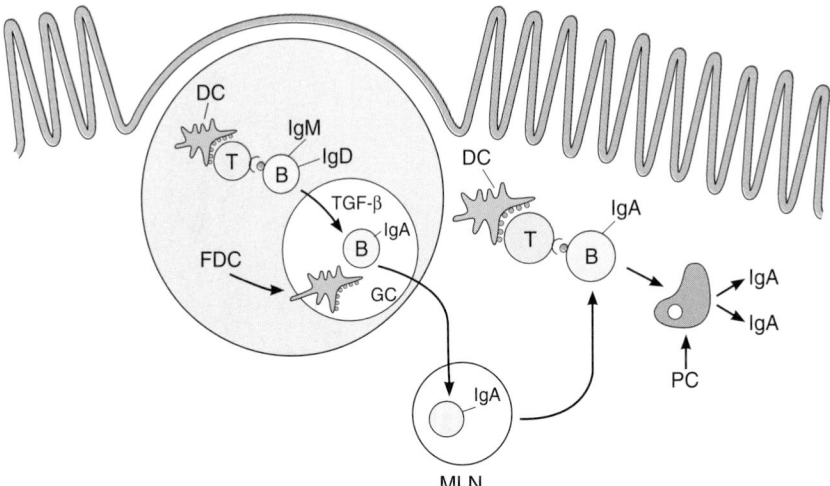

Figure 13–7. Regulation of IgA synthesis at mucosal sites. Dendritic cell (DC)-activated T cells interact with IgM/IgD B cells and induce class-switching to IgA B cells under the influence of transforming growth factor beta (TGFβ). IgA B cells in the germinal centers (GC) are inhibited from further differentiation by contact with antigen on the surface of follicular dendritic cells (FDC) until they migrate via the mesenteric lymph node (MLN) to the lamina propria. There, further contact with T cells expressing CD40L and cytokines (IL-5 and IL-6) leads to IgA plasma cell (PC) formation.

the IgA1 B cells that produce IgA in the marrow originate in the mucosa and secondarily colonize the marrow to form a separate (but subordinate) locus of IgA-producing B cells. In any case, the monomeric IgA1 arising from the bone marrow in humans may provide a selective advantage to this species because such IgA may be better suited than other forms of IgA to mediate the clearance of mucosal antigens from the circulation (as discussed earlier). In this regard, the monomeric IgA1 molecule may form smaller, less pathogenic complexes with circulating antigens than polymeric IgA yet retain the capacity to undergo removal via interaction with appropriate receptors in the liver.

PRODUCTION OF OTHER IMMUNOGLOBULINS IN THE MUCOSA

Immunoglobulins other than IgA also play a role in the mucosal immune system. Mucosal synthesis of IgM, which can also be transported across the epithelial cell via an SC-mediated mechanism, is measurable and physiologically significant. Its capacity to act as a mucosal immunoglobulin is underscored by the fact that it usually serves as an adequate replacement for IgA in individuals with selective IgA deficiency. Mucosal synthesis of IgG, on the other hand, is quite low in most mucosal areas, and IgG cannot be transported across the epithelium. Nevertheless, it

does have a mucosal role: it is synthesized in substantial amounts in the distal pulmonary tract and is thus an important antibody class in pulmonary secretions. IgE is also synthesized in mucosal tissues, particularly during parasitic infection or in relation to certain pathologic (allergic) states; however, there is no preferential localization of IgE B cells in the mucosa, and the number of B cells synthesizing IgE is small, as it is in other tissues.

REGULATION OF IgA SYNTHESIS AT MUCOSAL SITES

That IgA responses dominate the mucosal humoral response is a result of the fact that B cells in mucosal follicles develop into IgA-producing cells rather than into IgG-producing cells (Fig 13–7). A striking demonstration of this is contained in a recent study in which germ-free mice received reovirus orally and promptly developed germinal centers in Peyer's patches that contained IgA B cells exclusively, whereas systemic immunization of these mice with reovirus evoked IgG B cells in germinal centers of systemic lymphoid tissues.

The basis of preferential IgA B-cell development in Peyer's patches is not yet fully understood. One factor that has been identified is the presence of activated T cells that influence B cells to undergo IgA-specific isotype switching. Thus, it has been shown that T cells from Peyer's patches, but not T cells in the spleen, can induce IgM B cells to become IgA B cells. The properties of Peyer's patch T cells that lead to such IgA-specific switching are only now being identified. One such property is the ability to secrete TGFβ, which promotes IgA class switching. Another is the ability to express CD40 ligand, which interacts with CD40 on B cells and thus initiates B-cell switch differentiation and proliferation. Finally, one or more as-yet-unidentified surface proteins on Peyer's patch T cells may also be necessary for IgA switch differentiation; this possibility arises from the fact that T cells producing TGFβ and expressing CD40L are not unique to Peyer's patches even though IgA switch differentiation is limited to these sites. Recently, it has been shown that stimulation of B cells in vitro via CD40L, TGFβ and surface immunoglobulin (with anti-IgD) in the presence of IL-4 and IL-5 induces high levels of IgA switching. These data indicate that IgA switch differentiation can be achieved in vitro with sufficient B-cell stimulation; however, whether this is the necessary combination of factors causing preferential IgA switching in vivo remains to be determined.

IgA switch differentiation, as discussed earlier, is followed by further B-cell development into IgA memory cells or IgA plasma cells. This further development again depends on T cells, which act on B cells via cell–cell interactions or secretion of lymphokines. The cell–cell interactions are likely to include those involving OX40 on T cells and OX40-ligand on B cells, which have recently been shown to be capable of inducing lymphokine-independent memory cell and plasma cell development of postswitch IgG and IgA B cells. The lymphokines involved, on the other hand, include IL-5 and IL-6, which appear to be particularly important for the terminal differentiation of IgA B cells (as compared with IgG B cells) at least under some circumstances. Interestingly, interaction of antigens with surface IgA on postswitch IgA B cells results in cells that cannot be induced to undergo terminal differentiation; this is in direct contrast with the effect of antigen through surface IgM on unswitched B cells. Since IgA B cells in Peyer's patch germinal centers probably interact with antigens bound to follicular dendritic cells, antigen-mediated inhibitory effects may explain the lack of IgA plasma cell development in Peyer's patches, as noted earlier. Antigen-mediated inhibition can be reversed by a strong T-cell signal delivered via CD40L and perhaps other T-cell surface molecules. Thus, one might hypothesize that IgA B cells developing in Peyer's patches are initially suppressed by exposure to antigen in the germinal centers and are then reactivated following migration to the lamina propria area by CD40L-expressing activated T cells present at the latter site. This ensures that IgA B cells do not produce IgA until they arrive at effector sites where such production is needed.

MUCOSAL HOMING

A characteristic feature of the mucosal immune system is the capability of cells developing in the mucosal follicles to migrate to effector sites in the lamina propria underlying the mucosal surfaces (Fig 13–8). This selective homing serves to focus mucosal immune responses to mucosal tissues and accounts for the ability to expose one mucosal surface to anti-

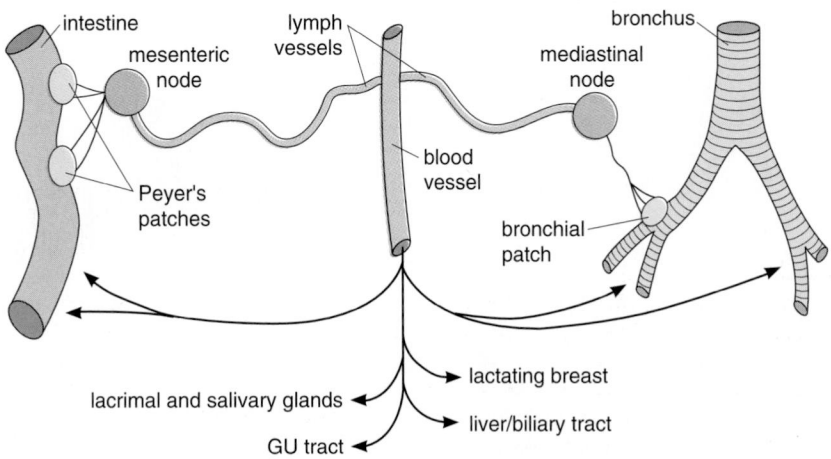

Figure 13–8. Cell traffic in the mucosal immune system. Cells originating in the mucosal follicles localize in subepithelial regions of many mucosal tissues. The ability to do so is governed by specific interactions between homing receptors on lymphoid cells and vascular addressins on endothelial cells genitourinary tract (GU tract).

gen (eg, the intestine) and then to measure specific IgA at other surfaces (eg, the lung).

The mucosal homing phenomenon has been defined most completely for IgA B cells that arise in mucosal follicles after having undergone class switching and differentiation into plasmablasts or IgA memory B cells in follicular germinal centers. While B-cell homing is directed to all mucosal sites, some regional preferences have been noted: thus, bronchial node-derived B cells have a greater tendency to home to the lungs than to the intestines, and Peyer's patch B cells have a greater propensity to home to the intestines than to the lungs.

Mucosal T lymphocytes also display a homing capability, but in this case, the migration is more promiscuous, and only some of the T cells of mucosal origin end up at mucosal sites. In addition, although most lamina propria T cells have probably originated in the Peyer's patches, a large fraction of IELs are bone marrow-derived cells that develop in the intraepithelial compartment itself. As in other homing phenomena, the specificity of mucosal homing is dictated by specific interactions between lymphocyte homing receptors and vascular addressins. Interactions between the $\alpha4\beta7$ integrin and its ligand (the endothelial addressin MAdCAM-1) are particularly important, but in all probability other integrin–addressin interactions also contribute to this process (see Chapter 3). Thus, one can postulate that a particular feature of B-cell and T-cell development in the mucosal follicular compartment is the acquisition of the $\alpha4\beta7$ integrin, which then mediates homing to the lamina propria.

Another integrin involved in localization of mucosal cells to mucosal sites is the $\alpha E\beta7$ integrin. This surface molecule is expressed on virtually all IELs and appears to be important in the passage of IEL into, or retention in, intraepithelial sites.

ORAL TOLERANCE

The antigenic milieu of the mucosal immune system differs from that of the systemic immune system in that mucosal immune cells are constantly exposed to antigenic substances, including those present in food or associated with the intestinal flora. Many of these substances would evoke unnecessary and potentially harmful immune responses were it not for a specialized mechanism, known as **oral tolerance,** by which the mucosal immune system is rendered unresponsive to oral antigens (Fig 13–9).

As a rule, oral tolerance develops to protein antigens and is a T-cell-mediated phenomenon. Polysaccharide antigens do not induce oral tolerance, though it should be noted that such antigens (which are generally T-cell-independent) typically evoke only low-level IgM antibody responses that have very low pathogenic potential. Other factors that influence the development of oral tolerance include antigen dose, the genetic makeup of the host, prior immunization, and the level of overall immunologic activation. In contrast, certain bacterial toxins, such as cholera toxin, act as **mucosal adjuvants** rather than inducing oral tolerance, as will be discussed later on.

Of the several mechanisms that have been shown to operate in the development of oral tolerance, perhaps the best established is the induction of suppressor T cells. In a now-classic series of experiments, it was shown that mice subjected to oral immunization with relatively small doses of antigen develop T cells in their Peyer's patches and spleen that, when transferred to a second animal, can suppress responses to the same antigen given parenterally in a form that ordinarily is immunogenic. While initial studies indi-

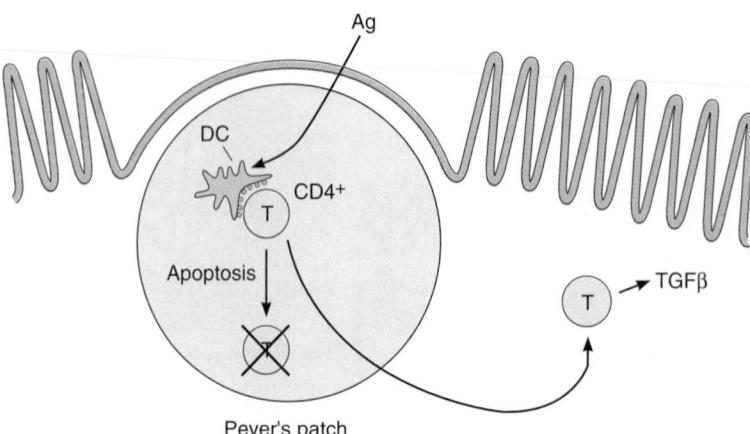

Figure 13–9. IInduction of oral tolerance. Protein antigens entering the Peyer's patches are captured by dendritic cells (DC), which then induce antigen-specific T cells to either undergo apoptosis (deletional mechanism) or differentiate into transforming growth factor beta (TGFβ)-producing suppressive T cells (suppressive mechanism).

cated that suppression was due to CD8 T cells, more recent studies have shown that CD4 T cells are also involved and may be the main suppressor cells. In addition, it has been established that the suppressor T cells operate in an antigen-nonspecific fashion by producing TGFβ and possibly other nonspecific suppressor factors. Because of this antigen-nonspecificity, oral tolerance induced by feeding one antigen can lead to suppression of responses against a second, parenterally administered antigen if the oral antigen is re-administered along with the parenteral antigen. Such "bystander" suppression could theoretically allow one to suppress a pathologic immune reaction by inducing oral tolerance with an antigen irrelevant to that reaction, provided, of course, that the suppressor cells induced by the irrelevant antigen can be delivered to the appropriate site.

A second mechanism of oral tolerance that has come to the fore involves induction of T-cell anergy, T-cell deletion, or both. Thus, it has been shown that mice fed relatively large amounts of antigen subsequently can be shown to lack cells capable of responding to that antigen, yet manifest little or no suppressor activity with respect to that antigen. Such deletional non-responsiveness is also seen in transgenic mice that have been manipulated genetically to express a particular T cell receptor (TCR) on their T cells rather than the normal array of TCRs. Such mice, when fed antigen, lose the baseline responsiveness to the antigen that would normally be present.

Further studies of such TCR-transgenic mice has yielded additional insight into the relationship between the suppressor and deletional mechanisms of oral tolerance. Feeding of a soluble protein to these mice elicits a T_H1- (ie, IFNγ-) dominated response in the Peyer's patches; only if this T_H1 response is inhibited (by systemic administration of antibodies to IL-12) do T cells producing TGFβ emerge. Thus, it can be postulated that feeding regimens which elicit weak T_H1 responses (such as feeding low doses of antigen, or feeding substances that induce primarily T_H2 responses) would favor development of T cells producing TGFβ. In contrast, regimens that elicit strong T_H1 responses (such as those containing high antigen dosages) do not favor development of TGFβ-producing cells. These new studies provide a rationale for the regulation of two main mechanisms of oral tolerance, as well as for the relationship of antigen dosage to these mechanisms.

The induction of oral tolerance is currently being evaluated as a potential treatment for certain autoimmune states. The approach is to administer a relevant antigen (such as collagen to those with rheumatoid arthritis, or myelin basic protein to those with multiple sclerosis) by the oral route in hope of inducing suppressor T cells which could migrate to involved tissues and secrete antigen-nonspecific suppressor substances that would inhibit the pathologic process.

ORAL TOLERANCE INDUCTION VERSUS ORAL IMMUNIZATION & IgA ANTIBODY PRODUCTION

If protein antigens are likely to induce oral tolerance, how does the mucosal immune system overcome such tolerance to mount protective IgA responses? One answer to this question—not yet completely proven—is that IgA responses are not induced unless the protein antigen is presented to the mucosal immune system in association with an adjuvant that allows for circumvention of oral tolerance. Evidence for this view comes from the observation that a fed protein does not elicit an IgA response (or any response) unless it is given along with an adjuvant, such as cholera toxin. This finding could mimic the situation of proteins present on the surface of pathologic bacteria or viruses that naturally express substances with adjuvant properties. Just how adjuvants work is still a matter of intense investigation. One attractive possibility is that they inhibit mucosal T_H1 (IFNγ) responses and thus, as noted earlier, favor development of T cells that produce TGFβ and other cytokines necessary for IgA class switching. Since TGFβ is far less inhibitory of IgA B cells than of other B cells or T cells, TGFβ secretion does not itself shut off IgA responses, although it may lead to "split tolerance" marked by augmentation of IgA responses and suppression of IgG responses, as observed in several studies. In addition, the adjuvant may at least temporarily prevent clonal anergy and deletion or, alternatively lead to the development of T cells that resist such anergy and deletion. The important "take-home" message, then, is that nontolerogenic stimuli, leading to IgA responses in the mucosal immune system, are naturally adjuvanted stimuli that stimulate a cache of T cells that are necessary for the IgA responses and resistant to the suppressive effects of oral tolerance.

BREAST MILK IMMUNOLOGY

An important aspect of mucosal immunity is the capacity of IgA B cells to enter the lactating breast and to secrete IgA, which is then transported into breast secretions (ie, the colostrum and milk). This is, in fact, a key means of intragenerational transfer of immunity and is thus a very tangible example of the importance of mucosal immune processes in mammalian survival.

IgA B cells home to lactating breast tissue following the secretion of certain gestational hormones that presumably act by inducing the expression of specific addressins on breast tissue endothelial cells. Within breast tissue, IgA B cells differentiate, and the IgA subsequently secreted is transported into milk via the SC transport mechanism. The concentration of IgA in initial breast secretions (colostrum) is extremely high (averaging 50 mg/mL, versus 2.5 mg/mL in adult serum) in the initial four postpartum days and then rapidly falls to serum levels. Such IgA secretion is accompanied by the secretion of other, less specific, host defense factors, such as lysozyme, lactoferrin, cytokines, and various antibacterial glycoproteins, glycolipids, oligosaccharides, and lipids. Together, these various soluble agents act as potent host defense components in the newborn gut.

The breast secretions are also rich in various cellular elements that contribute breast milk immunity. These include activated neutrophils and macrophages, which produce active oxygen radicals, and various proinflammatory cytokines, such as TNFα, IL-1β, and IL-6. In contrast, the lymphocyte content of breast secretions is relatively low, and whether such cells survive the environment of the infant intestine is open to question.

The various soluble and particulate immune elements present in breast milk secretion provide critical protection to the newborn against infectious diseases, particularly in the nonhygienic environments of less developed countries. In this regard, there are extensive data that breast feeding offers protection against the development of infant diarrhea, septicemia, lower res-

piratory tract infection, and necrotizing enterocolitis.

A final possible salutary effect of breast feeding relates to the ability of IgA to prevent absorption of certain environmental proteins early in life, at a time when the organism is susceptible to developing lifelong IgE-mediated allergic reactions. This possibility has, in fact, been used as an explanation for why early dietary exposure to certain antigens leads to allergy, or why transient IgA deficiency has been associated with atopy. It should be noted, however, that the data on this point are conflicting, and the precise role of breast feeding in allergy development remains to be defined.

CONCLUSION

The previous discussion provides ample evidence that the mucosae are home to a unique and separate part of the immune system. Given the fact that stimulation of this system can, on the one hand, lead to effective immunization against many important pathogens and, on the other hand, lead to tolerance induction and the prevention of autoimmunity, it is incumbent on us to continue to expand our knowledge of mucosal immune processes and thus to learn ways to manipulate them for our benefit.

REFERENCES

GENERAL

Croitoru R, Bienenstock J: Characteristics and functions of mucosa-associated lymphoid tissue. In: *Handbook of Mucosal Immunology,* Ogra PL (editor). Academic Press, 1994.

Kelsall BL, Strober W: Host defenses at mucosal surfaces. In: *Clinical Immunology Principles and Practice,* Rich R (editor). Mosby, 1996.

ANTIGEN-PRESENTING CELLS

Blumberg RS et al: Expression of a non-polymorphic MHC-class I like molecule CD1d, by human intestinal epithelial cells. *J Immunol* 1991;**147:**2518.

Kelsall BL, Strober W: Distinct populations of dendritic cells are present in the subepithelial dome and T cells regions of the murine Peyer's patch. *J Exp Med* 1996;**183:**237.

Panja A, Mayer L: Diversity and function of antigen-presenting cells in mucosal tissues. In: *Handbook of Mucosal Immunology,* Ogra PL (editor). Academic Press, 1994.

M CELLS

Tomohiro K, Owen RL: Structure and function of intestinal mucosal epithelium. In: *Handbook of Mucosal Immunology,* Ogra PL (editor). Academic Press, 1994.

INTRAEPITHELIAL LYMPHOCYTES

Lefrancois L: Basic aspects of intraepithelial lymphocyte immunobiology. In: *Handbook of Mucosal Immunology,* Ogra PL (editor). Academic Press, 1994.

MUCOSAL MAST CELLS

Befus AD et al: Mast cells from the human intestinal lamina propria. *J Immunol* 1987;**138:**2604.

LAMINA PROPRIA LYMPHOCYTES

Boirivant M et al: Hypoproliferative human lamina propria T cells retain the capacity to secrete lymphokines when stimulated via CD2/28 pathways. *Proc Assoc Am Physicians* 1996;**108:**56.

James SP, Zeitz M: Human gastrointestinal mucosal T cells. In: *Handbook of Mucosal Immunology,* Ogra PL (editor). Academic Press, 1994.

London SD: Cytotoxic lymphocytes in mucosal effector sites. In: *Handbook of Mucosal Immunology,* Ogra PL (editor). Academic Press, 1994.

IgA STRUCTURE & TRANSPORT

Mestecky J, McGhee JR: Immunoglobulin A(IgA): molecular and cellular interactions involved in IgA biosynthesis and immune responses. *Adv Immunol* 1987;**40:**153.

Mestecky J et al: Selective transport of IgA: cellular and molecular aspects. *Gastroenterol Clin North Am* 1991;**20:**441.

Sanderson IR, Walker WA: Mucosal barrier. In: *Handbook of Mucosal Immunology,* Ogra PL (editor). Academic Press, 1994.

Underdown BJ, Mestecky J: Mucosal immunoglobulins. In: *Handbook of Mucosal Immunology,* Ogra PL (editor). Academic Press, 1994.

REGULATION OF IgA SYNTHESIS

Coffman RL et al: Transforming growth factor-β specifically enhances IgA production by lipopolysaccharide-stimulated murine B cell lymphocytes. *J Exp Med* 1989;**170:**1039.

Defrance T et al: Interleukin-10 and transforming growth factor β cooperate to induce anti-CD40-activated naive human B cells to secrete immunoglobulin A. *J Exp Med* 1992;**175:**671.

Kawanish H et al: Mechanisms regulating IgA production in murine gut-associated lymphoid tissues. *J Exp Med* 1983;**157:**433.

McIntyre TM et al: Novel in vitro model for high-rate IgA class switching. *J Immunol* 1995;**154**(7):3156.

Weinstein PD, Cebra JJ: The preference of switching to IgA expression by Peyer's patch germinal center B cells is likely due to the intrinsic influence of their micro environment. *J Immunol* 1991;**147:**4126.

ORAL TOLERANCE

Mowat A: Oral tolerance and the regulation of immunity to dietary antigens. In: *Handbook of Mucosal Immunology,* Ogra PL (editor). Academic Press, 1994.

Weiner HL et al: Oral tolerance: Immunologic mechanisms and treatment of animal and human organ-specific autoimmune diseases. *Ann Rev Immunol* 1994;**12:**809.

Weiner HL et al: Treatment of autoimmune diseases by oral tolerance to autoantigens. *Adv Exp Med Biol* 1995;**371:**1217.

Whitacre CC et al: Oral tolerance in experimental autoimmune encephalomyelitis. III. Evidence for clonal energy. *J Immunol* 1993;**147:**2155.

MUCOSAL CELL HOMING

Phillips-Quaglita JM, Lamm ME: Lymphocyte homing to mucosal effector sites. In: *Handbook of Mucosal Immunology,* Ogra PL (editor). Academic Press, 1994.

Springer TA: Traffic signals for lymphocyte recirculation and leukocyte emigration: the multi step paradigm. *Cell* 1994;**76:**301.

BREAST MILK

Carlsson B, Hanson LA: Immunologic effects of breastfeeding on the infant. In: *Handbook of Mucosal Immunology,* Ogra PL (editor). Academic Press, 1994.

Goldman RM, Goldman AS: Immunologic components of milk: formation and function. In: *Handbook of Mucosal Immunology,* Ogra PL (editor). Academic Press, 1994.

Section II.
Immunologic Laboratory Tests

Clinical Laboratory Methods for Detection of Antigens & Antibodies

14

Daniel P. Stites, MD, R.P. Channing Rodgers, MD, James D. Folds, PhD, & John Schmitz, PhD

One of the major challenges for modern medicine is the translation of basic advances in immunochemistry and immunobiology into diagnostic and therapeutic procedures that will be useful in the practice of clinical medicine. In the clinical immunology laboratory, tests that use a great many of the recently elucidated principles of basic immunology can be performed on a wide variety of samples taken from patients. The results of these laboratory procedures are then used by practicing physicians in the diagnosis, treatment, and prognosis of clinical disorders. Furthermore, qualitative and quantitative analysis of immune responses has led to better understanding of the pathogenesis of many clinical disorders. This understanding in turn has stimulated further basic scientific research in immunology. In fact, observations made by clinical investigators in immunology have frequently dramatically changed the course of basic research in immunology and related fields. An example is the impetus given to research on T cells and B cells by careful clinical descriptions of patients with thymic aplasia and hypogammaglobulinemia.

Over the past three decades, immunologic laboratory methods have gradually become increasingly more refined and simplified. Because of their inherent specificity and sensitivity, these methods have now achieved a central role in the modern clinical laboratory. The goals of laboratory medicine are to improve the availability, accuracy, and precision of a body of medically important laboratory tests, to ensure correct interpretation, to facilitate data transmission, and to assess the significance and appropriateness of new tests introduced into clinical medicine. A better understanding of the methods used in the immunology laboratory should provide the student and practitioner of medicine with a useful guide for correct application and interpretation of this body of knowledge.

This chapter discusses tests for the detection of antigens and antibodies in clinical practice. One should distinguish between two separate uses of methods described. First, they can be used to detect immune responses and their pathology; second, they can use immunologic principles for quantitative and qualitative detection of antigens or antibodies. Most of the techniques described involve application in the clinical laboratory of the principles of immunochemistry. This chapter and the following one are not meant to be comprehensive laboratory manuals. Rather, the principles of the various immunologic methods and their application to selected clinical problems are reviewed. It is hoped that careful study of the chapters in this section in conjunction with the first section of this book will provide the reader with a solid background for an enhanced understanding of the detailed discussions of clinical immunology and descriptions of specific tests used in various disorders presented in clinical chapters that follow.

The topics covered in this chapter include the following:

1. Immunodiffusion
2. Electrophoresis and immunoelectrophoresis
3. Immunochemical and physiochemical methods
4. Binder–ligand assays
5. Immunohistochemical techniques (immunofluorescence)
6. Agglutination
7. Complement assays
8. Monoclonal antibodies and flow cytometry
9. Predictive value theory

IMMUNODIFFUSION

Immunodiffusion is used for the qualitative and quantitative analysis of antigens and antibodies in serum or other body fluids. The assay readout is the development of a precipitation reaction (the formation of an insoluble antigen–antibody complex from soluble antigen–antibody). Although the formation of

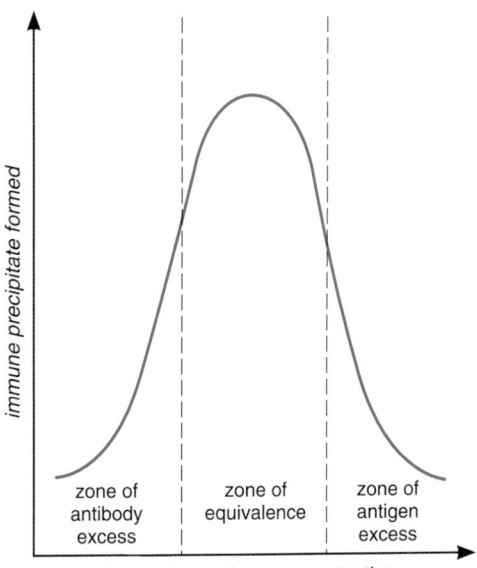

Figure 14–1. Antigen–antibody precipitin curve. Typical precipitin curve resulting from titration of increasing antigen concentration plotted against amount of immune precipitate formed. Amount of antibody is kept constant throughout.

antigen–antibody complexes in a semisolid medium such as agar is dependent on buffer electrolytes, pH, and temperature, the most important determinants of the reaction are the relative concentrations of antigen and antibody. This relationship is depicted schematically in Figure 14–1. Maximal precipitation forms in the area of equivalence, with decreasing amounts in the zones of antigen excess or antibody excess. Thus, formation of precipitation lines in any immunodiffusion system is highly dependent on relative concentrations of antigen and antibody. The **prozone phenomenon** refers to suboptimal precipitation that occurs in the region of antibody excess. Thus, dilutions of antisera must be reacted with fixed amounts of antigen to obtain maximum precipitin lines. The prozone phenomenon may be a cause of misinterpretation of immunoelectrophoresis patterns in the diagnosis of paraproteinemias when large amounts of antibodies are present. Prozone can also result in false-negative serologic tests other than precipitation, such as agglutination reactions.

Immunoprecipitation is a simple and direct means of demonstrating antigen–antibody reactions. The application of immunoprecipitation to the study of bacterial antigens launched the field of serology in the first part of the twentieth century. In 1946, J. Oudin described a system of single diffusion of antigen and antibody in agar-filled tubes. This important advance was soon followed by Ouchterlony's classic description of double diffusion in agar layered on slides. This method is still in use today and has many applications

in the detection and analysis of precipitating antigen–antibody systems.

Immunodiffusion reactions may be classified as single or double. In single immunodiffusion, either antigen or antibody remains fixed and the other reactant is allowed to move and complex with it. In double immunodiffusion, both reactants are free to move toward each other and precipitate. Movement in either form of immunodiffusion may be linear or radial. Specific examples are discussed in the remainder of this section.

Immunodiffusion has a clinical application in the quantitative and qualitative analysis of serum proteins, although this is now often done by more sensitive and automated methods, such as nephelometry, enzyme-linked immunosorbent assay (ELISA), or radioimmunoassay (RIA). Single radial diffusion in agar has largely been supplanted by these methods, which do not rely on immunoprecipitation or diffusion.

METHODS & INTERPRETATION

Double Diffusion in Agar

This simple and extremely useful technique (also called **Ouchterlony analysis**) is based on the principle that when antigen and antibody diffuse through a semisolid medium (eg, agar) they form stable immune complexes, which can be analyzed visually.

The test is performed by pouring molten agar onto glass slides or into Petri dishes and allowing it to harden. Small wells are punched out of the agar a few millimeters apart. Samples containing antigen and antibody are placed in opposing wells and allowed to diffuse toward one another in a moist chamber for 18–24 hours. The resultant precipitation lines that represent antigen–antibody complexes are analyzed visually in indirect light with the aid of a magnifying lens. When antigen and antibody are allowed to diffuse in a radial fashion, an arc that approximates a straight line is formed at the leading edges of the diffusing antigen and antibody. Examples of patterns produced in simple double diffusion are shown in Figure 14–2.

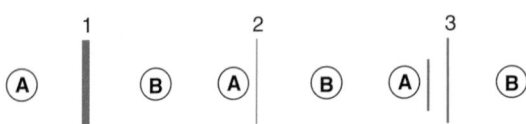

Figure 14–2. Reactions in simple double diffusion. In (1) antigen A and antibody B react equidistantly and intensely at equivalence. In (2) antigen A is present in reduced concentration or has not diffused as rapidly owing to size or charge, forming a precipitin line closer to the antigen well. In (3) a contaminant or impurity present in antigen A is reacting with antibody B.

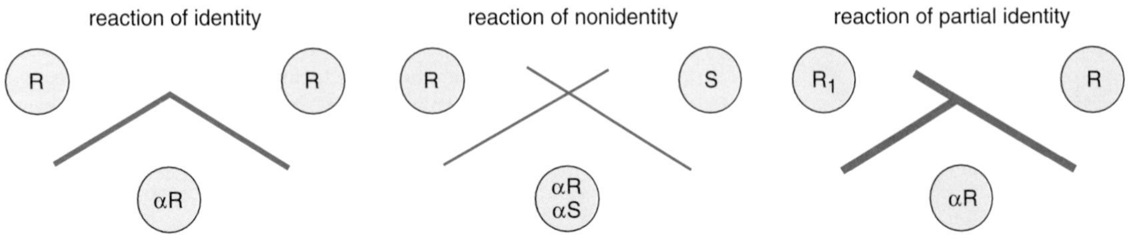

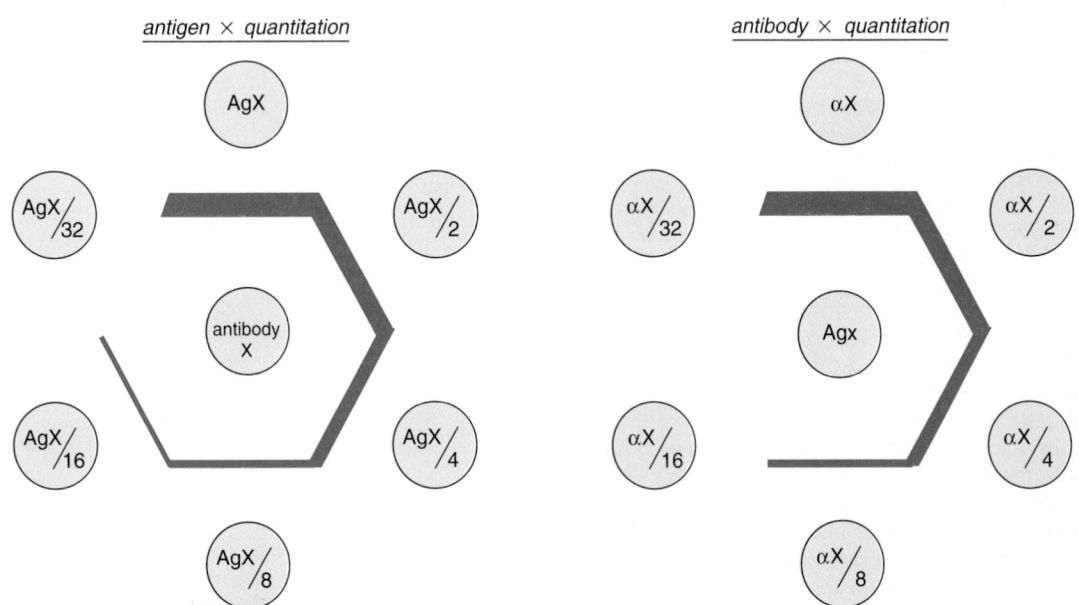

Figure 14–3. Reaction patterns in angular double immunodiffusion (Ouchterlony). R = antigen R, S = antigen S, R_1 = antigen R_1, αR = antibody to R, αS = antibody to S. Reaction of identity: Precisely similar precipitin lines have formed in the reaction of R with αR. Note that the lines intersect at a point. Reaction of nonidentity: Precipitin lines completely cross owing to separate interaction of αR with R and αS with S when R and S are noncross-reacting antigens. Reaction of partial identity: αR reacts with both R and R_1 but forms lines that do not form a complete cross. Antigenic determinants are *partially* shared between R and R_1.

Double diffusion is commonly performed by placing antigen and antibody wells at various angles for comparative purposes. The three basic characteristic patterns of those reactions are shown in Figure 14–3. In addition to these three basic patterns, more complex interrelationships may be seen between antigen and antibody. The formation of a single precipitation line between an antigen and its corresponding antiserum can be used as a rough estimate of antigen or antibody purity. The relative insensitivity of the test and the limitation of immunodiffusion to *precipitating* antigen–antibody reactions partly restrict the applications of this technique, however. It is useful in demonstrating the identity of serologic reactions to antigens from various infectious agents with antibodies of known positive reactivity.

Double immunodiffusion in agar can also be used for semiquantitative analysis in human serologic systems in which the specificity of the precipitation lines has already been determined. Such an analysis is performed by placing antibody in a central well surrounded circumferentially by antigen wells (Fig 14–4). Serial dilutions of antigen are placed in the surrounding wells, and the development of precipitation lines can be taken as a rough measure of antigen concentration. Alternatively, this form of analysis is very

Figure 14–4. Semiquantitative analysis of antigen and antibody by double immunodiffusion. Antigen X (AgX) is serially diluted and placed circumferentially in wells surrounding the central well containing antibody against antigen X. Precipitin lines form with decreasing thickness until no longer visible at dilution of 1:32 of antigen X. On the right, a similar pattern is generated but with serial twofold dilutions of antibody X (αX). Formation of a single precipitin line indicates that a single antigen–antibody reaction has occurred.

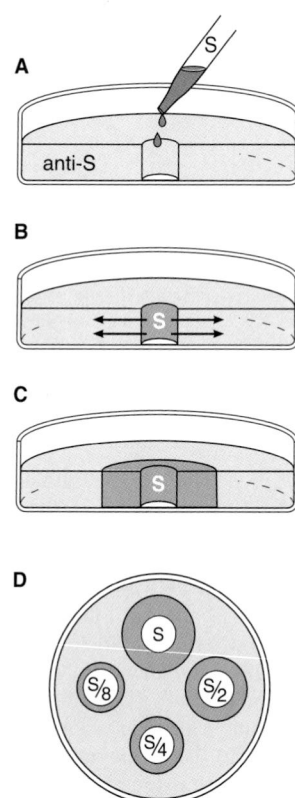

Figure 14–5. Single radial diffusion in agar (radial immuno-diffusion). **A:** Petri dish is filled with semisolid agar solution containing antibody to antigen S. After agar hardens, the center well is filled with a precisely measured amount of material containing antigen S. **B:** Antigen S is allowed to diffuse radially from the center well for 24–48 hours. **C:** Where antigen S meets corresponding antibody to S in the agar, precipitation results. After reaction proceeds to completion or at a timed interval, a sharp border or a ring is formed. **D:** By serial dilution of a known standard quantity of antigen S—S/1, S/2, S/4, S/8—rings of progressively decreasing size are formed. The amount of antigen S in unknown specimens can be calculated and compared with standard in the timed interval (Fahey) method (Fig 14–6).

useful in determining the approximate precipitating titer of an antiserum by simply reversing the location of antigen and antibody in the pattern (see Fig 14–4).

Double immunodiffusion is frequently used for the detection of antibodies to extractable nuclear antigens in patients with various connective tissue diseases. This method has proven to be a reliable technique for their detection. More recently, enzyme immunoassays have been used for this purpose and have been shown to be a more sensitive method for detection of these antibodies.

Single Radial Diffusion

Double immunodiffusion is only semiquantitative. In 1965, Mancini introduced a novel technique involv-

ing single diffusion for accurate quantitative determination of antigens. This technique grew out of the simple linear diffusion technique of Oudin by means of the incorporation of specific antibody into the agar plate. Radial diffusion is based on the principle that a quantitative relationship exists between the amount of antigen placed in a well cut in the agar–antibody plate and the resulting ring of precipitation. The technique is performed as diagrammed in Figure 14–5.

In the method described originally by Mancini, the *area* circumscribed by the precipitation ring was proportionate to the antigen concentration. This end point method requires that the precipitation rings reach the maximal possible size, which often requires 48–72 hours of diffusion. Alternatively, the single radial diffusion method of J. Fahey allows measurement of the rings prior to full development. In this modification, the logarithm of the antigen concentration is proportionate to the *diameter* of the ring.

A standard curve is experimentally determined with known antigen standards, and the equation that describes this curve can then be used for the determination of antigen concentration corresponding to any diameter size (Fig 14–6). The sensitivity of these methods is in the range of 1–3 µg/mL of antigen.

An important clinical application of single radial diffusion is in the measurement of serum proteins—for example, immunoglobulin concentrations. A monospecific antiserum directed only at Fc or H chain

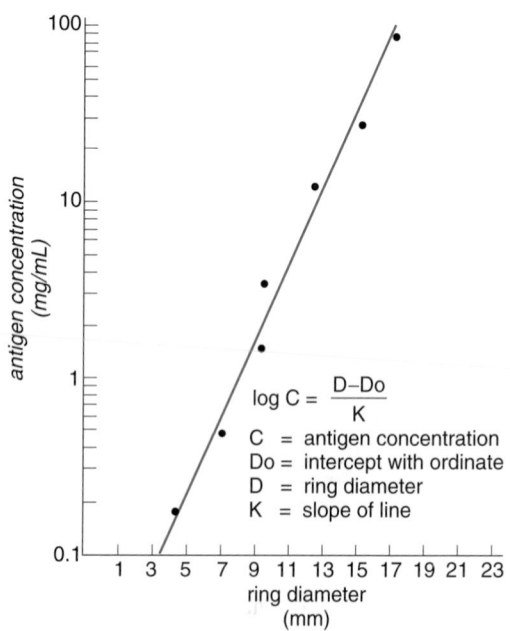

Figure 14–6. Standard curve for single radial diffusion. Relationship between ring diameter and antigen concentration is described by the line constructed from known amounts of antigen. Equation and curve for timed interval (Fahey) method.

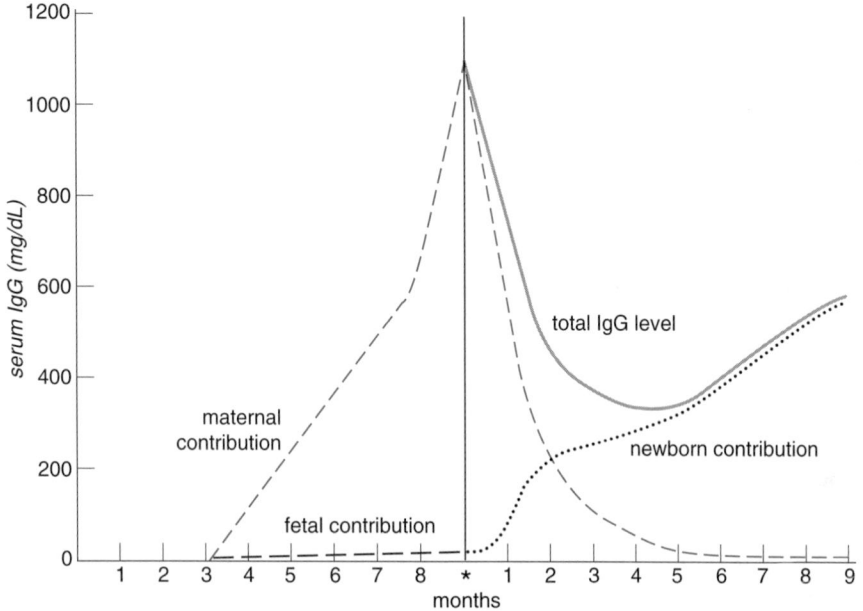

Figure 14–7. Development of IgG levels with age. Relationship of development of normal levels of IgG during fetal and newborn stages and maternal contribution. (Modified and reproduced, with permission, from Allansmith M et al: *J Pediatr* 1968;**72**:289.)

determinants of the immunoglobulin molecule must be incorporated into the agar to determine immunoglobulin concentrations, since L (light)-chain determinants are shared among immunoglobulin classes. Owing to the relatively low concentrations of IgD and IgE in human serum, this technique is used primarily to determine the other three immunoglobulin classes: IgG, IgA, and IgM. By decreasing the amount of specific anti-immunoglobulin antiserum placed in the agar, however, so-called low-level plates can be produced that have increased sensitivity for detection of reduced levels of serum immunoglobulins (IgG, IgA, IgM, and IgD).

There are a number of common pitfalls in the interpretation of single radial diffusion tests for immunoglobulin quantitation: (1) Polymeric forms of immunoglobulin such as occur in multiple myeloma or Waldenström's macroglobulinemia diffuse more slowly than native monomers, resulting in underestimation of immunoglobulin concentrations in these diseases. (2) High-molecular-weight immune complexes that may circulate in cryoglobulinemia or rheumatoid arthritis result in falsely low values by a similar mechanism. (3) Low-molecular-weight forms such as 7S IgM in sera of patients with macroglobulinemia, systemic lupus erythematosus, rheumatoid arthritis, or ataxia-telangiectasia may give falsely high values. This phenomenon results from the fact that monomeric IgM diffuses more rapidly than the pentameric IgM parent molecule, which is used as the standard. (4) Reversed precipitation may occur when the test human serum

contains anti-immunoglobulin antibodies. In such a circumstance, diffusion and precipitation occur in two directions simultaneously and may result in falsely high values. This phenomenon has been well documented in the case of subjects with IgA deficiency who have antibodies to ruminant proteins. These proteins cross the IgA-deficient intestinal mucosa, thereby gaining access to lymphatic tissues and stimulating anti-IgA responses. The problem of IgA quantitation in this circumstance can be avoided by using anti-immunoglobulin from rabbits (ie, a nonruminant species).

Although this assay is relatively simple to perform, great care must be taken to set it up since variations in the amount of sample placed in the well affect the final results. In addition, a consistent measuring technique must be used to obtain reproducible results. This assay provides the benefits of simplicity and lower cost; however, other, more automated, methods are available that allow a higher throughput, but at increased cost.

APPLICATIONS: SERUM IMMUNOGLOBULIN LEVELS IN HEALTH & DISEASE

Serum immunoglobulin levels are dependent on a variety of developmental, genetic, and environmental factors. These include ethnic background, age, sex, history of allergies or recurrent infections, and geographic factors (eg, endemic infestation with parasites results in elevated IgE levels). The patient's age is especially important in the interpretation of immunoglobulin levels. Normal human infants are born with very low levels of serum immunoglobulins that they have synthesized; the entire IgG portion of cord serum has been transferred transplacentally from the mother (Fig 14–7). If an infection occurs in utero, cord IgM and IgA are elevated. After birth, maternal IgG decays, resulting in a falling serum IgG level. This trend is reversed with the onset of significant autologous IgG synthesis. There is a gradual and progressive increase in IgG, IgA, and IgM levels until late adolescence, when nearly normal adult levels are achieved (Fig 14–8). Furthermore, it is clear that there is a great deal of variability in immunoglobulin levels in the healthy population (see Fig 14–8).

In routine practice, only IgG, IgA, IgM, and IgE levels are ordinarily measured. Abnormalities of serum IgD concentrations have not clearly been associated with specific disease states. In fact, this immunoglobulin is the major B-cell receptor for antigens and plays only a minor role as a circulating antibody. IgE levels, on the other hand, are useful in differential diagnosis of allergic, parasitic, and rare immunodeficiency states. Measurement of serum IgE levels requires sensitive methods such as RIA or ELISA. Measurement of serum IgG levels is particularly valuable in diagnosis and in monitoring immunoglobulin replacement in hypogammaglobulinemic patients.

Individual changes in serum immunoglobulin levels have been recorded in many diseases. A partial list of the instances of quantitative abnormalities in immunoglobulins is listed in Table 14–1. For a detailed discussion of immunoglobulin disorders, the reader is referred to Chapters 21 and 23 as well as other chapters in the clinical section of this volume.

ELECTROPHORESIS & IMMUNOELECTROPHORESIS

The heterogeneity in human serum proteins can be readily analyzed by electrophoresis. The separation of proteins in an electrical field was perfected in 1937 by Arne W. Tiselius, who used free or moving boundary electrophoresis. Owing to the relative complexity of this method, however, zone electrophoresis in a stabilizing medium such as paper or cellulose acetate has replaced free electrophoresis for clinical use.

In 1952, a two-stage method was reported that combined electrophoresis with immunodiffusion for the detection of tetanus toxoid by antiserum. Shortly thereafter, the now classic method of immunoelectrophoresis was introduced by C. Williams and P. Grabar and by M. Poulik. In this technique, both electrophoresis and double immunodiffusion are performed on the same agar-

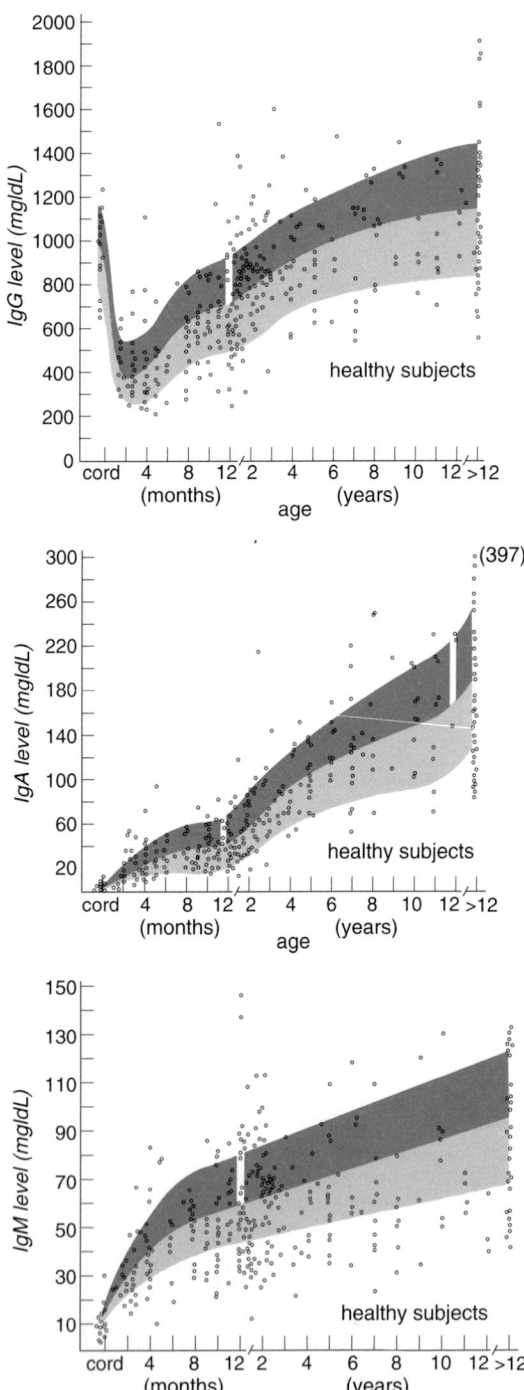

Figure 14–8. An example of variation of healthy subjects' serum levels of IgG, IgA, and IgM with age. Scattergrams of levels of IgG, IgA, and IgM in healthy subjects. Shaded areas are = 1 SD of the mean; each point represents one subject. (Reproduced, with permission, from Stiehm ER, Fudenberg HH: *Pediatrics* 1966;**37**:718.)

Table 14–1. Serum immunoglobulin levels in disease.

Diseases	IgG	IgA	IgM
Immunodeficiency disorders			
Combined immunodeficiency	↓↓↔↓↓↓	↓↓↔↓↓↓	↓↓↔↓↓↓
X-linked hypogammaglobulinemia	↓↓↔↓↓↓	↓↓↔↓↓↓	↓↓↔↓↓↓
Common variable immunodeficiency	↓↔↓↓↓	↓↔↓↓↓	↓↔↓↓↓
Selective IgA deficiency	N	↓↓↓	N
Protein-losing gastroenteropathies	N↔↓↓↓	N↔↓↓↓	N↔↓↓↓
Acute thermal burns	N↔↓↓↓	N↔↓↓↓	N↔↓↓↓
Nephrotic syndrome	N↔↓↓↓	N↔↓↓↓	N↔↓↓↓
Monoclonal gammopathies (MG)			
IgG (eg, G-myeloma)	N↔↑↑↑	N↔↓↓↓	N↔↓↓↓
IgA (eg, A-myeloma)	N↔↓↓↓	N↔↑↑↑	N↔↓↓↓
IgM (eg, M-macroglobulinemia)	N↔↓↓↓	N↔↓↓↓	N↔↑↑↑
L-chain disease (ie, Bence Jones myeloma)	N↔↓↓↓	N↔↓↓↓	N↔↓↓↓
Chronic lymphocytic leukemia	N↔↓↓↓	N↔↓↓↓	N↔↓↓↓
Infections			
Infectious mononucleosis	↑↔↑↑	N↔↑	↑↔↑↑
Acquired immunodeficiency syndrome (AIDS)	↑↑	↑↑	↑↑
Subacute bacterial endocarditis	↑↔↑↑	↓↔N	↑↔↑↑
Tuberculosis	↑↔↑↑	N↔↑↑↑	↓↔N
Actinomycosis	↑↑↑	↑↑	↑↑↑
Deep fungus diseases	N	N↔↑	N
Bartonellosis	↑	↓↔N	↑↑↔↑↑↑
Liver diseases			
Infectious hepatitis	↑↔↑↑	N↔↑	N↔↑↑
Laennec's cirrhosis	↑↔↑↑↑	↑↔↑↑↑	N↔↑↑
Biliary cirrhosis	N	N	↑↔↑↑
Chronic active hepatitis	↑↑↑	↑	N↔↑↑
Collagen disorders			
Systemic lupus erythematosus	↑↔↑↑	N↔↑	N↔↑↑
Rheumatoid arthritis	N↔↑↑↑	↑↔↑↑↑	N↔↑↑
Sjögren's syndrome	N↔↑	N↔↑	N↔↑↑
Scleroderma	N↔↑	N	N↔↑
Miscellaneous			
Sarcoidosis	N↔↑↑	N↔↑↑	N↔↑
Hodgkin's disease	↓↔↑↑	↓↔↑	↓↔↑↑
Monocytic leukemia	N↔↑	N↔↑	N↔↑↑
Cystic fibrosis	↑↔↑↑	↑↔↑↑	N↔↑↑

N = normal, ↑ = slight increase, ↑↑ = moderate increase, ↑↑↑ = marked increase, ↓ = slight decrease, ↓↓ = moderate decrease, ↓↓↓ = marked decrease, ↔ = range.
Source: Modified and reproduced, with permission, from Ritzmann SE, Daniels JC (editors): *Serum Protein Abnormalities: Diagnostic and Clinical Aspects.* Little, Brown, 1975.

coated slide. Immunoelectrophoresis has become an important tool for clinical paraprotein analysis as well as a standard method for immunochemical analysis of a wide variety of proteins. More recently, immunofixation electrophoresis and electroimmunodiffusion methods have been introduced. Various electrophoretic methods and examples of their uses in clinical immunodiagnosis are described in the following paragraphs.

ZONE ELECTROPHORESIS

Proteins are separated in zone electrophoresis almost exclusively on the basis of their surface charge (Fig 14–9). The supporting medium is theoretically inert and does not impede or enhance the flow of molecules in the electric field. Generally, paper, agarose, or cellulose acetate strips are used as supporting media. A major advantage of cellulose acetate, however, is the speed of completion of electrophoretic migration (ie, 60–90 minutes compared with hours for paper). Additionally, cellulose acetate is optically clear; microquantities of proteins may be applied; and it is adaptable to histochemical staining procedures. For these reasons, cellulose acetate or agarose is preferred as the supporting medium for clinical zone electrophoresis.

In the technique itself, serum or other biologic fluid samples are placed at the origin and separated by electrophoresis for about 90 minutes, using alkaline buffer solutions. The strips are then stained for protein and scanned in a densitometer. In the densitometer, the stained strip is passed through a light beam. Variable absorption due to different serum protein concentrations is detected by a photoelectric cell and reproduced by an analog recorder as a tracing (see Fig 14–9). Scanning converts the band pattern into peaks and allows for quantitation of the major peaks. Normal human serum is separated into five major

A

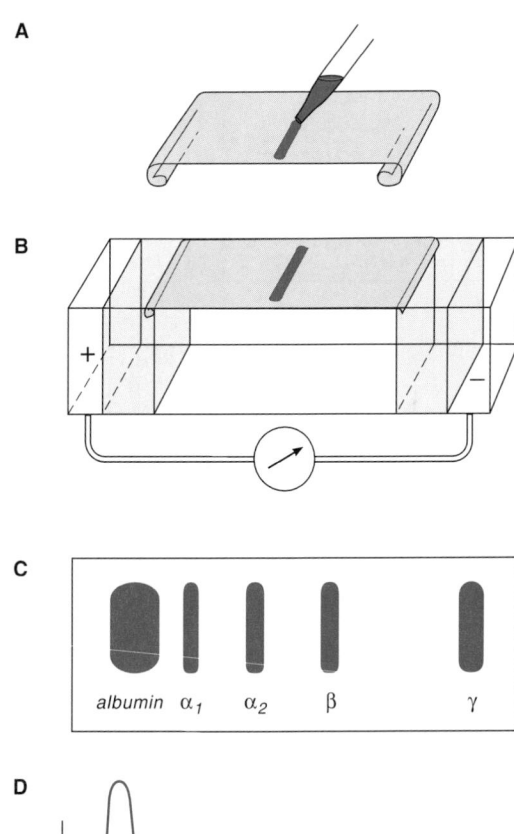

B

C

albumin   α₁   α₂   β   γ

D

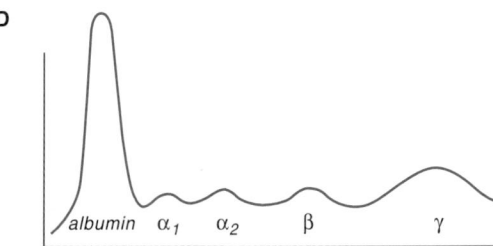

albumin   α₁   α₂   β   γ

Figure 14–9. Technique of cellulose acetate zone electrophoresis. **A:** Small amount of serum or other fluid is applied to cellulose acetate strip. **B:** Electrophoresis of sample in electrolyte buffer is performed. **C:** Separated protein bands are visualized in characteristic position after being stained. **D:** Densitometer scanning from cellulose acetate strip converts bands to characteristic peaks of albumin, α_1-globulin, α_2-globulin, β-globulin, and γ-globulin.

electrophoretic bands: albumin, α_1-globulin, α_2-globulin, β-globulin, and γ-globulin, by this method.

Applications

Zone electrophoresis is useful in the diagnosis of human paraprotein disorders such as multiple myeloma and Waldenström's macroglobulinemia (Fig 14–10). In these disorders, an electrophoretically restricted protein spike usually occurs in the γ-globulin region of the electrophoretogram. Since in zone electrophoresis the trailing edge of immunoglobulins extends into the β region and occasionally the α region,

spikes in these regions are also consistent with paraproteinemic disorders involving immunoglobulins.

A marked decrease in serum γ-globulin concentration such as occurs in hypogammaglobulinemia is sometimes detected by this technique (see Fig 14–10). Reduction in IgA or IgM to very low levels cannot be detected by this method, since they represent such a relatively small fraction of total serum immunoglobulins. Free light chains are readily detectable in urine when present in increased amounts such as in Bence Jones proteinuria of myeloma (Fig 14–11). Zone electrophoresis in agarose gels has also been useful in the diagnosis of certain central nervous system diseases with alterations in cerebrospinal fluid proteins (Figs 14–12 and 14–13).

Oligoclonal bands in cerebrospinal fluid with restricted electrophoretic mobility have been detected in about 90% of clinically definite cases of multiple sclerosis. Agarose electrophoresis gel in conjunction with measurement of cerebrospinal fluid IgG/albumin ratios makes possible a fairly high degree of specificity for diagnosis of multiple sclerosis (see Chapter 40 and Fig 40–3).

Abnormalities in levels of serum proteins other than immunoglobulins may also be detected by serum protein electrophoresis. Hypoproteinemia involving all serum fractions occurs during excessive protein loss, usually in the gastrointestinal tract. Reduction in albumin alone commonly occurs in many diseases of the liver, kidneys, or gastrointestinal tract or with severe burns. α_1-globulin decrease may indicate α_1-antitrypsin deficiency, and an increase may reflect acute-phase reactions occurring in many inflammatory and neoplastic disorders. An increase in α_2-globulins usually reflects the nephrotic syndrome or hemolysis with increased hemoglobin–haptoglobin in the serum. Because of its relative insensitivity, zone electrophoresis is almost always a presumptive screening test for serum protein abnormalities. Specific quantitative biochemical or immunologic tests must be performed to definitively identify the particular protein.

IMMUNOELECTROPHORESIS

Immunoelectrophoresis combines electrophoretic separation, diffusion, and immune precipitation of proteins. Both identification and approximate quantitation can thereby be accomplished for individual proteins present in serum, urine, or other biologic fluid.

In this technique (Fig 14–13), a glass slide is covered with molten agar or agarose in an alkaline buffer solution. An antigen well and antibody trough are cut with a template-cutting device. The serum sample (antigen) is placed in the antigen well and is separated in an electric field with a potential difference of approximately 3.3 V/cm for 30–60 minutes. Antiserum is then placed in the trough, and both serum and antinormal serum

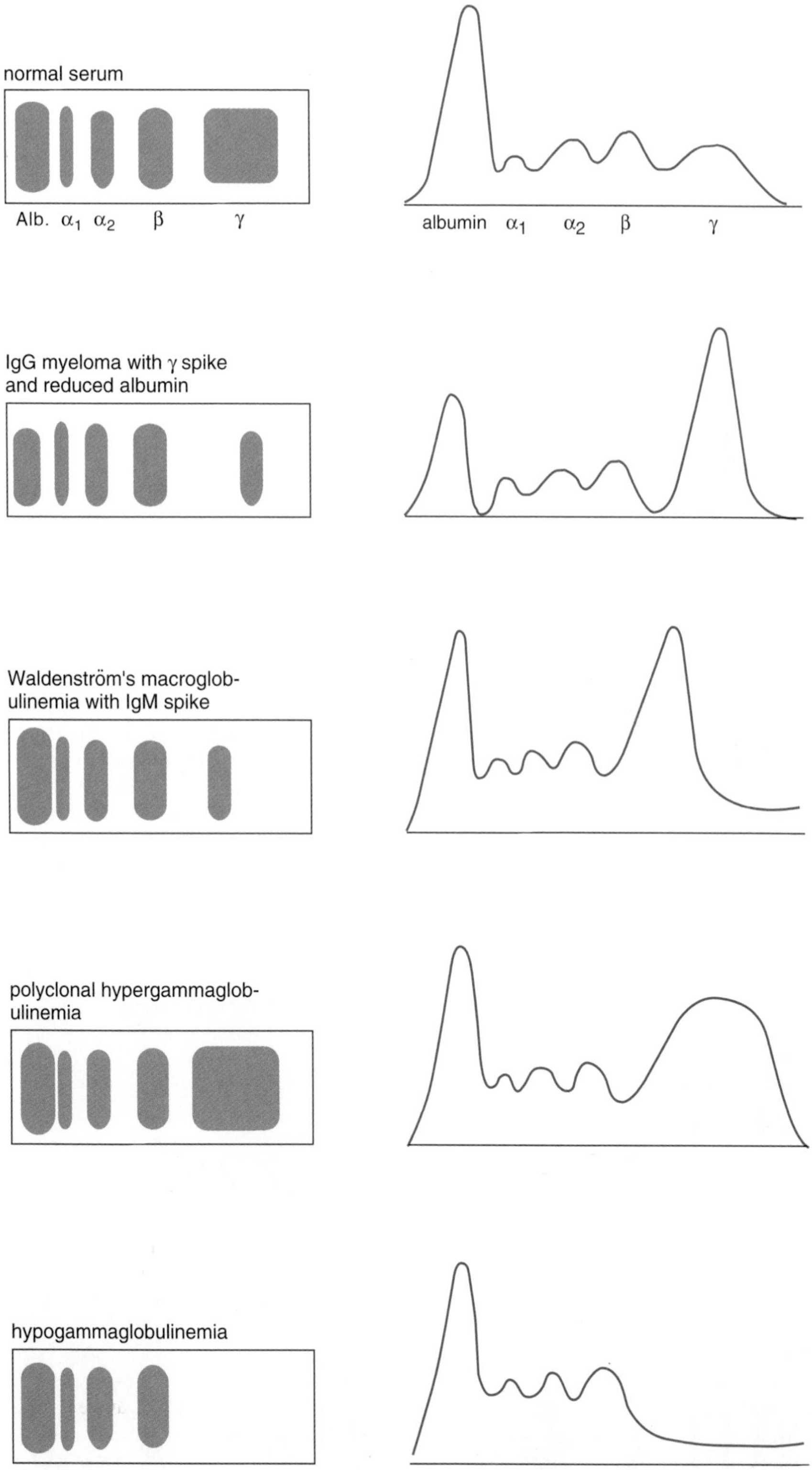

Alb.　α_1　α_2　β　γ

albumin　α_1　α_2　β　γ

IgG myeloma with γ spike
and reduced albumin

Waldenström's macroglob-
ulinemia with IgM spike

polyclonal hypergammaglobulinemia

hypogammaglobulinemia

Figure 14–10. Zone electrophoresis patterns of serum immunoglobulin abnormalities in various diseases.

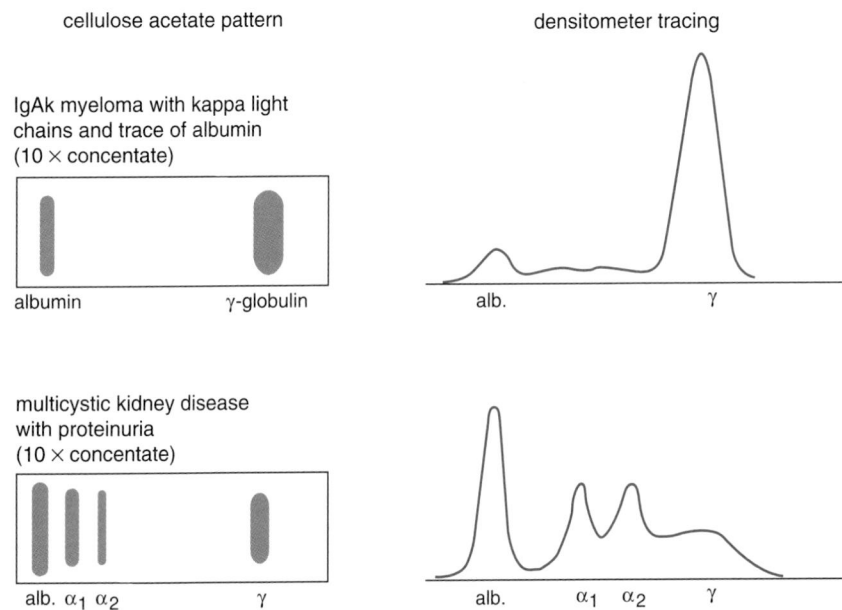

Figure 14–11. Zone electrophoresis patterns of urine abnormalities in various diseases.

bodies are allowed to diffuse for 18–24 hours. The resulting precipitation lines may then be photographed or the slide washed, dried, and stained for a permanent record.

A comparison of the relationship of precipitation lines developed in normal serum by immunoelectrophoresis and zone electrophoresis is shown in Figure 14–14.

Applications

In the laboratory diagnosis of paraproteinemias, the results of zone electrophoresis and immunoelectrophoresis should be combined. The presence of a sharp increase or spike in the γ-globulin region on zone electrophoresis strongly suggests the presence of a monoclonal paraprotein. It is necessary to perform immunoelectrophoresis, however, to determine the

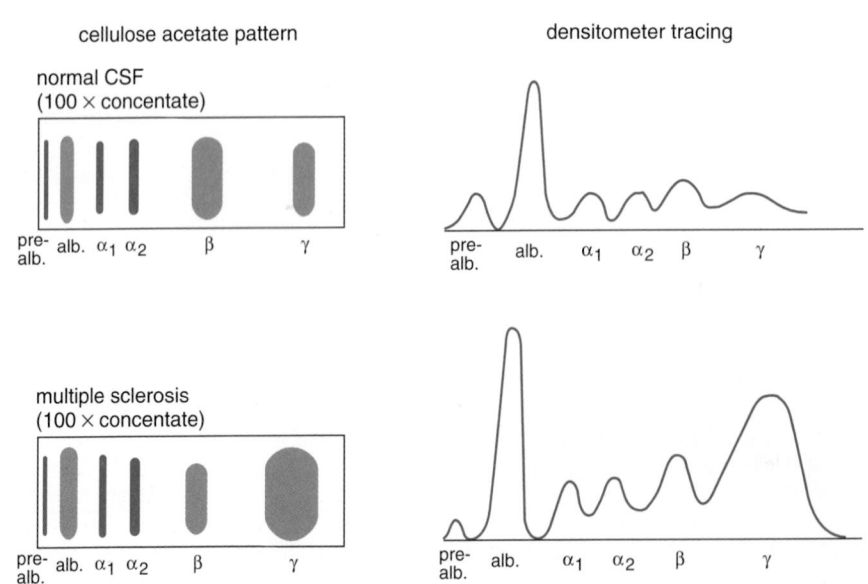

Figure 14–12. Zone electrophoresis patterns of cerebrospinal fluid from normal subject and multiple sclerosis patient.

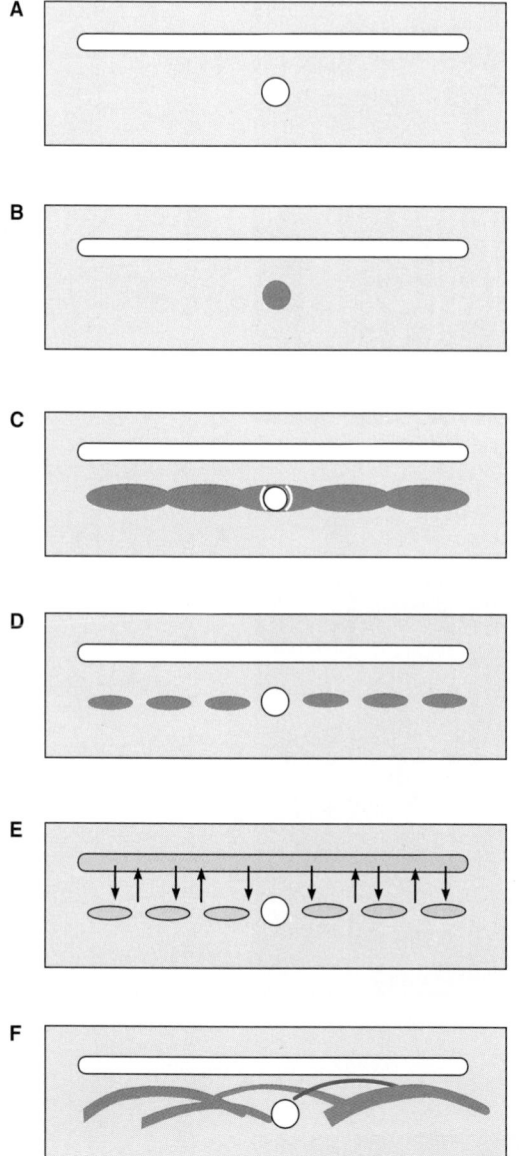

Figure 14–13. Technique of immunoelectrophoresis. **A:** Semisolid agar poured onto glass slide and antigen well and antiserum trough cut out of agar. **B:** Antigen well filled with human serum. **C:** Serum separated by electrophoresis. **D:** Antiserum trough filled with antiserum to whole human serum. **E:** Serum and antiserum diffuse into agar. **F:** Precipitin lines form for individual serum proteins.

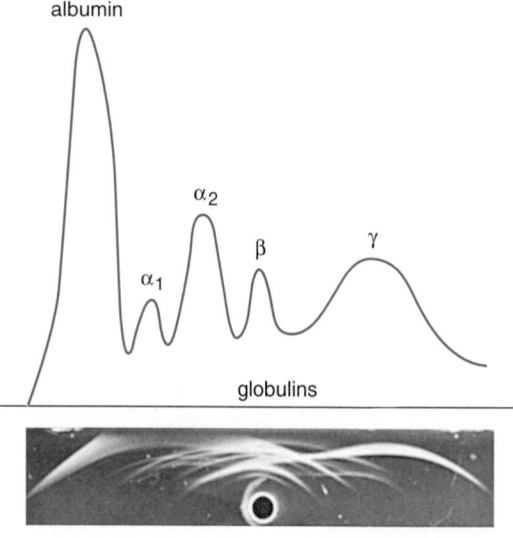

Figure 14–14. Comparison of patterns of zone electrophoresis and immunoelectrophoresis of normal human serum.

mune deficiency disorders can be analyzed with this technique. A further quantitative analysis, however, such as single radial diffusion, nephelometry, or RIA, should be performed for measurement of immunoglobulin levels.

Immunoelectrophoresis can be used to identify L chains in the urine of patients with plasma cell dyscrasias or autoimmune disorders. Thus, with specific anti-κ or anti-λ antisera, the monoclonal nature of Bence Jones protein in myeloma can be confirmed.

Antisera to "free light chains" (κ or λ) obtained from the urine of myeloma patients occasionally reveal antigenic determinants not present on chains "bound" to heavy chains in the intact immunoglobulin molecule. In H-chain diseases, fragments of the immunoglobulin H chain are present in increased amounts in the serum (see Chapter 45). It was by careful analysis of immunoelectrophoretic patterns that E. Franklin initially discovered the existence of this rare but extremely interesting group of disorders. Immunoelectrophoresis is also helpful in identifying increased amounts of proteins present in the cerebrospinal fluid in patients with various neurologic diseases.

Immunofixation Electrophoresis

This technique involves separation of proteins electrophoretically in a gel, followed by immunoprecipitation in situ with monospecific antisera (Fig 14–16). Nonprecipitated proteins are removed by washing and the immunoprecipitation bands revealed with a protein stain. This method has been employed clinically to identify C3 conversion products and to identify paraproteins. This latter application is especially helpful for low-level IgM or IgA components, which may

exact H-chain class and L-chain type of the paraprotein. Several examples of the use of immunoelectrophoresis in demonstrating the identity of human serum paraproteins are shown in Figure 14–15.

Determination of H-chain class and L-chain type distinguishes polyclonal from monoclonal increases in γ-globulin (see Fig 14–15). Additionally, decreased or absent immunoglobulins observed in various im-

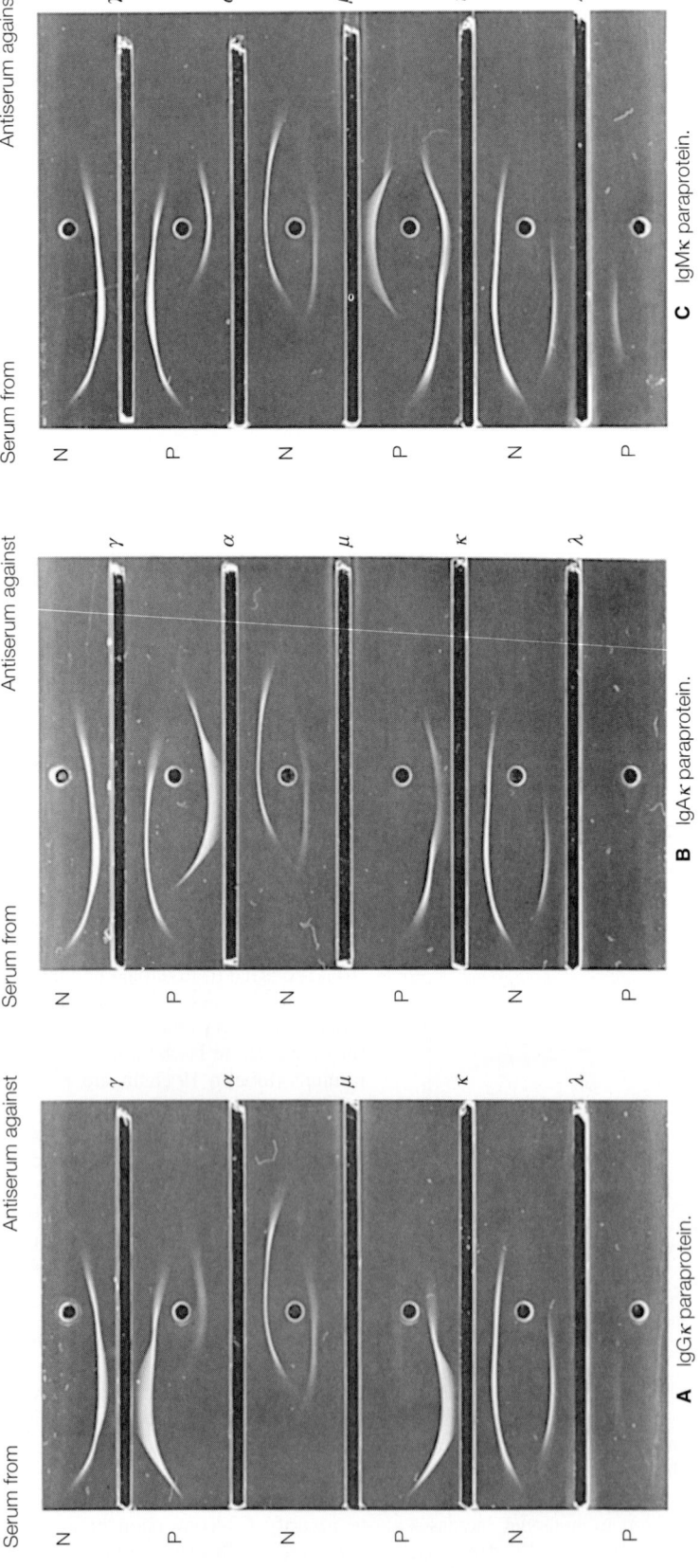

Figure 14–15. Immunoelectrophoresis patterns of serum in various diseases. *A:* IgGκ paraprotein. *B:* IgAκ paraprotein. *C:* IgMκ paraprotein.

A IgGκ paraprotein. **B** IgAκ paraprotein. **C** IgMκ paraprotein.

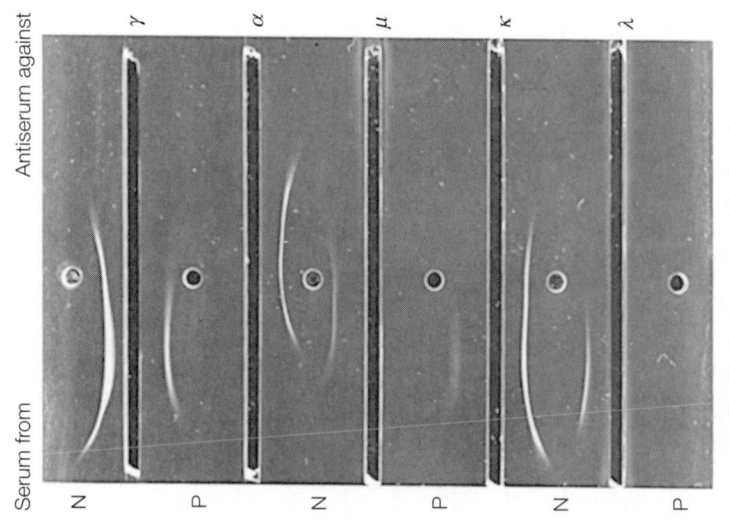

Serum from   Antiserum against

N

P

N

P

N

P

γ

α

μ

κ

λ

D Polyclonal hypergammaglobulinemia (increase in IgG, IgA, and IgM).

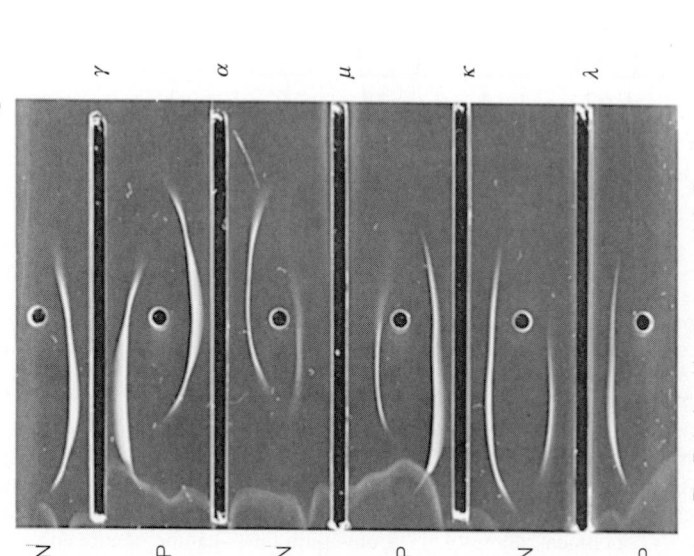

Serum from   Antiserum against

N

P

N

P

N

P

γ

α

μ

κ

λ

E Panhypogammaglobulinemia (decreased IgG, IgA, IgM).

Figure 14–15. *Continued.* ***D:*** Polyclonal hypergammaglobulinemia. ***E:*** Panhypogammaglobulinemia. Individual patterns of serum from normal individuals (N) and patients with various serum protein abnormalities (P). In each case, N and P sera are reacted against antisera which are monospecific for γ, α, and μ heavy chains and κ and λ light chains.

223

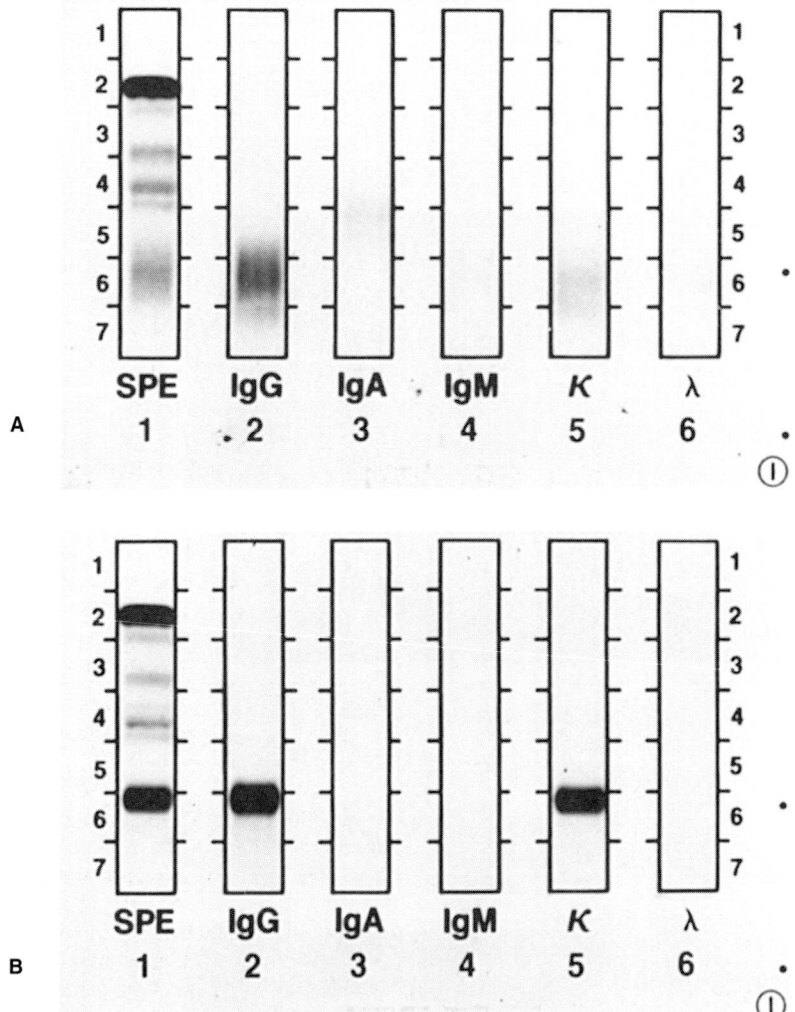

Figure 14–16. Immunofixation electrophoresis. **A:** Normal serum pattern. In lane 1 antibody to whole serum has detected normal serum proteins. In lanes 2–6 specific antibody to various light and heavy chains has detected the polyclonal immunoglobulins present in normal serum. The faint patterns for IgA, IgM, and κ reflect the relatively low concentrations of those molecules. **B:** IgG kappa paraprotein detected in serum from a patient with multiple myeloma. Note the very heavy IgG and kappa bands, which share the same position on the electropherogram. There is a reduction in other immunoglobulins, but other serum proteins are easily seen in lane 1.

be buried in an excess of normal IgG. There are several modifications of this basic method, such as overlay with radioactive or enzyme-linked antibodies, that markedly increase its sensitivity. In clinical laboratories, its main use is for resolution of serum proteins in difficult diagnostic problems in which results of routine methods are equivocal. It is commonly used as a substitute for immunoelectrophoresis.

ELECTROIMMUNODIFFUSION

In immunodiffusion techniques described earlier in this chapter, antigen and antibody are allowed to come into contact and to precipitate in agar purely by diffusion. The chance of antigen and antibody meeting, however—and thus the speed of development of a precipitin line—can be greatly enhanced by electrically driving the two together. The technique of electroimmunodiffusion is useful in the serologic diagnosis of infectious diseases by serum **antigen** detection. Although numerous variations have been described coupling electrophoresis with diffusion, only two have as yet achieved any degree of clinical applicability. These are **one-dimensional double electroimmunodiffusion** (counterimmunoelectrophoresis) and **one-dimensional single electroimmunodiffusion** (Laurell's rocket electrophoresis).

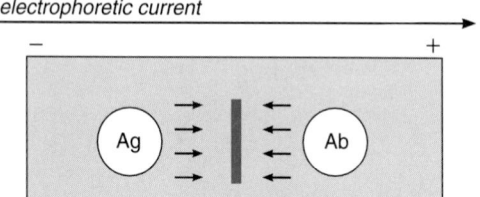

electrophoretic current

Figure 14–17. Double electroimmunodiffusion in one dimension. Antigen (Ag) and antibody (Ab) are placed in wells and driven together with an electric current. A precipitin line forms within a few hours after electrophoresis was begun.

One-Dimensional Double Electroimmunodiffusion

This method is also known as countercurrent immunoelectrophoresis, counterimmunoelectrophoresis, and electroprecipitation. The basic principle of the method involves electrophoresis of antigen and antibody in opposite directions simultaneously from separate wells in a gel, with resultant precipitation at a point intermediate between their origins (Fig 14–17).

The principal disadvantages of double diffusion without electromotive force are the time required for precipitation (24 hours) and the relative lack of sensitivity. Double electroimmunodiffusion in one dimension can produce visible precipitin lines within 30 minutes and is approximately 10 times more sensitive than standard double diffusion techniques. This technique is only semiquantitative, however. Some of the antigens and antibodies detected by double electroimmunodiffusion are listed in Table 14–2.

One-Dimensional Single Electroimmunodiffusion

This method is also known as rocket electrophoresis, or the Laurell technique. Its principal application has been to quantitate antigens other than immunoglobulins. In this technique, antiserum to the particular antigen or antigens one wishes to quantitate is incorporated into an agarose supporting medium on a glass slide in a fixed position so that antibody does not migrate. The specimen containing an unknown quantity of the antigen is placed in a small well. Electrophoresis of the antigen into the antibody-containing agarose is then performed. The resultant pattern of immunoprecipita-

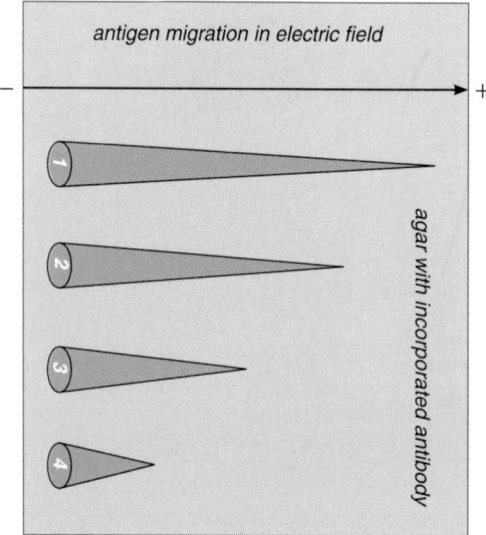

antigen migration in electric field

agar with incorporated antibody

Figure 14–18. Single electroimmunodiffusion in one dimension (rocket electrophoresis, Laurell technique). Antigen is placed in progressively decreasing amounts in wells numbered 1–4. Electrophoresis is performed, and antigen is driven into antibody-containing agar. Precipitin pattern forms in the shape of a "rocket." The amount of antigen is directly proportionate to the length of the rocket.

tion resembles a spike or rocket—hence the term *rocket electrophoresis* (Fig 14–18).

This pattern occurs because precipitation occurs along the lateral margins of the moving boundary of antigen as the antigen is driven into the agar containing the antibody. Gradually, as antigen is lost through precipitation, its concentration at the leading edge diminishes and the lateral margins converge to form a sharp point. The total distance of antigen migration for a given antiserum concentration is linearly proportionate to the antigen concentration. The sensitivity of this technique is approximately 0.5 μg/mL for proteins. Unfortunately, the weak negative charge of immunoglobulins prevents their electrophoretic mobility in this system unless special electrolytes and agar are employed. Several commercial systems are available for quantitating serum immunoglobulins and complement components by this technique.

IMMUNOCHEMICAL & PHYSICOCHEMICAL METHODS

Serum protein disorders can usually be effectively evaluated by immunodiffusion and electrophoretic methods. Occasionally, more detailed study of immunologically relevant serum constituents is necessary. In this section, we describe a number of the

Table 14–2. Examples of clinical applications of double electroimmunodiffusion.

Cryptococcus-specific antigen in cerebrospinal fluid
Meningococcus-specific antigen in cerebrospinal fluid
Haemophilus-specific antigen in cerebrospinal fluid
Fibrinogen
Cord IgM in intrauterine infection
Carcinoembryonic antigen (CEA)
α_1-Fetoprotein
Fungal precipitins

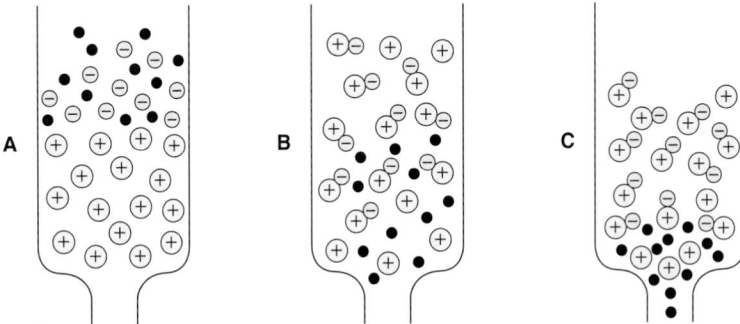

Figure 14–19. Principles of ion-exchange chromatography. Three stages of protein separation by ion-exchange chromatography are shown: **A:** The column bed is made up of a matrix of positively charged cellulose beads +. **B:** The negatively charged molecules ⊖ in the protein mixture bind to the column and are retained. **C:** The neutral molecules • pass between the charged particles and are eluted.

more complex immunochemical and physicochemical techniques that have proved to be important adjuncts in the characterization of serum protein and other disorders. These techniques may be available in the clinical laboratory. They include column chromatography; measurement of serum viscosity; and methods to detect cryoglobulins, pyroglobulins, and immune complexes.

CHROMATOGRAPHY

Chromatography is a technique of separating molecules, usually in a column, by partitioning them between a **liquid moving phase** and a **solid stationary phase,** which are in contact with each other. The sample containing materials to be separated is miscible with the moving phase. Chromatographic techniques are useful methods for protein fractionation and isolation of immunoglobulins. In these techniques, a sample is layered on the top of a glass cylinder or column filled with a synthetic gel and is allowed to flow through the gel. The physical characteristics of protein molecules result in retention in the gel matrix to differing degrees, and subsequent elution under appropriate conditions permits protein separation.

Ion-Exchange Chromatography

Ion-exchange chromatography separates proteins by taking advantage of differences in their electric charges. The functional unit of the gel is a charged group absorbed on an insoluble backbone such as cellulose, cross-linked dextran, agarose, or acrylic copolymers. Diethylaminoethyl (DEAE), a positively charged group, is the functional unit of anion exchangers used for fractionation of negatively charged molecules (Fig 14–19). Carboxymethyl (CM), a negatively charged group, is the functional unit of cation exchangers used for fractionation of positively charged molecules. Changing the pH of the buffer passing through the column affects the charge of the protein molecule. Increasing the molarity of the buffer provides more ions to compete with the protein for binding to the gel. By gradually increasing the molarity or decreasing the pH of the elution buffer, the proteins are eluted in order of increasing number of charged groups bound to the gel. DEAE-cellulose chromatography is an excellent technique for isolation of IgG, which can be obtained nearly free of all other serum proteins.

Gel Filtration

Gel filtration separates molecules according to their size. The gel is made of porous dextran beads. Protein molecules larger than the largest pores of the beads cannot penetrate the gel pores. Thus, they pass through the gel in the liquid phase outside the beads and are eluted first. Smaller molecules penetrate the beads to different extents depending on their size and shape. Solute molecules within the gel beads maintain a concentration equilibrium with solute in the liquid phase outside the beads; thus, a particular molecular species moves as a band through the column. Molecules therefore appear in the column effluent in order of decreasing size (Fig 14–20).

IgM can be easily separated from other serum immunoglobulins by gel filtration. Figure 14–21 shows the separation of the IgM and the IgG components of a mixed IgM–IgG cryoglobulin. Gel filtration is widely used also to separate H and L chains of immunoglobulins or to isolate pure Bence Jones proteins from the urine of patients with multiple myeloma.

Affinity Chromatography

Affinity chromatography uses specific and reversible biologic interaction between the gel material and the substance to be isolated. The specificity of the binding properties is obtained by covalent coupling of an appropriate ligand to an insoluble matrix, such as agarose or dextran beads. The gel so obtained is able to absorb from a mixed solution the substance to be isolated. After unbound substances have been washed

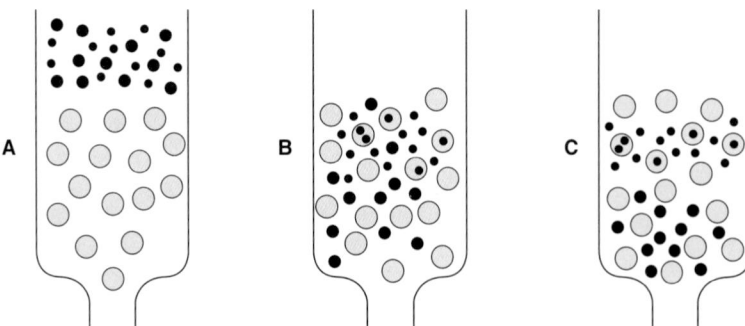

Figure 14–20. Principles of gel filtration chromatography. Three stages of protein separation by gel filtration are shown. **A:** Open circle ○ represents polymerized beads onto which a mixture of small • and large ● protein molecules is layered. **B:** The molecules enter and pass through the column at different rates depending primarily on size and are separated by a simple sieving process. **C:** Larger molecules are eluted while smaller ones are retained.

out of the column, the purified compound can be recovered by changing the experimental conditions, such as pH or ionic strength.

Antigen–antibody binding is one of the reactions that can be applied to affinity chromatography. When the gel material is coupled to an antigen, a specific antibody can be purified. Alternatively, when a highly purified antibody can be coupled to the gel, the corresponding antigen can be isolated.

Protein A is a protein, isolated from the cell wall of

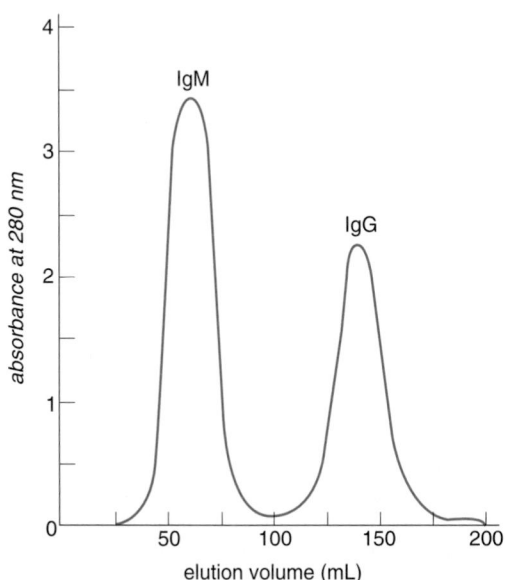

Figure 14–21. Separation of IgG-IgM mixed cryoglobulin by gel filtration. Two peaks are eluted from gel filtration column. The larger IgM molecules precede the smaller IgG molecules, which were dissociated by dissolving the cryoprecipitate in an acidic buffer prior to application to the column. The absorbance at 280 nm measures the relative amount of protein in various eluted fractions.

some strains of *Staphylococcus aureus,* that specifically reacts with IgG molecules of subclasses 1, 2, and 4. It is used as a specific ligand for isolation of IgG or for isolation of IgG3 from a mixture of IgG molecules of all subclasses. Protein G, from streptococcus binds all four subclasses of human IgG and thus provides a more complete removal of IgG from samples.

Cell separation can also be achieved by affinity chromatography. Subpopulations of T and B lymphocytes have been defined by characteristic surface markers (see Chapters 3, 8, 9, and 15) that can react with specific ligands. For example, B cells that bear surface immunoglobulins can be separated on an anti-immunoglobulin column. Immunoglobulin-positive cells are retained on the gel, and desorption is achieved by running through the column a solution of immunoglobulins that compete with the cells.

Currently, many of the chromatographic techniques described are done by high-performance (or pressure) liquid chromatography (HPLC). The principles are the same, but the moving phase is forced through a sealed column under pressure, resulting in a much more rapid, precise, and sensitive separation profile.

SERUM VISCOSITY

The measurement of serum viscosity is a simple and valuable tool in evaluation of patients with paraproteinemia. Normally, the formed elements of the blood contribute more significantly to whole-blood viscosity than do plasma proteins. In diseases with elevated concentrations of serum proteins, however, particularly the immunoglobulins, the serum viscosity may reach very high levels and result in a characteristic symptom complex—the hyperviscosity syndrome. Serum viscosity is determined by a variety of factors, including protein concentration; the size, shape, and deformability of serum molecules; and the hydrostatic state (solvation), molecular charge, and temperature sensitivity of proteins.

In clinical practice, serum viscosity is measured in an Ostwald viscosimeter. A few milliliters of serum are warmed to 37 °C and allowed to descend through a narrow-bore capillary tube immersed in a water bath at 27 °C. The rate of descent between calibrated marks on the capillary tube is recorded. The same procedure is repeated with distilled water instead of serum. The relative serum viscosity is then calculated according to the following formula:

$$\text{Relative serum viscosity} = \frac{\text{Rate of descent of serum sample (in seconds)}}{\text{Rate of descent of distilled water (in seconds)}} \quad (1)$$

Normal values for serum viscosity range from approximately 1.4 to 1.9. Similar measurements can be performed with plasma instead of serum. Fibrinogen present in plasma is a major determinant of plasma viscosity, however, and variations in this protein, especially in the presence of nonspecific inflammatory states, can markedly affect the results. For this reason, measurement of serum viscosity is preferred.

Serum viscosity measurements are primarily of use in evaluating patients with Waldenström's macroglobulinemia, multiple myeloma, and cryoglobulinemia. In myeloma, aggregation or polymerization of the paraprotein in vivo often results in hyperviscosity. In general, there is a correlation between increased serum viscosity and increased plasma volume. The correlation between levels of relative serum viscosity and clinical symptoms is not nearly as direct, however. Increased serum viscosity may interfere with various laboratory tests that employ flow-through devices, such as hematology counters and analyzers in clinical chemistry. Examples of disorders associated with increased serum viscosity are listed in Table 14–3.

CRYOGLOBULINS

Precipitation of serum immunoglobulins in the cold was first observed in a patient with multiple myeloma. The term *cryoglobulin* was introduced to designate a group of proteins that had the common property of forming a precipitate or a gel in the cold. This phenomenon was reversible by raising the temperature. Since those initial descriptions, cryoglobulins have

Table 14–3. Disorders associated with increased serum viscosity.

Waldenström's macroglobulinemia
Essential macroglobulinemia
Multiple myeloma
Cryoglobulinemia
Hypergammaglobulinemic purpura
Rheumatoid diseases associated with immune complexes or paraproteinemias
    Rheumatoid arthritis
    Sjögren's syndrome
    Systemic lupus erythematosus
    Human immunodeficiency virus (HIV) infection

been found in a wide variety of clinical situations. Purification and immunochemical analysis have led to classification of this group of proteins (Table 14–4). Type I cryoglobulins consist of a single monoclonal immunoglobulin. Type II cryoglobulins are mixed cryoglobulins; they consist of a monoclonal immunoglobulin with antibody activity against a polyclonal immunoglobulin (rheumatoid factor activity). Type III cryoglobulins are mixed polyclonal cryoglobulins with rheumatoid factor activity; that is, one or more immunoglobulins are found, none of which are monoclonal.

Technical Procedure for Isolation & Analysis

Blood must be collected in a warm syringe and kept at 37 °C until it clots. Serum is separated by centrifugation at 37 °C and then stored at 4 °C. When a cryoglobulin is present, a white precipitate or a gel appears in the serum after a variable period, usually 24–72 hours. The serum should be observed for 1 week, however, to make certain that unusually late cryoprecipitation does not go undetected. The reversibility of the cryoprecipitation should be tested by rewarming an aliquot of precipitated serum.

The cryoprecipitate can be quantitated in several ways. Centrifugation of the whole serum in a hematocrit tube at 4 °C allows determination of the relative amount of cryoglobulin (cryocrit). Alternatively, the protein concentration in the serum before and after cryoprecipitation may be compared. The precipitate formed in an aliquot of serum may be isolated and dissolved in an acidic buffer and the cryoglobulin level estimated by the absorbance at 280 nm.

After isolation and washing of the precipitate, the components of the cryoglobulin are identified by immunoelectrophoresis, immunofixation electrophoresis, or immunodiffusion. These analyses are performed at 37 °C, using antiserum to whole human serum and antisera specific for γ, α, μ, κ, and λ chains. In this way, cryoglobulins can ordinarily be classified into the three types described earlier. Additionally, antiserum to fibrinogen may be used to determine the presence of a cryofibrinogen precipitate.

Clinical Significance

Type I and type II cryoglobulins are usually present in large amounts in serum (often more than 5 mg/mL). In general, they are present in patients with monoclonal paraproteinemias; for example, they are commonly found in patients with lymphoma or multiple myeloma. Some, however, are found in patients lacking any evidence of lymphoid malignancy, just as are "benign" paraproteins. Type III cryoglobulins indicate the presence of circulating immune complexes and are the result of immune responses to various antigens. They are present in relatively low concentrations (usually less than 1 mg/mL) in rheumatoid diseases and chronic infections (see Table 14–4).

All types of cryoglobulins may be responsible for

Table 14–4. Classification of types of cryoglobulins and associated diseases.

Type of Cryoglobulin	Immunochemical Composition	Associated Diseases
Type 1 monoclonal cryoglobulin	IgM IgG IgA Bence Jones protein	Myeloma, Waldenström's macroglobulinemia, chronic lymphocytic leukemia.
Type II mixed cryoglobulin	IgM–IgG IgG–IgG IgA–IgG	Myeloma, Waldenström's macroglobulinemia, chronic lymphocytic leukemia, rheumatoid arthritis, Sjögren's syndrome, mixed essential cryoglobulinemia, hepatitis C.
Type III mixed polyclonal cryoglobulin	IgM–IgG IgM–IgG–IgA	Systemic lupus erythematosus, rheumatoid arthritis, Sjögren's syndrome, infectious mononucleosis, cytomegalovirus infections, acute viral hepatitis, chronic active hepatitis, hepatitis C, primary biliary cirrhosis, poststreptococcal glomerulonephritis, infective endocarditis, leprosy, kala-azar, tropical splenomegaly syndrome.

specific symptoms that occur as a result of changes in the cryoglobulin induced by exposure to cold. The symptoms include Raynaud's phenomenon, vascular purpura, bleeding tendencies, cold-induced urticaria, and even distal arterial thrombosis with gangrene.

Since type II and type III cryoglobulins are circulating soluble immune complexes, they may be associated with a serum sickness-like syndrome characterized by polyarthritis, vasculitis, glomerulonephritis, or neurologic symptoms. In patients with mixed essential IgM–IgG cryoglobulinemia, a rather distinctive syndrome may occur that is associated with arthralgias, purpura, weakness, and frequently lymphadenopathy or hepatosplenomegaly. This syndrome may be a sequela of hepatitis B infection. Glomerulonephritis is common. In some instances, it occurs in a rapidly progressive form and is of ominous prognostic significance.

Cryoglobulins may cause serious errors in a variety of laboratory tests by precipitating at ambient temperatures and thereby removing certain substances from serum. Complement fixation and inactivation and entrapment of immunoglobulins in the precipitate are common examples. Redissolving the cryoprecipitate usually does not fully restore activity to the serum, especially that of complement.

PYROGLOBULINS

Pyroglobulins are monoclonal immunoglobulins that precipitate irreversibly when heated to 56 °C. This phenomenon is different from the reversible thermoprecipitation of Bence Jones proteins and seems to be related to hydrophobic bonding between immunoglobulin molecules, possibly as a result of decreased polarity of the heavy chains. Pyroglobulins

may be discovered incidentally when serum is heated to 56 °C to inactivate complement before routine serologic tests. Half of the cases involve patients with multiple myeloma. The remainder occur in macroglobulinemia and other lymphoproliferative disorders, systemic lupus erythematosus, and carcinoma, and occasionally without known associated disease. They are not responsible for any particular symptom and have no known significance.

DETECTION OF IMMUNE COMPLEXES

The factors involved in deposition of immune complexes in tissues and production of tissue damage are discussed in Chapter 12. Subsequent chapters deal with the clinical manifestations of diseases associated with immune complexes, including rheumatic diseases (Chapter 33), hematologic diseases (Chapter 35), and renal diseases (Chapter 38). These clinical situations have in common the presence of detectable immune complexes in tissues or in the circulation.

Immune complexes are occasionally detected in tissues by standard immunohistochemical staining techniques with specific antisera.

There are many methods for detecting circulating immune complexes in serum, most of which rely on the binding of such complexes to various complement components. None of these methods are used in routine clinical laboratory practice.

In a few disorders, such as Lyme disease and HIV infection, antigen detection is hampered by its masking within immune complexes. Techniques to dissociate the antigen–antibody complexes have increased the apparent sensitivity of these antigen detection assays.

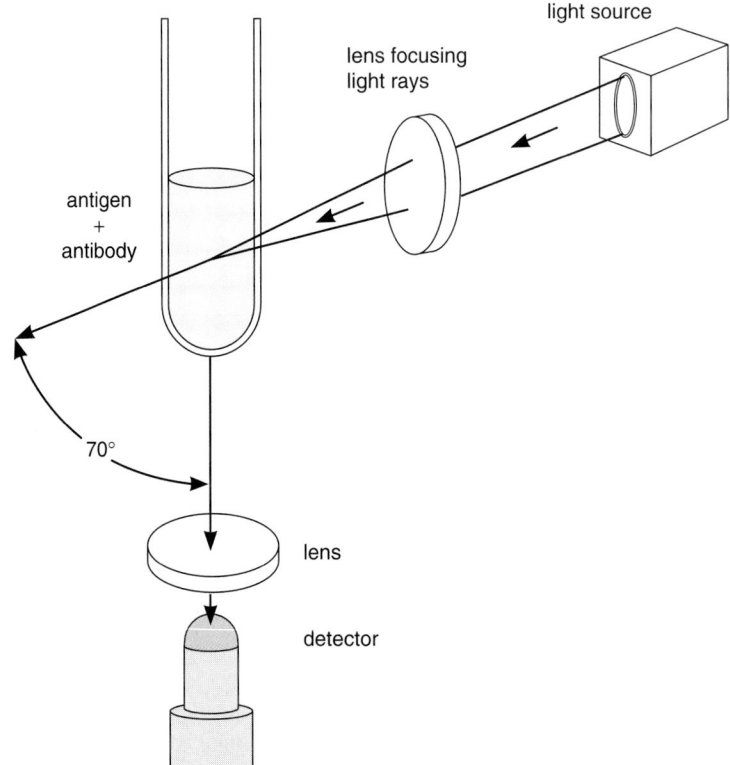

Figure 14–22. The principle of nephelometry for measurement of antigen–antibody reactions. Light rays from a laser or other high-intensity source are collected in the focusing lens and pass through the sample tube containing antigen and antibody. Light passing through the tube and emerging at a 70° angle is collected by another lens and focused into an electronic detector. This signal is converted to a digital recording of the amount of turbidity in the sample tube and can be mathematically related to either antigen or antibody concentration in the sample.

Clinical Usefulness

Initial enthusiasm regarding possible clinical benefits of measuring immune complexes has been tempered by their relative lack of diagnostic or prognostic specificity. Circulating complexes can occur in the absence of tissue deposition, and occasionally no serum complexes can be found despite tissue deposition. In addition, the considerable potential for uncovering causes of many idiopathic diseases by isolating and identifying the antigen in immune complexes has not yet been realized. Discrepancies among the results of various assays are common, and standards are generally lacking. Nevertheless, immune complexes have pathogenic roles depending on their size, immunoglobulin class, concentration, and affinity for cellular receptors.

NEPHELOMETRY

Nephelometry is measurement of light that is scattered from the main beam of a transmitted light source. This should not be confused with turbidimetry, which is the measurement of the decrease of light passing through a cloudy solution or suspension of material. In dilute solutions, the precipitation reaction between antigen and antibody produces increased reflection that can be measured by the scattering of an incident light. Devices to measure light scattering produced by reaction of diphtheria toxin and antitoxin were introduced by J. Libby in 1938, and this technique has received increasing application in the clinical laboratory.

Nephelometric determination of antigens is performed by addition of constant amounts of highly purified and optically clear specific antiserum to varying amounts of antigen. The resultant antigen–antibody reactants are placed in a cuvette in a light beam, and the degree of light scatter is measured in a photoelectric cell as the optical density (Fig 14–22). Accurate measurement of antigens can be made only in the ascending limb of the precipitin curve (see Fig 14–1), where there is a direct linear relationship between antigen concentration and optical density. Thus, for accurate determination of solutions with high antigen concentrations, the samples are diluted to various concentrations.

There are several different approaches to applying

nephelometry in the clinical laboratory. Automated immunoprecipitation employs a fluorometric nephelometer in line with a series of flow-through channels that allow for the measurement of multiple samples simultaneously. Laser nephelometers use a helium–neon laser beam as the light source and sensitive detection devices to measure forward light scatter. Introduction of various electronic filters near the detection device ensures a high signal-to-noise ratio and a relatively high degree of sensitivity. A modified centrifugal fast analyzer equipped with a laser light source has also been used for scatter measurements. This method has the potential advantages of speed, small amounts of reagents required, and versatility for other assays.

Nephelometry is theoretically a rapid and simple method for quantitation of many antigens in biologic fluids. Disadvantages of the technique include the relatively high cost of optically clear, potent antisera of uniform specifications; high background resulting from sera containing lipids or hemoglobin; and the need for multiple dilutions, especially for high antigen concentrations. Some of these potential sources of error, however, are inherent in other immunoquantitative methods. Many of these inherent disadvantages can be overcome by the use of **rate nephelometry.** In this technique, a nephelometer electronically subtracts the background signal from that of an unreacted serum sample. More precise measurement of turbidity is achieved by taking several measurements rapidly during the ascending phase of the precipitation reaction. The concentration of the analyte is proportional to the peak rate of immune complex formation, provided the reaction is in antibody excess. In samples with large amounts of analyte present, automated instruments check for antibody excess by delivering an aliquot of calibrator to a dilution of the patient sample. An increase in complex formation confirms antibody excess. Nephelometers that combine many of these features are commercially available and provide accurate and precise quantitation of a variety of proteins in a rapid fashion. The widespread use of such instruments—and nephelometric-grade reagents—has made this method cheaper and applicable to many immunochemical determinations.

BINDER–LIGAND ASSAYS

One of the most important analytical methods developed in the past quarter century is binder–ligand assay (also known as **ligand assay, competitive protein-binding assay,** and **saturation analysis**). The first ligand assay method was **radioimmunoassay (RIA),** developed by Berson and Rosalyn Yalow in 1959 to detect and quantify human insulin, using human anti-insulin antibodies. Their discovery that the

body manufactures antibodies against endogenous substances went against a fundamental dictum of the time, which held that the body could not make antibodies against itself. This discovery was in certain respects as important as the application of these antibodies to a new assay method. Simultaneously, F. Ekins developed an assay for human thyroid hormone by using thyroid-binding globulin isolated from a patient with elevated levels of this protein. The basic principle of his assay was the same, although it used a serum carrier protein rather than an antibody.

Since their inception, ligand assays have revolutionized disciplines within biology and medicine. Using these methods, one can quantify hormones, drugs, tumor markers, and allergens and antibodies associated with allergy. The rapid detection of bacterial and viral antigens and antibodies in infectious diseases such as hepatitis and AIDS is now routine. Concentrations on the order of the attomolar (10^{-18} mol/L) and below are now possible, a feat that was unimaginable when the first ligand assays appeared in the early 1960s.

THE ASSAY PROCESS

The chief goal of an assay is to determine the concentration of some molecule of interest, the **analyte.** Common to all ligand assays is the reaction of analyte with a binding protein, or **binder,** which is most often an **antibody.** In its role as a reactant with binder, the analyte is referred to as a **ligand** (small analyte molecules are also sometimes referred to as **haptens,** as they need to be conjugated to carriers to be rendered immunogeneic for the purpose of forming antibodies to be used for their detection).

The assay process consists of subjecting analyte-containing specimens to a series of physical and chemical processes that, taken together, are referred to as the **analytic method** of the assay. The final measurement resulting from the analytic method, or some computed value derived from it, is known as the **response.** The choice of an appropriate response is dictated by the statistical requirements of data reduction.

The number of possible analytic methods is large and continually growing, some involving multiple types of ligands or binders (or both). At the highest conceptual level, however, all properly performed ligand assays follow the same series of events:

1. **Calibration:** The use of specimens containing known amounts of analyte (**standards** or **calibrators**) to establish a relationship between what we actually measure (the response; for example, a reading of radioactivity or light intensity), and what we actually seek to measure—analyte concentration.
2. **Interpolation:** The use of the calibration relationship to estimate the concentrations corre-

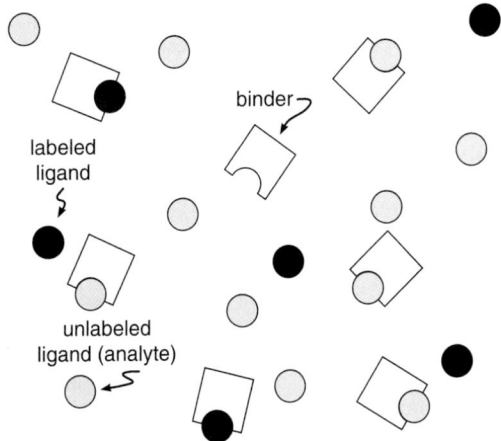

Figure 14–23. The binder–ligand reaction underlying radioimmunoassay (RIA).

sponding to the responses obtained for test specimens containing unknown amounts of analyte.

3. **Quality control:** Steps to assess and control the amount of error in the estimation of analyte concentration.

This process is described in full for the founding member of the ligand assay family, RIA, followed by descriptions of the broad principles underlying the analytic methods for other binder–ligand assay methods.

RADIOIMMUNOASSAY

Calibration

A. The Binder–Ligand Reaction: A number of reaction vessels are established, each containing a small fixed concentration of binder and a small fixed concentration of radioisotopically labeled analyte known as the **label,** or **tracer** (Fig 14–23). Varying known amounts of analyte are added to a series of these antibody–label mixtures (using premixed calibration standards). The central event in RIA is the competition between the label and the unlabeled analyte for binding sites on an antibody. According to the degree of completion of the binder–ligand reaction, the assay is said to be either an **equilibrium assay** (the reaction is complete), or a **disequilibrium assay** (the reaction is incomplete). The label is divided into two categories by the reaction: label that is bound to antibody (the **bound fraction**) and label that is free in solution (the **free fraction**). As the amount of analyte increases relative to the small fixed amount of label present, an increasing fraction of the label is free.

B. Partitioning and Separation: The bound and free fractions are subjected to a **partitioning step.** Partitioning methods that sequester the binder and binder–ligand complexes include **salting out** of protein (using ammonium or sodium sulfate), **protein**

denaturation/precipitation by solvent (such as methanol, ethanol, or acetone), and **precipitation** by polyethylene glycol or by a **second antibody** directed against the primary antibody. Immobilization of the binder to a **solid phase,** such as the assay reaction tube or a macroscopic particle, allows for rapid separation of bound and unbound label or analyte. Another method of removing the free fraction is by **adsorption** (using talc, charcoal, silica, ion-exchange resin, cellulose, cross-linked dextran beads [Sephadex], or fuller's earth). Following partitioning, the bound and free fractions are subjected to physical separation by decanting, centrifugation, or filtration, during which a small degree of mixing of bound and unbound fractions (misclassification) can occur.

C. Measurement of Response: In radioassays, the measurement method is **radioactive counting,** the method for which depends on the type of radiation emitted by the label. A **liquid scintillation counter** is used for alpha or beta emitters and a **solid crystal gamma counter** for gamma emitters. A commonly employed value for the response in RIA is the ratio of bound to total label, or B:T.

D. Creation of a Calibration Curve: The relationship between calibrator concentration and assay response is known as the **calibration curve.** Most currently encountered relationships are roughly symmetric sigmoid curves, when plotted using a logarithmic concentration axis (Fig 14–24).

This sort of curve can usually be characterized by the four-parameter logistic equation

$$y = [\frac{a - d}{a + (x/cb)}] + d \qquad (2)$$

where a is the upper asymptote, d is the lower asymptote, c is the concentration corresponding to the response $(a + d)/2$, and b is related to the slope at this point. Earlier workers used a simplified form of this equation, the **logit transformation,** which lends itself

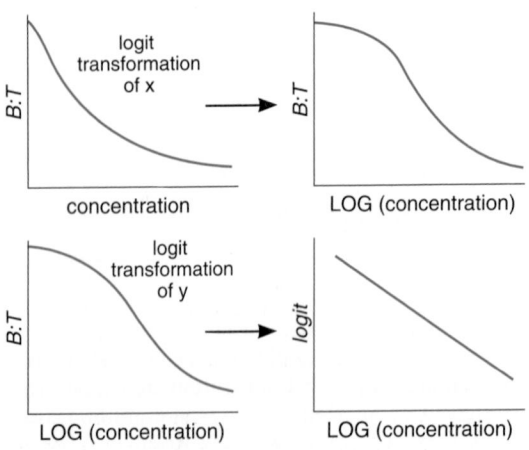

Figure 14–24. The logistic equation and the logit transformation. B:T = ratio of label bound to total label present.

to manual plotting. If one defines a new response value as $y' = (*y - d)/(a - d)$, the logit transformation proceeds as follows:

$$Y = logit(y') = \ln \left[\frac{y'}{1 - y'}\right] \qquad (3)$$

Note the similarity of this approach to that of the von Krogh equation discussed later in this chapter. If the data really follow a symmetric sigmoid on the log-linear plot, then a plot of Y versus log concentration is a straight line. The term b in the four-parameter logistic equation is simply the slope of the line in the logit-log coordinate system.

Interpolation of Test Concentrations

Once a calibration relationship is in hand, we are ready to estimate the concentration of analyte in **test specimens ("unknowns").** These specimens are processed just as the calibrators were, and a response is obtained. The calibration curve can be used to find the **concentration estimate** corresponding to the observed response; this process is known as **interpolation.**

Quality Control & Error Computations

Error is the unavoidable companion of any measurement process. Measurement errors can be divided into two categories: **random error** and **systematic (or bias) error.** There are numerous sources for random error in any analytic method (for example, minute fluctuations in reagent concentration, temperature, and detector efficiency); these sources compound to produce some level of random variability in the final assay concentration estimate. An assay result should be accompanied by statistically determined **confidence limits** to express the magnitude of random error. Such confidence limits define a zone within which a result would be expected to fall, at some stated level of probability, were the analysis to be repeated many times.

Bias errors arise from nonrandom occurrences. Examples include events that produce nonidentical chemical behavior between calibration and test specimens, such as the presence of nonanalyte chemical species that **cross-react** with components of the analytic method, or a colored substance that **interferes** with an assay spectrophotometric measurement. If cross-reacting or interfering substances are a potential problem, their behavior can be studied in advance. The most important component of quality assurance dealing with bias error is the use of **quality control specimens.** Drawn from stored pools of material similar in nature to actual test specimens (for example, human plasma), these specimens are analyzed repeatedly over time to ensure that the concentration estimates obtained for them have not shifted beyond limits accounted for by random error. The results for quality control pools are sometimes plotted on time charts known as **Shewhart** or **Levey Jennings** plots, or using a statistical graphing method known as the **cumulative sum** chart.

The goal of a good analytic design is to minimize all error. Some level of random error is inescapable, though bias errors can in principle (but rarely in practice) be corrected for if not eliminated. Quality control is intimately connected with the final product of an assay, which is generally not simply an analyte concentration estimate but rather a scientific or clinical decision based on the estimate. The goal is generally to answer a question such as "Is the analyte concentration larger (or smaller) than a given dangerous or therapeutic level?" or "Is the concentration larger or smaller than some previously measured concentration?" Such questions cannot be addressed without adequate quality control and statistical computation for assay results. In practice, this requires automated data reduction methods. With the increasing automation of all aspects of ligand assay procedure, it becomes difficult to assess the rigor of the statistical computations used by vendors, who are not always forthcoming with respect to this aspect of their product. Also, pressure to reduce assay cost tends to reduce the use of quality control specimens. There is little in the way of theory or experimental data to help guide the practitioner toward an optimal amount of quality control that balances the costs associated with quality control against the costs associated with making poor decisions based on inadequate quality control.

TYPES OF ANALYTIC METHODS

Radioisotopic Labels

The variety of analytic methods has burgeoned based on various modifications of the initial RIA scheme, arbitrarily divided according to their labeling methods.

A. Immunoradiometric Assay (IRMA): In this method, the binder (generally an antibody) is labeled rather than the ligand.

B. Sandwich Assay: There are numerous variations of this technique. In its most basic form, ligand reacts with an antibody that has been immobilized on a solid surface. Then a radiolabeled second antibody is added, which reacts with ligand at a different site. This method has the potential advantage of added chemical specificity owing to the use of two distinct antigenic sites (Fig 14–25).

Enzymatic Labels

A. Enzyme-Multiplied Immunoassay Technique (EMIT): The label consists of ligand conjugated to an enzyme, which remains active (Fig 14–26). Binding of antibody to the enzyme–ligand complex inactivates the enzyme; the presence of free ligand (analyte) competes with the enzyme–ligand complex for antibody, increasing the resulting enzymatic activity. Over a limited range, the enzyme activity is approximately proportionate to analyte concentration. This method has been widely employed for therapeutic drug monitoring.

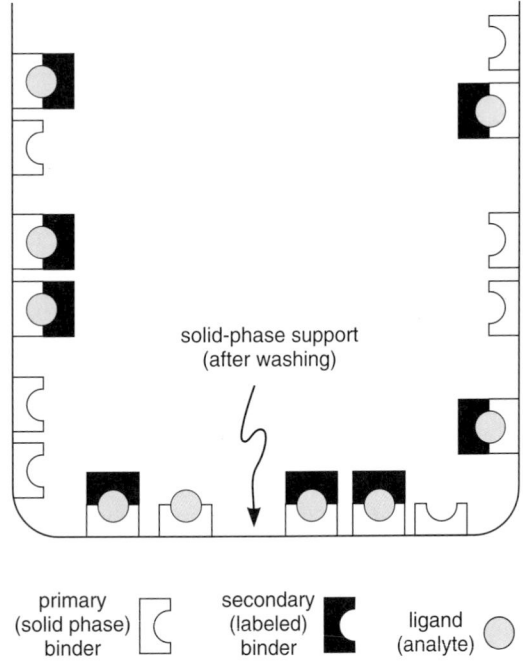

Figure 14–25. Sandwich assay.

primary
(solid phase)
binder

secondary
(labeled)
binder

ligand
(analyte)

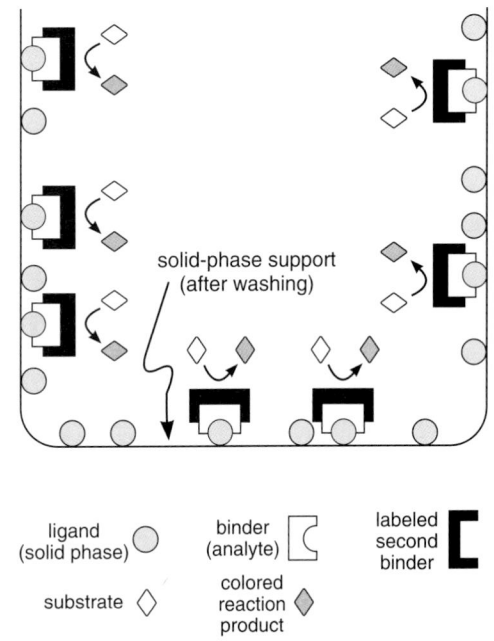

ligand
(solid phase)

binder
(analyte)

labeled
second
binder

substrate

colored
reaction
product

Figure 14–27. Enzyme-linked immunosorbent assay (ELISA).

B. Enzyme-Linked Immunoabsorbent Assay (ELISA):

This is an enzymatic variation on the sandwich assay method. In the standard indirect ELISA the goal is to detect antibody, so the roles of binder and ligand are reversed (Fig 14–27). The solid-phase component is an antigen. The antibody to be de-

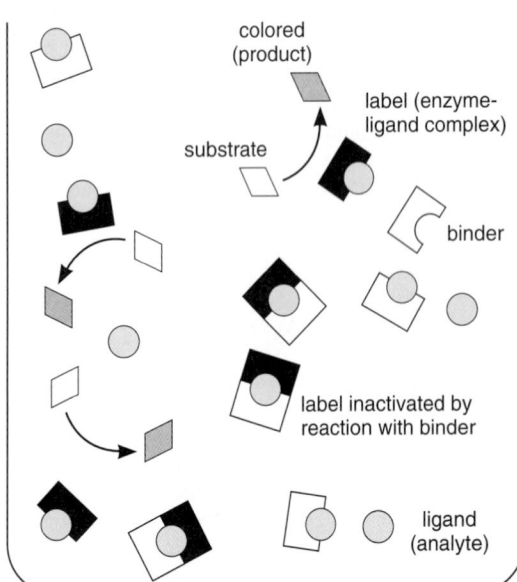

colored
(product)

label (enzyme-
ligand complex)

substrate

binder

label inactivated by
reaction with binder

ligand
(analyte)

Figure 14–26. Enzyme-mediated immunoassay technique (EMIT).

tected binds to this component, and then a second, enzyme-labeled antibody directed against the antibody to be detected is added. The substrate of the enzyme is added, producing a colored reaction product that is measured spectrophotometrically.

ELISAs are integral components of clinical immunology laboratories. Their high degree of sensitivity and lack of radioisotope use has made them popular means to qualitatively and quantitatively detect antigens and antibodies.

Numerous modifications of the basic ELISA described here are used to increase sensitivity and specificity and allow detection of specific antibody isotypes. An example of isotype specific ELISA is the mu-capture ELISA for detection of IgM specific antibodies to infectious agents. In this assay anti-IgM specific antibodies are absorbed in the wells of microtiter plates. Patient serum is added to the wells, and IgM antibodies are bound by the anti-IgM capture reagent. Next, a solution of purified antigen is added and, if pathogen-specific IgM antibodies are present, binds to the plate. After washing away unbound antigen, a second antibody to the antigen, labeled with an enzyme, is added. Next, the addition of substrate indicates the presence of pathogen-specific IgM antibodies if a color change occurs.

ELISAs are finding widespread use in the clinical laboratory not only because of their sensitivity and specificity but because they can be automated. Several automated systems are available that perform a variety of ELISA assays. The use of these automated ELISAs greatly increases the through-put of the laboratory.

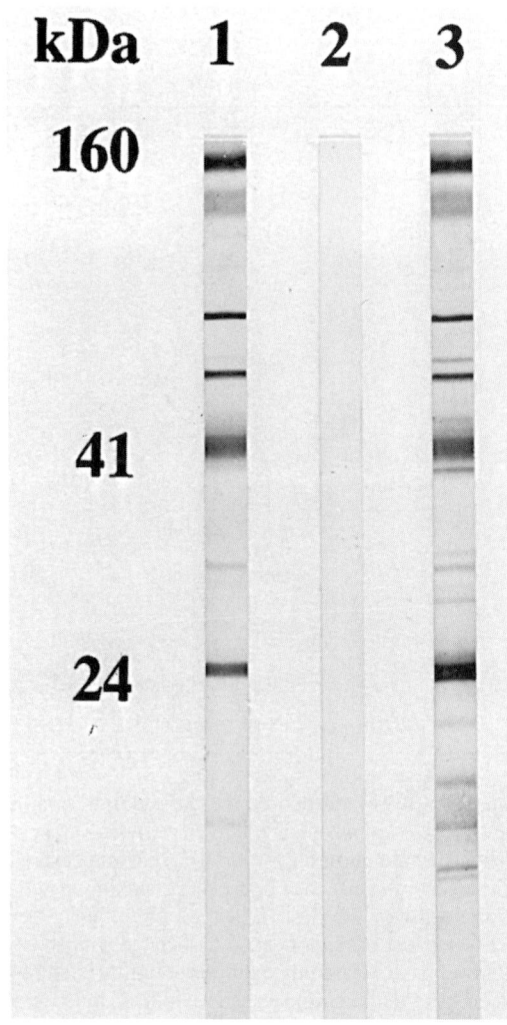

Figure 14–28. HIV Western Blot analysis of serum from a patient who tested repeatedly positive on the HIV ELISA screening assay. In lane 1, the positive control demonstrates bands of significance at 24, 41, and 160 kd. The negative control (lane 2) shows no reactivity. The patient's serum (lane 3) demonstrates reactivity with bands of 24, 41, 120/160 kd. The serum is thus considered reactive for antibodies to HIV because it meets the criteria of two out of three bands positive as 24, 41, or 120/160 kd.

C. Western Blot (WB): Using the combination of electrophoresis and ELISA one can determine the response to a variety of pathogen-specific proteins rather than reactivity to whole or solubilized organisms. This approach provides a very specific means to identify antibody reactivity. Response to pathogen-specific proteins can be differentiated from cross-reactive proteins that may not be useful diagnostically.

One of the most frequent uses of WB is for the confirmation of reactive serologic screening tests for HIV antibodies. Viral antigens are separated by sodium dodecyl sulfate-polyacrylamide gel electrophoresis (SDS-PAGE). Treatment of a viral lysate with SDS imparts a negative charge to the proteins. The viral proteins are then electrophoresed in a polyacrylamide gel. Because the proteins are negatively charged, when electrophoresed, they separate based on their molecular weight. Larger proteins remain at the top of the gel and smaller proteins migrate toward the bottom of the gel. For detection of antibodies to the HIV proteins, the proteins are transferred from the gel to a support matrix (eg, nitrocellulose). This "Western" transfer results in an exact copy of the gel pattern on the matrix. Detection of viral specific antibodies then proceeds as in the indirect ELISA described earlier. Reactions are read as positive when a line of precipitation or color forms at the correct molecular weight for a particular protein (Fig 14–28).

The ability to identify specific reactivity to individual proteins imparts a high degree of specificity to this technique. In addition, isotype-specific secondary antibodies can be used to detect IgG-, IgM-, or IgA-specific antibodies.

D. Microparticle Enzyme Immunoassay (MEIA): There are a number of variations of this recently developed automated method. In the simplest, an enzyme-labeled binder binds to the analyte, which in turn is bound to binder-coated microparticles. Initially free in solution during the foregoing chemical reactions, the microparticles are immobilized on glass fiber, and then the complex of primary binder, ligand, and labeled binder is exposed to substrate, producing a colored product. This can be seen to be an enzymatic variant of the sandwich assay.

Fluorometric Labels

A. Fluorescence Polarization Immunoassay (FPIA): The label is coupled by means of the analyte to a fluorescein derivative to form tracer molecules (Fig 14–29). When free in solution, tracer molecules tumble randomly and so rapidly that when ex-

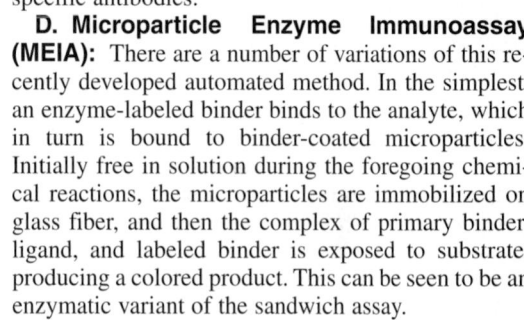

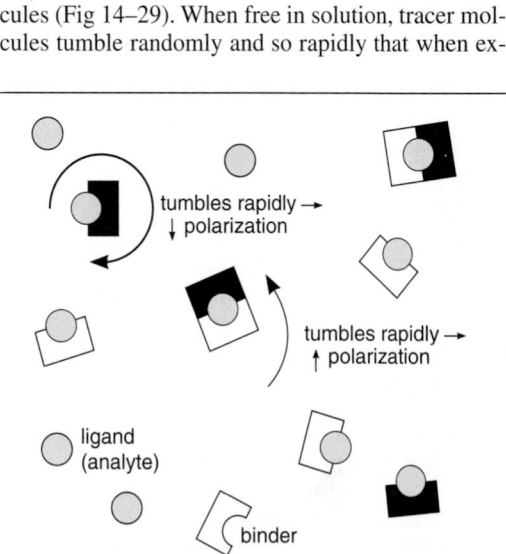

Figure 14–29. Fluorescence polarization immunoassay (FPIA).

cited by polarized light, emitted light is unpolarized. When the tracer is bound to an antibody, the tumbling is slowed and the emitted light is more polarized. The degree of polarization reflects the amount of label that is bound. Thus far, only small analytes have been measurable by this means.

Other Methods

Other methods employ liposomes or erythrocytes as solid supports, nephelometry for particle detection, metal atoms as labels (detected by atomic adsorption) and electron-spin resonance ("spin labeling"). Enzymes from the blood-clotting cascade have been employed to produce a colored product from a chromogenic substrate as a response. Solid-phase systems have been sped up by the use of ultrasound to enhance the reaction rate of ligand with immobilized binder. Magnetic solid-phase support for antibody has been used to facilitate separation of bound and free fractions in an automated RIA method and in a manual sandwich assay. Bacteriophages have been employed as labels, as have chemiluminescent substances (luminol and its derivatives). The latex agglutination assay is now commonly employed for the rapid detection of infectious agents. Microscopic latex spheres are coated with antibodies (or antigens), and agglutination (visible to the naked eye) is provoked by the presence of the corresponding antigen (or antibody). A technique called **biotin/avidin-enhanced immunoassay** increases the activity of labeled binder by chemically linking the binder to a large number of label molecules (enzymatic, radioisotopic, fluorometric, metallic, or other) that are part of an avidin–biotin complex. Time-resolved fluorescence with rare-earth labels such as europium has been employed to reduce the effects of nonspecific ("background") fluorescence.

Another technique, ultrasensitive enzymatic radioimmunoassay (USERIA) has also been used (Fig 14–30).

COMPARING THE ANALYTIC PERFORMANCE OF DIFFERENT METHODS

In the absence of analytic error, there would be no point in comparing assay methods, as they would all be capable of detecting any concentration of analyte under any circumstance. The presence of bias and random errors that are unique to a given analytic method places bounds on the capabilities of the technique.

The susceptibility of an assay method to various forms of systematic error can be experimentally characterized. For example, studies can be done using cross-reacting or interfering substances to determine the magnitude of their potential effect. The amount of bias is often a function of the analyte concentration as well as that of the cross-reacting or interfering sub-

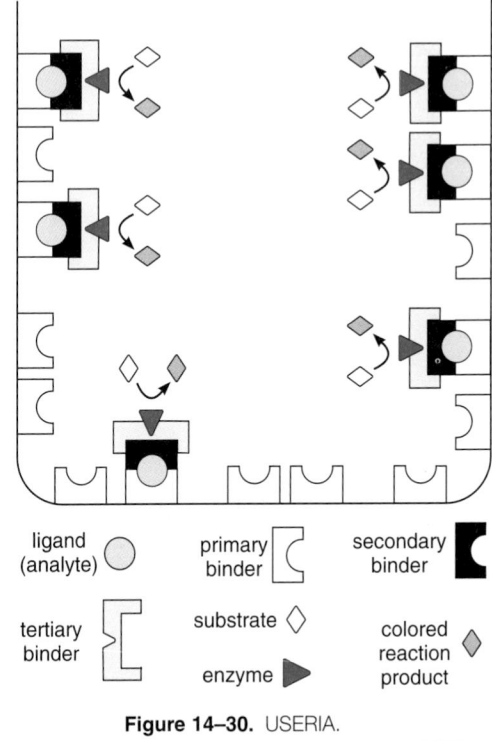

ligand (analyte)

primary binder

secondary binder

tertiary binder

substrate

enzyme

colored reaction product

Figure 14–30. USERIA.

stance. **Recovery studies** require the addition of varying known amounts of analyte to an analyte-free specimen. The amount of added material that is recovered can indicate the effect of nonspecific binding materials in the assay.

The amount of random error associated with an assay result is expressed by confidence limits, falling to either side of the estimate. The width of the confidence interval can be plotted against concentration to create an **imprecision profile.** Random error varies over the range of the assay, generally being lowest at some midrange value and increasing on either side. Random error determines the smallest amount of analyte that can be statistically distinguished from zero (the **lower detection limit,** sometimes referred to by the qualitative term **sensitivity**), as well as the **upper detection limit.** The zone between the lower and upper detection limits is the **valid analytic range** of the assay.

It is difficult to compare the analytic performance of different ligand assay methods, since the workers involved often provide inadequate numeric data. New methods are often accompanied by exaggerated claims. Use of a standardized data reduction method would allow more rigorous comparison of the merits of analytic performance.

One method of categorizing analytic methods has been to divide them into two basic categories, **limited reagent** (or **competitive**) methods and **excess reagent** (or **noncompetitive**) methods. RIA falls into the former category; labeled ligand and unlabeled ligand compete for a limited amount of binder. The best achievable sensitivity of a RIA is of the order of 10^{-14} mol/L (this represents about 6×10^6 molecules in 1 mL of solution). A sandwich IRMA is an example of the latter category; a massive excess of labeled second antibody is added to the solid-phase binder–ligand complex. Reagent excess methods are in principle capable of lower detection limits than limited reagent methods, but in practice IRMA has been associated with detection limits *above* those of RIA. ELISA has achieved detection limits one and two orders of magnitude smaller than RIA. There is a general trend away from earlier methods such as RIA to methods that are more readily automated (with particular interest in methods that do not require a physical separation step; this step is difficult to automate and can introduce substantial random error). No one universal method is available; it seems likely that an array of different methods will remain in use for different applications.

There are alternative chemical methods, such as HPLC, for many analytes. An important principle of ligand assay must be borne in mind—it measures the chemical (generally immunochemical) reactivity rather than the physiologic or functional activity of an analyte. This has sometimes been an advantage, where much new knowledge has been gained about the various forms of drugs and hormones capable of cross-reacting with the intended analyte.

IMMUNOHISTOCHEMICAL TECHNIQUES

IMMUNOFLUORESCENCE

Immunofluorescence can be applied as a histochemical or cytochemical technique for detection and localization of antigens in cells or tissues. Specific antibody is conjugated with fluorescent compounds without altering its immunologic reactivity, resulting in a sensitive tracer of tissue antigens. The conjugated antibody is added to cells or tissues and becomes fixed to antigens, thereby forming a stable immune complex. Unbound antibody is removed by washing, and the resultant preparation is observed in a fluorescence microscope. This adaptation of a regular microscope contains a high-intensity light source, excitation filters to produce a wavelength capable of causing fluorescence activation, and barrier filters to remove interfering wavelengths of light. When observed in the fluorescence microscope against a dark background, antigens bound specifically to fluorescent antibody can be detected by their bright color.

Fluorescence is the emission of light of one color, (wavelength) while a substance is irradiated with light of a different color. The emitted wavelength is at a lower energy level than the incident or absorbed light (Fig 14–31). Fluorochromes such as rhodamine or fluorescein used in clinical laboratories have characteristic absorption and emission spectra. Fluorescein isothiocyanate (FITC) is a chemical form of fluorescein that readily binds covalently to proteins at high pH primarily through ε-amino residues of lysine and terminal amino groups. Its absorption maximum is at 490–495 nm, and it emits its characteristic green color at 517 nm. Tetramethylrhodamine isothiocyanate, which emits red, has an absorption maximum at 550 nm and maximal emission at 580 nm (for rhodamine–protein conjugates). Consequently, different excitation and barrier filters must be used to visualize the characteristic green or red color of these fluorescent dyes. Generally, one wants to achieve an exciting wavelength nearly equal to that of the excitation maximum of the dye. Similarly, the barrier filter should remove all but the emitted wavelength spectrum. In practice, the actual brightness of fluorescence observed by the eye depends on three factors: (1) the ef-

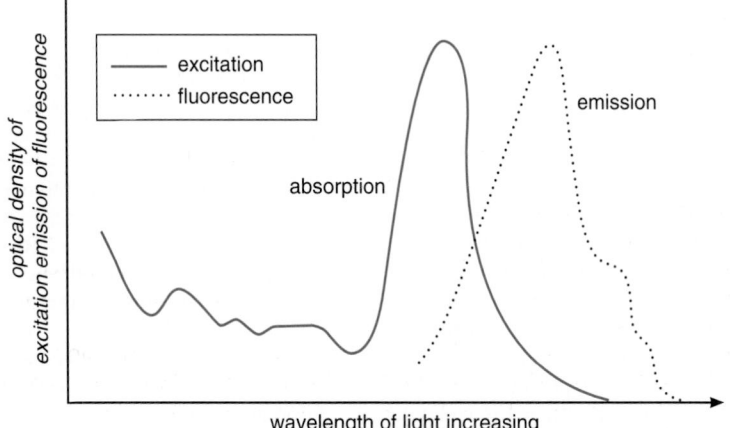

Figure 14–31. Absorption and emission spectra for a fluorescent compound.

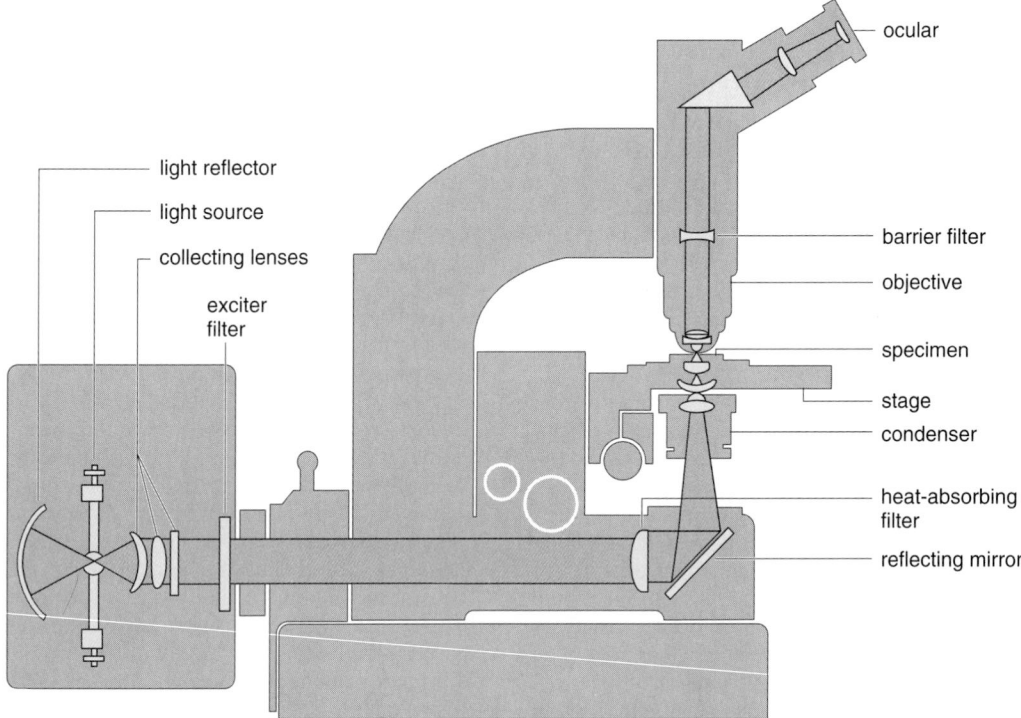

Figure 14–32. Fluorescence microscope with transmitted light. Light beam is generated by a mercury vapor lamp, reflected by a concave mirror, and projected through collecting lenses to the exciter filter, which emits a fluorescent light beam. A reflecting mirror directs the beam from underneath the stage, through the condenser into the specimen. A barrier filter removes wavelengths other than those emitted from the fluorescent compound in the specimen, and the fluorescence pattern is viewed through magnification provided by the objective and ocular lenses.

ficiency with which the dye converts incident light into fluorescent light; (2) the concentration of the dye in the tissue specimen; and (3) the intensity of the exciting (absorbed) radiation.

Microscopes used for visualizing immunofluorescent specimens are modifications of standard transmitted light microscopes (Fig 14–32). In 1967, J. Ploem introduced an epi-illuminated system that employs a vertical illuminator and a dichroic mirror. In this system (Fig 14–33) the excitation beam is focused directly on the tissue specimen through the lens objective. Fluorescent light emitted from the epi-illuminated specimen is then transmitted to the eye through the dichroic mirror. A dichroic mirror allows passage of light of selected wavelengths in one direction through the mirror but not in the opposite direction.

There are several distinct advantages to the Ploem system. Fluorescence may be combined with transmitted light for phase-contrast examination of the tissues, thereby allowing better definition of morphology and fluorescence. Also, interchangeable filter systems permit rapid examination of the specimen at different wavelengths for double fluorochrome staining, for example, red and green (rhodamine and fluorescein, respectively). This advantage in technique has resulted in superior sensitivity for examining cell membrane fluorescence in living lymphocytes.

Method & Interpretation

Virtually any antigen can be detected in fixed tissue sections or in live cell suspensions by immunofluorescence. It is the combination of high sensitivity and specificity, together with the use of histologic techniques, that makes immunofluorescence so useful. The steps involved in immunofluorescence include preparation of immune antiserum or purified antibodies, conjugation with fluorescent dye, and, finally, the staining procedure.

For immunofluorescence, an antiserum to the antigen one wishes to detect is raised in heterologous species. Pure monoclonal antibodies can be used and are prepared as described later on. Antisera should contain milligram amounts of antibody per milliliter. Specificity must exceed a level detectable in ordinary double diffusion or immunoelectrophoretic techniques. More sensitive methods available include hemagglutination inhibition, RIA, and ELISA. Unwanted antibodies present in either conjugates or antiglobulin reagents for the test can usually be removed with insoluble immunoabsorbents or avoided entirely by use of monoclonal antibodies.

After obtaining antiserum of high potency and appropriate specificity, the γ-globulin fraction can be prepared by ammonium sulfate precipitation and DEAE-cellulose ion-exchange chromatography. It is

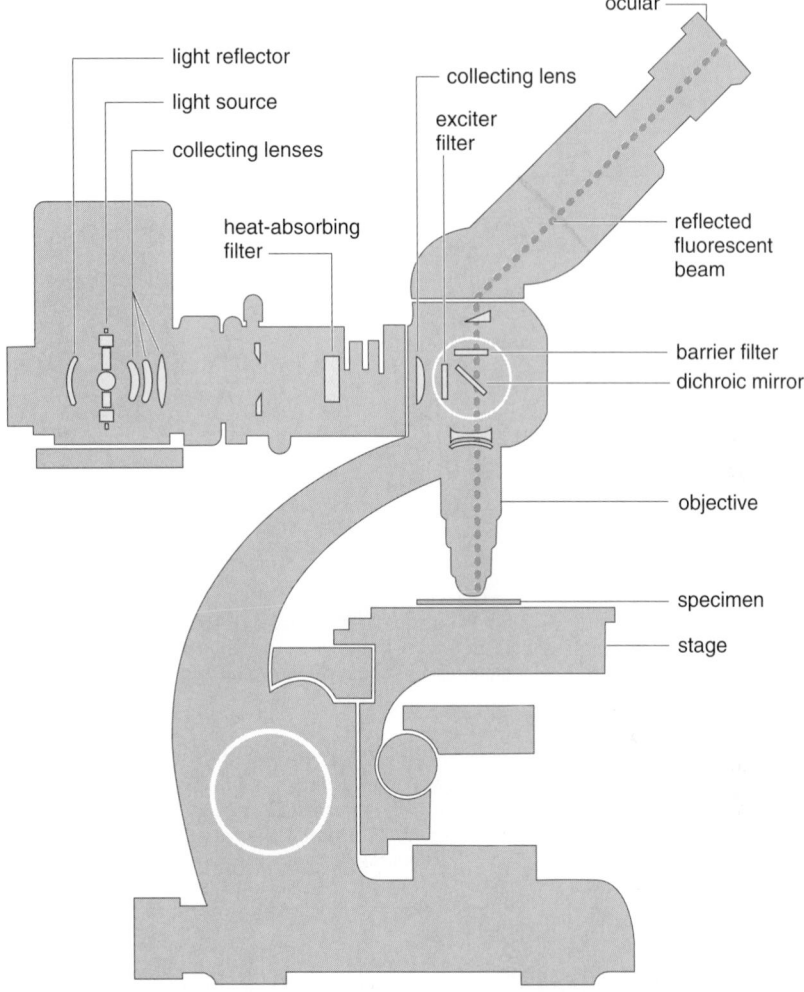

Figure 14–33. Fluorescence microscope with epi-illumination. The light beam is directed through the exciter filter and down onto the specimen. A dichroic mirror allows passage of selected wavelengths in one direction but not another. After reaching the specimen, the light is reflected through the dichroic mirror and emitted fluorescent light is visualized at the ocular.

necessary to partially purify serum γ-globulin, since subsequent conjugation should be limited to antibody as much as possible. This increases the efficiency of staining and avoids unwanted nonspecific staining by fluorochrome-conjugated nonantibody serum proteins that can adhere to tissue components.

Conjugation of γ-globulin depends largely on the particular dye to be combined with the antibody molecule. From a clinical laboratory standpoint, only fluorescein, rhodamine, and some phycobiliproteins have been used widely. Fluorescein, in the form of FITC, or rhodamine, as tetramethylrhodamine isothiocyanate, is either reacted directly with γ-globulin in alkaline solution overnight at 4 °C or dialyzed against γ-globulin. Unreacted dye is then removed from the protein–fluorochrome conjugate by gel filtration or exhaustive dialysis. If necessary, the resultant conjugate can be concentrated by lyophilization, pressure dialysis, or solvent extraction with water-soluble polymers. Thereafter, one must determine both the concentration of γ-globulin and the dye–protein or fluorescein–protein ratio of the compound. This is usually done spectrophotometrically with corrections for the alteration in absorbance of γ-globulin by the introduced fluorochrome. Many clinically useful antisera are commercially available already conjugated to fluorochromes.

Staining Techniques

A. Direct Immunofluorescence: (Fig 14–34) In this technique, conjugated antiserum is added directly to the tissue section or viable cell suspension.

B. Indirect Immunofluorescence: This technique allows for the detection of antibody in the serum. It eliminates the need to purify and individually conjugate each serum sample. The method is basically an adaptation of the antiglobulin reaction (Coombs'

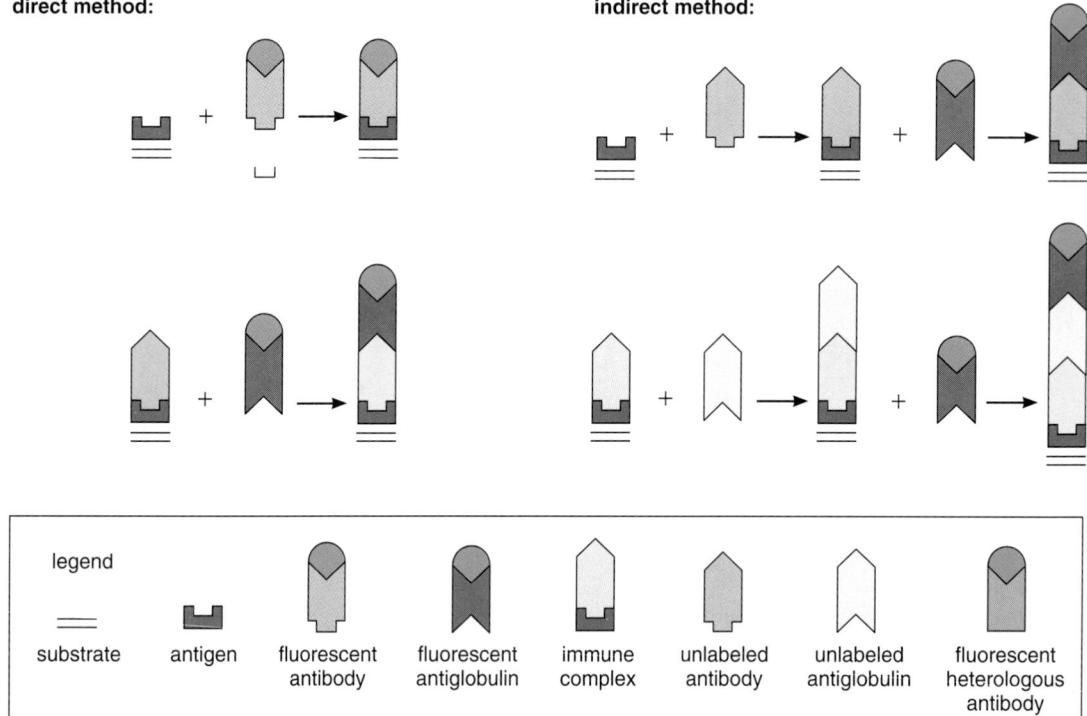

direct method:

indirect method:

legend

| substrate | antigen | fluorescent antibody | fluorescent antiglobulin | immune complex | unlabeled antibody | unlabeled antiglobulin | fluorescent heterologous antibody |

Figure 14–34. Mechanism of immunofluorescence techniques. *Direct Method **(Top):*** Antigen in substrate detected by direct labeling with fluorescent antibody. ***(Bottom):*** Antigen–antibody (immune) complex in substrate labeled with fluorescent antiglobulin reagent. *Indirect Method.* ***(Top):*** Incubation of antigen in substrate with unlabeled antibody forms immune complex. Labeling performed with fluorescent antiglobulin reagent. ***(Bottom):*** Immune complex in substrate reacted with unlabeled antiglobulin reagent and then stained with fluorescent antiglobulin reagent directed at unlabeled antiglobulin. (Modified and reproduced, with permission, from *Nordic Immunology,* Tilburg, The Netherlands.)

test) or double antibody technique (see Fig 14–34). Specificity should be checked as diagrammed and further established by blocking and neutralization methods (Fig 14–35).

Several additional variations in staining techniques have been used. These include (1) a conjugated anticomplement antiserum for the detection of immune complexes containing complement and (2) double staining with both rhodamine and fluorescein conjugates.

Immunofluorescence in which routine serologic procedures are used to detect antibody in human serum specimens has been widely applied (Table 14–5). Sensitivity is generally higher than with complement fixation and lower than with hemagglutination inhibition. Methods for detecting antibody by immunofluorescence include (1) the antiglobulin method, (2) inhibition of labeled antibody–antigen reaction by antibody in test serum, and (3) the anticomplement method.

C. Biotin–Avidin System: Avidin, a basic glycoprotein of MW 68,000, derived from egg albumin, has a remarkably high affinity (10^{15} kcal/mol) for the vitamin biotin. Biotin can easily be covalently cou-

pled to an antibody and then reacted with fluorochrome-coupled avidin. After reaction of antigen with unlabeled antibody, the biotin-labeled second antibody is added. Since many molecules of biotin can be coupled to an antibody, the subsequent addition of fluorochrome-labeled avidin results in a firm bond with exceedingly bright fluorescence. Other advantages are lack of nonspecific binding of fluorochrome-coupled avidin to various substrates and general use of avidin conjugates in binding to biotin-labeled antibodies regardless of their species of origin or isotype.

Quantitative Immunofluorescence

Quantitative immunoassays using fluorochrome-labeled antigens and antibodies are available. The amount of light of a given wavelength emitted from a fluorescent specimen can be precisely measured by a microfluorometer. A number of assay methods have been introduced commercially in the field of quantitative immunofluorescence. Fluorescent immunoassay systems can be used to measure IgG, IgA, and IgM; C3 and C4; and antinuclear and anti-DNA antibodies. Immunoglobulins are measured by competitive bind-

specificity tests

    direct method:

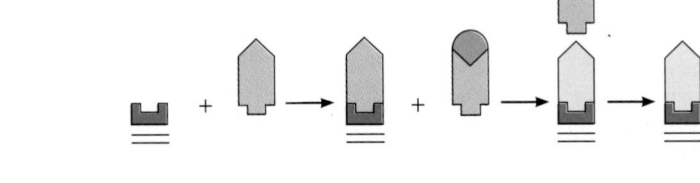

    indirect method:

blocking method

    (indirect method):

neutralizing method:

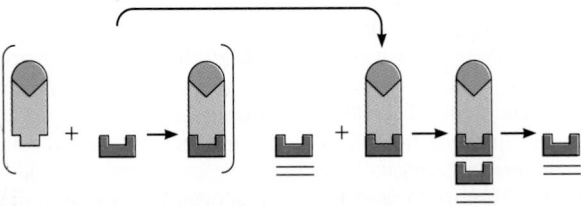

Figure 14–35. Specificity tests. *Direct method. (Left):* Substrate antigen fails to react with fluorescent antiglobulin reagent. No fluorescence results. *(Right):* Immune complex–substrate fails to react with fluorescent antibody directed against unrelated antigen. No fluorescence results. *Indirect method. (Top):* Unlabeled specific antiglobulin is replaced by unrelated antibody. In second step, fluorescent antiglobulin cannot react directly with antigen in substrate that has not bound specific antiglobulin. No fluorescence results. *(Bottom):* First step performed by reacting specific antibody with substrate antigen. In second stage, the specific conjugate is replaced by unrelated fluorescent heterologous antibody. No fluorescence results. *Blocking method.* Substrate antigen is incubated with unlabeled specific antibody prior to addition of specific fluorescent antibody. Decreased fluorescence results. *Neutralizing method.* Substrate antigen is incubated with specific fluorescent antibody after it is absorbed with specific antigen in substrate. No fluorescence results. Symbols are as in 14–34. (Modified and reproduced, with permission, from *Nordic Immunology,* Tilburg, The Netherlands.)

Table 14–5. Clinical applications of immunofluorescence.

Identification of T and B cells in blood
Detection of autoantibodies in serum (eg, antinuclear antibody [ANA])
Detection of immunoglobulins in tissues
Detection of complement components in tissues
Detection of specific, tissue-fixed antibody
Rapid identification of microorganisms in tissue or culture
Identification of chromosomes of specific banding patterns
Identification of tumor-specific antigens on neoplastic tissues
Identification of transplantation antigens in various organs
Localization of hormones and enzymes
Quantitation of serum proteins and antibodies

ing of labeled specific antiserum for free and solid-phase antigen. The free antigen is present in patients' serum, whereas the bound immunoglobulin is fixed to a polymeric hydrophobic surface. The amount of fluorescent antibody bound to the solid-phase antigen is measured in a specially designed microfluorometer and converted to milligrams per deciliter by reference to a standard curve.

Serum antibodies to various cellular antigens such as DNA or nuclei can also be measured by an indirect fluorescence technique. Substrate (eg, DNA) is fixed to the polymer surface in solid phase and incubated with test sera. A second fluorescein anti-immunoglobulin reagent is then bound to the first antigen–antibody complex and the amount of bound fluorescence measured fluorometrically (see Table 14–5).

OTHER IMMUNOHISTOCHEMICAL TECHNIQUES

Enzyme-Linked Antibody

In this method an enzyme is conjugated to antibody directed at a cellular or tissue antigen. The resulting conjugate is then both immunologically and enzymatically active. Use of these conjugates is entirely analogous to that for direct or indirect immunofluorescence techniques.

Horseradish peroxidase is usually the enzyme chosen for coupling to antibody. Tissues are first reacted directly with antibody-enzyme conjugate or directly with enzyme-linked antiglobulin reagent following incubation with unlabeled immune serum. Thereafter, the tissue is incubated with the substrate for the enzyme. The enzyme in this case is detected visually by formation of a black color after incubation with hydrogen peroxide and diaminobenzidine. One advantage of this method is that ordinary light microscopes may be used for analysis of tissue sections. Furthermore, enzyme-coupled antibody can be used for ultrastructural studies in the electron microscope.

Additional immunohistochemical techniques have been developed for localization of tissue or cellular antigens. One in particular, the peroxidase–antiperoxidase (PAP) method, has been used in surgical pathology for detecting enzymes and tumor-related antigens. This is a three-step method. First, fixed slides are stained with rabbit antiserum to a tissue antigen to be measured. Next, an antirabbit immunoglobulin that reacts with the first antibody is applied. Finally, an immune complex, consisting of rabbit antibodies to peroxidase combined with peroxidase, is added. This immune complex reacts with the antirabbit bridging antibody. A peroxidase substrate is added, which forms the colored reaction product.

Other techniques being developed include hapten-coupled antibodies, the use of staphylococcal protein A as an intermediate reagent, and systems with more than one immunoenzymatic reagent, that is, double staining. Fixation difficulties and standardization of readily available reagents still limit the wider application of these potentially powerful techniques.

Ferritin-Coupled Antibody

Ferritin, an iron-containing protein, is highly electron-dense. When coupled to antibody, it can be used for either direct or indirect tissue staining. Ferritin-coupled antibody–antigen complexes in fixed tissue can then be localized with the electron microscope. Other electron-dense particles, such as gold or uranium, can also be introduced chemically into specific antitissue antibodies. These reagents have also been applied in immunoelectron microscopy.

Autoradiography

Radioactive isotopes such as ^{125}I that can be chemically linked to immunoglobulins provide highly sensitive probes for localization of tissue antigens. The antigens are detected visually after tissue staining by overlaying or coating slides with photographic emulsion. The appearance of silver grains as black dots has been used for subcellular localization of antigen both at light microscopic and ultrastructural levels. Autoradiography has also been applied to detection of proteins or immunoglobulins synthesized by cells in tissue culture.

Miscellaneous Methods

A variety of other methods have been described for localization of antigens in tissues. Many have not found widespread clinical application. In most cases, these techniques depend on secondary phenomena that occur as a result of the antigen–antibody interaction. These methods include the following:

1. Complement fixation
2. Conglutinating complement absorption test
3. Antiglobulin consumption test
4. Mixed hemadsorption
5. Immune adherence
6. Hemagglutination and coated particle reaction
7. Immunoprecipitation

AGGLUTINATION

Agglutination and precipitation reactions form the basis of many techniques in laboratory immunology. Whereas precipitation reactions are quantifiable and simple to perform, agglutination techniques are only **semiquantitative.** Important advantages of agglutination reactions are their high degree of sensitivity and the ability to assess end points visually. The agglutination of either insoluble native antigens or antigen-coated particles can be applied to measurement of a large variety of analytes.

According to R. R. A. Coombs, the three main requirements in agglutination tests are the availability of a stable cell or particle suspension, the presence of one or more antigens close to the surface, and the knowledge that "incomplete" or nonagglutinating antibodies are detectable with modifications such as antiglobulin reactions.

Agglutination reactions may be classified as either direct or indirect (passive). In the direct technique, a cell or insoluble particulate antigen is agglutinated directly by antibody. An example is the agglutination of group A erythrocytes by anti-A sera. Passive agglutination refers to agglutination of antigen-coated cells or inert particles that are passive carriers of otherwise soluble antigens. Examples are latex agglutination (fixation) for detection of rheumatoid factor and agglutination of DNA-coated erythrocytes for detection of anti-DNA antibody. Alternatively, *antigen* can be detected by coating latex particles or erythrocytes with purified *antibody* and performing so-called reversed agglutination. Another category of agglutination involves spontaneous agglutination of erythrocytes by certain viruses. This viral hemagglutination reaction can be specifically inhibited in the presence of antiviral antibody. Thus, viral hemagglutination can be used either to quantify virus itself or to determine by inhibition the titer of antisera directed against hemagglutinating viruses.

Inhibition of agglutination, if carefully standardized with highly purified antigens, can be used as a sensitive indicator of the amount of antigen in various tissue fluids. Hemagglutination inhibition using passive hemagglutination reactions can be semiautomated in microtiter plates and is sensitive for measuring antigens in concentrations of 0.1–10 μg/mL. With appropriate modification, passive hemagglutination with protein-sensitized cells can detect antibody at concentrations as low as 0.01 μg/mL.

AGGLUTINATION TECHNIQUES

Direct Agglutination Test

Erythrocytes, bacteria, fungi, and a variety of other microbial species can be directly agglutinated by an-tibody. Tests to detect specific antibody are carried out by serially titrating antisera in twofold dilutions in the presence of a constant amount of antigen. Direct agglutination is relatively temperature-independent except for cold-reacting antibody, such as cold agglutinins. After a few hours of incubation, agglutination is complete, and particles are examined either directly or microscopically for evidence of clumping. The results are usually expressed as a titer of antiserum, that is, the highest dilution at which agglutination occurs. Because of intrinsic variability in the test system, a titer usually must differ by at least two twofold dilutions ("two tubes") to be considered significantly different from any given titer. Tests are carried out in small test tubes in volumes of 0.2–0.5 mL or in microtiter plates with smaller amounts of reagents.

Indirect (Passive) Agglutination Test

The range of soluble antigens that can be passively adsorbed or chemically coupled to erythrocytes or other inert particles has extended the application of agglutination reactions. Many antigens spontaneously couple with erythrocytes and form stable reagents for antibody detection (Table 14–6). When erythrocytes are used as the inert particles, serum specimens often must be absorbed with washed, uncoated erythrocytes to remove heterophilic antibodies that would otherwise nonspecifically agglutinate them. The advantages of using erythrocytes for coating are their ready availability, sensitivity as indicators, and storage capabilities. Erythrocytes can be treated with formalin, glutaraldehyde, or pyruvic aldehyde and stored for prolonged periods at 4 °C.

A list of general methods available for coating antigens to erythrocytes is presented in Table 14–7). Treatment of erythrocytes with tannic acid increases the amount of most protein antigens subsequently adsorbed. This higher density of coated antigen greatly increases the sensitivity of the agglutination reaction. Although highly purified antigens are required for immunologic specificity, slightly denatured or aggregated antigens coat tanned erythrocytes best.

Agglutination tests may be performed in tubes, microtiter plates, or on slides. In antisera with very high

Table 14–6. Substances that spontaneously adsorb to erythrocytes for hemagglutination.

Escherichia coli antigens
Yersinia antigens
Lipopolysaccharide from *Neisseria meningitidis*
Toxoplasma antigens
Purified protein derivative (PPD)
Endotoxin of *Mycoplasma* species
Viruses
Antibiotics, especially penicillin
Ovalbumin
Bovine serum albumin
DNA
Haptens (eg, dinitrochlorobenzene [DNCB])

Table 14–7. Methods used to coat fresh and aldehyde-treated red blood cells with various antigens and antibodies for passive hemagglutination assay.

Coupling Agent	Comments on Coupling	Antigens Commonly Coated
None	Simple adsorption	Penicillin, bacterial antigens, including endotoxins and exotoxins, viruses, and ovalbumin.
Tannic acid	Adsorption possibly caused by changes analogous to enzymes. Most popular; usually satisfactory but often difficult and unreliable.	A wide spectrum of antigens; serum proteins, microbial and tissue extracts, homogenates, thyroglobulin, and tuberculin proteins.
Bisdiazotized benzidine (BDB)	Chemically stable covalent azo bonds.	Proteins and pollen antigens.
1,3-Difluoro-4,6-dinitrobenzene (DFDNB)	Adsorption after modification of cell membrane.	Purified proteins and chorionic gonadotropin.
Chromic chloride (CrCl$_3$)	Proteins bound to erythrocytes by the charge effect of trivalent cations.	Proteins.
Glutaraldehyde, cyanuric chloride, tetrazotized O-dianisidine	Cross-linking and covalent coupling.	Various proteins and certain enzymes.
Tolulene-2,4-diisocyanate	Covalently bound.	Proteins.
Water-soluble carbodiimide	Covalently bound.	Proteins.

Source: Modified and reproduced, with permission, from Fudenberg HH: Hemagglutination inhibition: Passive hemagglutination assay for antigen–antibody reactions. In: *A Seminar on Basic Immunology.* American Association of Blood Banks, 1971.

agglutination titers, a prozone phenomenon may obscure the results. The prozone phenomenon produces false-negative agglutination reactions at high concentrations of antibody as a result of poor lattice formation and steric hindrance by antibody excess. The use of standard serial dilutions, however, eliminates this difficulty. Since IgM antibody is about 750 times as efficient as IgG in agglutination, the presence of high amounts of IgM can influence test results.

Flocculation is another type of complex formation assay. In contrast to agglutination or precipitation, however, the antigen–antibody complexes aggregate but remain in suspension. Reactions can be read with a microscope. This is the technique used in the Venereal Disease Research Laboratory (VDRL) for the screening test for syphilis.

HEMAGGLUTINATION INHIBITION

The inhibition of agglutination of antigen-coated red blood cells by homologous antigen is a highly sensitive and specific method for detecting small quantities of soluble antigen in blood or other tissue fluids. The principle of this assay is that antibody preincubated with soluble homologous or cross-reacting antigens is "inactivated" when incubated with antigen-coated erythrocytes. Thus, the test proceeds in two stages (Fig 14–36). Antibody in relatively low concentration is incubated with a sample of antigen of unknown quantity. After combination with soluble antigen, antigen-coated cells are added and agglutinated by uncombined or free antibody. (The degree of inhibition of agglutination reflects the amount of antigen present in the original sample.) Controls, including

samples of known antigen concentration and uncoated erythrocytes, must be used. This hemagglutination inhibition method has been used in the detection of hepatitis B surface antigen (HBsAg) in hepatitis and in the detection of factor VIII antigen in hemophilia and related clotting disorders, but its use has been primarily in research, not clinical laboratories.

CLINICALLY APPLICABLE TESTS THAT INVOLVE AGGLUTINATION REACTIONS

Antiglobulin Test (Coombs' Test)

The development of this simple and ingenious technique virtually revolutionized the field of immunohematology, and in various forms it has found widespread application in all fields of immunology. Antibodies frequently coat erythrocytes but fail to form the necessary lattice to produce agglutination. A typical example is antibody directed at the Rh determinants on human erythrocytes (see Chapter 16). The addition of an antiglobulin antiserum produced in a heterologous species (eg, rabbit antihuman γ-globulin), however, produces marked agglutination. Thus, the antiglobulin, or Coombs', test is used principally to detect subagglutinating or nonagglutinating amounts of antierythrocyte antibodies. More specific Coombs' reagents directed at immunoglobulin classes, however, such as anti-IgG, anti-IgA, or anti-L chains, may also be employed to detect cell-bound immunoglobulin. So-called nongamma Coombs' reagents, which are directed against various complement components, such as C3 or C4, may also produce erythrocyte agglutination in the case of autoim-

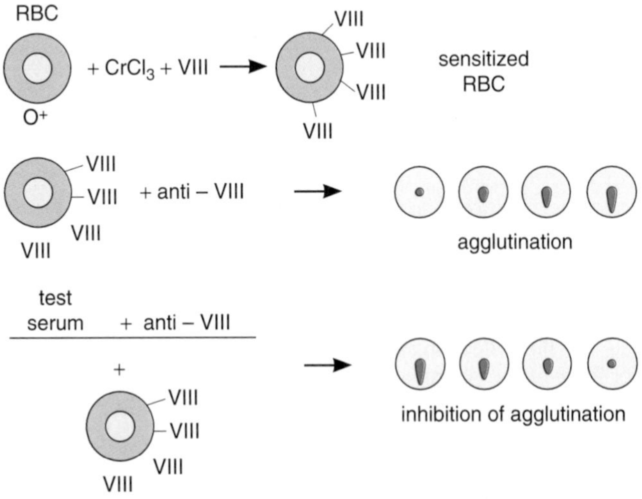

Figure 14–36. Hemagglutination inhibition. Human O-positive erythrocytes (RBC) are conjugated with coagulation factor VIII antigen by chromic chloride. The sensitized erythrocytes are reacted with specific antibody to factor VIII and are agglutinated. In the well of a V-shaped microtiter plate, agglutinated erythrocytes appear as discrete dots. Nonagglutinated cells form a streak when the plate is incubated at a 45° angle. Agglutination of sensitized red blood cells can be inhibited by the presence of homologous factor VIII antigen present in the test serum. With decreasing amounts of serum added to the test, the specific antibody agglutinates sensitized cells and forms a dot in the microtiter well. A semiquantitative estimation of the amount or titer of antigen in a test serum can be made in this way.

mune hemolytic anemia. In some instances of this disorder, only complement components are bound to the erythrocyte, and the regular antiglobulin reaction is negative. The **direct Coombs' test** detects γ-globulin or other serum proteins that are adherent to erythrocytes taken directly from a sensitized individual. The **indirect Coombs' test** is a two-stage reaction for detection of incomplete antibodies in a patient's serum. The serum in question is first incubated with test erythrocytes, and the putative antibody-coated cells are then agglutinated by a Coombs' antiglobulin serum. The major applications of Coombs' tests include erythrocyte typing in blood banks, the evaluation of hemolytic disease of the newborn, and the diagnosis of autoimmune hemolytic anemia.

Bentonite Flocculation Test

Passive carriers of antigen other than erythrocytes have been widely used in serology for the demonstration of agglutinating antibody. Wyoming bentonite is a form of siliceous earth that can directly adsorb most types of protein, carbohydrate, and nucleic acid. After adsorption, many antigens are stable on bentonite for 3–6 months. Simple flocculation on slides with appropriate positive and negative control sera indicates the presence of serum antibody. Bentonite flocculation has been employed to detect antibodies to *Trichinella,* DNA, and rheumatoid factor.

Latex Fixation Test

Latex particles may also be used as passive carriers for adsorbed soluble protein and polysaccharide anti-

gens. The most widespread application of latex agglutination (fixation) has been in the detection of rheumatoid factor. Rheumatoid factor is a pentameric IgM antibody directed against IgG (see Chapter 33). If IgG is passively adsorbed to latex particles, specific determinants on the IgG are revealed that then react with IgM rheumatoid factors. This method is more sensitive but less specific for rheumatoid factor than the Rose-Waaler test (see following section).

Rose-Waaler Test

This passive hemagglutination test is also used for the detection of rheumatoid factor. Tanned erythrocytes (usually from sheep) are coated with subagglutinating amounts of rabbit IgG antibodies specific for sheep erythrocytes. Human rheumatoid factor agglutinate these rabbit immunoglobulin-sensitized sheep erythrocytes by virtue of a cross-reaction between rabbit IgG and human IgG. The use of this test and latex fixation in the diagnosis of rheumatoid diseases (especially rheumatoid arthritis) is discussed in Chapter 33.

COMPLEMENT ASSAYS

Complement is one of the main humoral effector mechanisms of immune complex-induced tissue damage (see Chapter 11). Clinical disorders of complement function have been recognized for many decades, but their mechanism and eventual treatment have awaited elucidation of the complement sequence itself. The nine major complement components of the classic pathway (C1–C9), several from the alternative pathway, and various inhibitors can now be measured in human serum. Clinically useful assays of complement consist primarily of CH_{50}/AH_{50} or total hemolytic assays and specific functional or immunochemical assays for various components. Immunochemical means provide molecular concentrations in serum but do not provide data regarding the functional integrity of the various molecules.

It is worth emphasizing that the collection and storage of serum samples for functional or immunochemical complement assays present special problems as a result of the remarkable lability of some of the complement components. Rapid removal of serum from clotted specimens and storage at temperatures of $-70\ °C$ or lower are required for preservation of maximal activity.

Complement fixation or use, which occurs as a consequence of antigen–antibody reactions, provides a sensitive and useful means of detecting antigens or antibodies in serology.

HEMOLYTIC ASSAY

Specific antibody-mediated hemolysis of erythrocytes by complement is a relatively insensitive screening test for complement activity in human serum. It has limited usefulness, however, since a marked reduction in components is necessary to produce a reduction in the hemolytic assay. The hemolytic assay employs sheep erythrocytes (E), rabbit antibody (A) to sheep erythrocytes, and fresh guinea pig serum as a source of complement (C). Hemolysis is measured spectrophotometrically as the absorbance of released hemoglobin and can be directly related to the number of erythrocytes lysed. The amount of lysis in a standardized system employing E, A, and C describes an S-shaped curve when plotted against increasing amounts of added complement (Fig 14–37).

The curve is S-shaped, but in the midregion, near 50% hemolysis, a nearly linear relationship exists between the degree of hemolysis and the amount of complement present. In this range, the degree of erythrocyte lysis is very sensitive to any alteration in complement concentration. For clinical purposes, measurement of total hemolytic activity of serum is taken at 50% hemolysis level. The CH_{50} is an arbitrary unit defined as the quantity of complement necessary for 50% lysis of erythrocytes under rigidly standardized conditions of sensitization with antibody (EA). CH_{50} test results are expressed as the reciprocal of the serum dilution giving 50% hemolysis. Variables that can influence the degree of hemolysis include erythrocyte concentration, fragility (age) of erythrocytes, amount of antibody used for sensitization,

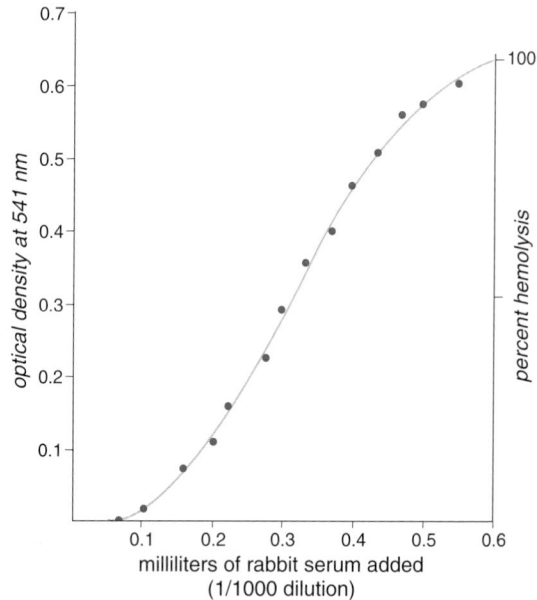

Figure 14–37. Relationship of complement concentration and erythrocytes lysed. Curve relating the percentage of hemolysis that results from increasing amounts of fresh rabbit serum (diluted 1:1000) as complement source is added to sensitized sheep erythrocytes (erythrocyte amboceptor [EA]). Hemolysis can be precisely determined by measuring the optical density of hemolysis supernates at 541 nm, the wavelength for maximal absorbance by hemoglobin.

nature of the antibody (eg, IgG or IgM), ionic strength of the buffer system, pH, reaction time, temperature, and divalent cation (Ca^{2+} or Mg^{2+}) concentrations.

The value for CH_{50} units in human serum may be determined in several ways. Usually, one employs the von Krogh equation, which converts the S-shaped complement titration curve into a nearly straight line.

The S-shaped curve in Figure 14–37 is described by the von Krogh equation:

$$X = K\left(\frac{Y}{1-Y}\right)^{1/n} \qquad (4)$$

where X = mL of diluted complement added;
Y = degree of percentage lysis;
K = constant, and
n = $0.2 \pm 10\%$ under standard E and A conditions.

It is convenient to convert the von Krogh equation to a log form that renders the curve linear for plotting of clinical results (Fig 14–38).

$$\log X = \log K + \frac{1}{n}\ \log \frac{Y}{1-Y} \qquad (5)$$

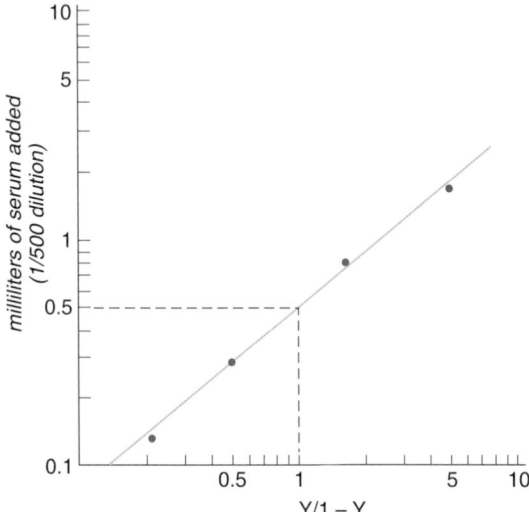

Figure 14–38. Determination of CH_{50} units from serum. Standard curve relating milliliters of serum 1:500 dilution to $Y/(1 - Y)$ from von Krogh equation. When $Y/(1 - Y) = 1.0$, the percentage of lysis equals 50%. In the example shown, 0.5 mL of 1:500 serum dilution has produced $Y/(1 - Y) = 1.0$ or 50% lysis. The CH_{50} value for this serum equals 1000, since 1 mL of serum would have 1000 lytic units.

The values of $Y/(1 - Y)$ are plotted on a log–log scale against serum dilutions. The reciprocal of the dilution of serum that intersects the curve at the value $Y/(1 - Y) = 1$ is the CH_{50} unit. Values for normal CH_{50} units vary greatly depending on particular conditions of the test employed. It should again be emphasized that the CH_{50} assay is relatively insensitive to reduction in specific complement components unless there is a congenital deficiency of a particular component, and the assay may in fact be normal or only slightly depressed in the face of significant reduction in individual components.

MEASUREMENT OF INDIVIDUAL COMPLEMENT COMPONENTS

Functional Assays

Activation of the entire complement sequence of C1–C9 must occur to produce lysis of antibody-coated erythrocytes (EA). Thus, a general scheme can be proposed to determine the level of activity of individual complement components. Initially, one must obtain pure preparations of each of the individual components. These pure components are then added sequentially to EA until the step is reached just prior to the component to be measured. The test sample is added, and the degree of subsequent erythrocyte lysis is then related to the presence of the later acting components. Of course, all proximal components must be supplied in excess to measure more distally acting in-

termediates. Alternatively, the presence of genetically defined complement deficiencies has made available to the laboratory a further source of specifically deficient reagents for estimating individual component activity. A description of the technique of functional assays for complement components and their inhibitors is found in the monograph by F. Rapp and T. Borsos.

Immunoassays for Complement Components

Antibodies can be prepared against most of the major complement components and complement inhibitors, which allows for immunochemical determination of complement components. Techniques that have been used for this purpose include electroimmunodiffusion (Laurell's rocket electrophoresis), single radial diffusion, rate nephelometry, and ELISA. Although immunologic assay of complement components is independent of their biologic function, alterations in the chemical composition of complement components during storage may alter their behavior in these immunoassays. For example, in storage, C3 spontaneously converts to C3c, which has a smaller molecular size than native C3. Thus, when single radial diffusion of the timed interval variety is used, stored serum gives falsely high estimates because more rapid diffusion produces a larger ring diameter. Crucial to accuracy in clinical laboratory tests for complement is reliability of standards. In general, commercial sera prepared from large normal donor pools are adequate. However, because complement components are thermolabile when stored above −70 °C, great care must be taken to ensure adequate refrigerated storage. In fact, the major source of error in complement determination is poor sample handling.

Measurement and significance of complement fragments or catabolic products are discussed in Chapter 11.

Significance of CH_{50} Units
A. Reduced Serum Complement Activity: Reduced amounts of serum complement activity have been reported in a variety of disease states (Table 14–8). The reduction in serum complement activity could be due to any one or a combination of (1) complement consumption by in vivo formation of antigen–antibody complexes, (2) decreased synthesis of complement, (3) increased catabolism of complement, or (4) formation of an inhibitor. Although complement has been demonstrated fixed to various tissues (eg, glomerular basement membrane) in association with antibody, tissue fixation of complement is apparently not an important mechanism in lowering serum complement activity. Isolated reduction in human serum levels of C1, C2, C3, C6, or C7 to 50% of normal only slightly reduces hemolytic activity. For this reason, many laboratories have switched from CH_{50} to a more simple immunochemical determination of the C3

Table 14–8. Diseases associated with reduced hemolytic complement activity.

Systemic lupus erythematosus with glomerulonephritis
Acute glomerulonephritis
Membranoproliferative glomerulonephritis
Acute serum sickness
Immune complex diseases
Advanced cirrhosis of the liver
Disseminated intravascular coagulation
Severe combined immunodeficiency
Infective endocarditis with glomerulonephritis
Infected ventriculoarterial shunts
Hereditary angioneurotic edema
Hereditary C2 deficiency
Paroxysmal cold hemoglobinuria
Myasthenia gravis
Infective hepatitis with arthritis
Allograft rejection
Mixed cryoglobulinemia (IgM–IgG)
Lymphoma

Table 14–9. Diseases associated with elevated serum complement concentrations.

Obstructive jaundice
Thyroiditis
Acute rheumatic fever
Rheumatoid arthritis
Periarteritis nodosa
Dermatomyositis
Acute myocardial infarction
Ulcerative colitis
Typhoid fever
Diabetes
Gout
Reiter's syndrome

level. In general, the reduction of the C3 level correlates positively with CH_{50} activity reduction. Alternative methods for detecting low levels of activation include the determination of complement split products. Immunochemical detection of C3d or Ba can be used for determination of classic and alternative pathway activation, respectively.

When screening for congenital deficiencies of various complement proteins, however, the CH_{50} and AH_{50} can provide useful information to localize the defect to the classic, alternative, or terminal pathway. Reduced CH_{50} activity in the presence of normal AH_{50} activity suggests a classic pathway deficiency. Reduced AH_{50} with normal CH_{50} suggests an alternative pathway deficiency. Defective CH_{50} and AH_{50} suggests a defect in the terminal pathway.

B. Elevated Complement Levels: Although complement levels are elevated in a variety of diseases (Table 14–9), the significance of this observation is unclear. The most likely mechanism is overproduction, which may be due to the behavior of complement components as acute-phase reactants.

The development of specific functional and immunologic methods for detecting complement components has led to the discovery of a variety of genetically determined disorders of the complement system. A discussion of the specific disease states that result from selective deficiency of the various complement components is found in Chapter 25.

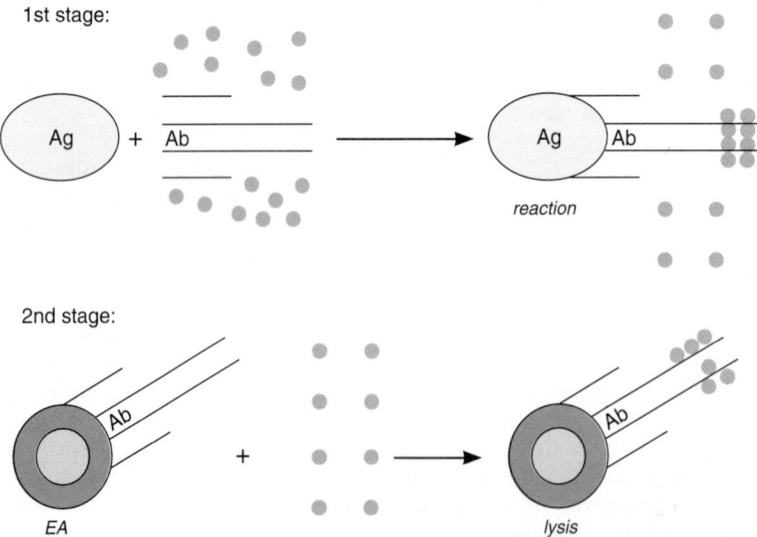

Figure 14–39. Principles of complement fixation. In the first stage, antigen (Ag) and antibody (Ab) are reacted in the presence of complement (●). The interaction of Ag and antibody fixes some but not all of the complement available. In the second stage, the residual or unfixed complement is measured by adding erythrocyte amboceptor (EA) which is lysed by residual complement. Thus, a reciprocal relationship exists between amounts of lysis in the second stage and antigen present in the first stage.

Table 14–10. Applications of complement fixation tests.

Hepatitis B surface antigen (HBsAg)
Antiplatelet antibodies
Anti-DNA
Immunoglobulins
L chains
Wassermann's test for syphilis
Coccidioides immitis antigen

COMPLEMENT FIXATION TESTS

The fixation of complement occurs during the interaction of antigen and antibodies. Thus, the consumption of complement in vitro can be used as a test to detect and measure antibodies, antigens, or both. The test depends on a two-stage reaction system. In the initial stage, antigen and antibody react in the presence of a known amount of complement and complement is consumed (fixed). In the second stage, hemolytic complement activity is measured to determine the amount of complement fixed and thus the amount of antigen or antibody present in the initial mixture (Fig 14–39). The amount of activity remaining after the initial antigen–antibody reaction is back-titrated in the hemolytic assay (see earlier discussion). Results are expressed as either the highest serum dilution showing fixation for antibody estimation or the concentration of antigen that is limiting for antigen determinations.

Extremely sensitive assays for antigen or antibody concentrations have been developed by using micro-complement fixation. These assays are too cumbersome and complex for routine clinical laboratory use, however.

Complement fixation tests (see Fig 14–39) have received widespread application in both research and clinical laboratory practice. Table 14–10 lists some of the applications of complement fixation for either antigen or antibody determination. It should be recalled that all complement assay systems involving functional tests can be inhibited by anticomplementary action of serum. This may result from antigen–antibody complexes, heparin, chelating agents, and aggregated immunoglobulins, such as in multiple myeloma.

MONOCLONAL ANTIBODIES

The production of monoclonal antibodies by somatic cell hybridization of antibody-forming cells and continuously replicating cell lines created a revolution in immunology. The technique of hybridoma formation described by H. Köhler and C. Milstein in 1975 has allowed preparation of virtually unlimited quantities of antibodies that are chemically, physically, and immunologically completely homogeneous since each antibody is synthesized from cells derived from a single clone. These molecules are then generally unencumbered by nonspecificity and cross-reactivity. In laboratory immunology, monoclonal antibodies are used to detect cellular and soluble antigens with RIA, ELISA, immunofluorescence assay (IFA), and flow cytometry. Some well-established immunochemical methods such as immunodiffusion and immunoelectrophoresis probably do not require the degree of specificity afforded by monoclonal antibodies. The narrow specificity of monoclonal antibodies for single epitopes can theoretically limit their applicability.

TECHNIQUE OF MONOCLONAL ANTIBODY PRODUCTION

Hybridomas, or somatic cell hybrids, can readily be formed by fusing a single cell suspension of splenocytes or lymphocytes from immunized mice or rats to cells of continuously replicating tumor cells, such as myelomas or lymphomas (Fig 14–40). The replicating cell line is selected for two distinct properties: (1) lack of immunoglobulin production or secretion, and (2) lack of hypoxanthine phosphoribosyl transferase (HPRT) activity. The cells are fused by rapid exposure to polyethylene glycol. Thereafter, three cell populations remain in culture: splenocytes, myeloma cells, and hybrids. The hybrids have the combined genome of the parent lines and eventually extrude chromosomes and acquire a diploid state. Selection for the hybrids is accomplished by awaiting natural death of the splenocytes. The myeloma cell line is killed, because in HAT medium, which contains hypoxanthine, aminopterin, and thymidine, HPRT cells cannot use exogenous hypoxanthine to produce purines. Aminopterin blocks endogenous synthesis of purines and pyrimidines, and the cells die. Hybrids begin to double every 24–48 hours, and colonies rapidly form.

The hybridoma cells are then cloned by limiting dilution methods, and supernates are assayed for antibody production, usually by ELISA or RIA. Recloning is performed to ensure monoclonality, and large numbers of cells are grown for antibody production. Extensive immunochemical and serologic studies are performed to ensure antibody specificity. Large quantities of antibody can be produced in serum-free tissue culture or in ascites fluid in syngeneic mice. Cells are stored in liquid nitrogen for further use.

Interspecies as well as intraspecies hybridomas can be produced and propagated in long-term culture. For use in human therapeutic research, mouse hybridomas have usually been employed, but these regularly produce antimurine antibody responses after infusions in humans. For this reason and for maximum specificity, human-to-human hybridomas have also been developed. Limitations in range of antibody specificities and technical difficulties in maintaining these hybridomas in culture need to be overcome.

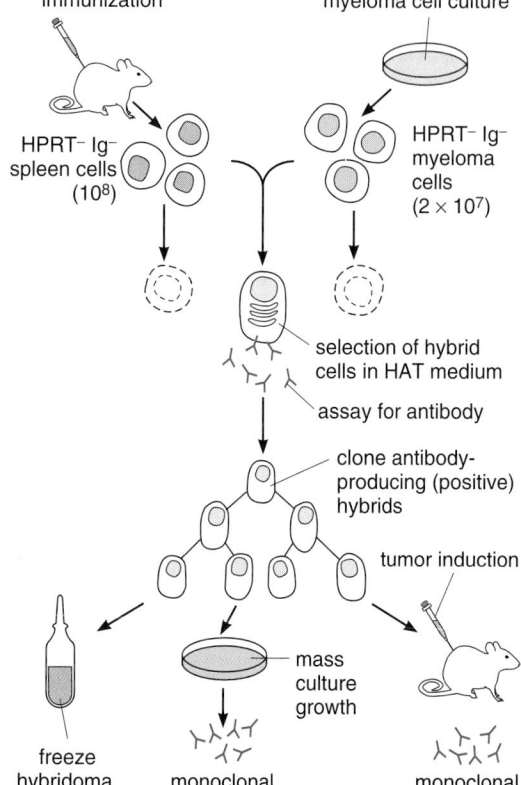

immunization

myeloma cell culture

HPRT⁻ Ig⁻
spleen cells
(10^8)

HPRT⁻ Ig⁻
myeloma
cells
(2×10^7)

selection of hybrid
cells in HAT medium

assay for antibody

clone antibody-
producing (positive)
hybrids

tumor induction

freeze
hybridoma
for future use

mass
culture
growth

monoclonal
antibody

monoclonal
antibody

Figure 14–40. Formation of hybridomas between mouse cells and myeloma cells. Mouse myeloma cells that do not produce their own immunoglobulins and lack hypoxanthine and phosphoribosyl transferase (HPRT) are fused to splenocytes from an immunized mouse with polyethylene glycol. The hybrid cells are selected in hypoxanthine–aminopterin–thymidine (HAT) medium. Unfused myeloma cells are killed by HAT, and unfused splenocytes die out. The hybridomas are cloned, and antibody is produced in tissue culture or by ascites formation. (Reproduced, with permission, from Diamond BA et al: Monoclonal antibodies: A new technique for producing serologic reagents. *N Engl J Med* 1981;**304:**1344.)

Table 14–11. Applications of monoclonal antibodies.

Diagnostic (Many achieved; some experimental.)
  Leukocyte identification
  Lymphocyte subset determination
  HLA antigen detection
    Individual specificities of A, B, C, DR loci
    Framework specificities
  Viral detection and subtyping (eg, influenza variants)
  Parasite identification
  Other microorganism detection
  Polypeptide hormone detection
  Relatedness of hormones (eg, hGH, hCS, hPRL)
  Detection of carcinoembryonic protein (eg, CEA, AFP)
  Detection of cardiac myosin for myocardial injury
  Typing of leukemias and lymphomas
  Detection of tumor-related antigens
  Immunohistochemical application in tissue sections

Therapeutic (Experimental; can be coupled to a toxin or radioisotope to enhance in vivo effects.)
  Antitumor therapy
    Individual tumor antigen-specific
    Anti-idiotype to surface immunoglobulin on B cell
      lymphomas
  Immunosuppression
    Organ transplantation
    Autoimmune and hypersensitivity diseases
    Treatment of GVH disease
  Fertility control
    Anti-hCG or antitrophoblast antibodies
    Drug toxicity reversal (eg, digitalis intoxication)

Abbreviations: hGH = human growth hormone; hCS = human chorionic somatomammotropin; hPRL = human prolactin; AFP = alpha-fetoprotein; GVH = graft-versus-host; hCG = human chorionic gonadotropin.

Some examples of application of monoclonal antibodies in immunology are listed in Table 14–11.

COMPARATIVE SENSITIVITY OF QUANTITATIVE IMMUNOASSAYS

A major limitation of all quantitative immunoassays is their sensitivity. Exact lower limits of analyte detection vary with avidity, concentration, lots of antisera, temperature, length of reaction, and other factors. Nevertheless, it is useful to consider the approximate limits of sensitivity of various methods

available in the clinical immunology laboratory. The most commonly employed techniques are listed in Table 14–12 in order of increasing sensitivity.

PREDICTIVE VALUE THEORY

When *any* test is used to make a decision, there is some probability of drawing an erroneous conclusion. Predictive value theory can be used to deal with this problem. An example of its application in the diagnosis of multiple sclerosis follows. This diagnosis is still made primarily by using the patient's history and physical findings. Several laboratory tests are also used as decision aids. One such test is the CSF IgG index, which is a ratio of ratios [CSF IgG:CSF albumin]:[serum IgG:serum albumin]. To simplify discussion, we have consolidated the patients into two groups: those with definite or probable multiple sclerosis, and all others. For every individual, two items of information are noted: (1) the diagnostic category (disease or no disease) and (2) the results of the laboratory test (normal or abnormal). This divides the results into four categories: **true-positives, true-negatives, false-positives,** and **false-negatives.** False-positive and false-negative results led to erro-

Table 14–12. Relative sensitivity of assays for antigens and antibodies.

Technique	Approximate Sensitivity (per dL)
Total serum proteins (by biuret or refractometry)	100 mg
Serum protein electrophoresis (zone electrophoresis)	100 mg
Analytic ultracentrifugation	100 mg
Immunoelectrophoresis	5–10 mg
Immunofixation	5–10 mg
Single radial diffusion	<1–2 mg
Double diffusion in agar (Ouchterlony)	< 1 mg
Electroimmunodiffusion (rocket electrophoresis)	< 0.5 mg
One-dimensional double electroimmunodiffusion (counterimmunoelectrophoresis)	< 0.1 mg
Nephelometry	0.1 mg
Complement fixation	1 µg
Agglutination	1 µg
Enzyme immunoassay (ELISA)	<1 µg
Quantitative immunofluorescence	<1 pg
Radioimmunoassay (RIA)	<1 pg

Source: Modified and reproduced, with permission, from Ritzmann SE: *Behring Diagnostics Manual on Proteinology and Immunoassays,* 2nd ed. Behring Diagnostics, 1977.

neous conclusions. The results can be presented as a two-by-two contingency table as in Table 14–13.

Several basic terms are used in predictive value theory. **Diagnostic sensitivity** (not to be confused with analytic sensitivity, discussed in the context of ligand assay) is defined as the fraction of diseased subjects with abnormal test results. **Diagnostic specificity** is defined as the fraction of nondiseased subjects who have a normal laboratory test. The **positive predictive value** is the fraction of abnormal tests that represent disease, and **negative predictive value** is the fraction of normal tests that represent the absence of disease. Computing these values for the data in Table 14–13, we find

$$\text{Diagnostic sensitivity} = \frac{54}{64} = 0.84 \qquad (6)$$

$$\text{Diagnostic specificity} = \frac{110}{129} = 0.85 \qquad (7)$$

$$\text{Positive predictive value} = \frac{54}{73} = 0.74 \qquad (8)$$

$$\text{Negative predictive value} = \frac{110}{120} = 0.92 \qquad (9)$$

Note that diagnostic sensitivity and specificity reveal something about the test, *given prior knowledge about the disease status,* whereas positive and negative predictive values estimate the *likelihood of disease, given the test result.* Clearly, it is the latter case that is of interest when trying to make a diagnosis. In this context, it is vital to realize that although diagnostic sensitivity and specificity are qualities of a test, positive and negative predictive values are determined by both test performance and the prevalence of the disease in the patient population under study. Prevalence is defined as the proportion of the population afflicted by the disease in question. For the patient population in Table 14–13, the prevalence was (64/193 = 0.33), or 33%. Table 14–14 illustrates the effect of prevalence by presenting data for the cerebrospinal fluid (CSF) index in which the sensitivity and specificity have remained the same as in Table 14–13, but the prevalence of disease has decreased 10-fold, to 3.3%.

The positive and negative predictive values are now

$$\text{Positive predictive value} = \frac{54}{334} = 0.16 \qquad (10)$$

$$\text{Negative predictive value} = \frac{1586}{1596} = 0.99 \qquad (11)$$

Note that although the negative predictive value has increased slightly, there has been a substantial drop in the positive predictive value. The latter effect is due to the presence of a large number of false-positives. For the population studied in Table 14–14 a positive test is associated with disease in only 16% of cases.

Predictive value theory applies only to dichotomous tests, that is, tests that are classified as normal or abnormal. In the case of the CSF index, this required the selection of some diagnostic cutoff that separates normal from abnormal values. The diagnostic sensitivity and specificity change as the cutoff is changed. More advanced decision theory provides more sophisticated tools for the analysis of tests reported as values from a continuous scale.

Table 14–13. A two-by-two contingency table.

Test Status	Disease Status		Totals
	Present	Absent	
Positive	54 (True-positives)	19 (False-positives)	73
Negative	10 (False-negatives)	110 (True-negatives)	120
Totals	64	129	193

Table 14–14. The effect of prevalence upon predictive value.

Test Status	Disease Status		Totals
	Present	Absent	
Positive	54 (True-positives)	280 (False-positives)	334
Negative	10 (False-negatives)	1586 (True-negatives)	1596
Totals	64	1866	1930

REFERENCES

GENERAL

Hudson L, Hay FC: *Practical Immunology,* 3rd ed. Blackwell, 1989.

IUIS/WHO Working Group: Use and abuse of laboratory tests in clinical immunology: Critical considerations of eight widely used diagnostic procedures. (Report of IUIS/WHO Working Group.) *Clin Exp Immunol* 1981;**46:**662.

Ritzmann SE (editor): *Protein Abnormalities.* Vol 1. *Physiology of Immunoglobulins.* Vol 2. *Pathology of Immunoglobulins.* Liss, 1982.

Rose NR et al: *Manual of Clinical Immunology,* 4th ed. American Society for Microbiology, 1992.

Voller A, Bartlett A, Bidwell D: *Immunoassays for the '80s.* University Park Press, 1981.

Weir DM (editor): *Handbook of Experimental Immunology,* 4th ed. 4 vols. Blackwell, 1986.

IMMUNODIFFUSION

Crowle AJ: *Immunodiffusion,* 2nd ed. Academic Press, 1973.

Deverill I, Reeves WG: Light scattering and absorption developments in immunology. *J Immunol Methods* 1980;**38:**191.

Ouchterlony O, Nilsson LA: Immunodiffusion and immunoelectrophoresis. In: *Handbook of Experimental Immunology.* Vol 1. Weir DM (editor). Blackwell, 1986.

Stiehm ER, Fudenberg HH: Serum levels of immune globulins in health and disease: A survey. *Pediatrics* 1966;**37:**715.

ELECTROPHORESIS

Andrews AT: *Electrophoresis: Theory, Techniques and Biochemical and Clinical Populations,* 2nd ed. Oxford University Press, 1986.

Cawley LP et al: *Basic Electrophoresis, Immunoelectrophoresis and Immunochemistry.* American Society of Clinical Pathologists Commission on Continuing Education, 1972.

Gockman N, Burke MD: Electrophoretic techniques in today's clinical laboratory. *Clin Lab Med* 1986;**6:**403.

Jeppsson JO et al: Agarose gel electrophoresis. *Clin Chem* 1979;**25:**629.

Kyle RA, Garton JP: Immunoglobulins and laboratory recognition of monoclonal proteins. Section III. Myeloma and related disorders. In: *Neoplastic Diseases of the Blood.* Vol 1, 2nd ed. PH Wiernik et al (editors). Churchill Livingstone, 1991, pp 373–391.

Ouchterlony O, Nilsson LA: Immunodiffusion and immunoelectrophoresis. In: *Handbook of Experimental Immunology,* 4th ed. Vol 1. Weir DM (editor). Blackwell, 1986.

Roberts RT: Usefulness of immunofixation electrophoresis in the clinical laboratory. *Clin Lab Med* 1986;**6:**601.

IMMUNOCHEMICAL
& PHYSICOCHEMICAL METHODS

Brouet JC et al: Biological and clinical significance of cryoglobulins: A report of 86 cases. *Am J Med* 1974;**57:**775.

Somer T: Hyperviscosity syndrome in plasma cell dyscrasias. *Adv Microcirc* 1975;**6:**1.

Whicher JT et al: Immunochemical assays for immunoglobulins. *Ann Clin Biochem* 1984;**21:**78.

Williams RC: *Immune Complexes in Clinical and Experimental Medicine.* Harvard Univ Press, 1980.

Winfield JB: Cryoglobulinemia. *Hum Pathol* 1983;**14:**350.

Binder–Ligand Assay

Ekins R, Jackson T: Non-isotopic immunoassay—an overview. In: *Monoclonal Antibodies and New Trends in Immunoassays.* Bizollon CA (editor). Elsevier, 1984, pp 149–163.

Kricka LJ: Selected strategies for improving sensitivity and reliability of immunoassays. *Clin Chem* 1994;**40:**347.

Rodgers RPC: Data analysis and quality control of assays: A practical primer. In: *Practical Immunoassay: The State of the Art.* Butt WR (editor). Dekker, 1984, pp 71–101.

Rodgers RPC: How much quality control is enough? A cost-effectiveness model for clinical laboratory quality control procedures (illustrated by its application to a ligand-assay-based screening program). *Med Decis Making* 1987;**7:**156.

Schall RF, Tenoso JH: Alternatives to radioimmunoassay: Labels and methods. *Clin Chem* 1981;**27:**157.

IMMUNOHISTOCHEMICAL TECHNIQUES

Colvin RB et al: *Diagnostic Immunopathology.* Raven Press, 1988.

Elias JM: *Immunohistopathology: A Practical Approach to Diagnosis.* ASCP Press, 1990.

Falini B, Taylor CR: New developments in immunoperoxidase techniques and their application. *Arch Pathol Lab Med* 1983;**107:**105.

Goldman M: *Fluorescent Antibody Methods.* Academic Press, 1968.

Kemeny DM: *A Practical Guide to ELISA,* Pergamon Press, 1991.

Nairn RC: *Fluorescent Protein Tracing.* 4th ed. Longman, 1976.

Robbins BA, Nakamura RM: Current status of fluorescent immunoassays. *J Clin Lab Anal* 1988;**2:**62.

AGGLUTINATION

Fudenberg HH: Hemagglutination inhibition. In: *A Seminar on Basic Immunology,* American Association of Blood Banks, 1971, pp 101–110.

Herbert WJ: Passive hemagglutination with special reference to the tanned cell technique. In: *Handbook of Experimental Immunology.* Weir DM (editor). Blackwell, 1978.

COMPLEMENT FUNCTION

Ahmed AEE, Peter JB: Clinical utility of complement assessment. *Clin Diag Lab Immunol* 1995;**2:**509.

Cruse JM, Lewis RE Jr: *Complement Today.* Karger, 1993.

Morgan BP: *Complement: Clinical Aspects and Relevance to Disease.* Academic Press, 1990.

Porcel JM et al: Methods for assessing complement activation in the clinical immunology laboratory. *J Immunol Methods* 1993;**157:**1.

Ross GD: *Immunobiology of the Complement System: An Introduction for Research and Clinical Medicine.* Academic Press, 1986.

Whaley W (editor): *Methods in Complement for Clinical Immunologists.* Churchill Livingstone, 1985.

MONOCLONAL ANTIBODIES

Beverley PCL: *Monoclonal Antibodies.* Churchill Livingstone, 1991.

Campbell AM: *Monoclonal Antibodies and Immunosensor Technology: The Production and Application of Rodent and Human Monoclonal Antibodies.* Elsevier, 1991.

Milstein C: Overview: Monoclonal Antibodies and four following chapters in section on Monoclonal Antibodies. In: *Handbook of Experimental Immunology,* 4th ed. Vol. 4. Weir DM (editor). Blackwell, 1986.

Peters JH, Baumgarten H: *Monoclonal Antibodies.* Springer Verlag, 1992.

Pinto A et al: New molecules burst at the leukocyte surface. A comprehensive review based on the Fifth International Workshop on Leukocyte Differentiation Antigens. *Leukemia* 1994;**8:**347.

PREDICTIVE VALUE THEORY

Gottfried EL, Gerard S: Selection and interpretation of laboratory tests and diagnostic procedures. In: *Textbook of Clinical Diagnostics in Medicine.* Samly AH et al (editors). Lea and Febiger, 1987, pp 19–38.

Griner PF et al: Selection and interpretation of diagnostic tests and procedures. *Ann Intern Med* 1981;**4:**553.

Hershey LA, Trotter JL: The use and abuse of the cerebrospinal fluid (CSF) profile in the adult: A practical evaluation. *Ann Neurol* 1980;**8:**426.

Sox HC Jr et al: *Medical Decision Making.* Butterworths, 1988.

Clinical Laboratory Methods for Detection of Cellular Immunity

Daniel P. Stites, MD, James D. Folds, PhD, & John Schmitz, PhD

The immune system in humans has been divided into two major parts: one involving humoral immunity (antibody and complement) and the other cellular immunity. In many ways this separation is artificial, and many examples of the interdependence of cellular and humoral immunity exist. Nevertheless, dividing the immune system into parts in this way provides a conceptual and practical framework for the laboratory evaluation of immunity in clinical practice.

In the preceding chapter we reviewed methods of detecting antibodies and methods that primarily employ antibodies for antigen detection. The role of a variety of distinct cell types (see Chapters 2 and 3) in immune mechanisms in normal and diseased persons has become measurable in the clinical laboratory. Immunocompetent cells, including lymphocytes, monocyte–macrophages, and granulocytes, are all involved in the delayed hypersensitivity reactions that are so important in immunity to intracellular infection, tumor immunity, and transplant rejection. The clinical laboratory investigation of the number and function of these cells is still beset by difficulties in test standardization, biologic variability, the imprecise nature of many assays, and the complexity and expense of the procedures. Nevertheless, several tests that are of value in assessing cellular function have emerged for clinical use. Many of these assays employ sophisticated immunochemical methods for detecting cellular antigens or markers. Of great importance is the advent of monoclonal antibodies to detect various leukocyte subsets. Molecular biologic techniques such as Southern blots have recently been employed to detect either immunoglobulin gene or T-cell receptor gene rearrangements as markers of specific B- and T-cell lineages. Thus, we are witnessing an increasing fusion of biochemistry and molecular biology with cellular immunology.

The present chapter reviews the tests that have medical application in the detection of cell types and their corresponding functions. The intention is not to provide a comprehensive laboratory manual of all cellular immunologic procedures but to familiarize the reader with the principles, applications, and interpretation of assays with clinical applicability. Our understanding of cellular immunity continues to expand, and technologic advances in methods for its assessment have been developed. In Chapter 17 special application of these and other tests for evaluating immune competence is described.

The topics discussed include (1) delayed hypersensitivity skin tests, (2) assays for T and B lymphocytes, (3) lymphocyte activation, (4) monocyte–macrophage assays, and (5) neutrophil function.

DELAYED HYPERSENSITIVITY SKIN TESTS

Despite the development of a multitude of complex in vitro procedures for the assessment of cellular immunity, the relatively simple intradermal test remains a useful tool, occasionally serving to establish a diagnosis. Delayed hypersensitivity skin testing detects cutaneous hypersensitivity to an antigen or group of antigens. When testing for an infectious disease, however, a positive test does not necessarily imply active infection with the agent being tested for. Delayed hypersensitivity skin tests are also of great value in the overall assessment of immunocompetence and in epidemiologic surveys. Inability to react to a battery of common skin antigens is termed **anergy,** and clinical conditions associated with this hyporeactive state are listed in Table 15–1.

Technique of Skin Testing

1. Lyophilized antigens should be stored sterile at 4 °C, protected from light, and reconstituted shortly before use. The manufacturer's expiration date should be observed.

Table 15–1. Clinical conditions associated with anergy.

I. Immunologic deficiencies
  Congenital
  Combined deficiencies of cellular and humoral
    immunity
  Ataxia-telangiectasia
  Nezelof's syndrome
  Severe combined immunodeficiency
  Wiskott-Aldrich syndrome
  Cellular
    Thymic and parathyroid aplasia (DiGeorge's
      syndrome)
    Mucocutaneous candidiasis
  Acquired
    Acquired immunodeficiency syndrome (AIDS)
    Sarcoidosis
    Chronic lymphocytic leukemia
    Carcinoma
    Immunosuppressive medication
    Rheumatoid diseases
    Uremia
    Alcoholic cirrhosis
    Biliary cirrhosis
    Surgery
    Hodgkin's disease and lymphomas
II. Infections
  Influenza
  Mumps
  Measles
  Viral vaccines
  Typhus
  Miliary and active tuberculosis
  Disseminated mycotic infection
  Lepromatous leprosy
  Scarlet fever
III. Technical errors in skin testing
  Improper antigen concentrations
  Bacterial contamination
  Exposure to heat or light
  Adsorption of antigen on container walls
  Faulty injection (too deep, leaking)
  Improper reading of reaction

Source: Modified, with permission, from Heiss LI, Palmer DL: Anergy in patients with leukocytes. *Am J Med* 1974;**56**:323.

2. Test solutions should not be stored in syringes for prolonged periods before use.
3. A 25- or 27-gauge needle usually ensures intradermal rather than subcutaneous administration of antigen. Multiple devices that deliver up to eight antigens simultaneously are also available, but these devices use a prick test, which has not been fully validated for delayed hypersensitivity skin testing. Subcutaneous injection leads to dilution of the antigen in tissues and thus can lead to a false-negative test.
4. The largest dimensions of both erythema and induration should be measured with a ruler and recorded at both 24 and 48 hours.
5. Hyporeactivity to any given antigen or group of antigens should be confirmed by testing with higher concentrations of antigen or, in ambiguous circumstances, by a repeat test with the intermediate dose.

Contact Sensitivity

Direct application to the skin of chemically reactive compounds results in systemic sensitization to various metabolites of the sensitizing compound. The precise chemical fate of the sensitizing compound is not known, but sensitizing agents such as dinitrochlorobenzene (DNCB) probably form dinitrophenylprotein complexes with various skin proteins. Sensitization with DNCB has been used experimentally in skin testing for delayed hypersensitivity in selected patients with suspected anergy. It is not a routine procedure and should be reserved for instances in which thorough delayed hypersensitivity testing with other antigens is negative. Concern regarding its possible toxicity and cross-sensitizing properties exist. Furthermore, its use as a diagnostic reagent is not currently approved by the FDA. Following application of DNCB to the skin, a period of about 7–10 days elapses before contact sensitivity can be elicited by a challenge dose applied to the skin surface. This sensitivity persists for years. The ability of a subject to develop contact sensitivity is a measure of cellular immunity to a new antigen to which the subject has not been previously exposed. Thus, the establishment of a state of cutaneous anergy in various disease states may be confirmed and extended by testing with DNCB.

Interpretation of contact sensitivity reactions depends on development of a flare, papular, or vesicular reaction at the site of challenge. Induration rarely occurs, since the test dose is not applied intradermally. In some clinical situations, a nonspecific depression in the inflammatory response can result in apparent anergy.

Patch testing is commonly employed by allergists and dermatologists to detect cutaneous hypersensitivity to various substances thought to be responsible for contact dermatitis. The test substance is applied in a low concentration and the area covered with an occlusive dressing. After 48 hours, the dressing is removed and the site examined for the presence of the inflammatory reaction previously described. False-positive reactions can result from too high a concentration of the test substance, irritation rather than allergy, and allergy to the adhesive in the dressing. False-negative tests usually result from too low a concentration of the test substance or inadequate skin penetration. The results of patch testing must be carefully weighed with the clinical history and knowledge of the chemistry of the potential sensitizing agent. (See also Chapters 26 and 30.)

Interpretation & Pitfalls

The inflammatory infiltrate that occurs 24–48 hours following intradermal injection of an antigen consists primarily of mononuclear cells. This cellular infiltrate and the accompanying edema result in induration of the skin, and the diameter of this reaction is an index of cutaneous hypersensitivity. A patient may also demonstrate immediate hypersensitivity to the same test antigen, that is, a coexistent area (wheal and flare) at 15–20 minutes and late-phase inflammation at 5–8 hours, but this usually fades by 12–18 hours (see Chapter 26). Induration of 5 mm or more in diameter is the generally accepted criterion of a positive delayed skin test. Smaller but definitely indurated reactions suggest sensitivity to a closely related or cross-reacting antigen. There is no definitive evidence that repeated skin testing can result in conversion of delayed hypersensitivity skin tests from negative to positive. With some antigens, however, intradermal testing can result in elevations of serum antibody titers and confuse a serologic diagnosis. For this reason, blood for serologic study should always be obtained before skin tests are performed.

False-negative results are obtained in patients receiving systemic corticosteroids and possibly other immunosuppressive or anti-inflammatory drugs.

Delayed hypersensitivity skin testing is of relatively little value in establishing the diagnosis of defective cellular immunity during the first year of life. Infants may fail to react because of lack of antigen contact with the various test antigens. Consequently, in vitro assay for T-cell numbers and function is much more useful in the diagnosis of congenital immunodeficiency disease (see Chapter 21–25). Genetic markers in the human leukocyte antigen (HLA) DR region are correlated with failure to respond to various tuberculin antigens.

Use of delayed and immediate hypersensitivity skin tests in diagnosis and management of allergies is discussed in Chapters 26–30.

Possible Adverse Reactions to Skin Tests

Occasional patients who are highly sensitive to various antigens have marked local reactions to skin tests. If unusual sensitivity is suspected, a preliminary test should be performed with diluted antigen. Reactions include erythema, marked induration, and rarely, local necrosis. Patch testing may rarely result in sensitization. Systemic side effects such as fever or anaphylaxis are uncommon. Injection of corticosteroids locally into hyperreactive indurated areas may modify the severity of the reaction. Similarly, the painful blistering and inflammation that sometimes occur following surface application of contact sensitizers can be reduced by topical corticosteroids.

ASSAYS FOR HUMAN LYMPHOCYTES & MONOCYTES

The era of modern cellular immunology began with the discovery that lymphocytes are divided into two major functionally distinct populations. Evidence for the existence of T (thymus-derived) and B (bone marrow-derived) lymphocytes in humans originated from studies of other mammalian and avian species and analysis of lymphocyte populations in immunodeficiency diseases. Extensive studies of cell surface molecules with monoclonal antibodies and in vitro functional assays have provided direct evidence for the existence of these major lymphocyte types and a third type called natural killer (NK) cells (see Chapter 3).

The terms *T lymphocyte* and *B lymphocyte* usually denote the two major classes of immunocompetent cells in peripheral blood. During embryonic development, T lymphocytes arise in the thymus, migrate to peripheral lymphoid organs (lymph nodes and spleen), and circulate in the blood. B lymphocytes mature during embryogenesis from this origin in sites that are a functional equivalent of the avian bursa of Fabricius. T lymphocytes function as effector cells in cellular immune reactions, cooperate with B cells to form antibody (helper function), and suppress certain B-cell functions (suppressor function). After appropriate antigenic stimulation, B lymphocytes differentiate into plasma cells that eventually secrete antibody. The notion that there is only one type of T cell or B cell has been found to be an oversimplification, since functionally distinct subclasses of T and B cells are now recognized. NK cells, a minor lymphocyte subpopulation, can also be assessed by cell surface markers and junctional assays (see Chapters 1–3).

Assays for T and B cells are currently in wide use in clinical immunology. Leukocytes are counted by microscopy or flow cytometry with specific antibodies to membrane antigens. The antibodies are conjugated either to fluorescent dyes or to enzymes that produce reactants. Such techniques can be applied either in tissue sections or in fresh suspensions of cells from blood, bone marrow, or other sites. Precise counting of T and B cells in human peripheral blood has made important contributions to our understanding of (1) immunodeficiency disorders, (2) autoimmune diseases, (3) tumor immunity, and (4) infectious disease immunity. It should be emphasized, however, that mere counting of T or B cells does not necessarily correlate with the functional capacity of these cells. At best, these assays provide a nosologic classification of immunocompetent cells; further evaluation of lymphocyte function usually should be performed to fully assess immunologic competence in clinical practice.

In 1983, the First International Workshop on Human Leukocyte Differentiation Antigens met and established a new nomenclature for immunologically defined cellular types and subtypes. They defined a series of **cluster of differentiation (CD)** types that define cellular antigens. In 1989, the fourth workshop refined and expanded this nomenclature. Definition of these CD types and relationship to other antigen or antibody designations are presented in Table 15–2. It should be emphasized that the CD nomenclature (also see CD table in Appendix A) continues to replace the more familiar, often proprietary, antibody designations, such as CD4 for T4 or Leu 3.

Table 15–2. T-cell differentiation antigens.

Cell Type Detected	CD Designation	Antibody Designation	Comments
Cortical thymocytes Langerhans' cells	CD1	Leu 6 T6	Early T-cell antigen also present on Langerhans' cells, associated with β_2-microglobulin and not present on peripheral T cells.
E rosette-forming cells T cells NK cells	CD2	Leu 5 T11	Pan-T-cell antigen SRBC receptor on T cells.
Mature T cells T cell antigen receptor	CD3	Leu 4	Also present on T cell in ALL and cutaneous T-cell lymphoma.
Helper/inducer T cells Monocytes	CD4	Leu 3 T4	Can be further subdivided into helper and inducer subsets. Weakly expressed on monocytes.
Pan-T and -B-cell subpopulation	CD5	Leu 1 T1 T101	B cells in CLL. B cells following marrow transplant. B cells secrete autoantibodies.
Mature T cells	CD6	T12	Malignant T cells.
Pan-T cells, thymocytes NK cells (some)	CD7	Leu 9 3A1	T-cell leukemias.
Suppressor/cytotoxic T cells NK cells (some)	CD8	Leu 2 T8	Can be further subdivided into cytotoxic and suppressor subsets.

Abbreviations: NK = natural killer; SRBC = sheep red blood cells; ALL = acute lymphoblastic leukemia; CLL = chronic lymphatic leukemia.

Separation of Peripheral Blood Mononuclear Cells for Lymphocyte & Monocyte Assays

Tests for human mononuclear cells are ordinarily performed on purified suspensions of blood cells. An accepted procedure for obtaining mononuclear cell suspensions is density gradient centrifugation on Ficoll-Hypaque. This method results in a yield of 70–90% mononuclear cells with a high degree of purity but may selectively eliminate some lymphocyte subpopulations. Mononuclear preparations obtained by this method are relatively enriched in *monocytes*. These cells must be distinguished from lymphocytes by morphologic characteristics, phagocytic ability, endogenous enzymatic activity, or cell surface antigens (see following section).

To avoid misinterpretation, results of tests for T-, B-, and NK cell markers on separated populations should generally be expressed as the number of cells per microliter of whole blood. Many published studies have indicated only the percentages of lymphocytes carrying a particular marker. Such a result could be due to an increase in the particular cell population or, alternatively, to a decrease in other populations. Thus, it is important that each laboratory establish standard absolute numbers of lymphocytes cells per microliter of whole blood from normal individuals.

Methods for assessing cellular phenotypes using whole unseparated blood have been developed. Cells are stained with fluorochrome-conjugated monoclonal antibodies, and erythrocytes are lysed. The residual washed leukocytes are counted by flow cytometry or fluorescence microscopy. The whole-blood method has the advantage of simplicity and has largely replaced the counting of separated mononu-clear cells. It is generally not useful for functional studies because of potential interference by erythrocytes or plasma proteins.

T-LYMPHOCYTE ASSAYS

Human T-Cell-Specific Markers

Production of heteroantisera to normal and malignant human T cells created the potential for direct immunochemical detection of cellular subpopulations by immunofluorescence and other sensitive techniques. With few exceptions, however, conventional antisera raised in animals to T-cell subsets have lacked sufficient specificity owing to extensive cross-reactivity and broad response to species-specific rather than lineage-specific antigens on the immunizing cells. Some degree of improvement in the quality of these reagents was achieved by use of naturally occurring human antibody derived from sera of patients with various autoimmune diseases or by use of purified or continuously cultured T-cell subpopulations. With the advent of monoclonal antibodies produced by murine hybridomas (see Chapter 14), however, a major breakthrough was achieved in identification of human T cells.

Monoclonal antibodies have been produced in many laboratories to class-specific and subclass-specific T-cell antigens. These antibodies are highly specific and sensitive reagents for detecting cells in suspensions or fixed tissue sections. An enormous proliferation of abbreviations for these sera has occurred simultaneously with their commercial availability. The use of CD terminology for some of these markers is compared with more common proprietary designations in Table 15–2 (see Appendix for more detailed listing of CDs). New antigens defining specialized subsets of T cells will continue to emerge for the current groupings.

A. Performance of Test:

1. Production of T-cell antibodies–T cells from various sources—especially thymocytes, purified peripheral blood T cells, T leukemia cells, or T cells from continuous culture—can be used for immunization of rodents and subsequent production of monoclonal antibodies (see Chapter 14). Specificity must be shown by positive reaction with T cells and negative reaction with B cells and other cell types.

2. Detection of T-cell antigens with specific antisera–Immunofluorescence or immunoenzyme staining of either live lymphocytes or frozen tissue sections is possible. Direct immunofluorescence is performed with fluorochrome-labeled immunoglobulin from hybridoma culture supernatants or purified antibodies from the hybridomas.

In vitro cytotoxicity of human T cells by specific antisera may also be used to estimate T-cell populations. Methods for assessing T-cell killing include trypan blue vital staining or ^{51}Cr release assay.

Methods to detect various CD molecules derived from either the surface or the interior of cells are being developed. Following lysis of mixed cell populations by detergents, the amounts of various CD molecules are quantified by enzyme-linked immunosorbent assay (ELISA), radioimmunoassay (RIA), or other immunoassays.

B. Interpretation: The percentage or absolute number of T cells or T-cell subsets is determined by their binding to various specific antibodies. Cells are counted by direct observation with a fluorescence or light microscope or by flow cytometry (see later discussion). Flow cytometry has essentially replaced microscopy in clinical laboratories as simpler and less expensive instruments are developed. The overwhelming advantages of objectivity, sensitivity, and speed make flow-cytometric analysis preferable to the tedious process of counting cells by microscopic observation.

T-Cell Subsets

Major subsets of T cells consist of helper and suppressor/cytotoxic types. Helper cells (CD4), however, consist of at least two phenotypically and functionally distinct subtypes: naive cells, which are CD4+CD45RA+, and memory cells, which are CD4+CD45R0+. These two subtypes of the CD4 class are recognized phenotypically by the simultaneous expression of CD4 molecules and other monoclonal antibodies for CD45RA and CD45R0. So far, no single reagent has been developed that can identify these populations.

Suppressor cells (CD8) can similarly be subdivided into so-called true suppressor cells (CD8+, CD11+),

which influence B cell antibody function, and cytotoxic T cells (CD8+, CD11–). Combinations of monoclonal antibodies are thus also used to detect these two important T-cell subsets.

Helper/Suppressor Cell Ratios (T_H/T_S Ratio)

Largely because of the interest and concern generated by the AIDS (acquired immunodeficiency syndrome) epidemic, many laboratories express results of helper/inducer and suppressor/cytotoxic T-cell counts as a ratio or quotient. Caution must be exercised in using this approach, since the ratio may vary depending on changes in either numerator or denominator or both. Also, standardization of normal values and the clinical significance of slight deviations from the reference range are not well understood. Diseases or conditions that have been reported to be associated with high or low helper/suppressor ratios are presented in Table 15–3. Obviously, this laboratory test is not diagnostic of any particular condition and has to be interpreted cautiously on the basis of the persistence or transience of the abnormality. In AIDS, for example, the reduction in the ratio seems to be permanent, whereas in some viral infections, such as cytomegalovirus, it is reversible.

The use of absolute numbers or, in some instances, percentages of CD4 and CD8 cells is preferred. CD4 numbers are useful in AIDS prognosis and monitoring treatment. Levels of CD8 cells are transiently elevated in many viral infections.

E Rosette-Forming Cells

Human T cells were formerly identified by their ability to bind sheep erythrocytes (SRBC) to form rosettes (Fig 15–1). Detection of this property, however, has largely been replaced by more sensitive

Table 15–3. Helper/suppressor cell ratios in human peripheral blood.

Decreased in	Increased in
SLE with renal disease	Rheumatoid arthritis
Acute cytomegalovirus infection	Type I insulin-dependent diabetes mellitus
Burns	SLE without renal disease
GVH disease	Primary biliary cirrhosis
Sunburn or ultraviolet solarium exposure	Atopic dermatitis
Myelodysplasia syndromes	Sézary syndrome
Acute lymphocytic leukemia in remission	Psoriasis
Recovery from bone marrow transplant	Chronic autoimmmune hepatitis
AIDS	
Herpes infections	
Infectious mononucleosis	
Measles	
Vigorous exercise	

Abbreviations: SLE = systemic lupus erythematosus; GVH = graft-versus-host; AIDS = acquired immunodeficiency syndrome.

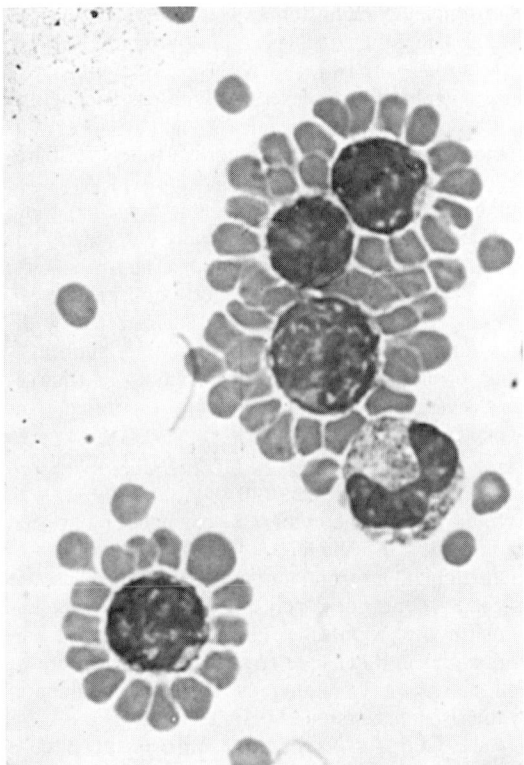

Figure 15–1. E rosette-forming cells. Lymphocytes from human peripheral blood that have formed rosettes with sheep erythrocytes. Such cells are T lymphocytes that bear the CD2 molecule. A granulocyte has failed to form a rosette. (Courtesy of M Kadin.)

binding of monoclonal antibodies that identify the SRBC receptor, designated CD2.

B-LYMPHOCYTE ASSAYS

B lymphocytes express a variety of cell surface molecules, which can be detected with either monoclonal antibodies or polyclonal antisera. Mature B cells express CD19, CD20, and HLA-DR. Immature B cells may express additional molecules such as CD10 (common acute lymphocytic leukemia antigen [CALLA]) (Table 15–4). Some B-cell tumors, particularly chronic lymphocytic leukemia, express CD5, and CD5-bearing B cells may produce autoantibodies in systemic lupus erythematosus and rheumatoid arthritis. The use of B-cell surface markers in tumor diagnosis is discussed in detail in Chapter 46.

Human B-Cell-Specific Markers
A. Performance of Test: Monoclonal antibodies labeled with fluorochromes or enzymes are used to detect cells bearing the mature B-cell markers CD19 and CD20. HLA-DR is also expressed on monocytes

Table 15–4. B-cell differentiation antigens.

Cell Type Detected	CD Designation	Comments
B-cell subset T cells	CD5	B-cell chronic lymphocytic leukemia. B-cell secretes autoantibodies.
Immature B cells	CD10	Pre-B cells. Granulocytes. Antigen is neural endopeptidase (encephalinase).
Immature and mature B cells	CD19	
B cell tumors	CD20	
Immature and mature B cells	CD21	Epstein-Barr virus.
B cells in mantle and germinal centers	CD22	

and activated on immature T cells. Fluorescence, or light microscopy in the case of enzyme-linked monoclonal antibodies, may be used, but flow cytometry is currently the preferred method. Additional markers for subsets of B cells are available (see Table 15–4) but have limited clinical utility. Plasma cells generally fail to express B-cell markers but have a set of their own (eg, PC1 + PCA – 1), which can be detected with monoclonal antibodies.

B. Interpretation: No functional information directly emerges from enumeration of B cells. Special problems exist with the use of nonmurine polyspecific antisera and Fc receptor binding (see later discussion).

Surface Immunoglobulin
B lymphocytes have readily demonstrable surface immunoglobulin. This surface immunoglobulin is synthesized by the lymphocyte and under ordinary conditions does not originate from serum; that is, it is not cytophilic antibody. Lymphocytes generally bear monoclonal surface immunoglobulin, or immunoglobulin of a single H-chain class and L-chain type.

A. Performance of Test: Polyspecific antisera against all immunoglobulin classes permit detection of total numbers of B cells in a blood sample. Alternatively, a mixture of anti-κ and anti-λ antisera detect total numbers of B cells. Monospecific antisera are developed by immunization with purified paraproteins and appropriate absorptions.

Tests for surface immunoglobulin-bearing B cells are performed by direct immunofluorescence with fluorochrome-labeled γ-globulin fractions derived from heterologous anti-immunoglobulin antisera or monoclonal antibodies. A major difficulty is to ensure the absence of all aggregated immunoglobulin in the test reagents (see later section).

Table 15–5. Surface immunoglobulin-bearing B lymphocytes in normal adult blood.

Surface Immunoglobulin	Mean % of Total Lymphocytes	Range
Total immunoglobulin	21	16–28
IgG	7.1	4–12.7
IgA	2.2	1–4.3
IgM	8.9	6.7–13
IgD[1]	6.2	5.2–8.2
IgE[2]	. . .	. . .
κ	13.9	10–18.6
λ	6.8	5–9.3

Source: Reproduced, with permission, from: WHO Workshop on Human T & B Cells. *Scand J Immunol* 1974;**3**:525.
[1] IgD and IgM are frequently expressed on the same cell.
[2] IgE cells are extremely rare.

Generally, small amounts of anti-immunoglobulin antisera are mixed with purified lymphocyte suspensions for 20–30 minutes at 4 °C. After removal of unbound immunoglobulin, the presence of surface immunoglobulin is determined by counting in a fluorescence microscope or by flow cytometry.

Table 15–5 summarizes data on the numbers of surface immunoglobulin-bearing B cells in normal subjects. In certain disease states, such as systemic lupus erythematosus, antilymphocyte antibody may be bound to B or T cells in vivo. To prove that surface immunoglobulin is a metabolic product of that cell, enzymatic removal and resynthesis of surface immunoglobulin may be performed in vitro.

B. Interpretation: The percentages of IgG-bearing lymphocytes are in fact considerably lower than previously reported. Falsely high levels are detected owing to formation of IgG/anti-IgG complexes at the cell surface with binding to B cells via the Fc receptor. When $F(ab)'_2$ anti-IgG reagents were prepared, the percentage of IgG-bearing cells was reduced from 5% to less than 1%.

The problem of binding of anti-immunoglobulin reagents to Fc receptors on B cells and monocytes is particularly severe with rabbit antihuman antisera. A recent study suggests that nonspecific binding is almost eliminated by use of goat or sheep antisera to human immunoglobulins. The use of monoclonal murine antibodies to H and L chains also avoids this problem. Most investigators agree that IgM and IgD are the predominant surface immunoglobulins on human peripheral B lymphocytes.

Cytoplasmic Immunoglobulins

In some lymphoid cancers, particularly Waldenström's macroglobulinemia, chronic lymphocytic leukemia, or B-cell lymphomas with leukemia, circulating lymphocytes with monoclonal intracytoplasmic immunoglobulins are detected (see Chapter 46). This immunoglobulin is usually identical to the molecule found on the surface of these cells and is occasionally present as a paraprotein in serum. Rarely, the intracellular immunoglobulin forms distinct crystals that appear as spindles or spicules within cytoplasm.

A group of patients with acute lymphocytic leukemias have been described with pre-B cells that express only intracytoplasmic IgM and no surface immunoglobulins at all. It is important to test for intracellular IgM, particularly in patients with so-called null cell acute lymphocytic leukemia, since the group with pre-B cell leukemia is probably a distinct clinical subgroup with a different course and prognosis. Most of these cells react with CD19 antisera as well.

Intracellular immunoglobulins are detected by direct immunofluorescence with specific antiheavy-chain or antilight-chain sera or acetone- or ethanol-fixed cytocentrifuged preparations of purified lymphocytes.

Functional B-Cell Assays

In the clinical laboratory, B-cell function has been traditionally measured by the assessment of immunoglobulin levels or antibody titers, since these are the end products of B-cell differentiation. Two additional in vitro approaches to assessing functional abnormalities in B cells are now available. These are B-cell activation by mitogens and immunoglobulin synthesis and secretion.

A. B-Cell Activation by Mitogens: B cells can be stimulated to proliferate by several mitogens. Pokeweed mitogen (PWM) functions with T-cell cooperation and is not a direct B-cell test. Staphylococcal protein A (Cowan 1 strain) (SAC), however, probably directly stimulates B-cell activation. Measurement of this B-cell attribute is analogous to phytohemagglutinin (PHA) or concanavalin A (Con A) stimulation described later for T cells.

B. Immunoglobulin Biosynthesis: B-cell activation by antigens or mitogens results in small but detectable quantities of polyclonal immunoglobulins. Following 7–10 days of culture, these products are measured by radioimmunoassay (RIA) or enzyme-linked immunosorbent assay (ELISA) methods. Alternatively, B cells that produce immunoglobulins can be quantified by the reversed hemolytic plaque assay. In this assay, erythrocytes are coated with goat or rabbit antihuman immunoglobulins. They are mixed with putative immunoglobulin-producing lymphocytes and semisolid agar, and complement is added. The presence of hemolytic plaques indicates the presence of immunoglobulin-producing cells.

B cells that have differentiated into plasma cells during an in vitro assay can be enumerated by staining for intracellular immunoglobulins by direct immunofluorescence in fixed smears of cultured cells.

The advantage of these in vitro B-cell function tests is that they allow for delineation of immunoregulatory defects involving T or B cells by substitution of various cell populations among healthy and diseased cell donors. These assays are not routinely available in most clinical laboratories.

FLOW CYTOMETRY

Biochemical and biophysical measurements on single cells have been performed for years, primarily using visual analysis in various types of microscopes. Many of the immunohistochemical methods described in Chapter 14—and the cellular analysis methods discussed earlier—have become increasingly refined through the development of flow cytometers. A detailed description of the myriad applications of this general technique is beyond the scope of our discussion here. In brief, flow cytometers are instruments capable of analyzing properties of single cells as they pass through an orifice at high velocity. Examples of measurements that can be made include physical characteristics such as size, volume, refractive index, and viscosity and chemical features such as content of DNA and RNA, proteins, and enzymes. Cell surface molecules are readily detected by immunofluorescence with monoclonal antibodies. These properties are detected by measuring light scatter, Coulter volume, and fluorescence. Instruments have been designed to analyze these properties and are combined with sophisticated electronics and computers. Another class of even more sophisticated instruments—cell sorters—combine analytic capacity with the ability to sort cells on the basis of various preselected properties. One type of sorter, the fluorescence-activated cell sorter, has found many applications in immunologic research. Flow cytometers are now routinely found in many clinical laboratories.

Cell Analysis by Flow Cytometry

Counting individual cells in complex mixtures is a tedious and imprecise technique even with monoclonal fluorescent antibodies and sophisticated microscopes. With the aid of a flow cytometer used as an analytic instrument, a single cell suspension may be analyzed for various measurements simultaneously at the rate of nearly 5000 cells per second. By combining light scatter or Coulter volume measurements with the powerful tool of fluorescently labeled monoclonal antibodies, subpopulations can be easily identified. A typical histogram produced by analysis of human T cells is shown in Figure 15–2. The number of cells under the curves can be determined and thereby the percentage of positive and negative cells in relation to an arbitrary threshold of fluorescent signal.

The use of two differently colored fluorochromes each coupled to a particular antibody allows simultaneous two-color immunofluorescence of individual cells. Flow cytometers have been developed that can excite two different dyes that absorb light at similar wavelengths but emit light in orange and green. One of the most frequent uses of flow cytometry is in the enumeration of CD4 cells in HIV-infected patients. Figure 15–3 demonstrates the approach to this task using dual-color flow-cytometric analysis. Using a whole-blood lysis methodology, the major cellular

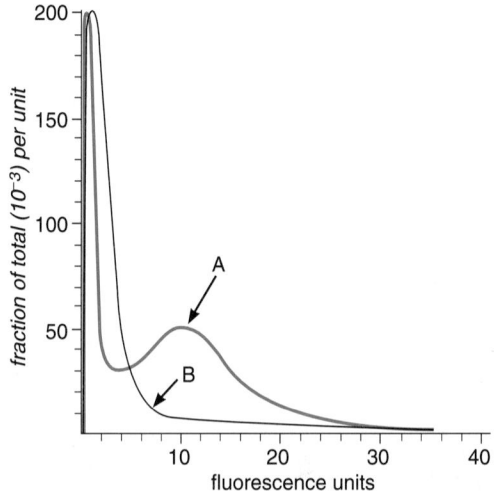

Figure 15–2. Single-color immunofluorescence histogram from flow-cytometric analysis of human T cells. **(A)** Human lymphocytes were stained with fluorescently labeled anti-T-cell antibody and **(B)** control nonreactive fluorescein isothiocyanate (FITC)-labeled antiserum. In both patterns, a high, sharp peak of autofluorescence from unstained cells is observed near the y-axis. However, in the curve labeled **(A)** stained with anti-T cell antibody, a significant peak appears at about 11 fluorescence units. No such increase in the number or intensity of fluorescent cells is observed in the control **(B)** peak. (Modified and reproduced, with permission, from: Melamed MR, Mullaney PF, Mendelsohn ML: *Flow Cytometry and Sorting.* Wiley, 1979.)

elements of the blood (lymphocytes, monocytes, granulocytes) can be discriminated. A bitmap gate can be drawn around the lymphocytes, excluding most other cell types, thus limiting further analysis to lymphoid cells. The expression of T, B, and other cell markers can then be analyzed on CD3-positive and -negative subpopulations by dual-color analysis.

Cells larger and smaller than lymphocytes can be "gated out" electronically so that the analysis concentrates solely on lymphocytes. With the addition of 90° light scatter, granulocytes can also be identified and gated out. This approach has allowed for the development of whole-blood methods for lymphoid cell analysis. This same type of approach can be used to determine the phenotype of malignant cells from patients with hematologic malignancies. This type of analysis can aid in the diagnosis, classification, and prognosis of these diseases (see Chapter 46). Figure 15–4 demonstrates the restricted expression of lambda light chains on cells from a patient with chronic lymphocytic leukemia. This expression of a single light-chain types confirms the monoclonal nature of this cell population.

Another frequently used application of flow cytometry is in the analysis of DNA ploidy and proliferative fraction. By staining nuclei with DNA-intercalating dyes, one can determine the percentage of cells in the

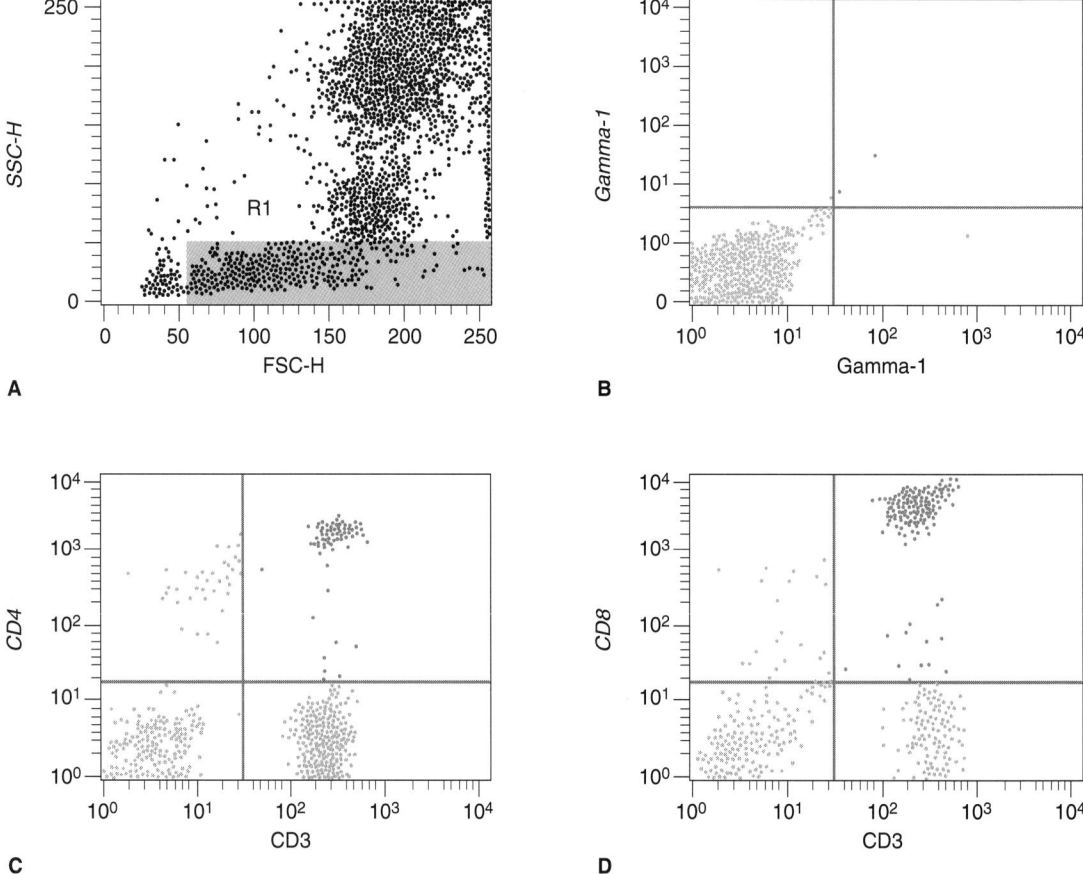

Figure 15–3. Dual-color flow-cytometric analysis of CD4 and CD8 expression on peripheral blood CD3 lymphocytes. Panel **A** shows the appearance of lysed whole blood displayed with forward (x-axis) and side scatter (y-axis). Lymphocytes (low forward and side scatter), monocytes (greater forward and side scatter relative to lymphocytes), and granulocytes (high side scatter) can easily be distinguished. An analysis gate (R1) is shown surrounding the lymphocyte population. Staining with isotype-matched, irrelevant monoclonal antibodies (**B**) serves as a control for nonspecific absorption of monoclonal antibodies (x-axis is FITC fluorescence, y-axis is phycoerythrin fluorescence). CD3 positive cells of the CD4 (T helper) type are identified in the upper right quadrant of panel **C,** and CD8 positive T cells are present in the upper right quadrant of panel **D.** The percentage of CD4 and 8 positive cells can be determined from these displays and, with the absolute lymphocyte count, the absolute CD4 and CD8 cell numbers can be determined. *Abbreviations:* FSC = forward scatter; SSC = side scatter.

various phases of the cell cycle (G_0/G_1, S, G_2/M). In addition, the presence of a cell population with an abnormal amount of DNA can be indicated by the presence of an aneuploid peak.

Fluorescence-Activated Cell Sorters

A single cell suspension is isolated from blood or other tissues and labeled with either fluorescent antibody or another fluorochrome dye such as ethidium bromide, which specifically stains DNA (Fig 15–5). The cells are forced under pressure through a nozzle in a liquid jet surrounded by a sheath of saline or water. Vibration at the tip of the nozzle assembly causes the stream to break up into a series of droplets, and the size of the droplets can be regulated so that each contains exactly one cell. The droplets are illuminated by the monochromatic laser beam and electronically

monitored by fluorescence detectors. Droplets that emit appropriate fluorescent signals are electrically charged in a high-voltage field between deflection plates and are then sorted into collection tubes. Rapid, accurate, and highly reproducible separation of cells is thereby accomplished. Viability and sterility can be maintained, so that cells can be not only analyzed but also cultured or assayed functionally.

Clinical Applications of Flow Cytometry

The flow cytometer has had many applications in immunology. A partial list includes the following: (1) analysis and sorting of subpopulations of T and B cells by monoclonal fluorescent antibodies; (2) separation of various classes of lymphoid cells through sorting by size or antibody marker; (3) separation of live from dead cells; (4) cloning of individual cells by

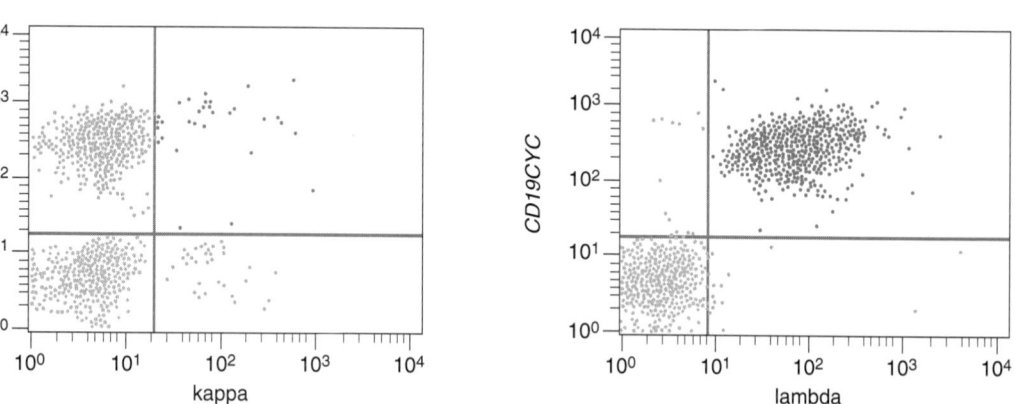

Figure 15–4. Dual-color flow-cytometric analysis of light-chain expression on cells from a patient with chronic lymphocytic leukemia. In panel **A** cells were stained with CD19 (*y*-axis) and anti-kappa (*x*-axis). The population of cells stains predominantly negative for kappa light chains. In panel **B** these cells were stained with CD19 (*y*-axis) and anti-lambda (*x*-axis). In this case, the majority of cells are seen to express lambda light chains. These findings support the monoclonal (restricted light-chain type) nature of this population of cells.

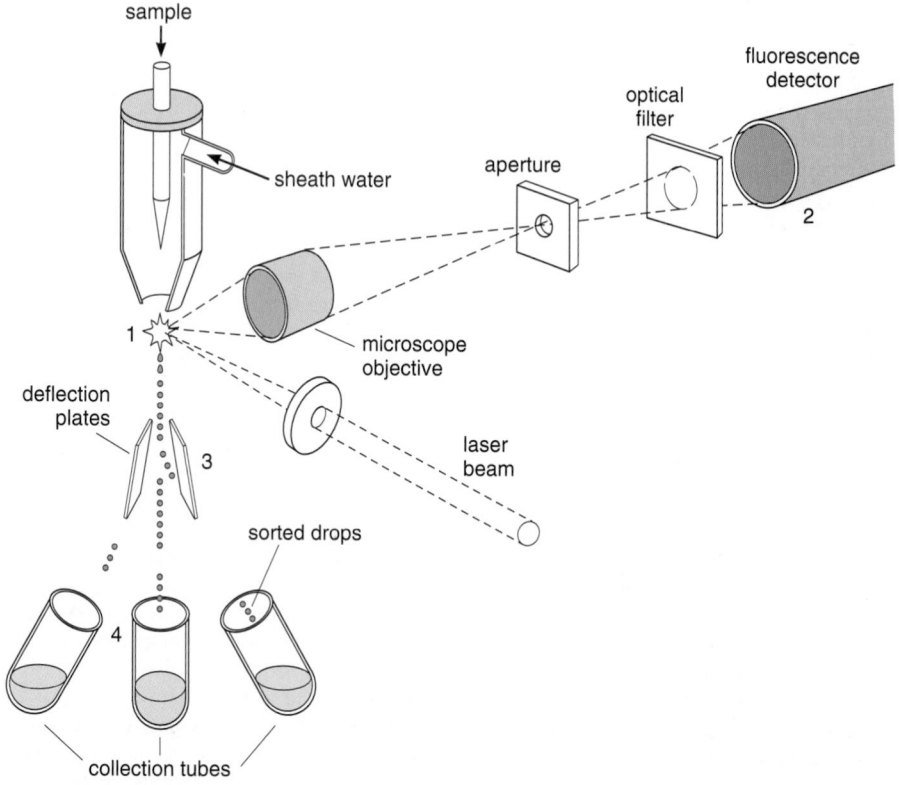

Figure 15–5. Cell purification by flow sorting. *1:* Fluorescently stained cells are forced out of a small nozzle in a liquid jet. *2:* Cellular fluorescence, measured immediately below the nozzle, is used to select the cells to be sorted. *3:* The jet is broken into droplets. Droplets containing selected cells are electrically charged in a high-voltage field between deflection plates. *4:* The charged droplets are electrically deflected into collection tubes. (Courtesy of Joseph Grey, PhD.)

Table 15–6. Clinical applications of flow cytometry.

Leukocyte phenotyping
  Diagnosis of congenital immunodeficiency diseases
  Assessment of prognosis of HIV-positive patients
  Monitoring of immunotherapy or chemotherapy in immuno-
    deficiency diseases
  Monitoring of immune reconstitution in bone marrow
    transplant recipients

Tumor cell phenotyping
  Diagnosis and classification of leukemias and lymphomas
  Determination of clonality of immunoglobulin-bearing cells
    from lymphomas and leukemias
  Differentiation of hematopoietic from nonhematopoietic
    tumors or cells
  Assessment of prognosis of cancers

DNA analysis
  Determination of aneuploidy
  Determination of cell cycle kinetics

Neutrophil function analysis

Other applications
  Reticulocyte counting
  Platelet-associated immunoglobulin detection
  Leukocyte crossmatching in transplant recipients
  Cytogenetics

introducing microtiter plates in place of collection tubes; (5) analysis of cell cycle kinetics by various DNA stains; and (6) detection of rare cells such as monoclonal B cells in the blood of lymphoma patients. Clinical applications are listed in Table 15–6. Computers are used to analyze multiple parameters measured simultaneously by the flow cytometer, including two-color fluorescence, forward-angle light scatter, and 90° light scatter. Sophisticated data analysis and presentation software are available to produce clinically applicable information.

LYMPHOCYTE ACTIVATION

Lymphocyte activation, or stimulation, refers to an in vitro correlate of an in vivo process that regularly occurs when antigen interacts with specifically sensitized lymphocytes in the host. Lymphocyte transformation is a nearly synonymous term used first by P. Nowell in 1960 and later by K. Hirschhorn and others to describe the morphologic changes that resulted when small, resting lymphocytes were transformed into lymphoblasts on exposure to the mitogen PHA. Blastogenesis refers to the process of formation of large pyroninophilic blast-like cells in cultures of lymphocytes stimulated by either nonspecific mitogens or antigens.

Lymphocyte activation is an in vitro technique commonly used to assess cellular immunity in patients with immunodeficiency, autoimmunity, infectious diseases, and cancer. Myriad complex biochem-

ical events occur in lymphocytes following incubation with mitogens (see Chapters 3 and 9). These are substances that stimulate large numbers of lymphocytes and do not require a sensitized host, as is the case with antigens. These biochemical events include early membrane-related phenomena, such as increased synthesis of phospholipids, increased permeability to divalent cations, activation of adenylate cyclase, and resultant elevation of intracellular cyclic adenosine monophosphate (cAMP). Synthesis of protein, RNA, and finally DNA occurs shortly thereafter. It is this last phenomenon, the increase in DNA synthesis, that eventually results in cell division and is the basis for most clinically relevant assays for lymphocyte activation. Convenience and custom have led clinical immunologists to use DNA synthesis rather than earlier events, such as calcium influx or phospholipid metabolism, as a marker for lymphocyte activation.

Although the relationship between lymphocyte activation and delayed hypersensitivity is not always absolute, the method has found widespread use in clinical immunology. The in vivo delayed hypersensitivity skin test is actually the result of a series of complex phenomena, including antigen recognition, lymphocyte–macrophage interaction, release of lymphokines and monokines, and changes in vascular permeability. In vitro methods such as lymphocyte activation are useful for studying cellular hypersensitivity, since they permit analysis of specific stages in the immune response. In addition, they avoid challenge of the patient with such potentially hazardous antigens as drugs, transplantation antigens, or tumor antigens. Lymphocyte activation measures the *functional* capability of T or B lymphocytes to proliferate following antigenic challenge and is therefore a more direct test of immunocompetence than merely enumerating types of lymphocytes.

Lymphocyte responses can be suppressed or augmented by a variety of nonspecific factors present in human serum. This humoral modulation of responses to antigens or mitogens should be clearly differentiated from intrinsic suppression of cellular reactivity. Therefore, it is essential to avoid culture of lymphocytes in serum that may contain inhibitory substances. Their presence may be excluded by careful questioning of serum donors about their medications. If it is suspected that an individual's serum contains an inhibitor of lymphocyte activation, controls should be done with carefully washed cells obtained from that individual and cultured in pooled normal serum. A partial list of serum suppressive factors and drugs that may influence in vitro lymphocyte responses is presented in Table 15–7. A note of caution is warranted regarding the significance of this heterogeneous group of substances. Despite clear demonstration of substances with in vitro effects on lymphocyte responses, their in vivo action, particularly in view of the high concentrations often used in tissue culture, remains a matter of speculation.

Table 15–7. Examples of lymphocyte suppressive factors in serum.

Serum proteins
  Albumin (high concentration)
  Specific antibodies to stimulating antigens
  Immunoregulatory globulin
  Alpha-1-acid glycoprotein
  Pregnancy-associated serum globulins
  C-reactive protein (CRP)
  Serum alpha globulin of amyloid (SAA)
  Alpha globulins in cancer, chronic infection, inflammatory
    diseases
  Alpha-fetoprotein (AFP)
  Low-density lipoprotein
  Antigen-antibody complexes
  HLA antibodies
  T-cell antibodies
  Normal serum inhibitors (poorly characterized)
Hormones
  Glucocorticoids
  Progesterone
  Estrogens
  Androgens
  Prostaglandins
Drugs
  Aspirin
  Cannabis
  Chloroquine
  Ouabain
Others
  Interferon
  Cyclic nucleotides
  Cytokines

METHODS & INTERPRETATIONS

Lymphocyte Activation by Mitogens

A number of plant lectins and other substances have been employed in assessing human lymphocyte function (Table 15–8). In contrast to studies in mice, there is no incontrovertible evidence that T or B lymphocytes are selectively activated by nonspecific mitogens. PHA and Con A are predominantly T-cell mitogens, whereas pokewood mitogen stimulates B cells. Neither lipopolysaccharide nor antiimmunoglobulin antibody appears to be a potent B-cell stimulant in humans. Staphylococcal protein A from *Staphylococcus aureus* cell walls is probably a specific stimulant of human B cells, possibly by triggering cells into DNA synthesis via the Fc receptor for IgG.

Anti-CD3 monoclonal antibody activates only those T cells that bear T-cell receptor complex (see Chapter 9).

Lymphocyte Culture Technique for Mitogen Activation

Lymphocytes are purified from anticoagulated peripheral blood by density gradient centrifugation on Ficoll-Hypaque. Cultures are set up in triplicate or more in microtiter trays at a cell concentration of approximately 1×10^6 lymphocytes per milliliter. The culture medium is supplemented with 10–20% serum—autologous, heterologous, or pooled human sera. Mitogens are added in varying concentrations on a weight basis, usually over a two to three log range. Cultures are incubated in a mixture of 5% CO_2 in air for 72 hours, at which time most mitogens have produced their maximal effect on DNA synthesis. DNA synthesis is measured by pulse-labeling the cultures with tritiated thymidine (^{3}H-Tdr), a nucleoside precursor that is incorporated into newly synthesized DNA. The amount of ^{3}H-Tdr incorporated relative to the rate of DNA synthesis is determined by scintillation counting in a liquid scintillation spectrophotometer. Scintillation counting yields data in counts per minute (cpm) or corrected for quenching to disintegrations per minute (dpm), which are then used as a standard measure of lymphocyte responsiveness. The cpm in control cultures are either subtracted from or divided into stimulated cpm, which yields a ratio commonly referred to as the stimulation index.

Obviously a multitude of technical as well as conceptual variables can affect the results of this sensitive assay system. These include the concentration of cells, the geometry of the culture vessel, contamination of cultures with nonlymphoid cells or microorganisms, the dose of mitogen, the incubation time of cultures, and the techniques of harvesting cells.

The degree of lymphocyte activation is also a function of the cellular regulatory influences present in the culture. Suppressor or helper T, B, and mononuclear cells are all capable of modifying the final degree of proliferation in the specifically stimulated cell population. Some mitogens, particularly Con A, are known to activate suppressor T cells, which may reduce the proliferative response in such cultures.

Of additional importance in lymphocyte activation are culture time and dose-response kinetics. Since clinically important defects in cellular immunity are rarely absolute, quantitative relationships in lymphocyte activation are crucial. This is especially true when comparing the reduction of responsiveness of normal control subjects with that of a group of patients with altered lymphocyte function. With the use of

Table 15–8. "Nonspecific" mitogens that activate human lymphocytes.

Mitogen	Abbreviation	Biologic Source	Relative Specificity
Phytohemagglutinin	PHA	*Phaseolus vulgaris* (kidney bean)	T cells
Concanavalin A	Con A	*Canavalia ensiformis* (jack bean)	T cells (different from PHA)
Antilymphocyte globulin	ALG	Heterologous antisera	T cells + B cells
Anti-CD3 (MAb)	CD3	Hybridoma supernatant	T-cell receptor-bearing cells
Staphylococcus protein A	SpA, SAC	*S aureus* (Cowan I strain)	B cells, T-cell-independent
Pokeweed mitogen	PWM	*Phytolacca americana*	B cells, T-cell-dependent
Streptolysin S	SLS	Group A streptococci	?(Probably T cells)

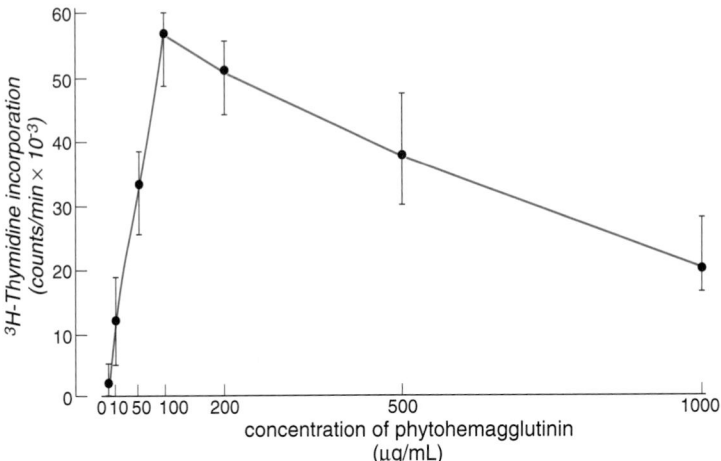

Figure 15–6. Dose-response curve for mitogen stimulation of 10^6 lymphocytes. Dose-response curve of a group of 10 normal adults whose peripheral blood lymphocytes were stimulated with varying concentrations of phytohemagglutinin for 72 hr. Lymphocytes were pulse-labeled with 2 μCi of tritiated thymidine 6 hr prior to harvesting. Counts per minute of tritiated thymidine incorporation were determined by liquid scintillation spectrometry and are plotted as the mean of 10 individual determinations ± 1 SD. A maximal response occurred at approximately 100–200 μg/mL of phytohemagglutinin.

microtiter culture systems and semiautomated harvesting devices, an attempt can be made to determine both dose- and time-response kinetics of either mitogen- or antigen-stimulated cultures (Figs 15–6 and 15–7).

Altered lymphocyte function can result in shifts in either time- or dose-response curves to the left or right. These shifts determine the optimal dose and optimal time of the lymphocyte response. Without such detailed analyses, it is usually impossible to accurately observe partial or subtle defects in lymphocyte responsiveness in various disease states. Cultures assayed at a single time with a single stimulant dose pe-riod are often grossly misleading.

Confusion may result from a nonstandardized format for presentation of data. Many laboratories present results of lymphocyte stimulation as a ratio of cpm in stimulated culture to those in control cultures—the so-called stimulation index. Others report "raw" cpm or dpm as illustrated in Figures 15–6 and 15–7. Neither method is entirely satisfactory. The stimulation index is a ratio, and marked changes can therefore result from changes in background or control cpm of the denominator. It is perhaps best to report data in both ways to permit better interpretations.

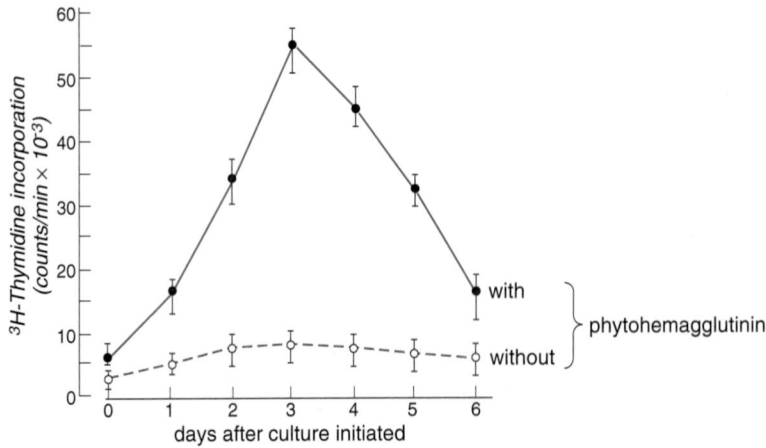

Figure 15–7. Time-response curve for mitogen stimulation of 10^6 lymphocytes. Time-response curve of peripheral blood lymphocytes from 10 normal adults stimulated in tissue culture for various lengths of time with an optimal concentration of phytohemagglutinin (100 μg/mL). Cultures were pulse-labeled with tritiated thymidine for 6 hr on the day of harvest. Maximal response occurred at 3 days after initiating the culture. Results are plotted as the mean ±1 SD of counts per minute.

Table 15–9. Antigens used to assess human cellular immunity in vitro.

PPD
Candida antigen
Streptokinase/streptodornase
Coccidioidin
Tetanus toxoid
Histoincompatible cells (MLC)
Trichophytin
Vaccinia virus
Herpes simplex virus

Abbreviations: PPD = purified protein derivative; MLC = mixed lymphoctyte culture.

Antigen Stimulation

Whereas mitogens stimulate large numbers of lymphocytes, antigens stimulate far fewer cells that are specifically sensitized to the antigen in question. In most instances, only T cells respond to antigens in this test. A wide variety of antigens have been employed in lymphocyte activation, many of them also being used for delayed hypersensitivity skin testing (Table 15–9). In general, normal subjects show agreement between the results of skin tests and antigen-induced lymphocyte activation. In many conditions, however, the in vitro technique is apparently a more sensitive index of specific antigen-mediated cellular hypersensitivity. Furthermore, in vitro tests for T-cell activation obviate the need for production of cytokines that produce dermal inflammation expressed as delayed hypersensitivity.

Lymphocyte Culture Technique for Antigen Stimulation

Culture methods are virtually identical to those described for mitogen stimulation. Additional factors to be considered include the possible presence in serum supplements of antibody directed against stimulating antigens. Antigen–antibody complexes may block or occasionally nonspecifically stimulate lymphocytes.

As in the case of mitogen-induced activation, time- and dose-response kinetics are crucial in generating reliable data. Representative examples of such curves are shown in Figures 15–7 and 15–8. In contrast to mitogen-induced lymphocyte activation, antigen stimulation results in lower total DNA synthesis. Furthermore, the time of maximal response does not occur until the culture has been allowed to continue for 5–7 days. Figure 15–9 clearly illustrates both the usefulness of and the necessity for performing careful time- and dose-response kinetics in assessing human lymphocyte function.

MIXED LYMPHOCYTE CULTURE & CELL-MEDIATED LYMPHOLYSIS

Mixed lymphocyte culture (MLC) is a special case of antigen stimulation in which T lymphocytes respond to foreign histocompatibility antigen on unre-

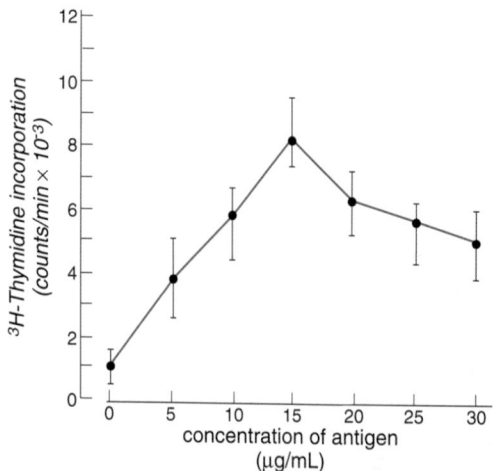

Figure 15–8. Dose-response curve for antigen stimulation of 10^6 lymphocytes. Dose-response curve of lymphocytes from 15 normal individuals were delayed hypersensitivity to the antigen. Cultures were harvested at 120 hours of culture after a 6-hour pulse with tritiated thymidine. Counts per minute were determined by scintillation spectrometry. Results are plotted as the mean ±1 SD from 15 skin test-positive subjects at various antigen concentrations. Maximum response is at 15 µg/mL of antigen.

lated lymphocytes or monocytes. This test is performed as either a "one-way" or "two-way" assay (Fig 15–10). In the one-way MLC, the stimulating cells are treated with either irradiation (≈ 2000 R) or mitomycin to prevent DNA synthesis without killing the cell. The

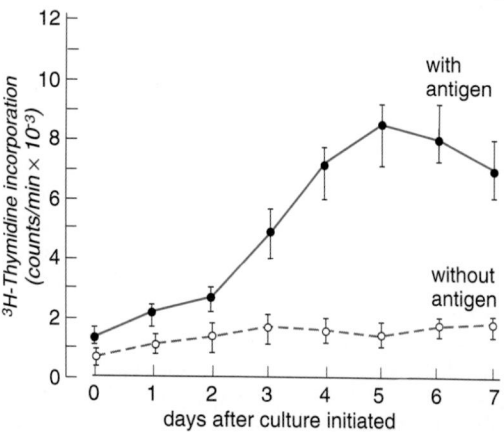

Figure 15–9. Time-response curve for antigen stimulation of 10^6 lymphocytes. Responses of peripheral blood lymphocytes from 15 normal adults with delayed hypersensitivity to the antigen. Cells were cultured as described in the legend to Figure 15–8. Antigen concentration for all cultures was 15 µg/mL. Maximal response occurred on days 5–7 of culture. Results are plotted as the mean ±1 SD for 15 individual determinations.

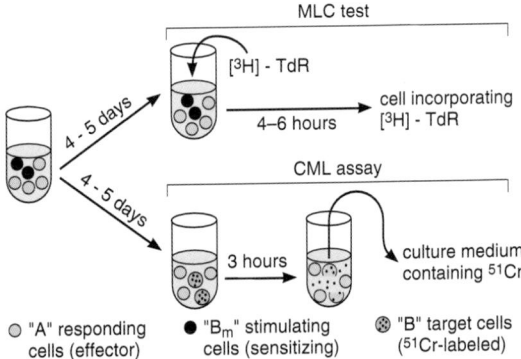

Figure 15–10. Mixed lymphocyte culture (MLC) and cell-mediated lympholysis (CML) assays schematically represented. Cells (black and white balls) from separate individuals are cultured. In MLC, DNA synthesis in responding (noninactivated) cell is measured. In CML assay, the ability of "A" cells to kill ⁵Cr-labeled "B" cells is measured. See the text for further explanation. [³H]-TdR, tritiated thymidine. (Reproduced, with permission, from Bach FH, Van Rood JJ: The major histocompatibility complex: Genetics and biology. *N Engl J Med* 1976:**295**:806, 872).

magnitude of the response is then entirely the result of DNA synthesis in the nonirradiated or nonmitomycin-treated cells. In the two-way MLC, cells from both individuals are mutually stimulating and responding, DNA synthesis represents the net response of both sets of cells, and the individual contributions cannot be discerned. The culture conditions, time of exposure, ³H-Tdr pulse labeling, and harvesting procedures are usually identical to those for antigen stimulation. Controls include coculture of syngeneic irradiated and nonirradiated pairs and coculture of allogeneic irradiated pairs. The first control provides baseline DNA synthesis, and the second ensures adequate inactivation by irradiation (or mitomycin) of the stimulator cells.

In the use of MLC as a test for T-cell function, difficulties in quantitation often arise owing to variations in stimulator cell antigens that determine the degree of genetic disparity between stimulator and responder cells. To overcome this difficulty and produce a more standardized test, frozen aliquots of viable pooled human allogeneic cells have been employed as stimulator cells.

The stimulating antigens on human cells are class II major histocompatibility (MHC) molecules encoded by the HLA-D locus (see Chapter 5). Responding cells are primarily T lymphocytes with obligate macrophage cooperation. B cells can also respond in MLC, since a marked increase in immunoglobulin synthesis can be detected. MLC may be used as a histocompatibility assay (see Chapter 17) and as a test for immunocompetence of T cells, particularly in immunodeficiency disorders (see Chapters 22 and 23).

Cell-mediated lympholysis (CML) is an extension of the MLC technique in which cytotoxic effector cells

generated during MLC are detected (see Fig 15–10). This test involves an initial one-way MLC culture followed by exposure of stimulated cells to ⁵¹Cr-labeled target cells specifically lysed by sensitized killer lymphocytes. These target cells are HLA-identical to the stimulator cells in MLC. Cytotoxicity is measured as the percentage of ⁵¹Cr released in specific target cells compared with the percentage of ⁵¹Cr released from control (nonspecific) target cells. Several lines of evidence indicate that cells that proliferate in MLC and killer cells that participate in CML assay are not identical. Killer cells are generated that have specificity for class I MHC antigens on target cells, whereas in class II MHC antigen differences determine the reaction. CML assays provide an additional measure of T-cell function and can be used to estimate presensitization and histocompatibility in clinical transplantation (see also Chapters 6, 17, and 57).

CLINICAL APPLICATION OF T- & B-CELL ASSAYS

Counting of T and B cells in peripheral blood and tissue specimens has limited application in both the diagnosis and investigation of pathophysiologic mechanisms of many disease states. Functional assays are even more limited in value primarily to studies of immune deficiency diseases. Current applications include the following.

1. Diagnosis and classification of immunodeficiency diseases (see Chapters 21–24 and 53).
2. Determination of origin of malignant lymphocytes in lymphocytic leukemia and lymphoma (see Chapter 46).
3. Evaluation of immunocompetence and mechanisms of tissue damage in autoimmune disease, such as systemic lupus erythematosus and rheumatoid arthritis (see Chapter 33).
4. Detection of changes in cellular immune competence in HIV and other infections that may be of prognostic value (see Chapter 53).
5. Monitoring of cellular changes following organ transplantation (see Chapter 57).

NATURAL KILLER (NK) CELLS

Natural killer (NK) cells can be enumerated by specific monoclonal antibodies using methods identical to those for T and B cells (see Chapters 3 and 19). Several monoclonal antibodies are available that detect either Fc receptors (CD16) or specific differentiation antigens (CD56, CD57) present on these cells. Some NK cells also express antigens from the CD2 T-cell family. Functional testing is done by measuring the ability of these nonimmune cells to kill special target cells such as erythroleukemia cell line K562.

Cytotoxicity is usually performed by using the ^{51}Cr release assay, similarly to cell-mediated lympholysis (see Fig 15–10). More recently, flow cytometric assays for determining NK activity have been developed. These assays correlate well with standard chromium release assays and in addition obviate the use of radioisotopes.

MONOCYTE–MACROPHAGE ASSAYS

The morphologic identification of normal peripheral blood monocytes in stained peripheral blood films is ordinarily quite simple. Monocytes are larger than granulocytes and most lymphocytes. They typically have round or kidney-shaped nuclei with fine, lightly stained granules. In suspension or even in tissue or blood specimens, however, additional markers may be required to differentiate monocytes from lymphocytes and primitive myeloid cells (see Chapters 1 and 2).

A reliable stain for monocytes is so-called nonspecific esterase, or α-naphthol esterase, which is present in monocytes but absent in most myeloid and lymphocytic cells. Monoclonal antibodies directed at specific differentiation antigens such as CD14 are available.

Functional attributes of monocytes are discussed in detail in Chapter 2. In the clinical laboratory, phagocytosis of particles or antibody-coated heat-killed microorganisms is useful for functional identification of monocytes.

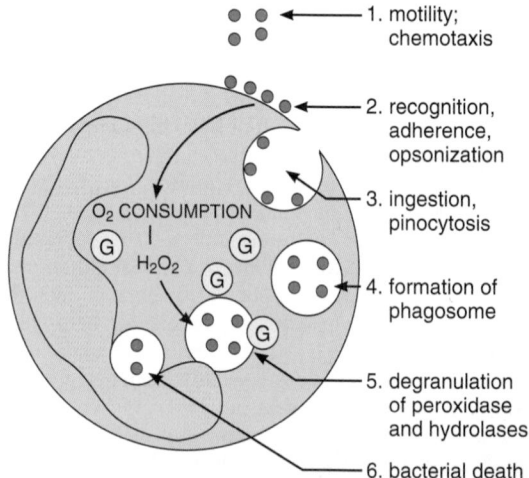

Figure 15–11. Steps in the progression of phagocytosis. Schematic representation of phagocytosis by a granulocyte. *1:* Bacteria attract phagocytic cells by chemotactic stimulus. *2:* Presence of opsonins (immunoglobulin and complement) facilitates recognition and surface attachment. *3:* Invagination of cell membrane with enclosed opsonized bacteria. *4:* Intracellular organelle, the phagosome, forms. *5:* Granules fuse with phagosomes and release enzymes into the phagolysosome. *6:* Bacterial death and digestion result. (Modified, with permission, from Baehner: Chronic granulomatous disease. In: *The Phagocytic Cell in Host Resistance.* Bellanti JA, Dayton DH [editors]. Raven Press, 1975, p. 175.)

NEUTROPHIL FUNCTION

Polymorphonuclear neutrophils (PMN) are bone marrow-derived leukocytes with a finite life span, which play a central role in defense of the host against infection. For many types of infections, the neutrophil plays the primary role as an effector or killer cell. In the bloodstream and extravascular spaces, however, neutrophils exert their antimicrobial effects through a complex interaction with antibody, complement, and chemotactic factors. Thus, in assessing neutrophil function, one cannot view the cell as an independent entity; its essential dependence on other immune processes, both cellular and humoral, must be taken into account.

Defects in neutrophil function can be classified as quantitative or qualitative. In quantitative disorders, the total number of normally functioning neutrophils is reduced below a critical level, allowing infection to ensue. Drug-induced and idiopathic neutropenia (see Chapter 35), with absolute circulating granulocyte counts of less than 1000/μL, are examples of this sort of defect. In these situations, granulocytes are functionally normal but are present in insufficient numbers to maintain an adequate defense against infection. In qualitative neutrophilic disorders, the total number of circulating PMNs is either normal or sometimes actually elevated, but the cells fail to exert their normal microbicidal functions. Chronic granulomatous disease is an example of this type of disorder (see Chapter 24). In patients with chronic granulomatous disease the normal or increased numbers of circulating neutrophils are unable to kill certain types of intracellular organisms.

Phagocytosis by PMN can be divided into five distinct and temporally sequential stages: (1) motility, (2) recognition and adhesion, (3) ingestion, (4) degranulation, and (5) intracellular killing (Fig 15–11). The microbicidal activity of the neutrophil is the sum of the activity of these five phases. The clinical syndromes resulting from defects in many of the various stages in phagocytosis are discussed in Chapter 24. The laboratory tests used in clinical practice to evaluate phagocytic function in humans with various diseases is discussed in terms of the five major steps in the process. It should be emphasized that for many neutrophil functions no standard assay exists; therefore, a variety of test choices depends on the local laboratory. The following sections include examples of useful clinical tests of neutrophil function.

TESTS FOR MOTILITY

Neutrophils are constantly in motion. This movement can be either random or directed. Random, or passive, motion is the result of **brownian movement.** In **chemotactic movement** the cells are actively attracted to some chemotactic stimulus. Chemotaxins are produced by complement activation (C3a, C5a, C567; see Chapter 11), by fibrinolysis (fibrinopeptide B), by microorganisms themselves (endotoxins), and by other leukocytes (lymphocyte chemotactic factor). Products of lipoxygenation of arachidonic acid, particularly leukotriene B_4 (LTB_4), are also chemoattractants. Relatively simple assays have been designed to assess leukocyte movement in vitro. An in vivo technique, the Rebuck skin window, preceded the development of in vitro assays and was one of the earliest methods developed for assessing leukocyte function.

Test for Random Motility

Random motility is tested for by the **capillary tube method.** Purified neutrophils in 0.1% human albumin solution at a concentration of 5×10^6 mL are placed in a siliconized microhematocrit tube. The tube is enclosed in a chamber specially constructed from microscope slides and embedded in adhesive clay. After being filled with immersion oil, the entire chamber is placed on the stage of a microscope. Motility is assessed by observing the leading edge of the leukocyte column in the microscope at hourly intervals. Measurements are expressed in millimeters of movement from the starting boundary of the packed leukocyte layer.

Test for Chemotaxis

Directional locomotion of neutrophils toward various chemotactic stimuli is quantitated by use of a Boyden chamber. Cells to be tested are placed in the upper chamber and are separated from the lower chamber containing a chemotactic substance by a filter membrane of small pore size. Neutrophils can enter the filter membrane but are trapped in transit through the membrane. After a suitable incubation period, the filter is removed and stained and the underside is microscopically examined for the presence of neutrophils.

Although this method is theoretically simple, there are numerous technical difficulties. These include nonavailability of filters of standard pore size, observer bias in quantitation of migrating neutrophils in the microscope, loss of cells that fall off or completely transverse the filter, and failure of many workers to standardize cell numbers and serum supplements.

An additional method for measuring chemotaxis and random motility has been recently developed. This technique involves the radial migration of leukocytes from small wells cut into an agarose medium in a Petri dish. In many respects, the method is similar to single radial diffusion (see Chapter 14). Generally, three wells are cut into agarose. The cell population in question is placed in the center well. A chemoattractant is placed in an outer well, and a control nonattractant is placed in the remaining well. After several hours of migration, the distance from the center of the well originally containing cells to the leading edges of the migrating cells is measured. In this way, the directed motility and the random motion can be quantitated. This method has achieved widespread application and in many laboratories has supplanted the somewhat more cumbersome Boyden's chamber technique.

TESTS FOR RECOGNITION & ADHESION

As the neutrophil in an immune host approaches its target, by either random or directed motility, it recognizes microorganisms by the presence of antibody and complement fixed to the surface of the microorganisms. Enhancement of phagocytosis (opsonization) occurs under these circumstances. Adherence and aggregation of neutrophils are promoted by a series of membrane glycoproteins.

The family of membrane glycoproteins that function as adherence molecules includes LFA-1 (lymphocyte function-associated antigen type 1), Mac-1 (macrophage 1) and p 150,95. These molecules all contain a common β subunit (CD18) and a unique α subunit. Mac-1 functions as a receptor for C3bi. Deficiencies of the β subunit have been described (see Chapter 23). Monoclonal antibodies to CD18 (the β subunit) are available, as well as those to specific α subunits: CD11a = LFA-1, CD11b = Mac-1, and CD11c = p 150,95. These molecules are present on granulocytes, monocytes, and some lymphocytes and can be readily measured by flow cytometry and immunofluorescence.

Tests to detect the presence of complement and antibody Fc receptors on neutrophils are rarely useful in clinical testing. The need for either antibody or complement (opsonins) coating of microorganisms for phagocytosis can be determined by employing sera devoid of either or both of these factors followed by an assay for ingestion and subsequent intracellular killing. Furthermore, IgG and complement receptors on neutrophils as well as mononuclear phagocytes can be readily detected by rosette formation with IgG-coated or complement-coated erythrocytes or by immunofluorescence with monoclonal antibodies.

TESTS FOR INGESTION

Ingestion of microorganisms by neutrophils is an active process that requires energy production by the phagocytic cell. Internalization of antibody-coated and complement-coated microorganisms occurs rapidly following their surface contact with neutrophils. Since subsequent intracellular events, that is, degranulation and killing, depend on the success of ingestion, tests for ingestion provide a rapid and relatively simple means of assessing the overall phagocytic process. Unfortunately, the term *phagocytosis* has often been used to denote *only* the ingestion phase of the process. Thus, terms such as *phagocytic index,* which refer to the average number of particles ingested, really should be considered measurements of ingestion rather than of phagocytosis.

All tests to measure the ability of neutrophils to ingest either native or opsonized particles involve one of two general approaches. Either a direct estimate is made of the cellular uptake of particles by assaying the cells themselves, or the removal of particles from the fluid or medium is taken as an indirect estimate of cellular uptake.

Methods for quantitation of the ingestion of particles by cellular assays include (1) direct counting by light microscopy; (2) estimation of cell-bound radioactivity after ingestion of a radiolabeled particle; (3) measurement of an easily stained lipid, such as oil red O, after extraction from cells, and (4) flow cytometric analysis of the uptake of fluorescently labeled particles.

One disadvantage of many of these assays is that particles adherent to the neutrophil membranes are included as ingested particles. Other elements that influence results in performing ingestion assays include the presence of humoral factors (opsonins) that enhance uptake, the presence of serum containing acute-phase reactants that depress uptake, the need for constant agitation or tumbling of cells and particles to maximize contact and subsequent uptake, the type or size of the test particle used, and, finally, the ratio of particles to ingesting cells. No well-standardized assay is currently available for estimating particle ingestion.

TESTS FOR DEGRANULATION

Following ingestion of particles or microorganisms, the ingested element is bound by invaginated cell surface membrane in an organelle termed the **phagosome.** Shortly thereafter, lysosomes fuse with the phagosome to form a structure called the **phagolysosome.** Degranulation is the process of fusion of lysosomes and phagosomes, with the subsequent discharge of intralysosomal contents into the phagolysosome.

Degranulation is an active process and requires energy expenditure by the cell. Thus, impairment of normal metabolic pathways of the neutrophil—especially oxygen consumption and the metabolism of glucose through the hexose monophosphate shunt—interferes with degranulation and subsequent intracellular killing.

A test for degranulation called frustrated phagocytosis has been developed and applied to the study of some neutrophil dysfunction syndromes. The frustrated-phagocytosis system (Fig 15–12) allows for

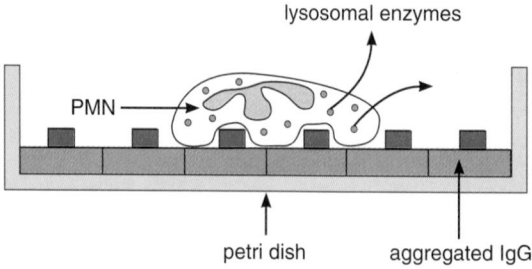

Figure 15–12. Assay of granulocyte degranulation by the "frustrated phagocytosis" method. The neutrophil is attached to aggregated IgG fixed to the bottom of a Petri dish. Lysosomal enzymes are discharged into supernatant as the cell attempts to phagocytose the IgG but is "frustrated." (Courtesy of S Barrett.)

examination of degranulation independently of in-gestion. Heat-aggregated γ-globulin or immune complexes are fixed to the plastic surface of a Petri dish so that they cannot be ingested. Neutrophils are placed in suspension in Petri dishes with and without attached aggregated γ-globulin. The cell membranes of the neutrophils are stimulated by contact between γ-globulin and appropriate cell membrane receptors. This process results in fusion of intraleukocyte granules (lysosomes) with the cell membrane. As a result, intralysosomal contents are discharged into the suspending medium. The rate of release of lysosomal enzymes, particularly β-glucuronidase and acid phosphatase, is taken as an estimate of the rate of degranulation. Nonspecific cell death or cytolysis can be estimated by measuring the discharge of lactate dehydrogenase (a nongranule enzyme) into the medium. This assay system has been used to demonstrate retardation in the degranulation rate by neutrophils from patients with chronic granulomatous disease.

TESTS FOR INTRACELLULAR KILLING

The primary function of the neutrophil in host resistance is intracellular killing of microorganisms. This final stage of phagocytosis is dependent on the successful completion of the preceding steps: motility, recognition, ingestion, and degranulation. A variety of intraleukocytic systems make up the antimicrobial armamentarium of the neutrophil (Table 15–10). Obviously, a defect in intracellular killing could be the result of any one or a combination of these functions. In clinical practice, however, two assays have received widespread use: the nitroblue tetrazolium dye reduction test and the intraleukocytic killing test. It is hoped that specific metabolic and antimicrobial assays for other intraleukocytic events will also become available in the future.

Table 15–10. Antimicrobial systems of neutrophils.[1]

Acidic pH of phagolysosome
Lysozyme
Lactoferrin
Defensins
Cathepsin G
Myeloperoxidase-halogenation system
Hydrogen peroxide
Superoxide radical
Hydroxyl radical
Singlet oxygen

[1] For a further description of these systems, see Lehrer RI, et al: Neutrophils in host defense. *Ann Intern Med* 1988;**109**:127, and Boxer LA, Morganroth ML: Neutrophil function disorders. *Disease-a-Month* 1987;**33**:681.

Nitroblue Tetrazolium Dye Reduction Test

Nitroblue tetrazolium (NBT) is a clear, yellow, water-soluble compound that forms formazan, a deep blue dye, on reduction. Neutrophils can reduce the dye following ingestion of latex or other particles subsequent to the metabolic burst generated through the hexose monophosphate shunt. The reduced dye can be easily measured photometrically after extraction from neutrophils with the organic solvent pyridine. The reduction of NBT to a blue substance thus forms the basis of the quantitative NBT test. The precise mechanism of NBT reduction is not known, but the phenomenon is closely allied to metabolic events in the respiratory burst following ingestion, including increased hexose monophosphate shunt activity, increased oxygen consumption, and increased hydrogen peroxide and superoxide radical formation. Since the generation of reducing activity in intact neutrophils parallels the metabolic activities following ingestion, NBT reduction is a useful means of assaying overall metabolic integrity of phagocytosing neutrophils. Failure of NBT dye reduction is a consistent and diagnostically important laboratory abnormality in chronic granulomatous disease. Neutrophils from these patients fail to kill certain intracellular microbes and fail to generate H_2O_2 or the superoxide radical.

Quantitative NBT Test

Isolated neutrophils are incubated in a balanced salt solution with latex particles and NBT. After 15 minutes of incubation at 37°C, the reduced dye (blue formazan) is extracted with pyridine and measured spectrophotometrically at 515 nm. The change in absorbance between cultures of cells that actively phagocytose latex particles and those that do not is taken as an index of neutrophil function. The test is strikingly abnormal in chronic granulomatous disease (see Chapter 24). Various modifications of the quantitative NBT test have been developed as screening tests for chronic granulomatous disease. Prominent among these are so-called slide tests in which neutrophils, latex, and NBT are placed in a drop on a glass slide and the reduction to blue formazan assayed under the microscope. It can be performed on a single drop of blood, but abnormal results should be confirmed with the more precise quantitative method described earlier.

Chemiluminescence

Neutrophils emit small amounts of electromagnetic radiation following ingestion of microorganisms. This energy can be detected as light by sensitive photomultiplier tubes, such as those in liquid scintillation counters. During the respiratory burst, H_2O_2, superoxide radicals, and singlet oxygen are generated. Singlet oxygen, a highly unstable and reactive species, combines with bacteria or other intralysosomal elements to form electronically unstable carboxy groups. As these groups relax to ground state, light energy is emitted. This entire process has been termed **chemiluminescence** and forms the basis of an important assay of neutrophil function. Similar to NBT, it requires all steps prior to actual bacterial killing to be intact. Recent studies show a precise correlation between light emissions and microbicidal activity. The oxidative steps in the biochemical pathways present in the neutrophil generate the chemiluminescence, which is easily detected in a liquid scintillation spectrometer with the coincidence circuit excluded.

In the test, neutrophils are incubated in clear, colorless balanced salt solution in the presence of an ingestible particle, such as latex or zymosan, in a scintillation vial. Luminol, an intermediate fluorescent compound, can be added to intensify the light emissions. The emission of photons of light is measured as cpm in a scintillation counter over the next 10 minutes at 2-minute intervals. Studies with this technique have revealed markedly reduced chemiluminescence in chronic granulomatous disease (patients and carriers) and in myeloperoxidase-deficient patients. This method appears to be somewhat more sensitive than the quantitative NBT test and can probably be performed on very small numbers of cells. Newer methods employ a sample of whole blood, greatly simplifying the procedure by obviating the granulocyte separation steps. Many laboratories are substituting it for NBT reduction as a screening test for neutrophil dysfunction and in detection of carriers of chronic granulomatous disease.

Flow Cytometry

The neutrophil oxidative burst that follows ingestion produces hydrogen peroxide, which oxidizes various intracellular components. If 2′, 7′, dichlorofluorescein diacetate, a small nonpolar dye, is present during incubation of neutrophils, it is cleaved by esterases and trapped inside the cell. Another dye, dihydrorhodamine (DHR) can also be used for this assay and behaves in a similar manner (Fig 15–13). Hydrogen peroxide oxidizes the compound to fluorescent dichlorofluorescein, which can be easily detected by flow cytometry in a gated population of neutrophils.

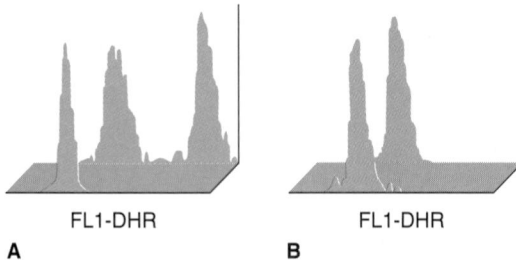

A   **B**

Figure 15–13. Three-dimensional flow-cytometric display of dihydrorhodamine (DHR) fluorescence in a patient with chronic granulomatous disease and his mother, a carrier. **A:** Fluorescent intensity of DHR (horizontal axis) of neutrophils from the mother. The peak in the foreground shows the histogram of unstimulated cells. After stimulation with pyridylmercuric acetate (PMA), two peaks are shown (background of panel **A**). The population to the left are neutrophils that did not reduce the DHR and thus show no increase in fluorescence. The peak to the right demonstrates an increase in fluorescence of PMNs that have reduced the DHR. In panel **B** it can be seen that the patient's PMNs do not reduce the DHR and thus there is no difference in fluorescence intensity of unstimulated (peak in foreground) versus PMA-stimulated cells (peak in background).

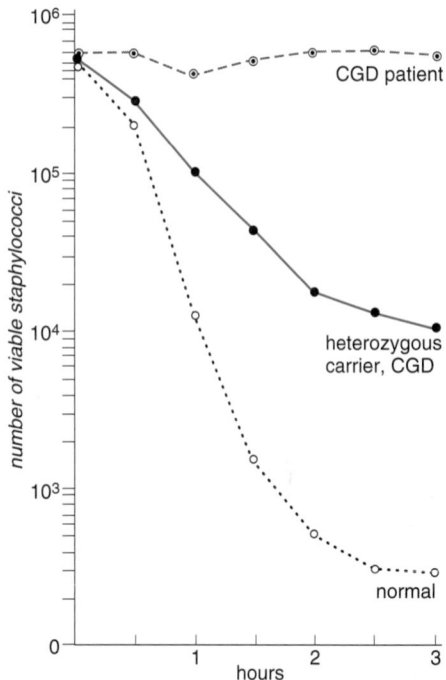

Figure 15–14. Bactericidal assay of granulocytes. Curves represent the number of viable intracellular organisms that survive after being ingested by granulocytes. Note the marked decline in bacterial survival in normal cells compared with reduced to absent killing by cells from patients and relatives with CGD (chronic granulomatous disease).

This technique allows for rapid, sensitive, and relatively reproducible detection of chronic granulomatous disease and generally facilitates discrimination between carriers and normal subjects. It has largely replaced the quantitative NBT tests in many laboratories.

Neutrophil Microbicidal Assay

Many strains of bacteria and fungi are effectively engulfed and killed by human neutrophils in vitro. Assuming that all of the stages of the phagocytic process that precede killing within the phagolysosome are intact, microbicidal assays are extremely useful tests for neutrophil function. As an example, the bactericidal capacity of neutrophils for the common test strain 502A of *Staphylococcus aureus* are described here in some detail.

Bacteria are cultured overnight in nutrient broth to make certain that they will be in a logarithmic growth phase. They are then diluted to give about five bacteria per neutrophil in the final test. Neutrophils are separated from whole heparinized blood by dextran sedimentation and lysis of erythrocytes with 0.84% NH_4Cl. Opsonin is provided as a 1:1 mixture of pooled frozen serum (−70 °C) and serum from freshly clotted blood. Bacteria, neutrophils, and opsonin are incubated in tightly capped test tubes and tumbled end over end at 37 °C. An aliquot of the entire mixture is sampled at zero time. After 30 minutes of incubation, antibiotics are added to kill extracellular bacteria. Aliquots of neutrophils with ingested organisms are sampled at 30, 60, and 120 minutes. Intracellular microorganisms are liberated by lysis of neutrophils by sterile water and the number of *viable* intracellular

bacteria is estimated by serial dilutions and plating of lysed leukocytes. Results plotted as in Figure 15–14 show that normal neutrophils result in an almost two-log reduction in viable intracellular *S aureus* cells 1 hour after incubation. Killing is virtually absent in cells from patients with chronic granulomatous disease and intermediate in heterozygous carriers.

By varying the test organism or the source of opsonin, this assay can be effectively used to measure a wide range of microbial activities and serum-related defects. Obviously, falsely "normal" killing is the interpretation of the results if cells fail to ingest organ-

Table 15–11. Disorders of neutrophil function.

Leukocyte adherence deficiency
Chronic granulomatous disease (X-linked or autosomal recessive)
Job's syndrome
Chédiak-Higashi syndrome
Myeloperoxidase deficiency
Glucose-6-phosphate dehydrogenase deficiency
Acute leukemia
Down's syndrome
Premature infants
Transient neutrophil dysfunction
    Acute infections
    Ataxia-telangiectasia
    Cryoglobulinemia

isms normally. Thus, an independent assay for microbial ingestion must be performed prior to the neutrophil microbicidal test.

Some diseases with defective microbicidal activity demonstrable with this assay are listed in Table 15–11. For further details, see Chapter 24.

REFERENCES

GENERAL
Hudson L, Hay FC: *Practical Immunology,* 3rd ed. Blackwell, 1989.

Mishell BB, Shiigi SM: *Selected Methods in Cellular Immunology.* W.H. Freeman, 1980.

Rose NR et al (editors): *Manual of Clinical Laboratory Immunology,* 4th ed. American Society for Microbiology, 1992.

Virella G et al: Diagnostic evaluation of lymphocyte functions of cell mediated immunity. *Immunol Series* 1993;**58:**291

Weir DM et al (editors): *Handbook of Experimental Immunology,* 4th ed. 4 vols. Blackwell, 1986.

DELAYED HYPERSENSITIVITY SKIN TESTS
Ahmed RA, Blose DA: Delayed hypersensitivity skin testing: A review. *Arch Dermatol* 1983;**119:**934.

Dannenberg AM: Delayed-type hypersensitivity and cell-mediated immunity in the pathogenesis of tuberculosis. *Immunol Today* 1991;**12:**228.

Frazer IH et al: Assessment of delayed-type hypersensitivity in man. A comparison of the "multitest" and conventional intradermal injection of six antigens. *Clin Exp Immunol* 1985;**35:**182.

Knapp W et al: *Leukocyte Typing IV.* Oxford, 1989.

Palmer DL, Reed WP: Delayed hypersensitivity skin testing: 1. Response rates in a hospitalized population. 2. Clinical correlates and anergy. *J Infect Dis* 1974;**130:**132, 138.

ASSAYS FOR HUMAN LYMPHOCYTES & MONOCYTES
Adams DO et al (editors): *Methods for Studying Mononuclear Phagocytes.* Academic Press, 1981.

Bray RA, Landay AL: Identification and functional characterization of mononuclear cells by flow cytometry. *Arch Pathol Lab Med* 1989;**113:**579.

Fletcher MA et al: Lymphocyte proliferation. In: *Manual of Clinical Laboratory Immunology,* 4th ed. Rose NR et al (editors). American Society for Microbiology, 1992, p. 213.

Lucey DR et al: Assessment of lymphocyte and monocyte function. In: *Clinical Immunology—Principles and Practice.* Vol. II. R Rich (editor-in-chief). Mosby, 1995, pp. 2124–2140.

Smith D, DeShazo RD: Delayed hypersensitivity skin testing. In: *Manual of Clinical Laboratory Immunology,* 4th ed. Rose NR et al (editors). American Society for Microbiology, 1992, p. 202.

LYMPHOCYTE ACTIVATION
Stobo JD: Mitogens. In: *Clinical Immunobiology.* Vol. 4. Bach FH, Good RA (editors). Academic Press, 1980, p. 55.

Weiss A, Imboden J: Cell surface molecules and early events involved in T lymphocyte activation. *Adv Immunol* 1987;**4:**1.

FLOW CYTOMETRY & CELL SORTING
Braylan RC, Benson NA: Flow cytometric analysis of lymphomas. *Arch Pathol Lab Med* 1989;**113:**627.

Fleisher TA, Marti GE: Flow cytometry. In: *Clinical Immunology: Principles and Practice.* Vol. II Rich RR (editor-in-chief). Mosby, 1995, pp. 2110–2123.

Keren DF: *Flow Cytometry in Clinical Diagnosis.* ASCP Press, 1989.

Kipps TJ et al: New developments in flow cytometric analysis of lymphocyte markers. *Clin Lab Med* 1992;**2:**237.

McCarthy RC, Fetterhoff TJ: Issues of quality assurance in clinical flow cytometry. *Arch Pathol Lab Med* 1989;**113:**658.

Papdopoulas NG et al: An improved fluorescence assay for the determination of lymphocyte-mediated cytotoxicity using flow cytometry. *J Immunol Methods* 1994;**177:**101.

Ryan DH et al: Flow cytometry in the clinical laboratory. *Clin Chem Acta* 1988;**171:**125.

NEUTROPHIL FUNCTION
Boxer LA, Morganroth ML: Neutrophil function disorders. *Disease-a-Month* 1987;**33:**681.

Horwitz MA: Phagocytosis of microorganisms. *Rev Infect Dis* 1982;**4:**104.

Lehrer RI et al: Neutrophils and host defense. *Ann Intern Med* 1988;**109:**127.

Synderman R, Gaetze EJ: Molecular and cellular mechanisms of leukocyte chemotaxis. *Science* 1981;**213:**830.

Vowells SJ et al: Flow cytometric analysis of the granulocyte respiratory burst: A comparison study of fluorescent probes. *J Immunol Methods* 1995;**178:**89.

Wade BH, Mandell GL: Polymorphonuclear leukocytes: Dedicated professional phagocytes. *Am J Med* 1983; **74:**686.

Yang KD, Hill HR: Neutrophil function disorders: Pathophysiology prevention and therapy. *J Pediatr* 1991;**119:**343.

Blood Banking & Immunohematology

16

Maurene Viele, MD, Elizabeth Donegan, MD, & Edith L. Bossom, SBB

The ability to successfully transfuse whole blood, or more specific blood components, has saved countless lives and supported the advance of modern surgery and cancer chemotherapy. The first lifesaving transfusion was performed less than 200 years ago by James Blundell in 1818. Today, more than 22 million blood components, prepared from approximately 14 million blood donations, are transfused in the USA annually. The safety of blood transfusion has steadily improved since the first US blood bank was founded in the 1940s. Techniques were developed to separate whole blood into its component parts (packed red blood cells, fresh-frozen plasma, and platelets) making one blood donation potentially available to treat as many as three patients. Many cases of intravascular volume overload, once a common side effect of transfusion, were prevented as patients could be transfused with only the particular component needed. Tests were developed and implemented to detect the infectious diseases recognized as transmitted in blood products. New molecular diagnostic techniques are now being investigated to improve the sensitivity of the tests used for donor blood analysis.

Nevertheless, transfusion continues to require the removal of blood from one human being for infusion into another. This "living transplant" carries with it the complexities of its human source and thereby brings with it the potential of undesirable side effects in the recipient. Some risks of transfusion are now known, and others have yet to be described. Consequently, the need for transfusion must be judged carefully in light of these risks.

BLOOD GROUPS

The first blood group system was described at the turn of the 20th century by Karl Landsteiner. He observed that erythrocytes from some individuals clumped when mixed with the serum of others but not with their own. Using this agglutination technique, he classified an individual's erythrocytes into four types: A, B, AB, and O. It is now recognized that A and B represent carbohydrate antigens on the erythrocyte. Group O individuals have neither of these antigens on their erythrocytes, whereas erythrocytes from AB individuals have both A and B antigens. The ABO system is the most important blood group system for transfusion purposes.

Knowledge about blood groups has expanded to include a diverse and numerous array of antigenic determinants on erythrocytes. Approximately 600 erythrocyte antigens are known, of which 195 belong to 23 recognized blood group systems. Each blood group system has members; each member may be composed of one or more different antigens. Each antigen is controlled by one gene. The antigenic determinants of a blood group are produced either directly (for proteins) or indirectly (for carbohydrates) by alleles at a single gene locus or at a gene locus so closely linked to one another that crossing over is extremely rare. For any antigen of a blood group, a single allele is present at that locus and other alleles are therefore excluded. A specific antigen on the erythrocyte surface is usually detected in the blood bank laboratory by reacting erythrocytes with sera known to contain antibodies reactive with that antigen. This test defines a phenotype. The number of antigenic determinants per erythrocyte and their ability to elicit an immune response vary from antigen to antigen.

ERYTHROCYTE ANTIGENS

H & ABO

Antigenic determinants of the H and ABO systems are carbohydrate moieties whose specificity resides in the terminal sugars of an oligosaccharide. On erythrocyte and endothelial surfaces, most of the antigens are bound to glycosphingolipids. Genetic control is via the production of transferase enzymes that conjugate terminal sugars to a stem carbohydrate. The H and

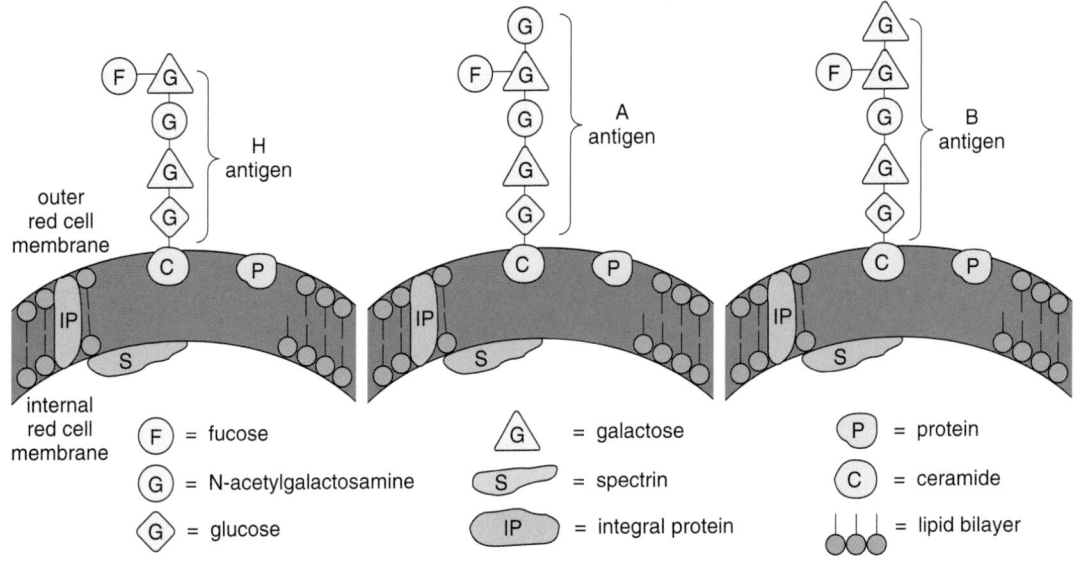

Figure 16–1. Chemical structure of A, B, and H blood groups.

ABO systems have separate gene loci and are independent of one another (Fig 16–1).

The H gene codes for a fucosyl transferase enzyme that adds fucose to precursor chains and completes the stem chain. The H gene is rarely absent; this phenotype (*hh*) is called O_h, or Bombay, type. In the absence of a complete stem chain, additional sugars cannot be added despite the presence of A or B transferase, and high-titer anti-H is produced.

The ABO blood groups are determined by allelic genes A, B, and O (Table 16–1). The A-group transferase conjugates *N*-acetylglucosamine to the completed stem chain. The B-group transferase conjugates a terminal galactose. The *O* gene produces no transferase to modify the blood group substance (see Fig 16–1).

Both groups A and B can be divided into subgroups. Many subgroups of A have been described, but most are rare. The most important are A_1 and A_2. Differences between subtypes of group A appear to be quantitative, that is, in the number of antigenic sites per erythrocyte surface. Of A blood, 78% is A_1 and 22% is A_2. A_1 cells carry about 1 million copies of A antigen on their surface, and A_2 cells carry 250,000 copies. AB blood can also be divided into A_1B and A_2B types. To detect weak variants of A, which may

go undetected in routine testing, blood grouping often includes the use of O serum that contains an anti-A capable of detecting these weaker forms, for example A_x. Although less frequently detected, subgroups of group B can also be distinguished. Subgroups of group B, like those of group A, demonstrate a continuum in the number of antigenic sites per erythrocyte.

The naturally occurring antibodies to groups A and B are thought to be stimulated by very common substances. Intestinal bacteria are known to have substances chemically similar to and therefore antigenically cross-reactive with A and B. Antibodies to A or B antigens (or both) are first detected in children at three to six months of age, peaking at 5–10 years of age and falling with age and in some immunodeficiency states.

Two other systems directly interact with the ABO and H systems: Lewis and secretor. Secretion of ABH substances in body fluids (saliva, sweat, milk, etc) is controlled by the allelic genes *Se* and *se*. These genes are independent of ABO and are inherited in a mendelian dominant manner. Eighty percent of people are *Se;* they secrete Lewis antigens in addition to ABH substances. Typing of body fluids for these antigens has been useful in forensic investigations.

Table 16–1. Routine ABO groupings.

			Frequency (%) in US Population			
Blood Group	Erythrocyte Antigens	Serum Antibody	White	Black	American Indian	Asian
O	H	Anti-A, Anti-B	45	49	79	40
A	A	Anti-B	40	27	16	28
B	B	Anti-A	11	20	4	27
AB	A and B	—	4	4	<1	5

Rh (Rhesus)

The Rhesus blood group system is second in importance only to the ABO system. Anti-Rh antibodies are the leading cause of hemolytic disease of the newborn and may also cause delayed hemolytic transfusion reactions.

Recent investigations have elucidated the genetic basis of the primary Rh antigens: D, C, c, E, e. The Rh locus on chromosome 1 consists of two adjacent structural genes designated *D* and *CcEe*. The *D* gene encodes the D polypeptide present on the erythrocyte in Rh-positive individuals. The *D* gene is completely absent in the genome of Rh-negative individuals, which explains why no D antigen counterpart (d) has ever been found in Rh-negative people. The *CcEe* gene encodes for both C/c and E/e proteins via alternative splicing events.

Previous theories explaining the genetic basis of the Rh system gave rise to different nomenclatures. In the Wiener nomenclature, multiple Rh alleles were designated as either *R* or *r* with one of many superscripts. *R* alleles produced the antigen Rh_o in a particular phenotype in addition to two other antigens; *r* alleles denote the absence of Rh_o in another phenotype. In the Fisher and Race system (Table 16–2), three allelic gene pairs were thought to commonly produce five antigens (the remaining antigens are rare variants). Each antigen (D, C, c, E, and e) has a corresponding designation in the Wiener system (ie, $D = Rh_o$, $C = rh'$, etc). *C* and *c*, as well as *E* and *e*, function as alleles. No d antigen was known so d describes the absence of D. The Rh antigens were believed to be inherited as two sets of three, one from each parent.

Clinically, Rh-positive (Rh+) means the presence of D (Rh_o) and Rh-negative (Rh−) indicates the absence of D (Rh_o). D is the most immunogenic of the Rh antigens. Slightly less than half of Rh+ people are homozygous for D. Because there are no antisera to detect the absence of D, determination of zygosity depends on family studies or gene amplification techniques. Roughly 15% of whites are Rh−. Rh− is less common in other races. Erythrocytes with less than the normal number of D antigen sites are described and designated weak D (previously termed D^u). A weak D can appear as D negative (Rh−) in testing if blood is typed only with routine anti-D antisera but are detected if the indirect antiglobulin test is used. Blood-banking standards require all donor blood to be tested using methods that detect weak D antigen. If weak D is detected, the blood unit is labeled Rh-positive and is transfused only to Rh-positive individuals. Standards do not require blood recipients to be tested for weak D because any patient typing Rh-negative will receive only Rh-negative blood.

Other Erythrocyte Antigens

Many of the remaining 20 blood group systems are rarely implicated in transfusion reactions. Antibodies to the Kidd, Duffy, Kell, and MNS systems, however, are known for their ability to cause hemolysis if antigen-positive blood is transfused into a sensitized recipient. The erythrocyte antigens more commonly involved in transfusion reactions are those that are both immunogenic and prevalent. Low-frequency antigens, even if highly immunogenic, have a low likelihood of being transfused. In general, hemolytic antibodies are IgG and react at 37 °C (body temperature). IgM antibodies rarely cause hemolysis.

Antibodies to Kidd antigens are a frequent cause of delayed hemolytic transfusion reaction and can cause hemolytic disease of the newborn (HDN). These antibodies are often difficult to identify in test systems because of poor reactivity. Four antigenic phenotypes have been described: Jk(a+ b−), Jk(a− b+), Jk(a+ b+), and Jk(a− b−). The Jk(a− b−) phenotype is rare except in some Pacific island populations.

The antigens of the Duffy system (Fy^a and Fy^b) are controlled by codominant alleles. Antibodies to Fy^a are more commonly associated with delayed hemolytic transfusion reactions than are those to Fy^b. Many blacks have a third allele, which produces the Fy(a− b−) phenotype. Duffy antigens on erythrocytes serve as receptors for the entry of *Plasmodium vivax* into the erythrocytes. Fy(a− b−) individuals who lack Duffy antigens are resistant to *P vivax* infection but not to *P falciparum* infection.

The Kell system, as first described, included the allelic pair *K* and *k*, k antigen being the more frequent. The system now includes two additional allelic pairs and several variants. The K antigen is highly immunogenic, with one of 20 individuals transfused with K+ cells developing antibody. Antibodies to Kell antigen cause hemolytic disease of the newborn, hemolytic transfusion reactions, and, occasionally, autoimmune hemolytic anemia. Individuals of the McLeod phenotype lack Kx antigen, which is a precursor in the synthesis of Kell antigens. Absence of Kx results in the depressed expression of k. These individuals have erythrocyte and neuromuscular system abnormalities. The McLeod phenotype is also associated with some cases of chronic granulomatous disease (see Chapter 24).

Table 16–2. Rh blood group terminology.

Fisher-Race	Wiener	Common Genotypes	
Rh-Positive		Caucasian	
DCe	R_1		R_1
DcE	R_2		R_2
Dce	R_0		r
DCE	R_z	Negro	
Rh-Negative			R_0
dce	r		R_1
dCe	r'		r
dcE	r''	Asian	
dCE	r^y		R_1
			R_2

METHODS FOR DETECTION OF ANTIGEN & ANTIBODIES TO ERYTHROCYTES

Antiglobulin Tests

Antibody or complement adsorbed onto erythrocytes is detected by using antibodies to human serum globulins (AHG). AHG reagents are produced either in animals or in tissue culture by using monoclonal antibody techniques (see Chapter 12). These reagents may be polyspecific (a mixture of antibodies to IgG, complement, and heavy and light chains) or monospecific (antibodies to specific immunoglobulin or components of complement). The direct antiglobulin test (DAT) detects antibody or complement coating the surface of erythrocytes, whereas the indirect antiglobulin test (IAT) identifies antibody in serum.

To perform the DAT (Fig 16–2) erythrocytes are washed with saline to remove unbound antibody or complement and then AHG is added. If antibody is present on the erythrocytes, the Fab portion of AHG attaches to the Fc portion of the erythrocyte-bound antibody. Bridging of AHG Fab molecules between erythrocytes results in visually detectable agglutination. A positive test requires a minimum of 200–500 antibodies per erythrocyte surface unless more sensitive methods are used. The DAT is used in the investigation of autoimmune or drug-induced hemolytic anemia, hemolytic disease of the newborn, and suspected hemolytic transfusion reactions.

The IAT detects **serum antibodies,** which can attach in vitro to erythrocytes (see Fig 16–2). This test differs from the DAT in that before an IAT is performed, the serum to be tested is incubated with washed erythrocytes so that serum antibody, if present, binds to erythrocyte antigen. The erythrocytes are then washed to remove any unbound globulin, and AHG is added. If agglutination is observed, serum globulins to

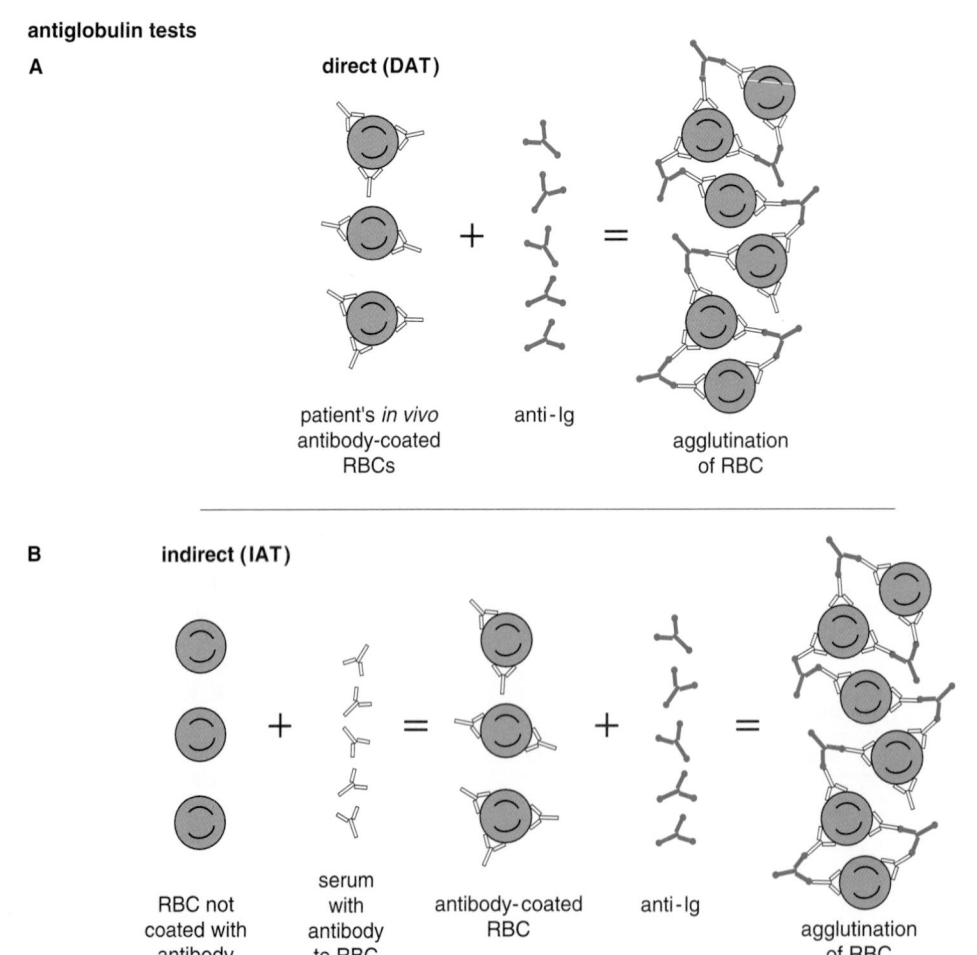

antiglobulin tests

A   **direct (DAT)**

patient's *in vivo* antibody-coated RBCs   anti-Ig   agglutination of RBC

B   **indirect (IAT)**

RBC not coated with antibody   serum with antibody to RBC   antibody-coated RBC   anti-Ig   agglutination of RBC

Figure 16–2. *A:* Schematic illustration of the technique for the direct antiglobulin test (DAT). ***B:*** Schematic illustration of the technique for the direct antiglobulin test (IAT).

erythrocyte antigens are present. The IAT is used by blood banks in three ways. First, to identify the presence and specificity of recipient serum antibody, serum is tested using panels of reagent erythrocytes with known antigens on their surface. Second, to select donor blood that is free of specific erythrocyte antigens, commercial reagents, containing known erythrocyte antibodies, are used to test donor blood for the absence of the antigen. Third, to confirm the absence of an antigen–antibody reaction, recipient serum is tested against donor blood cells (crossmatch).

Pretransfusion Testing

Blood is tested prior to transfusion to prevent clinically significant destruction of the transfused erythrocytes. Clinically significant antibodies are those that are known to have caused unacceptably shortened erythrocyte survival in vivo or frank hemolysis. Generally, they are antibodies that react at 37 °C (body temperature) and in the indirect antiglobulin test. Prior to transfusion, the recipient's erythrocytes and serum are tested for ABO and Rh_0 (D) types and for antibodies to erythrocyte antigens, often called the "type and screen." Additionally, the recipient's serum is tested for compatibility with the erythrocytes from the intended donor (crossmatch).

Type & Screen

ABO and Rh_0 (D) **types** are determined by mixing the recipient's erythrocytes with anti-A, anti-B, and anti-D antisera. The ABO group is then confirmed by testing the recipient's serum against commercial reagent A and B cells to detect isoagglutinins.

The recipient's serum is **screened** for alloantibodies that may not be demonstrated in the crossmatch. In antibody screens, suspensions of reagent O erythrocytes that contain known erythrocyte antigens on their surface are incubated at 37 °C with the recipient's serum. If antigen–antibody complexes are formed, hemolysis or agglutination of erythrocytes is observed. The screen is completed by the IAT and again observed for agglutination.

In the **crossmatch,** compatibility between donor and recipient is determined. Donor cells are combined with recipient serum, incubated, centrifuged, and observed for hemolysis or agglutination (called the "immediate spin" crossmatch). If the recipient either has a history of previous erythrocyte antibody or has had antibody detected during the antibody-screening procedure, the IAT must be performed before a crossmatch may be considered compatible.

These tests that detect antigen–antibody reactions with erythrocytes are performed most simply in saline solution. It is recognized that this causes some loss in test sensitivity for IgG antibodies owing to ionic repulsion forces between erythrocytes generated by clustering of Na^+ and Cl^- ions near erythrocyte surfaces. A variety of methods to increase the sensitivity of the IAT has been developed. These methods add albumin, LISS (low-ionic-strength solution), polybrene, or polyethylene glycol (PEG) to the test system. Reagent erythrocytes can also be treated with proteolytic enzymes to enhance the reactivity of some erythrocyte antigens (Rh and Kidd) and to abolish the reactivity of others (M, N, Fy^a, and Fy^b).

TRANSFUSION REACTIONS

Blood transfusion has become increasingly safe, but a variety of adverse reactions, only some of which are preventable, continues to occur (Table 16–3). Patients who are transfused must be monitored during infusion for immediate reactions and over time to detect delayed reactions.

Table 16–3. Transfusion reactions.

Cause	Incidence	Manifestations	Treatment
Erythrocyte antibodies Hemolytic (acute)	<0.02%	Fever, chills, hypotension. Pain in back or infusion site. Hemoglobin in blood and urine.	Stop transfusion; blood/urine to blood bank. Hydrate. Monitor hematocrit, liver, and renal function.
Hemolytic (delayed)		Lowered hematocrit, increased bilirubin; elevated LDH days to weeks posttransfusion.	Monitor hematocrit, also liver and renal function if severe.
Cytokines, WBC	<2%	Temp raised ≥1 °C, chills.	Stop transfusion: rule out hemolytic reaction blood/urine to blood bank; premedicate with antipyretics; give leukocyte-reduced products if available.
Donor WBC antibodies	<0.2%	Noncardiac pulmonary edema, bronchospasm.	Stop transfusion, treat symptoms.
Plasma proteins	2–3%	Itching, urticaria, rarely asthma, bronchospasm, anaphylaxis.	Stop transfusion; give antihistamines for urticaria; treat symptoms.

Abbreviations: WBC = white blood cells.

Hemolytic Reactions

The transfusion of incompatible blood may cause immediate hemolysis. Immediate hemolytic transfusion reactions, which are fatal in approximately 10–40% of cases, generally occur when ABO-incompatible blood is transfused. The cause is most often managerial or clerical error, such as transfusing patients with units intended for other recipients. Two thirds of these errors occur in areas other than the hospital blood bank. Incompatible transfusions involving other blood groups are usually less severe, but deaths have been reported. The most common presentation of a hemolytic transfusion reaction is fever or fever with chills. Other signs or symptoms are chest pain, hypotension, nausea, flushing, dyspnea, and hemoglobinuria. The hemolytic transfusion reaction may progress to shock, disseminated intravascular coagulation (DIC), and renal failure.

Delayed hemolytic transfusion reactions occur 3–10 days after transfusion and may be clinically undetected. This reaction occurs from an anamnestic immune response to transfused erythrocytes in a previously sensitized person with undetectable antibody in pretransfusion testing. Presenting symptoms are fever, anemia, and jaundice. The patient's transfused erythrocytes are coated with antibody demonstrated by a positive DAT. The antibody specificity is identified by removing it from the surface of the coated transfused erythrocytes by a procedure called elution. The eluted antibody is then tested against a panel of reagent erythrocytes by the IAT. The frequency of delayed hemolytic transfusion reactions is 1 per 4000 units of blood transfused. Mortality from delayed hemolytic transfusion reactions is uncommon.

Febrile Reactions

Until recently febrile nonhemolytic transfusion reactions (FNHTR) were thought to be caused by cytotoxic or agglutinating antibodies in the recipient, directed against donor leukocyte antigens. Leukocyte reduction filters used at the time of red cell or platelet transfusion decreased the amount of leukocytes transfused and should have eradicated FNHTRs. When this anticipated effect was not observed, researchers looked for other etiologies to explain the fever, chills, and rare rigors that describe a FNHTR. It was observed that during storage, cytokines (IL-1β, IL-6, TNFα) are released from leukocytes present in red cell and platelet components. These cytokines are known to have pyrogenic activity and thus may be the cause of this adverse reaction. FNHTR must be distinguished from fever associated with hemolytic transfusion reactions and from the high fever (>40 °C) and rigors associated with bacterial contamination of blood components. Only one in eight patients with a febrile reaction has another reaction on subsequent transfusion. Recurrent febrile reactions are often controlled with antipyretics, leukocyte-reduced components, or recently collected components.

Transfusion-Related Acute Lung Injury

High-titer leukocyte antibodies in either recipient or donor plasma can cause pulmonary edema (see Chapter 42). Donor antibodies bound to recipient granulocytes (or infrequently, recipient antibodies bound to donor granulocytes) activate complement. Complement activation leads to the sequestration of antibody–granulocyte complexes in the lung microvasculature. The presence of activated complement fragments and leukocyte enzymes or free radicals are thought to cause lung injury with resultant pulmonary edema. The sequelae are fever, dyspnea, and marked hypoxemia. The acute respiratory distress occurs within 1–6 hours of a transfusion and often requires aggressive respiratory support. Although some deaths have been reported, most patients with transfusion-related acute lung injury (TRALI) improve within 48–96 hours if promptly treated. The prevalence of TRALI, not widely documented, is approximately 1 per 625 patients transfused.

Allergic Reactions

Allergic reactions to transfusion are characterized by itching, hives, and local erythema. Rarely are they accompanied by cardiopulmonary instability. They are thought to be caused by infused plasma proteins and occur in 1–2% of transfusions. Patients with a history of allergy more frequently have allergic reactions to blood. Mild reactions can be treated with antihistamines, and the transfusion continued. Pretreatment with antihistamines often prevents recurrent allergic reactions. If the allergic reaction is severe, washed erythrocytes may be indicated. Anaphylactic reactions occur in some IgA-deficient recipients (see Chapter 21) after transfusion of as little as 10–15 mL of a blood component. Fortunately, these reactions are rare. The reaction is due to the IgA present in transfused plasma and is prevented by transfusing plasma-free or IgA-deficient components.

Other transfusion reactions include those caused by bacterial contamination of blood components, congestive heart failure due to intravascular volume overload, and artificially produced donor erythrocyte destruction prior to infusion. Erythrocytes may be destroyed by inadvertent overheating, freezing or mixing with nonisotonic solutions.

Transfusion-Transmitted Infection

Transfusion may be complicated by a variety of infectious microorganisms, only some of which can be detected by current donor-screening methods (Table 16–4). The most frequently reported posttransfusion infections in developed countries are hepatitis, cytomegalovirus (CMV), human immunodeficiency virus-1 (HIV-1), and human T-cell lymphotrophic virus I/II (HTLV-I/II). In certain countries, posttransfusion malaria and Chagas' disease are significant problems. Elimination of potentially infected blood

Table 16–4. Transfusion-transmitted infection.

Infection[1]	Risk/Unit Transfused
CMV infection	1:20–1:100
Hepatitis C	1:3300
Hepatitis B	1:200,000
HTLV-I/II	1:70,000
HIV-1 infection	1:650,000

Abbreviations: CMV = cytomegalovirus; HTLV-I/II = human T-cell lymphotrophic virus-I/II; HIV-1 = human immunodeficiency virus-1.
[1] Rare infections include syphilis, malaria, Epstein-Barr virus infection, delta hepatitis, brucellosis, Chagas' disease, babesiosis, and leishmaniasis.

depends on successful donor screening by medical history, aseptic blood collection, and adequate laboratory testing of the donated blood. The presence of hepatitis B surface antigen (HBsAg), antibody to hepatitis B core antigen (anti-HBc), antibody to hepatitis C virus (anti-HCV), anti-HIV 1/2, HIV-1 antigen, anti-HTLV I/II, and syphilis (STS) is currently tested in all US blood donors.

The prevalence of posttransfusion hepatitis (PTH) is estimated to be <1%. PTH is caused by hepatitis B virus in 5% of cases and by hepatitis C virus in 95% of cases. Of transfusion recipients who develop posttransfusion hepatitis, 50% develop chronic hepatitis; 10% of these develop cirrhosis. All blood components can transmit hepatitis, except those that can be pasteurized, such as albumin and other plasma proteins.

CMV is transmitted to CMV-seronegative transfusion recipients by leukocytes contaminating erythrocyte and platelet components. Whether transfusion of CMV-seropositive blood to CMV-seropositive recipients causes superinfection or other complications is unknown. Roughly 50% of blood donors are infected with CMV, which limits availability of CMV-negative blood. CMV disease causes significant morbidity and mortality in severely immunocompromised patients. When possible, CMV-seronegative blood should be given to low-birth-weight infants (<1250 g), CMV-seronegative pregnant women, and CMV-seronegative recipients of CMV-seronegative bone marrow or organ transplants.

HIV-1 infection due to transfusion is rare since implementation of donor HIV-1 antibody testing (March 1985). HIV-1 can be transmitted by erythrocytes, platelets, cryoprecipitate, fresh-frozen plasma, and possibly other blood components. The risk of infection by transfusion is now estimated to be about 1 in 650,000 per unit transfused. The virus can be transmitted by blood collected from donors who have been recently infected but don't yet have detectable levels of HIV antigen or antibodies (called the "window period") and who have not voluntarily excluded themselves from donating blood. Even though HIV-2 infection is rare in the USA, isolated cases are reported in parts of Europe and West Africa. Consequently, all US blood donations are screened for antibodies to both HIV-1 and HIV-2 as well as to HIV p24 antigen. Other retroviruses, HTLV-I and HTLV-II, are transmitted with 30% efficiency in cellular blood products. Prior to the availability of HTLV-I/II testing, one in 3500–5000 transfusion recipients were infected. HTLV-I is a rare cause of post-transfusion spastic paraparesis. It is known to cause a form of T-cell leukemia (see Chapter 46) and tropical spastic paraparesis in endemic populations. HTLV-II infection is not currently associated with a disease.

Other Diseases Transmitted by Transfusion

Epstein-Barr virus (EBV) may be transmitted by transfusion. In most cases it results in asymptomatic seroconversion, but it can cause a mononucleosis syndrome. Transfusion-acquired delta hepatitis requires the presence of both the hepatitis delta virus and hepatitis B virus in the blood donor for transmission to a recipient (see Chapter 49). Because effective donor screening for HBsAg eliminates almost all of these donors, the risk of transmitting this agent is low.

Posttransfusion syphilis is now rare. There is a low prevalence of syphilitic infection in blood donors, and all donors are screened for antibody. Since the organism does not survive cold storage for more than 48–72 hours, it can be transmitted only by fresh blood or platelets.

Malaria remains a disease of major worldwide importance. The parasite is present in erythrocytes of carriers sometimes for years after infection. There are no available laboratory tests that are simple and sensitive enough to screen the blood donor population. Therefore, blood banks in the USA rely on histories taken at the time of donation. Donors who have traveled to areas where malaria is endemic are deferred for 12 months.

Other parasitic diseases reported to be transmitted by blood transfusion include those caused by the microfilariae *Wuchereria bancrofti, Acanthocheilonema persians, Mansonella ozzardi, Loa loa,* and *Brugia malayi.* Chagas' disease can be transmitted by *Trypanosoma cruzi. Toxoplasma gondii* can cause toxoplasmosis in transfusion recipients, and *Babesia microti* can cause babesiosis. Leishmaniasis is also reported as a post-transfusion infection.

Transfusion-transmitted bacterial infections are often the result of inadequate decontamination of skin at the time of blood collection. Asymptomatic bacteremia in the donor or contamination of the blood during storage and handling may also be a cause.

Immunologic Mechanisms of Transfusion Reactions

Hemolytic transfusion reactions are caused by antigen–antibody complexes on the erythrocyte membrane. These complexes activate Hageman factor (factor XIIa) and complement and induce the production of several cytokines. Hageman factor activates the kinin system (see Chapter 11). Bradykinins thus generated increase capillary permeability and dilate arterioles, causing hypotension. Complement is activated and leads to intravascular hemolysis as well as to histamine release from mast cells. Hageman factor and free incompatible erythrocyte stroma activate the intrinsic clotting cascade, with consequent disseminated intravascular coagulation (DIC). Systemic hypotension with renal vasoconstriction and the formation of intravascular thrombi lead to renal failure. When complement activation is not complete, the reaction is less severe. Erythrocytes coated with C3b are cleared from the circulation by phagocytes, resulting in extravascular hemolysis, which takes place primarily in the liver.

Antileukocyte antibodies are either cytotoxic or agglutinating. These antibodies form complexes with antigens on leukocytes, activating complement. Activated complement generates vasoactive substances in the circulation. Endogenous pyrogens from destroyed granulocytes are also released into the circulation following cell lysis.

The mechanism of graft-versus-host disease depends on the engraftment of donor lymphocytes in the recipient. Donor lymphocytes recognize recipient tissue antigens as "foreign" and cause a clinical syndrome characterized by fever, skin rash, hepatitis, and diarrhea. Death may result. Engraftment can be prevented by irradiating lymphocyte-carrying blood components to preclude lymphocyte activation. Graft-versus-host disease occurs rarely in newborns undergoing exchange transfusion, patients with T-cell immunodeficiencies, and patients severely immunosuppressed by intensive chemo and irradiation therapy (see Chapter 58). There are rare reports of graft-versus-host disease following transfusion of blood from a haploidentical donor into an immunocompetent recipient. Consequently, designated blood donations collected from blood relatives are now irradiated before transfusion.

RH ISOIMMUNIZATION

The D antigen is a common, strongly immunogenic antigen, 50 times more immunogenic than the other Rh antigens. The prevalence of antibody formation to Rh$^+$ blood depends on the dose of Rh$^+$ cells: 1 mL of cells sensitizes 15% of individuals exposed; 250 mL sensitizes 60–70%. After the initial exposure to Rh$^+$ cells, weak IgM antibody can be detected as early as four weeks. This is followed by a rapid conversion to IgG antibody. A second exposure to as little as 0.03 mL of Rh$^+$ erythrocytes may result in the rapid formation of IgG antibodies.

The majority of potential transfusion reactions to Rh can be prevented by transfusing Rh$^-$ individuals with Rh$^-$ blood. Immunization and antibody formation to D antigen still occur owing to occasional Rh sensitization during pregnancy or to transfusion errors, particularly during emergencies. Immunization to other Rh antigens may occur because donor blood

is typed routinely for D but not for other Rh antigens.

Hemolytic disease of the newborn occurs with the passage of Rh$^+$ cells from the fetus to the circulation of the Rh$^-$ mother. Once anti-D antibody is formed in the mother, IgG but not IgM anti-D antibodies cross the placenta, causing hemolysis of fetal erythrocytes. Rh$^-$ mothers become sensitized during pregnancy or at the time of delivery as a result of transplacental fetal hemorrhage. Following delivery, 75% of women will have had transplacental fetal hemorrhage. Some obstetric complications increase the risk of transplacental fetal hemorrhage: antepartum hemorrhage, toxemia of pregnancy, cesarean section, external version, and manual removal of the placenta. Transplacental fetal hemorrhage can also occur following spontaneous or therapeutic abortion, amniocentesis, chorionic villus sampling (CVS), or percutaneous umbilical cord sampling (PUBS). Overall Rh immunization occurs in 8–9% of Rh$^-$ women following the delivery of the first Rh$^+$ ABO-compatible baby and in 1.5–2.0% of Rh$^-$ women who deliver Rh$^+$ ABO-incompatible babies.

Rh Prophylaxis

Rh immunization can now be suppressed almost entirely in antepartum or postpartum Rh$^-$ women if high-titer anti-Rh immunoglobulin (RhIg) is administered within 72 hours after the potentially sensitizing dose of Rh$^+$ cells.

The protective mechanism of RhIG administration is not clear. RhIG does not effectively block Rh antigen from immunosuppressive cells by competitive inhibition, since effective doses of RhIG do not cover all O antigen sites. Intravascular hemolysis and rapid clearance of erythrocyte debris by the poorly immunoresponsive liver is also unlikely. Although this mechanism appears to explain the 90% protective effect of ABO incompatibility between mother and fetus, RhIG-induced erythrocyte hemolysis is extravascular. Rh$^+$ fetal cells are removed primarily by highly phagocytic cells in the spleen and liver. The most likely mechanism is a negative modulation of the primary immune response thereby depressing antibody formation. Antigen–antibody complexes are bound to cells bearing Fc receptors in the lymph nodes and spleen. These cells presumably stimulate suppressor T-cell responses, which prevent antigen-induced B cell proliferation and antibody formation.

A prophylactic dose of 300 μg of RhIG intramuscularly prevents Rh immunization following exposure to up to 15 mL of Rh$^+$ erythrocytes, which corresponds to 30 mL of fetal whole blood. Initial recommendations were that 300 μg of RhIG be given to nonimmunized Rh$^-$ mothers within 72 hours after delivery of an Rh$^+$ infant. The postpartum dose of RhIG decreased the incidence of anti-D development to 1% in Rh$^-$ women giving birth to Rh$^+$ infants. To further decrease the chances of developing anti-D in this population of women, antepartum RhIG is also now administered at 28 weeks' gestation. A dose of RhIG is also indicated for an RRh⁻ woman after any terminated pregnancy, amniocentesis, CVS, PUBS, and fetal surgery or manipulation. Additional doses may have to be given in cases of massive transplacental fetal hemorrhage. The administration of RhIG to pregnant women has not been shown to have a detrimental effect on the fetus.

Large doses of RhIG can effectively suppress immunization following inadvertent transfusion of Rh⁺ blood into Rh⁻ patients if given within 72 hours of transfusion. Once Rh immunization is demonstrated by the IAT, administration of RhIG is ineffective.

BLOOD COMPONENT THERAPY

Improvements in the medical care of previously fatal illnesses has placed increasing demands on the blood supply. As the need for blood products has expanded, the pool of eligible blood donors has decreased due to more intensive screening and testing. The separation of a whole blood donation into its component parts (fresh-frozen plasma, platelets, and erythrocytes) has helped stretch a limited blood supply. The medical indication for the need to transfuse a patient with whole blood or one of its components is now more critically assessed. Members of the health care team recognize that although stringent screening and testing of blood donors occurs, blood transfusion is still not entirely safe and should be given judiciously (Table 16–5).

Erythrocytes

The indications for erythrocyte transfusion depend on the clinical state of the intended recipient. One unit of erythrocytes is expected to increase the nonbleeding adult's hemoglobin by 1 g/dL and to increase the hematocrit by 3%. After senescent and damaged erythrocytes are cleared, 70–80% of transfused erythrocytes survive normally.

During acute blood loss, 1 hour or more is required for equilibration of intravascular and extravascular fluids and an accurate assessment of the fall in the hemoglobin level. Generally, a loss of 20% of blood volume can be corrected with crystalloid (electrolyte) solution alone, which can then be supplemented with colloid (protein) solution. Whole blood is indicated if blood loss exceeds one third of blood volume. Operative blood loss of 1000–1200 mL rarely requires transfusion in an otherwise healthy adult. If increased oxygen-carrying capacity is required, erythrocyte transfusion is indicated.

A decreased hemoglobin level is tolerated better in a patient with chronic anemia than in a patient with acute blood loss. Patients with a slow decline in their hemoglobin level compensate for the decreased oxygen-carrying capacity by increasing their cardiac output. 2,3,-Diphosphoglycerate is also increased in patients with chronic anemia, shifting the oxyhemoglobin dissociation curve to the right. This rightward shift enhances oxygen release to the tissues.

Exchange transfusion of neonates is a special circumstance in which blood less than seven days old is required to ensure tolerable levels of plasma electrolytes and adequate levels of 2,3-diphosphoglycerate. Preferably, the blood should be irradiated to prevent

Table 16–5. Guidelines for component therapy.[1]

Component	Indications for Use
Red blood cells	Use to increase O_2-carrying capacity; 1 unit increases hemoglobin 1 g/dL in a 70-kg patient. Consider the degree of anemia, intravascular volume, and presence of coexisting cardiac, pulmonary, or vascular conditions. 1. If hemoglobin >10 g/dL, transfusion is rarely indicated. 2. If hemoglobin <7 g/dL, transfusion is usually indicated. 3. If hemoglobin is 7–10 g/dL, assess clinical status, mixed venous pO_2, and O_2 extraction ratio.
Platelets	Use to control or prevent bleeding due to low platelet count or abnormal platelet function; one concentrate increases platelet count by approximately 5000 platelets/μL. 1. Generally, patients with platelet counts <10,000–20,000 should receive platelets to prevent bleeding. 2. Actively bleeding patients with platelet counts <50,000 may benefit from platelets.
FFP	Used to increase clotting factors in patients with documented deficiencies (PT/PTT >1.5 × normal, 1 unit increases the level of any factor 2–3%. 1. FFP should not be used as a volume expander or nutritional source. 2. FFP is useful for treatment of factor II, V, VII, X, XI, or XIII deficiencies when specific concentrates are not available. 3. FFP is useful for patients with warfarin overdose who have life-threatening bleeding or who require emergency surgery. 4. FFP may be useful in massive blood transfusion (>1 blood volume within a few hours). 5. FFP is useful as a source of C1-esterase inhibitor in deficient patients with life-threatening angioedema and in patients with thrombotic thrombocytopenic purpura.

[1] Data from the following sources: Fresh frozen plasma—indication and risks, *JAMA* 1985;**253**:551; Platelet transfusion therapy, *JAMA* 1987;**257**:1777; and Perioperative red blood cell transfusion, *JAMA* 1988;**260**:2700.
Abbreviations: PT = prothrombin time; PTT = partial thromboplastin time; FFP = fresh-frozen plasma.

the rare occurrence of graft-versus-host disease.

All erythrocyte components should be administered through blood filters. Medications, especially solutions containing calcium or glucose, should not be infused with blood components.

Platelets

Platelets function to control bleeding by acting as hemostatic plugs on vascular endothelium. Platelet abnormalities that require platelet transfusion may be either quantitative or qualitative. The vast majority of platelet transfusions are given to supplement decreased numbers of circulating platelets due to suppressed production, pooling, or dilution.

Platelets are available as either platelet concentrates (recovered from a whole-blood donation) or as plateletpheresis (collected by using a cytopheresis instrument). The transfusion of one platelet concentrate is expected to increase the platelet count of a 70-kg adult by 5000–10,000/μL. A plateletpheresis is equivalent to six platelet concentrates because both have the same number of platelets. The survival of transfused platelets is decreased in patients who are actively bleeding; who have splenomegaly, fever, infection, or DIC; or who are sensitized to platelet antigens. The transfusion of ABO-incompatible platelets may be associated with slightly decreased platelet survival.

Transient thrombocytopenias, which are the result of treatment regimens for malignancy, are responsible for most platelet transfusions. Platelets are often transfused prophylactically to stable nonbleeding patients when their platelet counts fall below 20,000/μL. Platelets are frequently transfused therapeutically during bleeding episodes.

Platelets have a limited role in preventing bleeding in surgical patients. Platelet counts between 50,000 and 60,000/μL result in adequate hemostasis. In the event of massive transfusion (15–20 units of blood), the dilutional effect on the platelet count by transfused blood must be considered and corrected if necessary. Whole blood stored for more than 24 hours at 4 °C does not contain viable platelets. A functional platelet abnormality develops in proportion to the length of cardiopulmonary bypass during cardiac surgery. Intraoperative platelet counts of 100,000/μL are often adequate for hemostasis if cardiopulmonary perfusion is less than 2 hours.

Plasma Products

Fresh-frozen plasma (FFP), stored plasma, and cryoprecipitate are valuable sources of coagulation factors. Stored plasma and FFP may often be used interchangeably. Levels of factors V and VIII in stored plasma are half those in FFP, but levels of other factors are equivalent. Cryoprecipitate was initially produced to provide therapeutic doses of factor VIII and von Willebrand's factor. This use has been greatly supplanted by the development of recombinant or treated factor VIII, which have lower infectious risks to recipients. Cryoprecipitate is now most often used to treat bleeding in patients with fibrinogen less than 100 mg/dL.

FFP is used for treating isolated congenital factor deficiencies, with the exception of factor IX (for which it is relatively ineffective). It is also used to correct warfarin overdoses in patients with significant bleeding. Additional FFP uses are treatment of thrombotic thrombocytopenic purpura and C1 esterase inhibitor deficiency. Massively transfused patients with a prothrombin time or partial thromboplastin time greater than 1.5 times normal and platelet counts above 50,000/μL may benefit from FFP treatment. FFP or plasma should never be used for volume expansion, as colloid solutions without infectious risk are available (ie, albumin).

REFERENCES

American College of Physicians Clinical Guideline: Practice strategies for elective red blood cell transfusion. *Ann Intern Med* 1992;**116**:403.

Anderson KC, Weinstein HJ: Transfusion-associated graft-versus-host disease. *N Engl J Med* 1990;**323**:315.

Bowman JM: The prevention of Rh immunization. *Transfusion Med Rev* 1988;**2**:129.

Capon SM, Goldfinger D. Acute hemolytic transfusion reaction, a paradigm of the systemic inflammatory response: New insights into pathophysiology and treatment. *Transfusion* 1995;**35**:513.

Colin Y et al: Genetic basis of the RhD-positive and RhD-negative blood group polymorphism as determined by Southern analysis. *Blood* 1991;**78**:2747.

Heddle NM et al: The role of the plasma from platelet concentrates in transfusion reactions. *N Engl J Med* 1994;**331**:625.

Huestis DW et al: *Practical Blood Transfusion.* Little, Brown, 1988.

Issitt PD: *Applied Blood Group Serology,* 3rd ed. Montgomery Scientific, 1985.

Mollison PL: *Blood Transfusion in Clinical Medicine,* 9th ed. Blackwell, 1993.

Mourant AE et al: *The Distribution of Human Blood Groups and Other Polymorphisms,* 2nd ed. Oxford University Press, 1976.

Nance ST (editor): *Blood Safety: Current Challenges.* American Association of Blood Banks, 1992.

NIH Consensus Conference: Platelet transfusion therapy. *JAMA* 1987;**257**:1777.

NIH Consensus Conference: Perioperative red blood cell transfusion. *JAMA* 1988;**260**:2700.

NIH Consensus Conference: Fresh-frozen plasma. *JAMA* 1985;**253**:551.

Petz LD et al (editors): *Clinical Practice of Transfusion Medicine,* 3rd ed. Churchill Livingstone, 1995.

Pineda AA et al: Hemolytic transfusion reaction: Recent experience in a large blood bank. *Mayo Clin Proc* 1978;**53**:378.

Popovsky MA et al: Transfusion-related acute lung injury: A neglected, serious complication of hemotherapy. *Transfusion* 1992;**32**:589.

Sazama K: Reports of 355 transfusion-associated deaths: 1976 through 1985. *Transfusion* 1990;**30**:583.

Soland EM et al: Safety of the blood supply. *JAMA* 1995;**274**:1368.

Snyder EL (editor): *Transfusion Medicine Topic Update. Platelet Transfusion: A Consensus Development Conference.* Yale University, 1994.

Walker RH (editor): *Technical Manual for the American Association of Blood Banks,* 11th ed. American Association of Blood Banks, 1993.

Wallace EL et al: Collection and transfusion of blood and blood components in the United States, 1992. *Transfusion* 1995;**35**:802.

Welch HG et al: Prudent strategies for elective red blood cell transfusion. *Ann Intern Med* 1992;**116**:393.

17 Histocompatibility Testing

Beth W. Colombe, PhD

The human leukocyte antigen (HLA) system as we know it today has been defined largely by a single method, the complement-dependent lymphocytotoxicity test—a serologic assay. HLA antigens, encoded by the alleles of this genetic system, have been characterized through the reaction patterns of naturally occurring alloantibodies that bind to specific HLA antigens on target cells, fix complement, and then kill the cells. Through the discovery and testing of numerous alloantisera with lymphocytotoxic activity, the extensive polymorphism of the HLA system has been revealed. Table 17–1 lists the HLA antigens currently recognized by the World Health Organization.

The remarkable extent of HLA polymorphism has been revealed through the application of the new techniques of molecular biology. New alleles are being cataloged by the World Health Organization monthly. Now the serologically defined polymorphisms of the HLA system have a molecular basis in the variations that exist in the exact sequences of nucleotides of genomic DNA and the amino acid sequences of the HLA antigens themselves. As more alleles are being sequenced, a new image of increasing complexity and allelic variation is emerging. For example, there are now 9 variants of HLA B27, 17 of A2, 13 of B35, 22 of DR4, and so on. Whether such sequence differences have clinical significance remains to be determined. Despite these new advances, the majority of histocompatibility testing is still focused on the "classic" HLA specificities as defined serologically.

During the past 25 years, genetic and clinical studies have shown that HLA antigens are the major "transplantation antigens" that determine the compatibility of transplanted tissues and organs (Fig 17–1). Histocompatibility between individuals is based on the extent of matching of inherited HLA antigens and the degree of immunologic reactivity to these antigens in cellular and serologic cross-match testing. HLA matching and histocompatibility testing have an enormous practical influence on contemporary organ transplantation practices in clinical medicine.

HISTOCOMPATIBILITY TESTING & TRANSPLANTATION

The practice of testing for histocompatibility between an organ donor and the selected recipient is based on the presumption that tissue compatibility promotes graft acceptance and avoids immune rejection. The foundation for this assumption is the evidence that identical twins can accept and retain grafts from each other indefinitely, whereas grafts from all others are ultimately rejected in the absence of immunosuppressive therapy. Efforts to define the inherited basis for tissue compatibility have focused mainly on the HLA antigen system. It follows that the more comprehensive the identity of HLA antigens, the greater the histocompatibility of the graft with the recipient. Identification of HLA antigens is known as **tissue typing.** Serologic methods for tissue typing use antisera with reactivity directed toward specific HLA antigens. Cellular methods for tissue typing include the use of homozygous typing cells (HTC testing) and the mixed-lymphocyte culture (MLC) test. A state of histocompatibility between donor and recipient may also be inferred from absence of preformed antibodies and cytotoxic lymphocytes directed against the donor HLA antigens. Serologic testing for antidonor antibodies is called cross-matching; cellular testing is done by the direct cell-mediated lympholysis (CML) assay.

Table 17–2 is a flowchart that outlines a typical course of histocompatibility testing for a prospective kidney graft recipient. In the following sections, these various tests are described, including the interpretation of results and rationale for use.

RATIONALE FOR TISSUE TYPING FOR TRANSPLANTATION

Comparison of the tissue types of a donor and the potential (unrelated) recipient usually reveals some degree of antigen mismatching because of the exten-

Table 17–1. HLA antigen specificities.[1]

A	B	C	DR	DQ	DP
A1	B5	Cw1	DR1	Dq1	DPw1
A2	B7	Cw2	DR103	DQ2	DPw2
A203	B703	Cw3	DR2	DQ3	DPw3
A210	B8	Cw4	DR3	DQ4	DPw4
A3	B12	Cw5	DR4	DQ5(1)	DPw5
A9	B13	Cw6	DR5	DQ6(1)	DPw6
A10	B14	Cw7	DR6	DQ7(3)	
A11	B15	Cw8	DR7	DQ8(3)	
A19	B16	Cw9(w3)	DR8	DQ9(3)	
A23(9)	B17	Cw10(w3)	DR9		
A24(9)	B18		DR10		
A2403	B21		DR11(5)		
A25(10)	B22		DR12(5)		
A26(10)	B27		DR13(6)		
A28	B35		DR14(6)		
A29(19)	B37		DR1403		
A30(19)	B38(16)		DR1404		
A31(19)	B39(16)		DR15(2)		
A32(19)	B3901		DR16(2)		
A33(19)	B3902		DR17(3)		
A34(10)	B40		DR18(3)		
A36	B4005				
A43	B41		DR51		
A66(10)	B42				
A68(28)	B44(12)		DR52		
A69(28)	B45(12)				
A74(19)	B46		DR53		
A80	B47				
	B48				
	B49(21)				
	B50(21)				
	B51(5)				
	B5102				
	B5103				
	B52(5)				
	B53				
	B54(22)				
	B55(22)				
	B56(22)				
	B57(17)				
	B58(17)				
	B59				
	B60(40)				
	B61(40)				
	B62(15)				
	B63(15)				
	B64(14)				
	B65(14)				
	B67				
	B70				
	B71(70)				
	B72(70)				
	B73				
	B75(15)				
	B76(15)				
	B77(15)				
	B7801				
	B8101				
	Bw4				
	Bw6				

[1] Antigens as recognized by the World Health Organization. Antigens listed in parentheses are the broad antigens; antigens followed by broad antigens in parentheses are the antigen splits. Antigens of the Dw series are omitted.

sive polymorphism of the HLA antigen system. When nuclear family members are tissue typed for a living-related transplant, only 25% of full siblings are HLA identical to the transplant recipient, and parents and 50% of siblings are matched at one haplotype.

Cadaver donors are genotypically complete mismatches to the random recipient, although there is a finite probability of complete or partial phenotypic identity. If the phenotypes of the patient and the cadaver are composed of the more common antigens, such as HLA-A1, -A2, and -B8, and so on, the likelihood of HLA antigen matching increases.

A positive effect of HLA matching on kidney graft outcome has been clearly documented in reports from the two largest studies of renal transplant data: the UCLA Transplant Registry, Los Angeles, Calif, which has collected data on 106,000 transplants, and the Collaborative Transplant Study (CTS), Heidelberg, Germany, with data on 107,500 renal transplants. Both of these studies agree that the main factor that improves long-term (up to 10-year) renal allograft survival is donor–recipient matching for HLA antigens (Table 17–3). Table 17–3 indicates the decreasing graft survival obtained in primary renal transplants when the donor is HLA identical (sibling), one-half identical (parent), and completely mismatched and unrelated (cadaver).

Beneficial effects of HLA matching on short-term graft survival (1 year) are no longer apparent in the results from many individual transplant centers. Immunosuppression with cyclosporine has improved first-transplant graft survival of cadaver and living-related transplants to near that of HLA-identical transplants: approximately 80–85% after 1 year.

Matching for the splits (subtypes) of HLA antigens may be even more significant for graft outcome than simple matching of the "generic" HLA antigens (for example, matching for B51 or B52 rather than for the broad B5 antigen). As shown in Table 17–4, from a CTS review of 33,000 transplants, matching for A and B locus antigen splits in conjunction with HLA-DR shows a striking correlation with graft survival. Table 17–4 shows percent graft survival for patients with 0, 3, and 6 mismatches for HLA-A, -B, and -DR antigens and the estimated half-life survival time for those grafts. Well-matched grafts (0 mismatches) survive approximately 60% longer than do completely mismatched (6 mismatches) grafts (half-life of 12.3 and 7.5 years, respectively). Corroborative data is provided by the UCLA Transplant Registry showing graft half-lives of 20.3, 8.4, and 7.7 years for 0, 3–4, and 5–6 antigen mismatches, respectively.

Despite the dramatic improvement in 1-year survival, however, the ensuing rate of graft loss due to chronic rejection remains essentially unchanged; that is, half of cadaver grafts are still lost by 9 years, compared with 7.3 years in 1978. Thus, the use of cyclosporine has not established an operational state of long-term organ tolerance. It is estimated that if all kidneys were shared nationally, 25% of all waiting patients could be transplanted with kidneys with no HLA-A, -B, or -DR mismatches. These statistics argue in favor of sharing organs on a regional and national scale to promote the most beneficial usage of

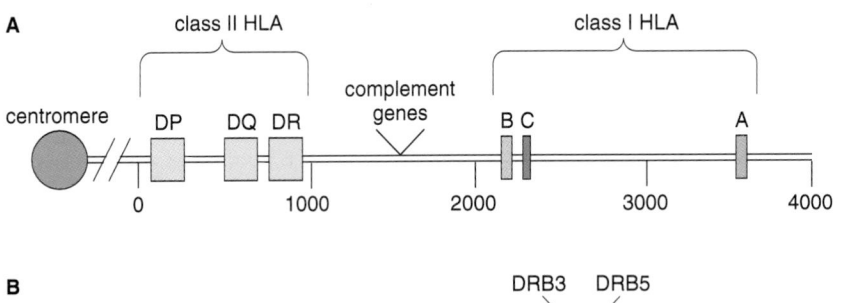

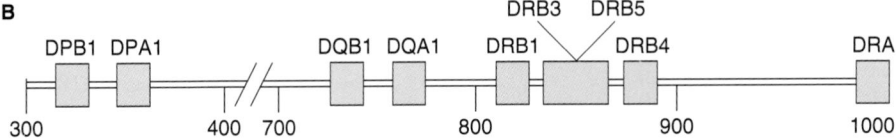

Figure 17–1. MHC genes on chromosome 6. **A:** Schematic representation of genes of the class I and II HLA regions. The region containing complement genes and genes for other factors, such as tumor necrosis factor (TNF), is indicated. **B:** Expanded view of class II HLA region showing genes for α and β chains of class II molecules. Pseudogenes have been omitted. The presence of genes for DRB3, DRB4, and DRB5 is dependent on the haplotype.

scarce organ resources. To achieve this end, the National Organ Transplant Act of 1987 established the United Network for Organ Sharing (UNOS). UNOS links local and regional transplant procurement centers with a national registry of waiting recipients and establishes mandatory criteria for selection of recipients based on a point system for the following attributes: quality of HLA matching, degree of sensitization (panel-reactive antibody [PRA]), time

Table 17–2. Flowchart of histocompatibility testing for the renal transplant patient.

A. Perform preliminary immunologic evaluation
  1. Patient
    HLA typing
    ABO/Rh typing
    Screening of serum for antibodies reactive with HLA
      antigens
    Testing of serum for autoantibodies
  2. Living related donors
    HLA typing
    ABO/Rh typing
    Crossmatch with serum of patient to detect antidonor
      antibodies
B. Select living related donor
  This is based on:
    ABO compatibility
    Best match for HLA antigens
    Negative preliminary crossmatch
  If there is no appropriate living related donor, then
C. Place patient on waiting list for cadaveric kidney
  Register patient with UNOS
  Screen serum samples for antibodies reactive to HLA
    antigens
D. Select appropriate recipient for cadaveric kidney
  HLA and ABO type cadaver donor
  Crossmatch cadaver with ABO-compatible recipients
  Select candidates having no antibodies to donor's HLA
    antigens and negative crossmatch
E. Transplant: living related and cadaveric donors
  Crossmatch with most recent patient sample preferably
    drawn immediately pretransplant

on the waiting list, medical emergency status, and geographic factors.

In heart transplantation, distribution of hearts based on HLA matching is impractical because of the lack of availability of the organ. Retrospective analysis indicates that HLA matching offers a benefit to graft survival, although there are few well-matched grafts to evaluate. For those prospective heart recipients who are sensitized to HLA antigens, a pretransplant crossmatch is routinely performed using preorgan-harvest donor blood where possible to minimize ischemia time of the heart. For liver transplantation, better HLA-matched livers are associated with fewer rejection episodes, but, paradoxically, liver graft survival results show no advantage from HLA matching and, possibly, a detrimental effect. Those patients who suffer recurrence of an autoimmune-type disease in the new, well-matched liver grafts presumably express the autoantigen better with shared rather than with disparate HLA antigens, thereby encouraging renewed disease. Some liver patients are transplanted despite positive crossmatches, whereas others receive no pretransplant testing. No consensus has been reached regarding the utility of crossmatching liver patients prior to transplant. Data on over 2100 pancreas plus kidney transplants from the UNOS transplant registry indi-

Table 17–3. Effect of HLA matching on long-term renal allograft survival.

Organ Donor	Number of Haplotypes Matched[2]	% Graft Survival (10 year)	Transplant Half-Life (years)
HLA-identical sibling	2	74	24
Parent	1	54	12
Cadaver[1]	0	40	9

Source: Data from Terasaki PI (editor): *Clinical Transplants 1992.* UCLA Tissue Typing Laboratory, 1993, p. 501.
[1] Recipient treated with cyclosporine.
[2] N = 40,765 transplants.

Table 17–4. Effect of HLA-A, -B, and -DR mismatches on primary renal graft survival.[1]

Number of Mismatches	Estimated 10-year Graft Survival(%)		Half-Life of Graft (years)	
	Study 1	Study 2	Study 1	Study 2
0	53	65	12.3	20.3
1–2	—	47	—	10.4
3–4	42	38	9.4	8.4
5–6	32	32	7.5	7.7

Sources: Study 1 data from G. Opelz: *Collaborative Transplant Study,* Newletter personal communication, May 1992; Study 2 data from Zhou & Cecka: in *Clinical Transplants,* 1993 (see References).
[1] Matching was done for split HLA-A and -B locus antigens.

cates the beneficial effect of matching for HLA antigens. Patients with technically successful transplants who were mismatched for 0 or 1 HLA antigens had significantly better ($p < .05$) 5-year graft survival than did those mismatched for from two to six HLA antigens. Preliminary data for cornea transplantation do show that patients with previously rejected transplants benefit from a well-matched transplant.

DETECTION OF SENSITIZATION TO HLA ANTIGENS

Exposure to HLA antigens can occur as a consequence of blood transfusions, prior organ grafts, or pregnancy. The resultant formation of specific antibodies to those antigens is termed "sensitization." Reexposure to the previously immunizing antigens on a new allograft can produce rapid humoral and cellular immune responses, leading to hyperacute or accelerated rejection. Detection of such preformed specific antibodies is of paramount importance in evaluating the state of initial histocompatibility between recipient and donor, especially in the face of known HLA antigen mismatches. Two standard procedures have been developed, both of which involve the exposure of lymphocytes to the patient's serum. Antibody screening tests a serum sample against a panel of HLA-typed lymphocytes for antilymphocyte reactivity; crossmatching tests the patient's serum against the lymphocytes of a selected prospective organ donor to detect donor-specific antibodies.

SEROLOGIC METHODS IN HISTOCOMPATIBILITY TESTING

The simplest and fastest methods for histocompatibility testing are serologic; that is, they used blood serum that contains antibodies to HLA antigens. Anti-HLA antibodies are highly specific for the individual structural determinants that characterize the different antigens of the HLA system. Thus, when sera containing HLA antibodies are mixed with lymphocytes, the antibodies bind only to their specific target antigens.

When the antigen–antibody complex is formed on the cell surface in the presence of complement, complement activation leads to cell lysis. Thus, cell death is an indicator of the shared specificity of antigen and antibody and is a "positive" test result. Detection of this identity between antibody and antigen provides the answer to most basic questions in histocompatibility testing: (1) What are the HLA antigens of a particular cell? When the antibody specificity is known, as for the HLA typing reagents, and the cell is of unknown phenotype, the positive test results with specific antisera identify the antigens of the cell. (2) Are there anti-HLA antibodies in a particular serum? When the serum is being tested for the presence of HLA antibodies, a positive test indicates antilymphocyte activity in the serum. From the pattern of reactions with a panel of HLA-typed cells, the specificity of the antibodies may be inferred. If the patient's serum reacts with the donor cell, the two individuals are incompatible.

Thus, through an iterative process of testing serum and typing cells, HLA antigens are defined, panels of typed lymphocytes are generated, and collections of HLA typing sera of known specificity are created.

TISSUE TYPING BY THE LYMPHOCYTOTOXICITY TEST

Tissue typing is accomplished by exposing the unknown cell to a battery of antisera of known HLA specificity. The typing sera are selected to give unequivocally strong positive scores to ensure reproducibility. When the cells are killed by the antiserum and complement, the cell is presumed to have the same HLA antigen as the specificity of the antibody.

Cell Isolation

Lymphocytes are the preferred cell type for HLA typing, antibody screening, and crossmatching. They are normally isolated from whole peripheral blood by buoyant density gradient separation (see Chapter 13), from buffy coat, or, in cadaveric testing, from lymph nodes and spleen. Care must be taken to prepare a cell suspension of excellent viability as well as one that is free of erythrocyte and platelet contamination. Although other cell types that bear HLA antigens, such as platelets, amniocytes, and fibroblasts, can be used for HLA typing in special circumstances, lymphocytes are the most responsive and reproducible target for the standard cytotoxicity assay.

Isolation of T and B lymphocytes by magnetic beads is now a useful method for basic tissue typing and crossmatching. The antibody-coated beads offer versatility, speed of cell recovery, and relative purity of the final cell preparation. Beads with anti-CD2 or anti-CD8 are used to isolate T cells and anti-CD19 for

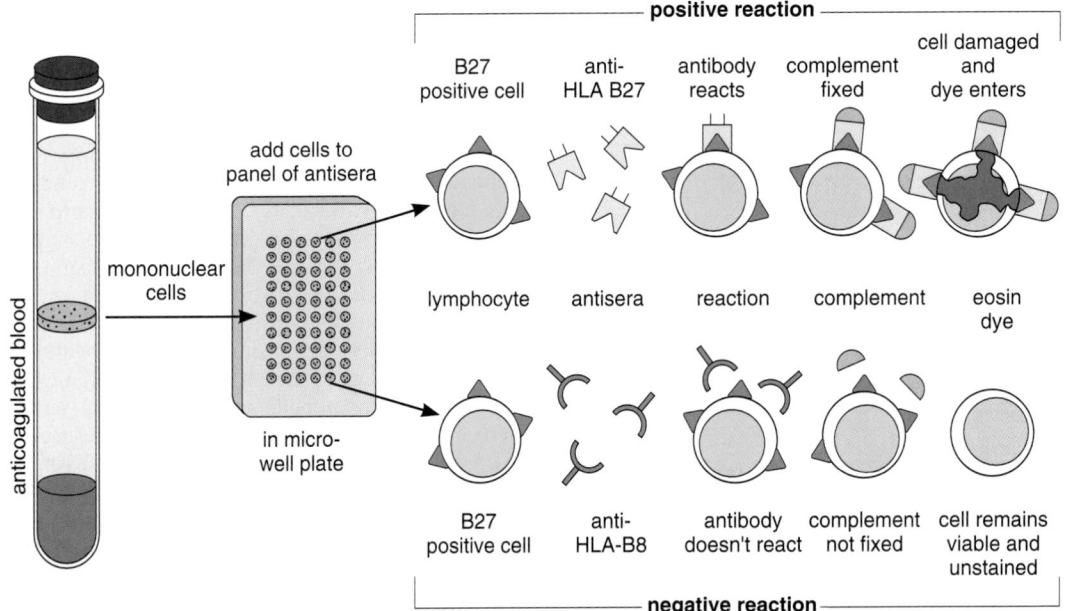

Figure 17–2. Microcytotoxicity testing for HLA antigens. PBL are isolated by Ficoll-Hypaque centrifugation and adjusted to 2×10^6 cells/mL. Then 1 µL of cells is added to each well of a tissue-typing plate that has been predispensed with a panel of HLA typing sera, each containing alloantibodies to specific HLA antigens. Illustrated are the reactions of HLA B27 cells with antisera specific for B27 **(upper)** and B8 **(lower)**. B27 antibodies bind to B27 antigens on the cell surface, the antigen–antibody complex activates and fixes serum complement, the cell membrane is damaged, and the cell dies. Eosin dye penetrates the dead cells, staining them dark red under phase-contrast microscopy, giving a positive test result. In contrast, the anti-B8 antibodies do not complex with the B27 antigen, the complement components are not activated, the cells remain undamaged, and eosin dye is excluded, resulting in a negative test. The cell is thus typed as B27-positive and B8-negative. Each test well is scored as percent dead cells (see Table 17–5) and the overall reaction pattern of the typing sera is interpreted to give the HLA antigen phenotype of the individual (see Table 17–6).

B cells. The beads can be used to obtain adequate numbers of cells from whole blood, buffy coats, or peripheral blood lymphocyte (PBL) preparations. Cells with bound beads also become more sensitive as targets, possibly due to disturbance of their cell membranes, and thus tests require less incubation time than the standard cytotoxicity assays.

The Complement-Dependent Lymphocytotoxicity Test: NIH Standard Method

Individual HLA antisera are predispensed in 1-µL quantities into the microtest wells of specifically designed plastic trays composed of 60 or 72 wells of 15-µL capacity. An array of anti-HLA sera is chosen with specificities covering the full range of known HLA antigens. Usually each antigen is represented by at least two antisera. Replicates of the test tray are stored frozen for later use. Into a thawed test tray, 2000 isolated lymphocytes are dispensed per well, and the tray is incubated for 30 minutes at room temperature to allow anti-HLA antibodies to bind to their specific target HLA antigens. Complement (5 µL) is added, usually as rabbit serum, and the tray is incubated for another 60 minutes. To visualize the dead and live cells

under phase-contrast microscopy, a vital dye, eosin Y, is added, followed by formalin to fix the reaction. Live cells exclude the dye and appear bright and refractile, but dead cells take up the dye and are swollen and dark (Fig 17–2). In an alternative method known as fluorochromasia, the cells are prelabeled with a fluorochrome such as fluorescein diacetate (green) prior to plating. When the cells are killed in the positive test, the fluorescein leaks out, and the cells "disappear." Positive results are compared with a negative well where all the cells are visible. A second fluorochrome of contrasting color such as ethidium bromide (red) may be added to visualize the dead cells.

Each test well is scored individually by inspection, with the percentage of dead cells per well being noted. The test is unequivocally positive when at least half of the cells are killed (Table 17–5).

Interpretation of the Tissue-Typing Test

An antigen is assigned by noting the patterns of reactivity of the individual sera and their specificities. The typing sera that reacted positively with the test cells should have antibody specificities in common. For an antigen to be assigned, the majority of sera of that specificity must be unequivocally positive. In

Table 17–5. Scoring the lymphocytotoxicity test for HLA typing.

% Dead Lymphocytes in Test Well	Score	Interpretation
0–10	1	Negative
11–20	2	Doubtful positive
21–50	4	Weak positive
51–80	6	Positive
81–100	8	Strong positive

phenotyping an individual for class I HLA, one expects to find patterns with two antigens each from the A, B, and C loci. When only a single antigen is identified at a locus, the individual may be homozygous for that allele, or the laboratory has failed to identify the second antigen, usually owing to inadequacies in the array of typing sera. Table 17–6 shows a representation of HLA-typing test results.

TISSUE-TYPING REAGENTS: HLA ALLOANTISERA

Sources of HLA-Typing Sera

The majority of HLA antisera are complex sera obtained from multiparous women. Maternal exposure to the mismatched paternal HLA antigens in the fetus gives rise to a polyclonal antibody response that frequently results in sera with multiple specificities.

Table 17–6. An example of HLA typing test results.[1]

Serum Name	Specificities	Score
A-001	A1	1
A-002	A1, A36	1
A-003	A1, A11	1
A-004	A2	1
A-005	A2, A28	6
A-006	A2, A28, B7	8
A-007	A3	8
A-008	A3	6
A-009	A3, A10, A11, A19	8
A-010	A11	1
A-011	A10, A11	1
A-012	A11, A1, A3 (weak)	4
B-001	B51, B52, B35	1
B-002	B51, B52	1
B-003	B51, B52, B53	1
B-004	B7, B42	8
B-005	B7, B27	8
B-006	B7, B55	8
B-007	B8	1
B-008	B8, B59	2
B-009	B44, B45, B21	6
B-010	B44, B45	8
B-011	B44	8
B-012	B45	1

[1] Interpretation: HLA phenotype is: A28, A3, B7, B44 (see Table 17–7).

Consequently, several different antisera are used to type for a specific antigen. It is not unusual for a laboratory to use typing trays composed of more than 200 different sera to type a single individual for HLA-A, -B, -C, and -DR, -DQ antigens.

Placental fluid, a mixture of serum and tissue fluids, has proved to be a valuable second source of alloantisera for tissue typing. Antibodies of high titer can be recovered from the fluid shed from fresh placentae that have been refrigerated for 24 hours after delivery. Attempts to immunize other animals, such as rabbits, for production of HLA antisera have largely failed. The xenoantisera reacted primarily with common human antigens such as the HLA-DR constant region. Thus, currently, the majority of HLA reagents are found among human sources by means of extensive serum-screening programs, a task undertaken by many tissue-typing laboratories. Through voluntary national and worldwide serum exchange programs, these reagents are distributed within the tissue-typing community for mutual benefit.

HLA antibodies are also found in the sera of patients exposed to HLA antigens through transfusions of blood and organ grafts. Generally, patients are not used as sources of HLA-typing sera, since the quantities obtainable would be limited by their medical conditions.

MONOCLONAL ANTIBODIES TO HLA ANTIGENS

Efforts in numerous laboratories have resulted in a limited production of monoclonal antibodies to HLA specificities. It was hoped that hybridoma cell lines (see Chapter 14) would produce inexhaustible quantities of monospecific antibodies to HLA antigens. In reality, many murine monoclonal antibodies have been directed against human monomorphic framework determinants or to common epitopes rather than to the private polymorphic determinants of the individual HLA antigens. Unfortunately, most murine monoclonal antibodies do not fix complement. Noncomplement-fixing antibodies can be used in assays that require only antigen binding, such as enzyme-linked immunosorbent assay (ELISA) and flow cytometry (see Chapters 14 and 15). Many monoclonal antibodies are reactive with more than one HLA specificity, indicating the existence of common antigenic determinants on HLA molecules.

SPECIFICITY OF HLA ANTIBODIES: PRIVATE & PUBLIC AND PANEL REACTIVE ANTIBODY LEVELS

An ideal HLA-typing serum would be monospecific, that is, would have specificity for a single HLA antigen; however, in reality, the observed alloantibodies in a single serum are usually polyspecific. An alloantiserum can contain antibodies to multiple determinants on the immunizing antigen(s). Some determinants are the classic HLA **private** specificities that characterize each HLA allele (see Table 17–1). Others are **public,** that is, are shared by several antigens that collectively constitute a cross-reacting antigen group (CREG group). Some complex sera can be rendered monospecific by dilution, whereas others lose all activity for all specificities simultaneously.

To determine the specificities of HLA antibodies, sera are tested against panels of cells of known HLA phenotype, a process termed "screening." The cell panel, usually from 40 to 60 cells, is preselected to provide a minimum of two to three representations of the most frequent HLA antigens. The antigens must be distributed among the cells so that the reaction pattern for one antigen is not entirely included within the pattern for a second antigen; for example, all of the HLA-A1 cells must not also be the only HLA-B8 cells. If they were, the reaction patterns for both antibodies would be identical and the determination of A1 or B8, or both, could not be made with certainty. When the sera react with a subset of the panel, the specificity of the antibody is deduced by inspecting the HLA phenotypes of the positive cells. Table 17–7 illustrates the type of reaction patterns obtained on reagent or patient serum screens. The percent panel reactive antibody (PRA) is calculated as the ratio of the number of positive cells to the number of total panel cells multiplied by 100. PRA is indicative of the extent of sensitization of the patient to HLA. Note that the antibody specificities of sera with high PRA cannot be determined. Special procedures must be used, such as dilution or treatment of the sera, or both, to determine antibody specificities.

TISSUE TYPING FOR CLASS II HLA ANTIGENS BY SEROLOGIC METHODS

Tissue typing for class II HLA antigens, HLA-DR and -DQ, is performed on lymphocyte preparations that are enriched for B lymphocytes. Special isolation procedures are required since approximately 80% of normal peripheral blood lymphocytes (PBL) are resting T cells that lack class II HLA antigens on their surface. The most popular method for isolation of B cells for DR typing uses immunomagnetic beads coated with anti-DR antibodies. The beads are mixed with isolated PBL, and surface DR antigens on the B cells bind to beads coated with antibody. The plastic beads have a magnetic core so that application of a magnet to the side of the reaction tube attracts and holds the cells stationary in the tube while the unattached cells are discarded. The isolated B cells are then washed, counted, and plated directly into DR-typing trays containing an array of antisera to DR antigens.

Table 17–7. An example of results of serum screening for class I HLA antibodies.[1]

Panel Cell HLA Antigens	Cytotoxicity Test Score for Patient Serum No:				
	1	2	3	4	5
A, A, B, B (locus)					
1, 2, 7, 60	1	1	8	1	8
2, 3, 8, 51	1	8	8	8	8
3, 29, 35, 44	1	8	1	6	8
30, 33, 55, 60	1	1	1	1	8
1, 30, 13, 51	1	1	1	8	8
24, 28, 35, 55	1	1	4	6	4
3, 28, 7, 44	1	8	4	1	6
2, 28, 35, 38	1	1	8	8	8

[1] PRA (panel-reactive antibody) was 0, 38, 50, 63, and 100%, for patient sera 1 through 5, respectively. PRA is calculated as (number of positive tests/number of cells tested) × 100. Analyzed antibodies were as follows (patient sera 1 through 5, respectively): None; A3; A2, weak A28; B51, B35; and Unknown (autoantibody?).

Prior to the use of immunomagnetic beads, the most common method for B-cell isolation was the adherence of B cells to nylon wool fibers. In this method, the PBL are passed through nylon-wool-packed columns made from plastic drinking straws or small syringes. The columns are filled with warm culture medium, and the cells are incubated in the wool for 30 minutes at 37 °C, allowing the B lymphocytes and macrophages to adhere to the fibers. The nonadherent T cells are then flushed out and saved for other tests. The B cells remaining are removed from the column by mechanical agitation of the wool and exposure to cooled medium. Nylon wool processing is normally used when large quantities of mixed lymphocytes must be processed for T- and B-cell lymphocyte testing, as in cadaver lymph node and spleen cell preparations. A minimum enrichment of 80% B cells is necessary for successful class II typing.

Antisera for Class II HLA Typing

Antisera for class II HLA tissue typing must be free of antibodies to class I HLA antigens. Unfortunately, the majority of HLA alloantisera contain mixtures of antibodies to class I and class II HLA antigens. Because their membranes have no class II antigens, pooled platelets are used as absorbents to clear HLA sera of any contaminating class I antibodies. Such manipulation of these sera can leave them diluted and operationally less reliable. Because B lymphocytes have more class I HLA antigens on their surface than do T cells, false-positive reactions from residual class I antibodies are possible. It is necessary that all absorbed class II antisera be thoroughly screened on T and B cells to ensure that absorption is complete. Overall, HLA-typing sera for class II antigens are of poorer quality and in shorter supply than are reagents for class I typing. Currently, very few sera for HLA-DP typing are available. The antigens of the DP locus have been defined mainly by cellular assays (see later section). Because of the paucity of good DR and DQ typing sera, serologic methods have had limited success in defining class II polymorphisms. Biochemical and molecular-biologic methods have provided significant new information. (See the section on molecular HLA typing.)

The complement-dependent cytotoxicity assay for class II HLA DR and DQ typing is performed with appropriate class II typing sera but is modified as follows: For cells isolated over nylon wool, initial incubation of cells and serum is performed at 37 °C or 22 °C for 60 minutes; after addition of complement, the mixture is incubated for 120 minutes at room temperature. The extended incubation times are used to promote binding of antibodies and complement. The temperature increase is used to avoid the false-positive reactions that can result from the binding of cold reactive nonspecific antibodies. When immunoabsorbent beads are used for class II typing, the incubation times are generally decreased by approximately one-half, possibly because of the weakening of the cell membrane by attachment to the beads.

Variability in Tissue-Typing Results

HLA-typing sera are not standardized by the usual practices of regulated quality control and licensure. The multiplicity of HLA antigens and the scarcity of the defining antisera make it impossible to license a standard reagent for each specificity. Each tissue-typing laboratory has the responsibility of obtaining the appropriate antisera and monitoring their performance. Typing sera are collected through serum exchange programs between laboratories, and new sera are discovered by means of extensive testing of sera from pregnant women, fluids recovered from placentae, and, occasionally, patient sera. Commercial typing trays are also available. Results with the laboratory's own serum trays may be compared with those of other collections of sera for confirmation of an HLA phenotype. All tissue-typing laboratories are required by the standards set by the American Society for Histocompatibility and Immunogenetics (ASHI) to control the quality of serologic and cellular reagents used for clinical testing. International and national quality control programs are available for typing, crossmatching, and serum analysis, and satisfactory performance is mandatory for ASHI accreditation of the laboratory.

A second variable in tissue typing is the serum complement, a reagent commercially available as the pooled serum from several hundred rabbits. Rabbit serum contains heterophile antibodies with antihuman lymphocyte activity that enhances its effectiveness in the cytotoxicity assay. Overabundance of these antihuman antibodies render the complement innately cytotoxic and therefore produces false-positive results. As with typing sera, the individual laboratory must screen its source of complement to find one that promotes strong serum reactions without causing non-specific toxicity. Because there is no standard complement source, it follows that the same serum tested in different laboratories has the potential of giving different results.

A third variable is the choice of method used to visualize the live and dead cells. Among these methods there are variations in incubation times and also in the definition of the end of the test period. Thus, in the exchange of typing sera between laboratories, it is important to note the method by which the serum was characterized.

CROSSMATCHING

The purpose of the crossmatch test is to detect the presence of antibodies in the patient's serum that are directed against the HLA antigens of the potential donor. If present, the antibodies signal that the immune system of the recipient has been sensitized to those donor antigens and is therefore primed to vigorously reject any graft bearing them. In the transplanted kidney, the main target of these antibodies is probably the HLA antigens on vascular endothelium of capillaries and arterioles. HLA antigen–antibody complexes on endothelium activate complement and lead to cell damage. Platelets then aggregate, eventually producing fibrin clots, which clog the vessels. This causes ischemic necrosis. Even weak, low-titer antibodies, particularly those directed against class I antigens, can contribute to graft rejection. Therefore, the ultimate goal of the crossmatch is a test of both great sensitivity and specificity for HLA antigens.

Crossmatching by Lymphocytotoxicity

A simple crossmatch by the standard cytotoxicity method (see earlier discussion) may be performed with donor PBL as targets. PBL crossmatches are usually included in the preliminary evaluation of potential living-related donors for renal graft recipients. PBL are normally about 80% T cells, which carry class I HLA antigens only, and 20% B cells and monocytes, which bear both class I and class II antigens. A strongly positive crossmatch by cytotoxicity (50% or more cell death per well) clearly indicates the presence of antibodies to class I antigens. However, 10–20% cell killing could result from an antibody specific for class II or could be due to a weak anticlass I antibody. To resolve the specificity of the antibody, crossmatching is then performed on cell preparations enriched for either T or B lymphocytes.

Crossmatching with Separated T & B Lymphocytes

A. T-Cell Crossmatches: T-cell crossmatches are performed at room temperature and also at 37 °C in some laboratories to avoid the binding of cold-reactive antibodies, presumed to be autoreactive. A positive T-cell crossmatch by any method contraindicates transplantation, no matter how weak the reaction level; that is, a reaction of 4+ (20–50% dead cells per well above background) is considered just as positive a result as 6+ or 8+ (51% dead cells or greater). Some laboratories even consider a reaction of 2 (10–20% dead over background) as a positive crossmatch result.

Several methods to improve the sensitivity of T-cell crossmatches by complement-dependent cytotoxicity have been developed. These include the following.

1. Extended incubation–The simplest modification in the cytotoxicity assay to increase sensitivity is to extend the incubation time of cells, serum, and complement.

2. The Amos wash step–This method interjects a wash step after the incubation of cells and serum and prior to the addition of complement to remove anticomplementary factors in the serum.

3. Antihuman globulin–The cytotoxicity of some antibodies may be enhanced by the addition of a second-step antibody, usually a polyclonal anti-human immunoglobulin (AHG) reagent.

B. B-Cell Crossmatches: Crossmatching for antibodies to class II HLA antigens requires the use of B lymphocytes as targets and the same extended incubation times as HLA-DR and -DQ serologic typing for nylon-wool isolated B cells. A positive B-cell crossmatch may result from antibodies binding to class I or class II HLA antigens. Moreover, B cells are a more sensitive indicator for weak class I antibodies, since they carry class I molecules in greater density than T cells do. Crossmatching by flow cytometry can readily distinguish between "true B" antibodies and weak class I antibodies of a positive B cell cytotoxicity crossmatch. The significance for transplant outcome of preformed antibodies to class II antigens is not yet clear. Successful transplantation into patients with low-titer anticlass II antibodies (titer of 1:1 or 1:2) has been reported, as has the acute rejection of grafts transplanted in the face of high-titer (1:8) antibodies. It is possible that the loss of grafts transplanted in the face of T-negative, B-positive crossmatches is due to the anticlass I component of these alloreactive sera.

C. Flow-Cytometry Crossmatching: Crossmatching by flow cytometry (FCC) (see Chapter 15) has been shown to be up to 100 times more sensitive than visual serologic methods for the detection of HLA antibodies on lymphocytes (Fig 17–3). In this crossmatching application, T cells can be separated from B cells electronically through the use of a fluoresceinated antibody to a T-cell surface antigen such as the CD3 T-cell receptor complex. An electronic "gate" can be created so that only the fluorescently labeled T cells are selected. Donor lymphocytes are incubated with patient's serum to allow binding of any antidonor antibodies. Antibody bound to the selected T-cell population is detected by addition of an antihuman IgG anti-Fc-specific F(ab')$_2$ antibody labeled with a fluorochrome of a different color from the T-

cell marking antibody (eg, green, if the anti-CD3 was red). The flow cytometer counts the number of labeled T cells and creates a histogram displaying the number of cells versus fluorescence intensity (Fig 17–4). Unlabeled cells lie near the origin, and labeled cells lie to the right of the origin on the x-axis. A shift to the right of the T-cell peak in the experimental test compared with the negative control indicates that anticlass I HLA antibody from the patient serum has bound to the donor T cells. FCCs can also be performed on gated B cells labeled with specific antibody to B-cell antigen.

FCC is generally performed with the most recent serum and a selection of historically reactive sera for all cadaver waiting list patients who have rejected prior transplants or who have high PRAs, and for patients with living related donors in the event of a negative T-cell and positive B-cell serologic crossmatch.

Occasionally, positive FCC crossmatches occur when both the serologic T- and B-cell crossmatches are negative. The nature of these antibodies is unknown and has been considered by some to be irrelevant to transplantation. For the unsensitized patient, such conclusions may be correct. For patients with high PRAs and those who have undergone previous transplants, however, caution (and further testing) is justified before the transplant is performed.

Crossmatching for Autoantibodies

In crossmatching patient serum for donor compatibility, it is most important to distinguish nonspecific antilymphocyte antibodies, referred to as autoantibodies, from the specific antidonor antibodies. The presence of autoantibodies is detected by the autocrossmatch, in which the patient's own serum and cells are combined in the standard cytotoxicity test. Autoantibodies can give a false-positive result in a donor crossmatch, leading to the erroneous disqualification of that donor. Alternatively, preexisting autoantibodies can mask the presence of specific antidonor antibodies. Autoantibody crossmatches are routinely performed in conjunction with all living-donor crossmatches for each serum that is tested. Auto FCC crossmatches are also recommended, particularly in the case of a negative serologic crossmatch coupled with an unexpectedly positive FCC. False-positive FCCs can occur when the patient has autoantibodies of undetermined specificity. Such autoantibody-positive FCCs are not considered contraindicative to transplantation.

CELLULAR ASSAYS FOR HISTOCOMPATIBILITY

In vivo, recognition of nonself antigens and destruction of cells bearing such markers is accomplished by

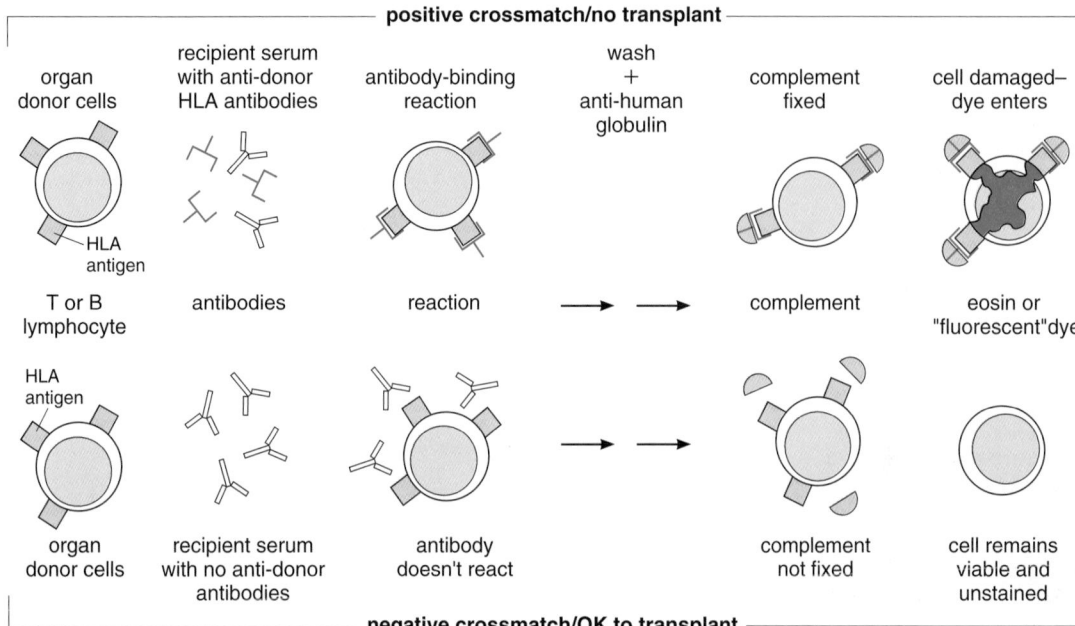

Figure 17–3. Lymphocytotoxicity T-cell crossmatch test for compatibility between recipient and donor. 1 μL of recipient serum is plated into multiple wells of a microtest plate. For sensitized patients, multiple sera of known PRA are plated. 2–3 × 10^6 donor T cells are added, and the test is incubated for 30–60 minutes. To increase sensitivity of the test, before complement is added, the sera are washed from the wells, leaving the cells behind. The addition of a second, developing antibody such as goat antihuman IgG (AHG) increases the sensitivity further. After several minutes of incubation with AHG, complement is added and the test incubated for another 60 minutes. A long complement incubation of up to 3 hours is sometimes performed instead of AHG addition. If the recipient serum contains antibodies that react with donor cells, the cells are killed and penetrated by dyes such as eosin or ethidium bromide, indicating a positive crossmatch. A positive serologic T-cell crossmatch is a contraindication to transplantation.

cells of the immune system. Some of the clinically relevant class II HLA antigens that can trigger the immune response are not readily detected by the serologic methods discussed previously. Instead, lymphocytes are used as discriminatory reagents for the HLA-Dw and -DP antigens and as indicators of histoincompatibility between donor and recipient. The functions of cellular recognition are used in the MLC, HTC, and primed lymphocyte typing (PLT) tests, and the dual functions of recognition and effector cell killing are used in the CML test.

MLC Test

The mixed lymphocyte culture (MLC) test (see Chapter 15) is also known as the mixed-lymphocyte reaction (MLR). When the lymphocytes of two HLA-disparate individuals are combined in tissue culture, the cells enlarge, synthesize DNA, and proliferate, whereas HLA-identical cells remain quiescent. The proliferation is driven primarily by differences in the class II HLA antigens between the two test cells.

On the basis of MLC testing, class II antigens were originally described as a series of lymphocyte-activating determinants, products of the HLA-"D" locus (-Dw1, -Dw2, etc). No D locus products have ever

been isolated, however, although several distinct "D region" loci (-DR, -DQ, and -DP) and their alleles have been identified. Dw "antigens" are now considered to be immunogenic epitopes formed by combinations of D region determinants that can be recognized by T cells. Distinct Dw types may represent unique haplotype combinations of various D region products.

Reactivity in MLC probably reflects the initial immune recognition step of graft rejection in vivo. The more immunogenic the D locus difference, the greater the cellular response in MLC and the more likely the rejection of the graft. Normally, both cells proliferate, forming the two-way MLC. To monitor the response of a single responder cell (the one-way MLC), the partner cell (stimulator) is inactivated by radiation or drugs (such as mitomycin C) that inhibit DNA synthesis (Fig 17–5). A maximum proliferative response usually occurs after incubation at 37 °C for 5–6 days. The culture is then pulsed with [^{3}H]thymidine for 5–12 hours to label the newly synthesized DNA. Finally, the cells are harvested, washed free of unbound radioactivity, and counted in a beta counter.

A properly composed MLC test includes a checkerboard of one-way combinations of each cell serving as both stimulator and responder with all other cells.

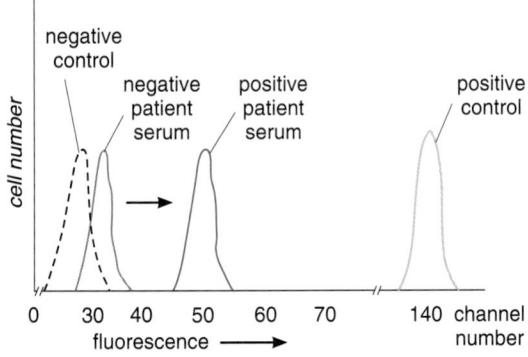

serum	mean channel no.	channel shift
negative control	27	—
negative patient	33	6
positive patient	50	23
positive control	140	113

Figure 17–4. Flow-cytometry crossmatch (FCC) with patient serum and donor T cells. A schematic composite tracing of an FCC fluorescence histogram illustrating representative peak positions for a negative and positive T-cell FCC crossmatch in relation to negative and positive control peaks. Peaks represent the number of cells (y-axis) at a given fluorescence level (x-axis) expressed as channel numbers. Donor lymphocytes are incubated with patient serum, and then a fluorescein isothiocyanate-labeled antihuman immunoglobulin is added, which fluorescently labels donor T cells that have bound patient antibody. When compared with the peak of T cells having no antibody bound, the fluorescent T-cell peak is brighter and shifted to the right on the x-axis. When the mean channel fluorescence of the T-cell peak shifts to the right by more than 10 channels on a 256-channel scale, the crossmatch is considered to be positive.

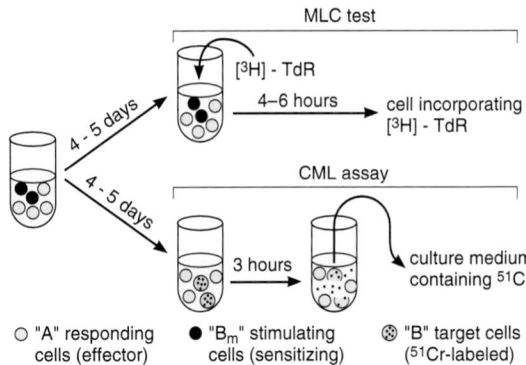

Figure 17–5. The MLC and CML tests. In the one-way MLC, responder PBLs are mixed 1:1 with irradiated stimulator cells and incubated at 37 °C in a humidified atmosphere with 5% CO_2. After 5 days, the culture is pulsed with [³H]thymidine ([³H]TdR) to label the nucleic acid in the responder cells. After 18 hours, cells are harvested and counted for internalized radioactivity. If the class II HLA antigens of the stimulator cells differ from those of the responder cells, the responder cells undergo blastogenesis, synthesize DNA, and proliferate. Increased sample radioactivity signals recognition of class II HLA differences. When responder and stimulator cells are class II-identical, the proliferative responses are less than 20% of the maximum response to the mismatched controls and less than 2% over autologous (background) controls. (Reproduced, with permission, from Bach FH, Van Rood JJ: The major histocompatibility complex: Genetics and biology. N Engl J Med 1976;**295**:806, 872.)

Each cell must be controlled for its ability to both stimulate and respond to HLA-mismatched cells. Normally, two to four unrelated control cells of known class II HLA type are tested individually with each family member. The maximum response of each cell is obtained by exposure to a pool of irradiated stimulator cells of diverse HLA types.

Autologous controls combining self with irradiated self are also run to normalize the response of each cell to stimulators. Each test should be run in triplicate. It is absolutely necessary to perform the entire familial MLC at one time owing to the inherent variability of individual cellular responses from day to day.

Results are expressed as a stimulation index (SI) or relative response (RR). The SI is the ratio of counts per minute of the test over the autologous test for that cell:

$$SI = \frac{\text{cpm of Responder vs Stimulator (irradiated)}}{\text{Responder vs Responder (irradiated)}}$$

A value of SI ≤2 is interpreted as HLA identity at HLA-D. The RR calculates the response in the experimental MLC relative to the maximum response of

that cell elicited by the pool. Counts per minute of both are corrected by subtraction of the autologous control for the responder cell.

$$RR = \frac{\text{Responder vs Stimulator (irradiated)} - \text{Autologous control}}{\text{Responder vs Pool (irradiated)} - \text{Autologous control}} \times 100$$
cpm of

MLC testing can be useful in selecting the most compatible (least stimulatory) organ donor if several nonidentical family members (matched for zero or one haplotype) are available. The donor who is the least stimulatory to the patient is the preferred organ donor. The results of an intrafamilial MLC can address such questions as (1) Are two serologically identical DR antigens also functionally identical? (2) Is the individual with only one identifiable DR antigen a homozygote, or is the DR "blank" really a second DR antigen that was missed in the serologic testing? (3) Are the serologically assigned class II antigens consistent with the MLC results? If apparently HLA-identical individuals are reactive, there may have been a genetic recombination event.

The MLC test is frequently used to confirm apparent HLA identity in the living related transplant situation and is especially useful if haplotyping could not be accomplished. When the HLA-identical recipient and donor are unrelated, as in voluntary bone marrow donation, MLC testing has been used to reveal hidden class II incompatibilities that could affect recipient tolerance to the graft and promote graft-versus-host disease. MLC testing has largely been replaced by DNA-based high-resolution typing for class II alleles. (see section on Histocompatibility Testing by Molecular-Biologic Methods).

HTC and PLT Testing

Individuals who are homozygous for a Dw type (HTCs—homozygous typing cells) can be used as stimulators in the MLC to "type" the responder cell in MLC tests. Lack of a response indicates identity of at least one of the responder cell's class II alleles with the stimulator HTC's Dw type.

The primed lymphocyte typing (PLT) test is a variation of the MLC that uses the unknown cell as the stimulator cell and, as a responder cell, one that has been previously exposed to a known stimulating antigen in a primary MLC, that is, the responder cell is "primed" to respond to that antigen on a second encounter. A response to the stimulator cell in the PLT test indicates that the stimulator cell bears the same antigen to which the PLT was primed and thus, that stimulator cell is typed for an HLA class II allele.

Both the HTC and PLT methods of typing have been replaced by high-resolution DNA-based typing for class II alleles in which a direct, rather than an inferential, identification of the allele is possible.

CML Test

In primary MLC testing, exposure to nonself class I and class MHC II antigens can result in the generation of cytotoxic T lymphocytes (CTL). CTL kill their targets through direct contact, probably by the release of toxic mediators that lead to cell lysis. CD4 and CD8 CTL can be found infiltrating kidney allografts during rejection and are considered to be imporant effector cells in graft loss (see Chapter 57). To test for the capacity to generate CTL, a primary MLC is run with the patient as the responder and prospective donor cells as inactivated stimulators. After the MLC, the patient's cells are harvested and then reexposed in culture to fresh donor target cells that have been loaded with ^{51}Cr (see Fig 17–5). Usually, the targets are preincubated with the mitogen phytohemagglutinin (PHA) for 6 days, since PHA-activated blast cells can incorporate more ^{51}Cr than resting lymphocytes can. CTL and targets are plated in effector/target-cell ratios of 100:1, 50:1, and 10:1. Control wells include targets alone to measure the spontaneous release of label and test wells containing target cells that are treated with detergent to release the maximum incorporated label. The test requires 4 hours of incubation in a humidified CO_2 atmosphere at 37 °C. At the conclusion, the supernatant of each test well is sampled and counted. In the experimental wells, the amount of ^{51}Cr released is corrected for the background level of spontaneously released label and compared with the maximum amount of label released:

$$\% \text{ Specific Release} = \frac{\text{cpm (Experimental)} - \text{cpm (Spontaneous)}}{\text{cpm (Maximum)} - \text{cpm (Spontaneous)}} \times 100$$

Elevated counts of 30–50% above spontaneous background are indicative of CTL activity.

Direct CML testing can be used to monitor post-transplant rejection by testing for the presence of activated circulating antidonor CTL. The patient's PBL are placed directly in culture with ^{51}Cr-labeled donor cells as targets. An elevated donor cell lysis compared with pretransplant levels is considered evidence of circulating CTL, which are particularly prevalent during rejection.

CML testing has applications in living related renal and bone marrow transplantation. The preferred kidney donor is the one who fails to stimulate the recipient to form CTL. In bone marrow transplantation, the recipient is at risk for immune attack by the marrow donor (graft-versus-host disease). The capacity of the prospective donors to form CTL against the recipient may be assessed through MLC plus CML testing.

A summary of the serologic and cellular methods for histocompatibility testing is presented in Table 17–8. All of these methods are in current use and are accepted as appropriate (in some instances mandatory) procedures for clinical histocompatibility testing.

HISTOCOMPATIBILITY TESTING BY MOLECULAR-BIOLOGIC METHODS

Introduction

The individual antigens of the classic HLA system have been identified through the binding patterns of antibodies in serologic tests and from the activation of lymphocytes by disparate MHC antigens in the mixed lymphocyte culture (MLC) test. With the advent of gene cloning and DNA sequencing, HLA antigen specificities are now known to derive from sequence differences localized to several hypervariable regions in the MHC molecules. These differences have arisen from intragene and intergene conversion events and have resulted in the complex polymorphism that characterizes the HLA system. In the HLA class II genes, the variable regions are found mainly in exon 2 of the coding regions, but polymorphic regions also exist in the introns and flanking regions of the genes. Class I polymorphisms are found in exons 2 and 3 and also in the introns. The exon-based variations in sequence are mainly localized to the floor of the MHC antigen-binding cleft and to the alpha-helical regions facing the T-cell receptor, locations strategic to the ability of

Table 17–8. Serologic and cellular methods used in histocompatibility testing.

Test	Test Type and Components	Time	Application
Tissue typing Complement-dependent lymphocytotoxicity	Serologic (HLA, antisera; complement; test cells)	3 h	Identification of class I and II HLA antigens.
Crossmatching PBL crossmatch	Serologic (recipient serum; donor cells; complement; AHG optional)	3 h	Detection of preformed anti-donor antibodies in patient serum.
T/B cell crossmatch	Serologic (purified donor T or B cells; recipient serum; AHG optional with T cells)	3–6 h	T cells: detection of anti-donor class I HLA antibodies; B cells: detection of antibodies to class I and II HLA.
MLC test	Cellular (donor and recipient cells combined in tissue culture)	6 d	Class II HLA antigen compatibility.
CML test	Cellular (patient cells from primary MLC; fresh donor stimulators as targets)	4 h	Detection of anti-donor CTL.
FCC	Serologic (patient serum; donor cells; fluorescent antihuman immunoglobulin)	3–4 h	Detection of very weak and non-cytotoxic antidonor antibodies.
Autocrossmatch	Serologic (patient PBL, T and B cells, and serum) and FCC.	3–4 h	Detection of nonspecific antilymphocyte antibodies (autoantibodies).
Screening Screening for class I HLA antibodies	Serologic (patient serum; panel of HLA-typed T cells or PBL	3 h × 60 cells	Detection of class I HLA antibodies; identification of antibody specificity.
Screening for class II HLA antibodies	Serologic (patient serum absorbed; B cell panel typed for HLA-DR, DQ)	4 h × no. of cells plus absorption time	Detection of class II HLA antibodies; identification of antibody specificity.

the immune system to recognize and respond to pathogenic (and possibly autoimmunogenic) endogenous and exogenous antigens.

HLA alleles share many of the same sequence motifs but in different combinations. Consequently, HLA class I and class II antigens can be thought of as a patchwork of combinations of these various sequence polymorphisms occurring on a background of shared (consensus) nucleotide base sequences. The long-observed phenomenon of crossreactivity of antisera and, more recently, the cross-hybridization of oligonucleotide probes, can be explained by the fact that several antigens can share the same sequence motifs. For example, the concept of the "public" (ie, held in common) HLA antigen specificity, such as antigens Bw4 and Bw6 that are associated with all HLA B locus specificities, is confirmed by finding a dimorphic amino acid sequence located at residues 77–83 in all B locus antigen sequences. There is an even greater degree of sharing of specific polymorphic sequences among the class I alleles, even occurring across the class I loci, making typing for class I alleles more technically demanding than for class II alleles. An important consequence of these shared sequence motifs is that certain heterozygous combinations of alleles cannot always be distinguished from a second, different combination. All DNA typing methods must take this into consideration when proposing schema for allele identification. Clearly, the most definitive HLA typing method would be to carry out a complete sequence analysis of the DNA of the HLA genes of

each individual. Undoubtedly, this will become the method of choice when automated sequencing technology becomes affordable and widely disseminated. Until then, alternative approaches are feasible that use knowledge of both the unique and the consensus sequences of HLA antigens.

Molecular typing offers several important advantages over serologic methods, as summarized in Table 17–9. The chief advantage is the ability to distinguish alleles that can be confounded by multispecific antisera. Antigens in cross-reactive groups (CREGs) such as DR5, -6, -8, and -12, are particularly problematic for serology but are easily distinguished by molecular typing. Similarly, when a phenotype contains two antigens from the same CREG group, such as B15 (which includes B62, B63, B46, B75, B76, etc), one antigen can mask the others by serologic reactivity, but usually the two are easily separable by molecular methods. The clinical utility of DNA-based HLA class II typing was clearly demonstrated by the improved renal graft survival of patients matched for transplant by HLA typing done by restriction fragment-length polymorphism (RFLP) as compared with patients typed by conventional serologic methods. Unrelated bone marrow transplantation absolutely requires identification of HLA antigens at the allele level, that is, high-resolution HLA typing, to avoid severe graft-versus-host disease. Similarly, investigations of the genetic susceptibility to disease are scrutinizing HLA antigens at the allele level. Knowledge of the molecular configuration of the HLA antigen-

Table 17–9. Comparison of HLA typing methods: DNA-based and serologic.

Method	Serologic	DNA:SSP/SSOP	DNA:SBT
Number of identifiable alleles			
HLA-A	21	21–62	62
HLA-B	43	43–125	125
HLA-C	10	10–35	35
HLA-DR	18	18–138	138
HLA-DQ	9	9–34	34
HLA-DP	—	6–61	61
Sample material	2–3 million live lymphocytes	Minute amount of DNA-containing biologic material	PCR product
Reagents	Alloantisera (supply exhaustible) some monoclonals	Synthetic oligonucleotide primers/probes (supply unlimited)	Synthetic primers (supply unlimited)
Power to identify new alleles	Very limited: depends on availability and specificity of sera	Limited: based on knowledge of sequences and on novel reaction patterns	Unlimited: new alleles identified by their sequences
Level of resolving power for known alleles	Generic level	Generic to allele level	Allele level
Detection affected by	Expression of HLA on cell surface	Quality of DNA, PCR reaction	Quality of DNA, PCR reaction
	Viability of test cells	Stringency of test conditions	

Abbreviations: SSP/SSOP = sequence-specific priming/sequence-specific oligonucleotide probing; SBT = sequence-based typing.

binding pocket can offer clues to the putative disease-associated antigen and suggest strategies for development of synthetic vaccines.

Methods of HLA Typing by DNA Analysis

Methods using DNA for HLA typing are characterized by the level of resolution of the antigen attainable, that is the capacity of either low (generic, serologic antigen level), medium (some alleles), or high (aiming at identification of all alleles) resolution. A new nomenclature has been developed to enumerate the alleles of the MHC loci. Table 17–10 illustrates the components of the HLA antigen names; first, the genetic locus is indicated (eg, HLA-A, -B, or DRB1) followed by the common or generic root of the antigen derived from serologic names if applicable (eg,

Table 17–10. Examples of revised nomenclature for HLA alleles.

HLA Allele	Locus Component	Generic Component[1]	Allelic Component	Serologic Equivalent
A*0201	A	02	01	A2
B*1510	B	15	10	B15
DRB1*0405	DRB1	04	05	DR4
DQB1*0501	DQB1	05	01	DQ5
DRB3*0202	DRB3	02	02	DR52

[1] Genetic nomenclature as applied to HLA alleles consists of the designation of the genetic locus, the common, "generic" name of the allele as defined by serology followed by the designation of the allelic subtype of the generic antigen.

"04" for DR4) followed by the subtype or allele (eg, "05," for DRB1*0405). Table 17–12 summarizes methods of DNA-based HLA typing in current use and highlights some relevant technical differences. The type of DNA used is either genomic (ie, DNA isolated from the cell nucleus) or the amplified product of the polymerase chain reaction (PCR), a process that produces multiple copies of a specific subregion of HLA DNA that was generated from isolated genomic DNA (see Chapter 18). The polymorphisms detected can be either **group-specific,** identifying sequences that are characteristic of a group of alleles (eg, the DR52-associated antigens DR3,-5,-6) or of the generic HLA allele (eg, DRB1*11 group, including DRB1*1101, -1102, -1103, etc.) or **allele-specific** (eg, specific for DNA sequences that identify the exact allele (eg, DRB1*0413). The latter is referred to as "high-resolution typing." Table 17–11 shows the current number of alleles of the class I and II loci, HLA-A, -B, -C, and DR, DQ, and DP loci. Table 17–11 shows the number of subtypes of the class II multilocus region. As a consequence of molecular typing, the number of HLA alleles has more than quadrupled from 100 to over 450 in the past 5 years. The complete DNA sequences have been determined for all of these alleles. New HLA alleles continue to be discovered as a consequence of these molecular methods, and an updated listing of new HLA alleles is now published monthly. The challenge of any high-resolution method is to be able to identify new alleles through unusual reaction patterns and to adapt the particular technique to identify the new alleles as they are discovered.

Table 17–11. Polymorphism of class II HLA alleles.

Locus	Antigen[1]	Number of Alleles	Nomenclature
DRB1	DR1	4	DRB1*0101 . . . . . *0104
	DR15 (DR2)	5	DRB1*1501 . . . . . *1505
	DR16 (DR2)	6	DRB1*1601 . . . . . *1606
	DR3	5	DRB1*0301 . . . . . *0305
	DR4	22	DRB1*0401 0422
	DR11 (DR5)	22	DRB1*11011 . . . . *1122
	DR12	3	DRB1*1201 . . . . . *1203
	DR13 (DR6)	22	DRB1*1301 . . . . . *1322
	DR14 (DR6)	21	DRB1*1401 . . . . . *1421
	DR7	1	DRB1*0701
	DR8	11	DRB1*0801 . . . . . *0811
	DR9	1	DRB1*09011
	DR10	1	DRB1*1001
DRB3	DR52	5	DRB3*0101 0105
DRB4	DR53	1	DRB4*0101
DRB5	DR51	6	DRB5*0101 0106
DQA1	. . .[2]	12	DQA1*0101 . . . . *0112
DQB1	DQ5 (DQ1)	4	DQB1*0501 . . . . *0504
	DQ6 (DQ1)	9	DQB1*0601 . . . . *0609
	DQ2	2	DQB1*0201 . . . . *0202
	DQ3	5	DQB1*0301 . . . . *0305
	DQ4	2	DQB1*0401 . . . . *0402
DPA1		6	DPA1*0101 . . . . . *0601
DPB1		61	DPB1*0101 . . . . *6101

[1] Equivalent antigens as defined serologically.
[2] No equivalent serologically defined antigens.

The first molecular method to be widely used to identify the generic (serologically defined) class II HLA antigens was based on restriction fragment-length polymorphisms (RFLP). The RFLP method has been largely supplanted mainly by sequence-specific priming (SSP) and sequence-specific oligonucleotide probing (SSOP). RFLP is still used in some typing strategies, however, as an adjunctive or simplifying approach for generic typing. SSP, SSOP, and, in some techniques, RFLP use the technology of the polymerase chain reaction.

HLA Typing by RFLP: The technique of RFLP (Fig 17–6) typing is based on the knowledge of the germline nucleotide sequences found in both coding (exons) and noncoding (introns and flanking) regions of class II HLA genes. Certain unique sequences serve as target sites for cleavage (cut sites) by bacterial restriction endonucleases. Such restriction sites are usually four or six bases in length, and more than 90 enzymes are known that can recognize a unique nucleotide sequence as a cut site. When isolated DNA is digested with a particular enzyme, the DNA of an HLA haplotype is cut into fragments of different lengths depending on the locations of the restriction cut sites. Thus, a new polymorphism, a fragment length, is created that is analogous to but not the same as the classic HLA serologic polymorphisms. Since most of the restriction sites lie in the introns of the HLA genes, however, the resulting fragments are not equivalent to the serologic polymorphisms. Subjecting the restriction digest fragments to gel electrophoresis separates them by size. The different

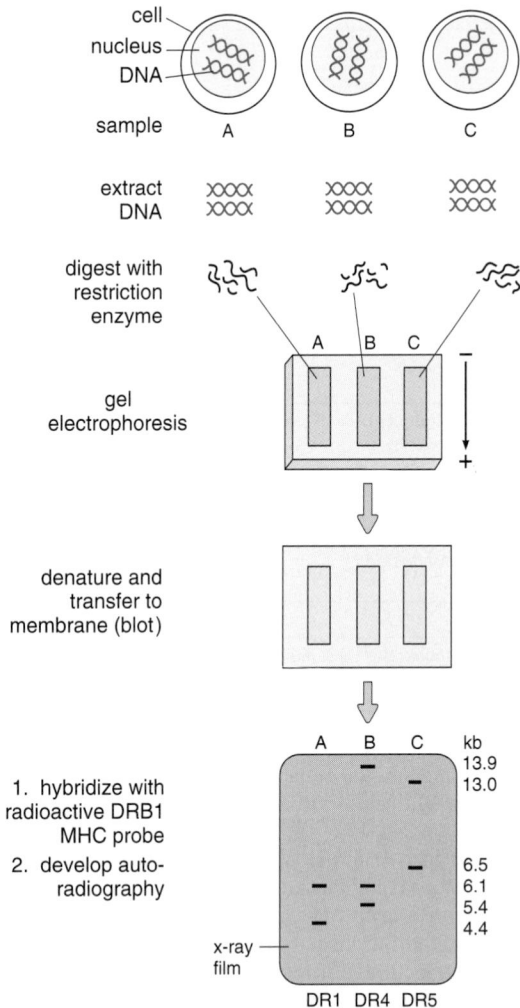

Figure 17–6. Tissue typing by RFLP. A comparison of RFLP tissue typing of three samples, A, B, and C, is shown. Genomic DNA is extracted from the cells and digested with selected restriction endonucleases. Digests are dispersed by agarose gel electrophoresis, the DNA is denatured into single strands, and the gel pattern of fragments is transferred to a support membrane by blotting (Southern blot). The DNA fragments are hybridized with a radiolabeled HLA locus-specific probe (eg, DRB1) that complexes with DNA nucleotide sequences. After autoradiography, the restriction fragments that have hybridized with the probe appear as patterns of isolated bands of specific size (kilobases; kb). Control digests containing fragments of known size permit sizing of the bands. Many HLA alleles have characteristic band patterns (fragment-length polymorphism) when digested with specific endonucleases. HLA antigens can be assigned from these patterns, as illustrated here for DR1, DR4, and DR5. (Reproduced, with permission, from Bidwell JL et al: A DNA RFLP typing system that positively identifies serologically well-defined and ill-defined HLA-DR and DQ alleles, including DRw10. *Transplantation* 1988;**45:**640.)

Table 17–12. Molecular histocompatibility testing techniques.

Name	Characteristic Reagents	Characteristic Processes	Polymorphisms Detected
RFLP	Bacterial restriction endonucleases	Southern blotting	Restriction fragment length
SSP	Sequence-specific PCR primers	PCR/gel electrophoresis	Generic to allele-level HLA antigens
SSOP	Sequence-specific oligonucleo-tide probes	PCR/hybridization of probes to PCR product	HLA alleles
SBT	Labeled primers/labeled sequence terminators	PCR/nucleotide sequencing of PCR product	Alleles at exact sequence level
Heteroduplex analysis	Denatured, single-strand DNA/Artificial universal hetero-duplex generator (UHG)	Reannealing of strands of DNA/electrophoresis of recombined DNA	DNA complexes characteristic of alleles

Abbreviations: RFLP = restriction fragment-length polymorphism; SSP = sequence-specific priming; SSOP = sequence-specific oligonucleotide probing; SBT = sequence-based typing.

sized fragments are visualized by probing with radioactive or colorimetrically labeled cDNAs that hybridize with the consensus sequences within the fragments. Band patterns are produced that are diagnostic for most of the generic level class II antigens. Locus-specific probes have been designed for the detection of the products of the different genetic subloci of DR, DQ, and DP, for example, DRB1, DQA1, DPB1, and so on. This process of enzyme digestion, transfer of the fragments to a membrane by blotting of the gel, and hybridization by labeled probes is known as **Southern blotting** (see Fig 17–6).

A. The Uses and Limitations of RFLP Typing: RFLP typing cannot identify the many class II alleles now known to exist (see Table 17–11). Its main use has been to confirm and clarify serologically assigned DR and DQ types and to identify generic DP alleles. The method is time-consuming, usually requiring from 1 to 2 weeks and requires at least 5–10 mm of DNA. It is limited in its ability to reveal both known and novel antigens because there may be no restriction enzymes capable of producing fragments to generate a unique band pattern for the allele. Several typing strategies have used RFLP in combination with SSP and SSOP to find a simplified method for DNA typing for low-volume laboratories that does not require the use of so many SSOPs (see section on SSOP typing). Group-specific and SSP products from PCR amplifications are digested with restriction enzymes and separated on gels, producing low to moderate resolution typing results. This method has been successfully applied to typing for DPA1 alleles.

Use of PCR in HLA Typing: The majority of molecular methods for HLA typing are based on the use of the polymerase chain reaction (PCR), as described in Chapter 18. PCR produces multiple copies of specifically targeted regions of DNA on chromosome 6 that contain the nucleotide sequences coding for HLA polymorphisms. The HLA genes exist in a single copy in the genome. Amplification of this DNA

is achieved through the PCR process, which can provide the necessary quantity for analysis by the methods of sequence-specific priming (SSP) sequence-specific oligonucleotide probing (SSOP) (discussed in later sections), and RFLP. PCR technology provides several advantages for molecular HLA typing (see Table 17–12). Only a minute quantity of sample is required to initiate the process, and living tissue is not necessary. Moreover, the reagents are synthetic and therefore unlimited in supply.

Currently, these methods are being applied mainly to class II HLA typing for bone marrow and solid organ transplantation. Because of the complexity of the class I alleles, PCR-based typing systems are still under development for HLA-A, -B, and -C locus (class I) antigens.

A. Types of PCR Amplification: The sequence of DNA to be amplified is determined by the composition of the PCR primers. That composition is determined by the level of HLA allele resolution desired and partly by any previous knowledge of the phenotype of the individual. For example, if the DR/DQ phenotype is unknown, then the primers chosen would amplify a segment of DNA that encompasses the entire range of DR and DQ genes, whereas if the subject were already known to be DR4-positive, the region chosen to be amplified would be particular to the DR4 group of alleles.

1. Generic, Group-Specific or Locus-Specific Amplification: Primers are directed at flanking sequences common to a group of alleles such as the DR4 group, or the alleles of the DRB3* (DR52) group or the HLA-C locus. The amplified product is a segment of DNA that contains sequence differences that characterize the alleles of the group. Several procedures may be applied to this product depending on the level of typing resolution desired. The product can be applied onto a membrane support and probed with oligonucleotides tailored to hybridize with, and thereby discriminate, these specific allelic differences (successful hybridization indicates the presence of that allele), or can be subjected to a second round of PCR (nested PCR) to achieve further allele discrimination by SSP, or can be treated with endonucleases to produce fragment for RFLP analysis.

2. Allele-Specific Amplification with Sequence-Specific Primers (PCR-SSP): Allele-specific PCR amplification is a simple and rapid method that has been very successfully applied to the identification of class II genes. Depending on the primers, identification of HLA antigens can be done at the generic (akin to the serologic resolution level, eg, DR15) or at the allele level (eg, DRB1*1502). This method uses the principle that PCR primers amplify a portion of DNA most efficiently when they anneal perfectly to their complementary flanking sequences. Primers based on sequences specific for the DR alleles have been designed so that under optimal conditions of annealing temperature, extension time, and reagent concentrations, amplified product is produced only when the exact fit of the primers has been made. In the amplification refractory mutation system (ARMS-SSP) a deliberate mismatch has been included in the primers near the 3′ residue to enhance specificity. Each sample contains an internal control of primers targeted to a consensus sequence to control for successful amplification. After amplification, the sample is run on a minigel and examined with ethidium bromide under ultraviolet light for the presence or absence of product. The presence of a product signifies the presence of the allele to which the primer was directed. Figure 17–7 summarizes this process. False-negatives can occur from incomplete annealing, whereas cross-reactivity and low-stringency conditions can give a false-positive amplification. SSP can easily identify the serologically defined DR antigens DR1-DR18. Some systems of SSP have been developed that are capable of high-resolution allele subtyping, which was previously possible only with SSOP typing methods. Not all combinations of heterozygosity can be distinguished. The success of PCR-SSP clearly depends on the stringency of the experimental conditions and the ability to design appropriate primers.

A major advantage of PCR-SSP typing is that with the proper equipment, highly accurate DR typing can be accomplished in several hours with minimal sample manipulation and at reasonable cost. Thus, molecular DR typing by this method will probably become the method of choice for class II typing in the pretransplant testing routine for cadaveric organ transplantation.

B. Typing for HLA Class I and Class II Antigens with Sequence-Specific Oligonucleotide Probes (SSOP): The PCR product obtained with primers for generic level or locus sequences can be further manipulated to reveal specific alleles within the amplified segment. The product can be probed with oligonucleotide probes specific for the sequence motifs that characterize the particular alle-

les, can be amplified by PCR again with more restrictive primers (nested PCR), or can be subjected to the RFLP process. Many SSOPs are required for clear resolution of HLA antigens at the allele level, which makes this method a more cumbersome and expensive procedure than SSP typing for low-volume laboratories.

1. Typing by SSOP: Oligonucleotide probes are short segments of single-stranded DNA, commonly 18–24 nucleotides long, each composed of a nucleotide sequence complementary to a particular polymorphic sequence motif found within the hypervariable regions of individual HLA alleles. These probes hybridize only to their exactly complementary sequences under stringent hybridization conditions (see Chapter 18). Even a single base pair difference causes the probes to break away from the pairing with the target DNA. This property of perfect sequence specificity gives this method of HLA typing the greatest power for resolution of HLA alleles.

Multiple probes are required to identify an HLA allele because of the sharing of sequence polymorphisms. The hybridization patterns with the panel of SSOPs identifies the specific allele in most instances. As the number of HLA alleles increases, so must the size of the SSOP panel so that all the possible hybridization patterns are demonstrable. Using the Eleventh International Histocompatibility Workshop collection of primers and probes for HLA class II typing, approximately 22 probes are required to identify an allele in the DR52-related group consisting of alleles of DR3, DR5, DR6 groups; DQB1 requires approximately 20, DQA1 17, and DR1 and DR2 each require 7 probes. Recent schemes for high-resolution typing for class I alleles currently require more than 39 probes for an initial generic screening followed by specific probes for individual alleles within the antigen group. As more alleles are discovered, this number will certainly increase. Some commercially available kits use fewer probes but consequently sacrifice completeness of allele coverage. The patterns produced by these probes identify the complex collection of polymorphisms that is characteristic of a particular allele. Table 17–13 shows the hybridization patterns for DR4 alleles using the Eleventh International Histocompatibility Workshop probes.

(a) The Dot-Blot Method of SSOP: In the initial PCR step, primer pairs are selected that amplify a region of DNA that contains sequences present in the antigen group of interest, for example, the DR4 group of alleles. Dots of amplified DNA product are allowed to adhere to a membrane in a "slot/dot-blot" fashion (Fig 17–8A), applying as many dots as there are probes. The blots are then cut into strips and each strip is exposed to a differently labeled probe. Probes can be labeled with radioactive or nonradioactive tags. Nonradioactive methods include the use of colorometric and luminescent dyes and are currently the method of choice. Hybridization conditions must be

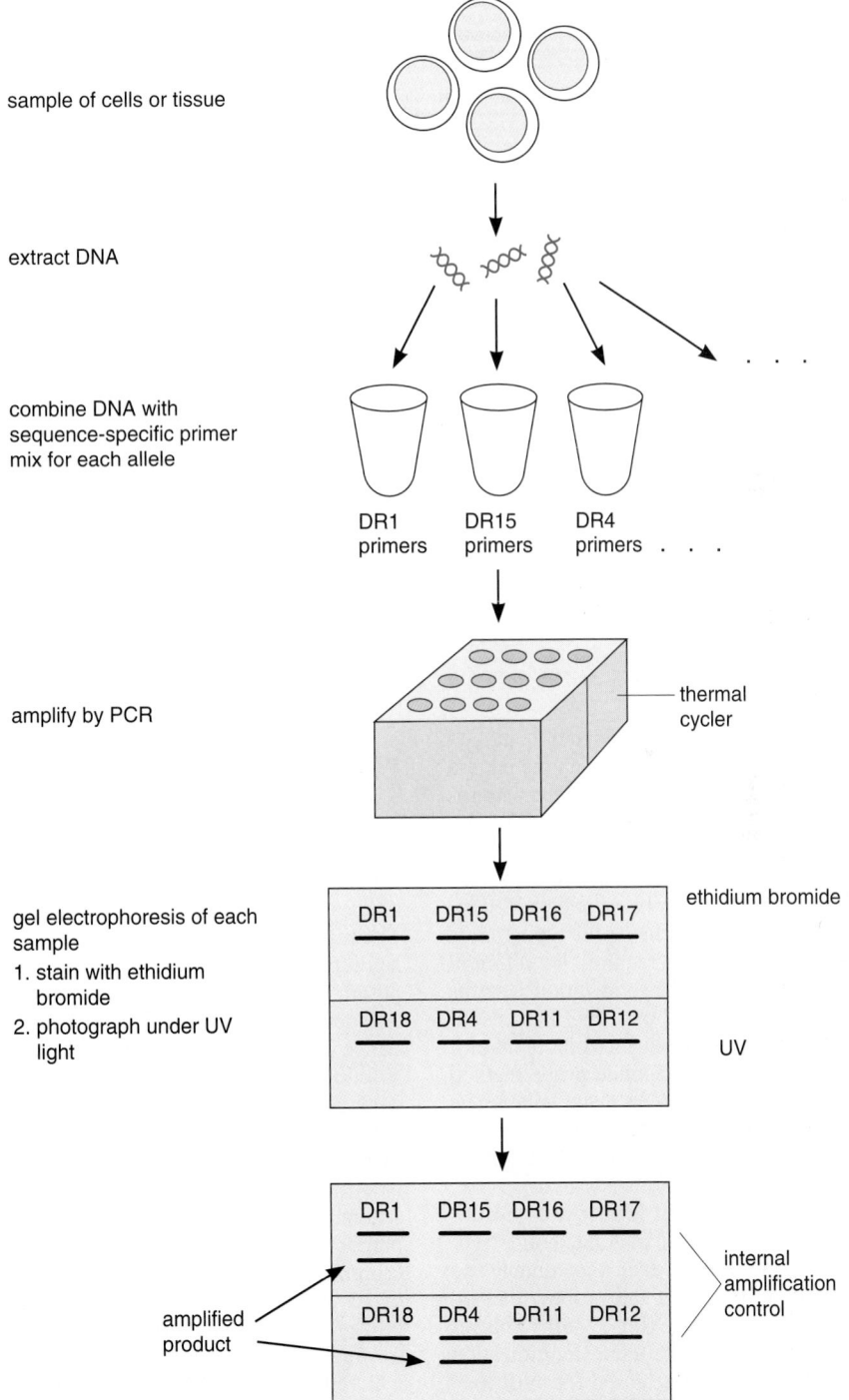

sample of cells or tissue

extract DNA

combine DNA with
sequence-specific primer
mix for each allele

DR1
primers

DR15
primers

DR4
primers . . .

amplify by PCR

thermal
cycler

gel electrophoresis of each
sample
1. stain with ethidium
   bromide
2. photograph under UV
   light

ethidium bromide

DR1   DR15   DR16   DR17

DR18   DR4   DR11   DR12

UV

DR1   DR15   DR16   DR17

DR18   DR4   DR11   DR12

internal
amplification
control

amplified
product

Figure 17–7. Typing for HLA class II by sequence-specific priming (SSP). DNA is extracted from the specimen (cells, tissue) and mixed with primers having specificity for the sequences characteristic of each of the alleles of the HLA class II locus being typed for (eg, loci such as DRB1, DRB3, DQB1, etc). Aliquots of the sample are placed in separate tubes, each containing a specific primer set, and amplified in the thermal cycler. The amplified products are electrophoresed and the gels stained with ethidium bromide and photographed under UV light. If the primers have hybridized with the sample DNA, a band is visible. The presence of the band indicates that the sample DNA had the sequence corresponding to the particular HLA allele. No amplification implies the absence of that particular allelic sequence in the sample DNA. All tubes contain an additional DNA template that hybridizes with all primers to serve as a control on PCR amplification success. This sample types as DR1, DR4 by SSP.

Table 17–13. Oligonucleotide hybridization patterns for DR4 alleles.[1]

DR4 Allele	Pattern with Oligonucleotide Probe:										
	WS 1004	WS 3701	WS 3704	WS 5701	WS 5702	WS 7001	WS 7005	WS 7006	WS 7007	WS 8601	WS 8603
0401	+		+	+			+			+	
0402	+		+	+					+		+
0403	+		+	+		+		+			+
0404	+		+	+		+					+
0405	+		+		+	+				+	
0406	+	+		+		+		+			+
0407	+		+	+		+		+		+	
0408	+		+	+		+				+	
0409	+		+		+		+			+	
0410	+		+		+	+					+
0411	+		+		+	+		+			+

[1] Hybridization patterns for alleles of the DR4 group which illustrate that class II molecules are composites of polymorphic sequences. Oligonucleotide probes are from the Eleventh International Histocompatibility Workshop.

optimized for each probe. After hybridization and development, the strips are reassembled, and the pattern of hybridization signals is compared with the patterns for known alleles. Figure 17–8A shows a result comparing signals from four individual samples being typed for DR4 alleles. The dot-blot technique is very labor-intensive because each probe must be added individually. For example, one scheme for typing class I alleles of the HLA-B locus requires 44 different probes. There are 84 resultant hybridization patterns that unambiguously identify 62 out of 93 B locus alleles in homozygous and heterozygous combinations.

HLA typing by the oligonucleotide probe method can reveal a new antigen when an unexplained new pattern of hybridization occurs. SSOP, however, can fail to detect a new sequence polymorphism if none of the probes can successfully hybridize with it.

(b) The Reverse Dot-Blot Method of SSOP Typing: A simpler method of oligonucleotide typing is to immobilize all the probes on a membrane and dot the amplified sample onto the probes, the so-called reverse dot blot technique (Fig 17–8B). This requires that all probes have the same hybridization conditions, a situation not yet achieved for most loci. In one schema, the probes are immobilized onto a membrane via their poly-dT synthesized tails, and the PCR product (amplicon) is labeled during the PCR process with biotin. After the applied amplicon hybridizes to the bound probe, streptavidin-horse radish peroxidase is then bound to the biotinylated probe-amplicon complex. After incubation with a chromogenic or chemiluminescent substrate, the developed color marks the pattern of probe hybridization and indicates the particular allele present.

C. Other HLA Typing Methods Involving PCR-Amplified Products

1. PCR-RFLP–Systems for class II typing have been devised that treat the PCR-amplified product with bacterial restriction enzymes and use gel electrophoresis to visualize the fragments produced. Alleles are identified by characteristic band patterns. The region to be amplified is chosen to be specific to a group of antigens, for example, the DQ1 group composed of DQ5 and DQ6 (group-specific priming). Aliquots of the resultant product are each digested with a different enzyme chosen for the presence of restriction sites within the amplified sequence. The resulting fragments are separated on polyacrilamide gels and stained with ethidium bromide. The fragment-length patterns that are visualized are characteristic for many but not all alleles. In some methods, a second round of restriction enzymes is used on the products of the first digestion to achieve further discrimination. This method is simpler than application of 10–30 (or more) oligonucleotide probes to immobilized PCR product but currently lacks the capacity for fine resolution of alleles.

2. HLA Typing by DNA Sequencing (Sequence-Based Typing—"SBT")–In this HLA-typing method, PCR products derived from the polymorphic regions of HLA class I and class II genes are directly sequenced to determine an HLA specificity. For the application of direct sequencing to histocompatibility testing, the most practical approach is to use the fluorescence-based automated sequencing technology now commercially available. The typing strategy involves a preliminary PCR step in which a sample of genomic DNA is amplified with primers selected to

dot/slot blot technique

A

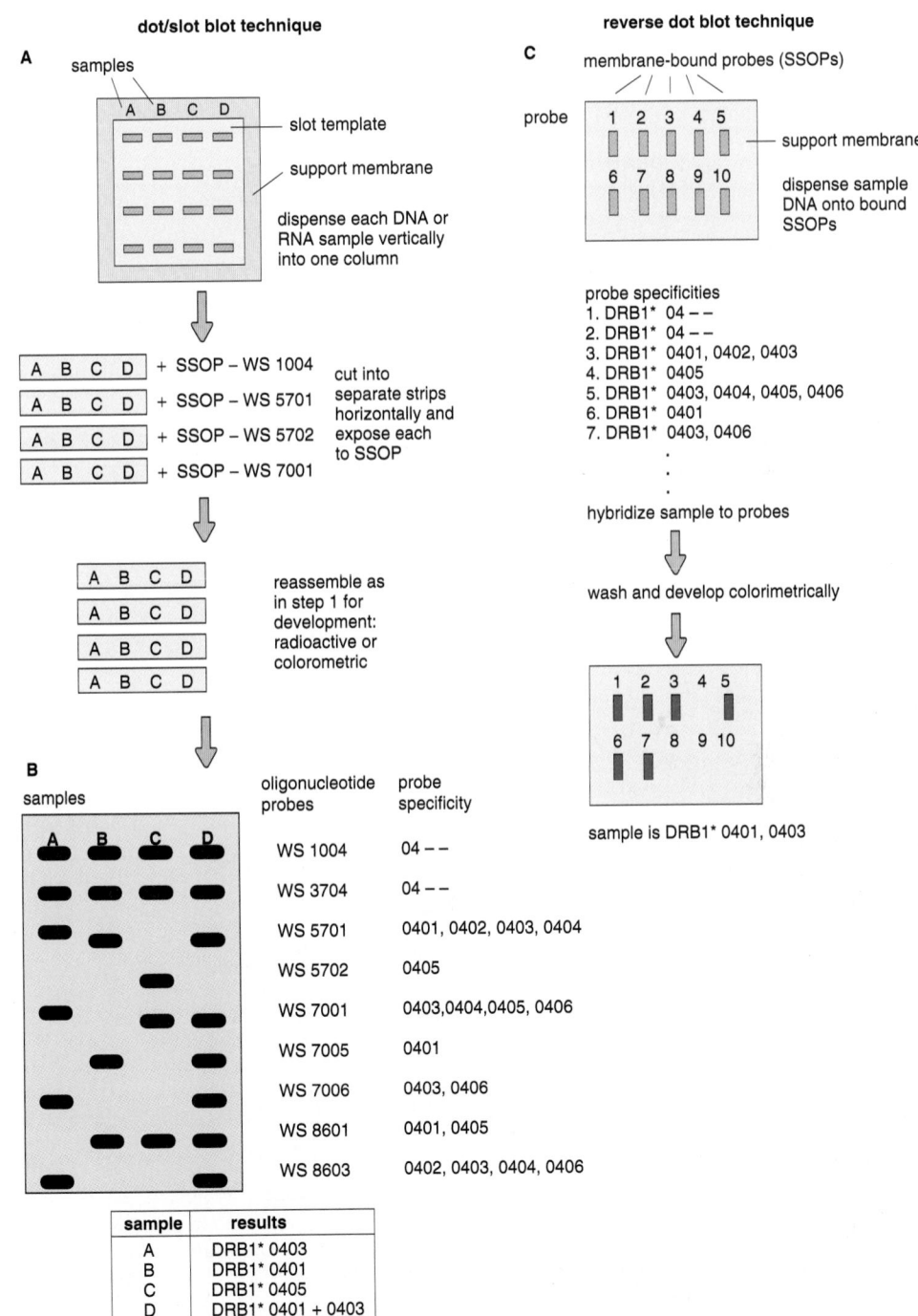

reverse dot blot technique

C

membrane-bound probes (SSOPs)

probe specificities
1. DRB1* 04 – –
2. DRB1* 04 – –
3. DRB1* 0401, 0402, 0403
4. DRB1* 0405
5. DRB1* 0403, 0404, 0405, 0406
6. DRB1* 0401
7. DRB1* 0403, 0406

hybridize sample to probes

wash and develop colorimetrically

sample is DRB1* 0401, 0403

oligonucleotide probes	probe specificity
WS 1004	04 – –
WS 3704	04 – –
WS 5701	0401, 0402, 0403, 0404
WS 5702	0405
WS 7001	0403,0404,0405, 0406
WS 7005	0401
WS 7006	0403, 0406
WS 8601	0401, 0405
WS 8603	0402, 0403, 0404, 0406

sample	results
A	DRB1* 0403
B	DRB1* 0401
C	DRB1* 0405
D	DRB1* 0401 + 0403

Figure 17–8. HLA typing by sequence-specific oligonucleotide probes. *(A):* Samples of DNA (or RNA) (A, B, C, or D) are dotted directly onto a support membrane by using a slotted template (the slot blot). Replicates of a single sample are placed into a single column of slots. After all samples have been dispensed, the membrane is cut horizontally into strips. Individual probes that are specific and diagnostic for individual HLA alleles, such as DR1 and DR2, are prepared. Each strip is hybridized with a different radiolableled sequence-specific oligonucleotide probe (SSOP). The probes hybridize only to an exactly complementary nucleotide sequence in the sample. *(B):* The membrane is reassembled and developed by autoradiography or colorimetrically. A band indicates the presence in the sample of the sequence of the corresponding HLA allele, and the antigen can be assigned, as illustrated here. *(C):* In the reverse dot-blot, the sequence-specific probes are bound to the membrane support, and the sample DNA is dotted onto the probes. Sample DNA is allowed to hybridize, the membrane is washed, and the hybridized probe-plus-sample DNA spots are developed by colorimetric methods.

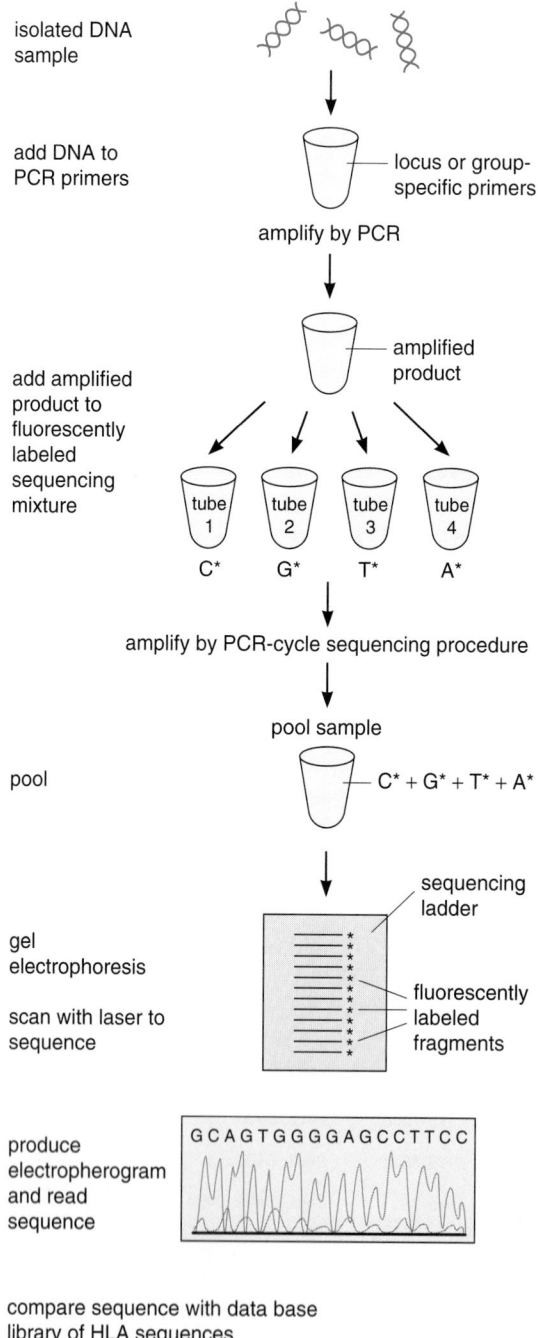

Figure 17–9. Automated DNA sequence-based HLA typing. DNA is isolated from a cell or tissue sample and amplified by PCR, using locus or group-specific primers. The amplified product is distributed into four tubes, each one a polymerase, dNTPs, and sequencing mixtures. Each of the four sequencing mixtures is labeled with a fluorescently tagged sequence terminator: tube 1 with labeled cytosine (C*), tube 2 with labeled guanine (G*), tube 3 with labeled thymine (T*), and tube 4 with labeled adenine (A*). The product is amplified by PCR to incorporate the labeled terminators. The four sample tubes are pooled and electrophoresed to form a sequencing ladder, which is scanned by the laser to generate the DNA sequence electropherogram. Software compares the sequence to the library of HLA antigen sequences and assigns the HLA antigens.

produce a group or a locus-specific product, for example, a product (or products) specific to the HLA-A locus that contains all the polymorphic sequences known to reside in the A locus. The resultant PCR products can be large, for example, more than 600 bp long; however, the chemistry available can sequence only 500–700 bases. Primer pairs are designed to amplify shorter regions within this first PCR product (nested PCR) so that these smaller segments can be sequenced in both 3′ to 5′ and 5′ to 3′ directions. Bidirectional sequencing provides confirmation of the accuracy of the sequence. Following the initial amplification, the template undergoes a PCR cyclic sequencing process. Two different labeling procedures are in use to produce fluorescently tagged sequence fragments: one in which the primers are labeled and the other in which the sequence terminators are labeled. In one schema (Fig 17–9), four separate sequence reaction tubes are prepared in which one of the four bases—T, A, C, or G—is labeled with a uniquely colored fluorescent dye. The generated DNA fragments are then pooled and subjected to gel electrophoresis to produce a ladder chromatogram. The ladders are automatically scanned for position (fragment size) and color by laser beam, and an electropherogram is produced showing position versus relative fragment intensity of fluorescence. The intensities of the peaks are examined with particular attention to the positions of known polymorphism. The nucleotide sequences are then compared with a library of HLA antigen sequences, and the antigens are assigned based on sequence identity. Occasionally, interpretation of the relative color intensities of the two bases at a given position either is ambiguous or one of the bases may be missed altogether. Such ambiguities are often resolvable by inspecting the counterdirection sequence. Of more concern is the likelihood that a heterozygous combination of alleles could produce the same sequence pattern. If serologic or DNA generic typing data is available, however, the field of candidate HLA antigens can be narrowed, and at least some of the ambiguities become irrelevant. Typing by sequencing is under intense development to improve the efficiency and convenience of the technology. It may be some time before the automatic sequencer replaces the basic serologic and DNA/PCR techniques, but the sequencing of DNA remains the ultimate defining technique for identification of known and new HLA alleles.

Molecular Testing Methods for Histocompatibility and Genetic Identity Determination

A. Heteroduplex Analysis Applied to Histocompatibility Testing: Molecular HLA typing per se may not be required when only a preliminary assessment of genetic identity is desired, as between serologically typed HLA-identical siblings or when multiple donors are available for unrelated bone marrow transplantation.

1. Heteroduplex Formation–Single-stranded conformational polymorphism (PCR-SSCP) is a rapid method that uses the property that denatured DNA strands reanneal into heteroduplexes (ie, to form a double helix in alternative combinations that are less than perfectly matched at all base pairs). If the individuals are genetically disparate for HLA alleles, mismatching at the polymorphic bases modifies the bending or increases the superhelical diameter of the DNA and causes a retardation in its electrophoretic mobility (see Chapter 18). When denatured DNA from two genetically disparate individuals is mixed, novel heteroduplexes form, generating new band patterns in electrophoresis. Thus, the genetic identity between two individuals can be quickly assessed by mixing PCR DNA from their HLA genes. Alternatively, a reference DNA for a single allele or a synthetic universal heteroduplex generator (UHG) molecule can be added to a PCR sample. This forms heteroduplex complexes that are unique for each allele, thus generating unique diagnostic bands and, thereby, a new polymorphism that must be carefully characterized.

2. VNTR and STR Typing–The human genome contains stretches of highly repetitious sequences, often occurring in clusters. The number of the repetitions in a cluster varies among individuals, giving a variable number of tandem repeats (VNTR). This polymorphism can be translated into fragments of variable length by PCR amplification with primers designed to amplify the region of repetition. VNTRs are typically 10–50 bases in length, and genetic polymorphisms of shorter sequences known as short tandem repeats (STRs) of 4–9 bp in length are also used for DNA "fingerprinting" (ie, identification of individual genomic DNA differences). VNTR and STR analysis is used as a genetic marker both in clinical and forensic applications. VNTRs can be analyzed by electrophoresis of either genomic or PCR-amplified DNA. Primers to flanking regions of the repetitive sequence cluster produce adequate PCR product for analysis even when the samples are minute or degraded. A most important clinical application of VNTR is the monitoring of engraftment of bone marrow transplant recipients when the marrow donor is HLA-identical to the patient. VNTR testing can reveal a chimeric state in which both the donor and the patient's original phenotypes can be found in the peripheral blood or bone marrow sample. Parentage testing can use either VNTR patterns or HLA allelic typing to determine exclusion of an alleged father in cases of disputed paternity.

Molecular HLA-typing methods provide the most accurate strategies for HLA class I and class II typing and the determination of genetic identity and compatibility. The challenge for molecular methods is the need to produce an HLA-typing result in a timely and cost-effective manner so that the benefits of precise molecular typing can be applied to the time-critical demands of organ donor testing for transplantation as well as for precise matching for bone marrow transplantation. There is every expectation that these requirements will be fully met within the decade.

REFERENCES

GENERAL

Arnett KL, Parham P: HLA class I nucleotide sequences, 1995. *Tissue Antigens* 1995;**46:**217.

Dyer P, Middleton D: *Histocompatibility Testing: A Practical Approach.* Oxford University Press, New York, 1993.

Marsh SGE, Bodmer JG: HLA class II region nucleotide sequences, 1995. *Tissue Antigens* 1995;**46:**258.

Phelan DL et al (editors): *ASHI Laboratory Manual,* 3rd ed. American Society for Histocompatibility and Immunogenetics, 1994.

Suzuki T (editor): *HLA 1991.* Oxford University Press, 1992.

SPECIAL METHODS

Böyum A: Separation of leukocytes from blood and bone marrow. *Scand J Clin Lab Invest* 1968;**21**(suppl):97.

Cook DJ et al: An approach to reducing early kidney transplant failure by flow cytometry crossmatching. *Clin Transplants* 1987;**1:**253.

Fuller TC et al: Antigenic specificity of antibody reactive in the antiglobulin-augmented lymphocytotoxicity test. *Transplantation* 1982;**34:**24.

Hirschberg H et al: Cell mediated lymphocytes: CML. A microplate technique requiring few target cells and employing a new method of supernatant collection. *J Immunol Methods* 1977;**16:**131.

Lee P, Garovoy MR: Flow cytometry crossmatching. The first 10 years. In: *Transplantation Reviews* 1994 (ed. N. Tilney, & P. Morris), Vol 8:1–14.

Rudy T, Opelz G: Dithiothreitol treatment of crossmatch sera in highly immunized transplant recipients. *Transplant Proc* 1987;**19:**800.

Terasaki PI et al: Microdroplet testing for HLA-A, -B, -C and -D antigens. *Am J Clin Pathol* 1978;**69:**103.

HLA AND TRANSPLANTATION

Mahoney RJ et al: The flow cytometry crossmatch and early renal transplant loss. *Transplantation* 1990;**49:**527.

Sutherland DER et al: Pancreas transplant results in United Network for Organ Sharing. In: *Clinical Transplants 1993.* Terasaki PI, Cecka JM (editors). UCLA Tissue Typing Laboratory, 1994, p. 47.

Terasaki PI et al: A ten-year prediction for kidney transplantation survival. In: *Clinical Transplants 1992.* Terasaki PI, Cecka JM (editors). UCLA Tissue Typing Laboratory, 1993, p. 501.

Zhou YC, Cecka JM: Effect of HLA matching on renal transplant survival. In: *Clinical Transplants 1993.*

Terasaki PI and Cecka JM (editors). UCLA Tissue Typing Laboratory, 1994, p. 499.

MOLECULAR-BIOLOGIC TECHNIQUES

Bein G et al: Rapid HLA-DRB1 genotyping by nested PCR amplification. *Tissue Antigens* 1992;**39:**68.

Bidwell J: Advances in DNA-based HLA-typing methods. *Immunol Today* 1994;**15:**303.

Bidwell JL et al: A DNA RFLP typing system that positively identifies serologically well-defined and ill-defined HLA-DR and -DQ alleles, including DRw10. *Transplantation* 1988;**45:**640.

Bugawan TL et al: A method for typing polymorphism at the HLA-A locus using PCR amplification and immobilized oligonucleotide probes. *Tissue Antigens* 1994;**44:**137.

Carrington M et al: Typing of HLA-DQA1 and DQB1 using DNA single strand conformation polymorphism. *Hum Immunol* 1992;**33:**208.

Coen DM: The polymerase chain reaction. In: *Current Protocols in Molecular Biology,* Supplement 16 15.0.3. Ausubel FM (editor) Greene Publishing, John Wiley & Sons, 1991.

Jeffreys AJ et al: Hypervariable "minisatellite" regions in human DNA *Nature* 1985;**314:**67.

Jeffreys AJ et al: Individual specific fingerprints of human DNA. *Nature* 1985;**316:**76.

Olerup O, Zetterquist H: HLA-DR typing by PCR amplification with sequence-specific primers (PCR-SSP) in 2 hours: An alternative to serological DR typing in clinical practice including donor-recipient matching in cadaveric transplantation. *Tissue Antigens* 1992;**39:**225.

Opelz G et al: *Transplantation* 1993;**55:**782.

Ota M et al: HLA-DRB1 genotyping by modified PCR-RFLP method combined with group-specific primers. *Tissue Antigens* 1992;**39:**187.

Petersdorf EW, Hansen JA: A comprehensive approach for typing the alleles of the HLA-B locus by automated sequencing. *Tissue Antigens* 1995;**46:**73.

Santamaria P et al: HLA class II "typing": Direct sequencing of DRB, DQB and DQA genes. *Hum Immunol* 1992;**33:**69.

Shaffer AL et al: HLA-DRw52-associated DRB1 alleles: Identification using polymerase chain reaction-amplified DNA, sequence-specific oligonucleotide probes, and a chemiluminescent detection system. *Tissue Antigens* 1992;**39:**84.

Molecular Genetic Techniques for Clinical Analysis of the Immune System

Tristram G. Parslow, MD, PhD

Genetic information in humans and most other organisms is encoded in the linear sequence of four nucleotide bases (abbreviated A, T, G, and C) along the strands of a DNA molecule. The sequence of the human genome is more than 3 billion DNA bases long, is divided among 23 chromosomes, and is present twice in each diploid nucleus. The human genome contains an estimated 100,000 genes, each comprising, on average, no more than a few thousand bases of coding sequence that specify a particular protein or structural RNA. The coding information of a typical human gene is rarely contained in a single, uninterrupted stretch of DNA but, instead, is divided into shorter coding segments called **exons,** which are separated by noncoding regions called **introns.** Individual genes are also widely separated from one another along the DNA, with noncoding sequences in between. Altogether, coding sequences are thought to make up only 5–10% of the human genome, and the function of the remaining sequences is, for the most part, unknown. The complete sequences of many human genes have been determined (by using techniques that lie outside the scope of this chapter), but the sequences that are known at present amount to only a tiny fraction of the entire genome.

During the past two decades, advances in nucleic acid chemistry and recombinant DNA technology have made it possible to analyze individual genes rapidly and precisely. The techniques involved are now commonplace in research and are gradually being adapted for use in clinical laboratories as well. DNA offers numerous advantages as a substrate for clinical analysis: it is a remarkably sturdy biomolecule that is fairly easy to handle; it can be obtained from either fresh or fixed tissue or blood specimens; and it can be manipulated and dissected in ways that are not possible with proteins. Most importantly, access to the information contained in DNA enables us to diagnose and investigate many disease processes at the most fundamental level. This chapter summarizes the basic concepts and practical techniques for ana-

lyzing DNA from clinical specimens, along with some specialized applications to the immune system. At the end of the chapter, related techniques for studying cellular RNA are briefly discussed.

NUCLEIC ACID PROBES

Underlying the complexity of DNA is a simple but profound symmetry. Each DNA molecule is composed of two linear strands of bases, which are bound to each other side by side and coiled to form a double helix (Fig 18–1). The two strands are held together by hydrogen bonding between adjacent bases: A on one strand always binds to T on the other, and similar binding occurs between G and C. In normal DNA, the two strands are said to be **complementary** in that every base is appropriately paired to the corresponding position on the opposite strand. Bases within a strand are held together by strong covalent bonds, but the base-pairing bonds between strands are relatively weak, so that the two strands can easily be separated (**"denatured"** or "melted apart") by heat or alkaline pH. When slowly returned to physiologic conditions, the strands reanneal spontaneously and in perfect alignment to re-form the original double-stranded helix.

This spontaneous pairing between complementary strands provides the basis for many of the techniques that are used to detect and characterize genes. These techniques employ short strands of known sequence as **probes** to detect strands with the complementary sequence. Probes of any desired sequence can readily be obtained in abundant quantities and at very high purity: single DNA strands up to about 100 bases long are easily prepared by using automated chemical synthesizers, whereas larger DNA sequences are generally introduced ("cloned") into bacteria to be replicated biologically. It is also possible to use probes made of RNA—a molecule that, for the purposes of this chapter, can be considered equivalent to single-stranded DNA—since these also anneal specifically

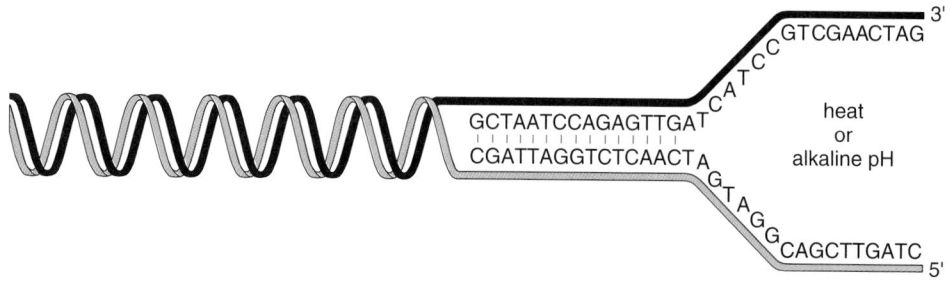

GTCGAACTAG 3'
C
C
A
T
GCTAATCCAGAGTTGAT
| | | | | | | | | | | | | | | | |
CGATTAGGTCTCAACT
A
G
T
A
G
G
CAGCTTGATC 5'

heat
or
alkaline pH

Figure 18–1. Structure of DNA. The molecule consists of two strands of covalently linked nucleotide bases, which are coiled around each other to form a double helix. The two strands are held together by relatively weak hydrogen bonds between bases. The strands dissociate from each other when exposed to heat or alkaline pH but spontaneously reassociate when returned to physiologic conditions.

to a complementary DNA strand. RNA probes are most often prepared enzymatically by cloning the corresponding DNA sequence and using this as a template for in vitro transcription, that is, producing a complementary RNA strand from the template DNA.

Cellular DNA can be isolated by chemical extraction from a blood or tissue specimen followed by enzymatic treatment to remove traces of contaminating RNA or protein. Unless special precautions are taken, the extremely long strands of chromosomal DNA are

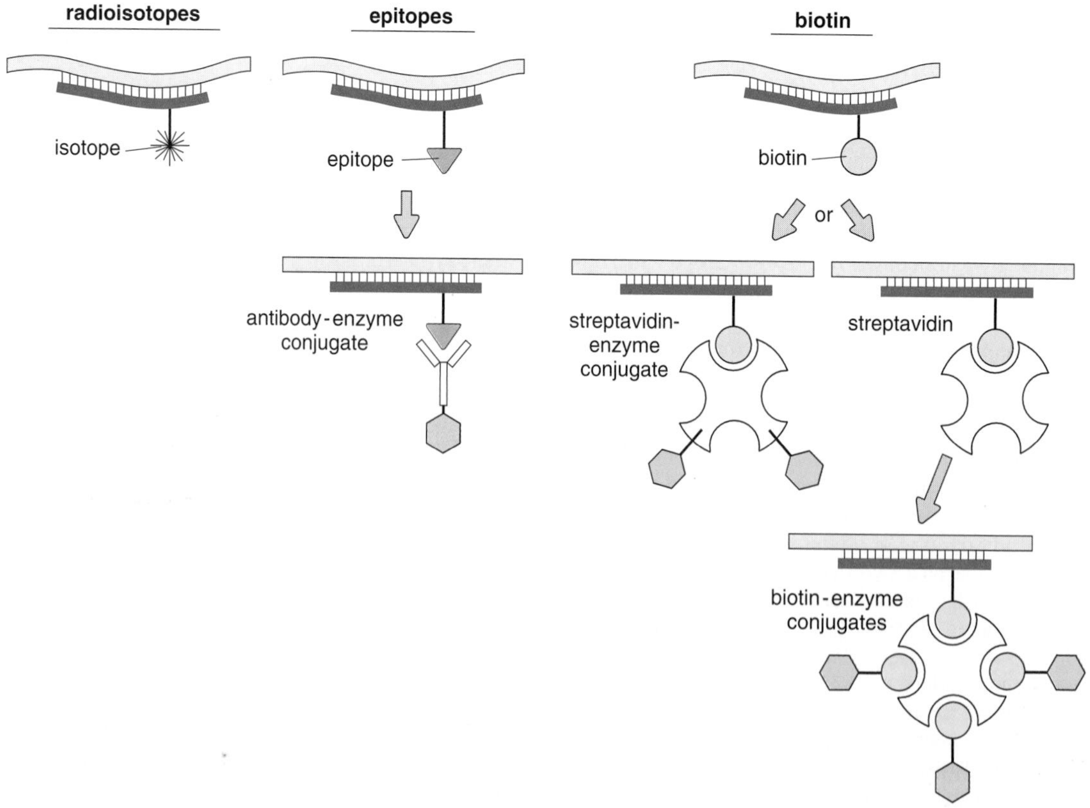

radioisotopes

isotope — ✳

epitopes

epitope — ▽

antibody-enzyme
conjugate

biotin

biotin — ◯

or

streptavidin-
enzyme
conjugate

streptavidin

biotin-enzyme
conjugates

Figure 18–2. Some methods for labeling and detecting DNA or RNA probes. Radioisotopes, small epitopes, or biotin can be incorporated covalently into one or more positions in a probe at the time of synthesis. The most commonly used radioisotopes for this purpose are ^{32}P and ^{35}S, which can be detected by autoradiography or scintillation counting. Probes labeled with epitopes or biotin can be detected by secondary labeling with an enzyme conjugated to a specific antibody or to the polyvalent biotin-binding protein, streptavidin. One variation on the latter technique uses unconjugated streptavidin alone, which is then detected by binding of a biotin–enzyme conjugate. The enzyme used most commonly in these procedures is alkaline phosphatase, which can readily be assayed by its ability to generate chromogenic or chemiluminescent products.

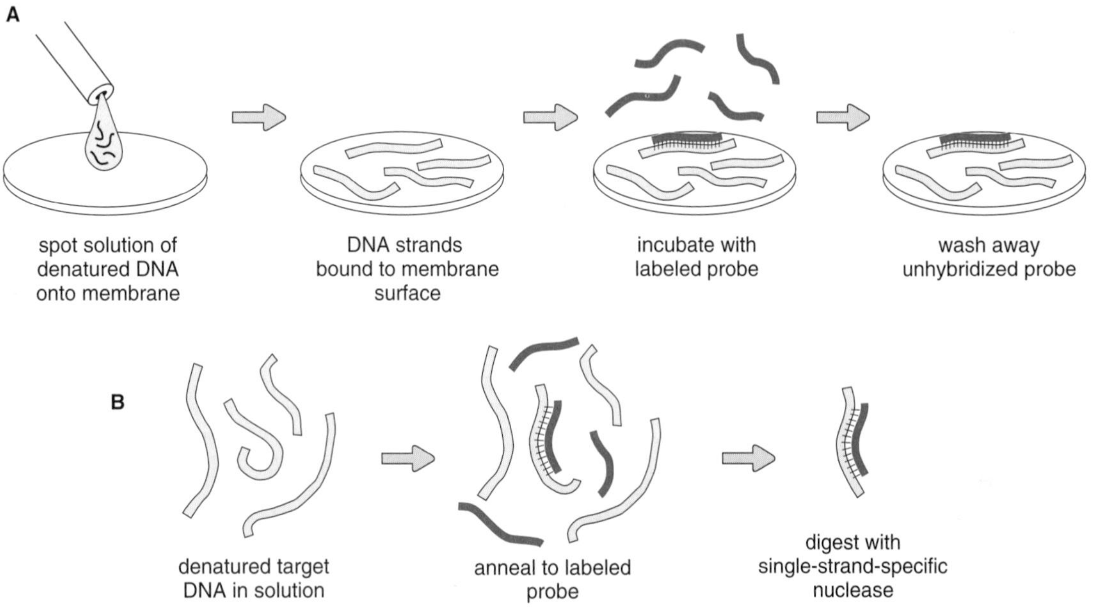

Figure 18–3. Two simple hybridization assays using nucleic acid probes. **A:** In the dot blot assay, denatured target DNA is attached to the surface of a nylon or nitrocellulose membrane and then incubated with a solution of labeled probe. **B:** In the nuclease protection assay, the reaction between probe and denatured target DNA takes place in solution; probes that have annealed to a target strand are detected by their ability to resist digestion by an enzyme (such as nuclease S1) that specifically digests single-stranded but not double-stranded nucleic acids.

usually sheared by mechanical forces into random fragments of roughly 50,000–100,000 bp during the purification process. To use a nucleic acid probe, this target DNA is first heated or exposed to alkali in order to separate the strands and then mixed with the labeled probe and returned to normal temperature and pH. As the molecules reassociate, some of the target strands anneal (**"hybridize"**) to the probe rather than to the unlabeled complementary strand, forming labeled duplexes. To maximize the likelihood that a target strand will anneal to the probe rather than to its original partner, the hybridization reaction is usually carried out with a great molar excess of probe. The stability of the complex formed by a probe and its target is influenced by many factors, the most important of which are temperature, salt concentration, the length and base composition of the probe, and the presence of any mismatched bases. Under the conditions used in most assays, two strands must share at least 16–20 consecutive bases of perfect complementarity to form a stable hybrid. The probability of such a match occurring by chance is less than one in a billion (10^{-9}). Thus, nucleic acid probes possess an extraordinary degree of specificity: a typical probe is capable of recognizing and binding selectively to a single copy of its complementary sequence among the 3 billion bp in the human genome. DNA or RNA probes can easily by tagged with radioisotopes, fluorochromes, or enzymatic markers prior to use (Fig 18–2) and can then act as "molecu-lar stains" that recognize and bind only to the exact complementary sequence.

HYBRIDIZATION ASSAYS

Several different methods can be used to test whether a DNA specimen contains sequences complementary to a particular probe. One common approach takes advantage of the fact that, under certain conditions (eg, when exposed to ultraviolet light or when heated in the presence of high salt), DNA strands can be made to bind tightly onto nylon or nitrocellulose membranes. In a procedure called **dot blot hybridization** (Fig 18–3A), a solution of target DNA is denatured, spotted onto the surface of such a membrane, and then treated so that the separated DNA strands adhere irreversibly to the membrane. When immobilized in this manner, the target strands remain accessible on the membrane surface but are prevented from reannealing with one another. The membrane is then incubated with labeled probes under conditions in which the probe does not adhere to the membrane but may hybridize with the target strands. Afterward, the filter is washed extensively to remove unhybridized probe. Any probe that has hybridized to the bound DNA can then be detected by autoradiography or enzymatic assay, depending on the particular label that it carries.

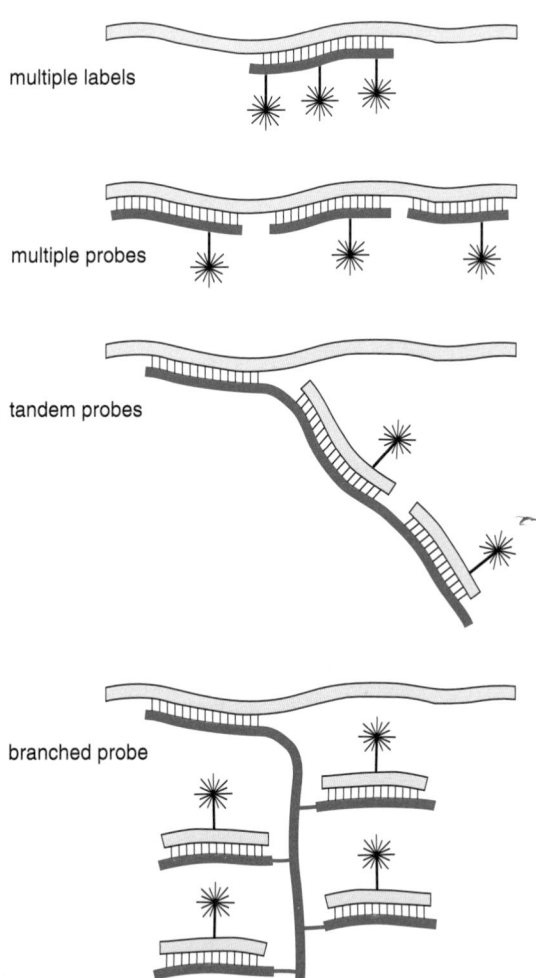

multiple labels

multiple probes

tandem probes

branched probe

Figure 18–4. Some approaches for increasing the sensitivity of nucleic acid hybridization assays. These can be used singly or in combination.

In an alternative approach, called a **nuclease protection** assay, target and probe DNAs are denatured, allowed to anneal together in solution, and then treated with an enzyme that specifically cleaves single-stranded but not double-stranded DNA. A probe survives this enzymatic digestion only if it has become stably hybridized to the target DNA (Fig 18–3B).

The interaction between probe and target occurs with one-to-one stoichiometry, and this tends to limit the sensitivity of hybridization assays. One way of maximizing the signal obtained is to incorporate multiple labels into a single probe, such as by radioactively labeling many bases in the probe (Fig 18–4). It may also be appropriate to use multiple probes that each recognize adjacent regions of a longer target sequence or to attach secondary probes onto a long, unhybridized "tail" on the primary probe (see Fig 18–4). A recent innovation is to attach short DNA side chains

onto the primary probe by means of synthetic chemistry, creating an artificial **branched DNA** molecule that can interact with many copies of a secondary probe. Still another approach is to use probes that form polyvalent complexes with an enzyme or fluorochrome marker, similar to those used in immunohistochemistry (see Chapter 14). For example, hybrids containing a probe that has been labeled with biotin can first be incubated with the polyvalent biotin-binding protein streptavidin and then secondarily tagged with many copies of a biotinylated marker enzyme (see Fig 18–2). The use of enzymatic detection systems that produce colored or chemiluminescent products can itself greatly amplify the signal obtained. Even when such measures are taken, however, about 10^4–10^5 copies of a target sequence must usually be present in a sample to be detectable by routine hybridization.

SOUTHERN BLOT

The simplest hybridization assays, such as the dot blot assay, indicate whether a particular sequence is present in the target DNA and may also give an estimate of its abundance. These assays are rarely used clinically, because easier and more sensitive tests can provide the same information (see the section, Target Amplification Techniques). Nucleic acid probes, however, offer special advantages when they are used in conjunction with **restriction enzymes,** a class of bacterial enzymes that cut both strands of a linear DNA molecule at specific short recognition sequences, usually 4–6 bp long. For example, the enzyme *Eco*RI cuts only within the sequence GAATTC, whereas the enzyme *Bam*HI cleaves only GGATCC. Each restriction enzyme therefore cleaves long target DNA molecules into specific smaller segments called **restriction fragments,** whose number and length are determined by the sequence of the substrate DNA.

Because of the enormous size and complexity of the human genome, cleaving human DNA with a restriction enzyme yields millions of unique restriction fragments ranging up to tens of thousands of bases long. Nevertheless, the fragment that carries any particular gene can readily be identified, provided that a DNA probe complementary to the gene is available. The technique used for this purpose (Fig 18–5A) is called the **Southern blot,** after its inventor, E. M. Southern. DNA extracted from a tissue or blood specimen is first cleaved with one or more restriction enzymes, and the resulting DNA fragments are then subjected to electrophoresis through an agarose gel, which separates them according to length. Afterward, the gel is immersed in alkali solution to melt apart the complementary strands of each fragment. A sheet of nylon or nitrocellulose is then pressed firmly against the gel; the denatured DNA fragments bind tightly to this sheet and are drawn out of the gel. When the sheet is peeled away, it retains on its surface the immobilized DNA

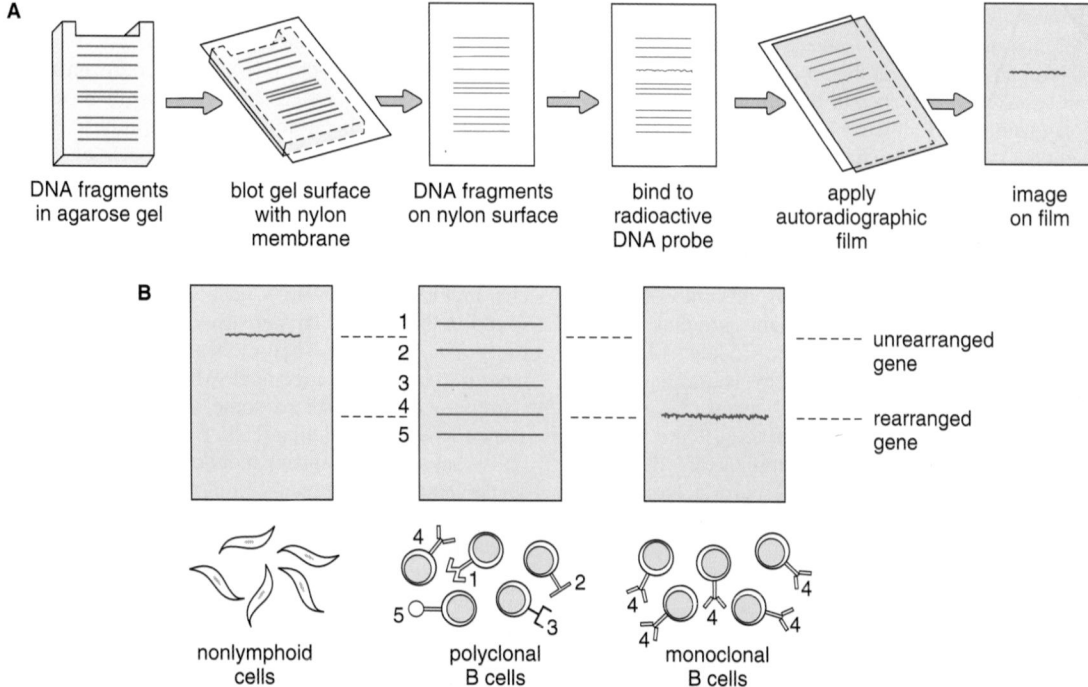

Figure 18–5. The Southern blot technique and an application of this technique to determining clonality of lymphoid cell populations. **A:** The blotting technique is described in the text; it can be used to determine the size of DNA restriction fragments that encompass a specific gene. **B:** DNA rearrangement in lymphocytes alters the sizes of fragments bearing the immunoglobulin or T-cell receptor genes: the sizes of the rearranged fragments are characteristic of each B-cell or T-cell clone. This provides a means of detecting B or T cells and of assessing the clonal composition of lymphoid populations. The approach is illustrated for B cells by using an immunoglobulin gene. DNA isolated from nonlymphoid cells contains only unrearranged immunoglobulin genes, whereas DNA from normal lymphocyte populations reveals many different rearranged genes—one from each of the many independent B-cell clones. Detection of only a single rearranged gene suggests that a lymphocyte population is monoclonal and therefore possibly malignant.

fragments, still arranged according to length as they had been in the gel but now exposed and accessible to further analysis. The sheet is then incubated with the labeled probe, which binds only to the fragment bearing its complementary sequence. Unbound probe is washed away, and the location of the remaining hybridized probe is determined by virtue of the label that it carries. The size of the bound target fragment can then be deduced from its location on the membrane, as this corresponds to the distance it migrated in the agarose gel.

The Southern blot reveals not only the presence of a particular sequence but also the size of the restriction fragment on which it lies. This size, in turn, is determined by the distribution of nearby restriction sites and so reflects the local DNA sequence.

GENE REARRANGEMENT ASSAY FOR LYMPHOCYTE CLONALITY

If all the cells in a population contain identical DNA, the restriction fragment carrying any given gene will have the same length in every cell, and all of these

fragments will appear together as a single band on a Southern blot. This is the case for most cellular genes, including the immunoglobulin (Ig) and T-cell receptor (TCR) genes of nonlymphoid cells. In lymphocytes, however, the Ig and TCR genes undergo specific rearrangements (see Chapter 7), which markedly alter the DNA sequences in and around these loci. Such rearrangements can be detected on the Southern blot by a shift in the size of the restriction fragment that carries an Ig or TCR gene. Moreover, because the size of the shifted fragment depends on the exact rearrangement that has occurred, it represents a unique and characteristic property of each lymphocyte clone—a molecular fingerprint that can be used to distinguish one lymphoid clone from another.

This provides a powerful means of estimating the clonal composition of lymphocyte populations (Fig 18–5B). In normal polyclonal lymphocyte populations, each of the innumerable clones contributes its own distinctively sized Ig or TCR fragment, but none of these is abundant enough to be detectable. Only when large numbers of clonally related cells are present do the rearranged genes appear in sufficient quantity to produce a detectable band. The presence of abnormally sized Ig or TCR bands on the Southern blot thus suggests the presence of a predominant clone of lymphoid cells, and this, in an appropriate setting, can be taken as evidence of lymphoid malignancy.

By using the Southern blot assay, clonal rearrangements of the Ig heavy-chain genes can be found in the neoplastic B cells in essentially all cases of B-cell lymphoma regardless of histologic type. The clinical utility of this approach is somewhat limited, however, because B-cell clonality can often be assessed more easily and cheaply by comparing the ratio of kappa (κ) and lambda (λ) light-chain proteins, using immunohistochemical stains (see Chapter 14). Nevertheless, the rearrangement assay is invaluable for demonstrating clonality in cases when malignant B cells either fail to express Ig protein or are heavily contaminated with polyclonal lymphocytes. Ig heavy-chain gene rearrangements are usually demonstrable in the lymphoid blast crisis of chronic myelogenous leukemia, in hairy cell leukemia, in "non-T, non-B" acute lymphoblastic leukemia, and in most null large cell lymphomas (see Chapter 46).

The analysis of TCR rearrangements has even greater potential usefulness, since no other practical method is available for assessing T-cell clonality. For technical reasons, most clinical assays focus on the TCR β-chain genes, which have been found to be clonally rearranged in nearly all cases of T-cell leukemia and lymphoma, including plaque- or tumor-stage mycosis fungoides, Sézary syndrome, and adult T-cell leukemia–lymphoma. The assay is especially useful for distinguishing reactive lymphadenopathy from T cell lymphoma (see Chapter 46).

Although Ig and TCR gene rearrangements are generally confined to the B- and T-cell lineages, respectively, the correlation is not absolute. Roughly 15% of poorly differentiated lymphoid malignancies harbor rearrangements of both TCR β- and Ig heavy-chain genes—an example of lineage infidelity. Ig light-chain rearrangements, which occur later in normal ontogeny than heavy-chain rearrangements (see Chapter 7), are more specific for the B lineage but less sensitive for detecting clonality. Absence of any rearrangements argues strongly that a tumor is not of lymphoid origin. Specimens from separate lymphomatous lesions in a single patient usually show identical rearrangements. Because the rearrangements in recurrent cancers are identical to those seen prior to treatment, the Southern blot technique offers special advantages in monitoring remission and recurrence, since it may reveal persistence of a malignant clone that is not yet detectable morphologically.

The Southern assay for lymphocyte clonality has several limitations. Although it is potentially more sensitive than histologic examination (a clonal subpopulation can be detected even when diluted 100-fold with polyclonal cells), this degree of sensitivity requires prior knowledge of the position of an abnormal band on the gel. Faint bands seen in a case being

analyzed de novo must be interpreted with great care, since they may represent technical artifacts. To minimize degradation of the DNA, fresh or frozen tissue must be used and processing must begin promptly. The method has been applied successfully to specimens obtained during fine-needle biopsies of lymph nodes, but obtaining sufficient DNA for a complete analysis generally requires a blood or tissue specimen that contains at least 25 million leukocytes.

It is also important to recognize that the TCR β locus includes far fewer V-gene segments than are found in the Ig loci. This greatly increases the probability that unrelated T-cell clones will coincidentally have the same rearrangement. Moreover, benign inflammatory responses to some antigens have been shown to use a particular TCR β V region preferentially and so might appear monoclonal by this assay. These facts may ultimately limit the validity of TCR rearrangements for diagnosing T-cell neoplasia. More fundamentally, it is not clear that monoclonality signifies malignancy in every case. Therefore, as with any other single test, results from gene rearrangement analyses must always be interpreted in the context of all other available clinical and laboratory data.

IN SITU HYBRIDIZATION

Another specialized hybridization technique, called **in situ hybridization,** is based on the ability of labeled probes to bind target DNA in thin tissue sections or cytologic smears (Fig 18–6). This technique reveals not only the presence of a specific sequence but also its spatial distribution within tissues or individual cells. In brief, cells or tissues attached to the surface of a glass microscope slide are fixed, incubated with a labeled probe, and then washed to remove unbound probe. The specimen is then coated with a thin layer of photographic emulsion or chromogenic substrate that reveals the location of any bound radiolabeled or enzymatically labeled probe. The assay is technically arduous and not very sensitive. It is sometimes used to detect abundant RNA species or viral DNA, which may be present in large amounts in a single infected cell. It is not well suited for examining most human genes, however, only two copies of which are present in each diploid cell.

TARGET AMPLIFICATION TECHNIQUES: POLYMERASE CHAIN REACTION

In the past, a major drawback of hybridization assays was their need for relatively large amounts of sample DNA to compensate for their low sensitivity. This problem has been surmounted in recent years by the development of powerful enzymatic techniques that can exponentially replicate specific DNA sequences in

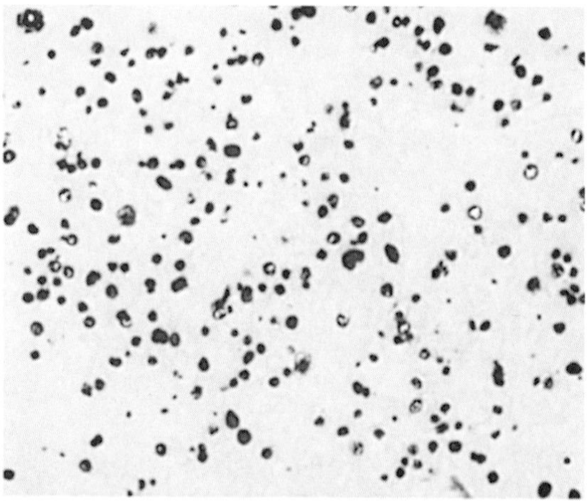

Figure 18–6. Detection of viral DNA in human cells by in situ hybridization. A lymph node biopsy specimen from a patient with Hodgkin's disease was fixed onto the surface of a glass slide and then hybridized with a biotinylated nucleic acid probe specific for sequences from Epstein-Barr virus. Hybridized probe was detected with streptavidin-conjugated alkaline phosphatase. The nuclei of cells that harbor the viral DNA stain darkly. (Courtesy of Lawrence M Weiss.)

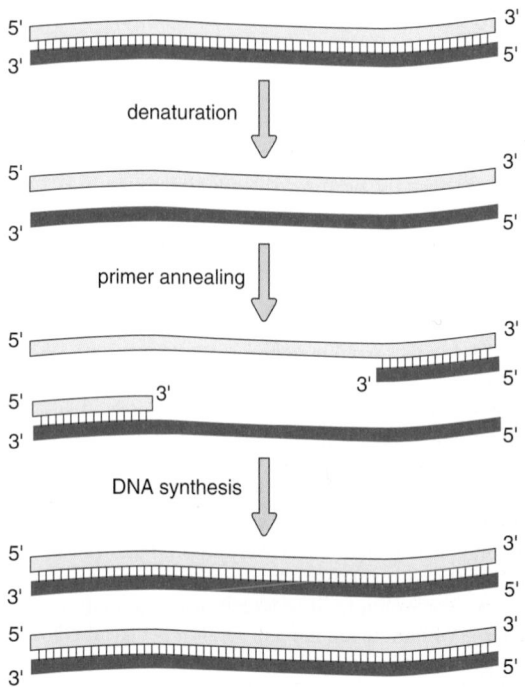

Figure 18–7. One cycle of DNA amplification by PCR. Each cycle consists of sequential heat denaturation, primer annealing, and DNA synthesis steps. Two different primers are used and must be oriented as shown with respect to each other. DNA synthesis is performed with a thermostable DNA polymerase and proceeds unidirectionally from each primer. After one cycle, the region between the primers has been duplicated. If the process is repeated, the number of copies of this region increases exponentially, doubling with each cycle until the supply of primers is exhausted.

the test tube. With these techniques, it is now possible to analyze vanishingly small samples that initially contain fewer than 10 copies of the sequence of interest. The new methods take advantage of the chemical properties of nucleic acids and of highly specialized enzymes that can repair and replicate DNA in vitro.

Every single-stranded DNA molecule has two ends, called the 5′ and 3′ ends, whose chemical and biologic properties differ. In double-stranded DNA, the two strands are always antiparallel (ie, their 3′ and 5′ ends are in opposite orientation to each other). Cellular enzymes known as **DNA polymerases,** which elongate these strands during DNA replication, can do so only by adding new nucleotide bases sequentially onto the 3′ end of a preexisting strand, which serves as a **primer.** Moreover, most DNA polymerases function only when the primer is annealed to a longer second strand, which serves as a **template** for DNA synthesis; the enzyme adds nucleotides in a sequence complementary to that of the template, producing a base-paired double helix.

These properties of DNA polymerases are exploited in a technique called the **polymerase chain reaction (PCR),** which can be used to replicate a particular region of target DNA selectively in vitro (Fig 18–7). Beginning with sample DNA from a very small number of cells, PCR can be used to synthesize multiple copies of a particular gene or gene segment that is present in those cells. PCR works best for copying regions less than about 2000 bp, and the DNA sequences flanking the region of interest must be known in advance. To use PCR, two short DNA primers (usually at least 16–20 bases long) are syn-

thesized whose sequences are complementary to those of the flanking regions but on opposite strands; the two primers must be chosen so that their 3′ ends are directed toward each other (see Fig 18–7). A vast molar excess of these primers is added to the sample DNA, which is then denatured by heating and allowed to anneal with the primers. A bacterial DNA polymerase is then added, which initiates synthesis at the 3′ end of each annealed primer and produces a new strand complementary to a portion of the adjacent template strand. Synthesis is continued for long enough that the newly synthesized strands extend through the entire region of interest. When the mixture is then denatured and reannealed again, each newly synthesized strand provides a new template for synthesis from the opposite primer. By repeated cycles of denaturation annealing, and synthesis, the region between the two primers is amplified exponentially, with the number of double-stranded copies of this region doubling at each cycle. Under ideal conditions, 220,000 copies should theoretically be produced from a single original after only 20 cycles of

PCR. This is enough copies to allow detection by routine hybridization techniques.

Automated, programmable instruments that can carry out the repeated thermal cycles necessary for PCR and that can accommodate multiple samples simultaneously are now widely available. The procedure is usually performed with **thermostable** DNA polymerases, isolated from thermophilic bacteria, since these can better withstand exposure to high temperature.

Perhaps the most common problem encountered when using PCR is cross-contamination: because the method is so sensitive, extreme care must be taken to avoid transferring even a trace of target DNA from one specimen to another. Another limitation of this technique arises from the fact that the bacterial polymerases frequently make errors when synthesizing new strands and so can introduce mutations that are not present in the original sample.

The basic technique of PCR amplification has been adapted in a great many ways to serve particular purposes. For example, it is widely used to facilitate detection of minute amounts of viral or bacterial DNA in clinical specimens, since it can often identify these microorganisms much more rapidly than conventional culture techniques. A similar approach can be used to monitor lymphoid cancers; if primers are chosen that selectively amplify only a uniquely rearranged Ig or TCR V/(D)/J gene segment in the malignant clone, this can be used as an extremely sensitive assay for detecting persistence or regrowth of that clone in blood or tissues after cancer therapy. Methods have been developed that allow **in situ PCR** on tissue sections so that cells harboring a distinctive DNA sequence, such as a viral genome, can be identified morphologically.

It is also possible to search for single-point mutations within a target sequence by testing PCR-amplified DNA for **single-strand conformational polymorphisms (SSCP).** For this purpose, the amplified product is treated with alkali to separate the DNA strands and is then quickly applied to an electrophoretic gel under nondenaturing conditions (Fig 18–8). Because the individual strands are not given the opportunity to reanneal with other strands, they tend instead to fold up on themselves by forming base pairs at short regions of intrastrand complementarity. Even subtle mutations can greatly affect the folding pattern and, hence, the three-dimensional shape of the folded strand, causing it to migrate anomalously on the gel relative to the normal sequence. One advantage of this technique is that it can detect many alternative mutations within an amplified region, even if their identities are not known in advance.

Other strategies for exponentially amplifying DNA have been described. For example, the **ligase chain reaction (LCR)** uses DNA-repairing enzymes, called **DNA ligases,** whose function is to link preexisting DNA strands together by covalently joining the 5′ end of one to the 3′ end of another. Ligases link two

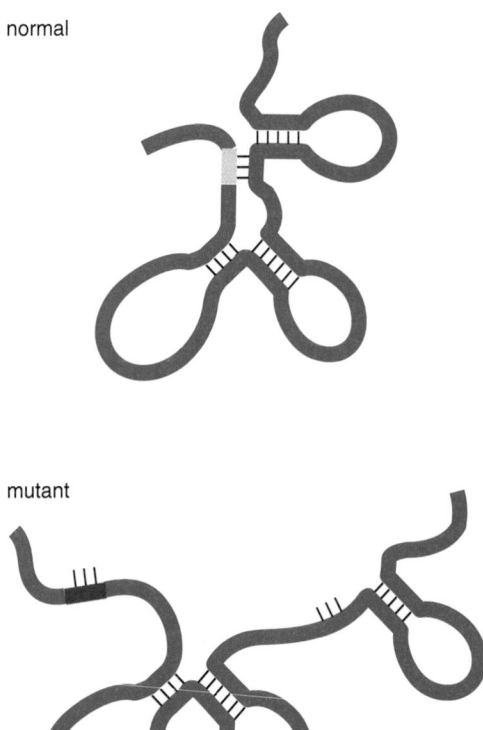

Figure 18–8. Single-strand conformational polymorphism. Under suitable conditions, a single strand of DNA often anneals with itself to form a complex folded structure due to regions of internal complementarity. Mutations may alter the folding pattern, and so change the electrophoretic mobility of the strand on a gel.

strands together only if they are already base-paired to a complementary strand that holds them in precise end-to-end alignment. LCR uses one pair of oligonucleotide strands whose sequences exactly match the two halves of the sequence of interest, along with a second pair of oligonucleotides whose sequences are complementary to the first (Fig 18–9). When denatured and allowed to reanneal to a target DNA, each pair of oligonucleotides binds to one of the target strands, and they are then permanently linked together by DNA ligase. At each subsequent cycle of denaturation and annealing, each linked pair of oligonucleotides can bring together the opposite pair, so that the number of linked pairs doubles with each cycle. LCR is usually performing with thermostable bacterial ligases and is somewhat more rapid than PCR, since no new DNA synthesis is required. The primers used are relatively short, which severely limits the size of the target sequence that can be examined. Since even a single base mismatch can prevent these short primers from annealing, however, the LCR is very well suited for detecting point mutations in target DNA.

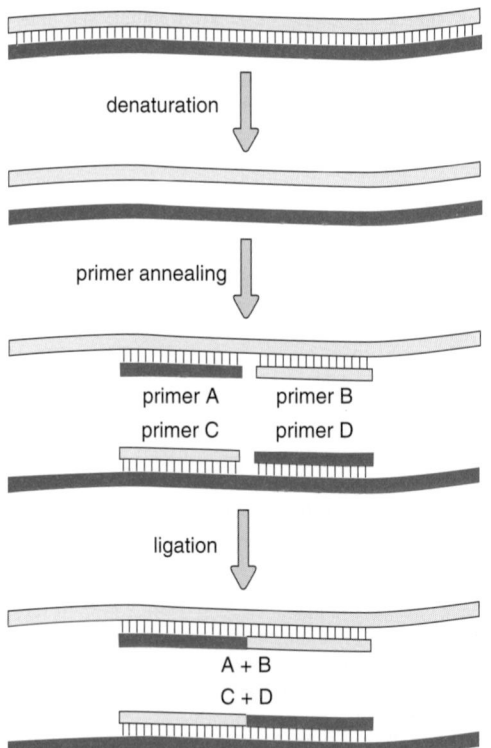

Figure 18–9. One cycle of DNA amplification by LCR. The process is similar to PCR, except that four different primers are required and a thermostable DNA ligase is used in place of DNA polymerase. With each cycle, pairs of primers bind to the target sequence and are then linked covalently by the ligase. In each subsequent cycle, a linked primer pair serves to bind the other two primers, so that the number of linked copies increases exponentially, doubling at each cycle.

METHODS OF ANALYZING RNA

DNA and RNA probes can also be used to analyze the RNAs from a clinical specimen, and this can be highly advantageous for some purposes. Whereas DNA analysis can reveal the presence and structure of a particular gene sequence, RNA analysis indicates whether, and how strongly, it is being expressed. Another important advantage is sensitivity: a cell that expresses a particular gene often contains hundreds of copies of the RNA derived from it, and this RNA may be readily detectable even though the gene itself is not. Techniques such as in situ or dot blot hybridization can easily be adapted to search for specific sequences in cellular RNA. In a modified form of the Southern blot, called the **Northern blot,** a mixture of cellular RNAs can be separated according to length by agarose gel electrophoresis, transferred to the surface of a nylon or nitrocellulose membrane, and then hybridized to a labeled nucleic acid probe to determine the size and abundance of any particular RNA species.

RNA analysis has some inherent limitations, however. Because expression of a given RNA varies widely depending on the lineage and physiologic state of a cell, it is critical to sample the right tissues at the right time. RNA is less durable than DNA (for example, it degrades rapidly and irreversibly at alkaline pH) and must be handled with correspondingly greater care. In addition, the number and types of enzymes that are available to manipulate RNA sequences are very limited. For some applications, it is necessary to begin by making a DNA copy of the target RNA, which then serves as the substrate for further analysis. For example, PCR amplification of RNA is carried out by a two-stage procedure known as **reverse transcriptase PCR (RT-PCR).** The first stage employs an enzyme called reverse transcriptase, which synthesizes a DNA strand complementary to the RNA of interest by using one of the PCR primers as its primer. This complementary DNA is then used, in the second stage, as the starting material for PCR amplification by a conventional thermostable DNA polymerase.

OVERVIEW & PROSPECTS

Tests based on nucleic acid technology are a relatively new addition to the armamentarium of the clinical immunology laboratory, and it is not yet clear to what extent they will supplement or replace conventional assays. They are particularly well suited to the detection of viruses and other microorganisms in tissue specimens, since such organisms can often be recognized and positively identified by their unique RNA or DNA sequences much more quickly and inexpensively than by culture. Hence, PCR-based tests have already assumed an important role in microbiologic diagnosis, and it seems likely that this role will increase in the future. Immunologically important organisms that are currently assayed in this manner include Epstein-Barr virus, human immunodeficiency viruses, and human T-cell leukemia viruses (see Chapters 46 and 53).

DNA-based assays are also very useful for detecting large-scale chromosomal deletions or rearrangements that occur at fairly constant locations in the genome and that characterize several types of hematologic malignancies. Examples include the Philadelphia chromosome of chronic myelogenous leukemia, the t(14,18) of follicular lymphoma, and the t(8,14) and related anomalies of Burkitt's lymphoma (see Chapters 7 and 46). Detection of these rearrangements can be a useful adjunct in diagnosis and also provides a simple means to monitor disease progression or to search for minimal residual disease after therapy. The Southern blot assay for lymphocyte clonality has similar potential utility and may be especially useful for evaluating poorly differentiated malignancies; however, it is currently too labor-intensive and technically demanding to be adopted by many clinical laboratories. Clonality assays based on PCR technology are being developed. In addition, PCR, LCR, and related techniques can detect extremely subtle DNA anomalies, including single-base point mutations, and are likely to be used increasingly for the diagnosis of congenital immunodeficiencies and of hereditary predispositions to cancer or other disorders.

REFERENCES

THEORY & PROTOCOLS

Barany F: Genetic disease detection and DNA amplification using cloned thermostable ligase. *Proc Natl Acad Sci USA* 1991;**88:**189.

Davey MP, Waldmann TA: Clonality and lymphoproliferative lesions. *N Engl J Med* 1986;**315:**509.

Engleberg NC, Eisenstein BI: Detection of microbial nucleic acids for diagnostic purposes. *Ann Rev Med* 1992;**43:**147.

Sambrook J et al (editors): *Molecular Cloning: A Laboratory Manual,* 2nd ed. Cold Spring Harbor, 1989.

Southern EM: Detection of specific sequences among DNA fragments separated by gel electrophoresis. *J Mol Biol* 1975;**98:**503.

SPECIFIC APPLICATIONS

Arnold A et al: Immunoglobulin-gene rearrangements as unique clonal markers in human lymphoid neoplasms. *N Engl J Med* 1983;**309:**1593.

Bakhshi A et al: Lymphoid blast crises of chronic myelogenous leukemia represent stages in the development of B-cell precursors. *N Engl J Med* 1983;**309:**826.

Cleary ML et al: Monoclonality of lymphoproliferative lesions in cardiac-transplant recipients. *N Engl J Med* 1984;**310:**477.

Cossman J et al: Gene rearrangements in the diagnosis of lymphoma/leukemia: Guidelines for use based on a multi-institutional study. *Am J Clin Pathol* 1991;**95:**347.

Flug F et al: T-cell receptor gene rearrangements as markers of lineage and clonality in T-cell neoplasms. *Proc Natl Acad Sci USA* 1985;**82:**3460.

Grody WW, Hilborne LH: Diagnostic applications of recombinant nucleic acid technology: Neoplastic disease. *Lab Med* 1992;**23:**19.

Reis MD et al: T-cell receptor and immunoglobulin gene rearrangements in lymphoproliferative disorders. *Adv Cancer Res* 1989;**52:**45.

Shibata D et al: Detection of specific t(14;18) chromosomal translocations in fixed tissues. *Hum Pathol* 1990;**21:**199.

Tawa A et al: Rearrangement of the T-cell receptor beta chain gene in non-T-cell non-B-cell acute lymphoblastic leukemia of childhood. *N Engl J Med* 1985;**313:**1033.

Waldmann TA: Rearrangements of genes for the antigen receptor on T cells as markers of lineage and clonality in human lymphoid neoplasms. *N Engl J Med* 1985;**313:**776.

Weiss LM et al: Clonal rearrangements of T-cell receptor genes in mycosis fungoides and dermatopathic lymphadenopathy. *N Engl J Med* 1985;**313:**539.

Weiss LM et al: Frequent immunoglobulin and T-cell receptor gene rearrangements in "histiocytic" neoplasms. *Am J Pathol* 1985;**121:**369.

Laboratory Evaluation of Immune Competence

19

Daniel P. Stites, MD, James D. Folds, PhD, & John Schmitz, PhD

The integrity of the human immune system depends on the presence of adequate numbers of functionally competent cells. These cells and their many secreted products interact in a complex manner to protect the host from invading microorganisms (for a summary, see Chapter 1). The several cardinal clinical manifestations of a failure in immune competence include (1) increased frequency of infections, (2) failure to clear infections rapidly despite adequate therapy, (3) dissemination of local infections to distant sites, and (4) occurrence of opportunistic infections. An increased risk of developing certain types of cancer may be a long-term consequence of immunodeficiency; however, the susceptibility to cancer in general and, particularly, the responsible mechanisms are still controversial (see Chapters 44 and 45). Similarly, development of autoimmunity could follow the loss of key suppressive regulatory influences within the immune system. Loss of such regulatory control can result in hypersensitivity or immune hyperfunction as a consequence of immunodeficiency (see Chapter 32).

UTILITY OF LABORATORY TESTS

A seemingly bewildering array of laboratory tests are available to finely dissect nearly every component of the immune response. Most assays have emerged from applications in basic or clinical immunology research. Relatively few such laboratory tests have developed established clinical reliability for diagnosis. To define a practical approach to clinical laboratory testing for immune competence, at least two key features of tests must be established: (1) sensitivity and specificity of the test for disease, and (2) technical accuracy of the testing procedure. Ideally, one needs to know predictive values that emerge from the sensitivities and specificities of the various tests in question (see Chapter 14). This usually requires extensive clinical investigation of large numbers of diseased patients and appropriate control subjects for each test.

Unfortunately, sometimes this information is often lacking or difficult to obtain (see Chapter 14). Applications of quality control procedures, internationally accepted reagent standards, and uniformly accepted laboratory techniques are in many instances lacking. Nevertheless, a variety of relatively useful and technically reproducible laboratory tests are available in many clinical immunology laboratories. Appropriate use of these tests can lead to a very complete profile of a patient's immune competence. Several important limitations regarding the application of laboratory tests, particularly in clinical contexts must be observed, however.

VARIABILITY OF TESTS

In contrast to its use for immunologic, epidemiologic, or other types of research, clinical laboratory testing for immunologic competence must always be interpreted in the context of a particular patient's history and physical examination. Ordinarily, the purpose of performing any laboratory test is to aid in diagnosis or treatment. Statistically speaking, abnormalities outside accepted reference ranges in laboratory tests in otherwise healthy individuals are to be expected. Many currently available tests have high inherent biologic and technical variability. The sources of biologic variability in test results include age, sex, race, diurnal variations, medications, nutritional status, intercurrent infections, and other less well-defined environmental factors. Technical variability is largely a function of instrumentation, reagents, and, especially, human error in sample labeling, preparation, and actual test performance. The presence of active disease, particularly of an infectious nature, can greatly influence immune system test results. In general, then, immune competence testing should be done during relatively disease-free intervals.

LIMITATIONS OF TESTING

Nearly all assays currently in clinical use are performed on blood cells or serum, even though blood is rarely, if ever, the main site of functional immunologic activity. Obviously, the results must be interpreted somewhat narrowly with respect to the circulating blood compartment as the source of test materials. The populations of the cells of lymphoid tissues, such as bone marrow, lymph nodes, and spleen, may not be accurately reflected by their populations in blood. For freely diffusible humoral proteins, such as most antibodies that are in equilibrium with extracellular fluid, blood levels directly reflect tissue levels and do not present a problem. Lymphocytes and monocytes, however, may be sequestered extravascularly or not distributed in blood in the same proportions as in other organs. IgM antibodies are generally restricted to the intravascular and intralymphatic spaces as a result of their molecular size. The additional limitation of in vitro artifacts and the relatively crude nature of currently available in vivo tests must also be considered. Thus, new, relatively noninvasive techniques to measure immune cell function and turnover in vivo are needed. Sampling cells or fluids from other sites, such as bronchoalveolar lavage fluid, cerebrospinal fluid, lymph nodes, mucosal sites and secretions, and skin, can give specialized insights into local immune competence in these organs. Obtaining such specimens is often difficult, however. Special problems of technical standardization, lack of homogeneity of samples (eg, bronchoalveolar lavage), lack of appropriate (age-matched) reference ranges, and continuous migration to and from these nonvascular sites make interpretation and measurement even more difficult. Stained tissue sections from biopsies allow for static cellular enumeration but are rarely if ever useful for making functional interpretations. Serum versus cerebrospinal fluid rations for albumin and IgG, for example, have been used to address the problem of compartmentalization and local antibody synthesis in the central nervous system (see Chapter 40).

In testing for immune competence, the clinical laboratory provides two types of quantitative information regarding various components of the immune system. These are (1) enumeration of various elements (eg, lymphocytes) and (2) functional competence of these elements, that is, the ability of T cells to proliferate in response to a particular recall antigen. A common pitfall in test interpretation is to confuse the mere *presence* of normal numbers or levels of a given immunologic element with *functional competence*. Thus, even though an individual's CD4 T-cell counts are within the laboratory's reference range, their normality should not be assumed unless functional studies are performed. In addition, most currently used laboratory tests for immune competence are not antigen- or epitope-specific. Thus, finding a normal serum concentration of IgG, for example, provides no information about specific antibodies to particular bacterial antigens. In practice it is, of course, not possible to assess immune competence to a specific antigen if the antigen is not available in a form that can be used in the test or if the precise in vivo chemical nature of the antigen is unknown.

Table 19–1. Indications for laboratory testing for immune competence.

Clinical diagnosis, therapeutic monitoring, or prognosis of[1]:
1. Congenital and acquired immunodeficiency diseases (see Chapters 20–25, 46, and 53)
2. Immune reconstitution following bone marrow or other lymphoid tissue grafts (see Chapter 57)
3. Immunosuppression induced by drugs, radiation, or other means (see Chapter 58) for transplant rejection, cancer treatment, or autoimmune diseases
4. Autoimmune disorders (see Chapter 33), as a possible adjunct to diagnosis (rarely useful) or to monitor therapy
5. Immunization (see Chapter 55), to monitor efficacy or immune status
6. Clinical or basic research

[1] Tests must be interpreted in the clinical context, particularly in conjunction with a thorough history and physical examination.

CLINICAL UTILITY OF TESTING

In which clinical situations are performance of laboratory tests for evaluation of immune competence indicated? Specific details of laboratory tests that are used for various diseases are included in the clinical chapters later in this volume. In general, these tests are useful in diagnosis, monitoring of treatment, and, occasionally, assessing prognosis in a limited group of clinical situations (Table 19–1). Most probably, additional applications will be defined in the future. Also, many additional tests and many other applications of the limited group of tests described later on can be found in the research investigations of immune disorders in contrast to clinical laboratory testing.

TESTING FOR IMMUNE COMPETENCE

NONSPECIFIC TESTING

Some simple approaches to the evaluation of immune competence take into account the age of the patient, the general clinical history, the history of infections, and physical abnormalities.

If the patient is an older infant, young child, or young adult, it may be possible to evaluate them initially for T-cell immunity by simply performing a complete blood count (CBC) and differential. This testing permits evaluation of the numbers and type of white blood cells present and the proportion of each.

Normal values are available for lymphocytes and neutrophils that are age-specific. Once it is known whether the lymphocytes are present in normal numbers, it is then possible to measure their function with a simple skin test for delayed hypersensitivity (DTH) (see Chapter 15). Skin testing is useful only in children who are old enough to have received vaccines or would have been exposed to a number of natural antigens. Generally, if a child responds to a recall antigen in a DTH reaction and has relatively normal numbers of lymphocytes, it is unlikely that the child has a T-cell immunodeficiency.

B-cell immunity can usually be evaluated, depending on the age of the patient, by quantitating the serum immunoglobulin levels. This is relatively inexpensive, and if IgG, IgA, and IgM are all present and within the normal range it usually indicates an intact B-cell system. If the total immunoglobulin levels are below the lower limits of normal, one should move on to evaluate whether the patient can respond to an antigenic stimulus. This may be difficult in infants younger than 6 months of age, but it can be evaluated easily in older children by measuring isohemagglutinin levels. These are natural antibodies to blood group antigens that appear by 1 year of age. Also, if the patient has received specific vaccinations against childhood diseases, it may be possible to measure antibodies against diphtheria or tetanus toxoids. In more difficult cases it may be necessary to move on to more specific testing.

SPECIFIC TESTING

A brief summary of one approach to testing basic elements of immune competence, including T cells, B cells, natural killer (NK) cells, complement, and phagocytes, is described. This is summarized in Table 19–2. There are obviously other tests available, and in some cases additional uses for the tests are described (see Table 19–4). The specific details of methods for detecting these elements and their functional states are presented in Chapters 14 and 15. "Normal" values or reference ranges for these tests are not given here because ordinarily they must be determined in individual laboratories.

T CELLS

Enumeration

The numbers and percentages of circulating T lymphocytes are maintained within fairly narrow limits by homeostatic mechanisms (Table 19–3). Since T cells have no morphologically distinguishing features, they can be counted only by detection of lineage-specific molecules or antigenic markers. For all T cells, the most universal among these markers is CD3, a major structural component of the T-cell receptor for

Table 19–2. Summary of immune competence testing.

Immune Cells	Detection or Enumeration	Function
T cells	FCM with MAbs for CD2, 3, or 5	Lymphocyte proliferation to mitogens or antigens, DHS skin test.
T-cell subsets	FCM with MAbs for CD4 (helper/inducer) and CD8 (suppressor/cytotoxic)	Functional assays for helper/suppression, cytotoxicity.
B cells	FCM with MAbs for CD19, 20, anti-H and anti-L chains	Serum immunoglobulins or subclasses, antibodies especially postimmunization.
NK cells	FCM with MAbs for CD16 or 56	K562 cellular cytotoxicity, ADCC.
Complement	Immunochemical component detection	CH_{50} or specific hemolytic assay for components.
Neutrophils	Morphologic or histochemical features by cell counter	Biochemical and microbicidal.
Monocyte–macrophages	Morphologic histochemical features or MAb to CD14	Biochemical and microbicidal.

Abbreviations: FCM = Flow cytometry; MAbs = monoclonal antibodies; DHS = delayed hypersensitivity; ADCC = antibody-dependent cellular cytotoxicity.

antigens. Other cell surface markers are either incompletely expressed or specific for subsets of T cells. CD5 is also present on a subpopulation of B cells; CD2 can also be found on some NK cells; and CD7 is only weakly expressed on some mature T cells.

Technical Considerations

For accurate enumeration, flow cytometry is currently clearly the method of choice (see Chapter 15). Monoclonal antibodies conjugated to fluorochromes directed at all known CD molecules on T cells are commercially available. Percentages of T cells in whole lysed blood are generally accurately determined by counting 10,000 cells per sample that are stained with fluorochrome-labeled monoclonal antibodies. Clearly, the accuracy of this technique is highly dependent on gating techniques to distinguish lymphocytes from other blood leukocytes. Manual counts of T cells by fluorescence microscopy are less desirable than flow cytometry, owing to the imprecision and laboriousness of cell-counting in a microscope. For calculation of absolute numbers of T cells, the percentage determined by immunofluorescence in a flow cytometer must be multiplied by the absolute lymphocyte count, usually determined by Coulter counting or manually in a hemacytometer. Lack of precision or accuracy in determining the absolute lymphocyte count from the leukocyte and differential

Table 19–3. Summary of major tests for T-cell immune competence.

Test	Technique	Parameters Measured	Limitations and Comments
Total T cells (numbers or percentages)	Flow cytometry with MAbs to CD2, CD3, or CD5	Percentage of cells bearing these epitopes in a particular gated mononuclear cell population	Need absolute lymphocyte count to convert to T-cell numbers; no functional or clonal antigen specific information.
T-cell subsets (numbers and percentages) Helper/inducer cells Suppressor/cytotoxic cells	Flow cytometry with MAbs to CD4, CD8, and CD3 simultaneously	Percentage of cells in mononuclear cell gate that bear these surface molecules	CD4 (but not CD3) also expressed on some monocytes; both subsets are functionally heterogeneous (eg, CD8 contains suppressor and cytotoxic T cells).
Lymphocyte proliferation to mitogens and allogenic cells	Lymphocyte culture with DNA synthesis detected by radioactive thymidine incorporation	Ability of polyclonal T cells to undergo activation to DNA synthesis	Does not define multiple possible defects in cellular physiology.
Antigens	Same	Clonal proliferation to epitopes	Avoids the need to perform skin test for DHS; relevant antigens may be unknown or unavailable for testing.

Abbreviations: MAbs = monoclonal antibodies; DHS = delayed hypersensitivity.

count is a major source of technical variability in determining T-cell counts.

Newly introduced flow cytometers can accurately determine absolute numbers of lymphocytes as well as immunofluorescently stained T cells. Recently, semiautomated instruments to quantitate CD4 and CD8 cells have become available for use. These instruments require little hands on time and correlate well with standard flow cytometric analyses. An added advantage is that a separate CBC and differential is not required for the determination of absolute counts. Techniques to measure total amounts of CD4, CD8, or other T-cell-specific molecules by solubilization with detergents followed by enzymed-linked immunosorbent assay (ELISA) have also been developed.

T-Cell Subsets

The two major T-cell subsets, CD4- and CD8-bearing cells, are enumerated by using fluorochrome-linked monoclonal antibodies and flow cytometry with lymphocyte gating (some monocytes also express low levels of CD4). It is now recommended that all such determinations be performed by simultaneous color analysis with anti-CD3 monoclonal antibodies labeled with a second flurorchrome to ensure exclusion of non-T cells. Simultaneous two-color analysis with additional monoclonal antibodies can resolve CD4 and CD8 into further subpopulations (see Chapter 15), but these finer distinctions are rarely of clinical value in assessing immune competence. One such example is the use of CD4 subsets in determining disease activity in multiple sclerosis by using the CD45R subset of CD4 cells, which decrease with disease activation, whereas CD45RO memory effector cells increase.

Functional Assays

A. All T Cells: Activation of T cells with non-specific plant lectins or anti-CD3 monoclonal antibodies results in a complex series of biochemical events culminating in cellular DNA synthesis. Phytomitogens, such as phytohemagglutinin, concanavalin A, and pokeweed mitogen, are used for this purpose. Also, allogeneic cells can be used as relatively nonspecific stimulants in a mixed-lymphocyte culture (MLC). Anti-CD3, which directly interacts with membrane T-cell receptors, can provide a particularly strong activation signal. Cellular responses are usually assessed by measuring radioactive thymidine uptake (see Chapter 15). Response to mitogen stimulation by these agents is macrophage-dependent but much less so than is the response to specific antigens.

B. T-Cell Subsets: CD4 and CD8 cells do not proliferate in response to monoclonal antibodies to these epitopes. Complex functional tests to assess helper, suppressor, or cytotoxic functions of these cells are still predominantly in the realm of research laboratories but are occasionally useful in clinical situations (see later section).

Antigen-specific T cells proliferate in response to soluble or cell-bound antigens in vitro (see Chapter 15). This test is particularly useful when one wants to avoid direct in vivo contact with potentially toxic antigens by patch testing or delayed hypersensitivity intradermal tests.

C. Delayed Hypersensitivity Skin Tests: The ability to mount cutaneous delayed hypersensitivity to intradermally or epidermally applied antigens (patch testing) depends on both specific antigen-reactive and other relatively noncommitted T cells. Antigen-stimulated T cells release mediators that affect vascular permeability, monocyte function and

Table 19–4. Additional tests for T-cell competence not regularly available clinically.

Lymphokine production
  IL-2, IL-3, IL-5
  Interferon gamma
  IL-4
  TNF
Receptors for lymphokines
  IL-1
  IL-2
Responsiveness to lymphokines
  IL-1
  IL-2
  IL-4
  Interferon gamma
Lymphocyte cytotoxicity
  MHC-restricted
  MHC-nonrestricted
  Antigen-specific
  Lectin (PHA)-dependent
  Antibody-dependent cell-mediated cytotoxicity (ADCC)
Helper/suppressor T-cell assays
  Polyclonal immunoglobulin synthesis (pokeweed mitogen-induced)
  Mitogen or antigen proliferation
  T-cell cytotoxicity
  Lymphokine release or effect

Abbreviations: IL = interleukin; MHC = major histocompatibility complex; PHA = phytohemagglutinin.

movement, and proliferation of other noncommitted T cells. These cytokines and cells all contribute to local erythema and induration characteristic of this response. Thus, the delayed hypersensitivity skin test is not a measure solely of T cells. Positive reactions to delayed hypersensitivity skin tests of one or more antigens, however, mean that broadly reactive T-cell immune competence is likely to be largely intact (see Chapter 15).

D. Flow Cytometric Assays. Recently the use of flow cytometric detection of cell surface activation antigens has been correlated with activation. These assays are new, however, and have not undergone rigorous evaluation.

Additional tests for T-cell function, which are not regularly available clinically, are listed in Table 19–4.

B CELLS

In contrast to assessing T-cell competence, tests for B-cell competence rely mainly on detecting the products of the B-cell/plasma cell series, that is, immunoglobulins. Specific assays for antibody directed at selected epitopes of microorganisms are also available (Table 19–5).

Enumeration

A variety of specific B-cell surface markers (CD antigens) that can be detected by monoclonal antibodies have been described. Initially, surface immunoglobulins using either H- or L-chain-specific antisera were used. More recently, monoclonal antisera that detect CD19 or CD20 have also been used relatively interchangeably as pan-B-cell markers. Additional antibodies that detect B cells from earlier stages of maturation or from other subsets are available (eg, CD22 and CD10) but are rarely useful in assessing B-cell competence in peripheral blood of adults or even children. The coexpression of CD5 on T cells and CD1 on dendritic cells and thymocytes restricts the usefulness of these markers for B-cell enumeration. Since plasma cells rarely circulate, antibodies directed at their special differentiation antigens (eg, PC-1 or PCA-1) are of use only in examining lymph nodes, spleen, bone marrow, or other lymphoid tissues. The typical morphologic features of plasma cells usually render them easily recognizable without immunohistochemical staining.

Technical Considerations

These are essentially the same as those discussed for T cells. Flow cytometry is the preferred method.

B-Cell Subsets

B cells at early stages of maturation (eg, pre-B cells) do express unique surface markers and cytoplasmic μ

Table 19–5. Summary of major tests for B-cell immune competence.

Test	Technique	Parameters Measured	Limitations and Comments
Total B cells (numbers or percentages)	Flow cytometry with MAbs to CD19 or CD20 or antibodies to H or L chains	Percentage of cells that express these epitopes in a particular gated mononuclear cell population	Need absolute count to convert to B-cell numbers; no functional or antigen-specific information.
Immunoglobulin concentrations (IgG, IgA, IgM)	Radial immunodiffusion or rate nephelometry with specific anti-H and anti-L chain antisera	Concentration of polyclonal immunoglobulin present in particular body fluid (eg, serum, cerebrospinal fluid, saliva)	No clonal or antigen-specific information; results are highly age-dependent.
Antibody to specific epitopes or microorganisms	ELISA, radioimmunoassay, agglutination, precipitation, etc (see Chapter 14)	Titers of antibody to a specific epitope or group of epitopes on antigen from microorganisms	Deliberate immunization with preantibody and postantibody titers useful; anti-A and anti-B are IgM isohemagglutinins.

Abbreviations: MAbs = monoclonal antibodies; ELISA = enzyme-linked immunosorbent assay.

chains. Detecting these cells is primarily of use in phenotyping B-cell cancers or investigating the detailed pathogenic cellular mechanisms of B-cell immunodeficiency diseases. Markers for other B-cell subsets can be detected, but their clinical utility is unknown. Clonal or antigen-specific B-cell detection has generally not been applied to assessment of clinical immunocompetence.

Functional Assays

The primary product of the B-cell/plasma cell series is antibody, and, as such, measurement of immunoglobulins or specific antibodies provides the major route for assessing the function of B-cell competence (see Chapter 14).

Immunoglobulin levels should be measured if a state of humoral immunodeficiency or B-cell failure is suspected. The use of less specific tests, such as protein electrophoresis or immunoelectrophoresis, which are only semiquantitative, is not recommended. These tests are used primarily in paraprotein diagnosis. Consideration of the patient's age is critical in interpreting immunoglobulin levels, since these levels are particularly susceptible to variation with age (see Chapter 14). Generally, IgG, IgA, and IgM levels are sufficient. Serum IgD levels are not useful in assessing immune competence, and, with the rare exception of the hyper-IgE syndrome with recurrent infections (see Chapter 24), IgE levels are also not helpful in diagnosis of immune deficiencies.

In some instances, particularly following deliberate immunization to test B-cell competence, specific antibody is measured. Sera should be collected and frozen prior to administration of antigen and then subsequently some days or weeks later when serum antibody responses to the antigen in question are known to be elevated in the blood. Antibody should then be measured in both preimmunization and postimmunization specimens simultaneously. This approach can be used to detect primary antibody responses to antigens such as keyhole limpet hemocyanin or recall antigens such as polyvalent pneumococcal antigens of *Streptococcus pneumoniae*, tetanus toxoid, or influenza virus vaccine. One should never expose a suspected or known immunodeficient patient to live or attenuated viral vaccine, since this may result in virus dissemination followed by disease and possibly death.

Isohemagglutinins, anti-A and anti-B, are IgM antibodies directed at naturally occurring microbial polysaccharides that cross-react with antigens of the human ABH blood groups (see Chapter 16). In individuals older than 1 year, their titer is approximately 1:4. In incompatibly transfused or in utero-sensitized individuals, ABH antibodies may also be of IgG or other classes besides IgM. Rarely, the Schick test in diphtheria-immunized individuals can be used to measure specific IgG antidiphtheria antibodies.

In vitro tests for immunoglobulin synthesis by mixed cultures of blood monocytes, T cells, and B cells have been extensively used in immunologic research. These tests depend on polyclonal immunoglobulin production induced by B-cell mitogens, such as pokeweed mitogen or staphylococcal protein A. By varying or eliminating selective T-cell subsets or monocytes, suppression, helper, or antigen-presenting functions can be assessed. Currently, such intricate B-cell functional assays have not achieved demonstrable routine clinical application.

IgG Subclasses

In some individuals with normal, reduced, or even elevated IgG levels, the level of one or more of the four IgG subclasses may be reduced (see Chapter 21). Since deficiency in some of these IgG subclasses, particularly IgG2, may be associated with recurrent infections, determination of their serum level is useful. Other possible indications and disease associations of IgG subclass deficiency are discussed in Chapter 21).

NK CELLS

NK cells represent a minor, or third, subpopulation (10–15%) of circulating peripheral blood mononuclear cells. Some appear as large granular lymphocytes. Functionally, these cells kill a variety of autologous and allogeneic target cells without prior sensitization or known restriction by human leukocyte antigens (HLA antigens). They are thought to provide defense against viral infections and possibly some tumors. Recently, a few patients with selective absence of NK cells and recurrent infections (particularly herpesvirus infections) have been described. Patients with Chédiak-Higashi syndrome also have defective NK cells (see Chapter 24). Research is under way to elucidate possible antitumor effects of NK cells stimulated by interleukin-2 (IL-2) or other lymphokines, as well as their modulation in the neuroimmunologic axis.

Enumeration

Monoclonal antibodies to specific cell surface CD antigens of NK cells include CD56 (NKH1) and CD16 (FcIgG). These are used to count NK cells by microscopy or flow cytometry.

Functional Assays

NK cells kill "NK-sensitive" target cells in vitro. An example of such a target cell is the erythroleukemia cell line K562. Cytolysis by measurement of ^{51}Cr lysis is the most common test to detect NK cell function (see Chapter 15). NK cells also mediate antibody-dependent cellular cytotoxicity (ADCC). Assays for ADCC employ cytolysis of ^{51}Cr-labeled target cells (eg, erythrocytes) that are coated with either human or rabbit antibodies which contain γ-Fc regions, which bind FcIgG receptors present on NK cells.

Although NK cell enumeration and functional assays have not yet achieved widespread application in clinical laboratories, there are newly described flow cytometric assays that use target cells and new fluorescent dyes that make the assays simple and rapid enough to fit into a clinical laboratory.

COMPLEMENT

Genetic and some acquired deficiencies of complement are associated with a breakdown in host resistance to microorganisms (see Chapter 25). Complement is involved in host defense mechanisms in several ways, including (1) as an opsonin (C3a), (2) in lysing microorganisms (C1–C9), (3) in chemotaxis (C5a), and (4) in altering vascular permeability (C3a, C4a, C5a). Thus, any evaluation of host defense failure clearly should include measurement of complement.

Screening for Complement Deficiencies

Defects in C1–C9, properdin, and complement-regulatory factors have all been described. For components C3–C9 (inclusive), determination of hemolytic complement activity (CH_{50}) (see Chapter 14) generally adequately screen for congenital lack of one of these components. In genetic defects of complement (eg, C6 deficiency) the entire activity of the protein is lost, and hence the lytic function of the entire sequence is blocked. Thus, CH_{50} values approach zero. In acquired deficiency, variable reductions in CH_{50} occur depending on selective loss of the critical components of the lytic pathway. Defects in the alternative pathway proximal to C3 must be tested immunochemically or with specialized functional assays not ordinarily available in most clinical laboratories.

Identification of Specific Component Defects

Genetic or acquired reductions in specific components of either the classic or alternative pathway can be measured by either specific functional or immunochemical assays for these components (see Chapters 11 and 14). Generally, specific antisera are used in the clinical laboratory in either radial diffusion or nephelometric tests. Reduction in the CH_{50} or specific components can be the result of hypercatabolism or underproduction, or both, depending on the disease state. Functional assays such as chemotaxis or opsonization are usually performed in conjunction with the evaluation of phagocytic function.

PHAGOCYTIC CELLS

Polymorphonuclear leukocytes, particularly neutrophils (PMN) and monocyte–macrophages, play a crucial role in host defense against nearly all microorganisms. From an evolutionary standpoint, this is the oldest and most primitive form of immunity, predating antibody or T-cell immunity by a considerable stretch of evolutionary development.

Enumeration

A. PMNs: PMNs are most readily counted by a routine leukocyte count and leukocyte differential. Although such counts can be made with a microscope, the use of automatic cell or Coulter counters provides much more accurate information. Morphologic assessments of neutrophils, particularly to assess maturity and granule content, also constitute an essential step in immune-competence evaluation. In cases of very low or high neutrophil counts, a bone marrow examination may be required to evaluate the integrity of granulocytopoesis.

B. Monocyte–Macrophages: Circulating monocytes can be counted by leukocyte counting and leukocyte differential similar to PMN. Histochemical stains, especially for nonspecific or α-naphthol esterase, are useful for identification. Monoclonal antibodies directed at CD14 or volume and light-scattering characteristics can be used to identify and count relative numbers of monocytes by flow cytometry.

Functional Assays

Granulocyte function includes a variety of stages outlined in Chapter 15. Screening for granulocytic function related to immune competence involves at least a biochemical assay for the hexose monophosphate shunt, such as nitroblue tetrazolium dye reduction, chemiluminescence, or dichlorofluorescein fluorescence by flow cytometry.

More extensive microbicidal assays can be used to confirm defects in neutrophil function or to detect specific lesions related to particular microorganisms. The principles and examples of these assays are discussed in Chapter 15. Monocyte function can be assessed by similar biochemical or microbicidal tests with isolated enriched monocytes (see Chapter 15).

REFERENCES

GENERAL

Primary Immunodeficiency Diseases: Report of WHO Scientific Group. *Immunodef Rev* 1992;**3**:83.

Buckley RH: Primary immunodeficiency diseases. In: *Fundamental Immunology*, 3rd ed. W. Paul (editor) Raven Press, 1993, pp. 1353–1374.

Van der Valk P, Herman C: Biology of disease: Leukocyte functions. *Lab Invest* 1987;**57**:127.

Virella G, Patrick C, Goust JM: Diagnostic evaluation of lymphocyte functions and cell-mediated immunity. *Immunol Ser* 1993;**58:**291.

T- AND B-CELL ASSESSMENT

Marti GE, Fleisher TA: Application of lymphocyte immunophenotyping in selected diseases. *Pathol Immunopathol Res* 1988;**7:**319.

Nicholson JKA: Using flow cytometry in the evaluation and diagnosis of primary and secondary immunodeficiency diseases. *Arch Pathol Lab Med* 1989;**113:**598.

DELAYED HYPERSENSITIVITY SKIN TESTS

Ahmed AR, Blose DA: Delayed hypersensitivity skin testing: A review. *Arch Dermatol* 1983;**119:**934.

NK CELLS

Richards SJ, Scott CS: NK cells in health and disease: Clinical functional phenotypes and DNA genotypic characteristics. *Leukemia Lymphoma* 1992;**7:**377.

Ritz J: The role of natural killer cells in immune surveillance. *N Engl J Med* 1989;**320:**1748.

IMMUNOGLOBULINS

French MAH: *Immunoglobulins in Health and Disease. Immunology and Medicine Series.* MTP Press, 1986.

Hamilton RG: Human IgG subclass measurements in the clinical laboratory. *Clin Chem* 1987;**33:**1707.

COMPLEMENT

Fries LF, Frank MM: Complement and relative proteins: Inherited deficiencies. In: *Inflammation: Basic Principles and Clinical Correlates,* 2nd ed. Gallin JI, Goldstein IM, Snyderman R (editors). Raven Press, 1992.

Ross SC, Denson P: Complement deficiency states and infections. *Medicine* 1984;**63:**243.

PHAGOCYTIC CELLS

Boxer LA, Morganroth ML: Neutrophil function disorders. *Disease-a-Month* 1987;**33:**681.

Yang KD, Hill HR: Assessment of Neutrophil function. In: *Clinical Immunology: Principles and Practice,* Vol. II. Rich RR (editor-in-chief). Mosby, 1995, pp. 2141–2156.

Section III.
Clinical Immunology

Mechanisms of Immunodeficiency 20

Arthur J. Ammann, MD, & E. Richard Stiehm, MD

Four major components of the immune system assist the individual in defending against a constant assault by viral, bacterial, fungal, protozoal, and non-replicating agents that have the potential to produce infection and disease. These systems consist of antibody-mediated (B-cell) immunity, cell-mediated (T-cell) immunity, phagocytosis, and complement. Each system may act independently or in concert with one or more of the others.

Deficiency of one or more of these systems may be congenital (eg, X-linked infantile hypogammaglobulinemia) or acquired (eg, acquired hypogammaglobulinemia). Deficiencies of the immune system may be secondary to an embryologic abnormality (eg, DiGeorge anomaly), may be due to an enzymatic defect (eg, chronic granulomatous disease), or may be of unknown cause (eg, chronic mucocutaneous candidiasis). The multiple causes of immunodeficiency are listed in Table 20–1.

In general, the symptoms and the physical findings of immunodeficiency are related to the degree of deficiency and the particular system that is deficient in function. General features are listed in Table 20–2. Features associated with specific immunodeficiency disorders are also listed in Table 20–2. The types of infections that occur often provide an important clue to the type of immunodeficiency disease present. Recurrent bacterial otitis media and pneumonia are common in hypogammaglobulinemia. Patients with defective cell-mediated immunity are susceptible to fungal, protozoal, and viral infections that may present as pneumonia or chronic infection of the skin and mucous membranes or other organs. Systemic infection with uncommon bacterial organisms, normally of low virulence, is characteristic of chronic granulomatous disease. Other phagocytic disorders are associated with superficial skin infections or systemic infections with pyogenic organisms.

Numerous advances continue to be made in the identification and diagnosis of specific immunodeficiency disorders (Table 20–3). Screening tests are available for each component of the immune system (Table 20–4). These tests enable the physician to diagnose more than 75% of immunodeficiency disorders. The remainder can be diagnosed by means of more complicated studies (see Chapters 14 and 15),

Table 20–1. Causes of immunodeficiency.

Genetic patterns
  Autosomal-recessive
  Autosomal-dominant
  X-linked
  Gene deletions and rearrangements

Biochemical and metabolic deficiency
  Adenosine deaminase deficiency
  Purine nucleoside phosphorylase deficiency
  Biotin-dependent multiple carboxylase deficiency
  Deficient membrane glycoproteins

Vitamin or mineral deficiency
  Biotin
  B_{12}
  Iron
  Vitamin A
  Zinc

Arrest in embryogenesis

Autoimmune diseases
  Passive antibody (maternal to fetus)
  Active antibody (antibody to T cells)
  Active T cell (anti-B cell)

Acquired immunodeficiency
  Postviral infection
  Posttransfusion
  Multiple transfusions
  Metabolic disorders
  Hemoglobinopathies
  Chronic infection
  Nutritional deficiency
  Drug abuse
  Medications
  Protein-losing states
  Maternal alcoholism
  Radiation therapy
  Immunosuppressive therapy
  Cancer
  Chronic renal disease
  Splenectomy
  Asplenia

Table 20–2. Clinical features associated with immunodeficiency.

Features frequently present and highly suspicious
  Chronic infection
  Recurrent infection (more than expected)
  Unusual microbial agents
  Incomplete clearing between episodes of infection or incomplete response to treatment

---

Features frequently present and moderately suspicious
  Skin lesions (eczema, cutaneous candidiasis, rash, seborrhea, alopecia, severe warts, etc)
  Diarrhea (chronic)
  Growth failure
  Hepatosplenomegaly
  Hematologic abnormalities
  Recurrent abscesses
  Recurrent osteomyelitis
  Evidence of autoimmunity
  Failure to thrive

Features associated with specific immunodeficiency disorders
  Ataxia
  Telangiectasia
  Short-limbed dwarfism
  Cartilage-hair hypoplasia
  Idiopathic endocrinopathy
  Partial albinism
  Thrombocytopenia
  Eczema
  Tetany
  Periodontitis
  Failure of umbilical cord to separate

---

which may not be available in all hospital laboratories. There are still a number of individuals with an immunodeficiency disorder in whom the precise etiology or mechanism of immunodeficiency is unknown. Nevertheless, with newer and more sophisticated tests, the carrier state and intrauterine diagnosis can be accomplished.

In addition to antimicrobial agents for the treatment of specific infections, new forms of immunotherapy are available to assist in the control of immunodeficiency or perhaps even to cure the underlying disease (Table 20–5). The usefulness of some of these treatment methods, such as bone marrow transplantation, is often limited by the availability of suitable donors although haploidentical, matched unrelated and umbilical cord blood stem cell transplants have enlarged the pool. The discovery of enzyme deficiencies (eg, adenosine deaminase deficiency) in association with immunodeficiency offers a potential new avenue of therapy by means of enzyme replacement. The most recent successful approach to treatment is that of gene therapy. Several patients with adenosine deaminase deficiency have been treated with their own cells transfected with the gene coding for adenosine deaminase.

Immunodeficiency disorders are discussed in the next four chapters under the following categories: antibody (B-cell) deficiency, cellular (T-cell) deficiency, combined T-cell and B-cell deficiency, and phagocytic dysfunction. Complement factor deficiencies are discussed in Chapter 25. AIDS is discussed in Chapter 53. In general, the terminology used for specific deficiencies is based on the classification proposed by a committee of the World Health Organization (see Table 20–3).

Table 20–3. Classification of primary immunodeficiency disorders.

Antibody (B-cell) immunodeficiencies
   X-linked agammaglobulinemia
   Transient hypogammaglobulinemia of infancy
   Common variable immunodeficiency
   Hyper-IgM immunodeficiency
   IgA deficiency
   IgM deficiency
   IgG subclass deficiencies
   Polysaccharide unresponsiveness
   Transcobalamin deficiency
   Immunodeficiency with thymoma

Cellular (T-cell) immunodeficiencies
   DiGeorge anomaly
   Chronic mucocutaneous candidiasis
   Biotin-dependent multiple cocarboxylase deficiency
   Natural killer cell deficiency
   Idiopathic CD4 lymphopenia

Combined B-cell (antibody) and T (cellular)-cell deficiencies
   Severe combined immunodeficiency (including X-linked SCID, Nezelof syndrome, etc)
   Combined immunodeficiency with T-cell membrane or signaling defects
   Wiskott-Aldrich syndrome
   Ataxia-telangiectasia
   Nijmegen breakage syndrome
   Immunodeficiency with short-limbed dwarfism/cartilage hair hypoplasia
   Immunodeficiency with enzyme deficiency; adenosine deaminase or nucleoside phosphorylase deficiency
   Graft-versus-host disease
   Bare lymphocyte syndrome
   Omenn syndrome
   Reticular dysgenesis
   X-linked lymphoproliferative syndrome

Phagocytic dysfunction diseases
   Neutropenic syndromes
   Chronic granulomatous disease
   Leukocyte glucose-6-phosphate dehydrogenase deficiency
   Chediak-Higashi syndrome
   Myeloperoxidase deficiency
   Specific granule deficiency
   Glycogen storage disease type 1b
   Hyper-IgE/Job's syndrome
   Leukocyte adhesion defect
   Schwachman syndrome
   Tuftsin deficiency
   Periodontitis syndromes

Table 20–4. Initial screening evaluation.

Antibody-mediated immunity
   Quantitative immunoglobulin levels: IgG, IgM, IgA
   Isohemagglutinin titer (anti-A and anti-B): measures IgM antibody function primarily
   Specific antibody levels following immunization

Cell-mediated immunity
   Leukocyte count differential: measures total lymphocytes
   Total T cells and T-cell subsets: measures total T cells, helper T cells, and suppressor T cells
   Delayed hypersensitivity skin tests: measure specific T cell and inflammatory response to antigens

Phagocytosis
   Leukocyte count with differential: measures total neutrophils
   Nitroblue tetrazolium (NBT), chemiluminescence, superoxide production: measures neutrophil metabolic function
   Natural killer cell number and function

Complement
   Total hemolytic complement

Table 20–5. Treatment of immunodeficiency.

Treatment	B-Cell Disorders	T-Cell Disorders	Phagocytic Disorders
Gamma globulin.	X-linked hypogammaglobuline-mia; acquired hypogamma-globulinemia; secondary hypogammaglobulinemia when associated with infection. Do not use in selective IgA deficiency.	Use only when absent antibody response is demonstrated. Not recommended for intra-muscular use in Wiskott-Aldrich syndrome.	Not recommended.
Hyperimmune gamma globulin, eg, varicella, HIV.	Use in above disorders when specific exposure has oc-curred.	May be used when specific exposure has occurred.	May be used when spe-cific exposure has oc-curred.
Frozen plasma by intravenous infusion. Largely replaced by intravenous gamma globulin. Risk of transmitting viral infections.	Replaced by gamma globulin.	Replaced by gamma globulin.	Not recommended.
Infusions of leukocytes.	Not recommended.	Not recommended.	Questionable value.
Infusion of erythrocytes.	Not recommended.	May be of benefit in certain en-zyme deficiencies associ-ated with immunodeficiency (adenosine deaminase, purine nucleoside phospho-rylase). Irradiate to prevent GVH disease. Largely re-placed by enzyme replace-ment.	Not recommended.
Bone marrow transplant.	Not recommended.	Treatment of choice for many conditions. Careful bone marrow donor selection im-perative.	Used successfully in chronic granulomatous disease and leukocyte adhesion defects.
Fetal thymus transplantation.	Not recommended.	DiGeorge anomaly. Rarely used at this time.	Not recommended.
Cultured thymus epithelium.	Not recommended.	Rarely used at this time.	Not recommended.
Thymosin, thymopentin, α_1 facteur thymique serique. (Investigational.)	Not recommended.	Limited evaluation to date. May enhance T-cell function in a variety of T-cell disorders, including DiGeorge anomaly. No effect in chronic candidi-asis or severe combined immunodeficiency.	Not recommended.
Adenosine deaminase polyethyl-ene glycol.	Not recommended.	Specific for adenosine deami-nase deficiency.	Not recommended.
Gene therapy.	Not used to date.	Used successfully in adeno-sine deaminase deficiency.	Not used to date.
Cytokines.	PEG-interleukin-2 for ADA de-ficiency.	PEG-interleukin-2 for ADA defi-ciency.	Interferon-gamma for chronic granulomatous disease. G-CSF for neutropenia.

Abbreviations: HIV = human immunodeficiency virus; PEG = polyethylene glycol; ADA = adenosine deaminase; GVH = graft-ver-sus-host disease; G-CSF = granulocyte colony-stimulating factor.

REFERENCES

Good RA, Pahwa RN (editors): The recognition of immunodeficiency disorders. (Symposium.) *Pediatr Infect Dis J* 1988;**7**(suppl):S2.

Stiehm ER: *Immunologic Disorders in Infants and Children,* 4th ed. WB Saunders, 1996.

Stiehm ER: New and old immunodeficiencies. *Pediatr Res* 1993;**33**(suppl):S2.

Symposium: Childhood immunodeficiency disorders: Diagnosis, prevention, and management. *Clin Immunol Immunopathol* 1986;**40**:1.

21

Antibody (B-Cell) Immunodeficiency Disorders

Arthur J. Ammann, MD & E. Richard Stiehm, MD

Antibody immunodeficiency disorders comprise a spectrum of diseases characterized by decreased immunoglobulin levels ranging from complete absence of all classes to selective deficiency of a single class or subclass. Cases of specific antibody deficiency also occur, particularly the inability to form antibody to polysaccharide antigens. The morbidity found in patients with antibody immunodeficiency disorders is dependent chiefly on the degree of antibody deficiency. Patients with hypogammaglobulinemia become symptomatic earlier and experience more severe disease than do patients with selective immunoglobulin deficiency. Screening tests for the specific diagnosis of antibody deficiency disorders are readily available in most hospital laboratories (see Table 20–4 and Chapter 14). They permit early diagnosis and prompt institution of appropriate treatment. Other procedures, such as quantitation of B cells in peripheral blood, determination of in vitro immunoglobulin production, and suppressor cell assays, may yield more precise diagnosis and insight into the cause or mechanism of the observed deficiency (Table 21–1). The exact role of these and other tests of B-cell function has not been established for most clinical conditions.

X-LINKED AGAMMAGLOBULINEMIA

Major Immunologic Features

- Symptoms of recurrent pyogenic infections usually begin by 5–6 months of age.
- IgG is less than 200 mg/dL, with absence of IgM, IgA, IgD, and IgE.
- B cells are absent in peripheral blood.
- Patients respond well to treatment with immunoglobulin replacement.

General Considerations

In 1952, Ogden Bruton described a male child with agammaglobulinemia, in what is now recognized as the first clinical description and precise diagnosis of

Table 21–1. Evaluation of antibody-mediated immunity.

Test	Comment
Protein electrophoresis	For presumptive diagnosis of hypogammaglobulinemia or to evaluate for paraproteins.
Quantitation of immunoglobulins	Best procedure for quantitation of IgG, IgM, IgA, and IgD.
Enzyme-linked immunosorbent assay (ELISA)	IgE quantitation.
Isohemagglutinins	For evaluation of IgM function. Expected titer of >1:4 after 1 year of age.
Specific antibody response	For evaluation of immunoglobulin function. Immunize with tetanus or diphtheria toxoid or pneumococcal polysaccharide. Do not immunize with live virus if immunodeficiency is suspected.
B-cell quantitation with monoclonal antibody	Normally 10–20% (total IgG-, IgM-, IgD, and IgA-bearing cells) of total circulating lymphocytes.
IgG subclass levels	Use for patients with IgA deficiency and symptomatic patients with normal IgG levels.

an immunodeficiency disorder. (The term *agammaglobulinemia* is used here to encompass cases with severe hypogammaglobulinemia as well.) The disorder is easily diagnosed by using standard laboratory tests that demonstrate marked deficiency or complete absence of all five serum immunoglobulin classes. Male infants with this disorder usually become symptomatic following the natural decay of transplacentally acquired maternal immunoglobulin at about 5–6 months of age. They suffer from severe chronic bacterial infections, which can be controlled readily with gamma globulin and antibiotic treatment. The prevalence of this disorder in the USA is not precisely known, but estimates in the United Kingdom suggest that it is one case per 100,000 population. Two female siblings with congenital hypogammaglobulinemia have been reported.

Immunologic Pathogenesis

Extirpation of the bursa of Fabricius in birds results in complete agammaglobulinemia. Several investigators think that the human equivalent of the bursa, the source of B-cell precursors, is the gastrointestinal tract-associated lymphoid tissue (tonsils, adenoids, Peyer's patches, and appendix), whereas others assign this role to stem cells in fetal liver and bone marrow. In X-linked infantile agammaglobulinemia, a stem cell population is presumed to be absent, resulting in the complete absence of B lymphocytes and plasma cells. Investigations have provided some evidence of pre-B cells in the marrow and peripheral blood of patients, however, suggesting that the defect may be at a later stage of B-cell differentiation. These pre-B cells do not secrete immunoglobulin. The genetic defect has recently been defined and consists of a deficiency of the enzyme B-cell progenitor kinase (BPK), a cytoplasmic tyrosine kinase. The gene encoding this enzyme is on the long arm of the chromosome at Xq22. This results in a more precise diagnosis, the ability to detect the carrier state, and eventual gene therapy.

The individual immunoglobulin isotypes are a result of immunoglobulin heavy (H)-chain diversity. The formation of individual H chains is a result of somatic rearrangement of variable (V), diversity (D), and joining (J) segment genes, as described in Chapters 7 and 8. In some forms of X-linked infantile agammaglobulinemia, a truncated μ chain is produced as a consequence of premature transcription prior to D-J segment rearrangement. A second form has been shown to be a result of failure of V_H gene rearrangement, resulting in the production of truncated μ and α H chains.

Clinical Features

A. Symptoms and Signs: Patients with X-linked infantile agammaglobulinemia usually remain asymptomatic until 5–6 months of age, at which time the passively transferred maternal IgG reaches its lowest level. The loss of protection from maternal antibodies usually coincides with the age at which these children are increasingly exposed to pathogens. Initial symptoms consist of recurrent bacterial otitis media, bronchitis, pneumonia, meningitis, dermatitis, and, occasionally, arthritis or malabsorption. Many infections respond promptly to antibiotic therapy, and this response occasionally delays the diagnosis of hypogammaglobulinemia. The most common organisms responsible for infection are *Streptococcus pneumoniae* and *Haemophilus influenzae;* other streptococci and certain gram-negative bacteria are occasionally

responsible. Although patients normally have intact T-cell immunity and respond normally to viral infections such as varicella and measles, there have been reports of paralytic poliomyelitis and progressive enterovirus encephalitis following immunization with live vaccines or exposure to wild virus. Fatal echovirus infection has been reported in patients with congenital agammaglobulinemia. The encephalitis in a few patients has responded to treatment with intravenous immunoglobulin. A relationship of echovirus infection, dermatomyositis, and agammaglobulinemia has been proposed. These observations suggest that some patients with agammaglobulinemia may also be unusually susceptible to some viral illnesses.

An important clue to the diagnosis of agammaglobulinemia is the failure of infections to respond completely or promptly to appropriate antibiotic therapy. In addition, many patients with agammaglobulinemia have a history of continuous illness; that is, they do not have periods of well-being between bouts of illness.

Occasionally, patients with agammaglobulinemia may not become symptomatic until early childhood. Some of these patients may present with other complaints, such as chronic conjunctivitis, abnormal dental decay, or malabsorption. The malabsorption may be severe and may cause retardation of both height and weight. Frequently, the malabsorption is associated with *Giardia lamblia* infestation. A disease resembling rheumatoid arthritis has been reported in association with agammaglobulinemia. This occurs principally in untreated infants or is an indication for more intensive therapy with immunoglobulin.

Physical findings usually relate to recurrent pyogenic infections. Chronic otitis media and externa, serous otitis, conjunctivitis, an abnormal degree of dental decay (Fig 21–1), and eczematoid skin

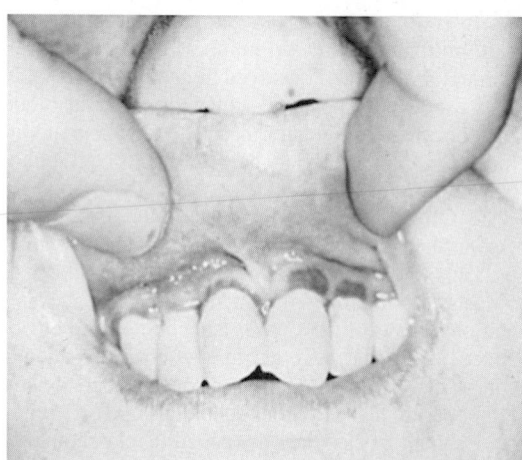

Figure 21–1. Early periodontal disease in a child with agammaglobulinemia. Recurrent ear infections and dental disease were the first manifestations of susceptibility to infection.

infections are frequently present. Despite the repeated infections, the tonsils and lymph nodes are absent and the spleen is of normal size.

B. Laboratory Findings: The diagnosis of X-linked infantile agammaglobulinemia is based on the demonstration of absence or marked deficiency of all five immunoglobulin classes. Although the diagnosis is suspected from serum protein electrophoresis and established by immunoelectrophoresis (see Chapter 14), specific quantitation of immunoglobulins is necessary, especially during early infancy. Total immunoglobulin levels are usually below 250 mg/dL. The IgG level is usually below 200 mg/dL, and IgM, IgA, IgD, and IgE levels are extremely low or undetectable. Rarely, patients have complete absence of IgG, IgA, IgM, and IgD but normal amounts of IgE. It is unusual for patients with agammaglobulinemia to have depressed levels of IgG and normal levels of IgM or IgA. Before a diagnosis of immunodeficiency is established in a patient with agammaglobulinemia, failure to make antibody following antigenic stimulation should be demonstrated. The diagnosis is difficult in infants under six months of age because of maternal IgG in the serum, but an absence of IgM, IgA, and B cells suggests the diagnosis.

Isohemagglutinins that result from natural immunization are normally present in infants of the appropriate blood group by 1 year of age. Titers of anti-A and anti-B should be greater than 1:4 in normal individuals. Antibody to a specific antigen may be measured following immunization, but a patient suspected of having an immunodeficiency disorder should never be immunized with live attenuated viral vaccine. Rarely, an intestinal biopsy to determine the presence or absence of plasma cells may be necessary to assist in the diagnosis in difficult cases. In X-linked infantile agammaglobulinemia, there are no plasma cells in the lamina propria of the gut. There is a complete absence of circulating B cells, with normal to increased numbers of T cells. T-cell immunity is intact. Delayed hypersensitivity skin tests are usually positive; isolated peripheral blood lymphocytes respond normally to phytohemagglutinin (PHA) and to allogeneic cells in mixed leukocyte culture (MLC).

C. Other Tests: X-ray of the lateral nasopharynx has been suggested as a method of demonstrating the lack of lymphoid tissue, but this rarely adds significant information to the findings on physical examination. X-rays of the sinuses and chest should be obtained at regular intervals to monitor the patient's course and to determine the adequacy of treatment. Pulmonary function studies should also be performed on a regular basis, when the patient is old enough to cooperate. Patients with agammaglobulinemia who have gastrointestinal tract symptoms should be investigated for the presence of *G lamblia* and other causes of malabsorption.

Immunologic Diagnosis

Total immunoglobulin levels are below 250 mg/dL; the IgG level is below 200 mg/dL, and IgM, IgA, IgD, and IgE levels are markedly reduced or absent. B cells are absent in peripheral blood, and there are no plasma cells containing immunoglobulins in tissue and lymph nodes. Lymph nodes are markedly depleted in B-cell-dependent areas. No antibodies are formed following specific immunization. T-cell numbers and functions are intact. Natural killer (NK) cell activity is normal.

Molecular Diagnosis

It is now possible to establish a genetic diagnosis of the tyrosine kinase gene defect.

Differential Diagnosis

A diagnosis of X-linked infantile agammaglobulinemia may be difficult to establish in the age range of 5–9 months unless new molecular techniques become available. By this time most infants have lost their maternal immunoglobulins and are susceptible to recurrent infections. The majority of normal infants during this time have IgG levels below 350 mg/dL but usually show some evidence of IgM and IgA production (usually >20 mg/dL). If the diagnosis appears uncertain, several approaches may be taken. Immunoglobulin levels may be determined again 3 months after the initial values. If there is an increase in IgG, IgM, or IgA, it is highly unlikely that the patient has agammaglobulinemia. Alternatively, the patient may be immunized with killed vaccines, and specific antibody levels determined. Patients suspected of having immunodeficiency should never be immunized with live vaccines. The most difficult diagnostic problem is the differentiation of prolonged physiologic agammaglobulinemia from X-linked infantile agammaglobulinemia. In the former, the agammaglobulinemia may sometimes be severe enough to require treatment, and immunoglobulin levels may be as low as those of patients with congenital agammaglobulinemia. Normal production of immunoglobulins may not occur until as late as 18 months of age in patients with physiologic agammaglobulinemia. In most instances these patients begin to produce their own immunoglobulin despite concurrent immunoglobulin administration. This is manifested by increasing levels of IgG as well as IgM and IgA. Since IgM and IgA make up less than 10% of commercial immunoglobulin, a gradual increase in these levels argues strongly against a diagnosis of congenital agammaglobulinemia. The best way to avoid mistaking congenital agammaglobulinemia for prolonged physiologic agammaglobulinemia in infants is to compare immunoglobulin levels with those in age-matched controls and to obtain sequential measurements of immunoglobulins at 3-month intervals during the first year of diagnostic uncertainty. Rarely, patients with human immunodeficiency virus (HIV) infection have agammaglobulinemia.

A number of familial syndromes of agammaglobulinemia and neutropenia have been described. The number is significant, and it is not certain whether this is an association or a secondary manifestation as a consequence of recurrent infection. In addition, some patients with X-linked agammaglobulinemia and growth hormone deficiency have been described.

Patients with severe malabsorption—particularly protein-losing enteropathy—may have severely depressed levels of immunoglobulins because of enteric loss. In most instances, a diagnosis of protein-losing enteropathy can be established by the demonstration of a concomitant deficiency of serum albumin. Occasionally, however, patients with severe malabsorption and primary agammaglobulinemia also lose albumin through the intestinal tract. Under these circumstances, a diagnosis can best be made by obtaining an intestinal biopsy. Patients with protein-losing enteropathy have normal numbers of plasma cells containing intracellular immunoglobulins in the gut and in other lymphoid tissues. These patients also have normal numbers of circulating B cells.

Polyarthritis may be a presenting feature in patients with agammaglobulinemia. Most patients with juvenile rheumatoid arthritis have elevated levels of immunoglobulins. Patients with arthritis and agammaglobulinemia usually respond promptly to immunoglobulin therapy. Patients with chronic lung disease should also be suspected of having cystic fibrosis, asthma, α-antitrypsin deficiency, or immotile cilia syndrome.

Treatment

Replacement immunoglobulin therapy consists primarily of the use of intravenous immunoglobulin. Although manufacturing techniques may vary for the different preparations that have been approved for clinical use, their compositions are similar. All contain almost exclusively IgG, with only trace amounts of IgM and IgA. Some preparations contain a more physiologic representation of the IgG subclasses and therefore may be useful in the treatment of IgG subclass deficiencies. All of the preparations may contain small amounts of other nonantibody proteins. Intramuscular immunoglobulin is prepared in a manner similar to that of intravenous immunoglobulin, but with the omission of chemical treatment steps that prevent it from aggregating or stimulating the complement pathway in vivo. Although intramuscular immunoglobulin is safe to use by local injection, it causes severe anaphylactoid reactions if given intravenously. Even though it is inexpensive to use and easy to administer, it has been largely replaced by intravenous immunoglobulin because larger amounts of the latter can be safely given to patients. The use of intramuscular immunoglobulin has been largely relegated to preventing hepatitis and other infectious diseases in normal individuals.

The starting dose of intravenous immunoglobulin is 200 mg/kg given intravenously once each month. The total amount given is dependent on the control of symptoms. Patients whose symptoms are not controlled on lower doses may have the total dose increased to as much as 400 mg/kg given on a monthly basis or even as frequently as every week. During an acute illness, such as meningitis or pneumonia, immunoglobulin may be given as frequently as every day if the patient fails to respond appropriately to antibiotics plus standard doses of immunoglobulin. If a patient with an acute illness has not received immunoglobulin for 2 weeks, it is advisable to provide a repeat maintenance dose. The maximum dose of intravenous immunoglobulin has not been defined, but certain factors should be considered when doses larger than 400 mg/kg are used or the frequency of administration is greater than once a week. Pulmonary function may be acutely impaired when large amounts of intravenous immunoglobulin are administered to children with pulmonary disease. Also, there are no data to suggest that giving excess amounts of passive antibody is therapeutically advantageous.

The half-life of intravenous immunoglobulin is between 15 and 25 days. Serum levels of IgG approaching normal can be achieved for the first 2–4 days following intravenous administration, but they return to abnormal values after 2–3 weeks. Weekly administration results in stabilization of levels, but this has not been shown to be of clinical benefit. Because there are limitations in the amount of immunoglobulin that can be given intramuscularly, this method of administration does not result in an increase in serum IgG levels.

Reactions to intravenous immunoglobulin are rare. Patients occasionally experience dyspnea, sweating, increased heart rate, or abdominal pain. In most instances these symptoms subside when the infusion rate is temporarily reduced.

Anaphylactoid reactions to immunoglobulin administration have been observed. These are not mediated through the IgE allergic pathway, since most patients with hypogammaglobulinemia do not form IgE antibodies. The chief causes of these reactions are aggregate formation in the immunoglobulin preparation and inadvertent intravenous administration of intramuscular preparations. Patients who have repeated reactions to immunoglobulin should first be treated with an alternative preparation obtained from a different commercial source. If reactions continue, it may be necessary to centrifuge the preparation to remove aggregates prior to administration.

Therapeutic immunoglobulin is prepared from pools of serum obtained from donors screened for absence of viruses causing hepatitis or acquired immunodeficiency syndrome (AIDS).

Additional therapy may be necessary in patients who fail to respond to maximum doses of immunoglobulin. Continuous use of antibiotics may be necessary. Prophylactic broad-spectrum antibiotics such as ampicillin in low to moderate doses may be effective in controlling recurrent infection. Physical therapy with postural drainage should be used for patients with chronic lung disease or bronchiectasis.

Occasionally, a patient with agammaglobulinemia may be discovered who has minimal or no symptoms. These patients should receive immunoglobulin therapy, even though they have not experienced repeated infection, to avoid future infections that may subsequently cause permanent complications.

Malabsorption, occasionally found in patients with agammaglobulinemia, usually responds to treatment with immunoglobulin. If *G lamblia* is found, the patient should be treated with metronidazole in doses of 35–50 mg/kg/day in three divided doses for 10 days (for children) or 750 mg orally three times a day for 10 days (for adults).

Complications & Prognosis

Although patients with congenital agammaglobulinemia have survived to the second and third decades, the prognosis must be guarded. Despite what may appear to be adequate immunoglobulin replacement therapy, many patients develop chronic lung disease. The presence of severe infection early in infancy may result in irreversible lung damage. Patients who recover from meningitis may have severe neurologic handicaps. Patients with severe pulmonary infection frequently develop bronchiectasis and chronic lung disease. Regular examinations and prompt institution of therapy are necessary to control infections and to prevent complications. Fatal echovirus infections of the central nervous system have been reported even in patients receiving immunoglobulin therapy. Some of these infections have been associated with dermatomyositis or arthritis. Some patients may develop leukemia or lymphoma. Vaccine-related poliomyelitis may occur. (Patients should not be immunized with live or killed vaccines.)

TRANSIENT HYPOGAMMAGLOBULINEMIA OF INFANCY

Under normal circumstances, maternal IgG is passively transferred to the infant beginning at week 16 of gestational life. At the time of birth, the serum IgG level in the infant is usually higher than that in the mother. IgA, IgM, IgD, and IgE are not placentally transferred under normal circumstances. In fact, the presence of elevated levels of IgM or IgA in cord blood suggests premature antibody synthesis, usually a sign of intrauterine infection. Over the first 4–5 months of life, there is a gradual decrease in the serum IgG level and a gradual increase in the serum IgM and IgA levels (Fig 21–2). The IgM level usually rises more rapidly than the IgA level. Almost all infants go through a period of agammaglobulinemia at approxi-

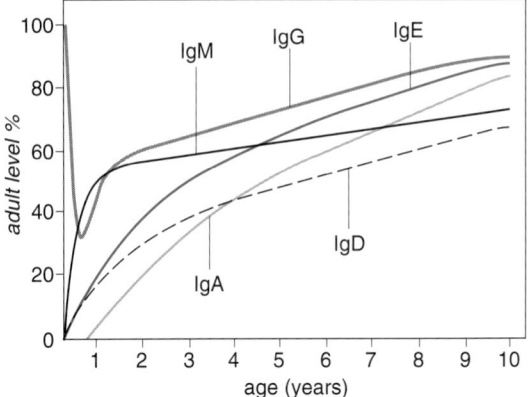

Figure 21–2. Development of serum immunoglobulins with increasing age. Levels are expressed as percentages of adult levels. Maternally acquired IgG levels decrease rapidly over the first 6 months of age. IgM levels increase more rapidly than IgA, IgD, and IgE levels.

mately 5–6 months of age. At this time, the serum IgG level reaches its lowest point (approximately 350 mg/dL), and many normal infants begin to experience recurrent respiratory tract infections. Occasionally, an infant may fail to produce normal amounts of IgG at this time, resulting in transient agammaglobulinemia, or so-called physiologic agammaglobulinemia. This effect may be more pronounced in infants born prematurely. The presence of normal serum levels of IgM and IgA argues strongly against a diagnosis of X-linked agammaglobulinemia. Some infants with transient agammaglobulinemia, however, may also fail to produce normal amounts of IgM or IgA.

Some studies may be of no diagnostic usefulness, since many infants fail to respond to immunization at this age and isohemagglutinin titers may be low. Patients with congenital agammaglobulinemia, however, lack circulating B cells, whereas children with physiologic agammaglobulinemia do not. If the patient is not experiencing severe recurrent infection, it is best to wait 3–5 months and repeat immunoglobulin measurements rather than to perform invasive procedures. In the presence of an increasing IgG, IgM, or IgA level, congenital agammaglobulinemia is unlikely. If the patient has been treated with immunoglobulin to prevent severe or recurrent infection, measurement of IgM and IgA levels assumes greater importance. Because commercial immunoglobulin contains primarily IgG, the administration of immunoglobulin does not affect serum levels of IgM and IgA. Increasing levels of these immunoglobulin classes indicate that the patient had transient agammaglobulinemia. Agammaglobulinemia may persist for as long as 2 years.

The cause of transient agammaglobulinemia is not known. A single study suggested that patients with transient agammaglobulinemia have normal numbers of B cells but a transient deficiency in the number and function of helper T cells.

Occasionally, these infants become sufficiently symptomatic that they must be treated just like those with X-linked infantile agammaglobulinemia. Immunoglobulin therapy may be required for as long as 18 months. Routine immunization should not be given during the period of transient agammaglobulinemia. The continued administration of immunoglobulin does not delay the development of normal IgG. Once a normal immune system has been established, the complete series of pediatric immunizations should be administered.

COMMON VARIABLE IMMUNODEFICIENCY (Acquired Hypogammaglobulinemia)

Major Immunologic Features
- Recurrent pyogenic infections occur, with onset at any age.
- There is increased incidence of autoimmune disease.
- The total immunoglobulin level is less than 300 mg/dL, with the IgG level below 250 mg/dL.
- B-cell numbers are usually normal.

General Considerations

Patients with common variable immunodeficiency present clinically like patients with X-linked infantile agammaglobulinemia, except that they usually do not become symptomatic until 15–35 years of age. In addition to increased susceptibility to pyogenic infections, they have a high prevalence of autoimmune disease. These patients also differ from those with congenital agammaglobulinemia in that they have a higher than normal prevalence of abnormalities in T-cell immunity, which in most instances progressively deteriorates with time. Common variable immunodeficiency affects both males and females and may occur at any age.

Immunologic Pathogenesis

The cause of common variable immunodeficiency is unknown. Most patients have an intrinsic defect in B cells. Peripheral blood lymphocytes from some patients with common variable immunodeficiency have an inhibiting effect on the immunoglobulin synthesis in cells from normal patients, suggesting that the course of this disorder may reside at the level of suppressor T cells. Other patients have diminished numbers of helper T cells. Some studies have shown a heterogeneity of arrested B-cell development ranging from normal proliferative B-cell responses and IgM-secreting cells to absent proliferative responses. Two enzymatic abnormalities have been described. In some patients there is a failure of glycosylation of the heavy-chain IgG. In others, a deficiency of 5'-nucleotidase

has been found. The latter abnormality is most probably secondary to alterations in T-cell:B-cell ratios rather than being a primary defect. An X-linked lymphoproliferative disorder associated with common variable immunodeficiency has been described following Epstein-Barr virus (EBV) infection. Genetic studies of common variable immunodeficiency have demonstrated an autosomal-recessive mode of inheritance in certain families in which abnormal lymphocyte metabolism and other forms of immunodeficiency, such as IgA deficiency, and specific major histocompatibility complex (MHC) haplotypes are found. In most instances, however, there is no clear-cut evidence of genetic transmission. An increased prevalence of other immunologic disorders, including autoimmune disease, has been observed in families of patients with common variable immunodeficiency. The presence of normal numbers of circulating peripheral blood B cells in most of these patients suggests that the disorder is a result of diminished synthesis or release of immunoglobulin rather than production of fewer cells synthesizing immunoglobulin.

Clinical Features

A. Symptoms and Signs: Recurrent sinopulmonary infection is the initial presentation of common variable immunodeficiency in most cases. These may be chronic rather than acute and overwhelming, as in X-linked infantile agammaglobulinemia. Infections may be caused by pneumococci, *H influenzae,* or other pyogenic organisms. Chronic bacterial conjunctivitis may be an additional presenting complaint. Some patients develop severe malabsorption prior to the diagnosis of agammaglobulinemia. The malabsorption may be severe enough to cause protein loss sufficient to produce edema. Giardiasis, cholelithiasis, and achlorhydria are additional findings.

Autoimmune disease has been a presenting complaint in some patients with common variable immunodeficiency. A rheumatoid arthritis-like disorder, systemic lupus erythematosus (SLE), thrombocytopenic purpura, dermatomyositis, hemolytic anemia, hypothyroidism, Graves' disease, and pernicious anemia have been reported in association with common variable immunodeficiency.

In contrast to patients with X-linked infantile agammaglobulinemia, those with common variable immunodeficiency may have marked lymphadenopathy and splenomegaly. Intestinal lymphoid nodular hyperplasia has been described in association with malabsorption. Other abnormal physical findings relate to the presence of chronic lung disease or intestinal malabsorption. Leukemia, lymphoma, and gastric carcinoma occur with increased frequency.

B. Laboratory Findings: Immunoglobulin measurements may show slightly higher IgG levels than are reported in X-linked infantile agammaglobulinemia. Total immunoglobulin levels are usually below 300 mg/dL, and the IgG level is usually below 250 mg/dL. IgM and IgA may be absent or present in significant amounts. The Schick test is useful to demonstrate a lack of normal antibody response, but it should be performed following booster immunization with diphtheria antigen. Blood group isohemagglutinins are absent or present in low titers (<1:10). The failure to produce antibody following specific immunization establishes the diagnosis in patients who have borderline immunoglobulin values. Live attenuated vaccines should not be used for immunization. Peripheral blood B lymphocytes are usually present in normal numbers in patients with common variable immunodeficiency, in contrast to their absence in patients with X-linked infantile agammaglobulinemia.

Although most patients with common variable immunodeficiency have intact cell-mediated immunity, a significant number demonstrate abnormalities as evidenced by absent delayed hypersensitivity skin test responses, depressed responses of isolated peripheral blood lymphocytes to PHA and allogeneic cells, and decreased numbers of T cells. Many patients also demonstrate reduced in vitro production of cytokines and interleukins (IL), including IL-2, IL-4, and IL-5, and interferon gamma. On the other hand, some patients have elevated levels of IL-4 and IL-6. Other patients have reduced CD4/CD8 ratios. NK cell activity is normal. A few patients have been found to have abnormal macrophage/T-cell interaction. Repetition of these tests is important, because the immunodeficiency appears to progressively involve cell-mediated immunity, resulting in additional immunologic deficiencies.

Biopsy of lymphoid tissue demonstrates a lack of plasma cells. Although some lymph node biopsies may reveal lymphoid hyperplasia, there is a striking absence of cells in the B-cell-dependent areas similar to that seen in congenital agammaglobulinemia.

C. Other Tests: Other tests that may be abnormal in these patients relate to associated disorders. The chest x-ray usually shows evidence of chronic lung disease, and sinus films show chronic sinusitis. Pulmonary function studies are abnormal. Patients with malabsorption may have abnormal gastrointestinal tract biopsies, with blunting of the villi similar to that seen in celiac disease. Studies for malabsorption may indicate a lack of normal intestinal enzymes and an abnormal D-xylose absorption test. Occasionally, autoantibodies are found in patients who have an associated autoimmune hemolytic anemia or SLE. Autoantibodies are not found in those with an associated pernicious anemia, but biopsies of the stomach demonstrate marked lymphoid cell infiltration.

Immunologic Diagnosis

The total immunoglobulin level is below 300 mg/dL, with the IgG level below 250 mg/dL. IgM and IgA may be absent or present in normal amounts. The antibody response following specific immunization is absent. Isohemagglutinins are depressed, and the

Schick test is reactive. The number of circulating peripheral blood B cells is usually normal but may be decreased.

Cell-mediated immunity may be intact or may be depressed, with negative hypersensitivity skin tests, depressed responses of peripheral blood lymphocytes to PHA and allogeneic cells, and decreased numbers of circulating peripheral blood T cells. The CD4/CD8 ratio may be reduced. The number of B cells in the peripheral blood may be normal or diminished. Occasionally, the number of null cells (lymphocytes lacking surface markers for either T or B cells) increases.

Differential Diagnosis

The clinical presentation of patients with X-linked infantile agammaglobulinemia and those with common variable immunodeficiency may be similar. This does not present a major clinical problem. Severe malabsorption in protein-losing enteropathy may cause agammaglobulinemia, but these patients always have a concomitant deficiency of serum albumin. Differentiating between protein-losing enteropathy and common variable immunodeficiency may be difficult under circumstances in which protein-losing enteropathy is accompanied by gastrointestinal loss of lymphoid cells. In both groups of patients, antibody responses and cell-mediated immunity may be impaired. When the presenting feature of common variable immunodeficiency is an autoimmune disease, there may be a delay in recognizing and treating the immune deficiency. In most instances, however, patients with autoimmune disease have normal or elevated immunoglobulin levels. Patients with chronic lung disease should also be investigated for cystic fibrosis, chronic allergy, α_1-antitrypsin deficiency, or immotile cilia syndrome. Patients with HIV infection may occasionally develop agammaglobulinemia. If HIV infection is suspected in a patient with hypogammaglobulinemia, HIV should be sought by means of viral culture or polymerase chain reaction (PCR) techniques rather than antibody testing.

Treatment

The treatment of common variable immunodeficiency is identical to that of X-linked infantile agammaglobulinemia (see Table 20–5). Immunoglobulin and continuous administration of antibiotics are usually required. Intravenous immunoglobulin at 200–400 mg/kg is given once each month. If symptoms are not controlled, the dose may be increased to 400 mg/kg per week or the original dose may be given more frequently. Immunoglobulin should always be given during an acute illness. During acute illnesses, it can be given weekly or daily. Patients should be monitored at regular intervals with chest x-rays and pulmonary function tests to determine the adequacy of therapy. Pulmonary physical therapy is an essential part of treatment in patients with chronic lung disease.

Specific treatment of malabsorption problems may be required. Some patients respond to treatment with immunoglobulin. In others, the malabsorption may be associated with secondary enzymatic deficiencies that resemble celiac disease. These patients may respond to dietary restrictions. If the malabsorption is associated with *G lamblia* infection, metronidazole therapy should be used.

Caution should be exercised in the treatment of associated autoimmune disorders. The use of corticosteroids and immunosuppressive agents in a patient with immunodeficiency may result in markedly increased susceptibility to infection. Splenectomy has been used in the treatment of agammaglobulinemia and hemolytic anemia, but the mortality rate from overwhelming infection is high.

Complications & Prognosis

Patients with common variable immunodeficiency may survive to the seventh or eighth decade. Women with this disorder have had normal pregnancies and delivered normal infants (albeit agammaglobulinemic until 6 months of age). The major complication is chronic lung disease, which may develop despite adequate immunoglobulin replacement therapy. An increased prevalence of malignant disease, including leukemia, lymphoma, and gastric carcinoma, has been observed. Patients who develop acquired T-cell deficiencies have increasing difficulty with infection characteristic of both T- and B-cell deficiencies.

IMMUNODEFICIENCY WITH HYPER-IgM

This syndrome, characterized by an increased level of IgM (ranging from 150 to 1000 mg/dL) associated with a deficiency of IgG and IgA, is relatively rare and in most instances appears to be inherited in an X-linked manner. Several cases have been reported, however, of an acquired form that affects both sexes. It has been postulated that in the normal individual there is a sequential development of immunoglobulins, initiated by IgM production and subsequently resulting in the production of IgG and IgA. Arrest in the development of immunoglobulin-producing cells after the formation of IgM-producing cells would be a possible cause. This hypothesis has been confirmed by several investigative groups who have shown that the X-linked form is associated with a genetic defect in the CD40 ligand on T cells. The normal sequence of IgM to IgG antibody production is dependent on the binding of the protein CD40 to the CD40 ligand on T cells. A defective ligand interferes with binding and antibody production. The hyper-IgM syndrome may be present congenitally or make a late appearance. It has also been reported in association with EBV. Inheritance may be X-linked or autosomal-dominant or recessive.

Patients present with recurrent pyogenic infections, including otitis media, pneumonia, and septicemia. *Pneumocystis carinii* pneumonia is a frequent initial infection. Some have recurrent neutropenia, hemolytic anemia, or aplastic anemia.

Laboratory evaluation reveals a marked increase in the serum IgM level, with absence of IgG and IgA. Isohemagglutinin titers may be elevated, and the patient may form antibodies following specific immunization. Detailed studies of cell-mediated immunity have not been performed, but some reports indicate that it is intact. Patients with this disorder may develop an infiltrating neoplasm of IgM-producing plasma cells.

Treatment is similar to that for X-linked infantile agammaglobulinemia (see Table 20–5). Because so few cases have been reported, it is difficult to determine the prognosis.

Since the genetic defect has been recognized, it should be easier to establish a diagnosis in utero and early in infancy. It should also be possible to detect the carrier state.

SELECTIVE IgA DEFICIENCY

Major Immunologic Features

- IgA level is below 5 mg/dL, with other immunoglobulin levels normal or increased.
- Cell-mediated immunity is usually normal.
- There is increased association with allergies, recurrent sinopulmonary infection, gastrointestinal tract disease, and autoimmune disease.

General Considerations

Selective IgA deficiency is the most common immunodeficiency disorder. The prevalence in the normal population has been estimated to vary between 1:800 and 1:600. Considerable debate exists about whether individuals with selective IgA deficiency are "normal" or have significant associated diseases. Studies of individual patients and extensive studies of large numbers of patients suggest that absence of IgA predisposes to a variety of diseases. The diagnosis of selective IgA deficiency is established by finding a serum IgA level of less than 5 mg/dL.

Immunologic Pathogenesis

The cause of selective IgA deficiency is usually not known. An arrest in the development of B cells has been suggested on the basis of the observation that these patients have increased numbers of B cells with both surface IgA and IgM or surface IgA and IgD. An associated IgG2 subclass deficiency has been found in some patients, and this has been used to explain the varied clinical manifestations related to antibody deficiency. Usually, the number of IgA B cells is decreased; however, the presence of normal numbers of circulating IgA-bearing B cells in many patients suggests that this disorder is associated with decreased synthesis or release of IgA or impaired differentiation to IgA plasma cells rather than with the absence of IgA B lymphocytes. Using the concept of sequential immunoglobulin production (IgM to IgG to IgA), selective IgA deficiency could result from an arrest in the development of immunoglobulin-producing cells following the normal sequential development of IgM to IgG. The variety of diseases associated with selective IgA deficiency may be the result of enhanced or prolonged exposure to a spectrum of microbial agents and nonreplicating antigens as a consequence of deficient secretory IgA. The continuous assault by these agents on a compromised mucosal immune system could result in an increased incidence of infection, autoantibodies, autoimmune disease, and cancer. Recently, an increased prevalence of HLA-A1, -B8, and -Dw3 has been found in patients with IgA deficiency and autoimmune disease.

Lymphocyte culture studies in IgA-deficient patients have demonstrated that IgA cells synthesize but fail to secrete IgA. Some individuals have suppressor T cells that selectively inhibit IgA production by normal lymphocytes.

Acquired IgA deficiency and susceptibility to sinopulmonary tract infections occur frequently in patients treated with phenytoin or penicillamine. In at least some instances, spontaneous recovery of IgA levels occurs when the drug is discontinued.

Clinical Features

A. Symptoms and Signs:

1. Recurrent sinopulmonary infection–The most frequent presenting symptoms are recurrent sinopulmonary viral or bacterial infections. Patients occasionally present with recurrent or chronic right middle lobe pneumonia. Pulmonary hemosiderosis occurs with increased frequency and may be erroneously diagnosed as chronic lung infection.

2. Allergy–In surveys of selected atopic populations the prevalence of selective IgA deficiency is 1:400–1:200, compared with a prevalence of 1:800–1:600 in the normal population. Although the reasons for this association are not known, the absence of serum IgA may result in a significant reduction in the amount of antibody competing for antigens capable of combining with IgE. Alternatively, patients who lack IgA in their secretions may more readily absorb allergenic proteins, thereby enhancing the formation of IgE antibodies. Allergic diseases in patients with selective IgA deficiency are often more difficult to control than the same allergies in other patients. Allergic symptoms in these patients may be "triggered" by infection as well as by other environmental agents.

An increase in circulating antibody to bovine proteins, sometimes associated with circulating immune complexes, including complexes with human antibody to bovine immunoglobulin, has been found in patients with selective IgA deficiency. This has been interpreted as providing additional evidence for abnormal gastrointestinal tract absorption. Removal of cow's milk from the diet, however, is usually not effective in ameliorating symptoms.

A unique form of allergy exists in these patients. Certain patients with selective IgA deficiency develop high titers of antibody directed against IgA. Anaphylactic reactions from infusion of blood products containing IgA occur in some of these patients. The prevalence of antibodies directed against IgA in patients, however, is much higher (30–40%) than the prevalence of such anaphylactic transfusion reactions. Most patients who have anti-IgA antibodies have not had a history of immunoglobulin or blood administration, suggesting that these antibodies are "autoantibodies" or that they arise from sensitization to breast milk, passive transfer of maternal IgA, or cross-reaction with bovine immunoglobulin from ingestion of cow's milk.

3. Gastrointestinal tract disease–An increased prevalence of celiac disease has been noted in patients with selective IgA deficiency. The disease may present at any time and is similar to celiac disease unassociated with IgA deficiency. Intestinal biopsies show an increase in the number of IgM-producing cells. An antibasement membrane antibody has also been found with increased incidence. Ulcerative colitis and regional enteritis have also been reported in association with selective IgA deficiency. Pernicious anemia has been found in a significant number of patients who also have antibodies to both intrinsic factor and gastric parietal cells.

4. Autoimmune disease–A number of autoimmune disorders are associated with selective IgA deficiency. They include SLE, rheumatoid arthritis, dermatomyositis, pernicious anemia, thyroiditis, Coombs-positive hemolytic anemia, Sjögren's syndrome, and chronic active hepatitis. Although the association of IgA deficiency and certain autoimmune disorders may be fortuitous, the increased prevalence of IgA deficiency in patients with SLE and rheumatoid arthritis (1:200–1:100) is statistically significant.

The clinical presentation of patients with autoimmune disease associated with selective IgA deficiency does not appear to differ significantly from that of individuals with the identical disorder and normal or elevated levels of IgA. Because patients with selective IgA deficiency are capable of making normal amounts of antibody in the other immunoglobulin classes, they usually have the autoantibodies that characterize the specific autoimmune disease (antinuclear antibody, anti-DNA antibody, antiparietal cell antibody, etc).

5. Selective IgA deficiency in apparently healthy adults–Patients with selective IgA deficiency are capable of making normal amounts of antibody of the IgG and IgM classes. Many are entirely asymptomatic, although long-term follow-up of some of these patients indicates that they may develop significant disease with time. The reasons for this are not clear, but some patients with selective IgA deficiency may have different exposures to pathogens and noxious agents in the environment.

6. Selective IgA deficiency and genetic factors—Both an autosomal-recessive and an autosomal-dominant mode of inheritance of IgA deficiency have been postulated. IgA deficiency appears with greater than normal frequency in families with other immunodeficiency disorders such as hypogammaglobulinemia. Partial deletion of the long or short arm of chromosome 18 (18q syndrome) or ring chromosome 18 has been described in selective IgA deficiency. Many patients with abnormalities of chromosome 18, however, have normal levels of IgA in their serum. Selective IgA deficiency has been reported in one identical twin but not the other. In a study of familial IgA deficiency, an association with HLA-A2, -B8, and -Dw3 was described. Other studies have shown an increase in association with HLA-A1 and -B8.

7. Selective IgA deficiency and cancer— Selective IgA deficiency has been reported in association with thymoma, reticulum cell sarcoma, and squamous cell carcinoma of the esophagus and lungs. Several patients with IgA deficiency and cancer also had concomitant autoimmune disease and recurrent infection.

8. Selective IgA deficiency and drugs— Phenytoin and other anticonvulsants have been implicated as a possible cause of some cases of selective IgA deficiency or hypogammaglobulinemia, and these patients are frequently symptomatic with recurrent sinopulmonary infections. Withdrawal of the drug does not always result in a return to normal IgA levels. In vitro production of IgA by peripheral blood lymphocytes in these patients may be normal or deficient. Deficient T-cell/B-cell interaction is found in some patients.

B. Laboratory Findings: Selective IgA deficiency is defined as a serum level of IgA below 5 mg/dL, with normal or increased levels of IgG, IgM, IgD, and IgE. Some patients with IgA deficiency may also have IgG2 subclass deficiency. Because there are a number of methods for measuring immunoglobulin levels, each laboratory should establish standards for detection of low IgA levels. B cells from these patients are capable of forming normal amounts of antibody following immunization. In most instances, absence of IgA in the serum is associated with absence of IgA in the secretions and with the presence of normal secretory component. Increased amounts of 7S IgM may be found in the serum and secretions. As discussed earlier, some patients have autoantibodies, including antibodies directed against IgG, IgM, and IgA. The number of circulating peripheral blood B cells (including IgA-bearing B cells) is normal. Increased numbers of suppressor T cells have been found in some patients.

Cell-mediated immunity is normal in most patients. Delayed hypersensitivity skin tests, the response of isolated peripheral blood lymphocytes to PHA and allogeneic cells, and the number of circulating T cells are normal. A few patients have low levels of T cells, diminished production of T-cell interferon, and decreased lymphocyte mitogenic responses.

Other laboratory abnormalities are those typical of the associated diseases. Individuals who have chronic sinopulmonary infection may have abnormal x-rays and abnormal pulmonary functions. Patients with IgA deficiency and celiac disease show appropriate pathology on gastrointestinal tract biopsies, impaired D-xylose absorption, and antibody directed against basement membrane in some cases. Patients with IgA deficiency and autoimmune disease have characteristic autoantibodies, such as anti-DNA, antinuclear, antiparietal cell, and a positive Coombs test. An increase in circulating immune complexes has been described.

Differential Diagnosis

Selective IgA deficiency must be distinguished from other more severe immunodeficiency disorders with a concomitant deficiency of IgA. Forty percent of patients with ataxia-telangiectasia have IgA deficiency. These patients usually have cellular immunodeficiency as well. If IgA deficiency is found during the first years of life, a definitive diagnosis may not be possible because the complete ataxia-telangiectasia syndrome may not be present until the patient is 4–5 years old. Other immunodeficiency disorders that have been associated with selective IgA deficiency are chronic mucocutaneous candidiasis and cellular immunodeficiency with abnormal immunoglobulin synthesis (Nezelof's syndrome) and selective deficiency of IgG2. A careful history should be obtained to rule out IgA deficiency secondary to drugs, especially anticonvulsants or penicillamine.

Treatment

Patients with selective IgA deficiency should not be treated with gamma globulin. Therapeutic gamma globulin contains only a small quantity of IgA, and this is not likely to reach mucosal secretions through parenteral administration. Furthermore, IgA-deficient patients are capable of forming normal amounts of antibody of other immunoglobulin classes. Finally, they recognize injected IgA as foreign, so that gamma globulin infusions in these patients enhance the risk of development of anti-IgA antibodies and subsequent anaphylactic transfusion reactions. There is as yet no means by which the deficient IgA can be safely replaced. Patients with combined IgA and IgG subclass deficiency with documented impaired antibody formation have been treated with gamma globulin, but its efficacy has yet to be documented. Patients with recurrent sinopulmonary infection should be treated aggressively with broad-spectrum antibiotics to avoid permanent pulmonary complications. Patients with

SLE, rheumatoid arthritis, celiac disease, and so on are treated in the same fashion as patients with the same diseases without IgA deficiency.

Transfusion reactions in patients with selective IgA deficiency may be minimized by several means. Packed washed (three times) erythrocytes should be used to treat anemia. Although this does not completely eliminate the possibility of a transfusion reaction, it does decrease the risk. Alternatively, patients may be given blood from an IgA-deficient donor whose blood type matches the recipient's. Preserving the patient's own plasma and erythrocytes for future use is recommended if possible. Patients should be encouraged to carry medical identification indicating they are IgA-deficient.

Complications & Prognosis

IgA-deficient patients have survived to the sixth or seventh decade without severe disease. Most individuals, however, become symptomatic during the first decade of life. Recognition of the potential complications and prompt therapy for associated diseases increases longevity and reduces the morbidity rate. Regular follow-up examinations are necessary for early detection of associated disorders and complications. A very few patients have developed normal IgA levels after years of IgA deficiency.

SELECTIVE IgM DEFICIENCY

Selective IgM deficiency is a rare disorder associated with the absence of IgM and normal levels of other immunoglobulin classes. IgM-bearing B cells are present in normal numbers. Some patients have decreased helper T-cell activity. Some patients are capable of normal antibody responses in the other immunoglobulin classes following specific immunization, whereas others respond poorly. Cell-mediated immunity appears to be intact, but the number of detailed studies to confirm this has been insufficient.

The cause of selective IgM deficiency is unknown. Increased suppressor T-cell activity specific for IgM has been described. The absence of IgM in the presence of IgG and IgA has yet to be explained, since it appears to contradict the theory of sequential immunoglobulin development. The disorder has been found in both males and females.

Patients with selective IgM deficiency are susceptible to autoimmune disease and to overwhelming infection with polysaccharide-containing organisms (eg, pneumococci, *H influenzae*). They may also have chronic dermatitis, diarrhea, and recurrent respiratory infections. Insufficient data are available to determine appropriate therapy. It would appear logical to treat these patients in a manner similar to the way an infant is treated following splenectomy, that is, either immediate antibiotic (penicillin or ampicillin) treatment of all infections or continuous antibiotic treatment. If patients are unable to form antibody to specific antigens, gamma globulin therapy should be given.

SELECTIVE DEFICIENCY OF IgG SUBCLASSES

Major Immunologic Features

- One or more IgG subclasses are deficient.
- T-cell immunity is normal.
- Patients have recurrent bacterial and respiratory infections.
- The condition is sometimes associated with other immunodeficiencies, such as selective IgA deficiency or ataxia-telangiectasia.

General Considerations

IgG antibodies exist in four isotypic variants identified by antigenic differences of the Fc portion of the immunoglobulin molecule. These are termed IgG1, IgG2, IgG3, and IgG4 and make up approximately 65, 20, 10, and 5% of the total serum immunoglobulin levels, respectively (Fig 21–3). IgG subclasses develop independently, with IgG1 and IgG3 maturing more rapidly than IgG2 or IgG4. Deletion of constant heavy-chain genes or abnormalities of isotype switching may result in deficiencies of one or more of the IgG subclasses with normal or near normal levels of total IgG.

Clinically, patients have recurrent respiratory tract infections and repeated pyogenic sinopulmonary infections with *S pneumoniae, H influenzae,* and *Staphylococcus aureus.* Some patients develop or present with evidence of autoimmune diseases, such as SLE or pulmonary hemosiderosis. As selective deficiency of IgG subclasses may be found in other immunodeficiency disorders, such as ataxia-telangiectasia or selective IgA deficiency, other features of immunodeficiency may predominate.

IgG1 deficiency is usually associated with other subclass deficiencies and low total IgG and thus, in truth have common variable immunodeficiency.

IgG2 deficiency is associated with recurrent sinopulmonary infections and an inability to respond to polysaccharide antigens (such as pneumococcal or *H influenzae* polysaccharide). The patient does respond normally, however, to protein antigens such as tetanus or diphtheria toxoid.

IgG2-IgG4 deficiency is usually found in individuals with recurrent infections or autoimmune disease who are either normoglobulinemic or hypergammaglobulinemic. A few healthy individuals with this deficiency have been described. It is also found in some patients with ataxia-telangiectasia.

IgG3 deficiency is found in a small percentage of individuals with recurrent infections who are screened by specific IgG subclass determinations for antibody deficiency. Familial occurrence of IgG3 deficiency has been reported.

A

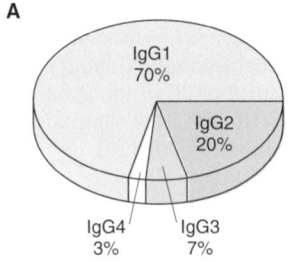

B

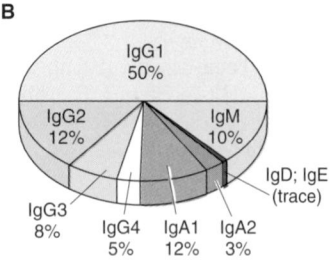

Figure 21–3. Normal distribution of serum immunoglobulins. **A:** Percentages of IgG subclasses relative to total IgG. **B:** Percentages of immunoglobulin classes and subclasses relative to total immunoglobulin.

IgG3 deficiency is also associated with recurrent respiratory infections or manifestations of autoimmune disease. IgG4 is low or absent in a significant number of asymptomatic (normal) individuals, however.

A diagnosis of one or more IgG subclass deficiencies is made by the finding of significantly low levels (<2SD below age-adjusted geometric means) of one or more IgG subclasses. For children older than 2 years, IgG1 levels should be <250 mg/dL, IgG2 <50 mg/dL, and IgG3 <25 mg/dL. The total IgG concentration may be normal, low, or elevated. The response to immunization may be variable, ranging from normal to a selective inability to respond to polysaccharide antigens. T cell immunity is usually intact.

Most patients with selective IgG subclass deficiency respond to treatment with immunoglobulin administered in a manner similar to that used in the treatment of hypogammaglobulinemia. The decision to commit a patient to lifelong treatment is a difficult one, however, and should not be based on immunoglobulin levels alone. Rather the antibody response following immunization and the clinical course should also be taken into account.

IMMUNODEFICIENCY WITH THYMOMA (Good's Syndrome)

Major Immunologic Features
■ Recurrent infections occur.
■ Acquired hypogammaglobulinemia may precede or follow thymoma.

General Considerations
Recurrent infection may be the presenting sign if the thymoma is associated with immunodeficiency. This takes the form of sinopulmonary infection, chronic diarrhea, dermatitis, septicemia, stomatitis, and urinary tract infection. Thymoma has also been associated with muscle weakness (when found in conjunction with myasthenia gravis), aplastic anemia, thrombocytopenia, diabetes, amyloidosis, chronic hepatitis, and the development of nonthymic cancer.

Patients with acquired hypogammaglobulinemia should be observed at regular intervals for the development of thymoma, which is usually detected on routine chest x-rays. Occasionally, the thymoma is detected prior to the development of immunodeficiency. Marked hypogammaglobulinemia is usually present. The antibody response following immunization may be abnormal. Some patients have deficient T-cell immunity as assayed by delayed hypersensitivity skin tests and response of peripheral blood lymphocytes to PHA. Increased activity of suppressor cells has been found in some patients. In patients who have aregenerative anemia, pure erythrocyte aplasia is seen on marrow aspiration. Thrombocytopenia, granulocytopenia, and autoantibody formation are occasionally observed. In 75% of cases, the thymoma is of the spindle cell type. Some tumors may be malignant.

In no instance has the removal of the thymoma resulted in improvement of immunodeficiency. This is in contrast to pure erythrocyte aplasia and myasthenia gravis, which may improve following removal of the thymoma. Intravenous immunoglobulin is beneficial in controlling recurrent infections and chronic diarrhea.

The overall prognosis is poor, and death secondary to infection is common. Death may also be related to associated abnormalities such as thrombocytopenia and aplastic anemia.

5′-NUCLEOTIDASE DEFICIENCY

There have been several reports of decreased activity of 5′-nucleotidase and immunodeficiency. This enzyme deficiency has been described in association with acquired hypogammaglobulinemia, X-linked hypogammaglobulinemia, Wiskott-Aldrich syndrome, AIDS, and selective IgA deficiency. 5′-Nucleotidase, however, may be a differentiation marker of lymphocytes—in particular B lymphocytes—and the deficiency may therefore reflect a diminished number of B cells or an abnormality of maturation in the peripheral circulation of these patients.

TRANSCOBALAMIN II DEFICIENCY

Several patients have been described with a deficiency of transcobalamin II, a vitamin B_{12} binding protein necessary for the transport of vitamin B_{12} into cells. These patients were found to have hypogamma-globulinemia, macrocytic anemia, lymphopenia, granulocytopenia, thrombocytopenia, and severe intestinal malabsorption. Vitamin B_{12} treatment resulted in the reversal of all of the manifestations of the disorder. Specific antibody synthesis occurred following administration of vitamin B_{12}.

REFERENCES

X-LINKED AGAMMAGLOBULINEMIA
Marx J: Tyrosine kinase defect also causes immunodeficiency. *Science* 1993;**259:**897.

Monafo V et al: X-linked agammaglobulinemia and isolated growth hormone deficiency. *Acta Paediatr Scan* 1991;**80:**563.

Rosen FS, Janeway CA: The gamma globulins. 3. The antibody deficiency syndromes. *N Engl J Med* 1966; **275:**709.

Tsukada et al: Deficient expression of a B cell cytoplasmic tyrosine kinase in human X-linked agammaglobulinemia. *Cell* 1993;**72:**279.

Van Maldergem L et al: Echovirus meningoencephalitis in X-linked hypogammaglobulinemia. *Acta Paediatr Scand* 1989;**78:**325.

COMMON VARIABLE IMMUNODEFICIENCY
Cunningham-Rundles C: Clinical and immunologic analyses of 103 patients with common variable immunodeficiency. *J Clin Immunol* 1989;**9:**22.

Eisenstein EM et al: Evidence for a generalized signaling abnormality in B cells from patients with common variable immunodeficiency. *Adv Exper Med Biol* 1995;**371B:**699.

Hermans PE, Diaz-Buxo JA, Stobo JD: Idiopathic late-onset immunoglobulin deficiency: Clinical observations in 50 patients. *Am J Med* 1976;**61:**221.

Jaffe JS et al: T cell abnormalities in common variable immunodeficiency. *Pediatr Res* 1993;**33**(suppl):S24.

Ochs H: Intravenous immunoglobulin therapy of patients with primary immunodeficiency syndromes. In: *Immunoglobulins: Characteristics and Uses of Intravenous Preparations.* US Department of Health and Human Services, 1981, p 14.

X-LINKED IMMUNODEFICIENCY WITH HYPER-IgM
Arrufo A et al: The CD40 ligand, gp39, is defective in activated T cells from patients with X-linked hyper IgM syndrome. *Cell* 1993;**72:**291.

Eskola J et al: Regulatory T-cell function in primary humoral immunodeficiency states. *J Clin Lab Immunol* 1989;**28:**55.

Ohno T et al: Selective deficiency in IL-2 production and refractoriness to extrinsic IL-2 in immunodeficiency with hyper-IgM. *Clin Immunol Immunopathol* 1987;**45:**471.

Stiehm ER, Fudenberg HH: Clinical and immunologic features of dysgammaglobulinemia type 1. *Am J Med* 1966;**40:**895.

SELECTIVE IgA DEFICIENCY
Ammann AJ, Hong R: Selective IgA deficiency: Presentation of 30 cases and a review of the literature. *Medicine* 1971;**50:**223.

Ferreira A et al: Anti-IgA antibodies in selective IgA deficiency and in primary immunodeficient patients treated with gamma-globulin. *Clin Immunol Immunopathol* 1988;**47:**199.

Oxelius VA et al: Linkage of IgA deficiency to Gm allotypes: The influence of Gm allotypes on IgA-IgG deficiency. *Clin Exper Immunol* 1995;**99:**211.

SELECTIVE IgM DEFICIENCY
Guill MF et al: IgM deficiency: Clinical spectrum and immunologic assessment. *Ann Allergy* 1989;**62:**547.

IgG SUBCLASS DEFICIENCY
Heiner DC: Recognition and management of IgG subclass deficiencies. *Pediatr Infect Dis J* 1987;**6:**235.

Inone R et al: IgG2 deficiency associated with defects in production of interferon gamma. *Scan J Immunol* 1995;**41:**130.

Ochs HD, Wedgwood RJ: Disorders of the B-cell system. In: *Immunologic Disorders in Infants and Children.* Stiehm ER (editor). Saunders, 1989, p 226.

Ochs HD, Wedgwood RJ: IgG subclass deficiencies. *Ann Rev Med* 1987;**38:**325.

Schur PH et al: Selective gamma-G globulin deficiencies in patients with recurrent pyogenic infections. *N Engl J Med* 1970;**283:**631.

IMMUNODEFICIENCY WITH THYMOMA
Hermaszewsk RA, Webster AD: Primary hypogammaglobulinemia: A survey of clinical manifestations and complications. *Quart J Med* 1993;**86:**31.

Soppi E et al: Thymoma with immunodeficiency (Good's syndrome) associated with myasthenia gravis and benign IgG gammopathy. *Arch Intern Med* 1985;**145:**1704.

Waldmann TA et al: Thymoma, hypogammaglobulinemia and absence of eosinophils. *J Clin Invest* 1967;**46:**1127.

T-Cell Immunodeficiency Disorders   **22**

Arthur J. Ammann, MD, & E. Richard Stiehm, MD

Immunodeficiency disorders associated with isolated defective T-cell immunity are rare. In most patients, defective T-cell immunity is accompanied by abnormalities of B-cell immunity. This reflects the collaboration between T cells and B cells in the process of antibody formation. Thus, almost all patients with complete T-cell deficiency have some impairment of antibody formation. Some patients with T-cell deficiency have normal levels of immunoglobulin but fail to produce specific antibody following immunization. These patients are considered to have a qualitative defect in antibody production.

Patients with cellular immunodeficiency disorders are susceptible to a variety of viral, fungal, and protozoal infections. These infections may be acute or chronic.

Screening tests utilized to evaluate T-cell immunity are listed in Table 20–4. The availability of additional tests for the evaluation of T-cell immunity (Table 22–1) permits more precise diagnosis in many instances.

CONGENITAL THYMIC APLASIA (DiGeorge Anomaly, Immunodeficiency with Hypoparathyroidism, Third and Fourth Pouch/Arch Syndrome)

Major Immunologic Features

- Congenital aplasia or hypoplasia of the thymus and parathyroid glands.
- Lymphopenia reflects a decreased number of T cells.
- T-cell function in peripheral blood is absent.
- Antibody levels and function are variable.
- Characteristic facial abnormalities.
- Congenital heart disease common.

General Considerations

DiGeorge anomaly is one of the few immunodeficiency disorders associated with symptoms immedi-

Table 22–1. Evaluation of cell-mediated immunity.

Test	Comment
Total lymphocyte count	Normal at any age: >1200/μL.
Delayed cutaneous hypersensitivity skin test	Used to evaluate specific immunity to antigens. Suggested antigens are *Candida*, mumps, tetanus toxoid, purified protein derivative.
Lymphocyte response to mitogens (PHA), antigens, and allogeneic cells (mixed leukocyte culture)	Used to evaluate T-cell function. Results are expressed as stimulated counts divided by resting counts (stimulated index).
Total T cells using monoclonal antibodies to CD3	Used to quantitate the number of circulating T cells. Normal: >60% of total lymphocytes.
Monoclonal antibody T cell subsets (CD4 and CD8)	Determines T-cell subsets, eg, helper/suppressor.
Cytokine production (IL-1, IL-2, lymphotoxin, tumor necrosis factor, etc)	Used to detect specific cytokine production from subsets of mononuclear cells as an index of function.
Cytotoxic function	Determines general and specific T-cell effector function.

Abbreviations: PHA = phytohemaglutinin; IL = interleukin.

ately following birth. The complete syndrome consists of the following features: (1) abnormal facies consisting of low-set ears, "fish-shaped" mouth, hypertelorism, notched ear pinnae, micrognathia, and an antimongoloid slant of eyes (Fig 22–1); (2) hypoparathyroidism with hypocalcemia; (3) congenital heart disease; and (4) cellular immunodeficiency. Initial symptoms are related to associated abnormalities of the parathyroids and heart and may result in hypocalcemia and congestive heart failure,

345

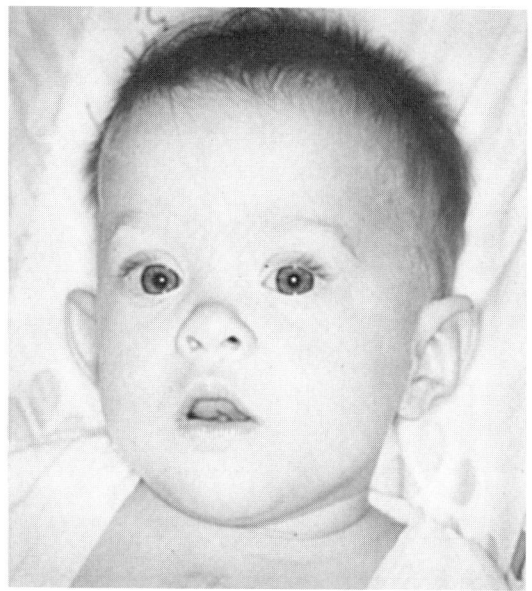

Figure 22–1. Infant with DiGeorge anomaly. Prominent are low-set and malformed ears, hypertelorism, and fish-shaped mouth. Also note the surgical scar from cardiac surgery.

respectively. If the diagnosis of DiGeorge anomaly is suspected because of these early clinical findings, confirmation may be obtained by demonstrating defective T-cell immunity. The importance of early diagnosis is related to *Pneumocystis carinii* prophylaxis

and attempts at reconstitution of T-cell immunity that can be achieved following fetal thymus transplant or bone marrow transplantation (see Table 20–5).

Immunologic Pathogenesis

During weeks 6–8 of intrauterine life, the thymus and parathyroid glands develop from epithelial evaginations of the third and fourth pharyngeal pouches (Fig. 22–2). The thymus begins to migrate caudally during week 12 of gestation. At the same time, the philtrum of the lip and the ear tubercle become differentiated along with other aortic arch structures. It is likely that DiGeorge anomaly is the result of interference with normal embryologic development at approximately 12 weeks of gestation. In some patients, the thymus is not absent but is in an abnormal location or is extremely small, though the histologic appearance is normal. It is possible that such patients have "partial" DiGeorge anomaly, in which hypertrophy of the thymus may take place with subsequent development of normal immunity. Abnormalities in chromosome 22 in >90% of patients occur, and deletions in chromosome 22 occur in some familial cases. The chromosome abnormalities may be related to congenital heart disease rather than immunologic defects. Fluorescent in situ hybridization studies are required to detect the chromosome abnormalities. Maternal alcoholism has been related to the DiGeorge anomaly.

Clinical Features

A. Symptoms and Signs: The most frequent presenting sign in patients with DiGeorge anomaly

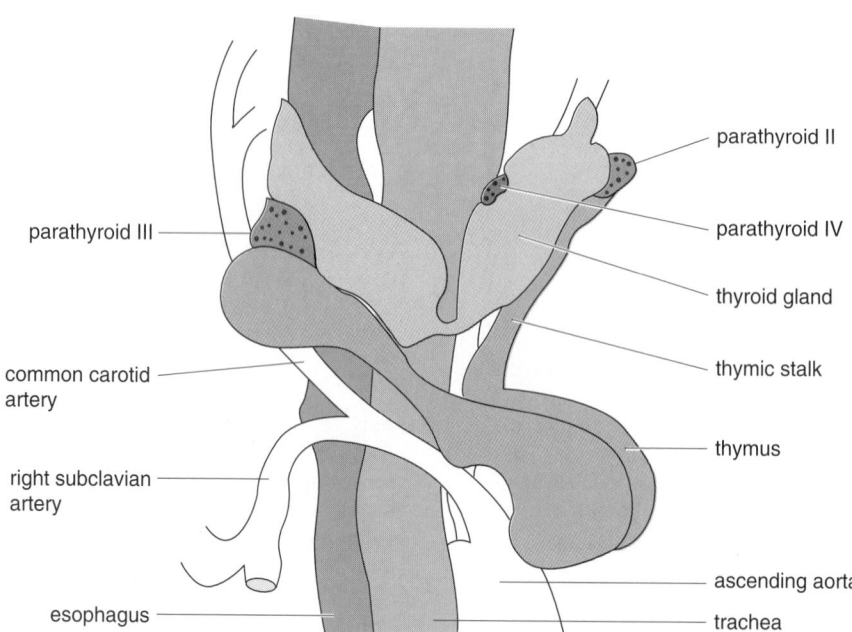

Figure 22–2. Embryologic development of the thymus and parathyroid glands from the third and fourth pharyngeal pouches.

occurs in the first 24 hours of life with hypocalcemia that is resistant to standard therapy. Various types of congenital heart disease have been described, including interrupted aortic arch, septal defects, patent ductus arteriosus, and truncus arteriosus. Renal abnormalities may also be present. Most patients have the characteristic facial appearance described earlier. Patients who survive the immediate neonatal period may then develop recurrent or chronic infection with various viral, bacterial, fungal, or protozoal organisms. Pneumonia, chronic infection of the mucous membranes with *Candida,* diarrhea, and failure to thrive may be present.

Spontaneous improvement of T-cell immunity occasionally occurs. These patients are considered to have "partial" DiGeorge anomaly, but the reason for the spontaneous improvement in T-cell immunity is not known. Patients have also been suspected of having DiGeorge anomaly on the basis of hypocalcemia and congenital heart disease with or without the abnormal facies but have been found to have normal T-cell immunity. Subsequently, these patients may develop severe T-cell deficiency.

B. Laboratory Findings: Evaluation of T-cell immunity can be performed immediately after birth in a patient suspected of having DiGeorge anomaly. The lymphocyte count is usually low (<1500/μL) but may be normal or elevated. In the absence of stress during the newborn period, a lateral-view x-ray of the anterior mediastinum may reveal absence of the thymic shadow, indicating failure of normal development. Delayed hypersensitivity skin tests to recall antigens are of little value during early infancy, because sufficient time has not elapsed for sensitization to occur. T cells are markedly diminished in number, and the peripheral blood lymphocytes fail to respond to phytohemagglutinin (PHA) and allogeneic cells.

Studies of antibody-mediated immunity in early infancy are not helpful, because immunoglobulins consist primarily of passively transferred maternal IgG. Although it is believed that some of these patients have a normal ability to produce specific antibody, the majority have some impairment of antibody formation. Sequential studies of both T-cell and B-cell immunity are necessary, since spontaneous remissions and spontaneous deterioration of immunity with time have been described.

A diagnosis of hypoparathyroidism is established by the demonstration of low serum calcium levels, elevated serum phosphorus levels, and an absence of parathyroid hormone. Congenital heart disease may be diagnosed immediately following birth and may be mild or severe. Other congenital abnormalities include esophageal atresia, bifid uvula, and urinary tract abnormalities.

Immunologic Diagnosis

T-cell immunity is usually absent at birth, as indicated by lymphocytopenia, depressed numbers of circulating T cells, and no response of peripheral blood lymphocytes to PHA and allogeneic cells. Normal T-cell immunity may develop with time particularly if the CD4 cell count exceeds 400/μL and there is some cellular response to mitogen stimulation, or previously normal T-cell immunity may become deficient. In some patients, studies of T-cell functions are variable and range from diminished T-cell numbers with normal function to a complete absence of T-cell immunity.

Many patients with DiGeorge anomaly have normal B-cell immunity as indicated by normal levels of immunoglobulins and a normal antibody response following immunization. Others, however, have low immunoglobulin levels and fail to make specific antibody following immunization. Live attenuated viral vaccines should not be used for immunization in these patients. Natural killer (NK) cell activity is normal.

Differential Diagnosis

Many infants with severe congenital heart disease and subsequent congestive heart failure develop transient hypocalcemia. These infants should be suspected of having DiGeorge anomaly. When the characteristic facial features are found in addition to the hypocalcemia and congenital heart disease an even stronger suspicion is present. Studies of T-cell immunity usually establish a diagnosis, except in infants with DiGeorge anomaly who have developed effective T-cell immunity with time. It is essential that all infants with congenital heart disease and hypocalcemia be monitored until they are at least 1 year old. The hypocalcemia associated with DiGeorge anomaly is usually permanent, in contrast to that seen in congenital heart disease with congestive heart failure. Congenital hypoparathyroidism is usually not associated with congenital heart disease. Both in this disorder and in DiGeorge anomaly, however, levels of parathyroid hormone are low to absent, and the patients are resistant to the standard treatment for hypocalcemia. Low parathyroid hormone levels may also be found in transient hypocalcemia in infancy. Two patients with DiGeorge anomaly are known to have had spontaneous remissions of their hypoparathyroidism.

Immunologic studies in DiGeorge anomaly and in severe combined immunodeficiency disease may be identical in the newborn period. The presence of hypocalcemia, congenital heart disease, and an abnormal facies differentiate DiGeorge anomaly from severe combined immunodeficiency disease.

Patients with the fetal alcohol syndrome may have similar facial and cardiac abnormalities to those in patients with DiGeorge anomaly, as well as recurrent infections associated with decreased T-cell immunity.

Treatment

Patients with T-cell deficiency should receive *Pneumocystis carinii* prophylaxis.

General care includes management of hypocalemia and correction of cardiac abnormalities.

The hypocalcemia is rarely controlled by calcium supplementation alone. Calcium should be administered orally in conjunction with vitamin D or parathyroid hormone.

Congenital heart disease frequently results in congestive heart failure and may require immediate surgical correction. If surgery is performed prior to the availability of a fetal thymus or bone marrow transplantation, blood transfusion products should be irradiated with 3000 R to prevent a graft-versus-host (GVH) reaction.

Fetal thymus transplantation was previously the treatment of choice. Human leukocyte antigen (HLA) matched bone marrow transplantation has also been successful. Both methods resulted in permanent reconstitution of T-cell immunity. The technique of thymus transplantation varied from local implantation in the rectus abdominis muscle to implantation of a thymus in a Millipore chamber. The thymus was also minced and injected intraperitoneally. Because patients with DiGeorge anomaly have been observed to develop a GVH reaction following administration of viable immunocompetent lymphocytes, fetal thymus glands older than 14 weeks of gestation were not used. Thymocytes from glands younger than 14 weeks of gestation lack cells capable of GVH reaction but can provide needed stem cells or thymic epithelial cells for further T-cell development. No attempts at immunologic reconstitution are warranted if T-cell immunity is normal. Some patients undergo spontaneous resolution of the T-cell immunodeficiency. Intravenous immunoglobulin therapy should be used if antibody deficiency exists and to control recurrent infection.

Complications & Prognosis

Prolonged survivals have been reported following successful thymus transplantation or spontaneous remission of immunodeficiency. Sudden death may occur in untreated patients or in patients initially found to have normal T-cell immunity. Congenital heart disease may be severe, and the infant may not survive surgical correction. Death from GVH disease following blood transfusions has been observed in patients in whom a diagnosis of DiGeorge anomaly was not suspected. Most patients with long-term survival have minimal heart disease.

CHRONIC MUCOCUTANEOUS CANDIDIASIS
(With & Without Endocrinopathy)

Major Immunologic Features

- Chronic candidial infection of the skin, nails, and mucous membranes with or without endocrinopathy.

- Delayed hypersensitivity skin tests to *Candida* antigen are negative despite chronic candidal infection.
- T-cell immunity to most antigens is intact.

General Considerations

Chronic mucocutaneous candidiasis affects both males and females. A familial occurrence has been reported in some instances, suggesting an autosomal-recessive or dominant inheritance. The disorder is associated with a selective defect in T-cell immunity, resulting in susceptibility to chronic candidal infection. B-cell immunity is intact, resulting in a normal antibody response to *Candida* and, in some patients, the development of autoantibodies associated with idiopathic endocrinopathies. The disorder may appear as early as 1 year of age or may be delayed until the second decade.

Various theories have been proposed to explain the association of chronic candidal infection and the development of endocrinopathy. Initially it was believed that hypoparathyroidism predisposed to candidal infection. Subsequently it was found that many patients developed severe candidal infection without evidence of hypoparathyroidism. A basic autoimmune disorder has been postulated, with the suggestion that the thymus also functions as an endocrine organ and that the thymus and other endocrine glands are involved in an autoimmune destructive process.

Clinical Features

A. Symptoms and Signs: The initial presentation of chronic mucocutaneous candidiasis may be either chronic candidal infection or the appearance of an idiopathic endocrinopathy. If candidal infection appears first, several years to several decades may elapse before endocrinopathy occurs. Other patients may present with the endocrinopathy first and subsequently develop the infection. Candidal infection may involve the mucous membranes, skin, nails, and, in older patients, the vagina. In severe forms, infection of the skin occurs in a "stocking-glove" distribution and is associated with the formation of granulomatous lesions (Fig 22–3). Patients are usually not susceptible to systemic candidiasis. Rarely, they may develop infection with other fungal agents.

Other symptoms are related to the specific endocrinopathy. Hypoparathyroidism is the most common and is associated with hypocalcemia and tetany. Addison's disease is the next most common. A variety of other endocrinopathies have been reported, including hypothyroidism, diabetes mellitus, hypogonadism, and pernicious anemia. Occasionally, there is a history of acute or chronic hepatitis. Additional disorders include pulmonary fibrosis, adrenocorticotropic hormone (ACTH) deficiency, keratoconjunctivitis, vitiligo, alopecia, enamel dysplasia, hematologic disorders, and myopathy.

B. Laboratory Findings: Studies of T-cell immunity reveal a specific although variable defect.

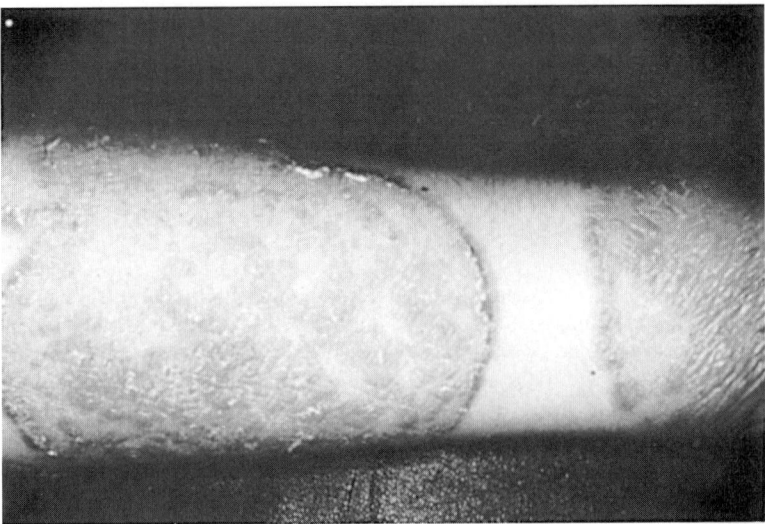

Figure 22–3. Chronic *Candida* infection in a patient with mucocutaneous candidiasis. Note the well-demarcated areas of involvement.

Patients usually have a normal total lymphocyte count. Peripheral blood lymphocytes respond normally to PHA, allogeneic cells, and antigens other than *Candida* antigens. The least severe T-cell defect is an absent delayed hypersensitivity skin test response to *Candida* antigen in the presence of documented chronic candidiasis. Other patients may have additional defects, including the inability to form migration inhibitory factor (MIF) or other cytokines in response to *Candida* antigens or the inability of lymphocytes to be activated by *Candida* antigens and decreased suppressor T-cell activity. B-cell immunity is intact, as demonstrated by the presence of normal or elevated levels of immunoglobulins, increased amounts of antibody directed against *Candida,* and autoantibody formation. Occasionally, selective absence of IgA or elevated levels of immunoglobulins may be observed. Plasma inhibitors of T-cell function and increased numbers of suppressor T cells have been reported in some cases. Isolated cases have been described with neutrophil chemotaxis or macrophage abnormalities.

Other laboratory abnormalities are related to the presence of endocrinopathies. Hypoparathyroidism is associated with decreased serum calcium levels, elevated serum phosphorus levels, and low or absent parathyroid hormone levels. Increased skin pigmentation may herald the onset of Addison's disease prior to disturbances in serum electrolytes. An ACTH stimulation test is useful to document the presence of Addison's disease. Other abnormalities of endocrine function include hypothyroidism, abnormal vitamin B_{12} absorption, and diabetes mellitus. Abnormal liver function studies may indicate chronic hepatitis. Occasionally, iron deficiency is present, which, when treated, results in improved resistance to the candidal infection. Autoantibodies associated with specific endocrinopathy are usually present before and during the development of endocrine dysfunction. They may be absent when complete endocrine deficiency is present. Patients should be evaluated on a yearly basis for endocrine function because the endocrinopathies are progressive.

Immunologic Diagnosis

Major aspects of T-cell immunity are normal, as indicated by a normal response of peripheral blood lymphocytes to PHA and allogeneic cells. Activation of lymphocytes and cytokine production in response to antigens other than *Candida* antigens is normal. T-cell numbers are normal. In some patients, only the delayed hypersensitivity skin test response to *Candida* antigens is absent. Other patients have absent cytokine production or an absence of lymphocyte activation by *Candida* antigens. Plasma inhibitors of cellular immunity may also occur. B-cell immunity is intact with normal production of antibody to *Candida*.

Differential Diagnosis

Children with chronic candidal infection of the mucous membranes may have a variety of immunodeficiency disorders. Detailed studies of T-cell immunity differentiate between chronic mucocutaneous candidiasis, in which there is a selective deficiency of T-cell immunity to *Candida* antigens, other disorders in which T-cell immunity may be completely deficient. Patients with DiGeorge anomaly (thymic aplasia and hypoparathyroidism) present early in infancy, whereas chronic mucocutaneous candidiasis with hypoparathyroidism is a disorder of later onset and progressive nature. Patients with late-onset idiopathic endocrinopathies should be considered to have chronic mucocutaneous candidiasis, even though candidal infection is not present at the time of diagnosis. These patients may develop chronic candidal infection as late as 10–15 years after the onset of endocrinopathy. Chronic candidiasis, especially involving the mucous membrane, may be associated with secondary immunodeficiency disorders due to immunosuppressive therapy or the human immunodeficiency virus.

Treatment

No treatment prevents the development of idiopathic endocrinopathy. The physician must be alert to the gradual development of endocrine dysfunction—particularly Addison's disease. Chronic skin and mucous membrane candidal infection is difficult to treat. Topical treatment with a variety of antifungal agents is only minimally successful for skin infection. Oral antifungals, such as ketoconazole, fluconazole, and miconazole, are the mainstay of therapy. Systemic therapy, when necessary, should first include fluconazole or miconazole.

Immunologic therapy has been of limited and questionable success and includes thymus transplantation, leukocyte infusions, transfer factor, and bone marrow transplantation. Courses of intravenous amphotericin B have resulted in improvement in a significant number of patients, but this form of treatment is limited by the renal toxicity of the drug. Oral clotrimazole is occasionally beneficial.

Complications & Prognosis

Patients may survive to the second or third decade but usually experience extensive morbidity. Individuals with severe candidal infection of the mucous membranes and skin develop serious psychologic difficulties. Systemic infection with *Candida* usually does not occur. Rarely, patients may develop systemic infection with other fungal agents. Hypoparathyroidism is difficult to manage, and complications are frequent. Patients may succumb at an early age from endocrinopathy, bronchiectasis, or chronic hepatitis.

NATURAL KILLER CELL DEFICIENCY

NK cells are non-B-cell/non-T-cell (CD3-negative) lymphocytes but have receptors for the Fc portion of the immunoglobulin molecule (CD16). In addition, they have the NKH-1 (CD56-positive, CD16-positive) determinant, which identifies the large granular lymphocyte population that NK cells resemble morphologically. NK cells spontaneously lyse a number of target cells, including tumor cells, but when activated by interleukin-2 (IL-2) or interferon gamma, they lyse a broad range of virus-infected cells. It is therefore believed that these cells play a role in host defense against cancer and microbial infection.

Deficiency of NK cells is not confined to a single defined immunodeficiency disorder, although there

are isolated case reports of what appear to be selective NK deficiencies. NK-cell deficiency has been documented in the Chédiak-Higashi syndrome, the X-linked lymphoproliferative syndrome, the chronic fatigue syndrome, and leukocyte adhesion defect (CD11/CD18 deficiency). NK-cell deficiency has also been detected in primary immunodeficiency diseases, primarily in severe combined immunodeficiency disease and other T-cell disorders, suggesting an association between NK- and T-cell defects.

Although NK-cell deficiency has been detected most consistently in the X-linked lymphoproliferative syndrome, which is associated with fatal Epstein-Barr virus infection, cancer, and hypogammaglobulinemia, there are reports of patients with recurrent severe infections with herpes viruses, including varicella, cytomegalovirus infection, and herpes simplex. Immunologic evaluation was normal, except for deficient NK-cell numbers and function. The peripheral blood mononuclear cells were unable to mediate spontaneous or IL-2-induced NK-cell functions. This case suggests that isolated defects in NK-cell function exist. No specific treatment to correct the NK-cell defect was attempted. Acyclovir was used to treat the acute infections, and the patient was maintained on intravenous immunoglobulin.

IDIOPATHIC CD4 LYMPHOCYTOPENIA

Idiopathic CD4 lymphocytopenia received considerable attention when first described because of a postulated association with an as yet unidentified virus possibly associated with human immunodeficiency virus (HIV-1 or HIV-2). After an exhaustive search, however, for a common etiology, such as HIV-1, HIV-2, or other virus, it was concluded that no common cause existed. Symptoms in patients varied from minimal abnormalities to individuals who succumbed to opportunistic infection. Both males and females were affected, and patients ranged in age from 17 to 70 years old. Follow-up of patients indicated that the defect was reversible in some. The syndrome can be differentiated from HIV-associated CD4 lymphocytopenia by the absence of evidence of HIV-1 infection, using HIV-1 polymerase chain reaction (PCR), or antibody testing, and the absence of hypergammaglobulinemia.

BIOTIN-DEPENDENT CARBOXYLASE DEFICIENCIES

Patients with infantile chronic mucocutaneous candidiasis, ataxia, alopecia, intermittent lactic acidosis, and increased excretion of β-hydroxypropionate, methylcitrate, β-methylcrotonylglycine, and 3-β-hydroxyisovalerate in the urine have been described. Immunologic abnormalities in both B-cell and T-cell function were found. A second (neonatal) form has been described that is associated with severe acidosis and multiple episodes of sepsis. An intrauterine diagnosis has been made, and intrauterine therapy with biotin has been given. Treatment with biotin, 10 mg/day, reduced the abnormal metabolites in the urine and reversed the alopecia, ataxia, and chronic candidiasis. Multiple biotin-dependent carboxylase deficiencies

may be one of several causes of the chronic mucocutaneous candidiasis syndrome with abnormal T-cell function or severe recurrent sepsis. Biotin deficiency and immunodeficiency may also be a result of nutritional deficiencies and has been found in patients receiving hyperalimentation without biotin supplementation and in individuals on diets high in avidin (raw eggs), which binds biotin and prevents absorption.

REFERENCES

THYMIC APLASIA WITH HYPOPARATHYROIDISM

Barrett DJ et al: Clinical and immunologic spectrum of the DiGeorge syndrome. *J Clin Lab Immunol* 1981;**6**:1.

DiGeorge AM: Congenital absence of the thymus and its immunologic consequences: Concurrence with congenital hypoparathyroidism. In: *Immunologic Deficiency Diseases in Man.* Bergsma D, McKusick FA (editors). National Foundation—March of Dimes Original Article Series. Williams & Wilkins, 1968.

Kurahashi H et al: Isolation and characterization of a novel gene deleted in DiGeorge syndrome. *Human Mol Genet* 1995;**4**:541.

Radford DJ et al: Spectrum of DiGeorge syndrome in patients with truncus arteriosis: Expanded DiGeorge syndrome. *Pediatr Cardiol* 1988;**9**:95.

CHRONIC MUCOCUTANEOUS CANDIDIASIS

Arulanantham K et al: Evidence for defective immunoregulation in the syndrome of familial candidiasis endocrinopathy. *N Engl J Med* 1979;**300**:164.

Herrod HG: Chronic mucocutaneous candidiasis in childhood and complications of non-*Candida* infection: a report of the Pediatric Immunodeficiency Collaborative Group. *J Pediatr* 1990;**116**:377.

Kirkpatrick CH: Chronic mucocutaneous candidiasis. Antibiotic and immunologic therapy. *Ann NY Acad Sci* 1988;**544**:471.

Kirkpatrick CH et al: Chronic mucocutaneous candidiasis: Model building in cellular immunity. *Ann Intern Med* 1971;**74**:955.

Mobacken H, Moberg S: Ketoconazole treatment of 13 patients with chronic mucocutaneous candidiasis: A prospective three-year trial. *Dermatologica* 1986; **173**:229.

NATURAL KILLER CELL DEFICIENCY

Biron CA et al: Severe herpes virus infections in an adolescent without natural killer cells. *N Engl J Med* 1989;**320**:1731.

Komiyama A et al: Impaired natural killer cell recycling in childhood chronic neutropenia and morphological abnormalities and defective chemotaxis. *Blood* 1985;**66**:99.

Ritz J: The role of natural killer cells in immune surveillance. *N Engl J Med* 1989;**320**:1789.

Stiehm ER: New and old immunodeficiencies. *Pediatr Res* 1993;**33**(suppl):S2.

IDIOPATHIC CD4 LYMPHOCYTOPENIA

Sneller MC et al: A unique syndrome of immunodeficiency and autoimmunity associated with absent T cell CD2 expression. *J Clin Immunol* 1994;**14**:359.

Smith DK et al: Unexplained opportunistic infections and CD4 T lymphocytopenia without HIV infection. An investigation of cases in the United States. *N Engl J Med* 1993;**328**:373.

BIOTIN-DEPENDENT MULTIPLE COCARBOXYLASE DEFICIENCY

Cowan MJ, Ammann AJ: Immunodeficiency associated with inherited metabolic disorders. *Clin Haematol* 1981;**10**:139.

Cowan MJ et al: Multiple biotin-dependent carboxylase deficiencies associated with defects in T cell and B cell immunity. *Lancet* 1979;**1**:115.

23

Combined Antibody (B-Cell) & Cellular (T-Cell) Immunodeficiency Disorders

E. Richard Stiehm, MD, & Arthur J. Ammann, MD

Combined immunodeficiency diseases are variable in cause and severity. Defective T-cell and B-cell immunity may be complete, as in severe combined immunodeficiency disease, or partial, as in ataxia-telangiectasia. The distinct clinical features of ataxia-telangiectasia serve to further differentiate the disorder from severe combined immunodeficiency disease and also suggest that these disorders do not have the same cause. Enzymatic deficiencies in the purine pathway have been described in association with combined immunodeficiency, and specific genetic mutations of single amino acids are responsible in many instances. These discoveries have provided additional evidence for a diverse origin of combined immunodeficiency disease.

Studies of both T-cell and B-cell immunity are necessary to completely evaluate patients with combined immunodeficiency disorders (see Tables 20–4, 21–1, and 22–1). In addition, analysis of erythrocyte and leukocyte enzymes (adenosine deaminase and nucleoside phosphorylase, respectively) can assist appropriate classification.

The onset of symptoms in patients with combined immunodeficiency diseases is usually early in infancy. These patients are susceptible to a very wide spectrum of microorganisms. Immunotherapy is frequently difficult and often not available.

RETICULAR DYSGENESIS

Reticular dysgenesis is a form of severe combined immunodeficiency in which there is an associated profound deficiency of myeloid elements of the hematopoietic system. As a result, marked leukopenia is present in addition to B- and T-cell immunodeficiency, and very early onset of infection. Bone marrow transplantation has been used successfully.

SEVERE COMBINED IMMUNODEFICIENCY (SCID)

Major Immunologic Features

- Onset of viral, bacterial, fungal, or protozoal infections before 6 months of age.
- X-linked, autosomal, and sporadic forms occur.
- T- and B-cell immunity are severely impaired.
- Several immunologic defects cause same clinical pattern.
- Bone marrow transplantation is the treatment of choice.

Several forms of severe combined immunodeficiency (SCID) result in an identical clinical picture. The immune defect, however, including the autosomal-recessive lymphopenic variants, has not been identified in most cases.

Among the defects identified, the interleukin **(IL)-2 receptor defect** is the best described as **X-linked combined immunodeficiency.** This results from mutations of the γ chain of the IL-2 receptor. This γ chain is also a component of the IL-4, IL-7, IL-9, and IL-15 receptors and several myeloid cytokine receptors.

Defective cytokine synthesis, including synthetic defects of IL-1, IL-2, and multiple cytokines, have been described. IL-2 therapy in the IL-2 deficiency was of some clinical benefit. **Nezelof's syndrome,** or cellular immunodeficiency with immunoglobulins, is not uncommon. In addition to profound T-cell deficiency, these patients have normal or high levels of one of more serum immunoglobulins but poor to absent antibody synthesis. Often these patients have a less severe course than other patients with SCID with survival into the teens. Nezelof's syndrome is a variant of SCID since all of these patients have significant thymic dysplasia.

Less common variants of combined immunodeficiency include isolated **CD8 deficiency,** associated with ZAP-70 kinase (a tyrosine kinase implicated in signal transduction) abnormality. Other surface receptor and tranduction defects have also been described (see later discussion). **Griscelli's syndrome** is a combined immunodeficiency in patients with fine silvery hair, hepatosplenomegaly, and lymphoid hyperplasia. They resemble patients with Chédiak-Higashi syndrome but without the giant granulocyte azurophilic granules. **CD7 deficiency** with SCID has been described. **OKT4 epitope** deficiency is quite common, identified by the absense of reactivity with the OKT4 monoclonal antibody to CD4 lymphocytes. CD4 cells are present when assessed by another monoclonal antibody (eg, Leu-3b). These patients have only mild susceptibility to infection.

The bare lymphocyte syndrome and immunodeficiency with purine enzyme defects are described later.

Treatment

Aggressive diagnostic measures are necessary to establish the cause of chronic infection before treatment can be instituted. Open lung biopsy or bronchoscopy should be performed if *Pneumocystis carinii* infection is suspected. Therapy includes pentamidine, trimethoprim-sulfamethoxazole, or both. Specific antibiotic treatment is necessary for suspected bacterial infection. Superficial candidal infection is treated with topical antifungal drugs, but systemic infection requires intravenous amphotericin B or other antifungals.

Complications must be avoided. Immunization with live attenuated virus should not be performed. Blood products containing potentially viable lymphocytes should be irradiated with 2500 R prior to administration (see the discussion of graft-versus-host [GVH] disease in the following paragraphs). Prophylactic trimethoprim-sulfamethoxazole should be used to prevent *P carinii* infection.

Intravenous immunoglobulin should be administered in doses of 100–400 mg/kg every 1–4 weeks, but this regimen does not correct the T-cell deficiency. Definitive treatment consists of bone marrow transplantation. The ideal donor is a human leukocyte antigen (HLA)-identical sibling. The donor and recipient must be matched by HLA typing and histocompatibility confirmed by a nonreactive mixed leukocyte reaction (MLR). Despite careful matching, a GVH reaction may develop. Transplantation of unmatched marrow results in a fatal GVH reaction.

The use of haploidentical (half-matched) marrow from a parent, prepared by removing mature T cells by lectins or by monoclonal antibody-complement combination can now be done at various centers. Many of these patients need to be immunosuppressed to ensure engraftment of the depleted marrow. This procedure is nearly as successful as HLA-identical transplantation. Another type of transplant is a matched unrelated donor, selected through the national registry of HLA-typed donors. Immunosuppression of the recipient is usually necessary.

Other considerations in bone marrow transplantation are the cytomegalovirus (CMV) and Epstein-Barr virus (EBV) status of the donor; antivirals are sometimes used to prevent CMV infection or EBV immunoproliferative disease. Prophylaxis with cyclosporin to prevent or minimize GVH is usually employed.

The benefit of thymic transplant or hormones or liver cells is unproven and no longer used.

COMBINED IMMUNODEFICIENCY WITH T-CELL MEMBRANE OR SIGNALING DEFECTS

Major Immunologic Features

- Phenotypic characteristics of other combined immunodeficiency disorders.
- Symptoms vary from mild to severe infections.
- Defects include structurally abnormal T-cell receptor or abnormal signal transduction.

T cells are activated following interaction with an antigen-presenting cell (APC), a step that is dependent on cell-to-cell contact. The T-cell receptor (TCR) binds to the major histocompatibility complex (MHC) of the APC, resulting in the expression of cytokine receptors and cytokine secretion. Multiple intracellular events, including the accumulation of phosphorylated substrates (especially tyrosine phosphorylation) and increases in concentrations of Ca^{2+}, also are necessary for cell activation. These events lead to secretion of cytokines, such as IL-2, tumor necrosis factor, interferon gamma, and transforming growth cell proliferation, and differentiation into cytotoxic cells.

Most patients have normal or near-normal T-cell numbers but deficient or absent proliferative responses to mitogens, antigens, or anti-CD3 monoclonal antibody. Most have moderate susceptibility to infection, but some patients have only mild susceptibility to infection. A defective TCR (such as the lack of the CD3 ζ chain) or an abnormality of signal transduction (such as a G-protein or a tyrosine kinase abnormality) have been identified in a few of these patients. Only a few research laboratories have the techniques established to evaluate these patients' biochemical defects.

BARE LYMPHOCYTE SYNDROME (Class II MHC Deficiency)

Major Immunologic Features

- Leukocyte class I or class II HLA antigens (or both) are absent or markedly decreased.
- Immunologic features are usually similar to those of combined immunodeficiency disease.

■ A few patients are asymptomatic or only minimally symptomatic.

General Considerations

Patients with the bare lymphocyte syndrome have deficient expression of HLA molecules with resultant combined immunodeficiency. A description of the HLA genes of the MHC on the short arm of chromosome 6, the families of cell surface proteins encoded by these genes, their expression on cells of the immune system, and their role in the immune response is found in Chapter 6.

The bare lymphocyte syndrome occurs primarily in families from the Mediterranean area and is often associated with consanguineous union. It is inherited in an autosomal-recessive manner. The first case was discovered by an inability to HLA type the patient's cells. From detailed investigation of subsequent patients, it is clear that the bare lymphocyte syndrome represents a collection of at least four genotypic abnormalities with differing phenotypic expressions. In all patients there is abnormally low or absent expression of class I or class II HLA antigens, or both. In patients with deficient cell surface class II antigens, both the presence and absence of the class II gene has been found. In some instances, when the gene is present, class II antigens can be induced following stimulation of cells in vitro with antigens or interferon gamma. In others, there is an abnormality of the transactivating class II regulatory gene (CIITA) that lies outside the major histocompatibility locus. In still others, there is a deficiency in a DNA-binding protein referred to as the X-box-binding protein (RF-X), implicated in regulation of class II gene transcription.

Clinical Features

A. Symptoms and Signs: Although a few individuals are entirely healthy, most have clinical features similar to those present in severe combined immunodeficiency. These include early onset of opportunistic infections, chronic diarrhea, recurrent viral infections, oral candidiasis, central nervous system viral infection, aplastic anemia, and growth failure.

B. Laboratory Findings: Lymphopenia with diminished T-cell numbers and function is found in severe cases. The response of peripheral blood lymphocytes to antigens is usually reduced, but the response to mitogens may be normal. B-cell numbers are normal or elevated, but hypogammaglobulinemia and decreased antibody function are present.

Immunologic Diagnosis

Routine typing for histocompatibility antigens reveals the absence or decreased expression of HLA class I or class II antigens, or both. An intrauterine diagnosis can be established in the presence of a family history by analyzing fetal blood cells or chorionic villus biopsy material. To assist in bone marrow trans-

plantation and matching, HLA genotyping has used typing with restriction enzyme fragments and specific HLA probes. The bare lymphocyte syndrome should not be confused with other combined immunodeficiency diseases since no other syndrome lacks HLA antigens. In rare instances, severe leukopenia associated with other forms of immunodeficiency may make HLA typing difficult.

Treatment

Severe forms of the bare lymphocyte syndrome require bone marrow transplantation. Determining an appropriate donor for transplantation may be difficult and may require special techniques such as DNA hybridization. Supportive therapy is similar to that for severe combined immunodeficiency, with the use of intravenous immunoglobulin and prophylactic trimethoprim-sulfamethoxazole.

OMENN SYNDROME
(Combined Immunodeficiency
with Eosinophilia)

This is an autosomal-recessive variant of combined immunodeficiency characterized by the early onset of a seborrheic pruritic skin eruption, hepatosplenomegaly, and lymphadenopathy. Eosinophilia is present, and the IgE is usually elevated. CD8 cytotoxic cells attacking the skin has been suggested as a possible immunologic abnormality. Engrafted maternal cells may be implicated in some patients. Bone marrow transplantation has been successful in treating this disorder.

WISKOTT-ALDRICH SYNDROME
(Immunodeficiency with
Thrombocytopenia & Eczema)

Major Immunologic Features

■ X-linked syndrome of eczema, recurrent pyogenic infection, and thrombocytopenia.
■ Decreased antibody responses to polysaccharide antigens with decreased IgM and elevated IgA and IgE level.
■ Decreased T-cell function with increased susceptibility to autoimmunity and malignancy.
■ Thrombocytopenia is characterized by small platelets.

General Considerations

Male infants with Wiskott-Aldrich syndrome (WAS) may become symptomatic early in life, with bleeding secondary to thrombocytopenia. Subsequently they develop recurrent bacterial infection in the form of otitis media, pneumonia, and meningitis. Eczema usually appears by 1 year of age. The disease is progressive, with increasing susceptibility to infection and cancer. At autopsy, the thymus and lymph node have an abnormal architecture, with depletion of lymphoid cells, poor follicle formation, and poor corticomedullary differentiation.

Immunologic Pathogenesis

Two of the earliest abnormalities are thrombocytopenia and hypercatabolism of immunoglobulin. There are several hypotheses linking thrombocytopenia, eczema, and recurrent infection. It has been suggested that abnormal α granules of platelets and macrophages occur in patients and carriers. Another suggestion is that the inability of patients to respond to polysaccharide antigens results in immunologic attrition. This, however, does not explain the thrombocytopenia or eczema. A 115-kd surface glycoprotein termed sialophorin (CD43) involved in lymphocyte activation and differentiation is decreased or absent on WAS lymphocytes; however, this is not the primary defect since CD43 is encoded on chromosome 16. Decreased expression of B-cell CD23 has been described. CD23 is involved in the differentiation of immune cells, inhibition of monocyte migration, B-cell proliferation, and IgE production. Thus, an abnormality of CD23 might result in many of the hematologic and immunologic defects described.

The gene for WAS has recently been identified on the X-chromosome; it encodes a protein termed Wiskott-Aldrich syndrome protein (WASP), which is expressed in lymphocytes, megakaryocytes, spleen, and thymus, but its function is not yet known.

Clinical Features

A. Symptoms and Signs: Recurrent infection usually does not start until after 6 months of age. Patients are susceptible to infection with capsular polysaccharide-type organisms (eg, *Pneumococcus, Meningococcus,* and *Haemophilus influenzae*), which cause meningitis, otitis media, pneumonia, and sepsis. As the patients become older, they become susceptible to infection with other types of organisms and may have recurrent viral infection. Eczema is usually present by 1 year of age and is typical in distribution (Fig 23–1) and often associated with other allergic manifestations. Thrombocytopenia is present at birth and may result in severe bleeding, particularly during episodes of infection. The bleeding tendency becomes less severe as the child becomes older.

B. Laboratory Findings: Thrombocytopenia is present at birth—a fact that is helpful in diagnosis. The platelet count may range from 5000 to 100,000/μL. Platelets are small in Wiskott-Aldrich syndrome, in contrast to most other disorders associated with thrombocytopenia. Megakaryocytes are present in the bone marrow. Anemia is frequently present and may be Coombs'-positive. An increased incidence of chronic renal disease has been reported.

Immunologic Diagnosis

The earliest immunologic abnormality is hypercatabolism of immunoglobulin G. Studies of B-cell

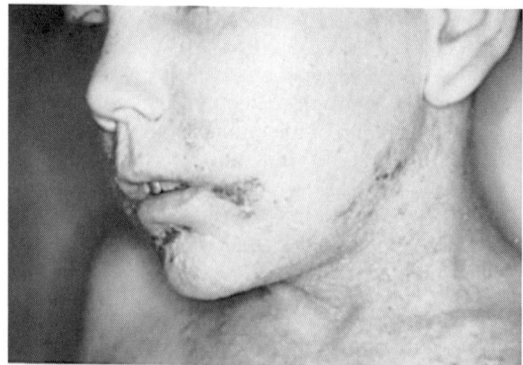

Figure 23–1. Chronic facial eczema in a child with Wiskott-Aldrich syndrome.

immunity demonstrate normal IgG levels, decreased IgM levels, increased IgA and IgE levels, or absent isohemagglutinin levels, normal numbers of B cells, and an inability to respond to immunization with polysaccharide antigen. Paraproteins are frequently observed. T-cell immunity is usually intact early in the disease but declines with advancing years.

Differential Diagnosis

When the complete syndrome is present, there is little doubt about the diagnosis. Idiopathic thrombocytopenia in a male child may be difficult to differentiate from Wiskott-Aldrich syndrome. In immune thrombocytopenia purpura (ITP), the immunoglobulins, isohemagglutinins, and response to polysaccharide antigens are normal. Small platelets favor the diagnosis of Wiskott-Aldrich syndrome. Unaffected male patients with eczema and recurrent infection have normal immunologic studies and normal platelet counts, although they may have elevated levels of serum IgA and IgE.

Treatment

Infections should be treated promptly and aggressively with antibiotics effective against the most common organisms. Corticosteroids should not be used to treat the thrombocytopenia, since they enhance the susceptibility to infection. Splenectomy has been fatal in this disease, but when combined with continuous antibiotic prophylaxis, may control both bleeding and infectious complications. Treatment of immunodeficiency is difficult. Intramuscular gamma globulin is contraindicated because of the thrombocytopenia and potential bleeding at injection sites, but intravenous gamma globulin can be given (see Chapter 21). Successful bone marrow transplantation with immunosuppression to achieve both a lymphoid and a hematopoietic cell engraftment is curative.

Complications & Prognosis

With aggressive therapy, the long-term prognosis has improved. Immediate complications are related to bleeding episodes and acute infection. Autoimmune phenomena such as vasculitis and Coombs'-positive hemolytic anemia may require corticosteroid therapy. As patients become older, they become susceptible to a wider spectrum of microorganisms. Chronic keratitis secondary to viral infection is frequent. Lymphoreticular cancers, especially of the central nervous system, occur in older patients. Myelogenous leukemia occurs more frequently in this disorder than in other immunodeficiency disorders.

ATAXIA-TELANGIECTASIA

Major Immunologic Features

- Clinical onset by 2 years of age.
- Complete syndrome consists of ataxia, telangiectasia, and recurrent sinopulmonary infection.
- Selective IgA deficiency, cutaneous anergy, and decreased T-cell function in most patients.
- Hypersensitivity to ionizing radiation with chromosome breakage.
- Predisposition to malignancies, including lymphoma, leukemias, and epithelial cell malignancies.
- Autosomal-recessive with abnormal gene ataxia-telangiectasia mutated (ATM) on 22q22–23.

General Considerations

Ataxia-telangiectasia, an autosomal recessive disorder, is associated with ataxia, telangiectasia, recurrent sinopulmonary infection, and abnormalities in both T- and B-cell immunity. The disorder was first considered to be primarily a neurologic disease; it is now known to involve the neurologic, vascular, endocrine, and immune systems.

Immunologic Pathogenesis

There is no unifying theory that explains the multisystem abnormalities present in ataxia-telangiectasia. It is unlikely that there is a fundamental immunologic defect. Rather, the multisystem abnormalities may be a result of a specific genetic defect that affects DNA repair and alters the function of many organ systems. Abnormalities that may result are abnormal collagen (deficient in hydroxylysine); elevated α-fetoprotein level, indicative of a defect in organ maturation; enhanced susceptibility of cells to radiation damage; and defective DNA repair. Clones of lymphocytes with structural rearrangements of band q11 of chromosome 14 and bands q32–35 and p13–15 of chromosome 7 have been consistently found. These chromosome markers may be found in malignant cell lines isolated from ataxia-telangiectasia patients. It is of interest that the structural rearrangements are at the locations that bear the TCR genes. Spontaneously occurring chromosomal translocations involving break points in T-cell receptor genes have been described and suggest a possible defect in recombination. The disorder is progressive, with both the neurologic abnormalities and the immunologic deficiency becoming more severe over time.

Clinical Features

A. Symptoms and Signs: The onset of ataxia may occur at 9 months to 1 year of age or may be delayed as long as to age 4 to 6 years. Telangiectasia is usually present by 2 years of age but has been delayed until 8 to 9 years of age. As patients grow older, additional neurologic symptoms develop, consisting of choreoathetoid movements, dysconjugate gaze, and extrapyramidal and posterior column signs. Telangiectasia may develop first in the bulbar conjunctiva and subsequently appear on the bridge of the nose, on the ears, or in the antecubital fossae (Fig 23–2). Recurrent sinopulmonary infections may begin early in life, or patients may remain relatively symptom-free for 10 years or more. There is increased susceptibility to both viral and bacterial infections. Secondary sexual characteristics rarely develop in patients at puberty, and most patients appear to develop mental retardation with time.

B. Laboratory Findings: Various degrees of abnormalities in T- and B-cell immunity have been described. Lymphopenia may be present. T-cell numbers may be normal or decreased, and the response of lymphocytes to phytohemagglutinin (PHA) and allogeneic cells may be normal or decreased. There usually is no response to delayed hypersensitivity skin tests. IgG2, IgG4, or IgA2 subclass deficiency is present in some patients. In other patients, IgE may be absent. Antibody responses to specific antigens may be depressed. CD4 cells are usually decreased and there are decreased α/β and increased γ/δ T cells. The number of circulating B cells is usually normal. Natural killer (NK) cell activity is normal.

Other laboratory abnormalities relate to associated findings. Abnormalities have been shown on pneumoencephalography and imaging studies of the central nervous system. Endocrine studies have shown decreased 17-ketosteroids and increased follicle-stimulating hormone (FSH) excretion. An insulin-resistant

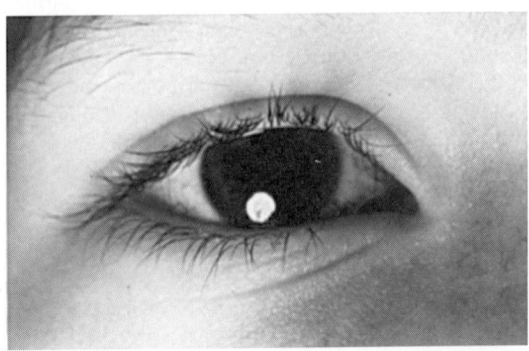

Figure 23–2. Telangiectasis of the conjunctiva and over the bridge of the nose in a child with ataxia-telangiectasia.

form of diabetes has been found. Cytotoxic antibodies to brain and thymus have been found. Many patients have elevated titers to EBV antigens. Elevated levels of α-fetoprotein are characteristic and help to differentiate this disorder from the Nijmegen breakage syndrome (see later section).

Immunologic Diagnosis

Selective IgA deficiency is found in 40% of patients with ataxia-telangiectasia. IgA2, IgG2, or IgG4 subclass deficiency has also been described. IgE deficiency and variable deficiencies of other immunoglobulins may also be found. The antibody response to specific antigens may be depressed. Variable degrees of T-cell deficiency are observed; these usually become more severe with advancing age.

Differential Diagnosis

If the onset of recurrent infection occurs before the development of ataxia or telangiectasia, it may be difficult to differentiate this disorder from cellular immunodeficiency with abnormal immunoglobulin synthesis. If a patient has a gradual onset of cerebellar ataxia unassociated with telangiectasia and immunologic abnormalities, it may take years before a diagnosis can be established with certainty. Usually, by the age of 4 years, the characteristic recurrent sinopulmonary infections, immunologic abnormalities, ataxia, and telangiectasia are present simultaneously. Because selective IgA deficiency is the most common immunodeficiency disorder detected and many patients with selective IgA deficiency have no associated symptoms, it may take several years before a diagnosis of ataxia-telangiectasia can be excluded. α-fetoprotein levels are normal in patients with IgA deficiency. Chromosomal instability is also present in the Nijmegen breakage syndrome.

Treatment

Early treatment of recurrent sinopulmonary infections is essential to avoid permanent complications. Some patients may benefit from continuous broad-spectrum antibiotic therapy. In patients who develop chronic lung disease, aggressive physical therapy is beneficial. Successful bone marrow transplantation has not been performed but probably would not benefit the neurologic problem. Fetal thymus transplantation and thymic hormone therapy have been used to treat a limited number of patients without clear evidence of efficacy. Intravenous immunoglobulin may decrease the number of infections if the patient has a severe antibody deficiency.

Attenuated viral vaccines should not be given. All blood products should be irradiated prior to administration.

Complications & Prognosis

Long-term survivors develop progressive deterioration of neurologic and immunologic functions. The

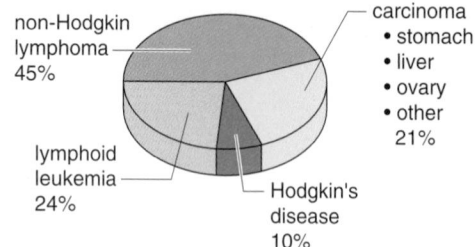

Figure 23–3. Relative percentages of cancers reported in patients with ataxia-telangiectasia.

oldest patients have reached the fifth decade of life. The chief causes of death are overwhelming infection and lymphoreticular or epithelial cell cancer (carcinoma of the stomach, liver, and ovaries). Leukemias, some with associated abnormalities of chromosome 14, have been reported in 24% of patients (Fig 23–3), and non-Hodgkin lymphomas have been reported in 45% of patients. As these patients reach the second decade, morbidity becomes severe, with chronic lung disease, mental retardation, and physical debility being the principal problems. Heterozygote carriers as well as family members have an increased incidence of cancer.

The Nijmegen Breakage Syndrome

The Nijmegen breakage syndrome is a distinct chromosomal instability syndrome characterized by microcephaly, growth retardation, susceptibility to infection and high risk of malignancy. As with ataxia-telangiectasia, the cells of patients with this syndrome are unusually sensitive to ionizing reduction leading to chromosome breakage; however, these patients do not have ataxia, telangiectasia, or elevated α-fetoprotein levels.

GRAFT-VERSUS-HOST DISEASE

Graft-versus-host (GVH) disease occurs when there is an unopposed attack of histoincompatible cells on an individual who is unable to reject foreign cells. The requirements for the GVH reaction are (1) histocompatibility differences between the graft (donor) and host (recipient), (2) immunocompetent graft cells, and (3) immunodeficient host cells. A GVH reaction may result from the infusion of any blood product containing viable lymphocytes, as may occur in maternal–fetal blood transfusion; intrauterine transfusion; therapeutic whole-blood transfusions or transfusions of packed erythrocytes, frozen cells, platelets, fresh plasma, or leukocyte-poor erythrocytes; or from transplantation of fetal thymus, fetal liver, or bone marrow. The onset of the GVH reaction occurs 7–30 days following infusion of viable lymphocytes. Once the reaction is established, little can be done to modify its course. In the majority of im-

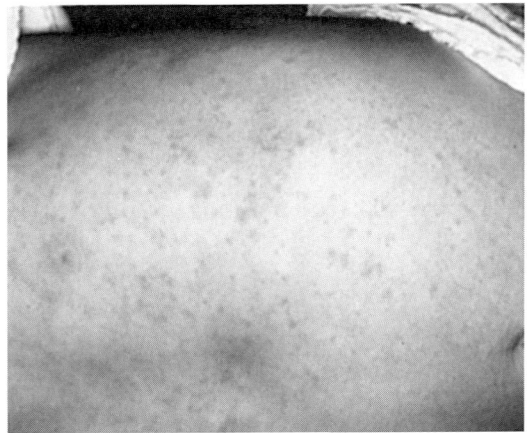

Figure 23–4. Maculopapular rash in early GVH disease in an infant with severe combined immunodeficiency disease.

munodeficient patients, a GVH reaction is fatal. The exact mechanism by which a GVH reaction is produced is not known. Biopsy of active GVH lesions usually demonstrates infiltration by mononuclear cells and eosinophils as well as phagocytic and histiocytic cells. The GVH reaction may appear in three distinct forms: acute, hyperacute, and chronic.

In the acute form of GVH reaction, the initial manifestation is a maculopapular rash, which is frequently mistaken for a viral or allergic rash (Fig 23–4). Initially, it blanches with pressure and then becomes diffuse. If the rash is persistent, it begins to scale. Diarrhea, hepatosplenomegaly, jaundice, cardiac irregularity, central nervous system irritability, and pulmonary infiltrates may occur during the height of the reaction. Enhanced susceptibility to infection is also present and may result in death from sepsis.

In the hyperacute form of GVH reaction, the rash may also begin as a maculopapular lesion, but then it rapidly progresses to a form resembling toxic epidermal necrolysis, usually associated with severe diarrhea. This has not been associated with staphylococcal infection. Clinical and laboratory abnormalities similar to those found in the acute form may be observed. Death occurs shortly after the onset of the reaction.

The chronic form of GVH reaction may be a result of maternal–fetal transfusion or attempts at immunotherapy with histocompatible bone marrow transplantation. The clinical and laboratory features may be markedly abnormal or only slightly so. Interference with normal nail growth results in a dysplastic appearance. Chronic desquamation of the skin is usually present. Hepatosplenomegaly may be prominent, along with lymphadenopathy. Chronic diarrhea and failure to thrive are common. Secondary infection is a frequent complication. On biopsy of skin or lymph nodes, histiocytic infiltration may be found, leading to an erroneous diagno-

sis of Letterer-Siwe disease. Patients with Letterer-Siwe disease have normal immunoglobulin levels and normal T-cell immunity, but patients with chronic GVH disease have severe immunodeficiency. Chronic GVH disease has also been confused with acrodermatitis enteropathica.

The diagnosis is suggested by the diffuse clinical abnormalities present in a patient who is known to have cellular immunodeficiency and who has received a transfusion of potentially immunocompetent cells in the preceding 5–30 days. The diagnosis is established by the demonstration of sex chromosome or HLA chimerism (Fig 23–5). On occasion, patients with known GVH disease fail to have detectable chimerism. Incubation of peripheral blood mononuclear cells with interleukin-2 may result in detectable chimerism.

Management

Prevention of GVH is essential. Patients with suspected T-cell immunodeficiency should receive only irradiated blood products (at least 2500 R) so as to prevent lymphocyte proliferation and resultant GVH disease. Blood products to be irradiated include whole blood, packed erythrocytes, lymphocyte-poor erythrocytes, platelets, and fresh and fresh-frozen plasma.

Following bone marrow transplantation when GVH is likely, the patients can be given cyclosporin or corticosteroids prophylactically for 3–6 months. Intravenous immunoglobulin therapy can ameliorate some of the symptoms of posttransplant GVH.

There is no adequate treatment of GVH disease once it is established. Corticosteroids serve to enhance the susceptibility to infection. Antilymphocyte globulin or anti-CD3 (OKT3) monoclonal antibody

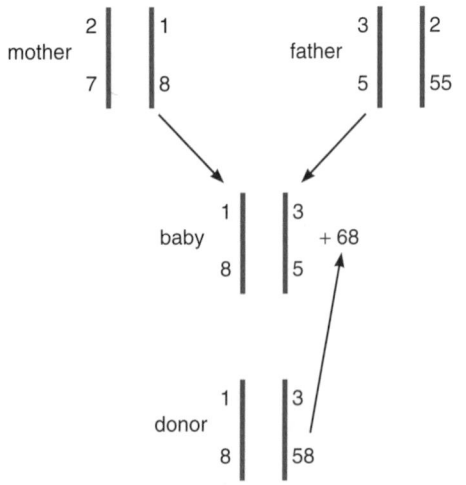

Figure 23–5. Inheritance of HLA antigens from the parents of a child with GVH disease and detection of additional antigen from the blood donor.

are of limited value. Cyclosporin and other immuno-suppressive agents may be useful. Experimentally, treatment with monoclonal antibody to tumor necrosis factor or interferon gamma reduces the severity of GVH disease.

Interestingly, GVH disease has not yet been described in patients with AIDS despite their severe T-cell immunodeficiency. This may be a result of HIV-1 infection of engrafting T cells, preventing the establishment of a graft.

SHORT-LIMBED DWARFISM WITH IMMUNODEFICIENCY AND CARTILAGE–HAIR HYPOPLASIA

Major Immunologic Features

- Skeletal dysplasia with dwarfism and fine hair.
- T-cell immunodeficiency with or without B-cell immunodeficiency.
- Autosomal recessive.
- Enhanced susceptibility to varicella-zoster infection.

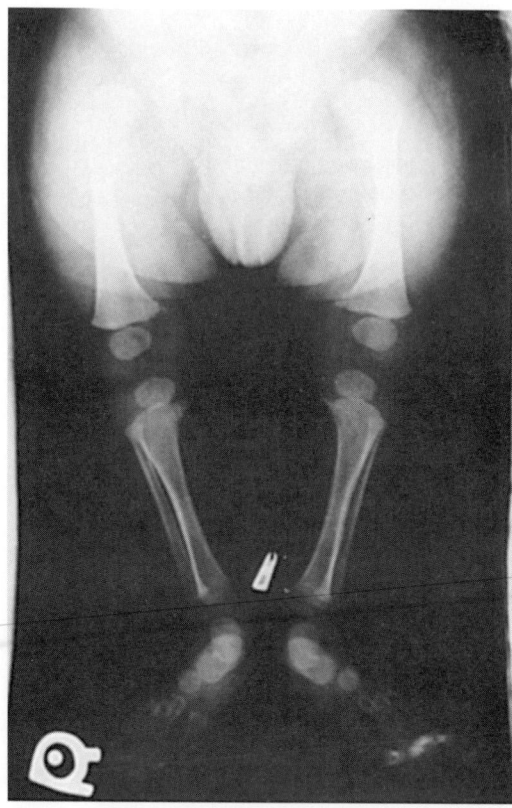

Figure 23–6. X-ray of extremities in a child with cartilage-hair hypoplasia and immunodeficiency. Note the redundant skin folds.

Short-limbed dwarfism with immunodeficiency is an autosomal recessive predominantly T-cell immunodeficiency associated with metaphyseal or spondyloepiphyseal dysplasia. Cartilage–hair hypoplasia is a variant in which fine, sparse hair is persistent.

Dwarfism is recognized at birth. The head size is normal and the hands are short and pudgy (Fig 23–6). There are redundant skin folds of the neck and limitation of elbow extension. The hair, if abnormal, is light, with a decreased diameter and lacking a central pigmental core. Neutropenia is not uncommon. Radiologic abnormalities consist of scalloping, irregular sclerosis, and cystic changes of the widened metaphyses (see Fig 23–6). Megacolon and malabsorption may occur.

Immunologic abnormalities can range from severe deficiency of B- and T-cell numbers and function (similar to severe combined immunodeficiency), a moderate T-cell immunodeficiency, or, occasionally, isolated B-cell deficiency with hypogammaglobulinemia.

Treatment is dependent on the degree of immunodeficiency. Intravenous immunoglobulin therapy is indicated for antibody deficiency. Successful bone marrow transplantation (HLA-identical and -haploidentical) has been accomplished. *Pneumocystis carinii* prophylaxis is indicated for patients with low CD4 numbers. Varicella-zoster immunoglobulin or acyclovir should be given following exposure to chicken pox. Varicella vaccine or other live virus vaccines are contraindicated.

IMMUNODEFICIENCY WITH ENZYME DEFICIENCY

ADENOSINE DEAMINASE & NUCLEOSIDE PHOSPHORYLASE DEFICIENCY

Major Immunologic Features

- Recurrent and severe viral, bacterial, fungal, and protozoal infections occur.
- There are varied degrees of T- and B-cell immunodeficiency.
- Purine enzyme activity is absent or reduced.

General Considerations

Patients with enzyme deficiency and immunodeficiency may have clinical and laboratory abnormalities identical to those of patients with immunodeficiency and normal enzyme activity. Enzyme deficiency as a cause of immunodeficiency probably accounts for less than 15% of immunodeficiency disorders at present. It is almost certain that additional enzyme deficiencies will be discovered.

Adenosine deaminase (ADA) and purine nucleoside phosphorylase are necessary for the normal catabolism of purines (Fig 23–7). Adenosine deaminase catalyzes

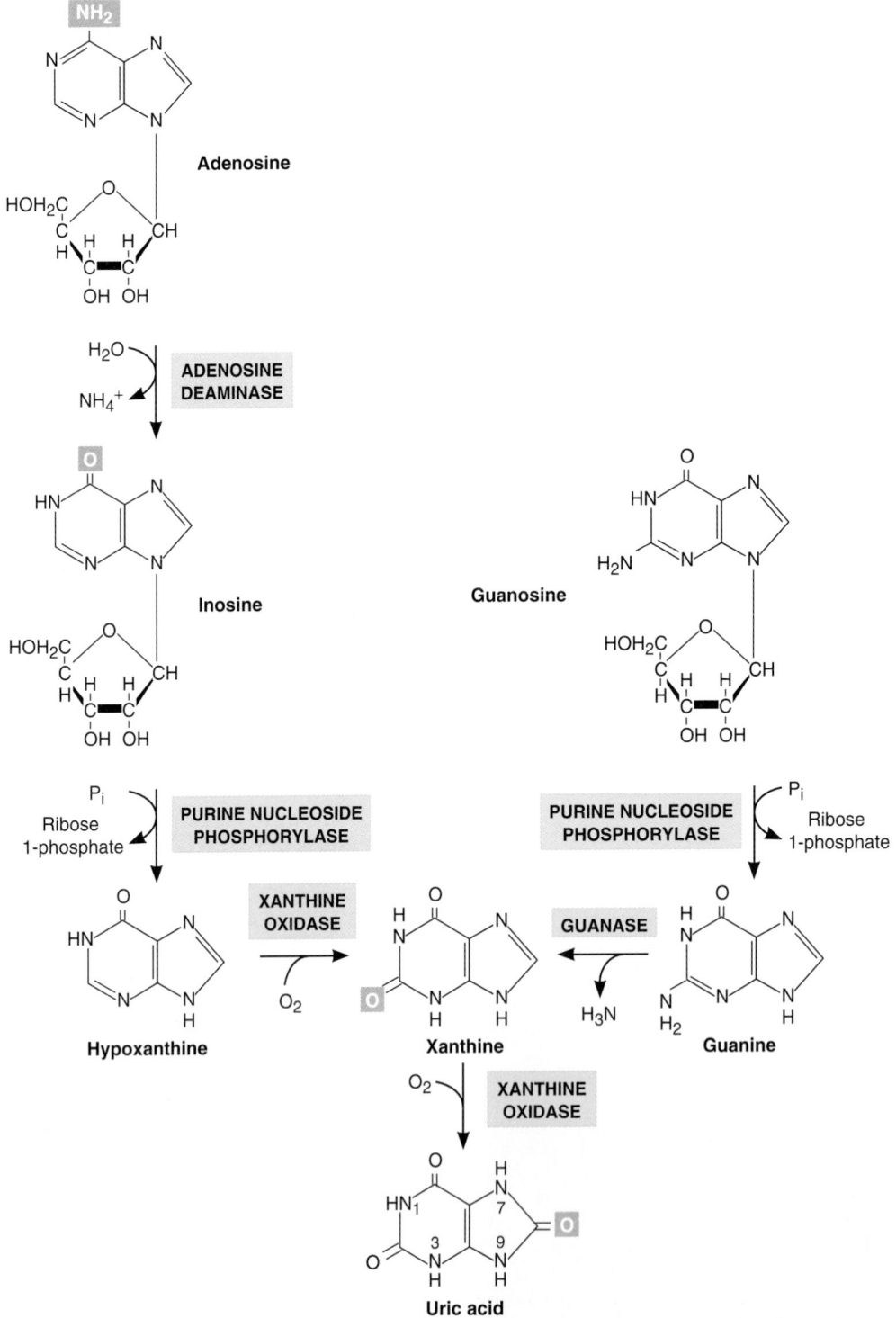

Figure 23–7. Schematic representation of purine metabolic pathway illustrating the critical role of adenosine deaminase and purine nucleoside phosphorylase. (Reproduced, with permission, from Murray RK et al: *Harper's Review of Biochemistry.* 22nd ed. Norwalk, CT, Appleton & Lange, 1990.)

the conversion of adenosine and deoxyadenosine to inosine and deoxyinosine. Nucleoside phosphorylase catalyzes the conversion of inosine, deoxyinosine, guanosine, and deoxyguanosine, to hypoxanthine and guanine. Several mechanisms have been postulated to explain the means whereby these enzyme deficiencies result in immunodeficiency. Experimental evidence indicates that adenosine, in increased amounts, may result in increased cyclic adenosine monophosphate (cAMP) activity, which is known to be associated with inhibition of lymphocyte function. Adenosine has also been shown to be toxic to cells in culture as a result of pyrimidine starvation. There is also evidence that exogenous adenosine can lead to the intracellular accumulation of S-adenosylhomocysteine, which acts as a potent inhibitor of DNA methylation. The most likely mechanism of inhibition of lymphocyte function, however, is a result of the accumulation of deoxyadenosine and subsequently deoxyadenosine triphosphate (deoxyATP), which results in inhibition of ribonucleotide reductase and subsequent depletion of deoxyribonucleoside triphosphates. In purine nucleoside phosphorylase deficiency, deoxyguanosine has been shown to result in the accumulation of deoxy-guanosine triphosphate (GTP). Again, this most probably results in inhibition of ribonucleotide reductase. These mechanisms have great importance in devising potential biochemical treatment for these disorders.

The degree of combined immunodeficiency is variable. The spectrum of immunologic aberrations varies from complete absence of T-cell and B-cell immunity, as observed in patients with severe combined immunodeficiency disease (85–90% of patients), to mild abnormalities of T-cell and B-cell function. Clinically, the phenotypic expression correlates with the degree of enzyme deficiency. Patients with the most complete form of enzyme deficiency have SCID. About 10–15% of patients have a delayed onset, some until 5–8 years of age. Routine neonatal screening has resulted in the detection of "partial" adenosine deaminase deficiency in immunologically normal individuals. Patients with enzyme deficiencies should be evaluated completely to determine the extent of the immunologic deficiency. As a result of the marked variability in immunodeficiency, there is considerable variation in the age at onset, severity of symptoms, and eventual outcome. Patients with adenosine deaminase deficiency and severe combined immunodeficiency may have radiologic abnormalities that include concavity and flaring of the anterior ribs, abnormal contour and articulation of posterior ribs and transverse processes, platyspondylisis, thick growth arrest lines, and an abnormal bony pelvis. Patients with nucleoside phosphorylase deficiency and T-cell immunodeficiency have normal bone x-rays, absent T-cell immunity, normal B-cell immunity, a history of recurrent infection, and autoantibody formation. They are susceptible to fatal varicella and vaccinia infections.

The mode of inheritance of these enzyme defects appears to be autosomal recessive. The carrier state can be demonstrated in both sexes by diminished adenosine deaminase or nucleoside phosphorylase activity. With the identification of the precise genetic defects in these disorders, intrauterine and carrier diagnosis will be more precise. The enzymes are absent in erythrocytes, leukocytes, tissues, and cultured fibroblasts in these patients. An intrauterine diagnosis of adenosine deaminase deficiency can be made. Patients may not be immunodeficient at birth.

The specific genetic defect(s) for both adenosine deaminase and nucleoside phosphorylase have been described. In most instances a mutation in a single nucleotide, which results in a single amino acid change, is responsible.

Treatment

Treatment of this disorder is similar to that of severe combined immunodeficiency or combined immunodeficiency. Several successful bone marrow transplants have been performed, with subsequent return of immunologic function. The patients' cells continue to have absent enzyme activity following transplantation.

Some patients with adenosine deaminase deficiency were benefitted by monthly infusions of irradiated erythrocytes as a source of ADA enzyme. Other patients have responded partially or not at all to such transfusions. Biochemical treatment of a single nucleoside phosphorylase-deficient patient with oral uridine was unsuccessful. Deoxycytidine therapy was attempted in a single patient without evidence of success.

Many ADA-deficient patients have been successfully treated with bovine ADA conjugated to polyethylene glycol (PEG–ADA) to prolong the half-life and reduce the immunogenicity of the enzyme. This treatment, given two or three times per week reduces the levels of toxic metabolites, and markedly improves B- and T-cell functions, particularly in patients who have some residual immunity.

Since 1990, several children and three newborns have received gene therapy for ADA deficiency. Their peripheral blood cells or their cord cells were transfected with the ADA gene and returned to the patients. Initial evaluation indicates that gene expression has occurred with some clinical benefit; however, these patients continue to receive PEG–ADA.

X-LINKED LYMPHOPROLIFERATIVE SYNDROME
(Duncan's Disease)

Major Immunologic Features

■ Exquisite susceptibility to Epstein-Barr virus (EBV) infection.

■ Most patients develop fatal infectious mononucleosis following EBV infection.

■ Others develop lymphoma, hypogammaglobuline-

mia, or aplastic anemia after EBV infection.
■ Bone marrow transplantation may be curative.

General Considerations

The X-linked lymphoproliferative (XLP) syndrome is characterized by a hereditary exquisite susceptibility to EBV infection. EBV infection can result in (1) severe progressive infectious mononucleosis, with liver failure and death; (2) infectious mononucleosis followed by lymphoproliferation; (3) immunodeficiency, lymphoma, or aplastic anemia. About 73% of patients develop fatal acute infectious mononucleosis. The mortality rate of XLP is 75% by age 10 and nearly 100% by age 40. The defective gene is on the long arm of the X chromosome (Xq25–26).

Immunologic abnormalities include inverted helper/suppressor T-cell ratios, deficient proliferative responses to mitogenic stimulation, defective interferon gamma production, and decreased NK-cell activity. B-cell abnormalities include hypogammaglobulinemia, failure to switch from IgM- to IgG-specific antibody following immunization with bacteriophage, and weak antibody responses to EBV antigens, especially to EBV nuclear antigen (EBNA). These abnormalities are found primarily in EBV-infected long-term survivors. In contrast, patients who are identified prior to EBV infection usually are immunologically normal, although some may have hypogammaglobulinemia.

Management

Intravenous immunoglobulin to prevent EBV infection has been used with limited success. Management once EBV infection has occurred is similar to other combined immunodeficiencies, that is, immunoglobulin, antibiotics, *Pneumocystis carinii* infection (PCP) prophylaxis, and so on. Antivirals against EBV (eg, acyclovir) are ineffective. Identification of at-risk uninfected carriers using DNA restriction fragment-length polymorphisms (RFLP) of genes at the XLP locus should be done so as to offer bone marrow or cord blood cell transplantation before EBV infection. Bone marrow transplantation, even after EBV infection, has been curative in a few patients, particularly if done before age 12.

REFERENCES

RETICULAR DYSGENESIS
Ownby DR et al: Severe combined immunodeficiency with leukopenia (reticular dysgenesis) in siblings: Immunologic and histopathologic findings. *J Pediatr* 1976;**89:**382.

SEVERE COMBINED IMMUNODEFICIENCY DISEASE
Castigli E et al: Severe combined immunodeficiency with selective T-cell cytokine genes. *Pediatr Res* 1993;**33:**52.
Chu ET et al: Immunodeficiency with defective T-cell response to interleukin 1. *Proc Natl Acad Sci USA* 1984;**81:**4945.
Conley ME: Molecular approaches to analysis of X-linked immunodeficiencies. *Ann Rev Immunol* 1992;**322:**1063.
Hong R: Disorders of the T cell system. In: *Immunologic Disorders in Infants and Children, 4th ed.* Stiehm ER (editor). WB Saunders, 1996, p 339.
Lawlor EJ et al: The syndrome of cellular immunodeficiency with immunoglobulins. *J Pediatr* 1974;**84:**183.
Pahwa SG et al: Heterogeneity of B lymphocyte differentiation in severe combined immunodeficiency disease. *J Clin Invest* 1980;**66:**543.
Pahwa R et al: Recombinant interleukin-2 therapy in severe combined immunodeficiency disease. *Proc Natl Acad Sci USA* 1989;**86:**5069.
Puck JM et al: The interleukin-2 receptor gamma chain maps to Xq13.1 and is mutated in X-linked severe combined immunodeficiency. *Hum Mol Genet* 1993;**2:**1099.

ATAXIA-TELANGIECTASIA
Baxter GD et al: T cell receptor gene rearrangement and expression in ataxia-telangiectasia B lymphoblastoid cells. *Immunol Cell Biol* 1989;**67:**57.
Boder E, Sedgwick RP: Ataxia-telangiectasia: A familial syndrome and progressive cerebellar ataxia, oculocutaneous telangiectasia and frequent pulmonary infection. *Univ South Cal Med Bull* 1957;**9:**15.
Savitsky K et al: A single ataxia telangiectasia gene with a product similar to PI-3 kinase. *Science* 1995;**268:**1749.
Swift M et al: Breast and other cancers in families with ataxia-telangiectasia. *N Engl J Med* 1987;**316:**1289.
Taylor AMR et al: Fifth International Workshop on Ataxia-Telangiectasia. *Cancer Res* 1993;**53:**438.

NIJMEGEN BREAKAGE SYNDROME
Weemaes CMR et al: A new chromosomal instability disorder: The Nijmegen breakage syndrome. *Acta Paediatr Scand* 1981;**70:**557.

WISKOTT-ALDRICH SYNDROME
Cooper MD et al: Wiskott-Aldrich syndrome: Immunologic deficiency disease involving the afferent limb of immunity. *Am J Med* 1968;**44:**489.
Derry JMJ et al: Isolation of a novel gene mutated in Wiskott-Aldrich syndrome. *Cell* 1994;**78:**635.
Parkman R et al: Complete correction of the Wiskott-Aldrich syndrome by allogeneic bone marrow transplantation. *N Engl J Med* 1978;**298:**921.
Shelly CS et al: Molecular characterization of sialophorin (CD43), the lymphocyte surface sialoglycoprotein defective in Wiskott-Aldrich syndrome. *Proc Natl Acad Sci USA* 1989;**86:**2819.
Simon HU et al: Defective expression of CD23 and autocrine growth-stimulation in Epstein-Barr virus (EBV) transformed B cells from patients with Wiskott-Aldrich syndrome (WAS). *Clin Exp Immunol* 1993;**91:**43.

Sullivan KE et al: A multi-institutional survey of the Wiskott-Aldrich syndrome. *J Pediatr* 1994;**125:**876.

IMMUNODEFICIENCY
WITH SHORT-LIMBED DWARFISM

Ammann AJ et al: Antibody mediated immunodeficiency in short-limbed dwarfism. *J Pediatr* 1974;**84:**200.

Lux SE et al: Chronic neutropenia and abnormal cellular immunity in cartilage-hair hypoplasia. *N Engl J Med* 1970;**282:**234.

Polmar SH, Pierce GF: Cartilage hair hypoplasia: Immunological aspects and their clinical implications. *Clin Immunol Immunopathol* 1986;**40:**87.

COMBINED IMMUNODEFICIENCY
WITH ENZYME DEFICIENCY

Giblet ER et al: Nucleoside phosphorylase deficiency in a child with severely defective T cell immunity and normal B cell immunity. *Lancet* 1975;**1:**1010.

Hershfield MS et al: Enzyme replacement therapy with polyethylene glycol adenosine deaminase in adenosine deaminase deficiency: Overview and case reports of three patients, including two now receiving gene therapy. *Pediatr Res* 1993;**33:**S42.

Levy Y et al: Adenosine deaminase deficiency with late onset of recurrent infections: Response to treatment with polyethylene glycol-modified adenosine deaminase. *J Pediatr* 1988;**113:**312.

Meuwissen HJ et al: Combined immunodeficiency disease associated with adenosine deaminase deficiency. *J Pediatr* 1975;**86:**169.

Bordignon C et al: Gene therapy in peripheral blood lymphocytes and bone marrow for ADA immunodeficient patients. *Science* 1995;**270:**470.

Blaese RM et al: T lymphocyte-directed gene therapy for ADA SCID: Initial trial results after 4 years. *Science* 1995;**270:**475.

BARE LYMPHOCYTE SYNDROME

Marcadet A et al: Genotyping with DNA probes in combined immunodeficiency syndrome with defective expression of HLA. *N Engl J Med* 1985;**312:**1287.

Reigh W et al: Congenital immunodeficiency with a regulatory defect in MHC class II gene expression lacks a specific HLA-DR promoter binding protein, RF-X. *Cell* 1988;**53:**897.

COMBINED IMMUNODEFICIENCY
WITH T-CELL MEMBRANE OR SIGNALING DEFECTS

Alarcon B et al: Familial defect in the surface expression of the T-cell receptor-CD3 complex. *N Engl J Med* 1988;**319:**1203.

Chatila T et al: An immunodeficiency characterized by defective signal transduction in T lymphocytes. *N Engl J Med* 1989;**320:**696.

Elder ME et al: Human severe combined immunodeficiency due to a defect in ZAP-70, a T cell tyrosine kinase. *Science* 1994;**264:**1596.

OMENN SYNDROME

Cederbaum SD et al: Combined immunodeficiency presenting as the Letterer-Siwe syndrome. *J Pediatr* 1974;**85:**466.

Omenn GS: Familial reticuloendotheliosis with eosinophilia. *N Engl J Med* 1965;**273:**427.

X-LINKED LYMPHOPROLIFERATIVE SYNDROME

Purtilo DT et al: Epstein-Barr virus infections in the X-linked recessive lymphoproliferative syndrome. *Lancet* 1978;**1:**798.

Seemayer TA et al: X-linked lymphoproliferative disease: Twenty-five years after the discovery. 1995;**38:**471.

GRAFT-VERSUS-HOST DISEASE

Glucksberg H et al: Clinical manifestations of graft-versus-host disease in human recipients of marrow from HLA-matched sibling donors. *Transplantation* 1974;**18:**295.

Kadowaki J et al: XX/XY lymphoid chimaerism in congenital immunological deficiency syndrome with thymic alymphoplasia. *Lancet* 1965;**2:**1152.

Sullivan KM et al: Cyclosporine treatment of chronic graft-versus-host disease following allogeneic bone marrow transplantation. *Transplant Proc* 1990;**22:**1336.

24   Phagocytic Dysfunction Diseases

E. Richard Stiehm, MD, & Arthur J. Ammann, MD

Phagocytic disorders may be divided into extrinsic and intrinsic defects. The **extrinsic** defects include opsonic abnormalities secondary to deficiencies of antibody and complement factors, suppression of the total number of neutrophils or granulocytes, suppression of phagocytic function by drugs, and suppression of the number of circulating neutrophils by autoantibody directed against neutrophil antigens. Other extrinsic disorders may be related to abnormal neutrophil chemotaxis secondary to complement deficiency or abnormal complement components.

Intrinsic disorders of phagocytic function include chronic granulomatous disease, several enzyme defects, glycogen storage disease type 1b, Chédiak-Higashi syndrome, and specific granule deficiency. Intrinsic disorders of directed phagocytic movement (chemotaxis) include the hyper-IgE/Job's syndrome, two leukocyte adhesion defects, Shwachman syndrome, tuftsin deficiency, and several syndromes with periodontitis. Defects of phagocytic movement may also occur secondary to diabetes mellitus, metabolic storage disease, splenic deficiency, malnutrition, immaturity, and burns.

Susceptibility to infection in phagocytic dysfunction syndromes may range from mild recurrent skin infections to severe, overwhelming, fatal systemic infection. Generally, these patients are susceptible to bacterial infection without difficulty with viral or protozoal infections. Some of the more severe disorders may be associated with overwhelming fungal infections.

Numerous tests can now be performed to evaluate phagocytic dysfunction (see Chapter 15). Screening tests are listed in Table 20–4, and definitive studies are listed in Table 24–1.

NEUTROPENIA

Neutropenia (circulating neutrophils <500 cells/mm^3), when persistent, is associated with a number of primary disorders, including congenital neutropenia (Kostmann's syndrome), cyclic neutropenia, glycogen storage disease type 1b, and myelokathexis (failure of release of neutrophils from the marrow). Acquired antibody-mediated autoimmune and isoimmune neutropenias have also been described. Neutropenia is common in several primary immunodeficiencies, including X-linked hyper-IgM, X-linked agammaglobulinemia, and reticular dysgenesis. Treatment with granulocyte colony-stimulating factor (G-CSF) is effective in reversing the neutropenia in some of these disorders.

CHRONIC GRANULOMATOUS DISEASE

Major Immunologic Features

- Susceptibility to infection with organisms normally of low virulence, such as *Staphylococcus epidermidis, Serratia marcescens, Aspergillus.*
- X-linked (65%) or autosomal-recessive (35%) inheritance.
- Onset of symptoms occurs by 2 years of age: draining lymphadenitis, hepatosplenomegaly, pneumonia, osteomyelitis, and abscesses.
- Diagnosis is established by abnormal nitroblue tetrazolium test, quantitative leukocyte killing curve, superoxide generation, or chemiluminescence.

General Considerations

Chronic granulomatous disease (CGD) is usually inherited as an X-linked disorder, with clinical manifestations appearing during the first 2 years of life. Three autosomal variants of the disease have also been described. All patients are susceptible to infection with a variety of normally nonpathogenic and unusual organisms. Characteristic abnormal laboratory studies detect both patients and female carriers of the disease. Female carriers are usually asymptomatic.

Table 24–1. Evaluation of phagocytosis.

Test	Comment
Nitroblue tetrazolium tests (NBT)	Used for diagnosis and screening of chronic granulomatous disease and for detection of carrier state.
Quantitative intracellular killing curve	Used for diagnosis of chronic granulomatous disease. Can be performed with organisms isolated from the individual patient.
Chemotaxis	Abnormal in a variety of disorders associated with frequent bacterial infection. Does not provide a specific diagnosis. Performed by using a Boyden chamber and a microscopic or radioactive technique to determine cell migration. Rebuck skin window provides a qualitative result in vivo.
Chemiluminescence	Abnormal in chronic granulomatous disease and myeloperoxidase deficiency.
Enzyme tests	Deficiencies of specific enzymes: glucose-6-phosphate dehydrogenase, myeloperoxidase.
Membrane glycoproteins	Deficient in leukocyte adhesion (integrin) disorders and associated with abnormal leukocyte adherence and movement.

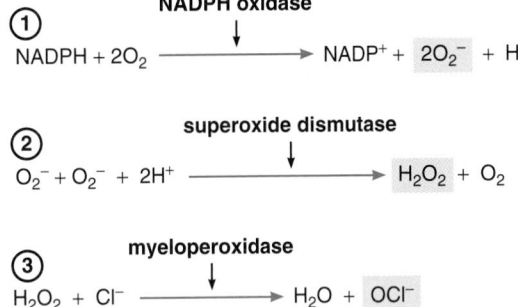

Figure 24–1. Respiratory burst resulting in the generation of superoxide (O_2^-), hydrogen peroxide (H_2O_2), and hypochlorite (OCl^-).

Early diagnosis and aggressive therapy have improved the prognosis for these patients.

Pathogenesis

There are four different genetic forms of CGD based on different biochemical abnormalities and patterns of inheritance. The functional defect, however, which occurs in the respiratory burst, is similarly abnormal in the various forms and results in characteristic clinical abnormalities. The normal respiratory burst in neutrophils and monocytes is triggered by opsonized microorganisms or other appropriate stimuli, resulting in an increase in intracellular oxygen consumption with conversion of oxygen to hydrogen peroxide, oxidized halogens, and superoxide and hydroxyl radicals (Fig 24–1). Patients with CGD are unable to generate a respiratory burst after stimulation of neutrophils and monocytes and are therefore unable to kill microorganisms.

The central enzyme in the respiratory burst is the oxidase of the reduced form of nicotinamide-adenine dinucleotide phosphate (NADPH). Without this enzyme, hydrogen peroxide, superoxide, and other microbicidal reactive oxygen species cannot be generated. NADPH is composed of a plasma membrane

cytochrome b_{588}, consisting of a 91-kd protein (gp 91-phox) and a 22-kd (p22-phox), and two cytosolic proteins, a 47-kd (p47-phox), and a 67-kd (p67-phox) component (gp = glycoprotein; p = protein; phox = phagocyte oxidase). Mutations of gp91-phox, termed the X91 variant, is responsible for the X-linked form of the disease, and constitutes 63% of the reported cases. Other variants are autosomal recessive, including mutations of (1) p47-phox (type A47, on chromosome 7, 33% of cases; (2) p22-phox (type A22, on chromosome 16, 5% of cases); and (3) p67-phox (type A67, on chromosome 1, 5% of cases). These types can be distinguished by Western blot analysis of leukocyte lysates using antibodies to the specific proteins.

Clinical Features

A. Symptoms and Signs: In the majority of patients, the diagnosis can be established before 2 years of age. The most frequent abnormalities are marked lymphadenopathy, infected skin lesions with ulcerations, hepatosplenomegaly, draining lymph nodes, and episodes of pneumonia. Other manifestations include rhinitis, conjunctivitis, dermatitis, ulcerative stomatitis, perianal abscess, osteomyelitis, chronic diarrhea with intermittent abdominal pain, esophageal stenosis, and intestinal and genitourinary tract obstruction. Chronic and acute infection occurs in lymph nodes, skin, lungs, intestinal tract, liver, and bone. A major clue to early diagnosis is the finding of normally nonpathogenic or unusual organisms. Organisms responsible for infection include *Staphylococcus aureus*, *S epidermidis*, *Serratia marcescens*, *Pseudomonas*, *Escherichia coli*, *Candida*, and *Aspergillus*.

B. Laboratory Findings: The most widely available diagnostic tests are the qualitative or quantitative nitroblue tetrazolium (NBT) test and chemiluminescence assays. Patient leukocytes have absent NBT dye reduction and reduced chemiluminescence, whereas carriers may have normal or reduced values. Patients with CGD are unable to kill certain intracellular bacteria at a normal rate. The leukocyte-killing curves for organisms to which these individuals are

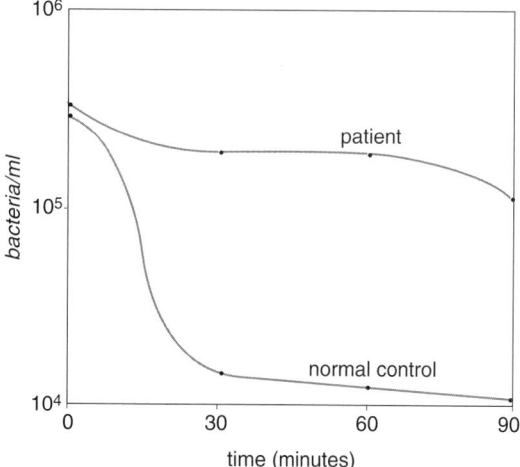

Figure 24–2. Bacterial killing curves in normal control and in patient with chronic granulomatous disease. The patient's phagocyte cells are unable to kill significant numbers of bacteria following an in vitro incubation period of 90 minutes.

susceptible usually indicate little or no killing over a period of 2 hours (Fig 24–2). Other abnormal findings include decreased oxygen uptake during phagocytosis and abnormal bacterial iodination. Natural killer (NK)-cell activity is normal.

The blood leukocyte count is usually elevated even if the patient does not have active infection. Hypergammaglobulinemia is present, and antibody function is normal. T-cell immunity is normal. Complement components may be elevated. During episodes of pneumonia, the chest x-ray is severely abnormal. Liver function tests may be abnormal as a result of chronic infection. Pulmonary function tests are usually abnormal following episodes of pneumonia and may not return to normal for several months. Several X-linked patients have the rare Kell blood type, K_0 (K null), allowing them to be sensitized to Kell antigens following blood transfusion. Histologic examination of the infected area often reveals an accumulation of pigmented histiocytes.

Immunologic Diagnosis

A diagnosis can be established by using the NBT dye reduction assay or quantitative chemiluminescence and confirmed by using specific bactericidal assays (see Chapter 13). These assays may also be used to identify the carrier state and to establish an intrauterine diagnosis. Both male and autosomal variants of CGD have abnormal test results. Chemiluminescence is the best method for detecting the carrier state. Intrauterine diagnosis can be accomplished by using fetal blood and NBT or chemiluminescence tests.

Differential Diagnosis

Few clinical disorders are confused with CGD. Leukocyte glucose-6-phosphate deficiency and

myeloperoxidase deficiency have clinical symptoms and laboratory features similar to those of CGD and an abnormal NBT test. Any child presenting with osteomyelitis, pneumonia, liver, abscess, or chronic draining lymphadenopathy associated with a normally nonpathogenic or unusual organism should be suspected of having CGD.

Treatment

Aggressive therapy is necessary for long-term survival and diminished morbidity. Blood cultures, aspiration of draining lymph nodes, liver biopsy, and open-lung biopsy should be used to obtain a specific bacterial diagnosis. Therapy should be instituted immediately, while results of cultures are pending. The choice of antibiotics should be appropriate for the spectrum of bacterial infections likely to be present. Treatment of infections with antibiotics must be prolonged, requiring 5–6 weeks of total therapy. Several investigators use prophylactic anti-infective therapy such as trimethoprim-sulfamethoxazole. *Candida* or *Aspergillus* infections require amphotericin B, or other antifungal drugs must be used. The ultimate survival of the patient is dependent on early and intensive therapy.

A double-blind placebo-controlled trial showed that interferon gamma (IFNγ) reduced the frequency and severity of infections in all types of CGD. The mechanism of action is unclear since NADPH oxidase activity is not affected; possibly macrophage nonoxidative defense mechanisms are enhanced. The usual dose is 60 µg/m² subcutaneously three times a week.

Therapy has also included the use of leukocyte infusions, but experience has been limited. Obstructive lesions respond to corticosteroids. A few successful bone marrow transplants have been performed.

Complications & Prognosis

Chronic organ dysfunction may result from severe or chronic infection. Examples are abnormal pulmonary function, chronic liver disease, chronic osteomyelitis, and malabsorption secondary to gastrointestinal tract involvement. Growth retardation is common. The mortality rate in CGD has been considerably reduced by early diagnosis and aggressive therapy. Survival into the second decade and beyond has been recorded. Female carriers have an increased incidence of systemic and discoid lupus erythematosus.

GLUCOSE-6-PHOSPHATE DEHYDROGENASE DEFICIENCY

Patients with glucose-6-phosphate dehydrogenase (G6PD) deficiency of their leukocytes have defective generation of hydrogen peroxide and susceptibility to *S aureus* and *E coli,* similar to patients with chronic granulomatous disease. The NBT test is abnormal, but the clinical severity is less than in CGD. This is a rare illness and is not present in patients with G6PD deficiency of erythrocytes.

CHÉDIAK-HIGASHI SYNDROME

Chédiak-Higashi syndrome is a multisystem autosomal recessive disorder. Symptoms include recurrent bacterial infections with a variety of organisms, hepatosplenomegaly, partial albinism, central nervous system abnormalities, and a high incidence of lymphoreticular cancers.

The characteristic abnormality of giant cytoplasmic granular inclusions in leukocytes and platelets is observed on routine peripheral blood smears under ordinary light microscopy. Additional abnormalities include elevated Epstein-Barr virus (EBV) antibody titers, abnormal neutrophil chemotaxis, decreased NK-cell activity, and abnormal intracellular killing of organisms (including streptococci and pneumococci as well as the organisms found in CGD). The killing defect is manifested in vitro by delayed intracellular killing. Oxygen consumption, hydrogen peroxide formation, and hexose monophosphate shunt activity are normal. Abnormal microtubule function, abnormal lysosomal enzyme levels in granulocytes, and proteinase deficiency in granulocytes have been described and are associated with increased levels of leukocyte cyclic adenosine monophosphate (cAMP). Abnormal leukocyte function in vitro has been corrected by ascorbate, but the results of treatment in vivo are contradictory. Improved granulocyte function in vitro has also been observed after treatment with anticholinergic drugs.

Definitive cure with bone marrow transplantation has been accomplished. Without transplantation, the prognosis is poor because of progressive increased susceptibility to infection and neurologic deterioration. Most patients die during childhood, but survivors to the second and third decades have been reported.

MYELOPEROXIDASE DEFICIENCY

Several patients with complete deficiency of leukocyte myeloperoxidase have been described. Myeloperoxidase is one of the enzymes necessary for normal intracellular killing of certain organisms. It catalyzes the oxidation of microorganisms by intracellular H_2O_2 in the presence of halides (see Fig 24–1). The leukocytes of these patients have normal oxygen consumption, hexose monophosphate shunt activity, and superoxide and hydrogen peroxide production. The intracellular killing of organisms is delayed, but may reach normal levels with increased in vitro incubation times. Chemiluminescence of leukocytes is decreased. Susceptibility to candidal and staphylococcal infections has been the chief problem,

but many patients are asymptomatic. The diagnosis can be established by using a peroxidase stain of peripheral blood. No specific treatment is available other than appropriate antibiotic therapy.

SPECIFIC GRANULE DEFICIENCY

This is an autosomal recessive disorder with recurrent mucous membrane and skin infections. The neutrophils are bilobed or kidney-shaped with absence of secondary granules by electron microscopy. As a result, they lack certain antimicrobial enzymes, such as lactoferrin and vitamin B_{12}-binding protein, but have normal levels of azurophilic granule proteins (eg, myeloperoxidase, lysozyme).

GLYCOGEN STORAGE DISEASE TYPE 1B

This is due to a defect in glucose-6-phosphate translocase with resulting hypoglycemia. Unlike patients with glycogen storage disease type 1a, type 1b patients have defects in neutrophil chemotaxis, intermittent neutropenia, a defective respiratory burst, and moderate increased susceptibility to bacterial infection.

HYPER IgE SYNDROME/ JOB'S SYNDROME

Major Features
- Recurrent staphylococcal infections of tissues and skin.
- Coarse facies.
- Exceptionally high serum IgE levels (>2000 IU/mL).
- Blood and tissue eosinophilia.
- Intermittent chemotactic defects.

These patients have an early onset of cutaneous infections and deep-seated staphylococcal infections, including pneumonia with pneumatocele formation; mastoiditis; and (less commonly) bone, joint, and visceral infection. The skin resembles recurrent severe eczema, but infection is more prominent and pruritis less common. Classical allergic features are rare. Many patients have coarse features (Fig 24–3). Some patients have osteopenia with frequent fractures. A few girls with red hair were described with "cold," nontender, cutaneous abscesses—a condition given the eponym of "Job's" syndrome. Job's syndrome is probably a mild form of the Hyper-IgE syndrome. Both sexes are affected and a few familial cases have been described; a clear genetic pattern has not emerged, however.

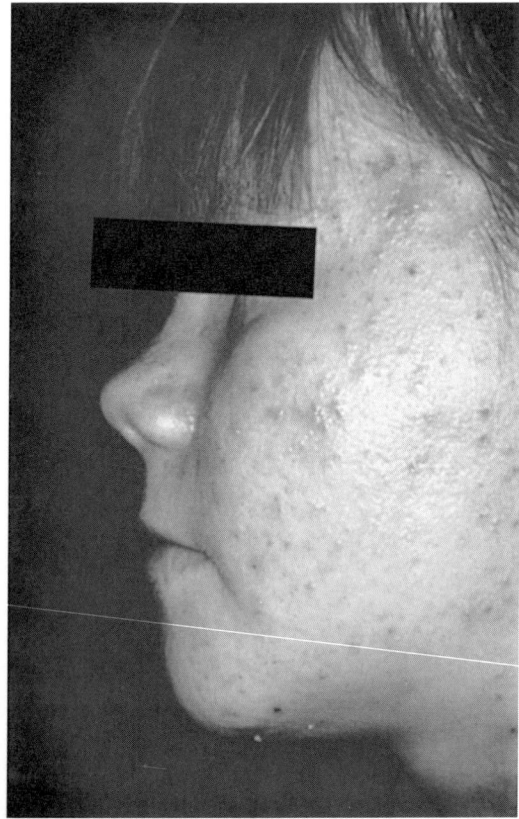

Figure 24–3. Coarse facial features, multiple small abscesses, and "saddle" nose in a female with Job's syndrome.

All patients have extremely elevated levels of serum IgE (>2000 IU/mL and up to 40,000 IU/mL) with blood and tissue eosinophilia. Serum IgD levels are also moderately increased. Other immunologic abnormalities include a variable chemotactic defect, (usually noted during infections), and decreased antibody and T-cell proliferative responses to antigens. IgG, IgM, and IgA levels are normal or elevated; CD3, CD4, and CD8 lymphocyte subsets are normal. The NBT test and complement levels are normal.

An immunoregulatory T-cell abnormality with excessive IL-4 production has been suggested as the immunologic defect. This explanation does not explain the propensity toward staphylococcal infection, however.

Treatment consists of optimal antistaphyloccocal antibiotic therapy given intravenously when infections are present. Continuous trimethoprim-sulfamethoxazole therapy is of value in controlling cutaneous infection. Levamisole was used without benefit. IFNγ and intravenous immunoglobulin (IVIG) have also been used with some anecdotal benefit.

LEUKOCYTE ADHESION DEFECT-TYPE 1 (LFA-1/Mac-1/p150, 95 [CD11/CD18] DEFICIENCY)

Major Immunologic Features
- Leukocytosis and delayed umbilical cord detachment.
- Autosomal-recessive mode of inheritance.
- Recurrent necrotic soft tissue infections and periodontitis.
- Defective leukocyte chemotaxis and cytoxic function (CTL, NK, and ADCC).
- Deficient expression of leukocyte adhesion proteins CD11a/CD18 (LFA-1), CD11b/CD18 (CR3, Mac-1) and CD11c/CD18 (p150,95).

General Considerations
Patients with leukocyte adhesion defect-type 1 (LAD-1) have recurrent pyogenic infections, often with onset in the first weeks of life. Common microbial agents of these infections include *Staphylococcus aureus, Pseudomonas aeruginosa, Klebsiella, Proteus,* and enterococci. Delayed separation of the umbilical cord is common (greater than 3 weeks). As patients become older, they develop recurrent skin infections, sinusitis, vaginitis, perianal abscesses, periodontal disease, tracheobronchitis, pneumonia, recurrent progressive necrotic soft tissue infections, and septicemia. The disease may be fatal in the first years of life, or it may follow a more protracted course, suggesting two clinical phenotypes: moderate and severe. The inheritance pattern of both is autosomal recessive.

The genetic basis of LAD-1 is mutations of the common beta subunit (CD18) of an integrin gene leading to deficiency of three leukocyte adhesion molecules, LFA-1(CD11a/CD18), CR3 or Mac-1(CD11b/CD18), and p150,95 or CR4(CD11c/CD18) (see Fig 24–4). These adhesion molecules are present on lymphocytes, monocytes, granulocytes, and large granular lymphocytes and permit cellular interactions, cell movement, and interaction with complement fragments.

Deficiency of these integrins results in several immunologic abnormalities. In vivo and in vitro chemotaxis of granulocytes and in vitro cell spreading are abnormal. Zymosan-induced chemiluminescence, but not phorbol myristate acetate-induced chemiluminescence, is abnormal. Cytotoxic responses, such as antibody-dependent cellular cytotoxicity, natural killer cytotoxicity, and cytotoxic T-lymphocyte cytotoxicity are abnormal, since all require cell interaction.

Treatment of LAD-1 is directed toward the specific infectious agents involved. As patients are infected with common pathogenic organisms but not with the opportunistic ones, they should respond to appropriate antibiotic therapy. Early aggressive treatment should be used, and prophylactic therapy should be given under certain circumstances, such as dental procedures. Bone marrow transplantation has been successful in

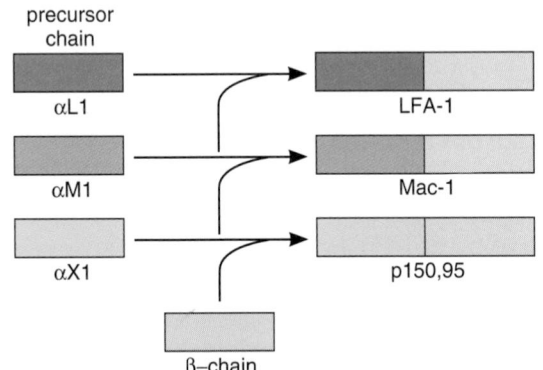

Figure 24–4. Comparative structure of leukocyte adhesion molecules, showing unique α chains and a common β chain.

many patients; indeed LAD-1 patients engraft readily, unlike most patients with phagocytic defects.

LEUKOCYTE ADHESION DEFECT TYPE 2

Two unrelated boys have been identified who have absence of a neutrophil receptor [Sialyl-Lewis X (CD15s)] for E-selectin, adhesion molecule on activated endothelial cells of blood vessels. This deficiency (leukocyte adhesion defect-type 2 [LAD-2]) results in a lack of neutrophil rolling and a chemotactic defect similar to that present in LAD-1. These boys have periodontitis, recurrent bacterial infections, and neutrophilia. Unlike LAD-1, CD11/CD18 expression on their leukocytes is normal.

SHWACHMAN SYNDROME

Patients with Shwachman syndrome have pancreatic insufficiency, malabsorption, dyschondroplasia, eczema, and recurrent infection. Patients have neutropenia and decreased neutrophil chemotaxis. The sweat test for cystic fibrosis is normal.

TUFTSIN DEFICIENCY

Tuftsin disease has been reported as a familial deficiency of a phagocytosis-stimulating tetrapeptide that is cleaved from a parent immunoglobulin-like molecule (termed leukokinin) in the spleen. Tuftsin also appears to be absent in patients who have been splenectomized. Local and severe systemic infections occur with *Candida, S aureus,* and *Streptococcus pneumoniae.* Tuftsin levels are determined only in a few specialized laboratories. There is no treatment, and the prognosis is uncertain. Gamma globulin therapy appeared to be beneficial in the two families in which it was tried.

PERIODONTITIS SYNDROMES

Several syndromes of severe periodontitis with chemotactic defects have been described, including localized juvenile periodontitis, rapidly progressive periodontitis, acute necrotizing ulcerative gingivitis, and the Papillon-Lefèvre syndrome (early-onset periodontitis with palmar–plantar hyperkeratosis). Each syndrome has a characteristic oral location, bacterial flora, and hereditary pattern.

REFERENCES

CHRONIC GRANULOMATOUS DISEASE
Baehner RL, Nathan DG: Quantitative nitroblue tetrazolium test in chronic granulomatous disease. *N Engl J Med* 1968;**287:**971.

Curnutte JT et al: Chronic granulomatous disease due to a defect in the cytosolic factor required for nicotinamide adenine dinucleotide phosphate oxidase activation. *J Clin Invest* 1988;**81:**606.

Hobbs JR et al: Chronic granulomatous disease 100% corrected by displacement bone marrow transplantation from a volunteer unrelated donor. *Eur J Pediatr* 1992;**151:**806.

International Chronic Granulomatous Disease Cooperative Study Group. A controlled trial of interferon gamma to prevent infection in chronic granulomatous disease. *N Engl J Med* 1991;**324:**509.

Johnston RB, Newman SL: Chronic granulomatous disease. *Pediatr Clin North Am* 1977;**24:**365.

Mills EL et al: X-linked inheritance in females with chronic granulomatous disease. *J Clin Invest* 1980;**66:**332.

Roos D: The genetic basis of chronic granulomatous disease. *Immunol Rev* 1994;**138:**121.

GLUCOSE-6-PHOSPHATE DEHYDROGENASE DEFICIENCY
Cooper MR et al: Complete deficiency of leukocyte glucose-6-phosphate dehydrogenase with defective bactericidal activity. *J Clin Invest* 1972;**51:**769.

MYELOPEROXIDASE DEFICIENCY
Lehrer RI, Cline MJ: Leukocyte myeloperoxidase deficiency and disseminated candidiasis: The role of myeloperoxidase in resistance to *Candida* infection. *J Clin Invest* 1969;**48:**1478.

Nauseef WM: Myeloperoxidase deficiency. *Hematol Oncol Clin North Am* 1988;**2:**577.

Parry MF et al: Myeloperoxidase deficiency. *Ann Intern Med* 1981;**95:**293.

CHÉDIAK-HIGASHI SYNDROME

Ganz T et al: Microbicidal/cytotoxic proteins of neutrophils are deficient in two disorders: Chédiak-Higashi syndrome and specific granule deficiency. *J Clin Invest* 1988;**82**:552.

Haliotis T et al: Chédiak-Higashi gene in humans. 1. Impairment of natural-killer function. *J Exp Med* 1980;**151**:1039.

Root RK et al: Abnormal bactericidal, metabolic and lysosomal functions of Chédiak-Higashi syndrome leukocytes. *J Clin Invest* 1972;**51**:649.

Stossel TP et al: Phagocytosis in chronic granulomatous disease and the Chédiak-Higashi syndrome. *N Engl J Med* 1972;**286**:120.

TUFTSIN DEFICIENCY

Constantopoulos A: Congenital tuftsin deficiency. *Ann NY Acad Sci* 1983;**419**:214.

Phillips JH et al: Tuftsin, a naturally occurring immunopotentiating factor. 1. In vitro enhancement of murine natural cell-mediated cytotoxicity. *J Immunol* 1981;**126**:915.

HYPER IgE/JOB'S SYNDROME

Buckley RH et al: Extreme hyperimmunoglobulinemia E and undue susceptibility to infection. *Pediatrics* 1972;**49**:59.

Claassen JL et al: Mononuclear cells from patients with the hyper-IgE syndrome produce little IgE when stimulated with recombinant interleukin-4 in vitro. *J Allergy Clin Immunol* 1991;**88**:713.

Davis SD et al: Job's syndrome. Recurrent, "cold," staphylococcal abscesses. *Lancet* 1966;**2**:1013.

Hill HR, Quie PG: Raised serum IgE levels and defective neutrophil chemotaxis in three children with eczema and recurrent bacterial infections. *Lancet* 1974;**1**:183.

Matter L et al: Abnormal immune response to *Staphylococcus aureus* in patients with *Staphylococcus aureus* hyper-IgE syndrome. *Clin Exp Immunol* 1986;**66**:450.

PERIODONTITIS SYNDROMES

Quie PG et al: Disorders of polymorphonuclear phagocytic system. In: Stiehm ER, *Immunologic Disorders in Infants and Children, 4th ed.* 1996, p. 443.

LEUKOCYTE ADHESION DEFECTS

Anderson DC, Springer TA: Leukocyte adhesion deficiency: An inherited defect in the Mac-1, LFA-1 and p150,95 glycoproteins. *Ann Rev Med* 1987;**38**:175.

Arnaout MA: Molecular basis for leukocyte adhesion deficiency. In: *Biochemistry of Macrophages and Related Cell Types,* Horton M (editor). Plenum, 1993, p 335.

Etzioni A et al: Recurrent severe infections caused by a novel leukocyte adhesion deficiency. *N Engl J Med* 1992;**327**:1789.

Fischer A et al: Bone marrow transplantation (BMT) in Europe for primary immunodeficiencies other than severe combined immunodeficiency: A report from the European Group for BMT and the European Group for Immunodeficiency. *Blood* 1994;**83**:1149.

GLYCOGEN STORAGE DISEASE-TYPE 1B

Kilpatrick L et al: Impaired metabolic function and signaling defects in phagocytic cells in glycogen storage disease type 1b. *J Clin Invest* 1990;**86**:196.

SHWACHMAN SYNDROME

Aggett PJ et al: An inherited disorder of neutrophil mobility in Shwachman syndrome. *J Pediatr* 1979;**94**:391.

SPECIFIC GRANULE DEFICIENCY

Ambruso DR et al: Defective bactericidal activity and absence of specific granules in neutrophils from a patient with recurrent bacterial infections. *J Clin Immunol* 1984;**4**:23.

Complement Deficiencies

25

Michael M. Frank, MD

As discussed in detail in Chapter 11, there are two major pathways of complement activation. In each pathway, peptides derived from several complement components assemble to form a complex enzyme capable of binding and cleaving C3, the principal component formed by complement activation. Once these pathways have joined at the level of the component C3, they proceed together to interact with C5, C6, C7, C8, and C9 to produce a lytic lesion when activated at a cell surface. These later-acting components have together been termed the membrane attack complex, since they form a C5b–9 complex that inserts into biologic membranes to cause lysis. There are a limited number of patients with a genetically controlled deficiency of one of the components of the classic, alternative, or terminal attack pathways. In addition, there are patients who are known to have defects in control proteins that regulate a number of steps in the cascade. The major clinical features of each are shown in Table 25–1. For the most part, the consequences of these defects can be predicted from a knowledge of the mechanisms of activation and the biologic activities of the various complement components.

In general, defects of components of the two pathways behave as autosomal-recessive traits. Individuals with one normal gene have about half-normal levels of the deficient proteins. Affected individuals are those with little or no gene product; they are the product of two heterozygous deficient parents. A few complement components composed of subunits are encoded by multiple genes. Individual independently inherited genes code for Clq, Clr, and C1s as well as C8 α-γ chain and C8 β chain. Inheritance of these also follows an autosomal-recessive pattern. Since there is a broad range of plasma concentrations for many of the components in normal individuals, it is not always possible to distinguish heterozygous individuals from normal individuals on the basis of their plasma complement component levels. In most cases, heterozygous individuals are phenotypically normal, except as noted later on. When

an individual with the homozygous phenotype is totally deficient in one of the proteins of the classic pathway or one of the terminal components, the lytic pathway is interrupted at the point at which that component must function and the complement titer (CH50) is zero; that is, the quantity of serum required to lyse an antibody-sensitized sheep erythrocyte is infinite. Similarly, with a defect in the alternative pathway components or terminal components, the alternative pathway titer is zero.

ALTERNATIVE PATHWAY COMPONENT DEFICIENCIES

The alternative complement pathway is believed to be the older pathway phyogenetically and to provide the first line of host defense to bacterial attack, before the host has had sufficient time to respond to the infection by developing antibody. For that reason it might be expected that defects in the early steps of the alternative pathway might predispose individuals toward serious infection. The individual's ability to bind and activate C3 to provide adequate opsonic and other complement functions is compromised, and such patients have frequent infections with virulent pathogens (eg, pneumococci, *Haemophilus influenzae,* and staphylococci). Relatively few such individuals have been reported. An increased incidence of neisserial infection, in addition to infections with high-grade pathogens, has been reported in properdin deficiency.

CLASSIC PATHWAY COMPONENT DEFICIENCIES

Since the alternative pathway provides a first line of defense against bacterial infection, one might expect that the deficiencies in the early steps of the classic pathway would not be associated with frequent

Table 25–1. Inherited complement and complement-related protein deficiency states.

Deficient Protein	Observed Pattern of Inheritance at Clinical Level	Reported Major Clinical Correlates[1]
C1q	Autosomal-recessive.	ACUD, PID
C1r	Autosomal-recessive.	ACUD
C1s	Found in combination with C1r deficiency.	ACUD
C4	Autosomal-recessive (two separate loci C4a and C4B).[2]	ACUD
C2	Autosomal-recessive, HLA-linked.	ACUD
C3	Autosomal-recessive.	ACUD, PID
C5	Autosomal-recessive.	Recurrent disseminated neisserial infections, SLE.
C6	Autosomal-recessive.	Recurrent disseminated neisserial infections.
C7	Autosomal-recessive.	Recurrent disseminated neisserial infections, Raynaud's phenomenon.
C8 (β chain or α-γ chains)	?Autosomal-recessive.	Recurrent disseminated neisserial infections.
C9	Autosomal-recessive.	PID
Properdin	X-linked recessive.	Recurrent pyogenic infections, fulminant meningococcemia.
Factor D	Autosomal-recessive.	Recurrent pyogenic infections.
C1 inhibitor	Autosomal-recessive.	Hereditary angioedema, increased incidence of several autoimmune diseases.[3]
Factor H	Autosomal-recessive.	Glomerulonephritis.
Factor I	Autosomal-recessive.	Recurrent pyogenic infections, ACUD.
CR1	Autosomal-recessive.[4]	Association between low erythrocyte CR1 and SLE, ACUD.
CR3	Autosomal-recessive.[5]	Leukocytosis, recurrent pyogenic infections, delayed umbilical cord separation.

Abbreviations: ACUD = autoimmune collagen vascular disease (SLE, glomerulonephritis); SLE = systemic lupus erythematosus; PID = propensity to infectious diseases.
[1] A significant number of individuals with complement deficiencies, especially of C2 and the terminal components, are clinically well. A significant number of patients with defects in C5–9 have had autoimmune disease.
[2] Individuals lacking C4A or C4B are designated "q0" (quantity 0). Thus, individuals can be C4Aq0 or C4Bq0. Such individuals are reported to have an increased incidence of autoimmune disease. Similarly, heterozygous C2 deficient individuals are reported to have an increased incidence of autoimmune disease.
[3] Includes approximately 85% of cases with silent alleles and 15% with alleles encoding for dysfunctional variant C1 inhibitor protein.
[4] Homozygosity for low (not absent) numerical expression of CR1 on erythrocytes is detectable in vitro and appears to be associated with SLE. An acquired defect in CR1 numbers may also be operative.
[5] Low but not absent leukocyte CR3 is detectable in both parents of most CR3-deficient children.

severe infections, and this is the case. Nevertheless, it has become increasingly clear, as the relatively few patients with defects in this portion of the cascade have been observed for more prolonged periods, that these individuals do not have normal host resistance. Patients with deficiency of early classic pathway components generally recover from infections well, but they are at a clear disadvantage when other defense mechanisms are inadequate. They are more likely to die of overwhelming infection than are persons with normal levels of all complement components. Mannose-binding protein, a protein with function similar to C1, is discussed in Chapter 11. Protein defects are associated with increased infection.

C3 & TERMINAL COMPONENT DEFICIENCIES

C3 is critical to both the classic and alternative pathways, and, as might be expected, patients with C3 deficiency are prone to develop overwhelming sepsis with high-grade pathogens. Patients with defects in the later acting terminal components respond quite well to most infectious agents. Their opsonic function, mediated by both the classic and alternative pathways, is intact; however, they have a much higher than normal frequency of disseminated meningococcal and gonococcal (neisserial) infections. Presumably, the lytic function of the late-acting components is required to defend adequately against these highly encapsulated organisms. It is interesting that neisserial infections in individuals with deficiencies in late-acting components follow a quite different course from those in non-complement-deficient individuals. These infections tend to occur in relatively older individuals, involve different groups of neisserial organisms (untypable and Y-type organisms), and are less likely to be lethal than infections that occur in normal individuals. Presumably, such complement-deficient patients synthesize antibody to the organisms, and this antibody provides partial but not complete protection. Individuals with no antibody to the organisms are far more likely to die of overwhelming sepsis than are individuals with antibody.

A large group of C9-deficient individuals has been discovered by mass screening in Japan. Careful studies have shown that this defect carries with it a small but clear increase in the incidence of infectious diseases. It should be recalled that lytic lesions usually can be formed in target cells by the action of the C5–C8 component. The function of C9 is to enlarge and stabilize the C5678 lytic lesion, but the action of C5–C8 on the infecting organism may be sufficient to protect against disease.

COMPLEMENT DEFICIENCIES & AUTOIMMUNITY

Patients missing proteins of the classic or alternative pathway, as well as some individuals with late component defects, have an unexpectedly high incidence of autoimmune disease, particularly systemic lupus erythematosus (SLE) and glomerulonephritis. It is currently believed that one of the biologic consequences of complement activation is to cause antigen–antibody complexes, once they have bound complement, to adhere to circulating erythrocytes via the erythrocyte complement receptor CR1. Presumably, such complexes, adherent to the erythrocyte surface, are less likely to escape from the circulation into the tissues, where they can cause tissue damage.

The genes for at least three complement proteins, C4, C2, and factor B, are located within the major histocompatibility locus on chromosome 6 in humans (class 3 histocompatibility genes). One of these genes, C4, normally exists in two copies on each chromosome, coding for two different gene products: C4A and C4B. These two proteins have biochemical differences, and they differ in their efficiency in mediating complement attack. It is quite common to find individuals missing one or more of the C4 alleles and others deficient in one of the C2 genes. Many investigators have found that such individuals who are heterozygous for the deficiency are more prone to develop the signs and symptoms of autoimmune disease than are normal controls. In particular, individuals missing the C4A alleles and designated C4Aq0 (for

C4A quantity 0) are far more likely to develop SLE. Because the C4B allele is much more active hemolytically and because the range of normal values is wide, these individuals can be identified only by specific characterization of the circulating protein by methods not available in most hospital laboratories.

COMPLEMENT REGULATORY FACTOR DEFICIENCIES

Regulatory proteins that control complement activation may also be deficient. The best studied and most common of these deficiencies is the partial deficiency of the control protein C1 inhibitor (C1INH). This protein functions to inactivate the subcomponents of C1, C1r, and C1s following their activation by stoichiometrically binding to the enzymatic sites on these proteins. The C1 inhibitor also acts to inactivate activated Hageman factor and its enzymatically active fragments, as well as those pathways activated by Hageman factor, the intrinsic clotting pathway (factor XI), the kinin-generating pathway (kallikrein), and the fibrolytic pathways (plasmin).

HEREDITARY ANGIOEDEMA

The disease of C1INH deficiency, hereditary angioedema, is characterized by recurrent attacks of edema of subcutaneous and submucosal tissues. It particularly affects the extremities and the mucosa of the gastrointestinal tract. Typically, attacks last for 1–4 days and are harmless, although when they involve the bowel wall they usually induce severe abdominal pain. Occasionally, attacks affect subcutaneous and submucosal tissue in the region of the upper airway. In this case they may be associated with respiratory obstruction and asphyxiation. Attacks are sporadic, but in some patients they may be induced by emotional stress or physical trauma. Although attacks usually begin in childhood, they seldom become severe until puberty.

Diagnosis is important, because patients respond poorly to the drugs usually used to treat episodic angioedema: epinephrine, antihistamines, and glucocorticoids. Diagnosis is established by the demonstration of low antigenic or functional levels of C1 esterase inhibitor. Such patients usually have normal levels of C1, low levels of C4 and C2, and normal levels of C3. The actual mechanism of angioedema formation is unknown; investigators have implicated both the complement- and kinin-generating systems in the production of attacks.

Two classes of drugs provide effective therapy. Plasmin inhibitors are fairly effective, although they do not correct the biochemical abnormality (low C4 and C2 levels), suggesting that their principal action is not the inhibition of enzymatic C1. Their mode of action is unknown. The second class of drugs that has proved useful is the group of anabolic steroids or impeded androgens. These agents, particularly the drug danazol, cause an increase in C1 inhibitor, presumably owing to increased synthesis. This leads to a rise in C4 and C2 levels toward normal, and in most patients the drug completely alleviates symptoms. All the useful oral androgens appear to have similar clinical activity, although the effect on levels of C1 inhibitor, C4 and C2 is much less striking with some.

Hereditary angioedema is different from most hereditary complement deficiency diseases in that it results from autosomal-dominant rather than recessive inheritance. Individuals with this disease have defective production of C1INH by one of the two genes present on chromosome 11. Approximately 85% of patients have one nonproductive gene and have one third to one half the normal levels of C1INH. The other 15% of patients have a gene mutation that leads to production of an abnormal C1INH product with no functional activity of the abnormal gene product. The precise defect for many of the mutations has been analyzed in great detail. The product of one normal gene does not appear to be sufficient to control activation of the various mediator pathways. Hereditary angioedema is treated effectively in most patients by administration of androgens or anabolic steroids. Although the mechanism of action of these drugs is not formally proven, they appear to act by inducing synthesis of the C1INH protein by hepatocytes, thereby correcting the defect. These drugs markedly diminish the frequency and severity of angioedema attacks. For unknown reasons, drugs that inhibit active plasmin are also therapeutically useful. They improve the clinical manifestations but do not correct the C1INH deficiency.

There are rare patients with an acquired form of C1 esterase inhibitor deficiency who present with clinical findings of recurrent angioedema similar to the patients with the inherited form of the disease. In most cases, this is due either to the formation of a monoclonal autoantibody to the C1INH protein that blocks normal C1 inhibitor function or to excessive activation of C1 with utilization of C1INH at a higher rate than the rate of resynthesis. The latter may occur during the course of an autoimmune disease such as SLE or may occur in the setting of a cancer, where it appears that the malignant cell synthesizes molecules that activate C1 and deplete C1 inhibitor. Interestingly, diseases associated with depletion of C1 inhibitor also often respond to treatment with anabolic steroids. Whereas patients with the inherited form of C1 esterase inhibitor deficiency have normal plasma levels of C1 and C3 and markedly depressed levels of C4 and C2, patients with the acquired form have profoundly depressed C1 titers, reflecting the marked activation and utilization of C1 that, in turn, depletes C1 inhibitor.

Patients have also been described who are deficient in the C3 regulatory factors H and I. These individuals also have a higher than expected incidence of infections, reflecting the fact that normal degradation of C3b does not occur, alternative pathway activation is poorly regulated, and C3 is abnormally consumed. Thus, these individuals act as if they were partially deficient in C3 and other alternative pathway regulatory factors. They also would be expected to have an abnormally high incidence of autoimmune disease.

COMPLEMENT RECEPTOR DEFICIENCIES

There are many cell membrane-bound complement regulatory factors. In general, inherited deficiencies of these proteins are rare. A group of children have been identified who fail to express the iC3b receptor (CR3) on their cell surface or who have low expression of the protein. These children fail to express the three CD11 membrane proteins. These three proteins have different α chains (CD11a, b, and c) and the same β chain (CD18), which is coded for by a gene on chromosome 21, and are members of an adhesion-promoting group of molecules termed **integrins.** The β chain is important in protein transport, and this inherited defect causes a failure to transport synthesized CD11/18 proteins to the cell surface. All of these children have phagocytes with defective cell–cell adhesion properties and defective adhesion to glass and other surfaces. The children show abnormal separation of the umbilical cord after birth and have frequent infections, often of the skin.

Acquired deficiencies of cell membrane-bound complement regulatory factors exist. The best studied is the group of defects associated with the acquired disease paroxysmal nocturnal hemoglobinuria (PNH). The regulatory proteins delay-accelerating factor (DAF), homologous restriction factor (HRF), and CD59 are bound to the cell by a glycosidic linkage rather than by a hydrophobic, membrane-spanning domain. The formation of this linkage is abnormal in patients with PNH, due to an abnormal synthetic enzyme. Phoshatidylinositol glycan class A (PIG-A) and all proteins bound to the cell by similar linkages are absent from progeny of a proportion of the marrow stem cells. Thus affected erythrocytes from PNH patients are missing some or all of the regulatory proteins that prevent formation of the membrane attack complex on autologous cells and are highly susceptible to complement-mediated lysis.

It has been reported that individuals with SLE have decreased numbers of CR1 on their cell surfaces as an inherited defect, but this point remains controversial. Clearly, the expression of CR1 on erythrocytes is an inherited trait, with some individuals showing larger numbers of receptors than others.

COMPLEMENT
ALLOTYPE VARIANTS

Many of the complement proteins exist in allotypic forms, with many inherited variants that can be detected by difference in their electrophoretic mobility. Some of these electrophoretic variants show a predilection for certain disease states, especially autoimmune disease. Whether this reflects a change in function of the complement protein caused by a mutation that leads to the electrophoretic variant or a linkage of the gene for one complement variant to other nearby disease-causing genes on the same chromosome that segregate together is not clear. Nevertheless, these cases of linkage disequilibrium have been well documented in population studies.

REFERENCES

GENERAL REVIEWS

Figueroa JE, Densen P: Infectious diseases associated with complement deficiencies. *Clin Microbiol Rev* 1991; **4:**359.

Frank MM: Complement in disease: Inherited and acquired complement deficiencies. In: *Samter's Immunologic Diseases, 5th ed.* Frank HH et al (editors). Little Brown, 1995, p 489.

Ross SC, Densen P: Complement deficiency states and infection: Epidemiology, pathogenesis and consequences of neisserial and other infections in an immune deficiency. *Medicine* 1984;**63:**243.

COMPLEMENT DEFICIENCY & INFECTION

Alper CA et al: Increased susceptibility to infection associated with abnormalities of complement-mediated functions and of the third component of complement (C3). *N Engl J Med* 1970;**282:**349.

Densen P et al: Familial properdin deficiency and fatal meningococcemia correction of the bactericidal defect by vaccination. *N Engl J Med* 1987;**316:**922.

Ellison RT et al: Prevalence of congenital or acquired complement deficiency in patients with sporadic meningococcal disease. *N Engl J Med* 1983;**308:**913.

C9 DEFICIENCY IN POPULATION STUDIES

Inai S et al: Deficiency of the ninth C1 component of complement in man. *J Clin Lab Immunol* 1979;**2:**85.

Nagata M et al: Inherited deficiency of the ninth component of complement; an increased risk of meningococcal meningitis. *Pediatr* 1989;**14:**260.

COMPLEMENT DEFICIENCY & AUTOIMMUNITY

Davies KA et al: Complement deficiency and immune complex disease. *Springer Semin Immunopathol* 1994; **15:**397.

GENETICS & HLA LINKAGE

Atkinson JP: Complement deficiency: Predisposing factor to autoimmune syndromes. *Clin Exp Rheumatol* 1989;**7:**95.

Colten HR: Genetics and synthesis of components of the complement system. In: *Immunobiology of the Complement System.* Ross GD (editor). Academic Press, 1986, p 163.

Howard PF et al: Relationship between C4 null genes, HLA-D region antigens, and genetic susceptibility to systemic lupus erythematosus in Caucasian and black Americans. *Am J Med* 1986;**81:**187.

HEREDITARY ANGIOEDEMA & ACQUIRED
C1 INHIBITOR

Alsenz J et al: Autoantibody-mediated acquired deficiency of C1 inhibitor. *N Engl J Med* 1987;**316:**1360.

Frank MM et al: Hereditary angioedema: The clinical syndrome and its management. *Ann Intern Med* 1976; **84:**580.

Frank MM et al: Epsilon aminocaproic acid therapy of hereditary angioneurotic edema: A double-blind study. *N Engl J Med* 1972;**286:**808.

Frank MM: Acquired C1 inhibitor deficiency. *Behring Inst Mitt* 1989;**84:**161.

Gelfand JA et al: Treatment of hereditary angioedema with danazol: Reversal of clinical and biochemical abnormalities. *N Engl J Med* 1976;**295:**1444.

Schapira M et al: Biochemistry and pathophysiology of human C1 inhibitor: Current issues. *Complement* 1985;**2:**111.

Tosi M: Molecular genetics of C1 inhibitor and hereditary angioedema. In: *Complement in Health and Disease,* 2nd ed. Whaley K et al (editors). Kluwer Academic, 1993, p 245.

CD11/CD18 DEFICIENCY

Anderson DC et al: The severe and moderate phenotypes of heritable Mac-1, LFA-1 deficiency: Their quantitative definition and relation to leukocyte dysfunction and clinical features. *J Infect Dis* 1985;**152:**668.

Petty HR, Todd RF 3rd: Receptor–receptor interactions of complement receptor type 3 in neutrophil membranes. *J Leuk Biol* 1993;**54:**492.

26

Mechanisms of Hypersensitivity

Abba I. Terr, MD

Allergy refers to certain diseases in which immune responses to environmental antigens cause tissue inflammation and organ dysfunction. The clinical features of each allergic disease reflect the immunologically induced inflammatory response in the organ or tissue involved. These features are generally independent of the chemical or physical properties of the antigen. The diversity of allergic responses arises from the involvement of different immunologic effector pathways, each of which generates a unique pattern of inflammation. The classification of allergic diseases is based on the type of immunologic mechanism involved. Table 26–1 compares the distinguishing features of allergic diseases. This chapter covers mechanisms, classification, and clinical evaluation of the allergic diseases.

DEFINITIONS

An **allergen** is any antigen that causes allergy. The term is used to denote either the antigenic molecule itself or its source, such as pollen grain, animal dander, insect venom, or food product. **Hypersensitivity** and **sensitivity** are often used as synonyms for allergy. **Immediate hypersensitivity** and **delayed hypersensitivity** are the terms formerly used to define antibody-mediated allergy and T-lymphocyte-mediated allergy, respectively.

Table 26–1. Comparison of allergy with other responses.

Disease	Mechanism	Antigen Source	Result
Allergy	Immunologic	Foreign	Disease
Immunity	Immunologic	Foreign	Prophylaxis
Autoimmunity	Immunologic	Self	Disease
Toxicity	Toxic	Foreign	Disease

PREVALENCE

Allergy is common throughout the world. The predilection for specific allergic diseases, however, varies among different age groups, sexes, and races. The prevalence of sensitivity to specific allergens is determined both by genetic predilection and by the geographic and cultural factors that are responsible for exposure to the allergen.

ALLERGENS

Any foreign substance capable of inducing an immune response is a potential allergen. Many different chemicals of both natural and synthetic origin are known to be allergenic. Complex natural organic chemicals, especially proteins, are likely to cause antibody-mediated allergy, whereas simple organic compounds, inorganic chemicals, and metals more frequently cause T-cell-mediated allergy. In some cases the same allergen may be responsible for more than one type of allergy. Exposure to the allergen may be through inhalation, ingestion, injection, or skin contact.

Allergies caused by certain allergens are encountered frequently in clinical practice, whereas others are rare. Examples of common allergens are the protein Amb a I in ragweed pollen and pentadecylcatechol in poison ivy. Sensitization of a specific individual to a particular environmental allergen is the result of a complex interplay of the chemical and physical properties of the allergen, the mode and quantity of exposure, and the unique genetic makeup of the individual.

SUSCEPTIBILITY TO ALLERGY

A clinical state of allergy affects only some of the individuals who encounter each allergen. The occurrence of allergic disease on exposure to an allergen requires not only prior sensitization but also other

Table 26–2. Factors that determine expression of disease in allergy.

Allergen Exposure	Allergic Sensitization	Target Organ Susceptibility	Clinical Disease	Type of Disease
– or +	–	–	–	No disease
+	+	–	–	Asymptomatic sensitivity
+	+	+	+	Allergic disease
– or +	–	+	+	Nonallergic disease

factors that detemine the localization of the reaction to a particular organ (Table 26–2). This is particularly evident in atopic allergy, where sensitization may cause disease localized to the nasal mucosa, the bronchial mucosa, the skin, the gastrointestinal tract, or a combination of two or more of these sites (see Fig 27–1). The nonimmunologic factors involved in the expression of clinical atopic disease are not yet known, although a disturbance in autonomic control, such as beta-adrenergic blockade or cholinergic hyperreactivity in the target tissue, has been postulated.

Most of the diseases in which allergy is expressed, (asthma, rhinitis, atopic dermatitis, contact dermatitis, anaphylaxis, and urticaria-angioedema) can occur in the absence of allergy. Recognition of these nonimmunologic diseases is important in differential diagnosis. In some cases, environmental triggers are nonspecific or cannot be identified. In other cases a specific environmental agent activates inflammatory mediators nonimmunologically. Examples of the latter phenomenon include direct mast cell release of histamine by opiate drugs, aspirin-induced asthma (possibly an aberrant metabolism of arachidonic acid), anaphylactoid reactions from radioiodinated contrast media, some instances of urticaria from eating shellfish and berries, and occupational isocyanate asthma. In these examples, no allergen-specific immunologic sensitivity has been shown to be responsible for the reaction, even though the disease occurs in only a limited percentage of the exposed population.

MECHANISMS & CLASSIFICATION OF ALLERGIC DISEASE

Allergy is an immunologic phenomenon. The disease results when an exposure to the allergen induces an immune response, referred to as "sensitization" rather than immunization (Fig 26–1A). Once sensitization occurs, an individual does not become symptomatic until there is an exposure to the allergen. Then the reaction of allergen with specific antibody or sensitized effector T lymphocyte induces an **inflammatory response,** producing the symptoms and signs of the allergic reaction (see Fig 26–1B).

Among the currently recognized pathways of immunologically induced inflammation (see Chapter 12), three different ones are responsible for the known allergic diseases: (1) the IgE/mast cell/mediator pathway, (2) the IgG or IgM immune complex/complement/neutrophil pathway, and (3) the effector T-lymphocyte/lymphokine pathway. Specific diseases associated with each of these processes are shown in Table 26–3 and are discussed in the following three chapters. A brief description of the immunologic mechanisms is given here. More detailed information can be found in the first section of this book.

THE IgE/MAST CELL/MEDIATOR PATHWAY

IgE antibodies have a unique configuration on the Fc portion of the molecule for fixation to mast cells and basophils (Fig 26–2). Fixation occurs at a high-affinity cell surface receptor, **FcεRI.** The allergic reaction is initiated when the polyvalent allergen molecule reacts with antibodies occupying these receptors. The result is a bridging of FcεRI, thereby altering the cell surface membrane. This, in turn, signals intracellular events causing release and activation of mediators of inflammation: histamine, leukotrienes, chemotactic factors, platelet-activating factor, and proteinases. Mast cell activation is modulated by intracellular cyclic nucleotides and is accompanied by cell degranulation. The released activated mediators act locally and cause increased vascular permeability, vasodilation, smooth muscle contraction, and mucous gland secretion. These biologic events account for the salient clinical features of the **immediate phase,** occurring in the first 15–30 minutes following allergen exposure. Over the succeeding 12 hours there is a progressive tissue infiltration of inflammatory cells, proceeding from neutrophils to eosinophils to mononuclear cells in response to other chemical mediators and biochemical events not yet fully delineated. The period of 6–12 hours after allergen exposure is designated the **late phase** of the IgE response and is characterized by clinical manifestations of cellular inflammation.

This mechanism is responsible for the atopic diseases, anaphylaxis, and urticaria. The reaction can be triggered by extremely small amounts of allergen.

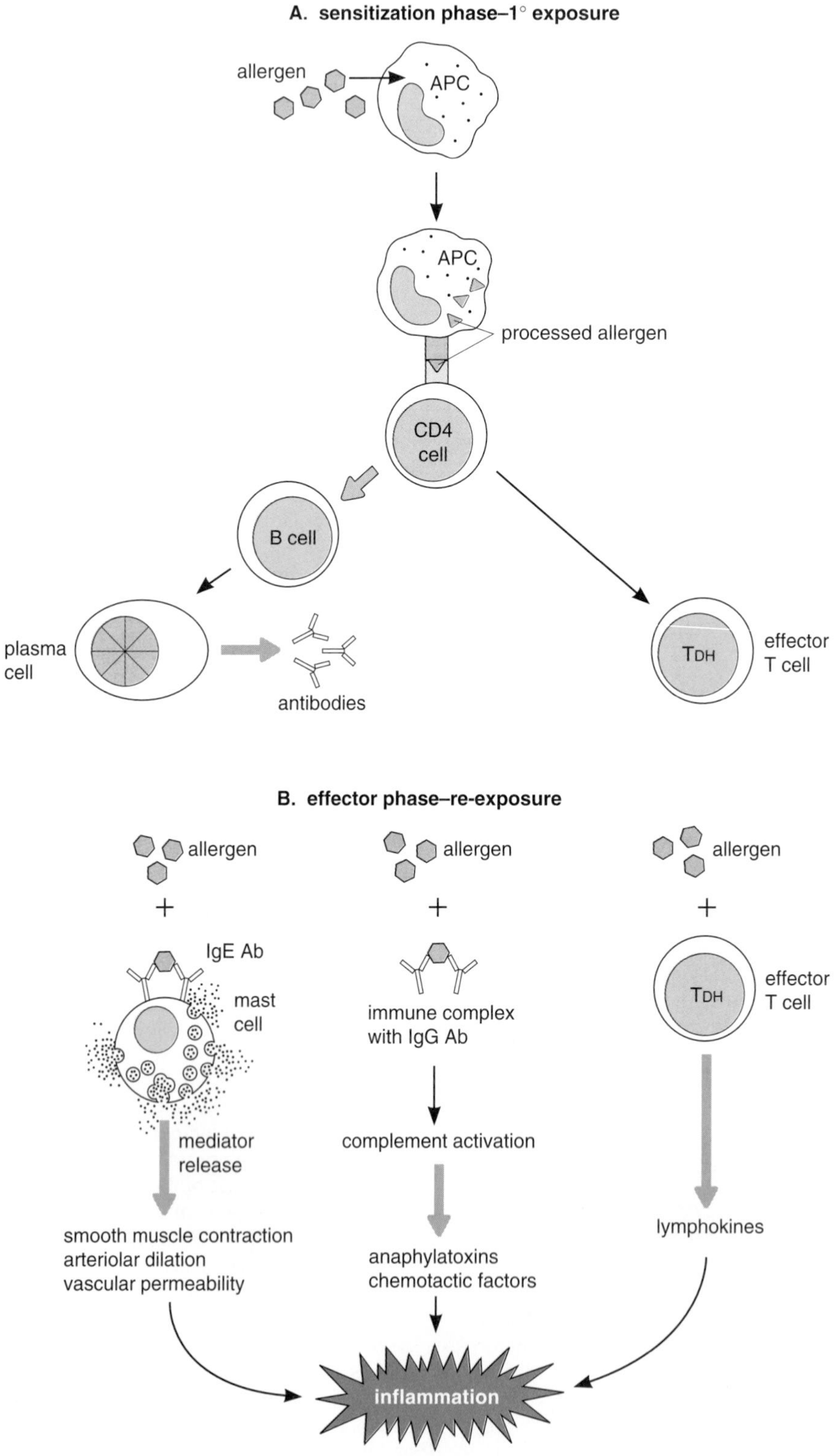

A. sensitization phase–1° exposure

B. effector phase–re-exposure

Figure 26–1. Role of the immune system in allergy. **A:** Sensitization phase, showing immunologic response to allergen from unsensitized (nonallergic) state to sensitized (allergic) state. **B:** Effector phase, showing reaction on reexposure of allergen to specific antibody or to specifically sensitized effector T cell.

Table 26–3. Classification of allergic diseases based on immunologic mechanisms.

1. **Allergic disease caused by IgE antibodies and mast cell mediators**
   a. Atopic diseases
      1. Allergic rhinitis
      2. Allergic asthma
      3. Atopic dermatitis
      4. Allergic gastroenteropathy
   b. Anaphylactic diseases
2. **Allergic disease caused by IgG or IgM antibodies and complement activation**
   a. Serum sickness
   b. Acute hypersensitivity pneumonitis
3. **Allergic disease caused by sensitized T lymphocytes**
   a. Allergic contact dermatitis
   b. Chronic hypersensitivity pneumonitis

Table 26–4. Immunologic pathways potentially capable of allergen–antibody activation.

1. Alternative complement pathway activation via IgA antibodies.
2. Anaphylatoxins (C3a, C5a, C4a) generated by classic or alternative pathway complement activation.
3. IgG4 antibody activation of mast cells for mediator release.
4. Complement activation of the kininogen-kallikrein-kinin system.

alveolitis). Because immune complexes in moderate antigen excess are the most efficient for activating C1q, relatively large quantities of allergens are required to initiate the reaction.

THE IgG OR IgM/COMPLEMENT/NEUTROPHIL PATHWAY

IgG or IgM antibodies form complexes with antigen, and such complexes cause tissue inflammation. This pathway contributes to the pathogenesis of many human diseases, including certain allergic diseases. Allergen–antibody complexes activate the complement system through the classic pathway via receptors on C1q for the Fc portion of the IgG or IgM antibody molecule. Complement activation generates anaphylatoxins and chemotactic peptides, which cause increased vascular permeability and infiltration of neutrophils. Activated neutrophils generate additional inflammatory and toxic products. Macrophages are also recruited and become activated, contributing further to tissue inflammation and injury.

This mechanism is responsible for the cutaneous Arthus reaction, serum sickness, and the acute phase of hypersensitivity pneumonitis (extrinsic allergic

THE EFFECTOR T-LYMPHOCYTE/LYMPHOKINE PATHWAY

Some allergic diseases are not mediated by antibody but, rather, by reaction of allergen with the effector T lymphocyte sensitized to the specific allergen from a prior exposure. The effector T cell has the CD4 phenotype, and when it encounters the allergen it is activated to generate lymphokines; this results in the accumulation over several days of a mononuclear cell infiltrate.

Other immunologic pathways leading to inflammation have been studied so far only at an in vitro level but have not yet been clearly identified as the primary pathogenetic mechanism of human disease. These potential mechanisms for allergy are listed in Table 26–4. They may play a secondary role in diseases caused by the three primary pathways already described.

CLINICAL EVALUATION

GENERAL CONSIDERATIONS

When allergy is suspected, the diagnostic process is aimed at determining whether the disease is caused by allergy and, if so, to identify the type of allergy and each of the responsible allergens. Many straightforward cases of seasonal hay fever caused by pollen or contact dermatitis caused by poison ivy can be diagnosed easily and quickly, but more complex or obscure allergic diseases require considerable detective work. History, physical examination, and appropriate laboratory tests are required, as in the diagnosis of any medical condition.

HISTORY

The history is essential. It is critically important to correlate results of specific allergy testing to the

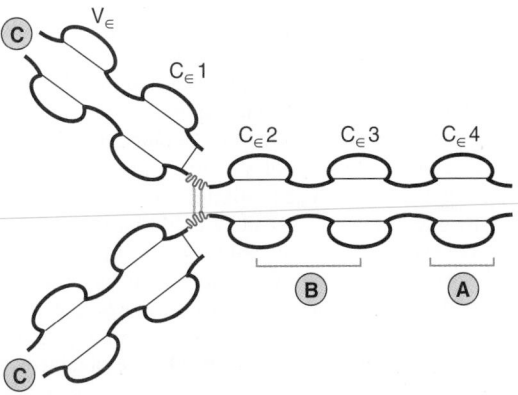

Figure 26–2. Schematic diagram of the IgE antibody molecule. ***A:*** The structure is similar to that of IgG, but there is an additional H-chain domain, accounting for its higher molecular weight. ***B:*** The regions of the molecule containing the site for fixation to mast cell FcεRI and ***C:*** the allergen-binding sites are indicated.

patient's history. Whenever allergy is suspected, the physician should be prepared first to obtain a detailed description of the symptoms and the timing and environmental locations associated with appearance and disappearance of those symptoms. Allergen exposure may occur through inhalation, ingestion, injection, or skin or mucous membrane contact. Variations in symptoms during the course of a day, week, month, and year and the association with home, work, school, or vacation trips are useful clues in diagnosis of the common inhalant and occupational allergies. When inhalant allergy is suspected, an environmental history should include details of work, hobbies, pets, and the influence of weather and climate on respiratory symptoms. A history of medication usage and dietary habits is relevant for possible ingested allergens. Drugs and insect bites and stings may cause allergy by injection. When allergic contact dermatitis is suspected, the physician should inquire especially about exposure to plants, perfumes, cosmetics, clothing, topical medications, work, and hobbies.

Other important historical data are the age of onset; the course of the illness; and the effect of hormonal factors, such as puberty, menstrual-cycle variations, and pregnancy. The influence of prior treatments, such as antihistamine drugs, antibiotics, and corticosteroids, may help to distinguish allergic from nonallergic conditions. The presence of other known allergies and results of prior allergy evaluations in the patient, as well as family history of allergy, may also be helpful.

Many allergists use standard questionnaires for part or all of the history. If the questionnaire is self-administered, the patient's answers should be reviewed by the physician.

PHYSICAL EXAMINATION

Allergic diseases are often episodic, because signs and symptoms depend on exposure to the allergen. Objective signs of allergy are therefore present when the physical examination is performed during the period of allergen exposure. A negative physical examination performed during a period of allergen avoidance does not mean that the patient does not have the allergy. The examination should be thorough enough to rule out other causes for the patient's symptoms. In allergic dermatoses the appearance, distribution, and extent of the skin lesions can direct the questioning to likely environmental sources of the allergen.

LABORATORY TESTING

A variety of laboratory tests are available to supplement the history and physical examination. There are procedures for quantitating the extent of functional and anatomic effects on a particular organ, for sampling fluids or tissues for evidence of disease, and for establishing the presence of specific immune responses.

1. TESTS OF AIRWAY FUNCTION

The standard pulmonary function tests quantitate the amount of obstructive airway and restrictive lung disease in patients with respiratory allergy. Reversible airway obstruction can be shown by bronchodilator response in a patient with current airway obstruction or by bronchoconstrictor response in a patient without baseline airway obstruction. Tests of nasal airway resistance are available but are not suitable for routine use. Tympanometry may aid in diagnosis of otitis media complicating allergic rhinosinusitis.

Airway hyperirritability in patients with asthma can be quantitated by bronchoprovocation tests with inhalation of certain chemicals (histamine, methacholine) or with physical stimuli (exercise). The former are more sensitive but may be positive in nonasthmatics under certain conditions, whereas the latter are more specific to asthma but less sensitive.

The usual measurement used for the various bronchoprovocation tests is a fall in 1-second forced expiratory volume (FEV_1), measured by spirometry. Increasing doses of aerosolized methacholine or histamine are delivered by nebulizer, and the provocative dose causing a 20% fall in FEV_1 is designated PD_{20}.

Physical challenges with exercise, cold dry isocapnic hyperventilation, or ultrasonically nebulized distilled water have also been standardized for detecting nonspecific bronchial hyperirritability. The mechanisms involved are not understood precisely, although these physical stimuli possibly stimulate bronchial mast cells to release mediators nonimmunologically, whereas histamine and methacholine act directly on bronchial smooth muscle. In all cases of nonspecific testing, maximal bronchoconstriction is achieved in about 5 minutes, with reversion to baseline in 15–20 minutes without a late-phase response (Fig 26–3). Rarely, methacholine may produce a prolonged, severe episode of asthma that requires treatment. The procedures can be performed in an outpatient setting, but emergency equipment should be available in the event of a severe induced asthma attack.

Any one of these tests can be used to assist in diagnosis of asthma in patients with a history of symptoms but negative tests for reversible airway obstruction. Under these conditions a negative methacholine challenge test rules out asthma. A positive test indicating airway hyperirritability, however, may be obtained in other conditions, such as (1) allergic rhinitis, especially during the pollen season; (2) following a viral respiratory infection or recent immunization with influenza or live measles vaccine; (3) in some relatives of asthmatics; and (4) in a small portion of the normal population. The test has been especially helpful in diagnosis and screening for potential occupational asthma.

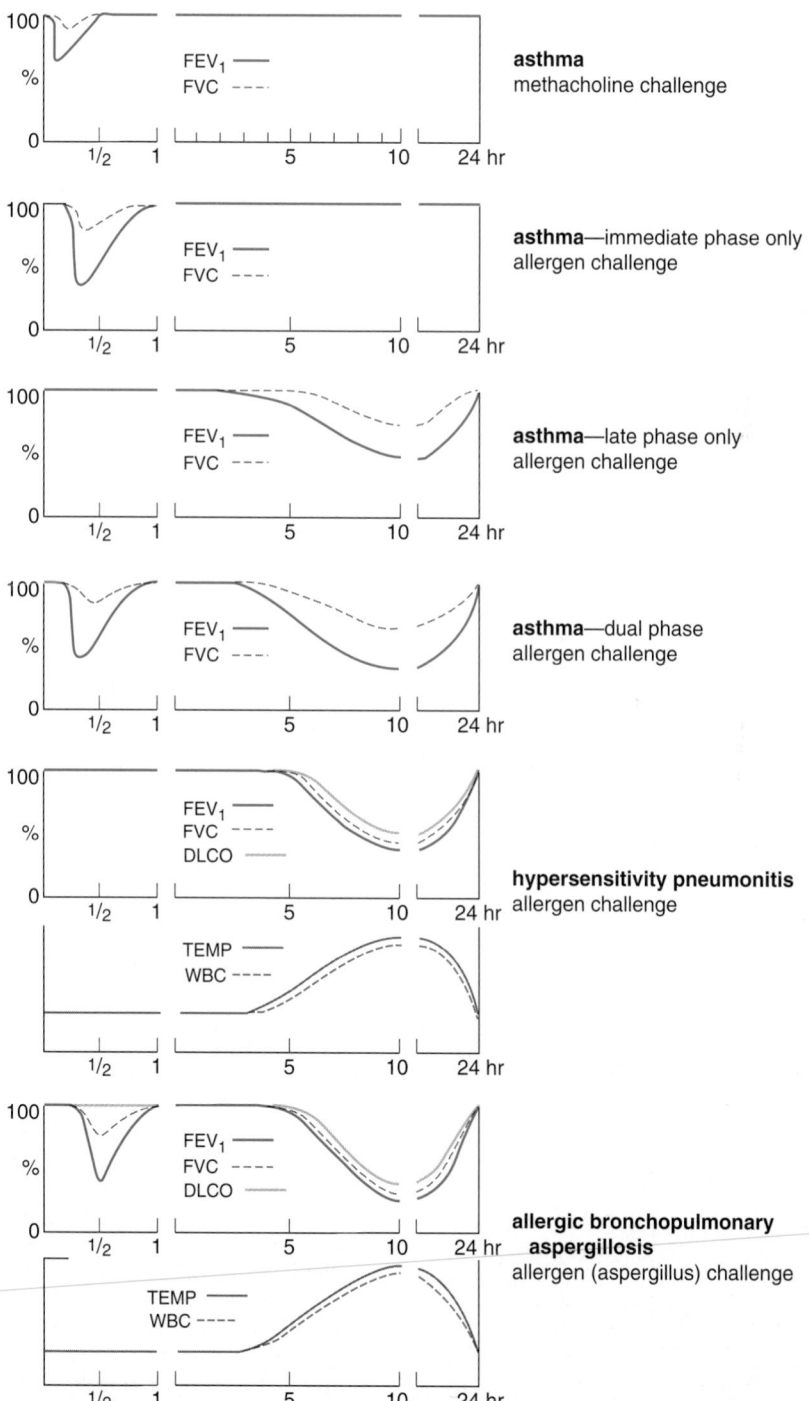

Figure 26–3. Bronchial provocation tests for detection of nonspecific bronchial hyperirritability (methacholine challenge) or immunologic reactivity (allergen challenge). Shown are the responses in patients with asthma (IgE antibody sensitivity), hypersensitivity pneumonitis (principally T-cell-mediated sensitivity), and allergic bronchopulmonary aspergillosis (combined IgE and IgG antibody sensitivities). *Abbreviations:* FEV$_1$ = forced expiratory volume in 1 second; FVC = forced vital capacity; DLCO = diffusing capacity for carbon monoxide; Temp = temperature; WBC = leukocyte count.

2. ANATOMIC TESTS

Visualization of paranasal sinuses, lungs, and the gastrointestinal tract may require x-ray, computed tomography, or endoscopy.

3. TISSUE DIAGNOSIS

When appropriate, samples of nasal or sinus secretions, sputum, bronchoalveolar fluid, gastrointestinal secretions, stool, or blood can be examined for inflammatory cell content. These studies, as well as histopathology of biopsy specimens from tissues of patients with suspected allergic disease, may confirm the type of inflammation associated with a particular type of allergic response, but they do not identify the causative allergen.

4. ALLERGY SKIN TESTING

A variety of skin test methods are used in the clinical diagnosis of each type of allergic disease. The skin test is a bioassay for the presence or absence of an immune response to a specific allergen that produces a visible transient skin lesion. The skin is a convenient organ to test, since it is equipped with all of the elements necessary for eliciting a localized controlled allergic reaction, even though the disease is targeted to another organ.

For diagnosis, skin testing occupies an intermediate position between in vitro tests, which demonstrate specific immune response only, and in vivo provocation tests, which demonstrate the ability of the diseased target organ to respond immunologically to the allergen. Skin tests require some skill in performance and interpretation, but they have many advantages. They are convenient, inexpensive, and safe if done properly. Results are available with no delay beyond the time required for the allergic response. There is no possibility of sample (ie, patient) error. Many suspected allergens can be tested simultaneously. Discomfort is usually minimal.

The principal disadvantage of skin testing is the need to discontinue certain inhibitory drugs. Occasionally, skin testing is prohibited for lack of available skin because of generalized dermatitis. The procedure may be unacceptable to some small children and adults. The potential for a systemic reaction or flare of the disease exists, but these are exceedingly unlikely with proper precautions.

Patch Tests

The patch test produces an allergic contact dermatitis on a small area of skin to which a known concentration of allergen is applied. It is therefore a true provocative test of the disease. In most cases of allergic contact dermatitis, the allergen is a chemical that couples to skin protein, yielding a hapten–protein conjugate. This conjugate then reacts with sensitized cutaneous T lymphocytes to liberate lymphokines, which produce localized cell-mediated inflammation at the site of contact with the test allergen.

A. Method: The concentration of allergen, usually a chemical, is determined by prior testing of several allergic and nonallergic subjects. It must be high enough to elicit a positive reaction in the former but not high enough to cause skin irritation in the latter. Two test methods are available. In the open-patch method a drop of acetone extract is applied to the skin. The acetone quickly dries, depositing the test chemical on the skin site, which is left uncovered and inspected after 48 hours. In the closed-patch method the allergen in petrolatum is applied to a pad taped to the skin. After 48 hours the pad is removed and the site is inspected. A positive test consists of erythema, papules, or vesicles. If the test is negative, the site should be examined again at 72 and 96 hours, because weak reactions may appear later. Multiple tests can be performed simultaneously. Preferred areas for testing are the back, forearms, or upper arms.

About 20 chemicals cause most cases of allergic contact dermatitis (see Chapter 30). Textbooks on contact dermatitis should be consulted for proper concentrations of many other known contact sensitizers.

Systemic corticosteroid drugs inhibit cell-mediated hypersensitivity and should be discontinued prior to testing. Antihistamines and other antiallergy drugs need not be discontinued.

B. Indications: The patch test is indicated for diagnosis of allergic contact dermatitis if the cause is not apparent by history and distribution of the lesions. When the disease is caused by a topical medication, cosmetic, or other product containing many chemical components, each one should be tested separately so that allergen elimination can be specific.

C. Adverse Effects: A strongly positive test in a patient with severe allergy may cause considerable itching and discomfort, in which case the patch should be removed in less than 48 hours. Patch testing during the active phase of contact dermatitis may exacerbate the disease. Whenever possible, the dermatitis should be cleared by treatment before the test is begun. Occasionally the test itself can induce sensitivity, so the selection of test allergens should be limited to those suspected clinically.

D. Photopatch Test: This is a test for photoallergic contact dermatitis. The procedure is identical to the patch test, except that the test site is exposed to ultraviolet light or sunlight after the patch is removed, and the reaction is read after 24 hours and again after 48 hours. A control site is a patch test to the allergen without light exposure.

Cutaneous Tests

The cutaneous test (prick test, puncture test, epicutaneous test) introduces into the dermis, at a single

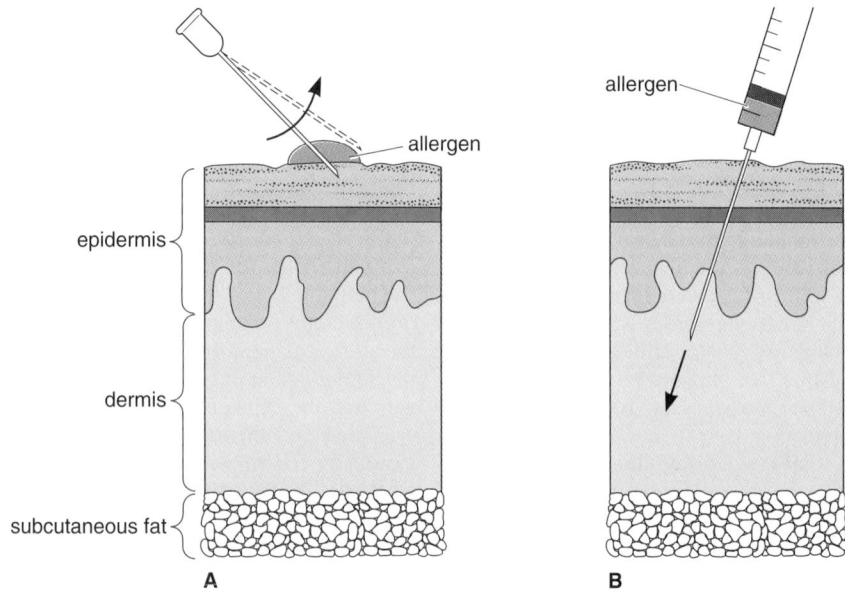

Figure 26–4. The technique of allergy skin testing. **A:** Cutaneous test. **B:** Intradermal test.

point, a minute quantity of allergen sufficient to react with IgE antibodies fixed to cutaneous mast cells for release of mediators to produce a visible wheal and erythema (Fig 26–4). It is the procedure least likely to produce systemic anaphylaxis, because of the small amount of allergen introduced into the skin. For the same reason it is also unlikely to elicit an Arthus or cell-mediated skin reaction.

For routine diagnosis in atopic and anaphylactic diseases, a single drop of concentrated aqueous allergen extract in buffered saline diluent at pH 6.0 is placed on the skin, which is then pricked lightly with a needle point at the center of the drop. After 20 minutes the reaction is graded and recorded as indicated in Table 26–5. A negative diluent control must be included. Positive controls of histamine or a nonspecific mast cell mediator-releasing agent such as codeine, or both, may be included. The skin of the back, volar aspect of the forearms, or upper arms can be used. Fifty or more allergens can be tested at one time on the back, but test sites should be at least 3.5 cm apart. A result of 2+ or greater is positive. A result of 0 or 1+ should be repeated by using the intracutaneous method. A late-phase reaction is not usually elicited by prick testing.

Another cutaneous testing method is the scratch test, in which a short linear scratch is made in the skin, to which the allergen is then applied. It is not recommended because it frequently causes nonspecific irritation, it is painful, and occasionally it causes scarring.

Any drug with antihistaminic (H_1-receptor blocking) activity must be discontinued for an appropriate period (24 hours or longer, depending on the drug) prior to testing. The new nonsedating antihistamines

have long half-lives and inhibit skin testing for weeks. Some drugs prescribed for other diseases, notably the tricyclic antidepressants, are potent antihistaminics. Corticosteroids, theophylline, sympathomimetic drugs, and cromolyn do not inhibit immediate skin test reactions and need not be withdrawn prior to testing.

Intradermal Tests

In the intradermal skin test (intracutaneous test), a measured quantity of allergen is introduced into the skin for detection of IgE-mediated (atopic or anaphylactic), IgG-mediated (immune complex), or effector T-lymphocyte-mediated (cellular or delayed hypersensitivity) responses (see Fig 26–4B). It is therefore used in diagnosis of several different types of allergic diseases.

Table 26–5. Wheal-and-erythema skin tests.

Test	Reaction	Appearances
Prick	Neg	No wheal or erythema.
	1+	No wheal; erythema <20 mm in diameter.
	2+	No wheal; erythema >20 mm in diameter.
	3+	Wheal and erythema.
	4+	Wheal with pseudopods; erythema.
Intracutan-eous	Neg	Same as control.
	1+	Wheal twice as large as control; erythema <20 mm in diameter.
	2+	Wheal twice as large as control; erythema >20 mm in diameter.
	3+	Wheal 3 times as large as control; erythema.
	4+	Wheal with pseudopods; erythema.

Intradermal tests should be applied to the arm only, so that a tourniquet can be used in the event of an unexpected systemic reaction. The allergen extract must be nontoxic and free of microbial contaminants. A tuberculin syringe with 27-gauge needle is used, and the volume to be injected depends on the immunologic effector mechanism under study.

For IgE-mediated sensitivities, the recommended volume ranges from 0.005 to 0.02 mL, but is usually 0.01 mL. Larger volumes are unnecessary and cause confusing results. In most cases, intradermal testing in suspected IgE-mediated diseases is performed only for allergens giving negative or at most 1+ responses to prior prick-testing (see previous section), since the intradermal test is approximately 1000 times more sensitive. The reaction is read in 20 minutes (see Table 24–4). A 1:500 (wt/vol) dilution of most common inhalant allergens is satisfactory for diagnosis of atopic allergy. A negative diluent control is necessary. A positive histamine or histamine release control, or both, is optional but recommended if the patient has recently taken antihistamines.

After the immediate wheal-and-erythema response subsides, a late-phase 6–12-hour reaction appears in some cases. The diagnostic significance of the late-phase skin reaction is currently uncertain.

Serial dilution titration is a semiquantitative form of intradermal testing in which 5- or 10-fold increasing concentrations of allergen extract are tested for each allergen until a positive result occurs. Skin test sensitivity correlates roughly with clinical target organ sensitivity, but the main purpose of serial titration is to determine a starting dose for immunotherapy that avoids the risk of systemic reaction. It is routinely used in testing for Hymenoptera insect venom anaphylaxis. Some physicians titrate atopic allergens in testing, but this is not recommended because it requires many more injections than the standard two-stage prick and single-dose intradermal test, which can be quantitated by the size of the reaction.

Antihistamine drugs inhibit the intradermal wheal-and-erythema skin test reactions, as discussed earlier.

Intradermal testing can be used to detect circulating IgG antibodies in a suspected Arthus reaction. The cutaneous Arthus reaction is grossly similar to the late-phase IgE antibody reaction in appearance and timing, except that there is no preceding immediate-phase wheal-and-erythema, and a high concentration of injection allergen is required to elicit a positive test. Immune-complex allergic reactions are infrequent in clinical practice (see Chapter 29), and IgG antibodies can usually be detected in vitro, so the Arthus skin test has not been standardized and is rarely used. A preliminary prick test should be done so that the procedure can be withheld if the patient has a significant (coincidental) IgE sensitivity to the allergen.

The tuberculin test is an intradermal test for cell-mediated hypersensitivity or immunity. It is performed by injecting 0.10 mL of the test allergen intradermally. There is a delayed (onset after 12 hours or more) response of erythema, induration, and tenderness. A positive test consists of induration 10 mm or greater in diameter at 48 hours. The test is not used in clinical diagnosis of cell-mediated allergies (see Chapter 12), but it is used extensively for detecting immunity in certain infections and in assessing cellular immunodeficiency (see Chapter 19).

Passive Transfer of the Skin Test

The immediate wheal-and-erythema skin test reaction in atopy or anaphylaxis can be transferred from the allergic patient to a nonallergic subject by injecting serum containing the IgE antibody from the former into the skin of the latter, proving an antibody causation for the disease. This is known as the **Prausnitz-Küstner** reaction. Cell-mediated skin test reactions, on the other hand, can be transferred by specifically sensitized effector T lymphocytes and not by serum antibodies. These serum or cell passive transfer procedures have been invaluable in research and have been used to a limited extent in the past for diagnosis. Their use in clinical practice is no longer justified, because of the risk of transmitting blood-borne microorganisms and the availability of the other testing methods discussed later on.

5. IN VITRO TESTS

The need for in vitro diagnostic tests for allergies that use blood (or occasionally other body fluids) stems from the potential danger, the perceived discomfort, and the subjectivity of in vivo tests. In vitro tests can provide precision, reproducibility, and efficiency. Blood samples can be stored so that serial testing of samples drawn at different times can be performed simultaneously under identical conditions. In vitro tests are especially well suited for large-scale population screening and for testing allergens that are potentially toxic or irritating. They are useful in situations in which in vivo testing is thwarted by other factors, such as the inability to do skin tests in a patient with extensive dermatitis or in an uncooperative child.

In vitro tests, however, frequently measure only isolated components of the complex events in an allergic reaction (Fig 26–5). The clinical expression of allergy requires not only an immune response (the sensitized state), but also a properly reactive target tissue or organ, and exposure to a sufficient amount of allergen. The reaction can be further modified by extraneous factors, such as age, endogenous endocrine hormone output, psychologic factors, and medications. All in vitro tests have limitations in sensitivity and depend on the quality of the allergen and reagents and on other technical factors. Results of any test must always be interpreted in the context of the history, physical examination, and other diagnostic procedures.

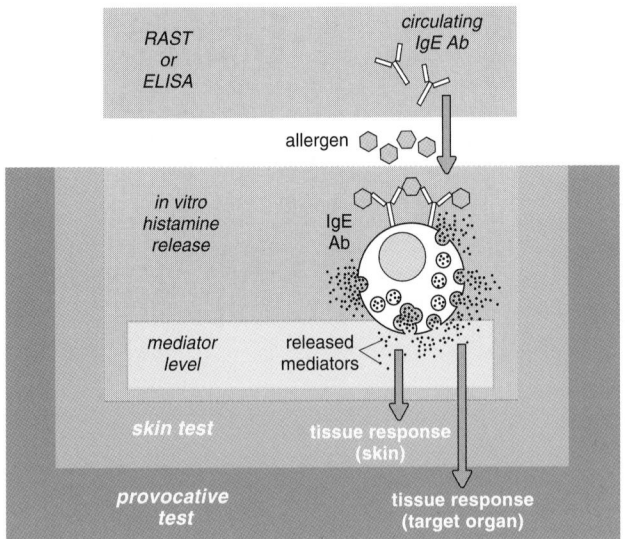
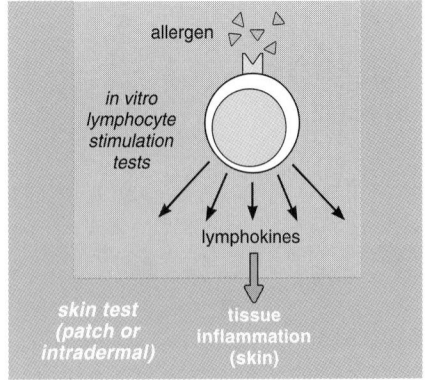

A   **B**

Figure 26–5. Schematic diagram showing the components of **A:** IgE-mediated and **B:** T-cell-mediated allergic reactions that are detected by various diagnostic procedures. *Abbreviations:* RAST = radioallergosorbent test; ELISA = enzyme-linked immunosorbent assay.

Tests for IgE Antibodies

Quantitative measurement of allergen-specific IgE antibodies in serum requires special methods to detect the extremely minute quantities (picograms per milliliter) found in allergic patients. The standard technique is the **radioallergosorbent test (RAST).** This is a two-phase (solid–liquid) system using an insolubilized allergen that is incubated first in the test serum to react with allergen-specific antibodies and then in radiolabeled heterologous antihuman IgE to detect the allergen-specific antibodies of the IgE isotype. The method is diagrammed and described in Figure 26–6. The test requires purified preparations of allergens and antihuman IgE. The RAST uses a cellulose disk as the insoluble immunosorbent to which protein allergens are coupled covalently with cyanogen bromide. There are a number of modifications of this method in which other immunosorbents and other detection labeling systems (various chemicals detected by fluorescence or colorimetry) are used.

Disadvantages of these in vitro methods are both biologic and technical. The quantity of serum IgE antibody is not necessarily a direct reflection of the biologically relevant mast cell-fixed antibody. The test result may be falsely positive in patients with a high total IgE level because of nonspecific binding of allergen to some immunosorbents, and it may be falsely low in desensitized patients with high levels of IgG antibody. Like all other allergy tests, results must be interpreted in the context of the clinical history and examination.

Tests for IgG Antibodies

These are discussed in Chapter 14.

Tests of Immune Complexes

These are discussed in Chapter 14.

Lymphocyte Stimulation

This is discussed in Chapter 15.

6. PROVOCATIVE TESTS

Occasionally it is desirable to test the target (respiratory, gastrointestinal, or cutaneous) tissue responsiveness to the allergen under controlled conditions. The patch test for immediate contact urticaria or delayed contact dermatitis is such a procedure. In the nasal provocation test, changes in nasal airway resistance and visible signs of congestion and rhinorrhea are observed after exposure to quantitative allergen challenge. Timed changes in bronchial airway flow rate or resistance are measured by bronchial provocation. Oral challenge with food or drug may be done to observe subjective gastrointestinal symptoms, appearance of skin eruptions, or objective changes in airway resistance.

A positive provocation test does not prove an immunologic basis for the disease, and except for patch testing, they are not used for routine diagnosis. Provocation testing is, however, an invaluable research tool for studying pathogenetic mechanisms and drug efficacy in allergic disease.

Allergen Bronchoprovocation Testing

Inhalational challenge with aerosolized allergen extracts to provoke a bronchial or pulmonary reaction

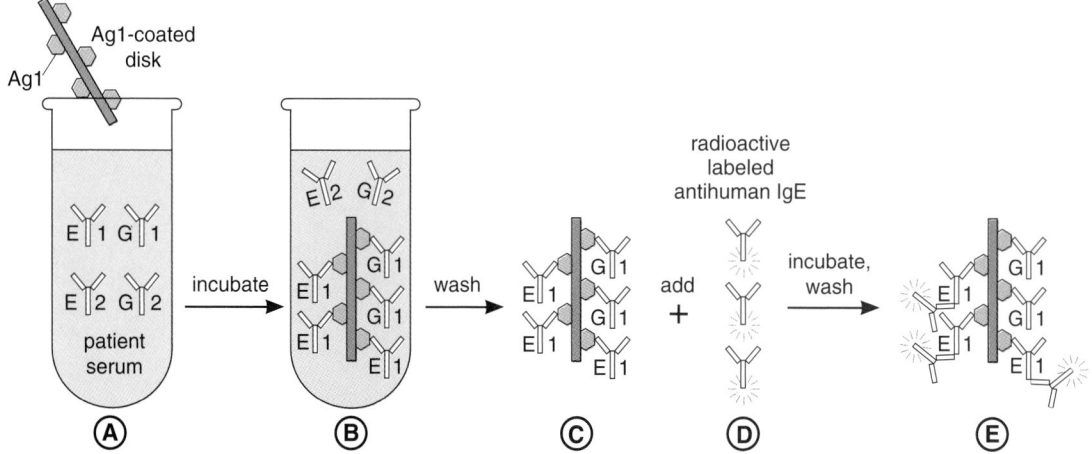

Figure 26–6. Diagram of radioallergosorbent test (RAST). **A:** A disk coated with the test allergen (Ag1) is incubated with serum of a patient with allergy to Ag1, as well as to other allergens (Ag2). **B:** IgE antibodies to Ag1 (E1) and IgG antibodies to the same allergen (G1) react with the Ag1-coated disk, whereas IgE and IgG antibodies (E2, G2) do not, and they remain in the serum. **C,D:** After being washed, the disk is incubated with a radiolabeled heterologous antibody to human IgE. **E:** After the disk is washed to remove unreacted labeled anti-IgE, the amount of radioactivity measured in a gamma counter is proportionate to the quantity of specific IgE antibody (E1) in the patient's serum. IgG antibodies to the same allergen (G1) on the disk do not react with the anti-human IgE antibody.

under controlled conditions in the laboratory is of limited use in clinical practice. It is applicable in testing for allergic asthma and hypersensitivity pneumonitis (see Fig 26–3).

The method of nebulizing and delivering known quantities of allergen extract is the same as for the methacholine challenge test (see earlier discussion). Aqueous allergen extracts in several dilutions are prepared in buffered saline. An initial titration skin testing is necessary to determine a safe starting dose for bronchial challenge.

For testing patients with allergic asthma, a measurement sensitive to acute airway obstruction is used, as in the methacholine challenge, and the dose-response result is presented in the same fashion. Usually the change in FEV_1 is expressed by determination of PD_{20}. Provocation tests have been done with the common inhalant atopic allergens, occupational allergens, and various chemicals. A fall in FEV_1 begins in 10 minutes or less, peaks at 20–30 minutes, and then returns to baseline. This immediate-phase asthmatic response occurs slightly later after allergen challenge than is the case for methacholine, histamine, or physical challenge. It is likely to be more severe and unpredictable, and it may require treatment with an inhaled bronchodilator drug. There may be a late-phase asthmatic response beginning at 4–6 hours, peaking at 8–12 hours, and clearing by 24 hours. Allergen challenges may cause isolated early or late responses, or both. Therefore, pulmonary function monitoring should be continued at hourly intervals after the immediate phase has subsided. Because of the possibility of late-phase responses, allergen bron-

choprovocation should be performed in a hospital with appropriate facilities for detecting and treating these reactions. A positive late-phase response may increase the patient's nonspecific bronchial hyperirritability for several days, so if a second allergen is to be tested, this should be done no sooner than 1 week later.

The **indications** for provocation testing in clinical practice are limited. For routine diagnosis of atopic asthma, bronchoprovocation with allergen gives results that correlate well with skin tests, but patients with only allergic rhinitis may also have a specific bronchial response to inhaled allergen extract. A positive test to a suspected causative agent of occupational asthma does not necessarily mean that the asthma is immunologic. For example, bronchoprovocation with isocyanates produces specific immediate and late asthmatic responses in workers with clinical isocyanate asthma, even though the illness does not correlate well with an IgE (or other) immune response to this chemical. Allergen bronchoprovocation may be useful to monitor desensitization therapy.

Allergen bronchoprovocation is especially helpful in cases of suspected hypersensitivity pneumonitis. The method of delivery of allergen is the same as in tests for asthma, but pulmonary function measurements should be sensitive to measures of restrictive lung disease. The fall in forced vital capacity (FVC) and diffusing capacity for CO, as well as fever and leukocytosis, begin 4–6 hours after challenge, reach maximum effect at 8 hours, and return to normal values by 24 hours in patients with acute hypersensitivity pneumonitis.

To quantitate and standardize allergen challenges, it is necessary to use aerosolized aqueous extracts. The procedure therefore does not simulate natural allergic asthma or hypersensitivity pneumonitis caused by particulate allergens, as in the case of pollen and mold asthma, in which the inhaled material is in the form of particles up to 60 μm in diameter. Particles of this size, when inhaled naturally, do not reach the tracheo-bronchial tree, in contrast to liquid aerosols 1–5 μm in diameter, which do so readily.

Nasal Provocation Testing

An objective quantitative test of nasal mucosal re-activity to allergen or nonimmunologic stimulus is not available for routine diagnosis because of technical difficulties in assessing nasal reactivity. Present methods of rhinomanometry for measuring nasal airway resistance are limited by artifacts and poor patient acceptance. Nasal airflow is subject to anatomic factors, atmospheric conditions, psychologic stimuli, and physiologic fluctuations. Quantitation of rhinorrhea, sneezing, or itching is crude and subjective. Nasal provocation testing has been useful in research but not in clinical practice.

Elimination Diet Testing

Dietary elimination and challenge with foods suspected of causing urticaria or exacerbating atopic dermatitis, asthma, and gastrointestinal or other symptoms are commonly used by allergists. The procedure is not standardized but, rather, is tailored to each individual diagnostic situation. Elimination diets aim to alleviate ongoing symptoms. One or more foods, depending on the patient's history, are eliminated until symptoms disappear. If symptoms are intermittent, a preliminary diet–symptom record may reveal the food(s) to be eliminated. If necessary, all natural foods are eliminated and nutrition is maintained by artificial diet, but restrictive diets should not be continued for more than 2 weeks. If symptoms clear, the eliminated foods are reintroduced one at a time to determine which food or foods provoke the allergic reaction or symptoms. A positive food challenge is repeated several more times for verification, but a single negative result generally rules out allergy to that food. There are no standard time limits for elimination or challenge, but, traditionally, most allergists accept a positive challenge within 2 hours to the same food on three successive trials as valid proof of a cause-and-effect relationship, although other information would be necessary to determine the mechanism. The clini-

cal features of the induced reaction and evidence by skin or in vitro test of the relevant immune response distinguishes allergic reactions from toxic, digestive, metabolic, or psychologic responses to the food.

These elimination challenge maneuvers are subjective and greatly prone to an erroneous diagnosis of food allergy because of physician and patient bias. A history of an acute allergic reaction to a single food allergen, supplemented if necessary by elimination and challenge testing and accompanied by IgE antibody detected by skin or in vitro test, is sufficient for diagnosis and therapeutic elimination of that food. In other situations in which delayed reactions, atypical or elusive symptoms and signs, and multiple suspect foods might lead to a nutritionally inadequate therapeutic elimination diet, the method of double-blind oral provocation testing should be employed.

Oral Provocation Testing

Double-blind food challenges are critical in defining the role of foods in allergic diseases. The procedure is simple and inexpensive enough to be used in clinical practice, although it is time-consuming. Patients with a history of anaphylaxis to a food should not be deliberately challenged.

Freeze-dried foods are packed into large opaque gelatin capsules. Each capsule can contain up to 600 mg of dry food. Lactose or a food to which the patient is not allergic can be used as a placebo control. The patient swallows a specified dose determined by the number of capsules and is observed for symptoms, signs, and an appropriate objective measure such as a pulmonary function test. The observation time and measurements are based on the history. The order and frequency of active and placebo challenges are determined by a double-blind protocol. If a severe reaction is anticipated, increasing doses are given, starting as low as 10 mg of dried food and increasing to an amount corresponding to the amount suspected to cause a reaction by history. As much as 8 g can be consumed in capsule form by most patients. Some foods can be disguised in flavored milk shakes. A negative double-blind food challenge should be confirmed by an open dietary trial of the same food, since freeze-drying and encapsulating the food could conceivably change its allergenicity. When properly performed, this procedure is a powerful tool for avoiding an unsubstantiated diagnosis of food allergy when the test is negative. It is important to remember that a positive response shows only an intolerance to the food and does not prove an allergic pathogenesis.

REFERENCES

GENERAL

deShazo RD, Smith DL (editors): Primer on allergic and immunologic diseases, second edition. *JAMA* 1992; **268:**2785. (Entire issue.)

Middleton E et al (editors): *Allergy: Principles and Practice,* 4th ed. Mosby, 1993.

Patterson R (editors): *Allergic Diseases: Diagnosis and Management,* 4th ed. Lippincott, 1993.

Samter M (editor): *Immunologic Diseases,* 5th ed. Little, Brown, 1994.

DIAGNOSIS

Adkinson NF: The radioallergosorbent test in 1981: Limitations and refinement. *J Allergy Clin Immunol* 1981;**67:**87.

AMA Council on Scientific Affairs: In vivo diagnostic testing and immunotherapy for allergy. Part I. *JAMA* 1987;**258:**1363.

AMA Council on Scientific Affairs: In vivo diagnostic testing and immunotherapy for allergy. Part II. *JAMA* 1987;**258:**1505.

AMA Council on Scientific Affairs: In vivo testing for allergy. Report II. *JAMA* 1987;**258:**1639.

Berstein M et al: Double-blind food challenge in the diagnosis of food sensitivity in the adult. *J Allergy Clin Immunol* 1982;**70:**205.

Bock SA et al: Appraisal of skin tests with food extracts for diagnosis of food hypersensitivity. *Clin Allergy* 1978;**8:**559.

Cockcroft DW: Bronchial inhalation tests. I. Measurement of nonallergic bronchial responsiveness. *Ann Allergy* 1985;**55:**527.

Cockcroft DW: Bronchial inhalation tests. II. Measurement of allergic and occupational bronchial responsiveness. *Ann Allergy* 1987;**59:**89.

Terr AI: In vivo tests for immediate hypersensitivity. *Ann Rev Med* 1988;**39:**135.

Townley RJ, Hopp RJ: Inhalation methods for the study of airway responsiveness. *J Allergy Clin Immunol* 1987;**80:**111.

The Atopic Diseases

27

Abba I. Terr, MD

GENERAL CONSIDERATIONS

Definition

Atopy refers to an inherited propensity to respond immunologically to many common naturally occurring inhaled and ingested allergens with the continual production of IgE antibodies. Allergic rhinitis and allergic asthma are the most common manifestations of clinical disease following exposure to these environmental allergens. Atopic dermatitis is less common. Allergic gastroenteropathy is still rarer and may be transient. Two or more of these clinical diseases can coexist in the same patient at the same time or at different times during the course of the illness. Atopy can also be asymptomatic (Fig 27–1).

Nonallergic rhinitis, asthma, and eczematous dermatitis occur in a significant number of patients without atopy, meaning in the absence of IgE-mediated allergy. There is a statistical association of elevated total serum IgE and blood and tissue eosinophilia with atopy, but these features are not always present in atopy, and they frequently occur in a variety of nonatopic conditions.

IgE antibodies also cause **nonatopic allergic diseases**—anaphylaxis and urticaria-angioedema (see Chapter 28)—and they are important in acquired immunity to parasites. A low level of IgE production to unknown antigens is present in the normal population.

Thus, the definition of atopy is restricted to a condition with certain specific immunologic and clinical features. Nevertheless, it is a condition that affects a significant portion of the general population, usually estimated at 10–30% in developed countries. The etiology of atopy involves complex genetic factors that are not yet well understood. Clinical disease requires both genetic predisposition and environmental allergen exposure.

Immunology

A detailed description of the immunopathogenesis of IgE-mediated diseases is given in Chapter 12. Both mast cells and basophils have high-affinity IgE cell membrane receptors for IgE (**FcεRI**). Mast cells are abundant in the mucosa of the respiratory and gastrointestinal tracts and in the skin, where atopic reactions localize. The physiologic effects of the mediators released or activated immunologically by these cells are responsible for the functional and pathologic features of the immediate and late phases of atopic diseases. The important mediators of IgE allergy are histamine, chemotactic factors, prostaglandins, leukotrienes, and platelet-activating factor.

In allergic rhinoconjunctivitis the reaction occurs entirely at the local tissue level. Contact with allergenic particles, such as pollen grains, fungus spores, dust, or skin scales from a pet, is followed promptly by absorption of soluble allergenic protein at the mucosal surface. There, the relevant IgE antibody on the mucosal mast cell reacts with allergen, causing prompt mediator release and clinical symptoms. It is not clear whether the bronchial reaction in asthma requires inhalation of smaller particles, such as pollen fragments, capable of reaching the lower respiratory airways, or whether allergic asthma is initiated by soluble allergen reaching the bronchial mucosa through the circulation. In atopic dermatitis, ingestion of allergenic food can flare the skin lesions, in which case exposure to the allergen must be via the circulation. The dermatitis can also be activated by direct topical exposure in instances of house dust mite allergy.

Atopic patients typically have multiple allergies; that is, they have IgE antibodies to, and symptoms from, many environmental allergens. As expected, the total serum IgE level is higher on average in the atopic population than in a comparable nonatopic population, although there is sufficient overlap that a normal serum IgE concentration does not rule out the diagnosis of atopy. In general, total IgE in serum is higher in patients with allergic asthma than in those with allergic rhinitis and higher still in those with atopic dermatitis. Some nonatopic diseases are associated with a high serum total IgE (Table 27–1). Although measurement

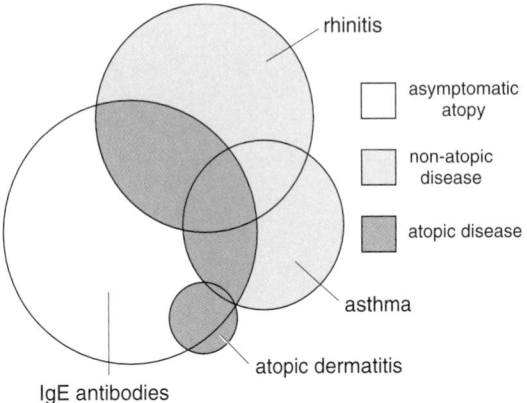

rhinitis

☐ asymptomatic atopy

▨ non-atopic disease

▨ atopic disease

asthma

atopic dermatitis

IgE antibodies

Figure 27–1. Interrelationships of atopy, atopic diseases, and IgE antibodies to environmental allergens.

of total serum IgE is not a dependable diagnostic indicator of atopy and does not identify specific IgE antibodies, several studies show that the amount of IgE in cord serum is a predictor of subsequent atopy.

Since mast cell-bound and not circulating IgE antibodies are functionally important in initiating atopic reactions on exposure to allergen, measurement of the total quantity of IgE fixed to high-affinity mast cell and basophil receptors (FcεRI) might be more relevant to atopy. There is no technique for making such a measurement currently, but estimates of skin mast cell-bound IgE by threshold-dilution skin testing with heterologous anti-IgE show that the tissue

Table 27–1. Diseases associated with elevated total serum IgE.

Disease	Possible Explanation of Elevated IgE
Allergic rhinitis.	Multiple atopic allergies.
Allergic asthma.	Multiple atopic allergies.
Atopic dermatitis.	Multiple allergies and linkage to a non-MHC gene.
Allergic bronchopulmonary aspergillosis.	Unknown; varies with disease activity.
Parasitic diseases.	IgE antibodies associated with protective immunity.
Hyper-IgE syndrome.	Unknown.
Ataxia-telangiectasia.	T-suppressor cell defect?
Wiskott-Aldrich syndrome.	Unknown.
Thymic alymphoplasia.	Unknown.
IgE myeloma.	Neoplasm of IgE-producing plasma cells; IgE is monoclonal.
Graft-versus-host reaction.	Transient T suppressor cell defect?

IgE level is much higher in atopic individuals than in the normal population.

It has been suggested that antibodies of the IgG4 subclass may also fix to mast cells and basophils. The mast cell affinity for IgG4 appears to be low, and evidence that IgG4 antibodies can trigger mediator release in the presence of allergens is controversial. There is no indication that human atopic disease pathogenesis involves IgG4 antibodies.

Etiology

The etiology of atopy is unknown. Epidemiologic, family, and twin studies, as well as animal experiments, provide substantial evidence that genetic factors are involved in the propensity for atopy, in the regulation of total IgE production, and in the production of IgE antibodies to specific epitopes. A genetic basis for the various disease manifestations is not established, however. Several family studies have shown associations of human leukocyte antigen (HLA) types with enhanced production of antibody of IgE (and other) isotypes to a particular allergen. Genetic control of the total level of serum IgE is independent of genes in the major histocompatibility complex (MHC).

One theory based on the study of in vitro IgE antibody production by blood lymphocytes suggests that atopic allergy may arise through abnormal regulation by T lymphocytes of the differentiation of B cells committed to IgE production into IgE antibody-secreting plasma cells. These regulatory T cells exert their effect through the secretion of protein IgE-binding factors that either enhance or suppress the differentiation of B cells.

A second theory suggests that the defect in atopy resides at the level of absorption of environmental allergens at respiratory and gastrointestinal surfaces prior to processing of the allergen for the immune response. The theory proposes that there is a normal protective mucosal barrier to exogenous antigens that is defective in atopy. Some support for this theory comes from the observation that levels of IgG antibodies to inhalant and food allergens are higher in atopic than nonatopic individuals, although these IgG antibodies are not believed to cause disease.

A third theory of atopy proposes a single defect for both the enhanced production of allergen-specific IgE antibodies and the hyperreactivity of target tissues to the mediators released from mast cells by IgE antibody. Immune cells and bronchial smooth muscle cells are both under autonomic control. Thus, an inherited (or perhaps acquired) **autonomic imbalance** such as beta-adrenergic blockade or cholinergic overactivity could account for both enhanced IgE antibody production and target organ hyperreactivity. There is no direct evidence for defective autonomic control of IgE antibody production in atopy, although there is some indirect evidence for functional beta-adrenergic blockade in the asthmatic airway and in atopic eczematous skin.

Substantial evidence points to the critical role of **cytokines** in the ability of CD4 T lymphocytes to induce IgE antibody production by B cells. Interleukin-4 (IL-4) enhances but gamma interferon (IFNγ) suppresses IgE responses. The currently popular paradigm recognizes two T_H cell subsets—T_H1 and T_H2—and that a reciprocal balance between the numbers of these cells locally in tissues influences the propensity for atopy and other diseases through the profile of cytokines that they synthesize and release. Extensive experimental evidence suggests that IgE production and atopic disease require the presence of IL-4, IL-5, IL-13, and granulocyte–macrophage colony-stimulating factor (GM-CSF) production by T_H2 cells. Thus, a fourth theory would involve up- or downregulation of these and other cytokines by as yet unidentified etiologic factors in atopy.

Environmental factors play a role in etiology. An accumulation of clinical experience suggests that the initial age of exposure to a particular food or pollen may determine the intensity of the subsequent IgE antibody response. A concurrent viral respiratory infection during environmental allergen exposure may have an adjuvant effect on both specific and total IgE production. Tobacco smoking may exert a similar effect. If the total level of serum IgE at the time of birth predicts future development of atopy, however, acquired factors would probably have only a secondary or permissive role.

Finally, the relationship between IgE-mediated atopic allergy and IgE-mediated immunity in **helminthiasis** offers an interesting opportunity to speculate about etiology. Atopic allergy is a prominent clinical problem in developed countries, which are largely free of helminthic infestation. In populations in which these infections are endemic, serum IgE levels are typically high because of ongoing IgE stimulation, and it can be assumed that tissue mast cells are chronically saturated with parasite-specific IgE antibodies. The IgE mast cell-mediated immune mechanism has a selective advantage for the host under these circumstances. In a population free of parasitic infections, however, the IgE immune system may be vestigial for immunity but still available to react adversely to innocuous environmental allergens.

ATOPIC ALLERGENS

The allergens responsible for atopic disease are derived principally from natural airborne organic particles, especially plant pollens, fungal spores, and animal and insect debris, and to a lesser extent from ingested foods. The ability of different pollens, molds, or foods to sensitize for IgE allergy varies, so that some of these environmental allergens are intrinsically more sensitizing than others, irrespective of the amount of exposure.

Table 27–2. Botanic classifications of pollinating plants frequently associated with atopic respiratory allergy.

Botanic Classification[1]	Common Names of Typical Plants
Division Microphyllophyta	Club mosses
Division Pteridophyta	Ferns
Division Pinophyta	
Subdivision Pinicae	Conifers
Division Magnoliophyta	Flowering plants
Class Liliopsida	
Subclass Commelinidae	Grasses, sedges
Subclass Arecidae	Palms, cattails
Class Magnoliopsida	
Subclass Hamamelididae	Nettles, beeches
Subclass Caryophyllidae	Chemopods, sorrels
Subclass Dilleniidae	Willows, poplars
Subclass Rosidae	Maples, ashes
Subclass Asteridae	Ragweeds, sages

Source: Adapted and reproduced, with permission, from Weber RW, Nelson HS: Pollen allergens and their interrelationships. *Clin Rev Allergy* 1985;**3**:291.
[1] Classification system of Takhtajan.

Pollen Allergens

The allergenic pollens are from wind-pollinated (anemophilous) flowering plants. There are far fewer of these plants than insect-pollinated (entomophilous) plants, but they discharge large numbers of lightweight, buoyant pollens that are dispersed over a wide area by wind currents. Within each local geographic area the common allergenic trees, grasses, and weeds pollinate during specific and predictable seasons, producing the corresponding seasonal respiratory symptoms in allergic patients.

The number of pollen-producing plants potentially capable of causing allergy is enormous, but those of proven allergenicity are limited. The major taxa and representative examples are listed in Table 27–2. Within each botanic subclass many species cause allergy. Natural, cultivated, and ornamental plants all may produce allergenic pollen. Plants with attractive flowers are generally insect-pollinated, producing small amounts of heavy pollen that does not become airborne, and thus they are usually not the cause of inhalant allergy.

Allergenic pollen grains are mostly spherical, 15–50 μm in diameter, and they can usually be identified morphologically by light microscopy (Fig 27–2). Air sampling for identifying and quantitating pollens is done by volumetric impaction devices such as the rotorod or rotoslide sampler (Fig 27–3). Several representative examples of pollen seasons are shown in Figure 27–4.

Mold Allergens

Fungi are multicellular eukaryotic organisms that are abundant and ubiquitous. They are saprophytic, growing on a variety of dead or decaying organic material, where they flourish in direct relation to temperature and humidity. They reproduce sexually or asexually, producing airborne spores, some of which are allergenic.

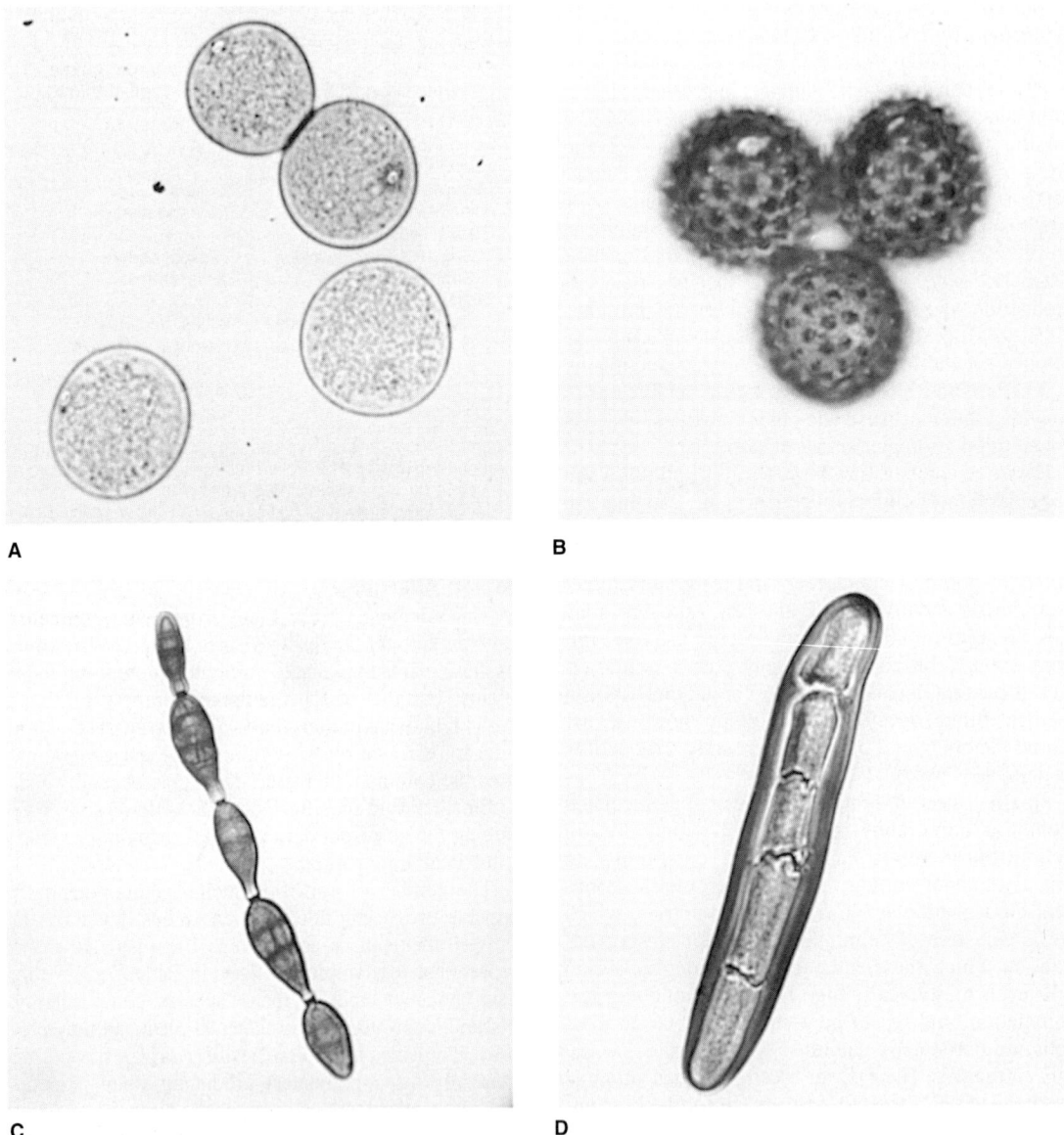

Figure 27–2. Photomicrographs of several common pollens. **A:** grass (30 µm in diameter); **B:** ragweed (20 µm in diameter); **C:** *Alternaria* mold spores (70 µm in length); **D:** *Helminthosporium* mold spores (80 µm in length). (Courtesy of William R Solomon, MD.)

Allergy to fungal spores is an important cause of disease in many atopic patients. Specific diagnosis, however, is hampered by the confusing taxonomic classification and nomenclature because of the enormous biologic complexity of fungi in their morphologic, reproductive, and ecologic behavior. It is difficult to obtain pure spores of many species for immunologic testing. Seasonal patterns of spores in air samples are poorly defined, making clinical correlation especially problematic. Mold spores range in size from 1 to 100 µm in diameter (see Fig 27–2). Volumetric impaction samplers that are used for

pollen counting are inefficient in trapping spores, so sampling by these devices does not yield quantitative data for spores. Table 27–3 lists some of the fungi most frequently associated with atopic allergy.

Arthropod Allergens

There are more than 50,000 species of mites. The house dust mites, *Dermatophagoides pteronyssinus* and *D farinae,* are the most common of all of the known atopic allergens. These tiny arachnids, barely visible to the naked eye, are found in house dust samples throughout the world but are most prevalent in

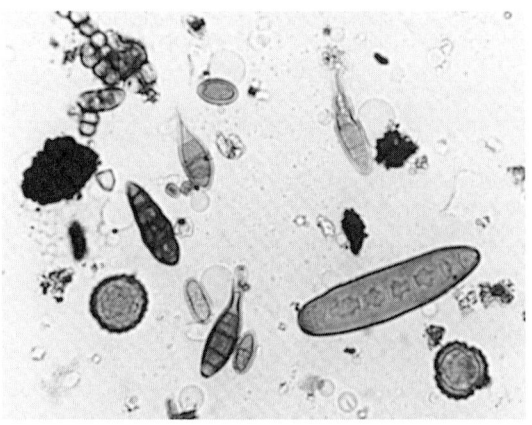

Figure 27–3. Typical "catch" of a volumetric air sampler showing pollen grains, mold spores, insect debris, plant particles, dust, and unidentified particles. (Courtesy of William R Solomon, MD.)

warm, humid climates. They are especially abundant in bedding, upholstery, and blankets, where their natural substrate, desquamated human skin scales, are likely to be found. The two species cross-react extensively but not completely. House dust contains other uncharacterized allergens, but they are of minor importance compared with *Dermatophagoides* spp. IgE antibodies and environmental exposure to these mite allergens correlate especially well with atopic asthma and atopic dermatitis, because exposure is by inhalation and dermal contact, respectively.

Other allergenic mites such as *Euroglyphus maynei, Lepidoglyphus destructor,* and *Acarus siro*—storage mites that infest grains—may cause occupational allergy in grain handlers.

Various species of cockroaches are insect pests in homes and restaurants, especially in large cities where there is overcrowding and poor hygiene. Several studies have now documented high rates of sensitivity to cockroach allergen among allergic patients in inner-city populations; this often occurs as an isolated allergy. Other "endemic" causes of respiratory allergy are the emanations and debris of certain insects that swarm in huge numbers seasonally in specific locales.

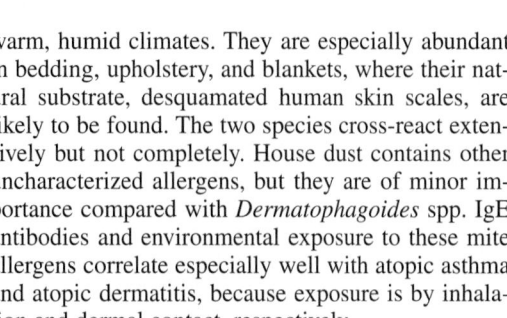

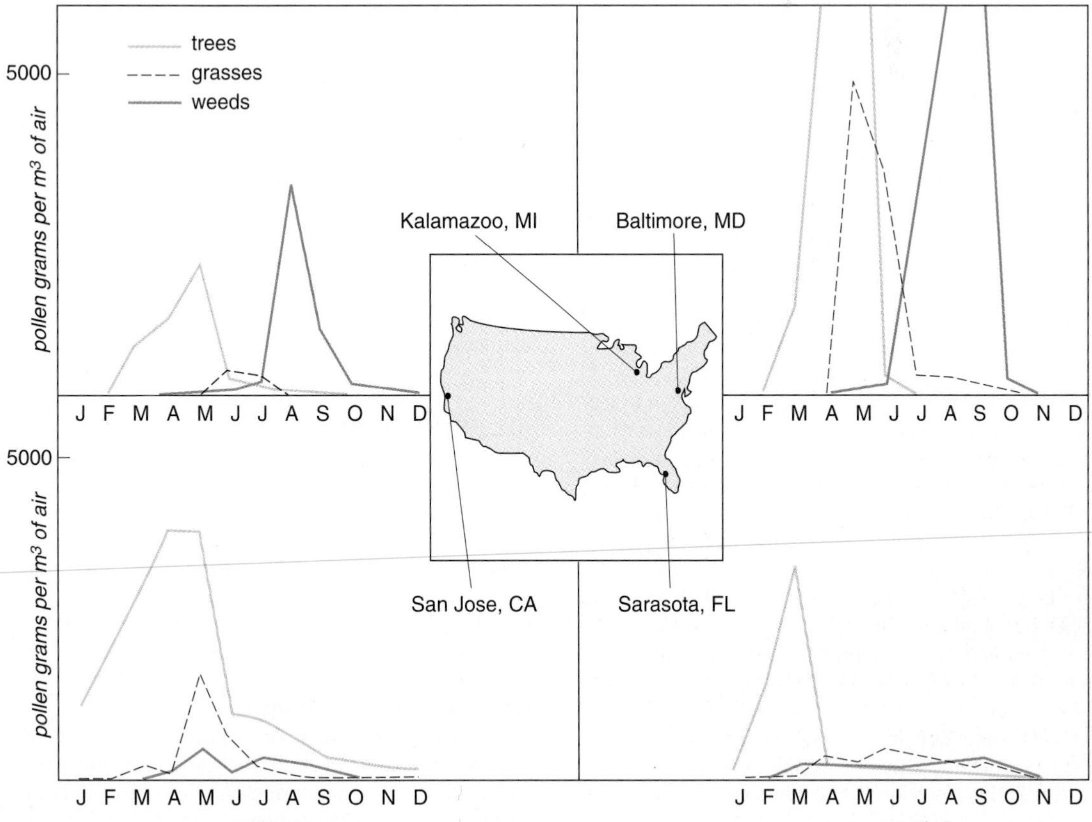

Figure 27–4. Representative examples of quantitative pollen counts at four different locations in the US during the same year (1984). Data from the American Academy of Allergy and Immunology Pollen and Mold Committee.

Table 27–3. Common fungal aeroallergens.

Basidiomycetes	*Botrytis*
Ustilago	*Helminthosporium*
Ganoderma	*Stemphylium*
Alternaria	*Cephalosporium*
Cladosporium	**Phycomycetes**
Aspergillus	*Mucor*
Sporobolomyces	*Rhizopus*
Penicillium	**Ascomycetes**
Epicoccum	*Eurotium*
Fusarium	*Chaetomium*
Phoma	

Table 27–4. Approximate equivalence of different methods for expressing allergen content in extracts used for testing and immunotherapy.

Method	Units
Weight/volume (W/V)	1:20
Protein nitrogen units/mL (PNU/mL)	10,000
Allergy units/mL (AU/mL)	100,000
Noon units/mL	100
Micrograms of protein/mL	100

Examples of such insects include caddis fly and mayfly at the eastern and western ends, respectively, of Lake Erie; the green nimitti midge, *Cladotanytarsus lewisi,* in the Sudan; and Lepidoptera in Japan.

Animal Allergens

Atopic allergy to household pets, especially cats and dogs, has always been easily recognized because patients sensitive to these animals experience immediate intense attacks of asthma when in the same house with an animal to which they are allergic. Other animals encountered in domestic, occupational, and recreational settings also cause allergy. The source of the allergen may be in the dander (horse, dog), saliva (cat), or urine (rodents).

Food Allergens

Allergenic components of foods can induce IgE antibodies that may be responsible for either atopic or nonatopic (anaphylactic) reactions. IgE antibodies to foods frequently exist in atopic patients without causing any reaction when the food is eaten. The factors that operate to convert asymptomatic sensitivity to symptomatic disease are currently unknown. IgG antibodies to many food antigens occur in most people, but they have no known pathogenic significance.

Virtually any food is capable of causing allergy on ingestion, and many have been shown to do so in isolated cases, but certain foods are more likely to be allergenic than others. Seafoods are a particularly prominent cause of allergy in areas where fish is a staple in the diet. Ingested crustaceans and mollusks are an important cause of anaphylaxis and anaphylactoid reactions. Legume, cow's milk, and egg white allergies are also common. Wheat, corn, chocolate, and citrus fruits, on the other hand, are often implicated in causing a variety of symptoms that are not characteristic of allergy in patients lacking IgE antibodies to these foods.

The allergenicity of a particular food protein can be changed by heating or cooking. A reaction can occur to the raw food only or to the cooked form only, or to both.

Occupational allergy, especially asthma from the inhalation of airborne food allergens, is a significant problem for many food handlers.

Allergen Extracts

Pollens, molds, foods, and animal and insect emanations are biologically complex materials made up of a mixture of numerous chemicals, many of which have allergenic potential. Aqueous extracts used in testing for IgE antibodies in allergic patients may contain a number of different allergens in addition to nonallergenic soluble compounds. There is an ongoing effort to isolate, purify, analyze, characterize, name, and standardize every important atopic allergen. To date almost 100 allergen proteins causing human IgE-mediated disease have been isolated and purified, and many have been cloned. Availability of these purified materials will help to resolve clinical problems such as cross-reactivity among plants or foods. Purified allergens are essential reagents for research studies on structure–function relationships and for genetic studies.

Crude aqueous extracts are useful for clinical testing and immunotherapy. For many years, standardization of extracts has been based on weight/volume or total protein content, neither of which reflects the allergen content accurately. Recently, standardization of allergen content either by skin test titration or by radioallergosorbent test (RAST) inhibition has been introduced, and the term "allergen unit" (AU) is now used to denote bioequivalence. A comparison of these methods is shown in Table 27–4.

ALLERGIC RHINITIS

Major Immunologic Features

- Allergic rhinitis is the most common clinical expression of atopic hypersensitivity.
- IgE-mediated allergy is localized in the nasal mucosa and conjunctiva.
- Pollens, fungal spores, dust, and animal danders are the usual atmospheric allergens.

General Considerations

Allergic rhinitis (also known as allergic rhinoconjunctivitis or hay fever) is the most common manifestation of an atopic reaction to inhaled allergens. More than 20 million persons in the US suffer from this disease. It is a chronic disease, which may first appear at any age, but the onset is usually during childhood or adolescence.

Epidemiology

Allergic rhinitis occurs in 10–12% of the US population. The prevalence and morbidity rate are influenced by the geographic distribution of the common allergic plants and dust mite. The disease affects both sexes equally. It persists for many years if untreated. It is never fatal, but it does cause considerable morbidity and time lost from school or work.

Clinical Features

A. Symptoms: A typical attack consists of profuse watery rhinorrhea, paroxysmal sneezing, nasal obstruction, and itching of the nose and palate. Postnasal mucus drainage causes sore throat, clearing of the throat, and cough. There is usually an accompanying allergic blepharoconjunctivitis, with intense itching of the conjunctivae and eyelids, redness, tearing, and photophobia. In some patients, conjunctivitis may occur in the absence of nasal symptoms. The disease occurs seasonally in patients with pollen allergy. It may be present year-round if the sensitivity is to a perennial allergen such as house dust, or there may be perennial symptoms with seasonal exacerbations in patients with multiple allergies. Diurnal variation may suggest a household allergen, and symptoms that disappear on weekends suggest an occupational allergy. Severe attacks are often accompanied by systemic malaise, weakness, fatigue, and, sometimes, muscle soreness after intense periods of sneezing. Fever is absent. Swelling of the nasal mucosa may lead to headache because of obstruction of the ostia of the paranasal sinuses.

B. Signs: Rhinoscopy shows a pale, swollen nasal mucosa with watery secretions. The conjunctivae are hyperemic and edematous. There may be eyelid swelling from edema. Lower eyelid ecchymoses—probably from eye-rubbing—are called "allergic shiners." These changes revert to normal when there is no allergen exposure and the patient is asymptomatic.

C. Laboratory Findings: Eosinophils are numerous in the nasal secretions, but this is not diagnostic, since nasal eosinophilia is found in some patients with nonallergic rhinitis and in those with asthma. Blood eosinophilia is present during symptomatic periods. The presence of any eosinophils in conjunctival scrapings, however, is probably diagnostic. Sinus imaging, tympanometry, and audiometry may be indicated if an associated sinusitis or otitis media is suspected.

Immunologic Diagnosis

The diagnosis of allergic rhinitis is established by the history and physical findings present during the symptomatic phase. Diagnosis of the specific allergic sensitivities in each case is then determined by skin testing for a wheal-and-flare response or by in vitro testing. Selection of allergens for detection of specific IgE antibodies by skin or in vitro test is based on the patient's history and on the known local environmental allergens.

Differential Diagnosis

Chronic nonallergic (vasomotor) rhinitis is a common disorder of unknown cause in which the primary complaint is nasal congestion, usually associated with postnasal drainage. It differs from allergic rhinitis by the absence of sneezing paroxysms or eye symptoms, and rhinorrhea is minimal. Congestion may be unilateral or bilateral, and it often shifts with position. Symptoms occur year-round and are generally worse in cold weather or in dry climates. The nasal mucosa is unusually sensitive to irritants such as tobacco smoke, fumes, and smog. Symptoms usually begin in adult life. The disease is more common among women, and it may begin during pregnancy. Examination shows swollen, erythematous nasal mucosa and strands of thick, mucoid postnasal discharge in the pharynx. Allergy skin tests are negative or unrelated to the symptoms. In nonallergic vasomotor rhinitis, the nasal secretions may or may not contain eosinophils, so nasal eosinophilia is not a reliable sign of allergy but may indicate a preasthmatic state. There is a good therapeutic response to decongestants and humidification, but antihistamines are usually not effective.

Rhinitis medicamentosa denotes the severe congestion that occurs from the rebound effect of excessive use of sympathomimetic nasal sprays or nose drops. In this disease, the mucosa is often bright red and swollen, but these changes are reversible with complete avoidance of nose drops or sprays, even if they have been used excessively for many years.

Infectious rhinitis is almost always due to a virus, and most patients with allergic rhinitis can distinguish their allergic symptoms from those of the common cold, which usually produces fever, an erythematous nasal mucosa, and an exudate in the nasal secretions that is polymorphonuclear rather than eosinophilic. Primary bacterial or fungal infections of the nasal passages are rare.

Some hormones may produce nasal congestion. This is common in pregnancy or with the use of oral contraceptive drugs. Nasal congestion occurs frequently in myxedema. Certain drugs produce nasal congestion (Table 27–5).

Anatomic obstructions may occur from foreign bodies in the nose, tumors, nasal septal deviation or spurs, and nasal polyps. Nasal polyposis is a constitutional condition independent of atopy and allergic rhinitis, but it is associated with asthma, aspirin sensitivity, sinusitis, and eosinophilia. Nasal polyps also occur in children with cystic fibrosis. Anatomic lesions are best detected by fiberoptic rhinoscopy after the application of a topical decongestant.

Vernal keratoconjunctivitis is a disease of unknown cause that usually affects children, producing giant papillary excrescences of the palpebral conjunctivae with symptoms of intense itching and a stringy exudate.

Table 27–5. Drugs that may cause nasal congestion.

Drug	Presumed Mechanism
Oral contraceptives	Unknown
Reserpine	Norepinephrine depletion
Guanethidine	Norepinephrine release blockade
Propranolol	Adrenergic blockade
Thioridazine	Beta-adrenergic blockade
Tricyclic antidepressants	Norepinephrine uptake blockade
Aspirin (rarely)	Idiosyncratic generation of vasodilating arachidonate metabolite?

The exudate contains eosinophils, mast cells, basophils, and plasma cells, suggesting an immunologic basis, but search for an allergic cause is usually unrewarding. Reversible giant papillary conjunctivitis is caused in some patients by the use of soft contact lenses.

Immunologic Pathogenesis

Soluble allergens from inhaled pollens, spores, and other aeroallergenic particles are rapidly eluted on contact with the moist mucous membranes of the nasal mucosa and conjunctivae. Contact with the corresponding IgE antibody on local mast cells and basophils releases the various mast cell-associated mediators described in Chapter 12. Symptoms of sneezing, rhinorrhea, congestion, and pruritus appearing within minutes are caused by the effects of endogenously liberated histamine, leukotrienes, and prostaglandin D_2 in the early-phase allergic response. Chemotactic factors produce an inflammatory exudate that produces the more persistent congestion and nonspecific tissue hyperirritability of the late-phase response. The hyperirritability lowers the nasal threshold to both allergic and irritant stimuli, such as temperature changes, irritant particles and gases, sunlight, and ingested alcohol, thereby accentuating the effect of other allergens and prolonging symptoms after cessation of the allergen exposure.

A significant number of patients with allergic rhinitis have a coexisting bronchial hyperreactivity in the absence of clinical signs of asthma. It is not known whether this is an intrinsic abnormality related to atopy or an acquired defect from allergen exposure, possibly a component of the late allergic response. The absence of symptomatic asthma may be explained by effective compensating homeostatic mechanisms that are defective or inoperative in asthmatic patients.

Treatment

Treatment consists of environmental measures to avoid allergen exposure, drugs, and desensitization. For any atopic disease, prophylactic treatment by avoidance of allergens is usually the most effective means of treatment. Avoidance is not always possible or practical, however, and so medications are needed to control symptoms. In some cases, the immune response itself can be altered by desensitization therapy.

A. Environmental Measures: Avoidance of an allergen is recommended on the basis of a clinical history of symptomatic allergy and not because of a positive skin test alone. Appropriate measures in individual cases may be the removal of household pets, control of house dust exposure by frequent cleaning, and avoidance of dust-collecting toys or other objects in the patient's bedroom. Air-cleaning devices with high-efficiency particle filters may be helpful. Dehumidification and repair of leaking pipes or roofs may be necessary to prevent mold growth. Avoidance of pollen and outdoor molds is not possible unless the patient is able to stay in an air-conditioned home or office. In some cases, the patient might arrange a vacation trip to a pollen-free area during the peak pollen season.

In cases of occupational allergy, every effort should be made to modify the patient's work routine and to employ industrial hygiene measures to avoid allergen exposure; however, if these measures fail, a change in the patient's job may be necessary.

B. Drug Treatment: Antihistamines are the most commonly used drugs in allergic rhinitis, although their use is restricted by side effects. New nonsedating antihistamines avoid the most troublesome side effects. Orally administered nasal decongestants may be helpful, either alone or in combination with antihistamines. Sympathomimetic and antihistaminic eye drops are useful for allergic conjunctivitis. Administration of cromolyn by nasal sprays or conjunctival drops four times daily is beneficial and is virtually free of any immediate or long-term toxicity.

Systemic corticosteroids can be extremely effective in relieving symptoms of allergic rhinitis, but since the disease is a chronic, recurrent, benign condition, these drugs should be used with extreme care. The patient with very severe symptoms lasting for only a few days or several weeks each year who does not respond to antihistamines can be given oral prednisone for 1 or 2 weeks in a dosage just high enough to suppress symptoms. Flunisolide or beclomethasone by nasal spray may be equally effective without causing significant systemic corticosteroid effects. Side effects of nasal burning and epistaxis from nasal corticosteroid sprays are more annoying than dangerous, but the potential for mucosal atrophy and septal perforation with prolonged use requires periodic monitoring. Corticosteroid eye drops should be used very sparingly for brief periods only to control acute severe allergic conjunctivitis, with careful monitoring by an ophthalmologist.

C. Desensitization: Allergen injection therapy has been shown in many prospective double-blind controlled trials to be effective in treating allergic rhinitis. Because of the length of treatment required and the potential danger of serious systemic reactions, injection treatment is used in patients whose symptoms are uncontrolled despite appropriate environmental measures and symptomatic medications. The procedure, which is discussed more fully in Chapter 56, must be individualized and coordinated with environmental and drug treatment to be most effective; therefore, it should be initiated and monitored by a trained allergist.

Complications

Sinusitis may complicate allergic rhinitis. The diagnosis of sinusitis is difficult because of frequent discrepancies between paranasal sinus symptoms and radiographic evidence of pathology. Mild sinus membrane thickening (less than 6 mm) is frequent in allergic rhinitis and could represent noninfectious allergic inflammation. Significant thickening, opacification, and air–fluid levels usually indicate an infectious sinusitis. Obstruction of the sinus ostia by swollen nasal membranes, whether caused by allergy, a common cold, or nonallergic vasomotor rhinitis, can cause secondary sinus infection, or the sinus mucosa per se may be a target organ in atopy.

Otitis media with or without effusion is common in children, and its causes are multifactorial, usually involving eustachian tube dysfunction and anatomic factors. The disease does not appear more frequently in atopic than in nonatopic children or adults. It is unlikely that inhaled allergen reaches the middle ear or eustachian tube, although tubal obstruction by swollen nasopharyngeal allergic mucosa or dysfunction caused by the allergic mediators could prolong or exacerbate the disease.

Nasal polyps are likewise observed with similar frequency in atopic and normal individuals. Although polyposis is not a complication of allergic rhinitis, management can be hampered by untreated nasal allergy, and vice versa.

Prognosis

Although no definitive studies have been done on the course of untreated allergic rhinitis, symptoms can be expected to recur or persist for many years if not for life. The severity of the symptoms depends on the degree of exposure to the allergen. A patient with a pollen allergy who moves to an area where that pollen-producing plant does not grow will no longer be symptomatic.

ASTHMA

Major Immunologic Features

- Allergic asthma is a manifestation of IgE-mediated allergy localized in the bronchus.
- Important immunologically released or activated mediators are histamine, leukotrienes, and eosinophil chemotactic factor.
- Hyperirritability of bronchial mucosa amplifies the bronchoconstricting effects of mediators.

Definition

Asthma (also known as reversible obstructive airway disease) is characterized by hyperresponsiveness of the tracheobronchial tree to respiratory irritants and bronchoconstrictor chemicals, producing attacks of wheezing, dyspnea, chest tightness, and cough that are reversible spontaneously or with treatment. The disease is chronic and involves the entire airway, but it varies in severity from occasional mild transient episodes to severe, chronic, life-threatening bronchial obstruction. There is an associated eosinophilia in the blood and in respiratory secretions. Episodes of asthma are triggered immunologically by allergen inhalation in patients with atopic allergy.

General Considerations

It is important to understand the role of atopic allergy in asthma. Asthma and atopy may coexist, but only about half of the asthmatic population has atopy and a smaller percentage of atopic patients have asthma. All asthmatic patients—regardless of the presence or absence of atopy—have the cardinal features that define asthma: airway hyperreactivity, reversible airway obstruction, and eosinophilia. In those with allergic asthma, attacks are triggered by allergen exposure as well as by other nonallergic factors.

Asthma and atopy are not wholly independent, however, because asthma occurs more frequently among atopic than among nonatopic individuals, especially during childhood. It is not known whether predisposition to the two conditions is genetically linked or whether atopy enhances the clinical expression of an undefined asthmatic predisposition. A recent large-scale epidemiologic study showed that, contrary to abundant previous evidence, there is a positive statistical correlation of asthma and IgE antibodies in all age groups. Nonetheless, by tradition and clinical usefulness, asthma is often classified into extrinsic and intrinsic subgroups.

A. Extrinsic Asthma: This is also known as allergic, atopic, or immunologic asthma. As a group, patients with extrinsic asthma generally develop the disease early in life, usually in infancy or childhood. Other manifestations of atopy—eczema or allergic rhinitis—often coexist. A family history of atopic disease is common. Attacks of asthma occur during pollen seasons, in the presence of animals, or on exposure to house dust, feather pillows, or other allergens, depending on the patient's particular allergic sensitivities. Skin tests show positive wheal-and-flare reactions to the causative allergens. Total serum IgE concentration is frequently elevated but is sometimes normal.

B. Intrinsic Asthma: This is also known as nonallergic or idiopathic asthma. It characteristically appears first during adult life, usually after an apparent respiratory infection, so that the term "adult-onset asthma" is sometimes applied. This term is misleading, because some nonallergic asthmatics first develop the disease during childhood and some allergic asthmatics become symptomatic for the first time as adults when they are exposed to the relevant allergen. Intrinsic asthma pursues a course of chronic or recurrent bronchial obstruction unrelated to pollen seasons or exposure to other allergens. Skin tests are negative to the usual atopic allergens. The serum IgE concentration is normal. Blood and sputum eosinophilia is present. Personal and family histories are usually negative for other atopic diseases. Other schemes for classifying asthma into subgroups, like aspirin-sensitive, exercise-induced, infectious, and psychologic, merely define external triggering factors that affect certain patients more so than others.

Epidemiology

Asthma is a worldwide disease that has been recognized for centuries, but prevalence figures vary, in part because of differences in definition and methods of case finding. It is a common disease, which affects approximately 5% of the population of Western countries. There is no reason to suspect that the rate in Asia and Africa is substantially different. Onset during childhood is predominantly before the age of 5 years, and it affects boys more than girls (by about 3:2). The childhood-onset form is usually of the allergic variety. Adult onset may be at any age, but typically it occurs in the fifth decade. Ordinarily it is of the intrinsic type, and it affects women more than men (by about 3:2).

Some recent studies suggest that the prevalence is increasing, but this may reflect better diagnosis and not a true change in incidence. Death caused by asthma—about 2000–3000 cases per year in the US—is relatively infrequent, but there are reports recently from several countries, including the US, of increasing asthma mortality rates and some evidence of increasing morbidity rates, despite substantial advances in symptomatic therapy.

Although not a major cause of mortality, asthma remains a leading cause for time lost from work and school.

Clinical Features

A. Symptoms: Asthma may begin at any age. It is characterized by attacks of wheezing and dyspnea that can range in severity from mild discomfort to life-threatening respiratory failure. Some patients are symptom-free between attacks, whereas others are never entirely free of airway obstruction. The asthmatic attack causes shortness of breath, wheezing, and tightness in the chest, with difficulty in moving air during inspiration but more so during expiration. Coughing is usually present, and with prolonged asthma the cough may produce thick, tenacious sputum that can be either clear or yellow. In children, coughing, especially at night, may be the only symptom to suggest the diagnosis. Fever is absent, but fatigue, malaise, irritability, palpitations, and sweating are occasional systemic complaints.

B. Signs: Physical examination during the attack shows tachypnea, audible wheezing, and use of the accessory muscles of respiration. The pulse is usually rapid, and blood pressure may be elevated. Pulsus paradoxus indicates severe asthma. The lung fields are hyperresonant, and auscultation reveals diminished breath sounds, wheezes, and rhonchi but no rales. The expiratory phase is prolonged. In a severe attack with high-grade obstruction, breath sounds and wheezing may both be absent. These are ominous signs, especially if accompanied by pallor and peripheral cyanosis, excitement or anxiety, and inability to speak. Chronic severe asthma in young children may lead to a structural barrel chest deformity.

C. Laboratory Findings: An increased total eosinophil count in the peripheral blood is almost invariably present unless suppressed by corticosteroids or sympathomimetic drugs. There is eosinophilia in nasal secretions. Sputum examination reveals eosinophils, Charcot-Leyden crystals, and Curschmann's spirals.

The chest x-ray may be normal during the attack or may show signs of hyperinflation, and there may be transient scattered parenchymal densities indicating focal atelectasis caused by mucus plugs in scattered portions of the airway. Total serum IgE is usually elevated in childhood allergic asthma and normal in adult intrinsic asthma, but this test lacks specificity in individual cases as a diagnostic screen for either asthma or atopy (Fig 27–5).

Pulmonary function tests show the abnormalities of airway obstructive disease. Flow rates and 1-second forced expiratory volume (FEV_1) are decreased, vital capacity is normal or decreased, and total lung capacity and functional residual capacity are usually normal or slightly increased but may be decreased with extreme bronchospasm. Following administration of

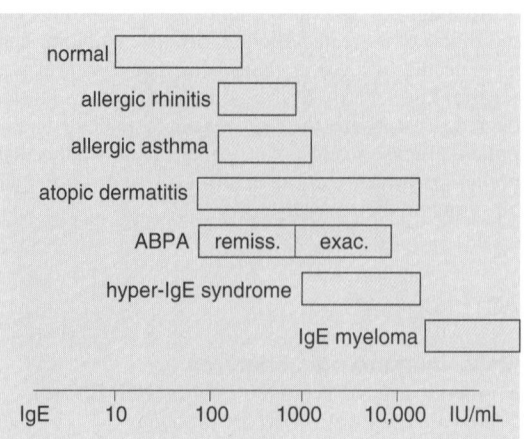

Figure 27–5. Total serum IgE levels in normal individuals and patients with various allergies and IgE disorders. *Abbreviations:* ABPA = allergic bronchopulmonary aspergillosis; remiss. = remission; exac. = exacerbation.

an aerosolized sympathomimetic bronchodilator, ventilation improves with significant increase in flow rates and FEV_1, indicating the reversible nature of the bronchial obstruction. The lack of response in a patient already receiving large doses of sympathomimetic drugs does not rule out reversibility, and the test should be repeated at a later date after improvement from such additional treatment as hydration, corticosteroids, and chest physical therapy.

Repeated tests of ventilatory function are helpful in the long-term management of asthma. Serial determinations of FEV_1, maximal expiratory flow rate, or peak flow rate are easily done in the office or clinic, and they often detect airway obstruction that may not be apparent to the patient or to the physician on auscultation of the chest.

Inexpensive peak flow rate measurement devices are valuable for daily monitoring at home and work. Information can be used to uncover possible allergens and irritants in the patient's environment and as early warning of a worsening condition requiring more intensive treatment.

Bronchial provocation testing has made a significant contribution to pathophysiologic and pharmacologic research in recent years. These procedures are not necessary for routine diagnosis but are helpful in special circumstances (see Chapter 26). Nonspecific bronchial hyperirritability can be demonstrated by using quantitative challenges with methacholine, histamine, cold air, or exercise. These tests of bronchial hypersensitivity are almost always positive in asthma, but they are not by themselves diagnostic of the disease, since bronchial hyperirritability occurs in a significant number of patients with allergic rhinitis, in normal subjects following viral respiratory infections, and in a small percentage of normal individuals. Since the procedure provokes an asthma attack, it should not be used in the presence of significant bronchial obstruction or if asthma can be diagnosed by other criteria.

Bronchial provocation by inhaling allergens to diagnose specific atopic sensitivities is sometimes useful in suspected occupational asthma, for which measurement of a dose-response effect under controlled conditions is desirable. This may be the case when the patient encounters several potential allergens at work. The patient should be monitored in a hospital for this procedure because of possible severe late-phase reactions.

Pathology

Autopsy on fatal asthma shows hyperinflation of the lungs, hypertrophy and hyperplasia of bronchial smooth muscle, and excessive mucus secretion. Death is usually caused by asphyxiation from mucus plugging the airways. Microscopic examination shows hypertrophy and hyperplasia of submucosal glands and bronchial smooth muscle, mucosal infiltration with an edematous and mixed cellular inflammatory response especially rich in eosinophils, and epithelial desqua-

mation within mucous plugs. Similar but less intense pathology exists during asymptomatic periods. The pathology therefore reflects both the early phase (smooth muscle contraction, edema, hypersecretion) and late phase (cellular inflammation) of the IgE-mediated allergic response. The gross and microscopic pathology of allergic asthma is indistinguishable from that of nonallergic asthma.

Immunologic Pathogenesis

The cause of asthma is not known. Pathogenesis of the asthmatic attack involves both allergic and nonallergic mechanisms. There is evidence that bronchoconstriction is mediated by an autonomic (vagal) reflex mechanism involving afferent receptors in the bronchial mucosa or submucosa that respond to irritants or chemical mediators and efferent cholinergic impulses, causing bronchial muscle contraction and hypersecretion of mucus. The mast cell-associated mediators (histamine, leukotrienes, prostaglandins, kinins, platelet-activating factor, and chemotactic factors) have properties that can explain the pathologic and functional abnormalities of the asthmatic attack. In the asthmatic patient, the afferent receptors appear to be sensitized to respond to a low threshold of stimulation. It has been proposed that the hyperirritable state of the bronchial mucosa results from defective functioning or blockade of its beta-adrenergic receptor, preventing a homeostatic bronchodilating response from endogenous catecholamines. Bronchial hyperirritability is enhanced further during the late phase of the asthmatic reaction.

The linkage between allergen–IgE antibody interaction and release, activation, and secretion of mediators from the mast cell is now firmly established. The means by which nonallergic stimuli such as irritants and viral infections stimulate mast cells is unknown at present, and it is possible that other cells and mediators are involved in nonallergic asthma.

The variety of nonspecific agents that initiate an asthma attack is extensive. Some of these factors are listed in Table 27–6. Some of these items have been shown to increase the underlying bronchial hyperirritability as well, making the patient more sensitive to the effects of other triggers.

Approximately 10% of asthmatic patients have **aspirin sensitivity.** In these patients, ingestion of aspirin is followed in 20 minutes to 3 hours by an asthmatic attack, which is caused by an idiosyncratic pharmacologic response to the drug. Other nonsteroidal anti-inflammatory drugs cause a similar reaction. These anti-inflammatory drugs inhibit cyclooxygenase, the initial enzyme in the synthesis of prostaglandins from cell membrane arachidonic acid, and the quantitative ability of these drugs to provoke asthma is directly related to their ability to inhibit cyclooxygenase, indomethacin being the most potent and acetaminophen the least. Nasal polyposis is common in aspirin-sensitive patients.

Table 27–6. Nonspecific triggers of asthma.

Infections
  Viral respiratory infections
Physiologic factors
  Exercise
  Hyperventilation
  Deep breathing
  Psychologic factors
Atmospheric factors
  SO_2
  NH_3
  Cold air
  O_3
  Distilled water vapor
Ingestants
  Propranolol
  Aspirin
  Nonsteroidal anti-inflammatory drugs
  Sulfites
Experimental Inhalants
  Hypertonic solutions
  Citric acid
  Histamine
  Methacholine
  Prostaglandin $F_{2\alpha}$
Occupational Inhalant
  Isocyanates

The mechanism of aspirin-sensitive asthma is idiosyncratic and not immunologic. Since aspirin and related compounds normally inhibit the cyclooxygenase pathway of biosynthesis of prostaglandin E_2 (a bronchodilator) from arachidonic acid, it is suspected that in this disease an idiosyncratic response to these drugs favors the local synthesis of either prostaglandin $F_{2\alpha}$ (a bronchoconstrictor) or leukotrienes via the lipoxygenase pathway.

The clinical significance of immediate and late phases of the IgE response is especially clear in asthma. Bronchospastic episodes that occur within minutes on exposure to the allergen and are promptly relieved by bronchodilators correspond to the immediate-phase response. Chronic asthma that is poorly responsive to beta-adrenergic agonists and theophylline, associated with enhanced nonspecific airway hyperirritability, and dependent on corticosteroids for reversal, is characteristic of the late-phase allergic response. Bronchial provocation challenge with many of the usual inhaled aeroallergens, such as pollens, fungi, and dust mite, produce dual early and late asthmatic reaction in untreated allergic asthma.

Exercise-induced and hyperventilation-induced bronchoconstriction in asthmatic patients is a consequence of water loss from the airway, which increases the osmolarity of fluid overlying the mucosal epithelial cells. This stimulates mast cells to release mediators, which, in turn, contract bronchial smooth muscle either directly or indirectly through vagal afferent receptor stimulation. Airway cooling, which occurs from inhaling cold air, exaggerates the effect of water loss.

The conceptual model of allergen–IgE antibody-induced allergic disease as discussed in Chapters 12 and

26 is well established. It requires direct contact of allergen with antibodies fixed to tissue mast cells, which then release mediators locally in the target tissues, where the inflammatory pathology and clinical symptoms and signs localize. In atopy the allergen molecule is often encountered as a component of an airborne particle, such as a pollen grain or mold spore. In allergic rhinconjunctivitis these particles easily impact on the target conjunctiva and nasal mucosa, completing the direct contact model. In allergic asthma, however, particles at the upper end of this size range are not ordinarily expected to penetrate as far as the tracheobronchial tree. Recent immunochemical air-sampling methods, however, have shown that pollen and spore fragments and even droplets containing allergen are inhaled as a significant portion of the ambient allergen load inhaled by the allergic patient.

The allergens commonly associated with allergic asthma and allergic rhinitis are generally similar. Individual patients, however, may tend to react with rhinitis to pollens and with asthma to molds and animal dander. Very young asthmatic children frequently have food-induced asthma without rhinitis.

Allergic asthma is the usual manifestation of IgE-mediated occupational disease. New occupational inhalant allergens are continually being discovered. A partial list is shown in Table 27–7. Occupational asthma may also arise from nonimmunologic sensitivity or irritation to many other substances that fail to induce IgE antibody or other immune responses. In these cases, the cause and pathogenesis are unknown, but possible mechanisms that have been suggested include toxic chemical injury to the bronchial mucosa, irritant stimulation of mast cells or vagal irritant receptors, and beta-adrenergic blockade. Patients with atopic allergy to specific allergens, such as animals, are obviously precluded from working in a job in which they are exposed to these allergens. Most cases of occupational asthma, however—both IgE-mediated and nonimmunologic—occur in nonatopic workers, showing that an unusual high-dose exposure to a potential allergen in an occupational setting can override the requirement for genetic predisposition of atopy.

Immunologic Diagnosis

The diagnosis of asthma is made by history, physical examination, and pulmonary function tests to show reversible bronchial obstruction. Blood and sputum examination for eosinophilia is confirmatory. Chest x-rays are useful primarily to exclude other cardiopulmonary diseases. The methacholine challenge test is reserved for instances in which the history is equivocal and pulmonary function is normal.

The history is the primary diagnostic tool for evaluating the presence of allergy and identifying the relevant allergens. In general, inhalant allergens that are important in allergic rhinitis are also implicated in allergic asthma. These include pollens, fungi, animal

Table 27–7. Occupational allergens causing IgE-mediated allergic asthma.

Allergen	Occupational Exposure
Animal products	
Cows, pigs, poultry, mice, hamsters, rabbits, rats, guinea pigs, bats, dogs, cats, horses.	Animal/insect breeders, laboratory workers, veterinarians, breeders.
Insect dusts	
Mealworms, storage mites, silk filatures, locusts, bees, cockroaches, flies.	Grain handlers, sewerage workers, beekeepers.
Sea creatures	
Crabs, shrimp, seasquirt body fluid, fish feed, *Echinodorus plamosus* larvae.	Processors, breeders.
Plant products	
Dusts, flours, cotton dust, grain dusts, grain flours.	Cotton mill and textile workers, grain elevator and bakery workers.
Fruits, seeds, leaves, pollens	
Castor beans, green coffee beans.	Coffee processors, seamen, laboratory workers.
Weeping fig, sunflower pollen, tobacco.	Producers, agricultural workers.
Organic dyes and inks	
Vegetable, dusts, gums, extracts	
Western red and eastern white cedar (plicatic acid), California redwood, exotic woods.	Carpenters, sawmill workers.
Colophony (abietic acid).	Electronics workers.
Microbial agents	
Alginates, fungal allergens, humidifier contaminants, protozoa, fungi, bacteria.	Biotechnology industry, laboratory, office workers.
Enzymes	
Subtilisin, papain, pineapple bromelain, pepsin, hog trypsin, pancreatic extracts.	Detergent manufacturers, pharmaceutical workers, food processors.
Therapeutic agents	
Antibiotics and related compounds, penicillins, cephalosporins, tetracycline, phenylglycine acid chloride, sulfonamides, spiramycin.	Pharmaceutical workers, poultry chick breeders.
Pharmaceuticals and related compounds	
α-Methyldopa, amprolium hydrochloride, cimetidine, furan-based binder, glycyl compound (salbutamol intermediate), psyllium (bulk laxative)	Pharmaceutical workers, nurses.
Piperazine	Medical and veterinary workers.
Sterilizing agents	
Chloramine, sulfone chloramides, hexachlorophene.	Abattoir, kitchen, hospital workers.
Inorganic chemicals	
Metal fumes and salts.	Metalworkers.
Aluminum, chromium, cobalt, fluoride, nickel, platinum, stainless steel, welding fumes, vanadium, zinc.	Chemical industry workers, metal refiners, platers, grinders, welders.
Ammonium persulfate.	Beauticians.
Organic chemicals	
Amines (diamines, ethanolamines, tetramines).	Chemical, electronic, plastic, rubber industry workers, photographers, beauticians, fur handlers.
Anhydrides (phthalic, tetrachlorophthalic, trimellitic), azobisformamide, azodicarbonamide.	Plastics industry workers, food wrappers.

Source: Modified and reproduced, with permission, from Butcher BT, Salvaggio JE: Occupational asthma. *J Allergy Clin Immunol* 1986;**78**:547.

danders, house dust, and other household and occupational airborne allergens. In young children and infants, allergy to foods may also cause asthma. History and physical findings of other atopic diseases—atopic dermatitis or allergic rhinitis—as well as a family history of atopy increase suspicion that asthma may involve atopic allergy. Skin testing for wheal-and-flare reactions verifies the specific sensitivities. Radioallergosorbent test (RAST) or other in vitro tests may be used in unusual situations when skin testing is contraindicated. Bronchoprovocation allergen testing is used primarily in difficult diagnostic cases of suspected occupational lung disease.

Differential Diagnosis

Chronic bronchitis and emphysema (chronic obstructive lung disease) produce airway obstruction that does not respond to sympathomimetic bronchodilators or corticosteroids, and there is no associated eosinophilia in the blood or sputum. In children, acute bronchiolitis, cystic fibrosis, aspiration of a foreign body, and airway obstruction caused by a congenital vascular anomaly must be considered. Benign or malignant bronchial tumors or external compression from an enlarged substernal thyroid, thymus enlargement, aneurysm, or mediastinal tumor may cause wheezing. Acute viral bronchitis may produce enough bronchial inflammation with symptoms of obstruction and wheezing that it may be termed asthmatic bronchitis. "Cardiac asthma" is a term used for intermittent dyspnea (resembling allergic asthma) caused by left ventricular failure. Carcinoid tumors may occasionally cause attacks of wheezing because of release of serotonin or activation of kinins produced by the neoplasm.

Treatment

Since the cause of asthma is unknown, cure of the basic defect, the hyperirritable bronchial mucosa, is not possible. The aim of treatment is symptomatic control. Environmental measures, drugs, and allergen desensitization may be required.

A. Environmental Control: Irritants such as smoke, fumes, dust, and aerosols should be avoided. If the diagnostic evaluation indicates allergy to animal danders, feathers, molds, or house dust, these should be eliminated from the house.

B. Drug Treatment:

1. Sympathomimetics–Beta-adrenergic bronchodilator drugs are effective and are used in the acute attack or for long-term management. Epinephrine has both alpha- and beta-adrenergic effects, but it has a long history of efficacy in acute asthma attacks. It acts rapidly and is given subcutaneously in a dose of 0.2–0.5 mL of 1:1000 aqueous solution. Its duration of action is short, so that if repeated injections are required, long-acting epinephrine (1:200 in suspension) or terbutaline can be used. Albuterol, pirbuterol, metaproterenol, and isoetharine are selective beta-adrenergic bronchodilators that are given by inhalation in aerosol. They are available as solutions to be administered by a hand-held nebulizer, in an intermittent positive-pressure breathing device, or in metered-dose pressurized inhalers, but patients must be cautioned that overuse can lead to paradoxic bronchial constriction and worsening of asthma. The beta-adrenergic drugs terbutaline, metaproterenol, and albuterol are available as oral sympathomimetic drugs for achieving sustained bronchodilation in chronic asthma. Side effects of nervousness, muscle twitching, palpitations, tachycardia, and insomnia can occur with all of them.

Salmeterol, an inhaled beta$_2$-adrenergic bronchodilator, is effective for long-term prophylaxis. It is not useful for relief of an acute attack, because of an extremely long latent period before its action takes place.

2. Xanthines–Theophylline and related compounds are especially effective as bronchodilators when used in combination with sympathomimetic drugs. Intravenous aminophylline, 250–500 mg, can be administered fairly rapidly in an acute asthmatic attack, and various oral forms of theophylline are available for long-term use. Absorption of theophylline varies with the drug preparation, the age of the patient, and other factors, such as smoking and heart failure. Serum theophylline determination should be utilized to obtain a therapeutic level of 10–20 µg/mL.

3. Corticosteroids–Glucocorticoids are remarkably effective in the treatment of asthma. Even when all other forms of treatment have failed, the response to adequate steroid treatment is so dependable that failure of response might be considered grounds for questioning the diagnosis of asthma. The therapeutic effect in asthma is anti-inflammatory, but the precise mechanism of action is unknown, and these drugs are just as effective in reversing asthma in nonallergic patients as in patients suffering allergen-induced attacks. Despite their effectiveness, however, systemic corticosteroids should not be considered primary drugs in the treatment of asthma, and in practice they should be given only when other forms of treatment prove inadequate. The dangers of long-term steroid therapy must be kept in mind by any physician prescribing the drugs.

Treatment is started at high dosage and continued until the obstruction is alleviated, with return of physical findings and flow rates to normal. The dose necessary to achieve this varies with the individual patient, but 30–60 mg of prednisone daily is usually sufficient. An occasional steroid-resistant patient may require a much higher dose because of an abnormally accelerated rate of drug catabolism. After complete clearing of the attack, the daily dose is reduced by slow tapering over many days or weeks to avoid a recurrence of asthma. Long-term alternate-day maintenance therapy minimizes adrenocortical suppression, but not all steroid-dependent asthma can be controlled in this fashion.

Beclomethasone dipropionate, triamcinolone acetonide, and flunisolide—highly potent corticosteroid drugs—are available in aerosolized form for inhalation. They are effective as long-term maintenance therapy for many steroid-dependent asthmatic patients. Many experts today recommend regular long-term inhaled corticosteroids as primary anti-inflammatory prophylaxis in virtually all asthmatic patients. Adrenocortical suppression and systemic side effects are usually slight. When they are used to replace a systemic steroid drug, the dosage of systemic drug must be tapered very slowly to avoid adrenal insufficiency. Inhaled corticosteroids are not useful for treatment of an acute asthma attack.

4. Cromolyn sodium–This drug is available as a powder administered in 20-mg doses by inhalation in a specially designed inhaler or micronized in a metered-dose inhaler. It is not a bronchodilator but is believed to inhibit the release of mediators of immediate hypersensitivity in the lung. It is administered as a long-term prophylactic treatment. It is more effective in younger patients with allergic asthma than in adults, and it frequently prevents exercise-induced bronchospasm. Cromolyn does not reverse an acute attack.

5. Other drugs–Antibiotics are used if secondary bacterial bronchitis or pneumonia occurs. Expectorants and hydration are helpful for thick, tenacious sputum. Inhaled ipratropium bromide, an anticholinergic drug with minimal side effects because of poor absorption, may help to eliminate the asthmatic cough.

Drugs that inhibit 5-lipoxygenase and therefore block the synthesis of leukotrienes and others that inhibit leukotriene receptors have been developed and are currently in clinical trials for treatment of asthma.

C. Desensitization: The effectiveness of injection treatment in pollen hay fever has been shown in several controlled studies, and most allergists believe that allergic asthma responds just as well (see Chapter 56).

D. Treatment of Status Asthmaticus and Respiratory Failure: A severe attack of asthma unresponsive to repeated injections of epinephrine or other sympathomimetic drugs, termed "status asthmaticus," is a medical emergency requiring immediate hospitalization and prompt treatment. Factors leading to this condition include respiratory infection, excessive use of respiratory-depressant drugs such as sedatives or opiates, overuse of aerosolized bronchodilators, rapid withdrawal of corticosteroids, and ingestion of aspirin in aspirin-sensitive asthmatic patients.

Immediate determination of arterial blood gases and pH with repeated measurements until the patient responds satisfactorily is necessary for optimal treatment. Injections of terbutaline or epinephrine are continued. If the patient has not been receiving oral theophylline, 250–500 mg of aminophylline may be given intravenously for 10–30 minutes initially, followed by slow intravenous drip with careful attention to toxic symptoms. Serum theophylline determinations are used to maintain the optimal therapeutic level of 10–20 µg/mL of serum. Intravenous corticosteroids are indicated if the patient has previously received steroids, if the attack was caused by aspirin, if excessive aerosolized bronchodilator was a factor in the attack, or if significant CO_2 retention exists. Intravenous hydrocortisone at 4 mg/kg or methylprednisolone at 1 mg/kg, repeated every 2–4 hours, should be given until the patient can be maintained on oral prednisone at 60–80 mg daily in divided doses.

Dehydration usually accompanies status asthmaticus and may give rise to inspissated mucus plugs that further impair ventilation. During the first 24 hours, up to 3–4 L of intravenous fluid may be necessary for rehydration. Oxygen should be supplied by tent, face mask, or nasal catheter to maintain arterial Po_2 at about 80–100 mm Hg. Expectorants and chest physical therapy are helpful adjuncts to eliminate mucus plugs. Sedatives should be avoided even in the anxious patient because of the danger of respiratory depression. Antibiotics are used only for concomitant bacterial infection.

Respiratory failure, indicated by an arterial Po_2 level above 65 mm Hg and arterial blood pH below 7.25, may requre mechanical assistance of ventilation in addition to all the measures already listed. This should be performed by a team of physicians, nurses, and technicians experienced in this form of respiratory therapy.

Complications & Prognosis

The disease is chronic, and its severity may change in an unpredictable fashion. Some children apparently "outgrow" asthma in the sense of becoming asymptomatic, but they may continue to show evidence of bronchial lability, and symptoms can reappear later in life. The acute attack can be complicated by pneumothorax, subcutaneous emphysema, rib fractures, atelectasis, or pneumonitis. There is no evidence that emphysema, bronchiectasis, pulmonary hypertension, and cor pulmonale result from long-standing uncomplicated asthma.

Allergic Bronchopulmonary Aspergillosis

This disease occurs almost exclusively in patients with a history of asthma who harbor *Aspergillus* endobronchially and who develop a heterogeneous form of hypersensitivity with both IgE and IgG antibodies to *Aspergillus* antigens (see Chapter 29).

ATOPIC DERMATITIS

Major Immunologic Features

- It often accompanies atopic respiratory allergy.
- The clinical course is usually independent of allergen exposure.
- Very high serum levels of IgE may occur.

Definition

Atopic dermatitis (also known as eczema, neurodermatitis, atopic eczema, or Besnier's prurigo) is a common chronic skin disorder specific to a subset of patients with the familial and immunologic features of atopy. The essential feature is a pruritic dermal inflammatory response, which induces a characteristic symmetrically distributed skin eruption with predilection for certain sites. There is frequent overproduction of IgE by B lymphocytes, possibly caused by abnormal T-lymphocyte regulation. Patients often have multiple IgE antibodies to environmental inhalant and food allergens, but the role of these allergens in the dermatitis is uncertain.

General Considerations

Atopic dermatitis is classified as a cutaneous form of atopy because it is associated with allergic rhinitis and asthma in families (and frequently in the same patient) and the serum IgE concentration is often high. The severity of the dermatitis, however, does not always correlate with exposure to allergens to which the patient reacts positively on skin testing, and allergy desensitization is not effective in this disease. There is evidence for an underlying target organ (ie, skin) abnormality that might be a metabolic or biochemical defect, possibly linked genetically to the high level of serum IgE. Some studies also suggest a partial deficiency in T-cell immunity. Atopic dermatitis may begin at any age. Onset at 3–6 months of age is typical, but it may first appear during childhood or adolescence and occasionally during adult life.

Clinical Features

A. Symptoms: The disease almost always begins in infancy or early childhood. Many cases clear by 2 years of age. Persistence into later childhood and adult life is marked by frequent cycles of remission and exacerbation. Itching is the cardinal symptom. It often worsens at night and is provoked by temperature changes, sweating, exertion, emotional stress, and embarrassment. There is a strong family history of atopy. Scratching and rubbing cause the typical eczematous skin eruption to flare. Itching is also exacerbated by irritants such as wool and by drying agents such as soap and defatting solvents. Ingestion of allergenic foods may cause acute exacerbations. The disease may improve spontaneously during the summer.

B. Signs: The skin is typically dry and scaly. Active skin lesions are characterized by intensely pruritic inflamed papules (prurigo), erythema, and scaling. Scratching produces weeping and excoriations. Chronic lesions are thickened and lichenified. Distribution of the lesions depends on age. In infancy, the forehead, cheeks, and extensor surfaces of the extremities are usually involved. Later, the lesions show a flexural pattern of distribution, with predilection for the antecubital and popliteal areas and the neck. The face, especially around the eyes and ears, is often affected when distribution is more widespread. Staphylococcal pustules are common. Stroking of the skin produces white dermographism, in contrast to the normal erythema and whealing of the triple response of Lewis.

C. Laboratory Findings: Elevated total serum IgE, sometimes extremely high, occurs in 60–80% of cases. A normal level does not rule out the diagnosis, however.

Epidemiology

Approximately 0.7% of the US population currently have active disease, but the prevalence in children is 4–5%, equally distributed between the sexes. Racial predilection and geographic distribution have not been studied.

Pathology

Grossly, the lesion begins acutely with an erythematous edematous papule or plaque with scaling. Itching leads to weeping and crusting, then to chronic lichenification. Microscopically, the acute lesion is characterized by intercellular edema, and the dermis is infiltrated with mononuclear cells and CD4 lymphocytes. Neutrophils, eosinophils, plasma cells, and basophils are rare, and vasculitis is absent, but

degranulated mast cells can be seen. The chronic lesion features epidermal hyperplasia, hyperkeratosis, and parakeratosis. The dermis is infiltrated with mononuclear cells, Langerhans' cells, and mast cells. There may be focal areas of fibrosis, including involvement of the perineurium of small nerves.

Immunologic Diagnosis

The history and physical examination are almost always sufficient to make the diagnosis. Marked elevation of serum IgE is confirmatory, but a normal IgE level does not rule out atopic dermatitis. Biopsy is usually not required.

Because of the uncertainty about specific allergic sensitivities in pathogenesis, skin or in vitro allergy tests usually produce positive results that may reflect concomitant respiratory allergies or asymptomatic sensitivities rather than causes of the skin disease. In some children with atopic dermatitis there may be positive skin tests to foods that cause acute exacerbation of eczema when those foods are given in a double-blind placebo-controlled oral challenge test. Blood T-lymphocyte subset counts are not useful in diagnosis.

Differential Diagnosis

Localized neurodermatitis (lichen simplex chronicus) and allergic or irritant contact dermatitis produce similar eczematous changes of the skin. Seborrhea and dermatophytoses are occasionally confused with atopic dermatitis. Pompholyx (dyshidrosis) with secondary eczema may simulate atopic dermatitis of the hands.

Immunologic Pathogenesis

There is an intrinsic skin abnormality in atopic dermatitis, perhaps analogous to the hyperirritable airway in asthma. Some evidence suggests hyperreactivity to cholinergic stimuli, which might relate to the reduced threshold of the itch response. Increased numbers of mast cells and increased histamine content in the skin have been reported, but the other mast cell-associated chemical mediators have not been thoroughly examined for a role in this disease. Blood basophil counts are normal. Injection of methacholine intradermally initially produces the expected wheal and erythema; this is followed in 2–5 minutes by blanching because of edema. This delayed-blanch response is typical but not diagnostic of atopic dermatitis.

A. Defective Lymphocyte Regulation: Much indirect information suggests a defect in cell-mediated immunity. Delayed hypersensitivity skin test responses to recall antigens, in vitro lymphocyte responses to mitogen and allergen, and the autologous mixed lymphocyte reaction have all been reported to be deficient. Decreased prevalence of naturally acquired and experimentally induced allergic contact dermatitis and increased susceptibility to herpes simplex virus, vaccinia virus, warts, molluscum contagiosum, and dermatophyte skin infections are consistent with a defect in the T-cell effector mechanism. Many studies have documented the association of high levels of IgE production in atopic dermatitis with the presence of a predominant population of T helper cells with the T_H2 cytokine profile. Other investigations have shown that excessive production of IgE by peripheral blood B lymphocytes in this disease can be accounted for by deficiency in CD8 T lymphocytes. It has been suggested that a defective CD4 helper T-lymphocyte population could explain the failure of CD8 T lymphocytes to function as suppressors of IgE production and to achieve sufficient cytotoxicity for effective immunity against secondary skin infections.

B. The Role of Allergy: Atopic respiratory diseases with hypersensitivity to environmental allergens, eosinophilia, elevated serum IgE levels, and a family history of allergy are frequently associated with atopic dermatitis. Nevertheless, it is often difficult to attribute the dermatitis to allergy. The skin lesions rarely flare during pollen seasons, although in some patients there is an association with exposure to house dust, animals, or other environmental allergens. More commonly, food allergy is implicated in the dermatitis in children. Milk, corn, soybeans, fish, nuts, and cereal grains are frequently implicated, but other foods may occasionally be important allergens also. Recent controlled food challenges have shown clear-cut exacerbations of the early inflammatory pruritic lesions in selected cases, although the responsible food cannot always be detected by skin testing.

C. Association with Systemic Disorders: Eczema indistinguishable from atopic dermatitis is found in children with phenylketonuria. The skin lesions of Letterer-Siwe disease are also very similar. Atopic dermatitis without allergy is a feature of several immunologic deficiency disorders, especially Wiskott-Aldrich syndrome, ataxia-telangiectasia, and X-linked hypogammaglobulinemia (see Chapters 20–22).

Treatment

Atopic dermatitis is a chronic disease requiring constant attention to proper skin care, environmental control, drugs, and avoidance of allergens when indicated. Because dry skin enhances the tendency to itch, frequent application of nonirritating topical lubricants is the most important preventive measure. Small areas of active eczema respond well to topical corticosteroids, but acute involvement of large areas of skin may warrant a brief course of systemic corticosteroids beginning with a high dose and tapering slowly after the acute eruption clears. Oral antihistamines help to control itching. If their sedative effect precludes use during the daytime, a bedtime dose helps to control involuntary scratching during sleep. Frequent bathing or washing, irritating fabrics such as wool, and harsh detergents should be avoided. The hands and fingernails must be kept clean to prevent secondary infection, and if infection does occur, an appropriate antibiotic should be prescribed.

Complications & Prognosis

Atopic dermatitis that persists beyond childhood has an unpredictable tendency to remit spontaneously, even after years of involvement. This is not related to the severity of involvement, the presence or absence of allergy, or treatment. Allergic rhinitis and asthma are not complications but, rather, additional manifestations of the underlying atopic disease.

The most frequent complication is secondary infection, almost always by *Staphylococcus,* as a result of scratching. In the past, the most serious complication was eczema vaccinatum from exposure to vaccinia virus by inadvertent vaccination or contact with a recently vaccinated person in the family or classroom. Eczema herpeticum is a similar condition caused by herpes simplex virus. Topical antibiotics or antihistamines may cause secondary contact dermatitis. Hand dermatitis occurs from excessive contact with water, soap, and solvents in the home and the workplace.

Ophthalmic complications include atopic keratoconjunctivitis, keratoconus, and atopic cataracts.

ALLERGIC GASTROENTEROPATHY

Major Immunologic Features

- Some atopic patients have localized IgE reactions in the gut to an ingested food.
- Gastrointestinal loss of serum proteins and blood may lead to edema and anemia.
- The condition is rare in adults; it is more common but transient in infants.

Definition

Allergic gastroenteropathy (also known as eosinophilic gastroenteropathy) is an unusual atopic manifestation in which multiple IgE food sensitivities are associated with a local gastrointestinal tract mucosal reaction. This produces acute gastrointestinal symptoms, eosinophilia, and gastroenteric loss of fluid, protein, and blood. Extraintestinal allergic symptoms, such as asthma and urticaria, may also be provoked by foods. Other atopic manifestations in the patient and family usually are present.

General Considerations

Allergic gastroenteropathy is the least common expression of atopy. Ingested food allergen reacting with local IgE antibodies in the jejunal mucosa liberates mast cell mediators, causing gastrointestinal symptoms shortly after the meal. Continued exposure to the food produces chronic inflammation, resulting in gastrointestinal protein loss and hypoproteinemic edema. Blood loss through the inflamed intestinal mucosa may be significant enough to cause iron deficiency anemia. In some patients, extraenteric manifestations of atopy may be produced by the same food allergen.

Epidemiology

Very few cases have been reported, but the disease has been described in infants, children, and adults. It is a very rare cause of gastrointestinal symptoms.

Immunologic Pathogenesis

The pathogenesis is that of atopy, as discussed earlier. The condition may occur more commonly in infants than in adults because of the much greater permeability of the infantile gastrointestinal mucosa to intact proteins. This may account for the transient nature of allergic gastroenteropathy in infants and young children.

The allergic reaction occurs locally in the upper gastrointestinal mucosa. Ingested food allergens react with IgE antibodies fixed to mucosal mast cells, thereby liberating mediators responsible for hyperemia, increased vascular permeability, and smooth muscle contraction. This results in acute symptoms, chronic loss of blood and plasma protein, and intestinal malabsorption.

Clinical Features

A. Symptoms and Signs: Nausea, vomiting, diarrhea, and abdominal pain occur within 2 hours after ingestion of the allergenic food, and these symptoms resolve on avoidance of the food. Rhinitis, asthma, or urticaria may accompany the intestinal symptoms. Chronic or repeated exposures to allergenic foods in undiagnosed disease may lead to blood loss anemia, abdominal distension, and voluminous foul stools from steatorrhea, edema from hypoalbuminemia, and systemic symptoms of anorexia, weight loss, and weakness. Children may experience growth retardation. Most patients have other manifestations of atopy, including atopic dermatitis, asthma, and allergic rhinitis, and there is usually a family history of atopy.

B. Laboratory Findings: Blood counts show hypochromic microcytic iron deficiency anemia and eosinophilia. Stool examination reveals gross or occult blood and Charcot-Leyden crystals. Serum albumin is low, and total serum IgE may be elevated. Gastrointestinal x-rays may show mucosal thickening and edema of the small bowel.

Immunologic Diagnosis

A history of chronic or recurrent gastrointestinal symptoms associated with specific foods in an atopic patient should raise a suspicion of this diagnosis, especially if there is accompanying evidence of gastrointestinal blood loss, iron deficiency anemia, intestinal malabsorption, protein-losing enteropathy, other manifestations of atopy, or high serum total IgE.

In reported cases the causative food allergens have been single or multiple. Milk is the usual cause in children. Nursing infants may react to food allergens in breast milk from the maternal diet. The suspected food allergens identified by history can be tested for IgE antibodies by a skin test or RAST. Tests for antibodies to other foods may uncover other allergies, but these should be confirmed by elimination and challenge, preferably performed double-blind. Peroral jejunal biopsy may be necessary in difficult cases.

Pathology

An eosinophilic inflammatory infiltrate in the lamina propria of the upper gastrointestinal tract mucosa is present following allergen exposure and resolves with allergen avoidance.

Differential Diagnosis

Gastrointestinal allergy is overdiagnosed. Patients with food-related gastrointestinal symptoms—even atopic patients—are much more likely to have nonallergic food intolerance. Primary gastrointestinal diseases, reactions to food contaminants, and psychologic food aversion must be considered. Inflammatory bowel diseases, intestinal lymphangiectasia, and primary immunoglobulin deficiencies may produce similar symptoms. In children, lactase and other carbohydrate enzyme deficiencies, phenylketonuria, pancreatic deficiency from cystic fibrosis, and maple syrup urine disease should be ruled out by appropriate tests.

Treatment

Elimination of the allergenic food from the diet is curative. In some cases of milk allergy, boiled milk may be tolerated if the protein allergen is heat-labile. Corticosteroid treatment usually inhibits the reaction, but long-term steroid therapy should be necessary only for patients who do not respond to the elimination diet. There are reports that oral cromolyn in a dose of 200–400 mg given before the allergenic food is eaten inhibits the gastrointestinal allergic reaction, but there are no long-term studies on this form of treatment.

Complications

The major complications of this disease are edema and anemia. Unlike intestinal lymphangiectasia, significant gastroenteric loss of plasma immunoglobulins and lymphocytes does not occur, so susceptibility to infection is usually not a problem. Persistent disease activity may lead to secondary reversible lactose intolerance. Malnutrition can result from undiagnosed disease.

Prognosis

The infantile form of allergic gastroenteropathy is usually transient, but the duration of the disease is unpredictable and is not related to severity of the reaction. No long-term follow-up studies on adults are available.

REFERENCES

GENERAL

Hopkin JM: Genetics of atopy. *Clin Exp Allergy* 1989;**19**:263.

Ishizaka K: IgE-binding factors and regulation of the IgE antibody response. *Ann Rev Immunol* 1988;**6**:513.

Leskowitz S et al: A hypothesis for the development of atopic allergy in man. *Clin Allergy* 1972;**2**:237.

Marsh DG et al: The epidemiology and genetics of atopic allergy. *N Engl J Med* 1981;**305**:1551.

ALLERGENS

Anderson JA, Sogn DD (editors): *Adverse Reactions to Foods.* NIH Publication no. 84–2442. US Department of Health and Human Services, 1984.

Anderson MC et al: A comparative study of the allergens of cat urine, serum, saliva, and pelt. *J Allergy Clin Immunol* 1985;**76**:563.

Korner WE et al: Fungal allergens. *Clin Microbiol Rev* 1995;**8**:161.

Platts-Mills TAE et al: Problems in allergen standardization. *Clin Rev Allergy* 1985;**3**:271.

Solomon WR: Aerobiology of pollinosis. *J Allergy Clin Immunol* 1984;**74**:449.

Weber RW, Nelson HS: Pollen allergens and their interrelationships. *Clin Rev Allergy* 1985;**3**:291.

Yunginger JW: Allergenic extracts: Characterization, standardization, and prospects for the future. *Pediatr Clin N Am* 1983;**30**:795.

ALLERGIC RHINITIS

Allansmith MR, Ross RN: Ocular allergy. *Clin Allergy* 1988;**18**:1.

Busse WW: Role of antihistamines in allergic disease. *Ann Allergy* 1994;**72**:281.

Druce HM, Kaliner MA: Allergic rhinitis. *JAMA* 1988;**259**:260.

Fireman P: Newer concepts in otitis media. *Hosp Pract* 1987;**22**:85.

Friedlaender MH: Ocular allergy. *J Allergy Clin Immunol* 1985;**76**:645.

Naclerio RM et al: Basophils and eosinophils in allergic rhinitis. *J Allergy Clin Immunol* 1994;**94**:1303.

Norman PS: Allergic rhinitis. *J Allergy Clin Immunol* 1985;**75**:531.

Meltzer EO: An overview of current pharmacotherapy in perennial rhinitis. *J Allergy Clin Immunol* 1995;**95**:1097.

Philip G, Togias AG: Nonallergic rhinitis. Pathophysiology and models for study. *Eur Arch Otorhinolaryngol Suppl* 1995;**1**:S27.

Todd NW: Allergy as a cause of otitis media. *Immunol Allergy Clin North Am* 1987;**7**:371.

ASTHMA

Barnes PJ: New concepts in the pathogenesis of bronchial hyperresponsiveness and asthma. *J Allergy Clin Immunol* 1989;**83**:1013.

Busse WW: The relationship between viral infections and the onset of allergic diseases and asthma. *Clin Exp Allergy* 1989;**19**:1.

Chan-Yeung M, Lam S: Occupational asthma. *Am Rev Respir Dis* 1986;**133**:686.

Chapman ID et al: The relationship between inflammation and hyperreactivity of the airways in asthma. *Clin Exp Allergy* 1993;**23**:168.

Cherniak RM: Continuity of care in asthma management. *Hosp Pract* 1987;**22**:119.

Fahy JV, Boushey HA: Controversies involving inhaled beta-agonists and inhaled corticosteroids in the treatment of asthma. *Clin Chest Med* 1995;**16**:715.

Fireman P: β_2-agonists and their safety in the treatment of asthma. *Allergy Proc* 1995;**16**:235.

Freedman AN: Models and mechanisms of exercise-induced asthma. *Eur Respir J* 1995;**8**:1770.

Hargreave FE et al: The origin of airway hyperresponsiveness. *J Allergy Clin Immunol* 1986;**78**:825.

König P: Inhaled corticosteroids—their present and future role in the management of asthma. *J Allergy Clin Immunol* 1988;**82**:297.

Lenfant C, Sheffer AL: Guidelines for the diagnosis and management of asthma. *J Allergy Clin Immunol* 1991;**88**(suppl):425. [Entire issue.]

Mathison DA et al: Precipitating factors in asthma: Aspirin, sulfites, and other drugs and chemicals. *Chest* 1985;**87**(suppl):S50.

McFadden ER: Therapy of acute asthma. *J Allergy Clin Immunol* 1989;**84**:151.

Ohman JL: Allergen immunotherapy in asthma: Evidence for efficacy. *J Allergy Clin Immunol* 1989;**84**:133.

Pattemore PK et al: Viruses as precipitants of asthma symptoms. I. Epidemiology. *Clin Exp Allergy* 1992;**22**:325.

Rachelefsky GS, Siegel SC: Asthma in infants and children—treatment of childhood asthma. Part II. *J Allergy Clin Immunol* 1985;**76**:409.

Siegel SC, Rachelefsky GS: Asthma in infants and children. Part I. *J Allergy Clin Immunol* 1985;**76**:1.

Spector SL: Leukotriene inhibitors and antagonists in asthma. *Ann Allergy* 1995;**75**:463.

Summer WR: Status asthmaticus. *Chest* 1985;**87**(suppl):S87.

Wasserfallen JB, Baraniuk JN: Clinical use of inhaled corticosteroids in asthma. *J Allergy Clin Immunol* 1007;**97**:177.

ATOPIC DERMATITIS

Burks AW et al: Atopic dermatitis and food hypersensitivity in children. *Allergy Proc* 1992;**13**:285.

Businco L, Sampson HA (editors): International symposium on atopic dermatitis: An update. *Allergy* 1989;**44**(suppl 9):1.

Charlesworth EN: Practical approaches to the treatment of atopic dermatitis. *Allergy Proc* 1994;**15**:269.

Friedmann PS et al: Pathogenesis and management of atopic dermatitis. *Clin Exp Allergy* 1995;**25**:799.

Hanifin JM: Atopic dermatitis. *J Allergy Clin Immunol* 1984;**73**:211.

Jones SM, Sampson HA: The role of allergens in atopic dermatitis. *Clin Rev Allergy* 1993;**11**:471.

Kapp A: Atopic dermatitis—The skin manifestations of atopy. *Clin Exp Allergy* 1995;**25**:210.

Leung DY: Atopic dermatitis: The skin as a window into the pathogenesis of chronic allergic diseases. *J Allergy Clin Immunol* 1995;**96**:302.

Morren MS et al: Atopic dermatitis: Triggering factors. *J Am Acad Dermatol* 1994;**31**:467.

ALLERGIC GASTROENTEROPATHY
Gryboski JD: Gastrointestinal aspects of cow's milk protein intolerance and allergy. *Immunol Allergy Clin North Am* 1991;**11**:773.

Hutchins P, Waler-Smith JA: The gastrointestinal system. *Clin Immunol Allergy* 1982;**2**:43.

Min K-U, Metcalfe DD: Eosinophilic gastroenteritis. *Immunol Allergy Clin North Am* 1991;**11**:799.

Scudamore HH et al: Food allergy manifested by eosinophilia, elevated immunoglobulin E level, and protein-losing enteropathy: The syndrome of allergic gastroenteropathy. *J Allergy Clin Immunol* 1982;**70**:129.

Anaphylaxis & Urticaria

28

Abba I. Terr, MD

The atopic diseases, discussed in the previous chapter, are characterized by a genetic predisposition to the production of IgE antibodies to common environmental antigens. Anaphylaxis and urticaria also are caused by **IgE antibodies,** but they lack the genetically determined propensity and the target organ hyperresponsiveness of atopy, and they have no special predilection for the atopic individual. The immunologic pathogenesis for all IgE-mediated diseases is the same, but separate consideration of atopic and nonatopic diseases is important clinically. There are differences in the allergens, mode of exposure to the allergen, genetic factors that influence etiology, diagnostic methods, prognosis, and treatment.

Allergic gastroenteropathy, described in Chapter 27, has features of anaphylaxis, but it is included in the chapter on atopic diseases because it occurs almost exclusively in patients with other atopic manifestations.

ANAPHYLAXIS

Major Immunologic Features
- Systemic anaphylaxis is the occurrence of an IgE-mediated reaction simultaneously in multiple organs.
- The usual causative allergen is a drug, insect venom, or food.
- The reaction can be evoked by a minute quantity of allergen and is potentially fatal.

General Considerations
A. Definitions: Anaphylaxis is an acute, generalized allergic reaction with simultaneous involvement of several organ systems, usually cardiovascular, respiratory, cutaneous, and gastrointestinal. The reaction is immunologically mediated, and it occurs on exposure to an allergen to which the subject had previously been sensitized. Anaphylactic shock refers to anaphylaxis in which hypotension, with or without

loss of consciousness, occurs. Anaphylactoid reaction is a condition in which the symptoms and signs of anaphylaxis occur in the absence of an allergen–antibody mechanism. In this case, the endogenous mediators of anaphylaxis are released in vivo through a nonimmunologic mechanism.

B. Epidemiology: Anaphylaxis has no known geographic, racial, or sex predilection. It occurs at the rate of 0.4 cases per million per year in the general population, although in the hospitalized patient population the prevalence is reported to be 0.6 per 1000 patients. The latter figure shows that medications and biologic products are a major cause.

C. Pathology: Grossly, urticaria and angioedema occur. The lungs are diffusely hyperinflated, with mucus plugging of airways and focal atelectasis. The microscopic appearance of the lungs is similar to that in acute asthma, with hypersecretion of bronchial submucosal glands, mucosal and submucosal edema, peribronchial vascular congestion, and eosinophilia in the bronchial walls. Pulmonary edema and hemorrhage may be present. Bronchial muscle spasm, hyperinflation, and even rupture of alveoli may be seen microscopically. An important feature of human anaphylaxis is edema, vascular congestion, and eosinophilia in the lamina propria of the larynx, trachea, epiglottis, and hypopharynx. Myocardial ischemia has been found in a high proportion of cases, probably secondary to shock. Occasionally, myocardial infarction occurs. A direct effect of anaphylaxis on the myocardium or coronary arteries has not been shown. The liver, spleen, and other visceral organs are often grossly congested and microscopically hyperemic and edematous. Eosinophils are found in the splenic sinusoids, liver, lamina propria of the upper respiratory tract, and pulmonary blood vessels. Pulmonary edema and intraalveolar hemorrhage may occur.

Death is usually attributable to asphyxiation from upper airway edema and congestion, irreversible shock, or a combination of these factors. Death occurring after many hours of shock may be from the effects of the late phase of the IgE allergic reaction or secondary to the failure of other organs.

D. Immunologic Pathogenesis: Anaphylaxis requires the presence of IgE antibodies and exposure to the allergen, but it is clear that it occurs in only a very small proportion of patients satisfying these requirements. In some cases the mode and quantity of allergen exposure are important. One example is the inadvertent injection of atopic allergens to atopic persons—a well-recognized risk of diagnostic skin testing and allergen immunotherapy. In most instances in which drugs, foods, or insect venoms are the cause, however, nonimmunologic potentiating factors, such as an increased reactivity of mast cells, basophils, or target organs, can only be surmised.

Anaphylaxis is the sudden systemic result of the allergen–IgE antibody mast cell-mediator release sequence detailed in Chapters 12 and 24. The result is a sudden profound and life-threatening alteration in functioning of the various vital organs. Vascular collapse, acute airway obstruction, cutaneous vasodilation and edema, and gastrointestinal and genitourinary muscle spasm occur almost simultaneously, although not always to the same degree.

E. Anaphylactic Shock: Hypotension and shock in anaphylaxis reflect generalized vasodilatation of arterioles and increased vascular permeability with rapid transudation of plasma through postcapillary venules. This shift of fluid from intravascular to extravascular spaces produces hypovolemic shock with edema (angioedema) in skin and various visceral organs, pooling of venous blood (especially in the splanchnic bed), hemoconcentration, and increased blood viscosity. Low cardiac output diminishes cardiac return and produces inadequate coronary artery perfusion. Low peripheral vascular resistance can lead to myocardial hypoxia, dysrhythmias, and secondary cardiogenic shock. Stimulation of histamine H_1 receptors in coronary arteries may cause coronary artery spasm. Some patients experience anginal chest pains and, occasionally, myocardial infarction during anaphylaxis. After a prolonged period of shock, organ failure elsewhere may ensue, particularly the kidneys and central nervous system. In some cases shock occurs rapidly before extensive fluid shifts would be expected to take place, suggesting that neurogenic reflex mechanisms might be involved.

F. Urticaria and Angioedema: Histamine and other mediators stimulate receptors in superficial cutaneous blood vessels, causing the swelling, erythema, and itching that characterize urticaria, a hallmark cutaneous feature of systemic anaphylaxis. Increased permeability of subcutaneous blood vessels causes the more diffuse swelling of angioedema, which may account for a substantial volume of fluid loss from the intravascular compartment.

G. Lower Respiratory Obstruction: Bronchial muscle spasm, edema and eosinophilic inflammation of the bronchial mucosa, and hypersecretion of mucus into the airway lumen occur in some patients with anaphylaxis and are indistinguishable from an acute asthmatic attack. Both histamine and leukotrienes have bronchoconstrictor activity, but the former affects the larger proximal airways preferentially, and the latter affects peripheral airways. Airway obstruction leads to impairment of gas exchange with hypoxia, further compounding the vascular effects of anaphylaxis. If this is left untreated, acute cor pulmonale and respiratory failure may occur.

H. Other Effects: Histamine acts on gastrointestinal and uterine smooth muscle, causing painful spasm. Hageman factor-dependent pathways may be activated by basophil and mast cell enzymes during anaphylaxis. One such enzyme has kallikrein activity and has been called basophil kallikrein of anaphylaxis, cleaving bradykinin from high-molecular-weight kininogen. Bradykinin has potent vascular permeability as well as vasodilating, smooth muscle-contracting, and pain-inducing properties, and it is occasionally found in anaphylactic states. Hageman factor activation of the intrinsic clotting mechanism may also explain some of the coagulation abnormalities found in systemic anaphylaxis.

Clinical Features

A. Symptoms and Signs: Exposure to the allergen may be through ingestion, injection, inhalation, or contact with skin or mucous membrane. The reaction begins within seconds or minutes after exposure to the allergen. There may be an initial fright or sense of impending doom, followed rapidly by symptoms in one or more target organ systems: cardiovascular, respiratory, cutaneous, and gastrointestinal.

The **cardiovascular** response may be peripheral or central. Hypotension and shock are symptoms of generalized arteriolar vasodilatation and increased vascular permeability producing decreased peripheral resistance and leakage of plasma from the circulation to extravascular tissues, thereby lowering blood volume. In some patients without previous heart disease, cardiac arrhythmias may occur. Without prompt treatment by intravascular fluid replacement, prolonged shock may lead to the secondary effects of hypoxia in all vital organs. Death can result from blood volume depletion and irreversible shock or from a cardiac arrhythmia.

The **respiratory** tract from the nasal mucosa to the bronchioles may be involved. Nasal congestion from swelling and hyperemia of the nasal mucosa and profuse watery rhinorrhea with itching of the nose and palate simulate an acute hay fever reaction. The hypopharynx and larynx are especially susceptible, and obstruction of this critical portion of the airway by edema is responsible for some of the respiratory deaths. Bronchial obstruction from bronchospasm, mucosal edema, and hypersecretion of mucus results in an asthma-like paroxysm of wheezing dyspnea. Obstruction of the smaller airways by mucus may lead to respiratory failure.

The **skin** is a frequent target organ, with generalized pruritus, erythema, urticaria, and angioedema. Angioedema often involves the eyelids, lips, tongue, pharynx, and larynx. The conjunctival and oropharyngeal mucosae are erythematous and edematous. Occasionally, urticaria persists for many weeks or months after all other symptoms have subsided.

Gastrointestinal involvement occurs because of contraction of intestinal smooth muscle and mucosal edema, resulting in crampy abdominal pain and sometimes nausea or diarrhea. Similarly, uterine muscle contraction may cause pelvic pain. Spontaneous abortion can result if the patient is pregnant.

Hemostatic changes can occur but are not often detected clinically. The intrinsic coagulation pathway is activated, resulting in the possibility of disseminated intravascular coagulation (DIC) and depletion of clotting factors. Thrombocytopenia may occur, possibly because platelets aggregated by platelet-activating factor (PAF) are sequestered from the circulation. In some cases, circulating heparin or other anticoagulants have been demonstrated.

Convulsions, with or without shock, have been reported rarely. In cases of fatal anaphylaxis, death usually occurs within 1 hour of onset.

B. Laboratory Findings: Laboratory tests are seldom necessary or helpful initially, although certain tests may be used later to assess and monitor treatment and to detect complications. Immediate emergency treatment should never be delayed pending results of laboratory studies. The blood cell counts may be elevated because of hemoconcentration. Eosinophil counts may be elevated but are usually normal or low because of the compensatory effect of endogenous or exogenous catecholamines and glucocorticoids. Chest x-ray shows hyperinflation, with or without areas of atelectasis caused by airway mucus plugging. The electrocardiogram may show a variety of abnormalities, including conduction abnormalities, atrial or ventricular dysrhythmias, ST-T wave changes of myocardial ischemia or injury, and acute cor pulmonale. Myocardial infarction may be evidenced by electrocardiographic and serum enzyme changes. Plasma histamine and serum tryptase levels may be elevated.

Clinical Diagnosis

The diagnosis of systemic anaphylaxis in a patient observed during an acute attack should be established or suspected as rapidly as possible by the symptoms and physical findings of hypotension, urticaria, angioedema, and laryngeal or bronchial obstruction, or any combination of these. Appropriate treatment should be instituted as soon as the condition is suspected. After the reaction is successfully treated, diagnostic efforts are directed to the cause.

Immunologic Diagnosis

The history is essential in determining the allergen responsible for an anaphylactic reaction. Skin testing or in vitro tests establish the presence of an IgE immune response to an allergen. This information is not in itself diagnostic but must be consistent with the history to establish the cause of the reaction. Ingestion of a food or drug; parenteral administration of a drug, vaccine, blood product, or other biologic material; or an insect sting occurring shortly (usually 1 hour or less) before the onset of symptoms raises suspicion that this is the cause. If the patient has experienced more than one episode, evidence of exposure to a common allergen should be sought.

Identification of the specific allergen may require persistent detective work. A reaction to drinking milk may be caused by penicillin contamination. A reaction to a viral vaccine may be caused by egg white from the egg embryo in which the virus was cultured. Occasionally, a reaction occurs after injection of two agents with anaphylactic potential (eg, penicillin and horse serum) or after a meal including several different "allergenic" foods, such as fish, legumes, nuts, or berries.

The diagnosis is confirmed by detecting the presence of **IgE antibody** to the suspected allergen. In most cases, the immediate wheal-and-flare skin test is the most reliable procedure, especially if the allergen is a protein. Systemic reactions to skin tests have occurred in highly sensitive individuals, so testing should be done initially by the cutaneous prick method. If the test is negative, intradermal testing to diluted sterile extracts of known potency can then be done.

To minimize the risk of anaphylaxis from the skin test itself, serial titration testing with 10-fold-increasing concentrations of allergen is recommended when testing with protein allergens. Table 28–1 lists several recommended starting concentrations.

Skin testing in cases of suspected Hymenoptera venom anaphylaxis has been shown to be reliable if freshly reconstituted lyophilized venom extracts are used for testing. Testing with standard food extracts may yield false-negative reactions if the allergen is labile. Prick testing with direct application of the food itself to the skin may yield a positive test, but some foods contain vasoactive chemicals that may produce false-positive reactions.

Skin testing with haptenic drugs is generally not reliable. Certain drugs cause nonspecific histamine release, producing a wheal-and-flare reaction in normal individuals (Table 28–2). Immunologic activation of mast cells requires a polyvalent allergen, so a negative skin test to a univalent haptenic drug does not rule out anaphylactic sensitivity to that drug.

Table 28–1. Starting intracutaneous skin test concentrations.

Allergen	Starting Concentration
Hymenoptera venoms	0.001 µg/mL
Insulin	0.001 U/mL
Horse serum	1:1000 dilution

Table 28–2. Drugs that cause nonspecific wheal-and-flare skin reactions.

Aspirin
Codeine
Curare
Histamine
Hydralazine
Meperidine
Morphine
Polymyxin B
Stilbamidine

Table 28–3. Some foods that cause anaphylaxis

Crustaceans	Seeds
Lobster	Sesame
Shrimp	Cottonseed
Crab	Caraway
Mollusks	Mustard
Clams	Flaxseed
Fish	Sunflower
	Nuts
Legumes	**Berries**
Peanut	**Egg white**
Pea	**Buckwheat**
Beans	**Milk**
Licorice	

IgE antibodies to major and minor penicillin allergy determinants are detected by wheal-and-flare skin tests. Penicilloyl-polylysine (6×10^{-5} M solution) elicits a positive skin test in most patients with "major determinant sensitivity," that is, a history of late urticaria or drug rash but not anaphylaxis. "Minor determinant sensitivity" indicates anaphylaxis to penicillin. The test mixture of minor penicillin allergy determinants is not presently marketed, although a skin test using penicillin G (1000 units/mL) is usually positive in persons with documented anaphylaxis. The test is not recommended if there is an unequivocal history of penicillin anaphylaxis, because of risk of anaphylaxis to the test.

In vitro tests to detect the presence of circulating IgE antibody may be helpful if the test is positive, but a negative result does not rule out anaphylactic sensitivity, because the high affinity of IgE antibodies for mast cell receptors may result in a level of circulating IgE antibodies too low for detection by in vitro methods. The radioallergosorbent test (RAST) is the most frequently used in vitro test for IgE antibody, but it can be used only for protein allergens. Technical factors account for a significant number of false-positive and false-negative results.

The presence of IgE antibodies, whether detected by a skin test or an in vitro test, does not diagnose the cause of anaphylaxis without correlation with the patient's history.

Allergens

The allergens responsible for anaphylaxis are different from those commonly associated with atopy. They are usually encountered in a food, a drug, or an insect sting. Foods and insect venoms are complex mixtures of many potential allergens. In only a few cases have the allergens been identified chemically. The same allergen or allergenic epitope may exist naturally in more than one food, drug, or venom, resulting in cross-reactivity.

A. Foods: Any food can contain an allergen that could cause anaphylaxis. Table 28–3 lists some of the more common ones. Peanuts, nuts, fish, and egg white lead the list in frequency.

B. Drugs: Any drug is capable of causing anaphylaxis, although the risk is minimal for most people. Table 28–4 lists drugs and diagnostic agents reported

to cause anaphylaxis in patients with drug-specific IgE antibody. Heterologous proteins and polypeptides are the most likely to induce this type of sensitivity. Most drugs used today are organic chemicals, however, which function immunologically as haptens. Anaphylaxis can occur from parenteral, oral, or topical drug administration. In some cases the amount needed to cause a systemic reaction can be extremely small; for example, a reaction in penicillin-allergic patients has been produced by minute amounts of penicillin in the milk obtained from penicillin-treated cows.

Anaphylaxis to blood and blood components may be caused by food allergens in donor blood or, rarely, by passive transfer of IgE antibodies to a food or drug when the transfusion recipient ingests that allergen shortly before or after the transfusion.

C. Insect Venoms: Anaphylaxis occurs from stings of Hymenoptera insects (Table 28–5), occasionally from biting insects such as deer flies, kissing bugs, and bedbugs, and rarely from snake venom. The venom of Hymenoptera insects is a complex biologic fluid containing several enzymes and other active

Table 28–4. Some drugs and diagnostic agents that cause anaphylaxis.

Heterologous proteins and polypeptides	Haptenic drugs
Hormones	Antibiotics
Insulin	Penicillin
Parathormone	Streptomycin
Adrenocorticotropic	Cephalosporin
hormone	Tetracycline
Vasopressin	Amphotericin B
Relaxin	Nitrofurantoin
Enzymes	Diagnostic agents
Trypsin	Sulfobromophthalein
Chymotrypsin	Sodium dehydrocholate
Chymopapain	Vitamins
Penicillinase	Thiamine
Asparaginase	Folic acid
Vaccines	Others
Toxoids	Barbiturates
Allergy extracts	Diazepam
Polysaccharides	Phenytoin
Dextran	Protamine
Iron-dextran	Aminopyrine
	Acetylcysteine
Acacia	

Table 28–5. Hymenoptera insects.

Honeybee (*Apis mellifera*)
Yellow jacket (*Vespula* spp)
Hornet (*Dolichovespula* spp)
Wasp (*Polistes* spp)
Fire ant (*Solenopsis* spp)

constituents. There are multiple allergens for human anaphylaxis, some specific to a particular species and others cross-reactive among species and genera. Allergens in honeybee venom include phospholipase A, hyaluronidase, phosphatase, and melittin.

The sting of a single insect is sufficient to produce a severe, even fatal anaphylactic reaction in sensitive patients. Sensitization occurs from prior stings, and if patients are allergic to a common or cross-reacting antigen they may have an anaphylactic reaction after being stung by any species of Hymenoptera insect. There is no evidence that other allergic diseases, including atopy and drug anaphylaxis, predispose to Hymenoptera anaphylaxis.

D. Other Allergens: Several cases of anaphylaxis have occurred in women during intercourse because of allergy to a glycoprotein allergen in seminal fluid. There is one report of a woman sensitized to exogenous progesterone administered as a drug. She subsequently had anaphylaxis to endogenous progesterone and was cured by oophorectomy.

Latex allergy is now a significant cause of anaphylaxis and contact urticaria among medical personnel and children with spina bifida or urogenital birth defects. The allergen is derived from the rubber tree *Hevea brasiliensis*. IgE antibodies in affected patients are detected best by skin test, and these patients must carefully avoid all sources of latex products.

Anaphylactoid Reactions

A reaction clinically and pathologically identical to anaphylaxis can occur without the participation of an IgE antibody and corresponding allergen. This phenomenon is called an anaphylactoid reaction. (The term "anaphylactoid" is sometimes used inappropriately to refer to a mild IgE-mediated anaphylactic reaction.)

A. Exercise-Induced "Anaphylaxis": A number of cases have been described. In some the reaction occurs only in association with eating, sometimes related to a specific food. During exercise the plasma histamine level rises, suggesting that nonimmunologic mast cell stimulation might be triggered by an endogenous factor, possibly endorphin. The reason for individual susceptibility is unknown, although a familial tendency has been reported, possibly because of a genetic defect. Many cases, however, are transient, suggesting a role for acquired factors.

B. Cholinergic Anaphylactoid Reaction. Exercise, emotions, and overheating provoke reactions in patients with this rare condition. The plasma histamine level rises when there is an increase in core body temperature. Patients may have a positive

methacholine urticarial skin test. A proposed mechanism is an abnormal reactivity of mast cells to the compensatory cholinergic response in thermoregulation when the core body temperature is elevated. This disease is an exaggerated form of cholinergic urticaria, described later in this chapter.

C. "Aggregate Anaphylaxis": Administration of gamma globulin for prophylaxis in patients with common variable immunodeficiency or other immunodeficiency diseases can cause anaphylactoid reactions. High-molecular-weight aggregated gamma globulin is probably responsible, since immunoglobulin aggregates can activate complement through the classic pathway. Ultracentrifugation of the preparation to eliminate aggregates prevents such reactions. Aggregated immunoglobulins generate anaphylatoxins C3a, C4a, and C5a from the parent complement components C3, C4, and C5, respectively, in a manner similar to the effect of antigen and corresponding specific IgG or IgM complement-activating antibodies. Anaphylatoxins are capable of activating mast cells for mediator release, thereby producing the anaphylactoid reaction.

D. Non-IgE Anaphylaxis: Some patients with selective absence of IgA produce IgG anti-IgA antibodies following transfusion of IgA-containing plasma in whole blood or blood products. In such patients, subsequent administration of transfused IgA may cause anaphylaxis, presumably from complement activation and anaphylatoxin generation by circulating complexes of IgA and anti-IgA. An alternative explanation would involve antibodies of the IgG4 subclass. Several laboratories have reported that IgG4 antibodies can activate mast cells for mediator release in the presence of antigen. There is no direct proof yet that IgG4 "short-term sensitizing" antibodies are involved in systemic anaphylaxis.

E. Anaphylactoid Reactions from Ionic Compounds: Radiographic iodinated contrast media, especially when used for intravenous pyelography or cholangiography, produce anaphylactoid reactions that are frequently mild, causing only hives or itching. They may be severe, however, causing shock. In one case in 100,000, these reactions are fatal. The reaction can occur on first exposure and does not necessarily recur on subsequent exposure. Attempts to demonstrate specific antibodies to the compounds have been unrewarding. The reaction may be related to the ionic nature of these compounds, since newer nonionic contrast media appear less likely to cause such reactions.

The antibiotic polymyxin B is also a highly charged ionic compound that causes anaphylactoid reactions in some patients.

F. Other Causes: Polysaccharides such as dextran, gums, and resins produce anaphylactoid reactions by unknown mechanisms, probably through direct mast cell activation. Certain drugs, especially the opiates, curare, and d-tubocurarine, behave similarly (Table 28–6).

Table 28–6. Drugs and additives that cause anaphylactoid reactions.

Nonsteroidal anti-inflammatory drugs
Aspirin
Aminopyrine
Fenoprofen
Flufenamic acid
Ibuprofen
Indomethacin
Mefenamic acid
Naproxen
Tolmetin
Zomepirac
Opiate narcotics
Morphine
Codeine
Meperidine
Mannitol
Radiographic iodinated contrast media
Curare and d-tubocurarine
Dextran

G. Idiopathic Anaphylaxis. A few patients experience recurrent attacks of anaphylaxis without evidence of exposure to an antecedent allergen. Exhaustive exploration of the history and careful observation of subsequent attacks sometimes reveal an unsuspected allergen, but most of these cases appear to be truly idiopathic. Recurrent idiopathic anaphylaxis, like idiopathic chronic urticaria-angioedema, occurs predominantly in women between 20 and 60 years of age.

Differential Diagnosis

Anaphylactic and anaphylactoid reactions are identical in presentation. The former is produced by an antigen–antibody reaction, whereas the latter is caused by nonimmunologic release of mediators, so that the distinction must be determined by demonstrating whether the causative substance is an allergen.

Anaphylactic shock must be differentiated from other causes of circulatory failure, including primary cardiac failure, endotoxin shock, and reflex mechanisms. The most common form of shock that simulates anaphylactic shock is vasovagal collapse, which may occur from the injection of local anaesthetics, particularly during dental procedures. In this case, there is pallor without cyanosis, nausea, bradycardia, and an absence of respiratory obstruction and cutaneous symptoms.

The Jarisch-Herxheimer reaction occurs several hours after antimicrobial treatment of syphilis or onchocerciasis. It is characterized by fever, shaking chills, myalgias, headaches, and hypotension. Unlike anaphylaxis, it can be prevented by pretreatment with corticosteroids.

Aspirin and nonsteroidal anti-inflammatory drugs affect a certain subset of asthmatic patients, producing an acute asthmatic reaction that may include nasal congestion, erythema, facial swelling, and shock. Sulfite additives in certain foods and drugs may affect some asthmatics with a similar anaphylactic-like reaction. These nonimmunologic phenomena are discussed in Chapter 27.

Treatment

Treatment of anaphylaxis and anaphylactoid reactions is the same. It must be started promptly, so a high index of suspicion is necessary, and the diagnosis must be made rapidly. Once anaphylaxis is suspected, **aqueous epinephrine,** 1:1000 solution, is injected intramuscularly or subcutaneously in a dose of 0.2–0.5 mL for adults or 0.01 mL/kg of body weight for children. The dose is repeated in 15–30 minutes, if necessary. If the reaction was caused by an insect sting or injected drug, 0.1–0.2 mL of epinephrine, 1:1000 solution, can be infiltrated locally to retard absorption of the residual allergen. When anaphylaxis occurs in a patient receiving a beta-adrenergic-blocking drug, the reaction may be especially resistant to epinephrine, so that higher doses may be required. A tourniquet should be applied proximally if the injection or sting is on an extremity. The patient should then be examined quickly but thoroughly to assess the involved target organs, so that subsequent treatment is appropriate to the physiopathologic abnormalities.

A. Shock: The patient should be recumbent with the legs elevated in Trendelenberg's position. An intravenous line, preferably by catheter, facilitates drug administration. Intravenous epinephrine can be given in a dose of 1–5 mL, 1:10,000 solution, for adults and 0.01–0.05 mL/kg for children if systolic blood pressure is below 60. Other vasopressor drugs, such as dopamine or glucagon, can be administered while blood pressure and pulse rate are being monitored. The specific treatment for shock, however, is fluid infused rapidly. Normal saline may be satisfactory, although as much as 6 L or more in 12 hours may be necessary. Initially, 1 L should be given every 15–30 minutes while vital signs and urine output are monitored. Plasma or other colloid solutions might be required. It may be necessary to monitor fluid replacement by measuring central venous pressure.

B. Laryngeal Edema: Examination of the airway for the presence of laryngeal obstruction should be done early. Establishing an effective airway is lifesaving. Passage of an endotracheal tube may be difficult because of the swelling. Puncture of the cricothyroid membrane with a 14- or 16-gauge short needle provides an airway, but it is too dangerous to attempt in a child. Cricothyrotomy is the preferred method if treatment must be done outside a hospital. In the hospital, surgical tracheostomy is preferred.

C. Bronchial Obstruction: The treatment is the same as for acute asthma. Intravenously, aminophyllin at 6 mg/kg in 20 mL of dextrose in water given over 10–15 minutes serves as a loading dose, to be followed by 0.9 mg/kg/h. If the patient is an asthmatic and is receiving theophylline currently, a lower dose is necessary, and theophyllin blood levels should be monitored. If bronchospasm persists, nebulized beta-adrenergic bronchodilators can be given by intermittent positive-pressure breathing. Hydrocortisone or methylprednisolone injections intramuscularly are used if the patient has recently received steroid therapy for asthma or for another condition. Oxygen by nasal catheter at 4–6 L/min is necessary in Pa_{CO_2} is less than 55 mm Hg. In the event of respiratory failure with Pa_{CO_2} above 65 mm Hg, intubation and mechanical assistance of ventilation are necessary.

D. Urticaria, Angioedema, and Gastrointestinal Reactions. These manifestations are not life-threatening and respond well to antihistamines. If they are mild, an oral antihistamine tablet is adequate. If they are severe, diphenhydramine, 50 mg (1–2 mg/kg for children), can be given intramuscularly or intravenously.

Monitoring treatment is vital in severe cases of anaphylaxis. Measurement of vital signs, examination of upper and lower airway potency, measurement of arterial blood gases, and electrocardiography are best accomplished in the emergency room or intensive care unit. All patients should be observed for 24 hours after satisfactory treatment, except in very mild cases.

Histamine H_2 receptor-blocking drugs, such as cimetidine or ranitidine, have been advocated as an adjunct to H_1 receptor antagonists, but their effectiveness has yet to be proven. Corticosteroid drugs have no antianaphylactic actions and should not be expected to alleviate the immediate acute life-threatening manifestations, although there may be special indications, as already noted. Complications such as cardiac arrhythmias, hypoxic seizures, and metabolic acidosis are treated in the usual way.

The management of anaphylaxis from a Hymenoptera insect sting is the same as for any anaphylactic reaction. In honeybee stings, the venom sac and stinger usually remain in the skin and should be removed promptly by scraping with a knife or fingernail. Local reactions usually require only cold compresses to ease pain and reduce swelling, but extensive local inflammation may require brief corticosteroid therapy.

Prevention

A. Avoidance. Once the diagnosis of anaphylaxis has been established and the cause has been determined, prevention of future episodes is essential. In the case of food or drug allergy, the allergen and potential cross-reacting allergens must be thoroughly avoided. Insect-sensitive patients should avoid outdoor food and garbage, flowers, perfumes, mowing the lawn, and walking barefoot outdoors. Pretreatment with antihistamines and corticosteroids prior to radiography requiring administration of a contrast medium reduces the risk of a reaction in patients who have experienced a prior radiographic anaphylactoid reaction. Patients with IgA deficiency who require blood products should be transfused from donors with absent IgA (see Chapter 21).

Any physician or nurse who administers drugs by injection should be prepared to treat a possible anaphylactic reaction by having appropriate drugs available, and patients should remain under observation for 15–20 minutes after any injection.

B. Anaphylaxis Kit: Patients with anaphylactic sensitivity to Hymenoptera insects or food should carry at all times a preloaded syringe of epinephrine in one of the commercially available preparations. Epinephrine or a beta-adrenergic drug in a metered-dose inhaler is not a reliable means of protection for anaphylactic shock.

C. Desensitization: Hymenoptera venom desensitization has been shown to be highly effective, as judged by responses to subsequent natural stings. Treatment is recommended for patients who have experienced systemic anaphylaxis after a sting and who have a significant positive skin test to one or more venoms. The maintenance dose for venom desensitization, 100 µg of each venom, is usually achieved in 12 weeks or less on a weekly, or "rush," schedule. It should be continued at intervals of 4–6 weeks indefinitely. Most patients maintain long-lasting protection after discontinuing the injections following a 5-year course of desensitization.

Insulin-allergic diabetic patients and the occasional penicillin-sensitive patient may require desensitization.

Complications

Death from laryngeal edema, respiratory failure, shock, or cardiac arrhythmia usually occurs within minutes after onset of the reaction, but in occasional cases irreversible shock persists for hours. Permanent brain damage may result from the hypoxia of respiratory or cardiovascular failure. Urticaria or angioedema may recur for months after penicillin anaphylaxis. Myocardial infarction, abortion, and renal failure are other potential complications.

Prognosis

It is usually assumed that in anaphylaxis each succeeding exposure results in a more severe reaction. Experience with cases of anaphylaxis to penicillin, Hymenoptera venom, and food indicates that this not necessarily the case, however. If sufficient time elapses without allergen exposure, there may be a decrease or loss of sensitivity in some patients. There is no method to predict changes in sensitivity, but it can sometimes be documented by periodic testing. Immunotherapy for stinging-insect sensitivity is strikingly effective in favorably altering the prognosis, and desensitization can occasionally abrogate penicillin anaphylaxis for a short time to permit the drug to be used safely. The prognosis must always be guarded by the knowledge that IgE immunologic memory may be lifelong. Anaphylactoid drug reactions follow various courses. Patients who react adversely to radiographic iodinated contrast media usually tolerate subsequent exposure to the same contrast medium without reaction, but statistically a reaction is more likely to occur in a patient who had experienced a prior reaction.

URTICARIA & ANGIOEDEMA

Major Immunologic Features
- Acute urticaria–angioedema is a cutaneous form of anaphylaxis.
- IgE-mediated allergies to foods or drugs are common causes.
- Chronic or recurrent disease is usually nonimmunologic and of unknown cause.

General Considerations
Urticaria (also known as hives) and angioedema (also known as angioneurotic edema) can be considered a single illness characterized by vasodilatation and increased vascular permeability of the skin (urticaria) or subcutaneous tissues (angioedema). It is a localized cutaneous form of anaphylaxis and is one of the manifestations of systemic anaphylaxis. The same **IgE antibody** mechanism is responsible for the pathogenesis of allergic urticaria–angioedema and for that of systemic anaphylaxis, and the causative allergens are very similar. Idiopathic (nonallergic) urticaria–angioedema is analogous to the anaphylactoid reaction. In contrast to anaphylaxis, urticaria is a benign condition and is much more common.

A. Epidemiology: Urticaria affects about 20% of the population, usually as a single or occasional acute attack.

B. Pathology: A variety of histopathologic lesions have been described, but these correlate poorly with the clinical presentation. They include edema, nonnecrotizing vasculitis, necrotizing vasculitis, perivasculitis, and a variety of different inflammatory reactions in the skin.

C. Pathogenesis: Urticaria and angioedema are the visible manifestations of localized cutaneous or subcutaneous edema from the increased permeability of blood vessels, probably postcapillary venules. Since injection of histamine into the skin produces the spontaneous wheal, erythema, and pruritus of a typical urticarial lesion, it is generally accepted that endogenous histamine liberation is the mechanism responsible for the disease. The fact that subcutaneous tissue is looser and contains fewer nerve endings explains the more diffuse swelling and less severe itching in angioedema. Elevated levels of histamine in venous blood draining areas of induced urticaria have been repeatedly demonstrated. Other mediators from mast cells, particularly leukotrienes, are also believed to contribute to the pathophysiology.

D. Immunologic Pathogenesis: Many cases of acute urticaria and angioedema have been shown to have an allergic cause. In these cases, allergen-specific IgE antibody fixed to local mast cells triggers mediator release or activation when allergen is encountered.

Other potential immunologic pathways for mast cell mediator liberation, for example, the complement-derived anaphylatoxin pathway, have not been shown to operate in this disease. Idiopathic urticaria–angioedema and the various physical urticarias described below lack an allergen–antibody etiology. The precise means by which cutaneous mast cells are stimulated under these circumstances is unknown.

Clinical Features
A. Symptoms and Signs: Urticaria appears as multiple areas of well-demarcated edematous plaques that are intensely pruritic. They are either white with surrounding erythema or red with blanching when stretched. Individual lesions vary in diameter from a few millimeters to many centimeters. They are circular or serpiginous. Regardless of the duration of the illness, individual lesions are evanescent, lasting from 1 to 48 hours. They may appear anywhere on the skin surface but often have a predilection for areas of pressure. Angioedema appears as diffuse areas of nondependent, nonpitting swelling without pruritus, with predilection for the face, especially the periorbital and perioral areas. Swelling can occur in the mouth and pharynx as well.

Acute urticaria lasts for a few hours or at most a few days and is most likely to be associated with an identifiable cause, including allergy, nonspecific drug effect, infection, or physical factors. Chronic or recurrent urticaria persists with a variable course over a period of many weeks to years. Urticaria and angioedema may appear together in the same patient.

B. Laboratory Findings: There are no abnormal laboratory tests, except for the specific procedures described in a later section.

Clinical Diagnosis
The diagnosis is immediately apparent on inspection of the skin.

Immunologic Diagnosis
A complete medical and environmental history and physical examination are usually necessary to determine the cause. Allergic urticaria may arise from exposure to allergens by ingestion or injection (most commonly), direct skin contact (less frequently), and inhalation (rarely). The discussion on common allergies in anaphylaxis earlier in this chapter applies to acute allergic urticaria.

Food allergy is diagnosed by careful dietary history, use of elimination diets, and appropriate food challenges. Drug allergy requires close scrutiny of the patient's recent drug history, elimination of suspected drugs, and occasionally deliberate challenge, although skin testing is helpful for certain drugs such as penicillin. The diagnosis of cold urticaria is made by applying an ice cube to the forearm for 5 minutes and observing localized urticaria after the skin has been rewarmed. Similar tests with application of heat, ultraviolet light, vibration, pressure, or water to a test area of the skin are appropriate if the history suggests these causes.

Cholinergic urticaria is suggested by the typical appearance of the lesions and exercise provocation. The methacholine skin test is positive in only one third of patients.

Diagnostic tests for parasitic or other infections, lymphomas or other neoplasms, or connective tissue diseases are generally indicated if the history and physical examination would have suggested such diseases in the absence of urticaria. It should be emphasized that in most cases of chronic recurrent urticaria, no cause is found even with the most diligent search.

Causes

A. Allergy: Ingestant allergens are much more frequent causes of urticaria than are inhalants. Any food or drug can cause hives. Occult sources of drugs including proprietary medications, such as laxatives, headache remedies, and vitamin preparations, must be considered. Food and drug additives are occasionally responsible. Insect sting allergy may cause urticaria without any other signs of systemic anaphylaxis.

B. Physical Causes: Dermographism, the whealing reaction that is an exaggerated form of the triple response of Lewis, occurs following scratching or stroking of the skin in 5% of the population. Another common phenomenon, unrelated to dermographism, is the appearance of hives after showering.

Cold urticaria may be induced locally by cooling of the skin on contact with cold. The hives often appear only upon rewarming. Occasionally generalized hives are provoked by cooling a portion of the body. Patients are in danger of shock when swimming in cold water. The diagnostic ice cube test was already described. Occasionally the reaction can be passively transferred by serum to the skin of an unaffected individual.

Familial cold urticaria is a rare autosomal-dominant disorder in which cold produces fever, chills, joint pains, and hives.

Urticaria and angioedema induced by heat, sunlight, water, or vibration are different syndromes and are rare. Pressure urticaria is a common feature of all forms of urticaria. Delayed-pressure urticaria resulting from prolonged sustained pressure producing painful swelling is a distinct entity, however.

Cholinergic urticaria is a disease of unknown cause in which small (1–3-mm) wheals with prominent surrounding flare appear after exercise, heat, or emotional stress. Elevated body temperature is necessary for the reaction, which is believed to be initiated by a cholinergic response that triggers mast cell release. Other symptoms, including hypotension and gastrointestinal cramping, may accompany the urticaria and angioedema.

C. Vasculitis: Urticaria is reported as a symptom in some patients with systemic lupus erythematosus (SLE), systemic sclerosis, polymyositis, leukocytoclastic vasculitis, palpable purpura, hypocomplementemia, or cryoglobulinemia, but there is as yet no clear explanation for the association.

D. Neoplasms: Urticaria or angioedema is occasionally reported in a patient with neoplasm, especially Hodgkin's disease and lymphomas, but a cause-and-effect relationship is difficult to document. Rarely, angioedema from C1 esterase deficiency is caused by a lymphoma. This is discussed in Chapter 25.

E. Cyclooxygenase Inhibitors: Aspirin and nonsteroidal anti-inflammatory drugs frequently precipitate acute or chronic urticaria. They also potentiate idiopathic urticaria or urticaria from other causes. The mechanism is unknown. There are many reports that food and drug additives, most notably tartrazine yellow dye and the preservative sodium benzoate, also cause or exacerbate hives, but the evidence is unimpressive.

F. Emotions: Precipitation of hives by emotional stress or other psychologic factors is a frequent clinical observation. Explanation of this phenomenon requires further study.

G. Idiopathic Urticaria–Angioedema: This category encompasses most cases of chronic urticaria–angioedema, because exhaustive diagnostic studies are unrevealing in the large majority of patients with recurrent urticaria lasting for more than 6 weeks.

Differential Diagnosis

The characteristic appearance of urticaria and angioedema, coupled with a history of rapid disappearance of the individual lesions, leaves little chance of incorrect diagnosis.

Multiple insect bites may evoke wheals, but careful inspection shows the bite punctum at the center of the lesion. Angioedema can be distinguished from ordinary edema or myxedema by its absence from dependent areas of localization and by its evanescent appearance.

Hereditary angioedema is a rare condition that produces periodic swelling and may be accompanied by abdominal pain and laryngeal edema. Urticaria does not occur in this disease. The disease is suspected when there is a similar family history of recurrent episodes unrelated to exposure to allergens. The diagnosis is made by finding decreased serum C4 and is confirmed by the absence of C1 esterase inhibitor activity in the serum. It is described in greater detail in Chapter 25.

Urticaria pigmentosa is an infiltration of the skin with multiple mast cell tumors that appear as tan macules which urticate when rubbed or stroked. It may be accompanied by visceral mast cell tumors (systemic mastocytosis).

Treatment

Urticaria caused by foods or drugs is treated by avoidance of the offending agents, although hyposensitization to a drug might be attempted in the rare instances in which no alternative drug is available. Urticaria associated with infection is self-limited if the infection is adequately treated. In cases of physical allergy, protective measures to avoid heat, sunlight, or cold must be advised.

Drug therapy is a useful adjunct in the treatment of all patients, whether or not the cause has been found, but a good response to symptomatic treatment should not deter the physician from efforts to find an underlying cause. Antihistamine drugs are the principal method of treatment, but they must be given in adequate dosage. H_1 receptor antagonists have a proven but inconsistent effectiveness in treating urticaria. The combined use of H_1 and H_2 receptor blockers is frequently recommended but of unproven value for this disease. Epinephrine injections may relieve hives transiently and should be used in treating angioedema involving the pharynx or larynx. Corticosteroids are usually ineffective and should not be used to treat urticaria of unknown cause.

Complications & Prognosis

Urticaria per se is a benign disease. Since allergic urticaria is a cutaneous form of anaphylaxis, it is possible that an excessive dose of allergen could result in life-threatening systemic anaphylaxis. This is also possible in certain cases of physical urticaria. Angioedema can obstruct the airway if localized in the larynx or adjacent structures.

REFERENCES

ANAPHYLAXIS

Briner WW Jr, Sheffer AL: Exercise-induced anaphylaxis. *Med Sci Sports Exerc* 1992;**24**:840.

Reisman RE, Lieberman P: Anaphylaxis and anaphylactoid reactions. *Immunol Allergy Clin North Am* 1992;**12**:501 (Entire issue).

Slater J: Latex allergy—what do we know? *J Allergy Clin Immunol* 1992;**90**:3.

Smith PL et al: Physiologic manifestations of human anaphylaxis. *J Clin Invest* 1980;**66**:1072.

Steiner DJ, Schwager RG: Epidemiology, diagnosis, precautions, and policies of intraoperative anaphylaxis to latex. *J Am Coll Surg* 1995;**180**:754.

Valentine MD: Insect venom allergy: Diagnosis and treatment. *J Allergy Clin Immunol* 1984;**73**:299.

Wiggins CA et al: Idiopathic anaphylaxis: Classification, evaluation and treatment of 123 patients. *J Allergy Clin Immunol* 1988;**82**:849.

Yunginger JW: Anaphylaxis. *Ann Allergy* 1992;**69**:87.

URTICARIA & ANGIOEDEMA

Hirschmann JV et al: Cholinergic urticaria. *Arch Dermatol* 1987;**123**:462.

Kauppinen I et al: Yearbook: Urticaria in children: Retrospective evaluation and follow-up. *Allergy* 1984;**39**:469.

Matthews KP: Urticaria and angioedema. *J Allergy Clin Immunol* 1983;**72**:1.

Soter NA, Wasserman SI: Physical urticaria/angioedema: An experimental model of mast cells activation in humans. *J Allergy Clin Immunol* 1980;**66**:358.

Wanderer AA et al: Clinical characteristics of cold-induced systemic reactions acquired in cold urticaria syndromes: Recommendations for prevention of this complication and a proposal for a diagnostic classification of cold urticaria. *J Allergy Clin Immunol* 1986;**78**:417.

Immune-Complex Allergic Diseases 29

Abba I. Terr, MD

This chapter discusses allergic diseases mediated by immune complexes of allergen with IgG or IgM antibodies. Activation of complement by immune complexes generates chemotactic and vasoactive mediators that cause tissue damage by a combination of immune-complex deposition, alterations in vascular permeability and blood flow, and the action of toxic products from inflammatory cells. The pathology of immune complexes has been extensively studied in animals, and the process is detailed in Chapter 13. Tissue injury caused by immune complexes is believed to occur also in certain nonallergic diseases discussed elsewhere in this book. These include systemic lupus erythematosus (see Chapter 33), vasculitis (see Chapter 36), glomerulonephritis (see Chapter 38), rheumatoid arthritis (see Chapter 33), and acute allograft rejection (see Chapter 57).

The classic immune-complex allergic diseases are the cutaneous **Arthus reaction** and systemic **serum sickness.** In allergic bronchopulmonary aspergillosis a two-phase immunologic mechanism is involved, in which immune complexes of *Aspergillus* antigens and IgG antibodies produce bronchial inflammation and bronchopulmonary tissue destruction in the presence of a concomitant IgE response to the allergen.

THE ARTHUS REACTION

In 1903, Nicholas-Maurice Arthus showed that the intradermal injection of a protein antigen into a hyperimmunized rabbit produced local inflammation that progressed to a hemorrhagic necrotic ulcerating skin lesion. Later investigations established that the Arthus phenomenon is a localized cutaneous inflammatory response to the deposition of immune complexes in dermal blood vessels. It therefore serves as a model system for all immune complex-mediated diseases.

Arthus reactions are rare in humans. Hemorrhagic necrosis at the site of injection of a drug or an insect bite or sting could suggest an Arthus reaction, but the distinction from a toxic reaction or secondary infection requires laboratory or immunohistochemical evidence of the presence of the relevant immune complexes. A limited form of the Arthus reaction occurs commonly at the site of allergy desensitization injections after sufficient doses of injected allergens have been given to generate IgG-"blocking" antibodies (see Chapter 56). Because the level of IgG antibodies achieved in allergy therapy is relatively low, the cutaneous and subcutaneous tissue inflammation produces only mild erythema and induration. This begins several hours after the injection and usually subsides in less than 24 hours.

The immunologic pathogenesis depends on antigen and antibody concentrations necessary to form immune complexes capable of initiating complement activation. Intermediate-size complexes activate complement most readily and therefore are the most damaging to tissues. Large insoluble complexes are rapidly cleared by the mononuclear phagocytes, whereas small complexes fail to activate complement receptors. Immune complexes activate complement through fixation of the Fc portion of antibody to the Fc receptor on C1q. C3a and C5a anaphylatoxins are liberated. These molecules activate mast cells to release permeability factors, permitting localization of the immune complexes along the endothelial cell basement membrane. Chemotactic factors from various complement components attract neutrophils. Neutrophils, macrophages, lymphocytes, and other cells with membrane Fc receptors are activated. The activated neutrophils are especially important in the Arthus reaction. They release toxic chemicals such as oxygen-containing free radicals, generate proteolytic enzymes from cytoplasmic granules, and phagocytose the immune complexes.

SERUM SICKNESS

Major Immunologic Features

- Serum sickness is a systemic immune-complex complement-dependent reaction to an extrinsic antigen.
- The severity of the disease is antigen dose-dependent.
- The typical reaction produced by heterologous serum can occur in milder forms from other drugs.

General Considerations

Serum sickness was a common disease in the pre-antibiotic era when heterologous antiserum was used as passive immunization in the treatment of a number of infectious and toxic illnesses. Today, specific "serum therapy" with heterologous (usually equine) serum or gamma globulin is restricted to passive immunization for a very few toxic diseases and the use of antilymphocyte or antithymocyte globulin for immunosuppressive therapy. Vaccines, other protein drugs, and bee stings may cause serum sickness. A mild serum sickness reaction is occasionally caused by nonprotein drugs, especially sulfonamides, penicillin, and cephalosporins.

A. Definition. Serum sickness is an acute, self-limited allergic disease caused by immune complex-activated complement-generated inflammation after injection of a protein or haptenic drug. The cardinal features are fever, dermatitis, lymphadenopathy, and joint pains.

B. Epidemiology. Serum sickness is caused by the therapeutic injection of foreign material that is potentially antigenic as well as therapeutic. Therefore, the prevalence of this disease depends on the prevalence of certain forms of medical treatment. Therapeutic injections or large quantities of heterologous serum produce serum sickness in proportion to the dose. The attack rate was approximately 90% when a 200-mL dose of horse serum was given. Fractionated gamma globulin is less likely than whole serum to cause the disease. There are no prevalence statistics available today, but reports of serum sickness are now uncommon.

C. Immunologic Pathogenesis: The pathogenesis of human serum sickness is believed to be similar to the mechanism of "one-shot" serum sickness produced experimentally in immunized rabbits (Fig 29–1). Following a single large dose of injected antigen there is a brief period of equilibration between blood and tissues followed by slow degradation of antigen over several days as the primary antibody response is initiated. Antibody synthesis leads to release of antibody into the circulation, where antigen–antibody complexes gradually form under conditions of moderate antigen excess. Intermediate-sized complexes deposit in small blood vessels in various organs, triggering the events previously described for the Arthus reaction. This gives rise to the clinical and pathologic manifestations of disease. Free antigen is

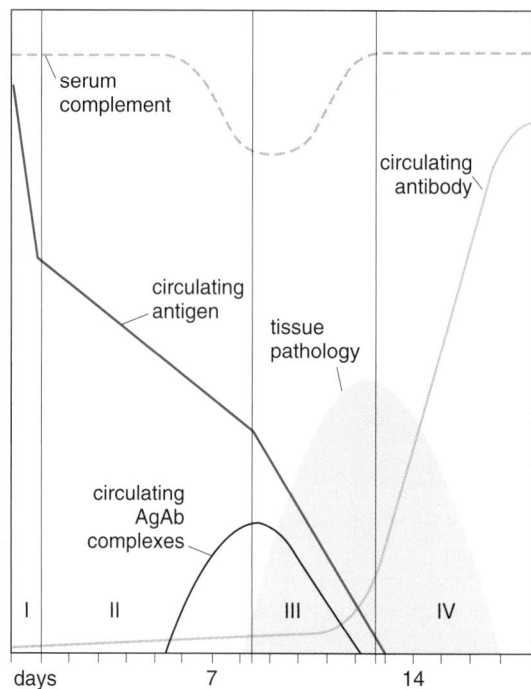

Figure 29–1. Immunologic events in experimental "one-shot" serum sickness in rabbits. The pathogenesis of human serum sickness is similar. A single high dose of antigen is given intravenously on day 0. **Phase I:** Equilibration of antigen between blood and tissues. **Phase II:** Primary antibody response. Near the end of this phase, antibody combines with antigen to form circulating immune complexes. **Phase III:** Tissue pathology and progression of clinical disease. Circulating complexes activate complement and deposit in tissues. The serum complement level falls transiently, and residual antigen is rapidly cleared from the blood. **Phase IV:** Remission. Antigen is no longer available, and the level of circulating antibody rises. No further immune complexes form, complement levels return to normal, pathologic lesions repair, and symptoms subside.

removed more rapidly from the circulation as antibody production and immune-complex formation increases. The circulating complexes then shift to antibody excess, thereby decreasing in size and clearing more rapidly. Finally, free antibody circulates, no further lesions appear, and healing takes place.

The optimal conditions for serum sickness occur during the primary antibody response of the previously immunized host. With subsequent exposures to the same antigen, the anamnestic antibody response facilitates rapid antigen clearance and greatly reduces the amount and persistence of immune complexes in the circulation.

Clinical Features

A. Symptoms and Signs: Primary serum sickness begins 4–21 days (usually 7–10 days) after initial exposure to the causative antigen. The first sign is often a pruritic rash, which may be urticarial, maculopapular, or erythematous. There may be angioedema, and the injection site usually becomes inflamed. Fever, lymphadenopathy, arthralgias, and myalgias complete the clinical presentation. Joint swelling and redness may occur, and occasionally there are headache, nausea, and vomiting. Recovery takes 7–30 days. Clinically significant cardiac or renal involvement is unusual. There may be neurologic manifestations, usually in the form of mononeuritis involving especially the brachial plexus. Rarely there may be polyneuritis, Guillain-Barré syndrome, or even meningoencephalitis.

Secondary serum sickness occurs in patients previously sensitized to the antigen. There is a short latent period of only 2–4 days, and the clinical course of the disease may be brief but the manifestations could be severe.

Serum sickness reactions to most drugs used today are much milder than the disease that was caused by horse serum injections.

B. Laboratory Findings: There is slight leukocytosis. Plasma cells in the bone marrow are increased in number and may appear in the blood. There may be eosinophilia, but this is not characteristic. The erythrocyte sedimentation rate is increased. Circulating immune complexes and reduced levels of serum complement components are often detected in disease caused by heterologous serum, but they are not usually detected in drug-induced serum sickness (for detection methods, see Chapter 14). Mild proteinuria, hematuria, and casts; transient electrocardiographic abnormalities; and pleocytosis are not unusual.

Immunologic Diagnosis

There is no specific diagnostic test. The diagnosis is made on the basis of a compatible history of typical symptoms at an appropriate interval after drug administration, along with the physical and laboratory evidence. The disease is almost always benign and self-limited, with good prospects for complete recovery, so invasive tests such as tissue biopsy are not indicated.

Serum IgG and IgE antibodies specific to the relevant antigen may be detected in the time course illustrated in Figure 29–1 if confirmation of the diagnosis is required.

Treatment

Treatment should be conservative and symptomatic. Aspirin and antihistamines are effective. A short high-dose course of oral corticosteroids is warranted if symptoms are severe.

Complications & Prognosis

Complications are rare. Occasionally laryngeal edema may cause respiratory obstruction. The neuritis rarely is permanent.

ALLERGIC BRONCHOPULMONARY ASPERGILLOSIS

Major Immunologic Features

■ Both IgE and IgG antibodies to *Aspergillus* are involved in the pathogenesis of pulmonary disease.
■ IgE antibodies are directed to spore allergens.
■ IgG antibodies are directed to mycelial allergens.
■ There is nonspecific elevation of serum IgE level during acute exacerbations of disease.

General Considerations

Allergic bronchopulmonary aspergillosis (ABPA) is an unusual but not rare illness that affects young atopic adults with allergic asthma. It is caused by a concomitant IgE and IgG antibody response to the ubiquitous fungus *Aspergillus fumigatus.* Airborne spores of this organism prevail both indoors and outdoors year-round in many geographic areas. The disease may occur in infants and children. It causes bronchiectasis and other destructive lung changes, but tissue damage can be prevented if the condition is diagnosed and treated properly.

A. Epidemiology: It is estimated that ABPA occurs in 1–2% of patients with asthma. Most cases have been reported in the USA and United Kingdom, but the disease probably occurs throughout the world. With rare exceptions, it is a disease of persons with atopic asthma, but it is also associated with cystic fibrosis. It has not been reported as an occupational disease. There is no known genetic predilection other than that related to atopy, and no human leukocyte antigen (HLA) association has yet been confirmed.

B. Immunologic Pathogenesis: *A fumigatus* is ubiquitous in the air and soil, and it may be found indoors where moisture and organic matter favor mold growth. Occasional cases are caused by *A ochraceous* or *A terreus.* Exposure to *Aspergillus* is universal, but there is no evidence that excessive environmental exposure causes the disease. High-dose exposure, however, may trigger acute attacks in the sensitized subject.

The pathogenesis of the disease is not entirely clear. There is consensus that ABPA is an allergic disease that requires both IgE and IgG antibodies to *Aspergillus* and that their corresponding immunologic effector mechanisms of inflammation result in the observed tissue damage (see Chapter 12). Inhalation of *Aspergillus* spores causes an immediate IgE-mediated bronchospastic reaction to an allergen in the spore, thereby trapping the organisms in the intraluminal mucus of the larger proximal bronchi. When the spores germinate and produce mycelia, the reaction of IgG antibodies to a different mycelial antigen produces tissue damage and inflammation, probably from immune complex-activated complement-derived products. Repeated episodes weaken the bronchial wall, leading to focal bronchiectasis. The significance of pathologic evidence of T-cell-mediated inflammation in disease pathogenesis is unknown. The inflammatory process extends to peribronchial lung parenchyma, causing acute inflammatory infiltrates and ultimately chronic parenchymal destruction and fibrosis.

C. Pathology: The disease is confined to the lungs, where pathologic effects are two-fold: those of the underlying asthma, and those associated with the acute inflammatory episodes and its sequelae. *Aspergillus* hyphae and inflammatory cells can be found in mucus plugs. The adjacent bronchial wall is infiltrated with mononuclear cells and eosinophils. A similar infiltrate affects peribronchial tissues, producing areas of interstitial pneumonia. There is a notable absence of granulocytic inflammation and vasculitis. Immunofluorescence studies have generally not shown immune-complex deposits in the lung, although these have been demonstrated in the late-onset skin test site in this disease (see later discussion). The reason for this discrepancy, which weakens the argument for immune-complex pathogenesis, is not clear, but it may reflect the timing of the biopsy studies. Areas of chronic inflammation show noncaseating granulomas. Bronchiectasis and pulmonary fibrosis are late effects in the disease. The pathology, like the clinical manifestations, is variable.

Clinical Features

A. Symptoms and Signs: The clinical picture of ABPA is that of asthma with superimposed acute episodes of fever, cough productive of mucus plugs, chest pains, and malaise. There may be hemoptysis. Other nonspecific symptoms include headache, arthralgias, and myalgias. Some patients present with chronic lung damage, which suggests that the acute inflammatory episodes may be asymptomatic. Physical findings are those of asthma, as well as rales in the presence of pulmonary infiltration.

B. Laboratory Findings: The diagnosis of ABPA is readily confirmed by objective evidence for the appropriate immune responses. Intradermal skin testing elicits an initial IgE antibody-mediated wheal-and-flare reaction to *A fumigatus* extract, followed by an Arthus reaction. Immunofluorescence at the height of the late response 6–12 hours after the intradermal injection reveals deposition of immunoglobulins and C3, distinguishing this response from a late-phase IgE reaction. Prick testing may not be sensitive enough to elicit the IgG antibody Arthus response, but it is usually sufficient for detecting the immediate IgE wheal-and-flare.

Serum precipitins to *Aspergillus* are found in about 70% of cases, and most of the remainder is positive if the serum is concentrated fivefold. IgG and IgE antibodies in serum can also be detected by radioallergosorbent test (RAST) or enzyme-linked immunosorbent assay (ELISA), but the extremely high sensitivities of these techniques results in low specificity for diagnosis of disease.

The total serum IgE level is characteristically high in ABPA, and the level varies directly with disease activity. The mechanism for this is not known, but IgE levels have important diagnostic and prognostic significance. The majority of the excess IgE cannot be accounted for by *Aspergillus*-specific antibody. Eosinophilia is present in blood and sputum, as it is in any case of asthma. Smear and culture of mucus plugs or sputum may yield the *Aspergillus* organism.

Pulmonary function testing reveals reversible airway obstruction, but the acute inflammatory episodes can be distinguished from simple asthma by reduction in diffusing capacity. In chronic disease, obstruction may be only partially reversible and a restrictive component may be prominent. Bronchial provocation testing with *Aspergillus* extract produces a dual immediate bronchospastic component followed by a late-phase obstructive–restrictive component accompanied by fever and leukocytosis (see Fig 26–3).

The chest x-ray may show a variety of abnormalities but it may also be normal. There is no pathognomonic radiologic finding in this disease. Abnormalities that do occur may be found in many other lung diseases. During the acute phase, mucus plugs may produce focal areas of atelectasis or even segmental or lobar collapse. The peribronchial inflammation appears as migratory infiltrates, especially in the upper lobes and hilar areas. Chronic disease from repeated acute insults can cause volume loss, particularly in the upper lobes. Bronchiectasis revealed by bronchography or tomography is saccular and proximal, less commonly cylindrical.

Clinical Diagnosis

The diagnosis of ABPA is made on the basis of certain clinical and laboratory findings. There is no single diagnostic test. Table 29–1 lists diagnostic criteria. The diagnosis is definite when all seven major criteria are met and probable when six are met. All major and minor criteria can be found in other illnesses, but the critical importance of a definitive diagnosis is that it alerts the clinician to the need for corticosteroid therapy to prevent irreversible pulmonary damage. Any patient with a history of asthma and recurrent pulmonary infiltrates not otherwise explained should be given a

Table 29–1. Diagnostic criteria for ABPA.

Major criteria
1. Episodic bronchial obstruction.
2. Peripheral blood eosinophilia.
3. Positive immediate skin reactivity.
4. Serum precipitating antibodies.
5. Elevated serum IgE.
6. History of pulmonary infiltrates.
7. Central bronchiectasis.

Minor criteria
1. *A fumigatus*-positive sputum culture.
2. History of expectorating brown plugs or flecks.
3. Arthus' (late) skin reactivity.

Source: Reproduced, with permission, from Slavin RG: Allergic-bronchopulmonary aspergillosis. *Clin Rev Allergy* 1985;**3:**167.

diagnostic skin test with *Aspergillus*. Absence of the immediate reaction virtually rules out ABPA, but if the test is positive, a search for serum precipitins and radiographic evidence of bronchiectasis is indicated.

Differential Diagnosis

A fumigatus can cause other respiratory diseases. Invasive aspergillosis is an opportunistic infection that may complicate immunosuppression caused by drugs or disease (as discussed in Chapter 58). Aspergilloma is a localized growth of the organism invading a lung cavity or cyst. It typically induces a very marked precipitating antibody response, with a negative Arthus skin test, probably because of antibody excess at the skin site. *Aspergillus* hypersensitivity pneumonitis is a rare cause of farmer's lung. Finally, the organism is an atopic allergen in some cases of allergic asthma.

The variable clinical and radiologic features of the disease mimic other pulmonary diseases, including asthma with periodic mucus plugging or intercurrent viral infections, tuberculosis, hypersensitivity pneumonitis, pulmonary infiltration with eosinophilia (PIE syndrome), mucoid impaction, and bronchocentric granulomatosis.

ABPA in Cystic Fibrosis

By using the criteria of Table 29–1, the diagnosis of ABPA is made more frequently in children with cystic fibrosis than in the atopic asthmatic population. It is difficult to be sure whether this reflects a fundamental predisposition or a secondary opportunistic effect. Both atopy and *Aspergillus* infections are prevalent in children with cystic fibrosis, setting the stage for the necessary immune response involved in the pathogenesis of ABPA. Markedly elevated and fluctuating serum IgE levels, eosinophilia, and dramatic x-ray resolution of infiltrates with corticosteroid treatment are important diagnostic clues that ABPA is present in this disease.

Treatment

A definitive diagnosis is important, because prompt high-dose systemic corticosteroid therapy causes prompt resolution of the acute allergic inflammatory episode and prevents the occurrence of long-term irreversible bronchial and parenchymal lung damage. The mechanism of the therapeutic effect can only be surmised, but it is probably anti-inflammatory rather than immunosuppressive. An initial dose of 60 mg of

prednisone daily in divided doses should be maintained until there is clinical and radiologic cure of the episode, after which a slowly tapering dose with maintenance at 20–30 mg once on alternate days should prevent relapses. It is useful to monitor total serum IgE levels, which fall during remissions and rise again with recurrences. There is some evidence that the serum IgE rise might precede the clinical exacerbation. Serial chest x-rays should also be part of the monitoring process.

The concurrent asthma is treated in the standard fashion, including desensitization if indicated. Injections of *Aspergillus* extract, however, should probably be avoided because this might theoretically enhance the IgG antibody response and hence worsen the disease. Inhaled corticosteroids are not indicated for acute attacks, but they can be used to control the asthma between attacks. Chest physiotherapy and inhaled bronchodilators are helpful adjuncts to improve expectoration of mucus plugs, but antifungal drugs are of unproven benefit.

Complications & Prognosis

Table 29–2 is a scheme for staging untreated disease. The course is variable and unpredictable and may depend on factors of environmental exposure, so that not all patients proceed through all stages. Nevertheless, early recognition and adequate treatment prevent deterioration in pulmonary function and subsequent development of chronic airway obstruction and restrictive disease with pulmonary fibrosis. Occasionally, aspergilloma develops in a bronchiectatic or emphysematous cyst in ABPA. Cor pulmonale is likely to occur in stage V disease.

Table 29–2. Proposed stages of increasing severity and chronicity in ABPA.

Stage	Description
I	Acute episode responsive to systemic corticosteroids.
II	Remission.
III	Recurrent exacerbations.
IV	Recurrent exacerbations with steroid-dependent severe asthma.
V	Pulmonary fibrosis, irreversible obstruction, advanced x-ray changes, cavitation and upper lobe contraction, severe bronchiectasis, emphysema.

Source: Reproduced, with permission, from Patterson, R et al: Allergic bronchopulmonary aspergillosis: Staging as an aid to management. *Ann Intern Med* 1982;**96:**286.

REFERENCES

SERUM SICKNESS

Bielory L et al: Human serum sickness: A prospective analysis of 35 patients treated with equine antithymocyte globulin for bone marrow failure. *Medicine* 1988;**67**:40.

Erffmeyer JE: Serum sickness. *Ann Allergy* 1986;**56**:105.

Naguwa SM, Nelson BL: Human serum sickness. *Clin Rev Allergy* 1985;**3**:117.

ALLERGIC BRONCHOPULMONARY ASPERGILLOSIS

Greenberger PA, Patterson R: Allergic bronchopulmonary aspergillosis and the evaluation of the patient with asthma. *J Allergy Clin Immunol* 1988;**81**:646.

Greenberger PA: Diagnosis and management of allergic bronchopulmonary aspergillosis. *Allergy Proc* 1994;**15**:335.

Knutsen AP, Slavin RG: Allergic bronchopulmonary aspergillosis in patients with cystic fibrosis. *Clin Rev Allergy* 1991;**9**:103.

Patterson R et al: Allergic bronchopulmonary aspergillosis: Staging as an aid to management. *Ann Intern Med* 1982;**96**:286.

Cell-Mediated Hypersensitivity Diseases

30

Abba I. Terr, MD

Certain allergic diseases are mediated by specifically sensitized effector T lymphocytes (T_{DH} cells) and not by specifically sensitized antibodies. The immunologic mechanism is often called **delayed hypersensitivity,** and it is also involved in immunity to infection by certain microorganisms, especially those that cause intracellular infections. This chapter discusses two very different T-cell-mediated allergic diseases: allergic contact dermatitis, which is very common, and hypersensitivity pneumonitis, which is quite uncommon but not rare.

Allergic contact dermatitis in its usual form is a pure form of T-cell hypersensitivity. (Occasionally, allergens that contact the skin or mucous membranes may elicit an IgE antibody response, especially urticaria but rarely systemic anaphylaxis.) **Hypersensitivity pneumonitis** is a clinically heterogenous disease that may assume several forms involving antibodies, T cells, or both, depending on factors of allergen dose and the form and duration of allergen exposure. It is included in this chapter because T-cell mechanisms are predominant in most clinically recognized cases.

ALLERGIC CONTACT DERMATITIS

Major Immunologic Features
- It is mediated by specifically sensitized T cells.
- It is caused most often by contact with haptenic chemicals.
- Patch testing is efficient and accurate in diagnosis.

General Considerations
A. Definition: Allergic contact dermatitis (also known as eczematous contact allergy) is an eczematous skin disease caused by cell-mediated hypersensitivity to an environmental allergen. Both sensitization and elicitation of the reaction involve contact of the allergen with the skin. Allergens causing the disease are numerous, and include both natural and synthetic chemicals.

B. Epidemiology: The disease occurs worldwide and affects both sexes and all age groups. The most common allergen, pentadecylcatechol, found in poison ivy and poison oak, affects 50% of the US population clinically and another 35% subclinically.

C. Immunologic Pathogenesis: Allergic contact dermatitis is mediated by cutaneous T-cell hypersensitivity. In this process, the Langerhans' cell, a skin macrophage, functions as the antigen-processing cell at the local site of allergen penetration. It is uncertain whether the site of origin of the sensitized T lymphocyte is the skin, the regional lymph nodes, or elsewhere. The dose of allergen necessary for sensitization varies widely. Once sensitization occurs, it lasts for years, if not for life, and is generalized. Reactions can be elicited anywhere on the skin. In some instances systemic reactions have been provoked when the allergen enters the body by ingestion or injection.

Many important sensitizing allergens are organic chemicals, and some are metals. It is assumed that they function as haptens, but the source and nature of the host carrier protein in the skin are unknown.

D. Pathology: The inflammatory response in allergic contact dermatitis is characterized by perivenular cuffing with lymphocytes, epidermal cell vesiculation and necrosis, appearance of basophils and eosinophils, interstitial fibrin deposition, and dermal and epidermal edema.

Clinical Features
A. Symptoms and Signs: The skin eruption appears acutely as erythema, swelling, and vesiculation. In severe cases there may be extensive blistering, scaling, and weeping. In chronic milder disease, papules and scaling are more prominent. The lesion is pruritic or frankly painful if severe. The rapidity of onset after contact is directly proportionate to the degree of sensitivity and may range from 6 hours to several days.

The location of the eruption on the skin is helpful in diagnosing the cause. Certain areas of skin, such as the eyelids, react more easily than others, such as the palms. Metal dermatitis, usually caused by sensitivity to nickel, appears in discrete patches corresponding to the area of contact with jewelry, watches, or metal objects on clothing. A variety of allergens, such as dyes and fabric finishes, are found in clothing, causing a skin eruption on areas of skin covered by the apparel. Volatile allergens affect exposed areas, usually the face and arms. *Rhus* dermatitis from poison oak or poison ivy produces an especially severe disease with prominent vesicles and bullae, and there are characteristic streaks of vesicles corresponding to brushing of the skin by the plant leaves.

B. Laboratory Findings: There are none.

Allergens

The list of known allergens is enormous and theoretically unlimited. All types of chemicals can produce this disease, but metallic inorganic compounds and organic chemicals are the most likely, in contrast to the protein allergens that dominate in the other types of allergic conditions. The reason for this is unknown but is probably associated with the unique handling of foreign materials by the skin. The most common contact allergens are listed in Table 30–1.

Clinical Diagnosis

The diagnosis of allergic contact dermatitis is suggested by the physical appearance of the eruption and distribution of lesions. By history, reactions may appear suddenly, or they may present as a chronic, low-grade, smoldering dermatitis. The history must then be directed to monitoring exposures in the home, work, and recreational environment for possible allergens.

Immunologic Diagnosis

The diagnosis is confirmed by **patch testing,** a time-honored, well-standardized procedure that is both an immunologic skin test and a provocation test that reproduces the disease "in miniature." Standard patch test allergens in concentrations that elicit allergic but not irritant reactions are available commercially for a number of the common contact sensitizers (see Table 30–1). Reactions are read in 48 hours for localized eczema at the patch test site (Table 30–2). Patch testing to the common allergens used in routine screening has an overall sensitivity of 77% and a specificity of 71%, which is acceptable for a bioassay. Weak (1+) reactions have poorer reproducibility than stronger ones.

Differential Diagnosis

Eczema refers to a general pattern of response of the skin to a variety of injurious stimuli. Scratching of the skin from any pruritic dermatosis can cause eczematization. The most common causes are atopic dermatitis; localized or generalized neurodermatitis; skin infection by bacteria or fungi; primary contact irritation by chemicals, foods, saliva, sweat, or urine; and dyshidrosis.

Table 30–1. Common contact allergens and concentrations.

Benzocaine 5%
Mercaptobenzothiazole 1%
Colophony 20%
p-Phenylenediamine 1%
Imidazolidinyl urea 2%
Cinnamic aldehyde 1%
Lanolin alcohol 30%
Carba mix 3%
Neomycin sulfate 20%
Thiuram mix 1%
Formaldehyde 1%
Ethylenediamine dihydrochloride 1%
Epoxy resin 1%
Quaternium 15 2%
p-tert-Butylphenol formaldehyde resin 1%
Mercapto mix 1%
Black rubber mix 0.6%
Potassium dichromate 0.25%
Balsam of Peru 25%
Nickel sulfate 2.5%

Treatment

The disease responds to systemic **corticosteroids,** which should be given as early as possible. Small localized areas of involvement can be treated with a topical steroid cream. Applications of cool, wet dressings containing Burow's solution (aluminum acetate) are helpful for treating acute lesions. Chronic lichenified dermatitis requires a potent fluorinated steroid ointment with an occlusive dressing. Extensive areas of involvement or severe bullous lesions should be treated with a brief oral burst of high-dose prednisone or with intramuscular triamcinolone or methylprednisolone. An antibiotic may be indicated for secondary infection. Antihistamines are generally not effective for controlling the pruritus.

Prognosis

A cure is to be expected in the case of acute allergic contact dermatitis if the allergen is identified correctly and avoided. Exposure to a cross-reacting allergenic chemical, however, may cause a recurrence. Chromate allergy tends to be chronic, despite avoidance.

Prevention

The only means of prevention of the dermatitis in a sensitized patient is avoidance. The Landsteiner-Chase phenomenon of tolerance to contact sensitivity in guinea pigs by prior oral ingestion of allergen has no practical application in humans. Some pa-

Table 30–2. Patch test interpretation.

Result	Interpretation
–	Negative reaction.
?	Doubtful reaction, macular erythema only.
+	Weak (nonvesicular) reaction: erythema, infiltration, possibly papules.
++	Strong (edematous or vesicular) reaction.
+++	Extreme (spreading, bullous, ulcerative) reaction.

tients with mild nickel sensitivity can tolerate jewelry that is treated with a protective coating. *Rhus* dermatitis can probably be lessened, if not prevented, if the skin is thoroughly washed with water immediately after contact.

Desensitization with oral or injected *Rhus* extract or pentadecylcatechol has advocates in clinical practice, but there is, as yet, no sound evidence of effectiveness. Some patients appear to lose sensitivity after repeated natural exposure, a phenomenon known as "hardening," but this also remains to be documented.

PHOTOALLERGIC CONTACT DERMATITIS

Major Immunologic Features
- Allergen requires activation by ultraviolet light.
- Immunologic mechanism is identical to that of allergic contact dermatitis.

General Considerations
A. Definition: Photoallergic contact dermatitis is an uncommon eczematous skin disease caused by cell-mediated hypersensitivity to certain environmental chemicals that require sunlight activation to render them allergenic. The skin eruption appears on sun-exposed areas of the skin only.

B. Epidemiology: The disease has been associated primarily with drugs or chemical constituents of topical products, such as soaps, cosmetics, and topical drugs. It therefore appears from time to time in epidemic form when a new product is introduced. The epidemic subsides when the product is withdrawn from the market once the photosensitivity potential is discovered.

C. Immunologic Pathogenesis: The mechanism is identical to ordinary allergic contact dermatitis, except that the causative chemical agent must be activated by the ultraviolet component of sunlight to become allergenic. The mechanism of allergen activation is unknown. Two theories have been proposed. Ultraviolet radiation may cause an alteration in tertiary structure to generate the necessary allergen epitope, or, alternatively, free radicals generated by ultraviolet light may be necessary for binding of the hapten chemical to skin carrier protein.

D. Pathology: The pathology is indistinguishable from that of allergic contact dermatitis.

Clinical Features
The dermatitis varies in its clinical appearance from an exaggerated sunburn to typical eczema to a severe vesiculobullous dermatosis. The distribution corresponds to sunlight exposure, but severe reactions may involve partially covered areas of skin as well. The eruption caused by a topically applied sensitizer is limited to the area of application.

Table 30–3. Some topical agents causing photoallergic and phototoxic reactions.

Photoallergic	Phototoxic
Drugs	Drugs
Sulfonamides	Sulfonamides
Phenothiazines	Phenothiazines
Soaps containing halogenated salicylanilides	Plant oils
	Psoralens
Sunscreen agents	Coal tar and its derivatives in
p-Aminobenzoate esters	dyes, perfumes, and
Benzophenones	other synthetics
Fragrances	Acridine
	Anthracene
	Phenothrene

Clinical Diagnosis
The disease is diagnosed by the combination of dermatitis in a sun-exposed distribution and a history of concurrent exposure to a known or suspected photoallergic sensitizer. A high index of suspicion facilitates diagnosis.

Immunologic Diagnosis
Photopatch testing is a modification of the standard patch test. The suspected agent is applied in the standard fashion for patch testing, and then the site is exposed to artificial ultraviolet light or sunlight. A test site not exposed to light is used as a control. The appearance of an eczematous eruption at the light-exposed site only is a positive test.

Differential Diagnosis
Certain chemicals and drugs produce dermatitis in sun-exposed areas of skin in all individuals, provided that sufficient amounts of the compound accumulate in the skin and that there is exposure to a particular wavelength of ultraviolet light. These are called phototoxic reactions and are not mediated immunologically. Differential diagnosis also includes ordinary contact dermatitis, sunburn, and other causes of photosensitivity.

Allergens
Some of the important drugs and chemicals that cause photoallergic and phototoxic contact dermatitis are listed in Table 30–3. Some drugs taken systemically produce photodermatitis.

Treatment
Avoidance of the sensitizing agent and sunlight and treatment with topical corticosteroids are usually sufficient. Systemic corticosteroids may be required in severe cases.

Prognosis
Occasionally the dermatitis persists despite avoidance measures. The reason for this is unknown.

HYPERSENSITIVITY PNEUMONITIS

Major Immunologic Features

- Primary pathogenetic mechanism involves the effector T cell.
- Antibody precipitins are useful to establish exposure to the allergen.
- Allergens are frequently components of biologic organisms or their products.

General Considerations

Hypersensitivity pneumonitis (also known as **extrinsic allergic alveolitis**) has been known as an occupational disease for well over two centuries, but it was only recently recognized as an allergic disease. It was first thought to be a pulmonary Arthus reaction caused by immune complexes of inhaled allergen and precipitating IgG antibodies, but persuasive evidence from clinical, pathologic, epidemiologic, and experimental studies has shown that the disease is mediated predominantly by T-lymphocyte (cellular) effector mechanisms. It shares some pathologic features with sarcoidosis and the pneumoconioses, but it differs from the former disease by having a recognized environmental cause and from the latter group of diseases by its immune responses to inhaled material. Hypersensitivity pneumonitis, like allergic asthma, is produced by inhaled allergens, and in fact there are allergens that can cause either disease. IgE antibodies, however, play no known role in the pathogenesis of hypersensitivity pneumonitis.

A. Definition: Hypersensitivity pneumonitis is an allergic disease of the lung parenchyma with inflammation in the alveoli and interstitial spaces induced immunologically by acute or chronic inhalation of a wide variety of inhaled materials. The disease may present in an acute, subacute, or chronic form. It is not currently possible to ascribe all features of the illness to a single immunologic mechanism. There is evidence for several different immune pathways that operate separately or concurrently, but the most compelling evidence favors allergen-specific cell-mediated hypersensitivity as the mechanism of pathogenesis. Interstitial pneumonitis is the primary clinical manifestation for all forms of the disease.

B. Epidemiology: Cases have been reported worldwide. The disease is most frequently associated with occupational allergens, which determine its prevalence and geographic, age, and sex distribution. Males aged 30–50 years are therefore usually affected. Farmer's lung, the prototype and most widely reported form of hypersensitivity pneumonitis, is caused by thermophilic actinomycetes, usually from warm, moist, moldy hay, and therefore the disease predominates in wet regions and especially among dairy farmers. Several surveys suggest that 2–4% of farmers have been affected. Bird handler's disease (also known as bird fancier's lung, pigeon breeder's disease, and bird breeder's disease) has been diagnosed in 15–21% of exposed individuals. Humidifier lung disease occurs in 23–71% of those exposed to contaminated humidifiers. Many published reports identify a single case or a small epidemic in a workplace. Once recognized, elimination of the environmental source of the allergen eliminates the disease.

C. Allergens: Hundreds of sources of allergens have been reported to cause hypersensitivity pneumonitis, usually in single cases. Some of the more common ones are shown in Table 30–4. The exact allergenic molecule has been isolated only infrequently, but these include a variety of heterologous proteins and organic or inorganic compounds. In many cases the chemical identification has been made by serologic or skin testing in the affected patient. As explained later, precipitins and skin tests may be epiphenomena, so definitive identification of the allergen requires bronchial provocation testing. (See the section on Immunologic Diagnosis.)

The allergens come from a variety of environmental sources. The most common ones are microorganisms, especially bacteria and fungal spores, and animal products, such as feathers and particles of dried excreta. The few industrial chemicals so far identified with this disease have been highly reactive ones, such as isocyanates and acid anhydrides. Many cases have been associated with inhalation of a product such as inhaled dust from a food or droplets of contaminated water without identification of the source, although microbial contamination is usually suspected.

To date most reported cases have been **occupational,** because these are more likely to be acute illnesses from high-dose exposure easily traced to the workplace by a history of an epidemic in a particular occupational site. The relatively few instances of disease caused by **domestic** exposure have been traced to thermophilic actinomycetes, fungi, mites, amebae, pet birds, and unknown organisms in contaminated water of home or automobile air conditioners, heaters, vaporizers, and evaporative air coolers. These tend to cause chronic and insidious pulmonary impairment. Physicians should be aware of this potential cause of "idiopathic" pulmonary fibrosis.

The allergen must be inhaled in a form, such as an aerosol or particle, that is capable of reaching the alveoli during normal respiration. Particulates, whether in the form of an organic dust or microorganism, must be less than 3 μm in diameter.

Many of the allergens associated with hypersensitivity pneumonitis have biologic properties, in addition to allergenicity, that may be important in causing disease. The thermophilic actinomycetes, which are classified in the same botanical order as *Mycobacterium tuberculosis,* contain immunologic adjuvants for both antibody synthesis and cell-mediated immunity. Many of the allergens can activate alveolar macrophages and the alternative complement pathway nonimmunologically. The role of these properties in disease pathogenesis is being actively investigated.

Table 30–4. Allergens causing hypersensitivity pneumonitis.

Allergen	Source	Disease
Bacteria		
Thermophilic actinomycetes	Contaminated hay or grains	Farmer's lung
	Contaminated bagasse	Bagassosis
	Mushroom compost	Mushroom worker's lung
Bacillus subtilis	Contaminated walls	Domestic hypersensitivity pneumonitis
Streptomyces albus	Contaminated fertilizer	*Streptomyces* hypersensitivity pneumonitis
Fungi		
Aspergillus spp	Moldy barley	Malt worker's lung
	Moldy tobacco	Tobacco worker's lung
	Compost	Compost lung
Aureobasidium, Graphium spp	Redwood bark, sawdust	Sequoiosis
	Contaminated sauna water	Sauna worker's lung
	Contaminated humidifier	Humidifier lung
Cryptostroma corticale	Maple bark	Maple bark disease
Penicillium casei	Moldy cheese	Cheese worker's lung
Sacchoromonospora viridis	Dried grass	Thatched roof disease
Various undetermined puffball spores	Moldy dwellings	Domestic hypersensitivity pneumonitis
	Mold in cork dust	Suberosis
	Lycoperdon puffballs	Lycoperdonosis
Alternaria, Penicillium spp.	Wood pulp, dust	Woodworker's lung
Insects		
Sitophilus granarius (wheat weevil)	Infested flour	Wheat miller's lung
Organic chemicals		
Isocyanates	Various industries	Chemical worker's lung
Miscellaneous		
Pituitary snuff	Medication	Pituitary snuff taker's lung
Coffee bean protein	Coffee bean dust	Coffee worker's lung
Rat urine protein	Laboratory rats	Laboratory worker's lung
Animal fur protein	Animal pelts	Furrier's lung
Unknown	Contaminated tap water	Tap water hypersensitivity pneumonitis

D. Pathology: The histopathology of hypersensitivity pneumonitis depends on the stage of disease. Very few patients have been examined in the acute phase immediately after exposure. Such patients show involvement of centrilobular respiratory bronchioles, alveoli, and blood vessels with intense infiltration by granulocytes, monocytes, and plasma cells. There is Arthus-like vasculitis of alveolar capillaries. Some studies show bronchiolar destruction. There is alveolar wall thickening but without necrosis. Immunofluorescence studies show deposition of immunoglobulins, C3, and fibrin in and around affected blood vessels. Thus, any role of precipitating antibodies causing immune-complex deposition and complement-mediated Arthus-like vasculitis, alveolitis, and terminal bronchiolitis would be restricted to the early acute illness after allergen exposure.

The subacute phase, beginning within 3 weeks of exposure, is characterized by noncaseating granulomas in the interstitial spaces accompanied by lymphocytes and plasma cells with only occasional eosinophils and no vasculitis. Mild bronchiolitis obliterans is seen in 50% of cases.

Chronic disease is characterized by persistence of the subacute pathology. There are lymphocytes in alveolar walls, and interstitial fibrosis accompanies the granulomatous and mononuclear interstitial and alveolar inflammation. There is no eosinophilia, and immunofluorescence shows no immunoglobulin or complement deposits. Monoclonal antibody reagents reveal the presence of activated macrophages and T lymphocytes, predominantly CD8 cells.

The histopathology of hypersensitivity pneumonitis is not pathognomonic, with the possible exception of histiocytes with foamy cytoplasm surrounded by lymphocytes, which are seen in the chronic phase.

E. Pathogenesis: The allergic pathogenesis of hypersensitivity pneumonitis was first suspected in farmer's lung because of the granulomatous interstitial inflammation, a hallmark of T-cell-mediated immunity. The discovery of precipitating antibodies to extracts of thermophilic actinomycetes in these patients' sera, however, led to a persisting concept that this is an immune-complex disease, even after many studies showed that precipitins correlated with exposure to allergens and not necessarily to the presence of pulmonary disease. As explained earlier, an Arthus mechanism could be operative in the acute form of hypersensitivity pneumonitis. However, the clinical manifestations, pathology, disease induced in animal models, epidemiologic data, and recent investigations of bronchoalveolar lavage samples all point to a more complex mechanism of disease involving specific cell-mediated immunity, immunoregulatory and immunogenetic factors, and nonspecific biologic effects of the inhaled material, but only a minor role, if any, for circulating antibodies. The disease is primarily a function of the local pulmonary mucosal cellular immune system, which is poorly reflected in peripheral blood samples. The role of mucosal IgA has not been fully explored. Both IgA and IgG antibodies are present in bronchoalveolar lavage fluid in proportion to allergen exposure, but IgA and not IgG antibody titers are higher in patients than in exposed persons without disease.

Unlike IgE-mediated diseases, allergen exposure by inhalation must be either intensive and massive or prolonged. It has been calculated that a farmer working with moldy hay may inhale 750,000 fungal spores per minute.

In experimental disease in animals, inhalation of soluble antigens produces a very mild disease or an acute hemorrhagic Arthus alveolitis analogous to human illness in workers exposed occupationally to high doses of trimellitic anhydride or isocyanate who develop high-titer circulating and alveolar-fluid antibodies and a restrictive infiltrative pulmonary disease with hemoptysis and anemia. On the other hand, the typical human hypersensitivity pneumonitis is best reproduced in animals by inhalation of particulate antigens that elicit alveolitis and interstitial granulomas, specific local and systemic cell-mediated hypersensitivity, activation of alveolar macrophages, local lymphokine production in alveolar fluid, and precipitins. Allergen inhalation challenge responses can be passively transferred by sensitized lymphocytes, and the disease can be inhibited with corticosteroids, with antimacrophage serum, and by neonatal thymectomy, all of which are consistent with cellular hypersensitivity.

Experiments in mice shed some light on the development and variability of the human disease. By using high- and low-responder strains, it has been shown that the disease is associated with a deficiency in allergen-specific suppressor T lymphocytes in the lung. The deficiency is determined by a dominant gene or genes linked to the immunoglobulin V_H haplotype but not to H-2 (analogous to human HLA) genes. Repeated exposure to the allergen causes a phenomenon of desensitization, with disappearance of infiltrates, refractoriness to disease by other, unrelated allergens, and cell-mediated anergy in some animals but not others. The anergic state is caused by an allergen-nonspecific suppressor macrophage, whose presence is controlled by a single recessive gene. Animals lacking this gene have sustained granulomatous disease and have failed to develop anergy. These intriguing experiments stress the role of genetic factors of immunoregulation that probably also control susceptibility to and expressions of the disease in humans.

Many of the allergens identified with this disease have intrinsic biologic effects that may be important in pathogenesis. These include adjuvant properties causing nonspecific immune stimulation, activation of macrophages, and nonimmunologic activation of the alternative complement pathway.

Clinical Features

A. Symptoms: Clinical patterns are wide-ranging, but they may be classified into acute, subacute, and chronic forms. Acute reactions are characterized by single or multiple episodes of dyspnea, cough, malaise, fever, chills, and chest pain. Each episode begins 4–8 hours after a high-dose allergen exposure and clears within 24 hours. Weight loss and hemoptysis are rare. Subacute disease begins insidiously over a period of weeks, resulting in cough, dyspnea, and weight loss. The cough is initially dry and later productive. Dyspnea may become progressively profound, and there may be cyanosis. Chronic disease occurs from low-dose continuous exposure, as in the case of hypersensitivity to a single bird in the home. Fatigue and weight loss may be the first indication of illness. Gradual progressive dyspnea may be overlooked or denied until it is noticed at rest.

B. Signs: During acute reactions, the temperature is elevated to as high as 39.5°C. The patient appears acutely ill, with tachypnea and tachycardia. There are bilateral crackling rales, especially at the lung bases, and occasional rhonchi and wheezes, but the lungs may be clear. In chronic disease, breath sounds are diminished and there may be a prolonged expiratory phase if an obstructive component is present.

C. Laboratory Findings: In acute disease there is usually slight leukocytosis without eosinophilia. The erythrocyte sedimentation rate is normal or mildly elevated. In chronic disease, serum immunoglobulin levels may be slightly increased and low-titer rheumatoid factor and antinuclear antibody may be present.

Pulmonary function tests performed during the acute phase of the disease reveal a reversible restrictive pattern with reduced lung compliance and reduced diffusing capacity. Arterial blood gases show hypoxemia. The spirometric findings in chronic disease are those of irreversible restriction with or without an accompanying obstructive component due to bronchiolitis obliterans. In some patients there may be an additional element of bronchial hyperirritability.

Chest x-ray findings are highly variable. During an acute episode, the presence of multiple bilateral small nodules sparing the apices and bases is the typical pattern. This indicates the presence of interstitial inflammation and an alveolus-filling infiltrate. Less common findings are patchy pneumonia or a normal x-ray. In chronic disease a fibrotic linear pattern with or without nodules increases in intensity toward the periphery. There may be a loss of volume that is most marked in upper lobes, honeycombing, and cor pulmonale-induced cardiac enlargement. The disease does not cause pleural effusion or thickening, hilar adenopathy, calcification, cavitation, atelectasis, or coin lesions.

The classification just described should not obscure the fact that hypersensitivity pneumonitis is highly variable and that individual cases can be "atypical." Clinical manifestations depend on the chemical and physical properties of the allergen and the frequency and intensity of exposure, as well as on host factors. Clinical descriptions have been dominated by occupational syndromes such as farmer's lung, bagassosis, and bird handler's disease. Many unique case reports have been published with quaint names and unusual allergen sources, such as New Guinea thatched roof lung (contaminated thatch), paprika slicer's lung (*Mucor stalonifer*), Bible printer's lung (contaminated ink), and coptic lung (mummy cloth wrappings).

Clinical Diagnosis

The history is important, as in any allergic disease. Because of the variable nature of hypersensitivity pneumonitis and wide range of environmental sources for the allergens, the diagnosis requires a high degree of suspicion. Any patient with a history of recurrent pneumonia of uncertain etiology, "idiopathic" restrictive or fibrotic lung disease, or unexplained pulmonary abnormality on chest x-ray is a prime suspect. The environmental, especially occupational, history is essential for providing clues for possible causative allergens.

There are no pathognomonic signs from physical examination, routine laboratory tests, or chest x-rays. Even pulmonary function testing may not show evidence of the restrictive abnormality during asymptomatic periods between acute attacks of early disease. Lung biopsy is likewise not pathognomonic, since histopathology is similar to that of other interstitial diseases, but it is useful mainly to rule out other diagnoses.

Immunologic Diagnosis

Serum antibodies are not usually involved in disease pathogenesis, but their presence nevertheless at least establishes the fact of exposure. There are usually large quantities of **precipitating antibodies,** especially in early or acute disease, but they may disappear after a prolonged period of allergen avoidance. Ouchterlony analysis is usually adequate to detect precipitins (see Chapter 14). The more sensitive radioimmunoassay, radioallergosorbent test (RAST), enzyme-linked immunosorbent assay (ELISA), and complement fixation test procedures lack specificity for diagnostic purposes. Serum complement component levels are normal or occasionally increased with acute allergen exposure.

When precipitating antibodies are present in serum, an intradermal skin test elicits a cutaneous Arthus reaction, characterized by localized diffuse edema and mild inflammation and erythema appearing at 4–6 hours and subsiding completely by 24 hours. Commercial test antigens are available for extracts of fungi and diluted avian serum. Many crude extracts of allergens known to cause this disease, such as thermophilic actinomycetes, are too irritating for skin testing. The Arthus skin test, like the precipitin test, is an indication of exposure and is not by itself diagnostic of the disease.

Bronchial provocation testing with allergen extract currently has the highest sensitivity and specificity for diagnosis, but it is an experimental procedure because of technical limitations and danger. It should be done in a hospital with 24-hour monitoring. A reversible restrictive lung defect begins at 4–6 hours, peaks at 8 hours, and resolves by 24 hours. Although the timing of response is similar to a late-phase asthmatic response, the abnormality in pulmonary function is different (see Fig 26–3).

Examination of bronchoalveolar lavage fluid for humoral and cellular components has been reported to date for only a few cases of subacute disease. The procedure is still experimental, and the diagnostic usefulness is unknown.

A simpler alternative to bronchial provocation is "on-site" challenge to observe changes in symptoms, lung auscultation, pulmonary functions, and chest x-ray by trial exposure of the patient to the suspected environment (eg, home or work) after an adequate period of avoidance. If an acute reaction is provoked, the site must be investigated to uncover the causative allergen. Environmental assessment might require the specialized services of engineers, microbiologists, or others.

Differential Diagnosis

Pulmonary mycotoxicosis (atypical farmer's lung) is a disorder caused by acute massive exposure to moldy silage. The disease is characterized by fever, chills, and coughing that last for several days to a week. There are diffuse infiltrations on chest x-ray and fungal organisms in alveoli and bronchioles, but no serum precipitins. The cause is unknown, but the illness is probably a toxic pneumonitis from a fungal product. Recurrent infectious pneumonias, other causes of interstitial lung disease, asthma, allergic bronchopulmonary aspergillosis, and pneumoconioses must also be differentiated from hypersensitivity pneumonitis.

Treatment

Systemic corticosteroid therapy is indicated for resolution of acute reactions and for terminating and reversing severe or progressive disease. The drug should not be used as an alternative to avoidance of the allergen, but it may be necessary to protect the patient by suppressing inflammation if the allergen source has not been identified. Inhaled corticosteroids are not indicated.

Complications

Respiratory failure and cor pulmonale may result from chronic disease. Bronchiolitis obliterans may lead to irreversible obstructive pulmonary disease. Death from respiratory failure is possible during any phase of the disease.

Prognosis

Prognosis for recovery is good in the acute or subacute stages once the cause has been identified and avoided. Some patients with bird handler's disease, however, have progressive pulmonary insufficiency even with complete avoidance of birds. On the other hand, farmers can continue to have some exposure to thermophilic actinomycetes without progressive illness as long as the acute febrile symptomatic attacks are avoided.

Prevention

Avoidance is the only means of preventing this disease. Effective treatment therefore requires a specific immunologic diagnosis whenever possible, since the same allergen may be found in different environments (Table 30–4). The purpose of avoidance is prevention of irreversible lung disease.

Occupational preventive measures are obvious for the currently recognized causes. Proper workplace hygiene, filters and masks where appropriate, and other measures should be employed. Diseases caused by allergens in homes, automobiles, and offices are best prevented by physician awareness of the disease.

REFERENCES

ALLERGIC CONTACT DERMATITIS

Adams RM: *Occupational Skin Diseases,* 2nd ed. Grune & Stratton, 1989.

Huntley AC (editor): Allergic contact dermatitis. *Clin Rev Allergy* 1989;**7:**345. (Entire issue.)

Nethercott J: The positive predictive accuracy of patch tests. *Immun Allergy Clin North Am* 1989;**9:**549.

Rietschel RL, Fowler JF, Jr: *Fisher's Contact Dermatitis,* 4th ed. Lea & Febiger, 1995.

HYPERSENSITIVITY PNEUMONITIS

Fink JN: Hypersensitivity pneumonitis. *Clin Chest Med* 1992;**13:**303.

Novey HS (editor): Hypersensitivity pneumonitis. *Clin Rev Allergy* 1983;**1:**449. (Entire issue.)

Salvaggio JE: Hypersensitivity pneumonitis. *J Allergy Clin Immunol* 1987;**79:**558.

Salvaggio JE: Recent advances in pathogenesis of allergic alveolitis. *Clin Rev Allergy* 1990;**20:**137.

Sharma OP, Fujimura N: Hypersensitivity pneumonitis: A noninfectious granulomatosis. *Semin Respir Infect* 1995;**10:**96.

Drug Allergy

31

H. James Wedner, MD

Adverse reactions to therapeutic agents are a significant problem in the practice of medicine. The spectrum of such reactions comprises (1) side effects, toxic reactions, and drug interactions that are the result of unwanted pharmacologic properties of the drug(s) in question; (2) idiosyncratic reactions, which occur in a variable proportion of the population and the cause of which is unknown; and (3) immunologic reactions, which depend on the ability of the drug, or its hydrolysis or biotransformation products, to induce a humoral or cellular immune response. Reactions resulting from an immunologic mechanism, such as drug allergy, constitute a substantial portion of all adverse drug reactions. Although this chapter is concerned with immunologic mechanisms, other causes must be considered when treating patients with adverse reactions to drugs, because different mechanisms may produce similar clinical presentations. It is imperative that the underlying mechanism be established since the therapeutic approach differs depending on the type of reaction that has occurred.

Drug allergy is sometimes defined as any reaction that results from an immune mechanism but other times is limited to reactions mediated by IgE antibody directed against the drug or one of its metabolic products. This chapter discusses all immunologically mediated drug reactions and then concentrates on those resulting from IgE antibody-dependent release of mediators from sensitized mast cells and basophils and those caused by the nonimmunologic release of mediators from mast cells and basophils. The latter have been called "anaphylactoid," or "pseudoallergic," reactions. They are important because the symptoms of allergic and pseudoallergic reactions are identical.

IMMUNOLOGIC BASIS OF DRUG ALLERGY

General Considerations

Although the frequency of reactions to different drugs varies widely, it is probable that any drug is capable of inducing humoral or cellular immune responses. In the majority of cases, the resulting immune state is not detrimental. For example, a large proportion of individuals treated with intravenous penicillin develop IgG antibodies to penicillin or penicillin biotransformation products. In the vast majority of instances, these antibodies do not result in either a clinical drug reaction or a decrease in the effectiveness of the drug. This is also true for patients treated with bovine or porcine insulin. Thus, the demonstration of antibodies or sensitized T cells directed against a drug or one of its biotransformation products does not indicate that this immune response necessarily results in an adverse drug reaction.

Drugs are capable of inducing allergic reactions by any of the hypersensitivity mechanisms discussed in Chapter 26, that is, Type I (IgE-mediated), Type II (cytotoxic antibody-mediated), Type III (immune complex-mediated), and Type IV (T effector cell-mediated) mechanisms. To induce these reactions, a drug must be immunogenic. Some drugs are large polypeptides or proteins and, therefore, are intrinsically immunogenic in their native state. These include insulin, pituitary snuff (used as a source of antidiuretic hormone), heterologous antisera and antivenins, L-asparaginase, factor VIII, and a number of vaccines. A few relatively low molecular weight drugs, such as polymyxin, appear to be immunogenic without tissue conjugation. Although the exact mechanism is currently unknown, immunogenicity is probably related to the ability of these drugs to form long-chain polymers. Most drugs are of low molecular weight, however, and they are in and of themselves nonimmunogenic. Only when the drug is capable of interacting with tissue proteins and serving as a hapten does it induce an immune response.

Metabolic Biotransformation and Haptenation

The ability of any drug to induce an immune response depends on the tissue reactivity of that drug. Drugs that easily form covalent bonds are more immunogenic than those that are relatively unreactive. Most haptenic drugs conjugate to tissue protein via a covalent bond. In rare cases, the bond may be noncovalent but of sufficient affinity for the drug–protein complex to remain intact during antigen processing and presentation. It is not necessary, however, that the native drug be highly reactive, since its hydrolysis or biotransformation products may serve as the hapten. For this reason, a thorough knowledge of the biotransformation products of a drug is critical in the evaluation of drug allergies. Unfortunately, this information is not available for most drugs, thereby limiting the ability to predict immunogenicity of a given drug and, as discussed later on, the ability to test for the presence of a drug allergy.

Early studies of patients with known allergy to penicillin demonstrated that only a small percentage of these patients reacted to the drug itself (benzylpenicillin); the majority reacted to the penicilloyl moiety, which is generated by the cleavage of the β-lactam ring, and others reacted to the penilloate group generated by the cleavage of the five-membered thiazolidine ring (Fig 31–1). This led to the development of accurate methods for detecting allergy to penicillin and other β-lactam drugs, as discussed later on.

Similarly, only a small percentage of patients allergic to sulfonamides react by skin tests to the native drug, so skin testing is not an accurate predictor of allergic reactivity for this class of drugs. On the other hand, Prausnitz-Kustner passive transfer of serum from sulfonamide-allergic patients to nonallergic individuals results in a wheal-and-flare at the site of the injection when the recipient ingests the drug. This suggests that metabolism of the drug results in a reactive molecule that, on conjugation to circulating proteins, is capable of interacting with and activating the locally sensitized mast cells. In clinical practice, passive transfer testing using recipient human volunteers is not feasible, although passive transfer to primates, such as rhesus monkeys, whose mast cells bind human IgE, can be used if necessary.

The immune response generated by certain drugs that are highly tissue-reactive may be directed not to the drug or its metabolic by-products nor to the host tissue but rather to a new antigenic determinant that forms from the combination of the drug with a specific tissue protein. This is the mechanism of thrombocytopenia following the ingestion of quinine, an antimalarial drug. In this case, the patient produces an IgG antibody with specificity for quinine bound to the surface of the platelet. The quinine–platelet interaction has generated a new antigenic determinant that does not cross-react with other blood cells or tissues. The exact immunologic mechanisms of most other tissue-specific drug reactions are currently unknown.

Finally, the interaction between a drug and a tissue protein (or other tissue component) may alter a site on the protein molecule distant from the actual binding to the drug. This altered tissue protein can then be recognized as foreign by the immune system, serving as an immunogen for either humoral or cell-mediated immune responses. This mechanism is of some

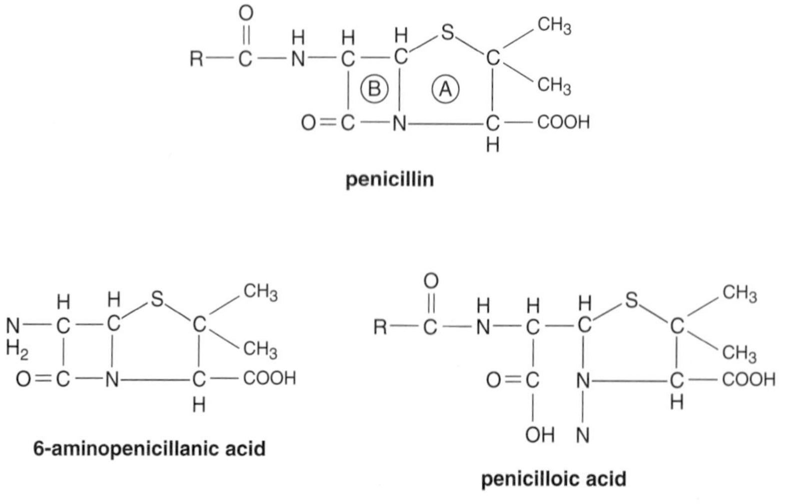

Figure 31–1. Penicillin and two allergenic biotransformation products. **A:** Thiazolidine ring. **B:** β-lactam ring.

importance, since the antibodies or any cytotoxic T cells generated may be capable of recognizing not only the altered protein but also the protein in its native state, thereby serving as the mechanism for some types of drug-induced autoimmunity. A good example of this phenomenon is the systemic lupus erythematosus syndrome associated with the drug hydralazine. Although in most cases the signs and symptoms of drug-induced lupus or other drug-induced autoimmune disease revert promptly following removal of the drug, some may persist long after the drug has been withdrawn. The various modes of hapten—carrier interaction in drug allergy are illustrated in Figure 31–2.

Other Factors in Drug Allergenicity

Certain drugs generate a humoral immune response, whereas others more commonly induce T-cell immunity. The factors that govern the type of immune response generated by a given drug are unknown but probably include (1) the chemical nature of the drug, (2) the route of presentation (ingestion, injection, or application to the skin), and (3) the genetic makeup of the individual.

The site of presentation of the drug markedly influences both the ability of the drug to induce an adverse immunologic reaction and the type of reaction. In general, drugs are far more likely to induce an immune reaction when they are given parenterally (subcutaneously, intramuscularly, or intravenously) than when given orally or applied to the skin. For example, IgE and IgG antibodies to penicillin or its derivatives are produced in a greater proportion of individuals treated intravenously than in those treated orally even when comparable doses of the drug are given.

The route of presentation may also determine the type of immune response (antibody or T cell) associated with a given drug. For example, antihistaminic drugs are rarely allergenic when given by the oral or parenteral route but frequently induce T-cell sensitization when applied topically to the skin, causing allergic contact dermatitis. This may be the result of the interaction of the drug or drug metabolite protein conjugate with highly active professional antigen-presenting cells (Langerhans' cells) present in the skin.

The prevalence of allergic reactions to drugs is greater in acquired immune deficiency syndrome

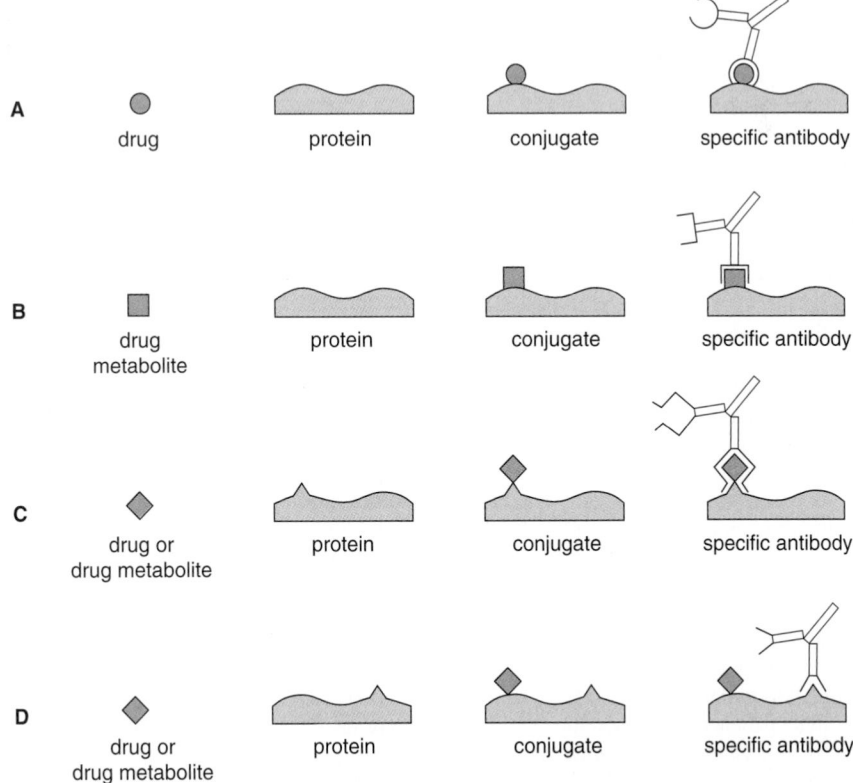

Figure 31–2. The interaction of a drug with tissue protein may result in antibodies (shown) or T cells directed against various determinants. **A:** The specific antibodies are directed against the native molecule. **B:** The antibodies are directed against a hydrolysis or biotransformation product of the drug. **C:** The antibodies are directed against a new determinant formed by the interaction of the drug or drug metabolite and the protein. **D:** Conjugation of the drug or its metabolites results in a conformational change in the tissue protein, which is then recognized as foreign by the immune system.

(AIDS) than in other diseases, presumably because of human immunodeficiency virus (HIV)-induced immune dysregulation. It has been demonstrated, for example, that AIDS patients have CD8 T cells, which are capable of T-cell help and secrete a cytokine profile similar to T_H2 of CD4 cells (IL-4, IL-5, and IL-10). These CD8 cells would then be capable of directing the synthesis of IgE antibodies to drugs. This could explain the increased incidence of drug allergy even though CD4 T_H2 cells are absent or present in very low numbers. In some patients with AIDS, CD8 helper cells may be particularly active, accounting for a Job-like syndrome (hyper-IgE, eosinophilia, skin rash, and frequent skin infections).

This is especially so for trimethoprim-sulfamethoxazole and other sulfonamides and their congeners. The spectrum of reactions covers a wide variety of allergic manifestations, including fever, rash, anaphylaxis, Stevens-Johnson syndrome, toxic epidermal necrolysis, and hematologic and hepatic disturbances. It should be pointed out, however, that in the majority of AIDS patients the reaction to sulfonamide-containing drugs is not that of a classic drug allergy but probably more like a toxic reaction, particularly in those patients who experience hepatic or hematologic alterations. The successful treatment of these reactions by rapid or slow desensitization protocols (see later on) does not preclude a nonallergic mechanism.

Clinical Manifestations

An adverse reaction to a drug can be considered as allergic if (1) the patient has antibodies or sensitized T cells with specificity for the drug, a drug metabolite, or a drug–tissue conjugate, and (2) the clinical features of the reaction are consistent with recognized immunologically induced inflammation (see Chapter 26). In some instances, the adverse reaction occurs promptly after the introduction of a drug and appears to be immunologic, but extensive testing fails to demonstrate drug-specific antibodies or T cells. This might be explained by failure to identify the appropriate antigen. Drug fever is an example of this phenomenon. A number of drugs are commonly associated with episodic or persistent fever, which remits on withdrawal of the drug and recurs promptly when the drug is readministered. Although it has long been suspected that drug fever is an immunologic phenomenon, studies to date have failed to provide a convincing immunologic mechanism.

Other factors may play a role in the induction or expression of drug allergy. For example, there is emerging evidence that patients who develop Stevens-Johnson syndrome (erythema multiforme major) or toxic epidermal necrolysis are more likely to have a slow *N*-acetylator genotype than normal controls or patients who experience less severe forms of this disease (erythema multiforme minor).

As noted earlier, any type of hypersensitivity reaction may cause drug allergy. In some cases, the type of immune response determines the location of reaction. For example, the vast majority of T-cell-mediated reactions produce dermatitis. Repeated application of the drug to the skin induces a T-cell response and causes allergic contact dermatitis localized to areas of skin in contact with the drug. Ingestion or injection of the drug generally causes a diffuse eczematoid dermatitis or, less commonly, erythema multiforme of either the minor or major (Stevens-Johnson syndrome) type, toxic epidermal necrolysis, or, in rare cases, erythema nodosum.

The manifestation of drug allergy mediated by antibody depends to a great extent on the type of antibody. Reactions attributed to IgE antibodies include organ-specific symptoms involving the skin (pruritus, urticaria, or angioedema), GI tract (nausea, vomiting, or diarrhea), or pulmonary system (wheezing or shortness of breath). The reaction may be generalized (ie, systemic anaphylaxis). IgG antibodies to drugs result in cytotoxicity to one or more organs or immune complex deposition with complement-mediated inflammation. These may be tissue-specific, as discussed previously, or they may be generalized, with multiple organ involvement (serum sickness).

DIAGNOSIS OF DRUG ALLERGY

Ideally, the diagnosis of drug allergy is made by in vivo or in vitro testing with the drug or its reactive metabolites. For this reason, the most important aspect of the diagnostic evaluation is an accurate and comprehensive history, with special attention paid to three areas: the nature of the symptoms, the drug history, and the temporal relationship between the institution of drug therapy and the onset of the reaction.

Nature of Symptoms

The nature of the symptoms helps to differentiate immunologic reactions from toxic or idiosyncratic reactions and nonimmunologic side effects. Drug allergy must also be distinguished from diseases that might have similar symptoms. For example, patients with systemic lupus erythematosus often present with symptoms resembling those of an allergic drug reaction. On the other hand, allergic drug reactions may simulate other illnesses.

Drug History

A history of prior drug use and adverse reactions may reveal that a current allergic response is caused by the same or similar class of drug. A drug reaction may appear after many years of use, but this is rare. Diagnosis is especially difficult in the patient with an adverse reaction while taking multiple medications.

Certain drugs, however, such as antibiotics, cause allergic reactions more frequently than others (eg, digitalis glycosides).

Temporal Relationship

The temporal relationship between the institution of drug therapy and the onset of the reaction is an important diagnostic clue. Patients who are already sensitized react more rapidly than those with a new sensitivity. Following administration of the drug, IgE antibody reactions generally start within 30–60 minutes, Arthus reactions in 6–24 hours, and allergic contact dermatitis in 48–72 hours, and serum sickness in 7–10 days. It is unlikely, but not impossible, for a patient who has been on a drug for a long period to develop a de novo sensitization to that drug or to develop a reaction to a drug after therapy with that agent has been discontinued.

In Vivo Tests

It is sometimes possible to confirm a suspected allergic drug reaction by using in vivo testing.

A. Patch or Skin Tests: In vivo testing includes prick or intradermal skin testing for IgE sensitivity, patch testing for delayed-type hypersensitivity, and provocative-dose challenges. The wheal-and-erythema skin test cannot be used to diagnose IgE-mediated allergy to drugs that nonspecifically release the mediators of anaphylaxis from mast cells. A partial list of such drugs is found in Chapter 28. When testing skin sensitivity to a new drug or drug class, it is imperative to perform control testing on nonexposed volunteers to determine the concentration of drug that does not induce a nonspecific wheal and flare reaction.

When performing skin tests for IgE-mediated drug allergy or patch tests for allergic contact dermatitis, the immunogenic form of the drug (native drug or metabolite) must be used. Usually, however, the true immunogen is not known, in which case the native drug is used at a concentration that has been shown not to induce nonspecific reactions. In the case of an immediate wheal-and-flare skin test response to a drug, one assumes that the drug is metabolized in the skin, binds to tissue proteins, and then becomes reactive with mast cell-bound IgE. A positive reaction is highly predictive of IgE antidrug. A negative reaction means either that no specific IgE exists or that there was not appropriate drug biotransformation to become immunogenic, and thus, a negative skin test does not rule out drug allergy. For patch testing, the drug must be used at a concentration low enough to be nonirritating to the skin.

B. Provocative Tests: The provocative-dose challenge is a method whereby the patient is given increasing doses of the drug and observed for signs of an allergic response, at which point the drug is withdrawn. Because this method is not without danger, it is reserved for instances when no alternative therapy is available and when the benefit of the drug far outweighs the potential harm; it must be performed only where adequate facilities and personnel are available to treat acute medical emergencies.

In Vitro Tests

In vitro tests are designed to identify the presence of either the antibody of sensitized T cell that reacts with the drug determinant. For IgE antibody-mediated reaction, the radioallergosorbent test (RAST) or enzyme-linked immunosorbent assay (ELISA) is applicable when the antigenic determinant is known and available. Lack of knowledge of the determinant for most drugs has limited this type of testing. A RAST or ELISA is available for detecting IgE antibodies to the major (penicilloyl) determinant of penicillin allergy or several of the minor determinants (see later discussion). Recently an ELISA for identifying allergy to the sulfonamide group has been developed. The sensitivity and specificity of these tests, however, has not been well characterized. Tests for IgG or IgM antibodies are available for only a limited number of allergenic drugs and are not yet clinically useful.

For the suspected cell-mediated reaction to drugs, lymphocyte activation assays have been used (see Chapter 15). These test the ability of the drug or a drug-protein conjugate to induce the proliferation of T lymphocytes. Lymphocyte activation analysis is relatively simple to perform; however, the 3–5 days necessary to complete the test and the need for appropriate cell culture facilities have limited its use in clinical practice.

TREATMENT OF DRUG ALLERGIES

Since there are only a few drugs for which accurate in vivo or in vitro testing is available, a suspected drug reaction must often be treated without such confirmation. Any drug not necessary for the care of the patient is discontinued. For drugs that cannot be eliminated, an alternative drug with similar pharmacologic properties but a different, noncross-reactive, chemical structure should be substituted. In cases when no alternative drug is available and the allergic reaction is mild, and not life-threatening, such as skin pruritus or urticaria, it may be possible to continue the drug and treat the patient symptomatically. If possible, the drug should be discontinued temporarily for a short time to confirm that it was the cause of the reaction and then reintroduced.

PENICILLIN ALLERGY

Penicillin and the other β-lactam antibiotics are a frequent cause of all types of immunologic drug reactions, including IgE-mediated single-organ (eg, urticaria) or multiple-organ (systemic allergic reactions or anaphylaxis) disease, serum sickness, T-cell-mediated contact dermatitis, and antibody-mediated cytolysis. By far the most common and potentially dangerous penicillin reactions, however, are those resulting from the production of specific IgE. As a group, the β-lactam antibiotics are the most common cause of IgE-mediated allergic reactions to drugs. This class of drugs includes the penicillins, the cephalosporins, the cephamycins, the penems, and the monobactams (Fig 31–3). The penicillins have a β-lactam ring conjugated to a five-membered thiazolidine ring. They differ from the cephalosporins in that the latter class has a six-membered rather than a five-membered sulfur-containing ring. The cephamycins are similar to the cephalosporins but have a methoxy group attached to the β-lactam ring. Penems are a large class that resembles the penicillins, with the exception that the five-membered ring contains a carbon or oxygen in place of the sulfur. Finally, the monobactams are the only class of drug that does not have a second ring conjugated to the β-lactam ring.

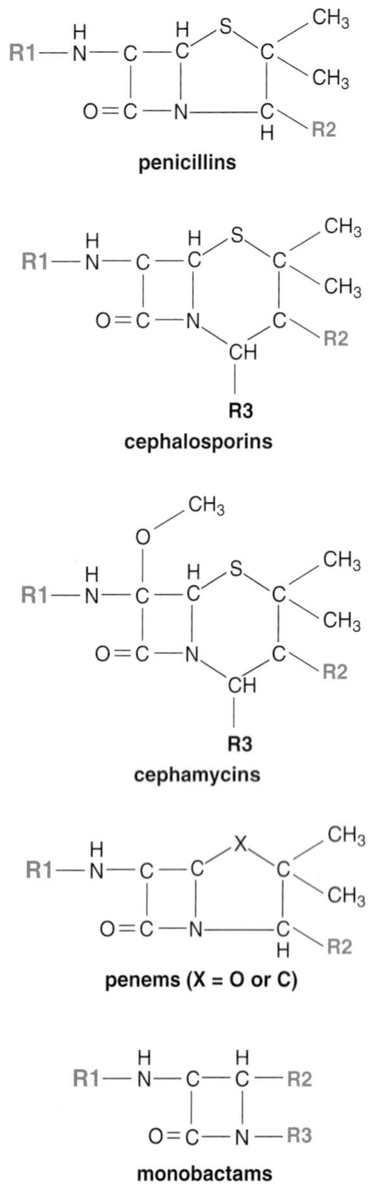

Skin Testing

Specific skin test reagents are available to evaluate patients with suspected penicillin allergy. Skin testing with penicillin G alone is effective in demonstrating allergic reactivity in only a small percentage of sensitive patients. Conjugation of penicillin to protein following cleavage of the β-lactam ring (penicilloyl group), however, has provided a skin test reagent that shows a positive correlation with clinical allergic sensitivity in more than 75% of all penicillin-allergic individuals. For this reason, the penicilloyl group has been termed the "major determinant." Fewer patients react with unconjugated penicilloic acid (7%) or with penicillin G (6%). These two molecules are presumed to conjugate to tissue proteins in the skin, thereby providing determinants other than the penicilloyl group. They are called the "minor determinants." In practice, penicilloyl-polylysine is used to test for the major determinant because poly-D-lysine is a relatively nonimmunogenic molecule. This reagent is available commercially. The minor determinants, however, are not yet available commercially, although methods for their production and use have been published.

There are a number of protocols for skin testing in cases of suspected penicillin allergy. In one protocol, penicillin G and penicilloic acid are prepared at a concentration of 3.3 mg/mL and diluted 1:100 and 1:10,000. Penicilloyl-polylysine is used at a concentration of 6×10^{-5} mol/L. Skin prick testing is performed first with the most dilute concentration and then with the more concentrated solution if there is no reaction to the first test. If the prick test is negative, intradermal testing (0.02 mL) is performed in a similar fashion. The patient is considered to be allergic to penicillin if there is a positive skin test to any of the reagents at any dilution.

The penicillin skin test has proven to be highly predictive. In one study of more than 1500 skin tests, only a single patient with negative skin tests had an acute anaphylactic reaction when given penicillin in full therapeutic doses. Patients who have a positive skin test are at risk for a systemic allergic reaction; in several studies the reaction rate was more than 25%. Thus, patients who are skin test-positive will need to be desensitized before full therapeutic doses of this drug can be used.

A number of factors have been shown to correlate with skin test positivity to penicillin. For example, 100% of patients who reported a previous anaphylactic reaction to penicillin were skin test-positive, and 75% of patients with serum sickness had positive tests. In our studies, more than 40% of patients with other symptoms of an immunologic response to peni-

Figure 31–3. Core structures of the five groups of β-lactam antibiotics. R1, R2, R3, side chains; X, oxygen atom or CH₂ in penems.

cillin were skin test-positive, although other studies have reported a significantly lower percentage. Skin test positivity correlates with the time course of the reaction during penicillin therapy. Immediate reactions in previously sensitized patients and reactions appearing 7–10 days after the institution of drug therapy in previously unsensitized patients are associated with the highest percentage of positive skin tests.

The time elapsed since the reported allergic reaction is also critical. Skin tests may be negative for several days or weeks after a systemic reaction before becoming positive. The tests remain positive over the next several years and then gradually decline, so that by 10 years following a reaction, fewer than 10% of history-positive patients are still skin test-positive. This demonstrates that although drug-induced IgE may persist over a relatively long period, the IgE levels will eventually decline in the absence of further antigenic stimulation.

Patients who present a history of penicillin allergy but are skin test-negative can be given penicillin in full therapeutic doses with no greater risk of reaction than those without a history of penicillin allergy. Several studies have demonstrated that patients with a positive history and negative skin tests who are treated with oral penicillin or its analogues are rarely resensitized, and, therefore, skin testing following oral therapy is not necessary. In contrast, patients who receive high-dose intravenous penicillin are frequently (70%) resensitized and, therefore, should be retested at 6–8 weeks following the cessation of therapy.

It has been estimated that at least 250 patients in the United States die each year from anaphylactic reactions to parenteral penicillin. By contrast, only six cases of anaphylactic death were reported from oral penicillin, and the number of reported nonfatal anaphylactic reactions from oral penicillin is less than 100. For this reason, we have chosen to use the oral route for penicillin desensitization.

Desensitization to Penicillin

The desensitization procedure is reserved for patients with a history of penicillin allergy in whom the skin test is positive or cannot be performed. There should be no alternative antibiotic available, and the infection should be serious enough to risk the dangers of anaphylaxis from the treatment. If the patient meets these criteria, one of several protocols can be used. In one protocol, the patient is given increasing doses of oral phenoxymethyl penicillin (chosen because of its excellent and predictable absorption from the gut), beginning at 100 U and progressing until 400,000–800,000 U (250–500 mg) has been given. The drug is then given intravenously. This procedure has been performed in more than 100 patients, and in only 2 instances has it failed because of unacceptable reactions. In about one third of patients, there is a minor skin reaction, but these reactions have not precluded achieving desensitization.

Others have preferred to use an intravenous desensitization. This method, in general, has a higher reaction rate but is effective, particularly when no oral form of the drug is available. Until recently, this has been the case for patients sensitive to the third-generation cephalosporins (see later discussion). Oral preparations of the third-generation cephalosporins should be used for desensitization when available.

Cross-Reactions with Other β-Lactams

The chemistry of penicillin metabolites has been well studied, and the chemical structure of the allergenic epitopes is now established. Similar studies have not been carried out for the related β-lactam antibiotics. Therefore, cross-reactivity of antipenicillin IgE antibodies with the other β-lactam antibiotics has been evaluated only by in vitro tests, such as RAST or ELISA inhibition, or by clinical studies. Although many of the data are speculative, some generalizations can be made. Natural or semisynthetic penicillins tend to cross-react with one another. In addition, the cross-reactivity between penicillin and the first-generation cephalosporins appears to be relatively high (greater than 50%), particularly in patients with extreme sensitivity. The cross-reactivity between penicillin and the second- and third-generation cephalosporins is significantly lower than for the first-generation drugs (Table 31–1). There is some cross-reactivity, however, and there are reports of at least three anaphylactic deaths resulting from the use of every second- and third-generation cephalosporin available in the United States. Only the monobactams appear to lack cross-reactivity with penicillin.

The problem of cross-reactivity among the various β-lactam antibiotics has now been evaluated by RAST or ELISA inhibition analysis. This work has shed some light on the mechanisms of cross-reactivity. In general, most IgE antibodies to the second- or third-generation cephalosporins or the penems are directed against the side chains and not the β-lactam ring. Many of these patients also have an IgE directed toward the β-lactam ring, but this is a separate and distinct antibody species. Indeed, there is now evidence

Table 31–1. Major groups of cephalosporins.

First Generation	Second Generation	Third Generation
Cephalothin	Cefamandole	Cefotaxime
Cephapirin	Cefuroxime	Ceftizoxime
Cefazolin	Cefonicid	Ceftriaxone
Cephalexin[1]	Ceforanide	Ceftazidime
Cephadrine[1]	Cefaclor[1]	Cefoperazone
Cefadroxil[1]	Cefoxitin	Moxalactam
	Cefotetan	Cefixime[1]
	Cefprozil[1]	Cefpodoxime
	Cefuroxime	proxetil[1]
	acetil[1]	
	Cefmetazole	

[1] Oral agents.

to suggest that a patient with a documented penicillin allergy is at greater risk for an allergic reaction to the alternative β-lactam antibiotics because these patients are more likely to produce IgE against haptens and do not show a true antigenic cross-reactivity. For these individuals who have antiside chain IgE, however, there is the possibility of cross-reactivity between different core molecules with similar side chains. For example, aztreonam and ceftazidime contain the same side chain. Similarly, piperacillin and cephapyrizone contain identical side chains.

Recently, a group of ampicillin or amoxicillin allergic patients who produce antiside chain IgE, in the absence of anti-β-lactam IgE has been reported. These patients have been detected by positive skin reactivity to ampicillin or amoxicillin but negative skin tests to penicilloyl-polylysine, penicilloic acid, or penicillin G, and this has been confirmed by in vitro testing. Interestingly, these side chain reactors appear to be more liable to develop T-cell reactions than those who react only to the β-lactam ring. These patients are also of interest because they do not have allergic reactions to penicillin, semisynthetic penicillins, or first-generation cephalosporins that do not contain the amoxicillin or ampicillin side chains.

SULFONAMIDE ALLERGY

The sulfonamide drugs cause acute allergic reactions in a significant percentage of patients. This class of drugs is used for a variety of therapeutic uses; it includes such sulfonamide antibiotics as sulfisoxazole and sulfamethoxazole, the diuretics furosemide and hydrochlorothiazide, and the angiotensin-converting enzyme (ACE) inhibitor captopril. The frequency of cross-reactivity among members of this class of drugs is not known. Patients sensitized to one sulfonamide may or may not react when treated with other sulfonamides. Skin testing is unreliable in confirming or rejecting the clinical history of an allergic reaction. Therefore, patients with a history of sensitivity to one member of this class should avoid all sulfonamide drugs. Alternative antibiotics are readily available: ethacrynic acid can be substituted for furosemide, and benazepril, enalapril, fosinopril, lisinopril, moexipril, quinapril, and ramipril, alternative ACE inhibitors, or another class of antihypertensive drug can be used to replace captopril.

Recently, an ELISA has been developed that uses sulfonamide conjugated with human serum albumin as antigen, but the test has yet to be studied in a sufficient number of patients to be used with confidence for diagnosis of sulfonamide allergy.

Experience with desensitization has burgeoned in the past several years due to the high incidence of sulfonamide sensitivity in HIV-positive patients, particularly those with AIDS. In this group of patients, both rapid (<12 hours) and slow desensitization protocols

have been described. The experience with desensitization by either type of protocol has been favorable so that most AIDS patients can be maintained on trimethoprim-sulfamethoxazole for long periods. Whether the success rate is due to the altered immune system of the AIDS patient or because most of the reaction is toxic rather than immunologic in nature remains to be determined.

For other patients with sulfonamide sensitivity, the published experience with desensitization procedures is very limited, and severe immediate reactions have been reported. Desensitization for sulfonamide-containing drugs should therefore be considered only in the very rare situations when a sulfonamide antibiotic is the only effective treatment for a life-threatening disease. Sulfonamides can cause severe skin reactions such as Stevens-Johnson syndrome, which are not amenable to desensitization. Thus, the potential danger from the administration of sulfonamides to sensitive individuals is significantly greater than for penicillin.

INSULIN ALLERGY

Insulin is a frequent cause of allergic reactions. Both IgG and IgE antibodies may be induced by therapeutic insulin, but these antibodies may or may not cause allergic reactions. Several syndromes are related to anti-insulin antibodies, however. Insulin allergic reactions may be local or systemic, and their onset can be either immediate or delayed. The immediate local reaction is mediated by IgE antibodies. It generally consists of local swelling and erythema, and, in contrast to other IgE-mediated reactions, it is often painful rather than pruritic. The delayed local reaction that occurs 4–12 hours following injection, however, is an Arthus reaction resulting from IgG anti-insulin antibodies. Immediate and delayed systemic reactions are both IgE-mediated. The majority of patients who have developed clinically significant anti-insulin IgE antibody have had an interruption in therapy. Patients who are obese have an increased incidence of insulin allergy.

The relationship of clinical cross-reactivity to the amino acid sequences of insulins from different animal species is not clear. Patients may be sensitized to either bovine insulin, which differs from human insulin by three amino acids in the α chain, or to porcine insulin, which differs from human insulin by a single amino acid in the β chain (Fig 31–4). Some patients are sensitized to proinsulin, which contaminates many insulin preparations. Most patients sensitive to animal insulin(s) react not only to the bovine and porcine varieties but also to human insulin. This is a true cross-reactivity, because insulin-sensitive patients who are treated with recombinant human insulin will also react. Patients treated exclusively with recombinant human insulin, however, do not develop either IgE or IgG antibodies.

amino acid sequence variations

	A-chain position 8 9 10	B-chain position 30
human	Thr-Ser-Ile	Thr
pig, dog, sperm whale	Thr-Ser-Ile	Ala
cattle, goat	Ala-Ser-Val	Ala

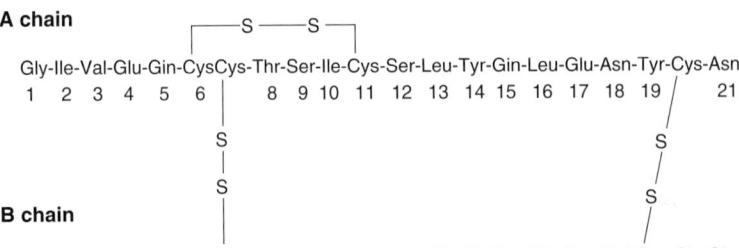

Figure 31–4. Covalent structure and variations of human and animal insulins. (Reproduced, with permission, from Ganong WF: *Review of Medical Physiology,* 14th ed. Appleton & Lange, 1989.)

The treatment of all allergic reactions to insulin must be balanced with the transient nature of these reactions. The patient may be assured that these reactions are rarely fatal and, in most instances, will disappear in a short time.

Treatment of patients with local reactions to insulin is largely symptomatic. The use of oral antihistaminics or concomitant injection of the antihistamine with the insulin is effective in most cases. For very severe reactions, insulin can be injected with corticosteroids (dexamethasone is preferred because it is compatible with most insulin preparations); however, the dose of corticosteroid must be relatively low (0.75 mg of dexamethasone or equivalent) to avoid steroid-induced gluconeogenesis.

For immediate systemic reactions, single-component (preferably human) insulin should be tried first. If the patient reacts to this preparation, then skin testing with human insulin, followed by rapid desensitization, generally to human insulin, is usually effective. It is preferable to have the patient discontinue insulin for several days prior to the desensitization, if possible.

Several studies have demonstrated that there is a rapid decline in the anti-insulin IgE levels in desensitized patients. The mechanism for this decline is not known. Patients who undergo desensitization to insulin, however, must be cautioned that there should not be lapses in therapy, because this may lead to reappearance of IgE antibodies and a severe allergic reaction when insulin therapy is resumed.

Patients with high levels of anti-insulin IgG antibodies may be insulin-resistant. The treatment of insulin resistance is beyond the scope of this chapter, and the reader is referred to standard texts.

MULTIPLE DRUG ALLERGY SYNDROME

Recent studies describe a group of patients who have true IgE-mediated allergy to multiple unrelated drugs and antibiotics. The immunologic basis for the multiple drug allergy syndrome is not clear. It would appear that this group of patients is genetically programmed to react to haptenated proteins with greater frequency than the normal population. Their offspring have a multifold increased incidence of drug allergy compared with children of parents with no drug allergy. The exact step (eg, antigen presentation, T-cell reactivity, B-cell reactivity) that is altered in these patients has not been elucidated. They can, however, be desensitized with the same ease as other allergic patients.

PSEUDOALLERGIC REACTIONS

Certain drugs can release mediators of anaphylaxis from mast cells or circulating basophils by nonimmunologic means. These drugs are therefore capable of causing significant reactions in a certain portion of the treated population. Although IgE antibodies are not involved, the symptoms of anaphylactic and anaphylactoid reactions are identical (see Chapter 28). Radiocontrast media, particularly the ionic forms or those with higher osmolality, are perhaps the best examples of drugs that cause pseudoallergic reactions. Other common drugs include aspirin and other nonsteroidal anti-inflammatory drugs (NSAIDs), curare and its derivatives, the opiate analgesics, and some local anesthetics. The reason for the susceptibility of only a portion of the treated population to nonimmunologic urticaria and anaphylactoid reactions to these drugs is not known.

Several strategies have been developed for safe administration of drugs that cause pseudoallergic reactions. For patients who have previously reacted to radiocontrast media, pretreatment with H_1 and H_2 receptor-blocking antihistamines and corticosteroids has proven highly effective. Patients with sensitivity to aspirin or other NSAIDs are best treated by avoiding these drugs.

For patients who have a history of reaction to local anesthetics, skin testing followed by provocative dose challenge is very effective. The local anesthetics belong to one of two classes: those containing a *para*-aminobenzoic acid ester group and those lacking this structure. The "ester" group (which includes procaine and tetracaine) tend to be more potent at direct degranulation of mast cells and also are cross-reactive within the group. By contrast, the local anesthetics lacking an "ester" do not cross-react with the ester group or with themselves. They are significantly less potent as direct mediator-releasing agents. We usually perform skin tests using preparations that are preservative-free and that contain no β-adrenergic agonist. The former can cause an IgE-mediated reaction, whereas side effects of the latter may simulate an allergic reaction. Following skin testing by the epicutaneous and intradermal route, a single agent is selected, and 0.1-mL, 0.5-mL, and, if desired, 1.0-mL subcutaneous injection are administered. Failure of the patient to react to any of these test doses demonstrates that the patient can safely receive that local anesthetic in the future.

CONCLUSIONS

Immunologically mediated drug hypersensitivity constitutes a significant proportion of the overall spectrum of adverse reactions to drugs. The entire spectrum of immune responses to antigens is encountered in drug allergy. Although the proportion of treated patients who react to a given drug or class of drugs varies widely, it is likely that any drug is capable of inducing an adverse immunologic reaction, and so any drug must be considered as a possible cause of an individual patient's reaction.

The majority of drugs in use today are haptens and, therefore, must conjugate to tissue protein in vivo to be immunogenic. Unfortunately, the actual immunogen is not known for most drugs. This has made the development of accurate in vivo or in vitro tests difficult. Thus, for most drug classes, an accurate clinical history is the only diagnostic test for suspecting a particular drug as the cause of a patient's reaction. When the history suggests a candidate, its effect can then be confirmed by testing. When testing is not possible, drug withdrawal and, if necessary, rechallenge will confirm the patient's sensitivity.

It is only in a minority of situations that continuation of or reintroduction of the drug is necessary. In this case, pretreatment protocols, provocative challenge, and drug desensitization procedures are available. The best treatment for drug allergy, however, is the use of a different drug with similar pharmacologic properties but different chemical (ie, antigenic) structure.

REFERENCES

Adverse reactions to radiocontrast media. *Invest Radiol* 1980;**15**(suppl 6):S1. (Entire issue).

Bayard PJ et al: Drug hypersensitivity reactions and human immunodeficiency virus disease. *J Acquired Immune Defic Syndr* 1992;**5**:1237.

Carrington DM et al: Studies of human IgE to a sulfonamide determinant. *J Allergy Clin Immunol* 1987;**79**:442.

Evans R, III et al: Current concepts in allergy: Drug reactions. *Curr Probl Pediatr* 1991;**21**:185.

Hansbrough JR et al: Anaphylaxis to intravenous furosemide. *J Allergy Clin Immunol* 1987;**80**:538.

Jick H, Derby LE: A large population-based follow-up study of trimethoprim-sulfamethoxazole, trimethoprim and cephalexin for uncommon serious drug toxicity. *Pharmacotherapy,* 1995;**15**:428.

Levine BB, Zolov DM: Prediction of penicillin allergy by immunological tests. *J Allergy* 1969;**43**:231.

Moreno F et al: Studies of the specificities of IgE antibodies found in sera from subjects with allergic reactions to penicillins. *Int Arch Allergy Immunol* 1995;**108**:74.

Parker CW et al: Hypersensitivity to penicillanic acid derivatives in human beings with penicillin allergy. *J Exp Med* 1982;**115**:821.

Ring J: Pseudoallergic reactions. In: *Allergy: Theory and Practice,* 2nd ed. Korenblat PE, Wedner HJ (editors). Grune & Stratton, 1989.

Sullivan TJ et al: Desensitization of patients allergic to penicillin by orally administered beta-lactam antibiotics. *J Allergy Clin Immunol* 1982;**69**:275.

Sullivan TJ et al: Skin testing to detect penicillin allergy. *J Allergy Clin Immunol* 1981;**68:**171.

Volz MA, Nelson HS: Drug allergy. Best diagnostic and treatment approaches. *Postgrad Med* 1990;**87:**137.

Wedner HJ: Adverse reactions to drugs. In: *Current Pediatric Therapy,* 12th ed. Gellis SS, Kagan BM (editors). WB Saunders, 1986, pp 640–646.

Wedner HJ: Protocols for penicillin desensitization. In: *Allergy: Theory and Practice.* Korenblat PE, Wedner HJ (editors). Grune & Stratton, 1984, p 423.

Weiss ME: Drug allergy. *Med Clin North Am* 1992;**76:**857.

Mechanisms of Disordered Immune Regulation

Cornelia M. Weyand, MD, PhD, & Jörg J. Goronzy, MD, PhD

Enormous progress has been made over the last decades in understanding the mechanisms of normal immune responses. A functioning immune system is absolutely crucial to an individual's survival. Immune responses are not always protective in nature, however, but can be associated with tissue destruction and disease. Unraveling what goes wrong in immune reactions considered to cause autoimmune diseases remains one of the biggest challenges of modern immunology. For none of the human diseases classified as autoimmune disorders do we have a complete concept of pathogenic mechanisms. This is partially related to the complexity of syndromes caused by pathologic immune responses. It is very unlikely that a singular immunologic abnormality leads to the sequelae of a tissue-destructive immune reaction. The combination of multiple abnormalities in the immune system, the contribution of nonimmune cells and tissues, a variety of genetic risk determinants, and random environmental factors may all be necessary to induce what clinically presents as a pathologic immune response.

NORMAL IMMUNE RESPONSES: FUNDAMENTAL PRINCIPLES

All available evidence indicates that pathologic immune processes in autoimmune disease use immune cells and mediators similar to those in protective immune reactions. It is therefore important to understand the fundamental properties of the normal immune system before analyzing the abnormalities leading to disease.

The tissue of immune system is unique in that its cells are able to travel to all parts of the body to recognize and eliminate foreign intruders, malignant cells, and agents that could harm the body. To do so, the immune system has a set of fundamental properties that distinguishes it from all other organ systems (Table 32–1).

Table 32–1. Fundamental principles of normal immune responses.

- T and B lymphocytes express clonally distributed receptor molecules that recognize subtle structural differences and are highly specific.
- The repertoire of receptor molecules is highly diverse to provide a fit for an enormous spectrum of antigens.
- Mature T cells are restricted by self-MHC determinants, recognize exogenous antigenic peptides, and are self-tolerant.
- The immune system memorizes the recognition of specific antigens. On reexposure the response is faster and more vigorous.
- Immune responses are self-limited. Antigen recognition leads to clonal expansion of specific lymphocytes. Growth of selected lymphocytes is provided by mechanisms of clonal downsizing.

Antigen-Specific Recognition

To recognize all potential antigens, the immune system has a receptor structure that can specifically bind and recognize subtle structural differences through clonal selection. This feature allows the immune system a focused response to an unwanted antigen and minimizes the chance for an antigen to escape immune recognition.

Diversity of the Lymphocyte Repertoire

Antigen-specific recognition is achieved through the availability of an enormous spectrum of reactive lymphocytes. The diversity of the lymphocyte repertoire is threatened whenever individual lymphocyte specificities expand and form clonogenic populations. Malignant diseases of T and B cells are the most extreme form of clonal outgrowth.

Discrimination of Self Versus Nonself

The ability of the immune system to distinguish self from nonself is not genomically encoded, and therefore not inherited, but rather it must be learned in a complex chain of events. Lymphocytes carrying receptors reactive to self-determinants are eliminated, but lymphocytes with receptors fitting non-self antigens are selected. Abnormalities in the generation and maintenance of self-tolerance have been considered one of the major mechanisms causing autoimmunity.

Immunologic Memory

Exposure of the immune system to an antigen leaves an imprint, or in other words, lymphocytes "memorize" prior antigen-specific stimulation. Although the molecular details leading to memory are not understood, immunoprotection depends on the immune system's ability to respond faster and more vigorously when reexposed to an antigen. The ability to prime immune responses, however, also has negative aspects because unwanted immune responses can be equally amplified.

Self-Limitation

Specific stimulation of the antigen receptor leads to lymphocyte proliferation. If unopposed, this would eventually result in an increasing number of immunocytes or reduced diversity (or both). It is therefore essential that immune reactions be self-limited. Only recently has it become clear that antigen stimulation of antigen receptors on T cells not only triggers proliferation but induces programmed cell death (apoptosis). Clonal expansion on antigen contact is thus linked to clonal downsizing. Temporary activation of responding lymphocytes with subsequent return to the resting state is another mechanism guaranteeing discontinuation of immune responses.

AUTOIMMUNITY

The currently accepted paradigm predicts that a normal immune system has the remarkable ability to respond to any possible foreign antigenic determinant while ignoring the world of self antigens. Paul Ehrlich expressed this concept as the "horror autotoxicus theory." Since then it has been assumed that immune-mediated diseases result from specific recognition of host antigens. The assumption that immunocytes are not allowed to become activated when their receptor fits to a self component has survived several decades, but it has become clear that the rules imposed on the immune system are not as simple as first predicted. It is still true that the pool of mature lymphocytes in a given individual includes a vast variety of receptor types, each with the potential to specifically react to unwanted antigens. At the same time self-antigens do not elicit a similar response. The distinction between self and nonself, however, appears not to be absolute, and increasing evidence points to an important contribution of self-recognition in a functional immune system.

The Phenomenon of Self-Tolerance

The immune system is constantly exposed to self antigens without inducing lymphocyte stimulation—a

Table 32–2. Self-Tolerance.

- Is antigen specific.
- Is not inherited but somatically acquired.
- Is achieved through clonal deletion of self-reactive lymphocytes and through clonal anergy of potentially autoreactive T and B cells.
- May be overcome leading to autoaggressive immune recognition.

phenomenon called self-tolerance (Table 32–2). Self-tolerance is not an inherited feature of the immune system but the result of several mechanisms designed to distinguish between lymphocytes with the potential to bind to self-components and those with much higher binding specificity for antigenic determinants expressed by foreign antigens. Initially the immune system generates diversity by combining highly polymorphic gene segments to form receptor molecules. The formation of the receptor repertoire is a random process and is followed by a selection procedure that sorts lymphocytes into those with self-reactivity and those lacking self-reactivity. Since self-tolerance is somatically acquired, it is subject to failure, particularly with the complexity of events necessary to create a pool of lymphocytes that are ready to attack any foreign antigen but ignore self proteins.

Tolerance, like immune recognition, is antigen-specific, and the major mechanisms clonally delete or anergize unwanted lymphocytes. Clonal deletion of T cells probed for their antigen specificity is only possible because immature lymphocytes have a different reaction pattern to antigen stimulation than mature lymphocytes do. The biochemical signals that lead to clonal deletion or clonal anergy of unwanted cells are not exactly understood. For clonal deletion and clonal anergy, antigen contact and triggering of the specific receptor molecule is necessary. The two mechanisms, however, are fundamentally different. Clonal deletion is a consequence of activation-induced cell death and is irreversible. Clonal anergy may be a reversible process since the cells continue to be available but are functionally paralyzed.

Antigen specificity mediated through a clonally distributed receptor molecule, and thus antigen-specific tolerance, is restricted to T and B lymphocytes. Other cells of the immune system, and many cell types involved in autoimmune reactions, lack this remarkable feature. Antibody responses facilitated by B lymphocytes generally depend on help provided by T lymphocytes. This central role of T cells in the immune response makes them an ideal target for tolerance induction. Elimination of T cells specific for self antigens should be sufficient to prevent anti-self-reactivity. Indeed, tolerance to self proteins is mainly controlled through the elimination or the functional impairment of autoreactive T cells. This central role of T lymphocytes in the maintenance of self-tolerance has made the T cell a focus of interest in the investigation of human autoimmune diseases.

Mechanisms of Tolerance Induction in T Lymphocytes

Mature T cells are self-tolerant, self-major histocompatibility complex (MHC)-restricted, and responsive to foreign antigens. They derive from an enormous collection of immature T cells that originate in the bone marrow, pass through the thymus to acquire the phenotype of a fully functional T cell, and are then selected for a receptor molecule that does not bind to self components but has an optimal fit for a unwanted antigen presented in the context of self-MHC. Induction of self-tolerance is one of the major achievements of thymic education and it cannot be viewed as an isolated process. Rather, it is an integral part of the events leading to the selection of an impressively large pool of functional T lymphocytes.

The earliest cells of the T-cell lineage develop from stem cells in the bone marrow and express neither typical T-cell markers nor T-cell receptors (TCRs). After settling into the thymus, they undergo expansion, rearrange TCR genes, and begin to express surface markers, such as CD4 and CD8. Gene segments used to create TCR are spatially separated in the germline and have to be brought together through a somatic rearrangement process (Fig 32–1). Through the action of recombinases, variable (V), diversity (D), and joining (J) gene segments are rearranged and, after deletion of noncoding sequences, are connected to a constant (C) gene element. For α-β TCRs, the β-chain locus is rearranged first followed by the construction of the α-chain gene. Although the rearrangement process is very similar for both, α chains lack integrated D segments. The spectrum of TCR genes formed by this rearrangement process is large and is estimated to include 10^{10}–10^{15} possible combinations. This level of diversity is generated by a combination of different mechanisms, such as:

- V, D, and J segments are represented in the germline in multiple forms.
- Up to 80 different BV genes are available for recombination.

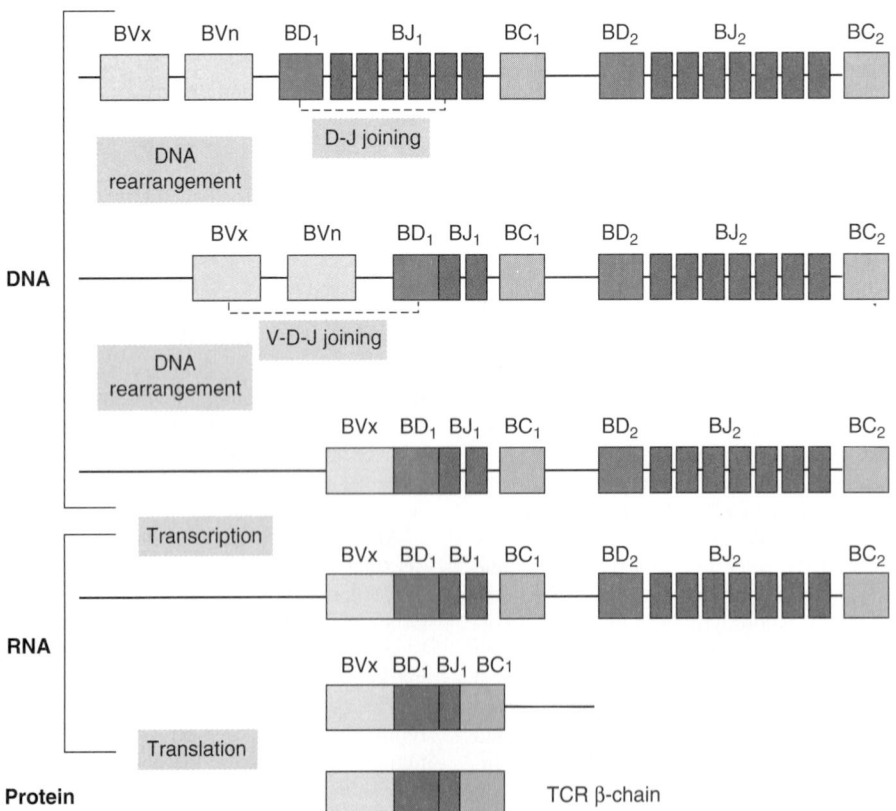

Figure 32–1. Somatic rearrangement of TCR gene segments. In the genomic germline configuration, TCR genes are nonfunctional. During thymic development, genes are rearranged to form functional TCR α, β, γ, and δ chains. This process is shown for the β chain. The D- and J-gene segments are first joined, followed by joining of a V-gene segment to the D-J element. Joining is imprecise, and the joining region is modified by several mechanisms to generate diversity.

- Combinatorial diversity is introduced by bringing together different V, D, and J genes in a patchwork-like manner.
- Junctional diversity adds significantly to the multitude of TCR constructs. Through the action of terminal deoxyribonucleotidyl transferase, nontemplated nucleotides are added at the V-D, D-J, and V-J junctions. Also, the joining of germline-encoded gene segments is imprecise (junctional flexibility), and nucleotides can be lost in the process. Finally, D-gene segments are often translated in all three reading frames, adding additional diversity to the region of the TCR molecule, which is considered the "active center" of the receptor molecule.
- The diversity of the final receptor molecule is multiplied by the pairing of polymorphic α and β chains, which are combined as dimers on the cell surface.

It is obvious that this process of creating a highly diverse repertoire of TCR genes must also result in receptor molecules that either do not fit to the ligand or are reactive to self-antigens. Both problems are addressed by the subsequent process of thymic selection in which T cells are sorted based on their receptor specificity (Fig 32–2).

Positive Selection: Mature T cells are activated when their receptor specifically binds to a complex formed by the host's MHC molecules and a processed antigenic peptide. One of the goals of thymic selection must therefore be to choose thymocytes expressing receptor molecules with a fit for self-MHC determinants. T cells with affinity for self-MHC are allowed to survive while all other T cells are eliminated. This selection step results in a pool of T cells that are self-MHC-restricted but still includes T cells with the potential to react to self antigens. It is currently believed that positive selection functions by preventing programmed cell death. In that model, thymocytes are prone to die unless they are rescued. Binding of the TCR to self-MHC molecules could provide the signals necessary to counteract programmed cell death and thus permit the survival of a self-MHC-restricted T-cell repertoire.

Negative Selection: To establish self-tolerance, the pool of thymocytes needs to be cleared from self-reactive T cells. During negative selection, T cells with receptor molecules binding with high affinity to the bimolecular complex of self peptides and self-MHC are eliminated. It is assumed that clonal deletion and clonal anergy are used to achieve this goal. Subsequently, only T cells should be left that have specificity for foreign antigens, are restricted by self-MHC molecules and are self-tolerant. These thymocytes acquire the phenotype of mature T cells, pass through the thymic medulla, and populate secondary lymphoid tissues until they are needed to defend the host. Although biochemical signals leading to thymocyte selection are not completely understood, there is evidence that negative selection is an apoptosis-dependent phenomenon. High-affinity binding of thymocyte

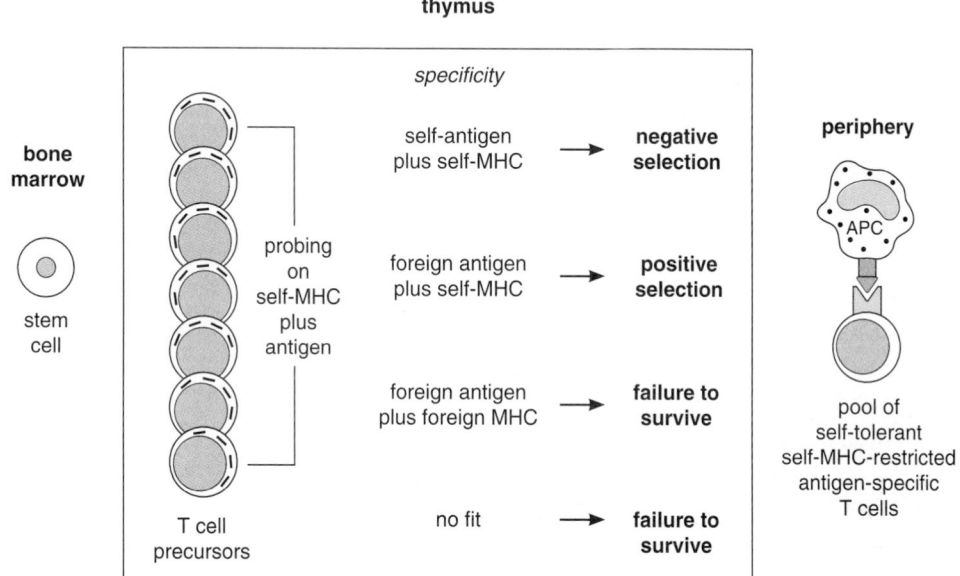

Figure 32–2. Thymic selection. Thymocytes that express functional TCR chains are selected on self-MHC and self antigen in the thymus. Autoreactive T cells that recognize self antigens with high avidity are deleted. Positive selection ensures that only T cells that have the ability to recognize antigen in conjunction with the self-MHC molecules mature and leave the thymus. T cells expressing TCR molecules that are not able to interact with self-MHC molecules undergo apoptosis by default.

TCR to self antigens is assumed to cause activation-induced apoptosis. The consequences of TCR triggering might thus be different for immature thymocytes and mature T cells.

Despite the progress made in understanding the thymic education of T cells, many questions remain unanswered. The thymus undergoes involution in postpubertal years and it is not clear whether or not other lymphoid tissues are taking its place. It is also not understood how the T-cell repertoire can be cleared of all self-reactive cells since it is unlikely that the total spectrum of self antigens can be probed in the thymus. The complexity of events has raised the question of how fool-proof the induction of thymic tolerance can be. It appears logical that a security net is necessary to catch all those T cells that leak through the thymus and have the potential for self-reactivity.

Peripheral Tolerance: Mature T lymphocytes are not resistant to tolerance induction but can still be rendered antigen-nonreactive. Different mechanisms have been described through which peripheral T-cell nonresponsiveness can be achieved. The best known condition for rendering T cells nonfunctional is anergy induction. To undergo complete activation, T cells require two signals. The first signal is provided by the TCR-binding antigen. The second signal derives from the interaction of costimulatory molecules expressed on the T-cell surface and the antigen-presenting cells. Pairing of the CD28 molecule with the CD80/86 ligand is considered a crucial part of T-cell activation. If T cells recognize antigen in the absence of appropriate costimulatory signals, they enter a state of anergy characterized by survival, but inability to proliferate when reexposed to antigen. Anergic T cells lack the production of interleukin-2 (IL-2). This form of T-cell tolerance is reversible and obviously depends strongly on the conditions of antigen contact.

The conditions of antigen exposure have long been known to determine whether the host will develop a productive immune response or remain nonresponsive. High doses of aqueous protein antigens (high-dose tolerance) administered systemically, protein antigens given orally (oral tolerance), and repetitive doses of low concentrations of antigens (low-dose tolerance) have all been shown in experimental systems to be tolerogenic.

Similarly, antigen-presenting cells may not only be innocent bystanders, but may be able to modulate the nature of the T-cell response. Besides positive signals, accessory cells could also provide negative signals and thus paralyze antigen-specific T cells.

Recently, more emphasis has been put on the microenvironment in which antigen exposure occurs. Particularly in the inflammatory infiltrates characterizing autoimmune reactions, several cell types interact and multiple cytokines are produced in situ. Exposure to IL-2 could prevent the induction of T-cell anergy. Alternatively, the balance between proinflammatory and anti-inflammatory cytokines might well affect the outcome of T cell–antigen contact.

It is becoming increasingly clear that antigen recognition by the host's T cells is not a simple process with a single outcome. Quantitative (how vigorous is the response) and qualitative (which T cells are recruited in a particular response) aspects ultimately determine whether an immune response is beneficial or harmful. The type and the amount of antigen is as important as the port of entry and the accessory cells involved. Under certain circumstances, nonresponsive T cells might serve the host better than a prompt T-cell response. Besides tolerance achieved through the major mechanisms of clonal deletion and clonal anergy, other regulatory mechanisms, such as the action of T cells with suppressor function and T-cell antibody interactions (idiotypic regulation), may contribute to the shaping of the final outcome of normal and pathologic immune responses.

Mechanisms of Tolerance Induction in B Lymphocytes

Induction of self-tolerance in B lymphocytes is less well investigated than the equivalent in T cells (Table 32–3). There is evidence that clonal deletion and clonal anergy exist for B cells. Generally, tolerance

Table 32–3. Tolerance mechanisms in T and B lymphocytes.

T cells	B cells
Tolerance-inducing antigen dose low	high
Persistence of tolerant state long term	short term
Tissue site of tolerance induction Thymus (central tolerance) Periphery (peripheral tolerance)	Bone marrow (central tolerance) ? Periphery (peripheral tolerance)

Tolerance-sensitive cell type
Recognition of antigen with high affinity in the thymus
    Clonal deletion (apoptosis)
Recognition of antigen in the absence of costimulation
    in the periphery
    Clonal anergy (inhibition of IL-2 transcription)
	Recognition of antigen with high affinity clonal deletion (apoptosis)
	
	Recognition of antigen in the absence of T-cell help (mechanism
	    unknown)

induction in B cells requires higher doses of antigen and is relatively short-lived.

Compared with central tolerance induction in the thymus preserving useful T cells and deleting autoreactive T cells, immature B lymphocytes are more sensitive to tolerance induction. During an early stage of B-cell development, when B cells express only surface IgM, interaction with self antigens leads to B-cell death or anergy. In later B-cell development, once IgM and IgD are present on the cell surface, antigen encounter results in B-cell proliferation. The site of tolerance induction is probably the bone marrow.

It has been assumed that peripheral tolerance mechanisms for mature self-responsive B cells are functional ones. Again, in analogy to anergy induction in T cells, when T-cell activation is initiated in the absence of costimulatory signals, B cells become nonresponsive if exposed to self components in the absence of T helper cell signals. Transgenic mouse models have been used to examine B-cell anergy. In these models, B cells enter a state of reversible anergy that is accompanied by reduced levels of membrane IgM.

Since B cells depend on T-cell help in their response to most antigens, including self antigens, T-cell tolerance is important to keep anti-self B-cell responses silenced. B-cell tolerance has to be maintained for T-cell-independent antigens. Also, anti-self B cells probably do survive and can produce autoantibodies of low affinity and low concentration. As long as no T-cell help is provided, these autoantibodies may not reach disease relevance.

MODELS OF AUTOIMMUNITY

Considering the development of the immune system, it appears surprising that antiself-reactivity is the exception and not the rule. It has been argued that the complete depletion of autoreactive lymphocytes cannot be achieved because too many specificities would have to be eliminated and the immune system would be left deficient. The recent observation that HLA molecules are regularly filled with peptides derived from self antigens has reignited the discussion about whether antiself-responses are an integral part of the immune system. This argument has been carried to the extreme stating that all immune responses are reactive to self components, that the immune system has a clearing function for dead and unwanted tissue components, and that recognition of foreign antigens is more of a side product resulting from antihost recognition events directed at altered host components.

Indeed, for none of the human autoimmune diseases has the pathogenesis been understood. Approaches to human autoimmune diseases have been dominated by the paradigm that due to a yet unknown antigenic stimulus, prior tolerant lymphocytes break the state of tolerance and initiate an immune response. Tissue-destructive events are understood as the consequences of

an ongoing immune process that has lost the cardinal feature of self-limitation due to the induction of memory responses specific for host antigens. This paradigm has led to the development of animal models, most of which function by exposure of the animal to a defined antigen closely related to a self antigen and study of the subsequent immune reaction. Unfortunately, there is no good evidence that such disease-inducing antigens do exist in human diseases, challenging the usefulness of these animal models for the understanding of human autoimmune disorders.

Almost any organ system of the body can be affected by a syndrome classified as an autoimmune disease. Thus, pathology of autoimmunity constitutes a wide spectrum of entities. Histomorphology also describes a wide variety of findings with the common denominator of tissue infiltrates composed of mononuclear cells and tissue destruction. Despite this heterogeneity, autoimmune syndromes share certain features and follow certain rules that provide some insight into their pathogenesis.

Principles of Autoimmunity

Normal Autoimmunity: Autoimmunity is not necessarily a sign of disease. Autoantibodies, particularly when produced in low titers, are frequently detected in normal individuals. The presence of autoantibodies as an isolated finding is insufficient to establish the diagnosis of an autoimmune syndrome. As an example, rheumatoid factors, antibodies to IgG determinants typically found in patients with rheumatoid arthritis, regularly accompany normal immune responses but are of low titer and short-lived. It has been suggested that they might be an important and necessary component of normal immune responses.

More Than One Immune Abnormality Is Required to Induce Autoimmune Disease: It certainly would be a simplified view of autoimmune disease to expect a single abnormality underlying the disease process. It is much more likely that more than one mechanism in a patient is dysregulated before an immune response acquires pathologic significance.

Heterogeneity of Tissue-Destructive Mechanisms: Classically, tissue-infiltrating cells in autoimmune inflammation include multiple different cell types. Besides antigen-specific lymphocytes, nonspecific phagocytes, granulocytes, fibroblasts, and others are part of the lesion. Expecting a single process of tissue aggression would be oversimplified. Also, the attacked tissue responds to the injury with a series of events counteracting or amplifying tissue destruction. The concerted action of several cell types in destroying intact tissue might give a pathognomonic histomorphology, such as granulomatous inflammation.

Diversity of Initiating Agents: The paradigm that a disease-inducing antigen breaks tolerance and thus causes an autoimmune disease has dominated our approach to this type of syndrome over the last decades. Despite intense searches, such an antigen has not been identified in any of the human autoimmune entities. The simple reason might be that for most disorders such an antigen does not exist. This paradigm has continued to be appealing due to the simplicity and straightforwardness of postulating an infectious origin of these mysterious diseases. It might be a more productive approach to hypothesize that several agents can initiate an immune response that in the microenvironment of the affected tissue and the genetic background of the patient finally leads to pathology.

The Multifactorial Pathogenesis of Autoimmunity: Emerging data are most compatible with the concept that autoimmune diseases develop in hosts with multiple inherited risk factors combined with environmental contributions. Single components are insufficient to induce the disease state. Rather, complex genotypes, somatic events, and random environmental risk determinants interact to reach the threshold for disease. The combinations of disease-relevant components might actually differ from patient to patient, thus adding additional complexity to the pathogenesis. From a clinical point of view such a disease model would much better fit the experience that autoimmune diseases are characterized by heterogeneity in clinical pattern, course, and treatment response.

Unraveling the pathologic events leading to such diverse entities as inflammatory joint disease, insulin-dependent diabetes mellitus, or multiple sclerosis remains a challenge for the next generation of investigators. The following section outlines hypothetical models that integrate the accumulated knowledge of how normal immune responses function and how alterations could result in pathologic immune reactions (Table 32–4).

Models

Failure of Thymic Education: Removal of self-reactive lymphocytes from the T-cell repertoire is achieved during thymic selection through clonal deletion and clonal anergy. Escape of autoresponsive T cells from the thymus could supply harmful T cells to the peripheral lymphoid tissue.

Recent evidence has been presented suggesting that thymic selection events might be distinct in patients with rheumatoid arthritis (RA). By comparing the TCR repertoire of T cells that recently emigrated from the thymus, RA patients could be clearly distinguished from human leukocyte antigen (HLA)-matched controls. The composition of the T-cell repertoire might well have disease relevance if it includes T cells with a distinct functional profile.

Breakdown of Peripheral Tolerance: Peripheral tolerance is often regarded as a security system to prevent activation of self-reactive T cells that have leaked through the thymus. As already outlined, anergy induction involves TCR triggering in the absence of appropriate costimulatory signals. It is easy to imagine that this mechanism could be overcome.

Table 32–4. Models of autoimmunity.

Model 1. Failure of thymic education

Autoreactive T cells that normally are clonally deleted in the thymus by negative selection escape and populate the periphery.

Model 2. Breakdown of peripheral tolerance

Lymphocytes with the potential of autorecognition are usually silenced by peripheral tolerance mechanisms that let them survive but render them functionally incapable. Anergy induction may fail, allowing self-reactive lymphocytes to become active.

Model 3. Antigen-nonspecific lymphocyte activation

Antiself lymphocytes could be released from anergy by nonspecific activation through polyclonal stimulation, superantigens, and so on.

Model 4. Molecular mimicry

Due to sequence homologies, immunogenic peptides derived from exogenous antigens could induce immunity to self-determinants.

Model 5. Abnormalities in lymphocyte interactions

Cross-regulation of lymphocyte subsets via mediators, antibodies, and so on could fail due to functional impairment of one component of the cellular network.

Supply of excess IL-2 has been shown to inhibit anergy induction. In an inflammatory infiltrate, IL-2 could derive from surrounding T cells and thus counteract attempts to paralyze antigen-specific T cells. Under normal conditions self-reactive T cells should encounter self peptides in the absence of costimulatory signals. In tissues infiltrated by inflammatory cells, however, HLA molecules and other costimulatory molecules are regularly upregulated. Inflamed tissue might actually provide ideal conditions for breaking peripheral tolerance. Although this model has appeal, no concrete data have been presented implicating this mechanism in autoimmune disease.

Antigen-Nonspecific Lymphocyte Activation: Systemic autoimmune disorders such as systemic lupus erythematosus are characterized by the production of a wide array of autoantibodies, suggesting the involvement of a diverse group of lymphocytes. Polyclonal stimulation of lymphocytes has been discussed as an underlying process. More recently, a new type of T-cell-stimulatory antigens has been evaluated, the so-called superantigens. Superantigens are frequently derived from bacteria and are highly active in very low concentrations. By binding to TCR Vβ chains, they effectively activate T cells while circumventing the requirement for antigen triggering of the receptor. Large populations of T cells, potentially including silenced antiself-reactive T cells, can be stimulated. Superantigens have been implicated in the pathogenesis of Kawasaki disease, toxic shock syndrome, and rheumatoid arthritis. Whether superantigen stimulation of T cells is related to breaking tolerance or simply causes the massive release of mediators that cause disease manifestations remains unclear.

Molecular Mimicry: A favored hypothesis explaining the emergence of antihost response has been the molecular mimicry concept. This model implies that an immunogenic peptide in a foreign antigen exhibits sequence similarity to a self peptide. Once an immune response has been primed and established against the foreign antigen, T-cell specificities could be activated that cross-react on self determinants. Sequences of viruses and bacteria have been searched for stretches resembling self components. It can be predicted that sharing of short sequence motifs is not an infrequent event, and the identification of sequences shared by exogenous and endogenous antigens should be frequently seen. Exogenous antigens could potentially initiate an antiself-response with pathologic relevance, but convincing experimental data applying the concept to human disease have not emerged.

Abnormalities in Lymphocyte Interactions: This model emphasizes the functional commitment of T cells besides their specificity. Based on their lymphokine profile, T cells have been classified into T_H1 and T_H2 cells. T_H1 cells secrete IL-2 and interferon gamma (IFNγ) and can downregulate T_H2 cells. Conversely, T_H2 cells release IL-4 and IL-10 and can suppress the function of T_H1 cells. This cross-regulation opens the possibility for biasing immune responses to certain functional pathways. Currently it is believed that inflammatory responses and autoimmune responses are often related to a T_H1 functional commitment. Autoimmunity could thus emerge in a host with impaired T_H2 function. $T_H1$ness and $T_H2$ness is partially determined by the nature of the antigen, the antigen-presenting cell, and the local concentration of cytokines, such as IL-4 and IL-12. Therefore not only the availability of antigen-specific precursor cells but also the when and where of the immune reaction becomes important. Besides cytokine interactions, other types of cell–cell or cell–mediator interactions could equally contribute in modulating the outcome of an antigen-driven immune response.

GENETIC SUSCEPTIBILITY FOR AUTOIMMUNE DISEASES

A major change and a potential for fundamental progress in our understanding of autoimmunity has come from the realization that genetic risk determinants play a cardinal role in disease pathogenesis. Interestingly, it turns out that autoimmune diseases follow genetic rules similar to those for other common diseases, such as hypertension and ischemic heart disease, which are not assumed to have immunologic abnormalities. Typical features of complex genetic diseases include incomplete penetrance, genetic variance, and the involvement of multiple disease genes. The "classical" genetic diseases are caused by a mutation in a single disease gene and are

Table 32–5. Genetic risk factors in autoimmune diseases.

Immune Response Genes
Polymorphic HLA sequences.
Complement genes.
T-cell receptor genes (?)
Immunoglobulin genes (?)
Cytokine genes.
Genes controlling antigen processing and presentation.

Nonimmune Genes
Genes regulating programmed cell death (eg, *fas* in lpr mice).
Genes regulating response to tissue injury (?)
Genes regulating tissue repair (?)

inherited in mendelian fashion, whereas genetic traits of common diseases are more complex. In most of these disorders, disease genes in the sense of a mutated allele are probably nonexistent. Rather, the emerging concept postulates that patients inherit multiple (possibly frequent) genetic risk factors, each of which is normal if considered alone. In combination, these genetic factors add up to significant disease risk sufficient to tip the balance toward pathology.

Clinicians have long employed the knowledge that autoimmune syndromes run in families. The increased probability of siblings developing an autoimmune disorder when compared with the general population provides evidence for genetic risk and suggests clustering of susceptibility factors in families. Shared environmental exposure could similarly contribute to risk. Clearly, autoimmune diseases do not follow simple mendelian recessive or dominant inheritance. How many disease genes exist and how they interact must be addressed for each individual autoimmune disease. Not all of the disease genes will be related to functions of the immune system (Table 32–5). The identification of nonimmune response genes will broaden the approach to autoimmune diseases dramatically and will allow the focus of interactions between nonimmune cells and the immune system.

A set of principle rules is emerging for the genetics of diseases such as autoimmune diseases, which include that

- Different genotypic combinations may underlie a similar clinical phenotype.
- Genetic risk determinants appear not to be independent, but interact. It can be assumed that disease genes differ in their effect.
- An individual becomes affected if the threshold on a liability scale is reached.
- Flexibility exists for individual phenotypes. Disease risk could be modulated by environmental factors that could alter the risk profile of an individual. Incomplete concordance rates among monozygotic twins are often used to estimate the influence of noninherited components. A basic assumption is that monozygotic twins are genetically identical, but this is not the case.

Particularly, somatic events in the immune system introduce differences among germline-identical donors. Shaping of the T-cell and B-cell repertoire is an excellent example of acquired immune characteristics, which have functional influence, depend partially on the pregiven genomic information, but are determined to a certain degree by stochastic events.

■ Finally, individual genetic risk determinants interact with one another and with the genetic background (epistatic interactions). These interactions can be synergistic or introduce protective effects.

HLA Disease Association

Initiated by a serendipitous finding in the early 1970s, it is now firmly established that genes of the HLA region influence susceptibility for a large group of diseases (Table 32–6). Most of the HLA-associated diseases are classified as autoimmune disorders. Principally, HLA disease association means that the frequency of a defined HLA allele is significantly increased in patients with a certain disease when compared with ethnically matched controls. The HLA region is composed of multiple closely linked genes, the products of which are essential in the control of immune functions. Specifically, HLA molecules combined with immunogenic peptides are the ligands of immature and mature T cells, and they determine when, where, and if T-cell receptors are triggered. Although a great deal of information has been collected on the potential role of HLA molecules in the disease pathogenesis of pathogenic autoreactivity, the precise contribution of these polymorphic molecules remains uncertain.

Several principles of HLA-associated diseases have been worked out, some of which might be transferable to non-HLA genetic risk factors:

1. The disease risk imposed by the inheritance of a certain HLA haplotype varies from disorder

Table 32–6. Genetic association of autoimmune diseases with HLA haplotypes.

HLA Allele	Disease	Relative Risk[1]
DR1	Rheumatoid arthritis	?
DR2	Multiple sclerosis	4
DR2	Systemic lupus erythematodes	3.5
DR3	Systemic lupus erythematodes	3
DR3	Sjögren's syndrome	10
DR3	Celiac disease	12
DR3	Insulin-dependent diabetes mellitus	5
DR3	Chronic active hepatitis	14
DR4	Rheumatoid arthritis	6
DR4	Insulin-dependent diabetes mellitus	6.5
DR4	Pemphigus vulgaris	24
DR4	Giant cell arteritis	?
DR3/4	Insulin-dependent diabetes mellitus	20
B27	Ankylosing spondylitis	90

[1] Relative risk estimates the degree of risk for a carrier of the HLA allele compared with individuals negative for the HLA allele. Data apply to caucasoids.

to disorder but never reaches 100%. Whatever HLA molecules contribute to pathologic events, it cannot absolutely depend on one allelic polymorphism.

2. Most individuals who inherit a disease-associated allele will never develop the disease.

3. Disease specificity in the genetic association exists to a certain degree. Different HLA polymorphisms accumulate in patient populations with distinct disease entities.

4. Disease risk has been associated with the polymorphic residues clustered in the antigen-binding site of the HLA molecule, emphasizing the effect of antigen selection and presentation on disease susceptibility.

5. In some HLA-associated diseases the inheritance of not only one but both haplotypes influences disease risk. Gene dosing raises the possibility of alternative roles of HLA molecules since antigen binding is usually not affected by the density of HLA molecules on the cell surface.

6. Recent evidence indicates that more than one HLA component is involved in conferring disease susceptibility. This is particularly the case for insulin-dependent diabetes mellitus but probably also applies to other HLA-associated syndromes. This phenomenon emphasizes the complexity of genetic traits in these diseases and provides an explanation for phenotype heterogeneity in clinical manifestations.

7. In family studies the risk of non-HLA-identical sibs of patients is still higher, emphasizing the role of non-HLA components.

Naturally, the fundamental question is how polymorphic sequences expressed by HLA molecules can influence an individual's risk of developing an autoaggressive immune response and how the clinical picture can be determined by these molecules. Several hypotheses have been explored, none of which have been proven. It is more than likely that the influence of HLA genes varies for different diseases and that separate mechanisms will be found for distinct syndromes.

Hypothesis 1: The dominant paradigm has implied that disease-associated HLA molecules have a particularly high or low affinity for peptides derived from a yet-to-be-determined disease-causating antigen. The HLA–peptide complex would either induce a vigorous T-cell response combined with tissue injury or would fail to stimulate a T-cell response and encourage chronic antigen persistence. In this hypothesis HLA molecules would serve as critical initiation factors in the disease process. Experimental data suggest that this may not be the case in all diseases. Recent evidence collected in RA patients indicates that the disease-associated HLA molecules function as progression factors and determine the severity of the disease. Their presence in the initiation of the pathologic immune response appears to not be required. The data challenge the "peptide selection" model and ask for alternative explanations.

Hypothesis 2: Polymorphic sites encoded by HLA genes resemble sequences expressed by exogenous antigens, such as infectious organisms. Since the carrier of particular HLA molecules develops self-tolerance, the individual would have a hole in the repertoire that renders it susceptible to chronic infection. Positivity for defined HLA alleles would then be linked with immunodeficiency toward peptides mimicked by the HLA.

Hypothesis 3: Disease-associated HLA molecules influence the risk for autoimmunity by shaping the TCR repertoire. During thymic selection events, certain HLA dimers bias the selection process toward certain specificities. The composition of the TCR repertoire determines the nature of normal and pathologic immune responses. Evidence that thymic selection events might indeed be distinct in patients compared with controls has recently been presented in RA.

Hypothesis 4: Genes in linkage disequilibrium, rather than HLA genes, are disease-relevant. Interestingly, cytokine genes and genes defining transporter genes involved in antigen presentations have been mapped close to the HLA region. Data regarding their disease association have so far been inconclusive.

The Role of Non-HLA Genes in Autoimmunity

Family studies have documented that the HLA region is only one of several genetic factors defining disease risk for patients with autoimmune diseases. Efforts are aimed at identifying additional disease genes and have been successful for insulin-dependent diabetes mellitus.

Gene mutations predisposing the host to autoimmune phenomena have so far been described for the complement genes. Several mutated complement genes have been found in patients with SLE. Sequence polymorphisms in the TCR gene loci have been suspected of increasing risk, but conclusive data are missing. Similarly, genes encoding for immunoglobulin molecules would be excellent candidates in a search for non-HLA disease genes.

Potentially interesting genes applicable to human disease may be located by the analysis of animal models. Recently, the inherited defects causing the lpr and gld genotypes have been isolated. The *fas* gene, which is defective in lpr mice and the fas ligand which is nonfunctional in gld mice are intimately involved in apoptosis. The lack of apoptosis can obviously lead to an array of immune dysfunctions and eventually cause autoimmune manifestations. It will be important to investigate the role of apoptosis mechanisms in human autoimmune disorders. Similarly, knockout mice have allowed the identification of genes that are involved in controlling lymphoproliferation and autoimmunity.

Host Responsiveness as a Component of Autoimmunity

It is naive to assume that autoimmune diseases are solely the result of abnormal immune responses. Recognition of self as well as foreign antigens does not occur without the involvement of the microenvironment in which the antigen is made available to specifically and nonspecifically interacting immune cells. Besides professional antigen-presenting cells, many different cell types can acquire the capability to incorporate, process, and present immunogenic peptides. Also, cytokines that regulate the function of lymphocytes are frequently derived from nonimmune cell types. If the immune system recognizes an antigen in a defined microenvironment, and in the case of disease states this happens to be frequently the case outside of lymphoid tissue, the affected organ is not just an innocent bystander. Ongoing immune reactions lead to mediator release, which induces a prompt reaction of the surrounding tissue. Similarly, injured tissue secretes products, including autoantigens, that affect the immune response. While extending the view from immune cells and their products to the tissue reactivity pattern can be productive in understanding tissue tropism and tissue-specific disease manifestations, it adds considerable complexity to the pathogenesis of autoimmune diseases.

It has been suggested that the immune system has a major function in surveying tissue integrity. Antiself-responses would then be defined as beneficial as long as they serve to remove necrotic tissue or help in tissue repair. If this is the case, autoimmune diseases could result from dysregulation of such clearing and repair mechanisms rather than from the initial recognition of a self antigen caused by selective loss of self-tolerance.

Tissue infection, ischemia, malignancy, and necrosis could all play a permissive role in attracting immune cells into an organ. The original infectious agent might not any longer be the stimulator but rather tissue-derived self antigens could drive the immune process. Alternatively, it has been suggested that neoantigens are formed under these circumstances and that tolerance against such antigens has not been established. Ultimately the spectrum of immunogenic peptides recognized by T cells in the infiltrate and the epitopes recognized by antibodies built in the infiltrate provide information about initiating and perpetuating mechanisms causing immune-mediated disease.

MECHANISMS OF IMMUNE-MEDIATED TISSUE DESTRUCTION

In the last two decades research into autoimmune mechanisms has focused on the role of T lymphocytes and the loss of self-tolerance. This is mainly due to the presumed central and regulatory position of T cells in immune reactions. T cells, however, are not always the major players in the pathologic events underlying clinical disease. Other effector mechanisms are probably equally important, and the relative contribution of different immune pathways changes from syndrome to syndrome. Traditionally, immunologic diseases have been classified based on the principal pathogenic mechanism responsible for cell and tissue injury.

Type I: Immediate Hypersensitivity

IgE antibodies have been identified as the primary immune mechanism causing this type of immunologic disease. Mast cells bind IgE antibody, and when exposed to antigen they promptly release mediators, facilitating the clinical manifestations of allergy. To date, IgE antibodies have not been unequivocally implicated in autoimmune disease.

Type II: Antibody-Mediated Diseases

The potential of antibodies to injure tissue has been extensively studied and has dominated the view of pathogenic autoreactivity for several decades. Autoantibodies recognizing soluble or cell surface antigens can initiate multiple pathways, eventually leading to tissue injury. Bound antibodies can activate the complement cascade or may induce the phagocytosis or lysis of antibody-coated structures. By-products generated through in situ complement activation serve as powerful chemoattractants and recruit inflammatory cells into the tissue. Occasionally, autoantibodies are specific for cell surface molecules that are normally triggered by physiologic ligands such as hormones. In this circumstance, autoantibodies can either mimic or block such signals and lead to clinicopathologic manifestations.

Type III: Immune Complex-Mediated Diseases

Complexes formed by specific antibodies and antigens can be deposited into the tissue and cause an intense inflammatory reaction. Deposition of such complexes in blood vessels has been associated with vasculitis. The classical forms of immune complex-mediated diseases are acute and chronic serum sickness and the Arthus reaction. Serum sickness represents the systemic variant of this disease, whereas the Arthus reaction is localized. Characteristic features of immune complex-mediated tissue injury includes necrosis, often in the form of fibrinoid necrosis, and dense cellular infiltrates composed mainly of neutrophils. In the localized form the histomorphology is dominated by vasculitis with necrosis.

Type IV: T-Cell-Mediated Immunologic Diseases

In the last 15 years the emphasis of pathologic immune reactions causing tissue destruction shifted from the autoantibody-producing B cell to the autoreactive T cell. The theory that autoimmunity is a T-cell-driven phenomenon was boosted when it became clear that self-tolerance is mainly established by the depletion of antiself T-cell specificities. The assumption that many human autoimmune diseases are T-cell diseases has been fostered by the demonstration that T cells constitute the dominant cell type in the tissue lesions and that T cells with antiself-antigen reactivity can be isolated from affected patients.

T cells can cause tissue injury through two major mechanisms, which essentially resemble their normal effector functions. CD8 T lymphocytes recognize antigen in restriction to HLA class I molecules, particularly viral antigens or antigens derived from intracellular infectious agents, and lyse the infected cell. Cell lysis can probably lead to considerable tissue necrosis. CD4 T cells function mainly by secreting lymphokines, which can recruit and activate macrophages. Activated macrophages are able to produce hydrolytic enzymes, reactive oxygen derivatives, lipid mediators, and nitric oxide, all of which have a high potential for attacking tissue structures. T-cell-derived lymphokines also boost the synthesis of proinflammatory cytokines by macrophages or other cells accumulated in the infiltrate. Even the induction of repair mechanisms and tissue-remodeling mechanisms are partially under T-cell control. Although the pathologic lesions in T-cell-mediated immune responses vary, the interaction of tissue-infiltrating T cells with activated macrophages is a hallmark of a wide spectrum of diseases thought to be caused by delayed-type hypersensitivity. Current concepts favor the idea that at least some of the T cells in the lesions are specific for the disease-causative antigen, although conclusive data from human disease has not emerged.

SUMMARY

The diagnosis of an autoimmune disease is made in about 2.5% of the population. Essentially, any organ system can be affected by pathologic immune reactions, creating a wide spectrum of clinical disorders that have more distinguishing than shared features. The common denominator of autoimmune syndromes is tissue destruction caused by an ongoing immune response. Understanding of the fundamental principles in normal immune reactions have centered the interest on pathologic T-cell reactivity. Despite intense research, the exact pathogenesis of any of the autoimmune diseases has not been clarified. Primary theories proposed to explain the induction of pathogenic autoreactivity concede that the immune system is the principal mediator of disease. One hypothesis favors a failure of central tolerance as the crucial abnormality breaking self-tolerance and thus permitting self-recognition with harmful consequences. Other models implicate dysfunction of peripheral tolerance mechanisms as the major contributing factor. Similarly, abnormalities in the immune network are cited as primary pathogenic processes. Recently the focus of interest has shifted to the genetics of autoreactivity. Evidence is emerging that multiple genetic risk determinants interact to create disease susceptibility. Genes regulating immune functions but also genes controlling other cellular functions may independently contribute to reach the liability threshold and cause the disease phenotype. The reactivity pattern of the microenvironment providing the site for the chronic immune response might be a major regulatory component of the pathologic events. Emerging concepts in autoimmunity stress the complexity of abnormalities, challenges the concept of a single, easily correctable dysfunction, and extend the view to non-immune cellular functions.

REFERENCES

NORMAL IMMUNE RESPONSE: FUNDAMENTAL PRINCIPLES

Ada GL, Nossal G: The clonal-selection theory. *Sci Am* 1987;**257:**62.

AUTOIMMUNITY

Ashton-Rickardt PG, Tonegawa S: A differential-avidity model for T-cell selection. *Immunol Today* 1994;**15:**362.

Davis MM: T cell receptor gene diversity and selection. *Ann Rev Biochem* 1990;**59:**475.

Goodnow CC: Transgenic mice and analysis of B-cell tolerance. *Ann Rev Immunol* 1992;**10:**489.

Johnson JG, Jenkins MK: The role of anergy in peripheral T cell unresponsiveness. *Life Sci* 1994;**55:**1767.

Linsley PS, Ledbetter JA: The role of the CD28 receptor during T cell responses to antigen. *Ann Rev Immunol* 1993;**11:**191.

Miller JF, Morahan G: Peripheral T cell tolerance. *Ann Rev Immunol* 1992;**10:**51.

Parker DC: T cell-dependent B cell activation. *Ann Rev Immunol* 1993;**11:**331.

Tonegawa S: The molecules of the immune system. *Sci Am* 1985;**253:**122.

von Boehmer H, Kisielow P: Self-nonself discrimination by T cells. *Science* 1990;**248:**1369.

MODELS OF AUTOIMMUNITY

Kotzin BL et al: Superantigens and their potential role in human disease. *Adv Immunol* 1993;**54:**99.

Matzinger P: Tolerance, danger, and the extended family. *Ann Rev Immunol* 1994;**12:**991.

Mosmann TR, Coffman RL: T_H1 and T_H2 cells: Different patterns of lymphokine secretion lead to different functional properties. *Ann Rev Immunol* 1989;**7:**145.

Oldstone MB: Molecular mimicry and autoimmune disease. *Cell* 1987;**50:**819.

Sinha AA et al: Autoimmune diseases: The failure of self tolerance. *Science* 1990;**248:**1380.

Steinberg AD et al: Systemic lupus erythematosus. *Ann Intern Med* 1991;**115:**548.

Trinchieri G: Interleukin-12: A proinflammatory cytokine with immunoregulatory functions that bridge innate resistance and antigen-specific adaptive immunity. *Ann Rev Immunol* 1995;**13:**251.

Walser-Kuntz DR et al: Mechanisms underlying the formation of the T cell receptor repertoire in rheumatoid arthritis. *Immunity* 1995;**2:**597.

Weyand CM, Goronzy JJ: Pathogenesis of rheumatic arthritis. *Med Dis Clin North Amer.* In press.

GENETIC SUSCEPTIBILITY FOR AUTOIMMUNE DISEASES

Aitman TJ, Todd JA: Molecular genetics of diabetes mellitus. *Baillieres Clin Endocrinol Metab* 1995;**9:**631.

Albani S et al: Positive selection of autoimmunity: Abnormal immune responses to a bacterial dnaJ antigenic determinant in patients with early rheumatoid arthritis. *Natur Med* 1995;**1:**448.

Davies KA et al: Complement deficiency and immune complex disease. *Springer Sem Immunopathol* 1994;**15:**397.

Honeyman MC et al: Analysis of families at risk for insulin-dependent diabetes mellitus reveals that HLA antigens influence progression to clinical disease. *Mol Med* 1995;**1:**576.

Mountz JD et al: Autoimmune disease. A problem of defective apoptosis. *Arthritis Rheum* 1994;**37:**1415.

Waterhouse P et al: Lymphoproliferative disorders with early lethality in mice deficient in Ctla-4. *Science* 1995;**270:**985.

Weyand CM et al: The influence of HLA-DRB1 genes on disease severity in rheumatoid arthritis. *Ann Intern Med* 1992;**117:**801.

Willerford DM et al: Interleukin-2 receptor α chain regulates the size and content of the peripheral lymphoid compartment. *Immunity* 1995;**3:**521.

33

Rheumatic Diseases

Kenneth E. Sack, MD, & Kenneth H. Fye, MD

Many of the major rheumatologic disorders are autoimmune in nature. Therefore, a thorough understanding of the mechanisms of the immune response is essential to an understanding of these diseases. Of particular importance is information in Chapter 32, which describes mechanisms of disordered immune regulation. This chapter discusses the rheumatologic diseases with proved or hypothesized immunologic pathogenesis.

SYSTEMIC LUPUS ERYTHEMATOSUS

Major Immunologic Features
- Antinuclear antibodies are present.
- Antidouble-stranded DNA or anti-Sm antibodies are present.
- Serum complement levels are depressed.
- Immunoglobulin and complement are deposited along glomerular basement membrane and at the dermal–epidermal junction.
- Numerous other autoantibodies are present.

General Considerations
Sir William Osler described the systemic manifestations of systemic lupus erythematosus (SLE) in 1895. Prior to that time, lupus was considered to be a disfiguring but nonfatal skin disease. It is now known to be a chronic systemic inflammatory disease that follows a course of alternating exacerbations and remissions. Involvement of multiple organ systems occurs during periods of disease activity. The cause of SLE is not known. The disease affects predominantly females (4:1 over males) of childbearing age; however, the age at onset ranges from 2 to 90 years. It is more prevalent among nonwhites (particularly blacks) than whites.

Immunologic Pathogenesis
The discovery of the lupus erythematosus (LE) cell phenomenon (see the section on Immunologic

Diagnosis) marked the start of the modern era of research into the pathogenesis of SLE. This initial clinical observation led to the finding of multiple antinuclear factors, including antibodies to DNA, in the sera of patients with SLE. Further studies of renal eluates from patients with SLE established the importance of DNA-containing immune complexes in the causation of lupus glomerulonephritis. Reduced serum complement and the presence of antibodies to double-stranded (ds) DNA are hallmarks of active SLE, distinguishing this entity from other lupus variants.

Autoantibodies directed against numerous nonnucleic acid antigens also occur in patients with SLE. Many of these autoantibodies fix complement and thereby damage target tissues. For instance, the hemolytic anemia and thrombocytopenia characteristic of SLE are often caused by antierythrocyte and antiplatelet antibodies. Lymphocytotoxic antibodies (with predominant specificity for T lymphocytes) occur in many patients with SLE. The pathogenetic significance of lymphocytotoxic antibodies is unclear. Autoantibody formation in SLE is in part genetically determined; for example, patients with human leukocyte antigen (HLA)-DR2 epitopes are more likely to produce anti-ds-DNA antibodies, those with HLA-DR3 produce anti-SS-A and anti-SS-B antibodies (Table 33–1), and those with HLA-DR4 and HLA-DR5 produce anti-Sm and anti-RNP antibodies. Family studies have demonstrated a genetic susceptibility to the development of SLE.

Autoantibody formation is partially prevented through the action of regulatory T lymphocytes called suppressor T cells. Although the mechanism of suppression is unknown, such suppressor T cells probably play an important role in immunologic tolerance and self–nonself discrimination. A defect in suppressor T-cell activity has also been observed in humans with SLE; however, this defect may be due to anti-T-cell antibody activity and may not represent a primary suppressor T-cell deficiency.

SLE, like many rheumatic disorders, occurs pre-

Table 33–1. Antinuclear antibodies.

Pattern	Antigen	Associated Diseases
Peripheral	Double-stranded DNA	SLE
Homogeneous	DNA-histone complex	SLE, occasionally other connective tissue disease
Speckled	Sm (Smith antigen)	SLE
	RNP (ribonucleoprotein)	Mixed connective tissue disease, SLE, Sjögren's syndrome, scleroderma, polymyositis
	SS-A (Ro)	Sjögren's syndrome, SLE
	SS-B (La)	Sjögren's syndrome, SLE
	Jo-1	Polydermatomyositis
	Mi-2	Dermatomyositis
	Sci-70	Scleroderma
	Centromere	Limited scleroderma
	RANA (rheumatoid-associated nuclear antigen) (nuclear antigen induced by EBV)	Rheumatoid arthritis
Nucleolar	Nucleolus-specific RNA	Scleroderma
	PM-Scl	Polymyositis

Abbreviations: EBV = Epstein-Barr virus; SLE = systemic lupus erythematosus.

dominantly in women. Studies have demonstrated that estrogens enhance anti-DNA antibody formation and increase the severity of renal disease in animal models. Androgens have an opposite effect on both anti-DNA antibody production and renal disease.

Pathology

Numerous pathologic changes are characteristic of SLE:

1. The verrucous endocarditis of Libman-Sacks consists of ovoid vegetations, 1–4 mm in diameter, which form along the base of the valve and, rarely, on the chordae tendineae and papillary muscles.
2. A peculiar periarterial concentric fibrosis results in the so-called "onion skin" lesion seen in the spleen.
3. A pathognomonic finding in SLE, the "hematoxylin body," consists of a homogeneous globular mass of nuclear material that stains bluish purple with hematoxylin. Hematoxylin bodies occur in the heart, kidneys, lungs, spleen,

lymph nodes, and serous and synovial membranes. It should be emphasized that patients with fulminant SLE involving the central nervous system, skin, muscles, joints, and kidneys may not have any distinctive pathologic abnormalities at autopsy.

Clinical Features

A. Symptoms and Signs: SLE presents no single characteristic clinical pattern. The onset can be acute or insidious. Constitutional symptoms include fever, weight loss, malaise, and lethargy. Every organ system may become involved.

1. Joints and muscles–Polyarthralgia or arthritis is the most common manifestation of SLE (90%). The arthritis is symmetric and can involve almost any joint. It may resemble rheumatoid arthritis, but bony erosions and severe deformity are unusual.

Avascular necrosis of bone is common in SLE. The femoral head is most frequently affected, but other bones may also be involved. Corticosteroids, which are major therapeutic agents in SLE, may play a role in the pathogenesis of this complication. Myalgias, with or without frank myositis, are common.

2. Skin–The most common skin lesion is an erythematous rash involving areas of the body chronically exposed to ultraviolet light. A few patients with SLE develop the classic "butterfly" rash. In some patients with systemic disease, discoid lupus erythematosus occurs. This rash may resolve without sequelae or may result in scar formation, atrophy, and hypopigmentation or hyperpigmentation. A nonscarring skin lesion termed subacute cutaneous lupus erythematosus occurs predominantly in patients with anti-SS-A antibodies. In addition, bullae, patches of purpura, urticaria, angioneurotic edema, patches of vitiligo, subcutaneous nodules, and thickening of the skin may be seen. Vasculitic lesions, ranging from palpable purpura to digital infarction, are common. Alopecia, which may be diffuse, patchy, or circumscribed, is also common. Mucosal ulcerations, involving both oral and genital mucosa, occur in about 15% of cases.

3. Polyserositis–Pleurisy, with chest pain and dyspnea, is a frequent complication of SLE. Although one third of cases have pleural fluid, massive effusion is rare. Pericarditis is the commonest form of cardiac involvement and can be the first manifestation of SLE. The pericarditis is usually benign, leading only to mild chest discomfort and a pericardial friction rub, but severe pericarditis with tamponade can occur. Isolated peritonitis is extremely rare, although 5–10% of patients with pleuritis and pericarditis have concomitant peritonitis. Manifestations of peritonitis include abdominal pain, anorexia, nausea and vomiting, and, rarely, ascites.

4. Kidneys–Renal involvement is a frequent and serious feature of SLE. Seventy-five percent of patients have nephritis at autopsy. The study of renal tissue by light microscopy, immunofluorescence, and electron microscopy has revealed five histologic lesions associated with rather distinctive clinical features. (1) Mesangial glomerulonephritis manifests as hypercellularity and the deposition of immune complexes in the mesangium. This is a benign form of lupus nephritis. (2) In focal glomerulonephritis, segmental proliferation occurs in less than 50% of glomeruli. Immune complexes are found in the mesangium and in the subendothelium of the glomerular capillary. Focal glomerulonephritis is often a benign process, but it may progress to a diffuse proliferative lesion. (3) Diffuse proliferative glomerulonephritis is characterized by extensive cellular proliferation in more than 50% of glomeruli. Immunofluorescence reveals subendothelial deposits of immune complexes. This process frequently leads to renal failure. (4) In membranous glomerulonephritis, glomerular cellularity is normal, but the capillary basement membrane is thickened. Immune complexes occur mainly in subepithelial and intramembranous areas. This lesion may be associated with the development of the nephrotic syndrome. (5) Sclerosing glomerulonephritis is defined by an increase in mesangial matrix glomerulosclerosis, capsular adhesions, fibrous crescents, interstitial fibrosis with tubular atrophy, and vascular sclerosis. This lesion portends a poor prognosis and is not responsive to drugs.

It must be emphasized that a benign renal lesion may evolve into a more serious one.

Systemic hypertension is a common finding in acute or chronic lupus nephritis and may contribute to renal dysfunction.

5. Lungs–Pleuritic chest pain occurs in about 50% of patients with SLE. Pleural effusions are less common, are typically unilateral, and resolve quickly with treatment. Clinically apparent lupus pneumonitis is unusual. When a pulmonary infiltrate develops in a patient with SLE, particularly one being treated with corticosteroids or immunosuppressive drugs, infection must be the first diagnostic consideration. Restrictive interstitial lung disease is the commonest form of parenchymal involvement. It may be asymptomatic and detectable only by pulmonary function tests. The chest x-ray is usually normal but may show "plate-like" atelectasis or interstitial fibrosis with "honeycombing." Other pulmonary manifestations include pulmonary hypertension, alveolar hemorrhage, pneumothorax, hemothorax, and vasculitis.

6. Heart–Clinically apparent myocarditis occurs rarely in SLE but when present may result in congestive heart failure. The verrucous endocarditis of SLE, with the characteristic Libman-Sacks vegetations, is usually asymptomatic and diagnosed only by echocardiography or at autopsy. Thickening of the aortic valve cusps with resultant aortic insufficiency can occur. Coronary artery disease, possibly related to corticosteroid therapy, is commonly recognized.

7. Nervous system–Disturbances of mentation and aberrant behavior, such as psychosis or depres-

sion, are the commonest manifestations of central nervous system involvement. Convulsions, cranial nerve palsies, aseptic meningitis, migraine headache, transverse myeltitis, peripheral neuritis, and cerebrovascular accidents may also occur.

8. Eyes–Ocular involvement is present in 20–25% of patients. The characteristic retinal finding (the cytoid body) is a fluffy white exudative lesion caused by focal degeneration of the nerve fiber layer of the retina secondary to retinal vasculitis. Scleritis is also a manifestation of ocular vasculitis. Corneal ulceration occurs in conjunction with Sjögren's syndrome (see item 12).

9. Gastrointestinal system–Gastrointestinal vasculitis can occur in SLE. Manifestations include abdominal pain, diarrhea, and hemorrhage. Pancreatitis, cholecystitis, acute and chronic hepatitis, and protein-losing enteropathy may be seen.

10. Hematopoietic system–See (section B) Laboratory Findings.

11. Vascular system–Small-vessel vasculitis commonly occurs in active SLE. Cutaneous manifestations of small-vessel disease include splinter hemorrhages, periungual occlusions, finger pulp infarctions, and atrophic ulcers. Small-vessel vasculitis may also cause a "stocking-glove" peripheral neuropathy. Medium-vessel arteritis, involving arteries 0.5–1 mm in diameter, also occurs in SLE. Manifestations range from bowel infarction to mononeuritis multiplex to cerebrovascular accidents. Hypercoagulation leading to arterial and venous occlusive disease is seen in patients with antiphospholipid antibodies (see item 13). Raynaud's phenomenon occurs in 15% of patients with SLE.

12. Sjögren's syndrome–Up to 30% of patients with SLE develop the sicca complex (keratoconjunctivitis sicca, xerostomia).

13. Drug-induced lupus-like syndrome–Certain drugs may provoke a lupus-like picture in susceptible individuals. The most commonly implicated drugs are hydralazine and procainamide, but quinidine, chlorpromazine, methyldopa, isoniazid, and phenytoin are also known to produce this syndrome. Typical manifestations of drug-induced lupus are arthralgias, arthritis, rash, fever, and pleurisy. Nephritis and central nervous system involvement are rare. The disease usually remits when the offending drug is discontinued. Antihistone and antisinglestranded DNA antibodies are typical of drug-induced lupus.

B. Laboratory Findings: Anemia is the most common hematologic finding in SLE. Eighty percent of patients present with a normochromic, normocytic anemia due to marrow suppression. A few develop Coombs'-positive hemolytic anemia. Leukopenia and thrombocytopenia are common. Urinalysis may show hematuria, proteinuria, and erythrocyte and leukocyte casts. The sedimentation rate is typically high in active SLE. Serologic abnormalities are described in the section on Immunologic Diagnosis. The synovial fluid in SLE is yellow and clear, with a low viscosity. The leukocyte count usually does not exceed 4000/μL, most of which are lymphocytes. The pleural effusion of SLE is typically a transudate with a predominance of lymphocytes and a total leukocyte count of no more than 3000/μL. A hemorrhagic pleural effusion is very rare. In central nervous system lupus, the cerebrospinal fluid protein concentration is sometimes elevated, and there is occasionally a mild lymphocytosis.

C. X-Ray Findings: Chest-x-ray may reveal cardiomegaly (due to either pericarditis or myocarditis), pleural effusion, plate-like atelectasis, or interstitial fibrosis with a "honeycomb" appearance. Joint x-rays may show soft tissue swelling and mild osteopenia but rarely show erosions.

Immunologic Diagnosis

A. Proteins and Complement: Most patients with SLE (80%) have elevated α_2- and γ-globulins. Hypoalbuminemia is occasionally present. The serum complement is frequently reduced in the presence of active disease because of increased use due to immune complex formation and to reduced liver synthesis of complement components. Individual complement components, including C3 and C4, and total hemolytic complement activity may be decreased during disease activity. The serum of patients with active SLE occasionally contains circulating cryoglobulin consisting of IgM/IgG aggregates and complement.

B. Autoantibodies:

1. LE cell phenomenon–The phenomenon of LE cells was first described in the bone marrow of patients with SLE. It reflects the presence of IgG antibody to deoxyribonucleoprotein. This relatively cumbersome and insensitive technique is only of historic interest, however.

2. Antinuclear antibodies–Immunoglobulins of all classes may form antinuclear antibodies (ANA). Six different morphologic patterns of immunofluorescent staining have been described, four of which have clinical significance (Fig 33–1 and Table 33–1).

a. The "homogeneous" ("diffuse," or "solid") pattern is the morphologic expression of antihistone antibodies and occurs in patients with systemic or drug-induced lupus erythmatosus. In this pattern, the nucleus shows diffuse and uniform staining.

b. The "peripheral" ("shaggy," or "outline") pattern denotes the presence of anti-ds-DNA antibodies. The outline pattern is best seen when human leukocytes are used as substrate. It is characteristic of active SLE.

c. The "speckled" pattern reflects the presence of antibodies directed against non-DNA nuclear constituents. The anti-ENA (extractable nuclear antigen) assay detects antibodies against two saline-extractable nuclear antigens, the Sm (Smith) antigen and RNP (ribonucleoprotein) antigen. Antibodies against the Sm antigen are characteristic of SLE. High titers of anti-

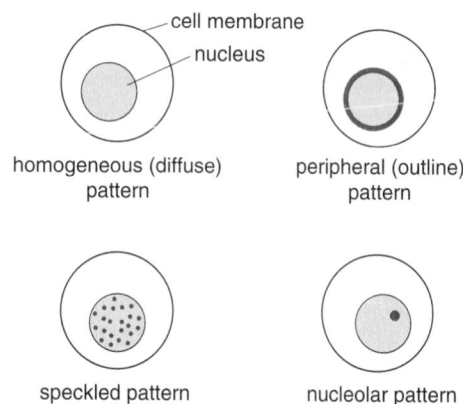

Figure 33–1. Patterns of immunofluorescent staining for antinuclear antibodies.

RNP antibodies are the hallmark of mixed connective tissue disease, but low-titer anti-RNP antibodies may occur in SLE.

d. The "nucleolar" pattern is caused by the homogeneous staining of the nucleolus. It has been suggested that this antigen may be the ribosomal precursor of ribonucleoprotein. This pattern is rare in SLE and most often associated with scleroderma or polymyositis–dermatomyositis.

A positive ANA test must be interpreted with caution because (1) the serum of a patient with any rheumatic disease may contain many autoantibodies to different nuclear constituents, so that a "homogeneous" pattern may obscure a "speckled" or "nucleolar" pattern; (2) different antibodies in the serum can be present in different titers, so that by diluting the serum one can change the pattern observed; (3) the stability of the different antigens is different and can be changed by fixation or denaturation; and (4) the pattern observed appears to be influenced by the types of tissues or cells used as substrate for the test.

The ANA test is occasionally positive in normal individuals, in patients with various chronic diseases, and in the aged. Absence of ANA is strong evidence against a diagnosis of SLE.

3. Anti-DNA antibodies and immune complexes–Three major types of anti-DNA antibodies can be found in the sera of lupus patients: (1) antisingle-stranded or, "denatured," DNA (ss-DNA); (2) antidouble-stranded, or "native," DNA (ds-DNA); and (3) antibodies that react to both ss-DNA and ds-DNA. These antibodies may be either IgG or IgM classes. High titers of anti-ds-DNA antibodies are characteristic of SLE. In contrast, anti-ss-DNA antibodies are not specific and can be found in other autoimmune diseases, such as rheumatoid arthritis, chronic active hepatitis, primary biliary cirrhosis, and drug-induced lupus. Antibodies to DNA can be quantitatively measured by RIA or ELISA techniques (see Chapter 12). Complement-fixing and high-avidity anti-ds-DNA antibodies may be associated with the development of renal disease. The amount of antibody correlates well with disease activity, and the antibody titer frequently decreases when patients enter remission.

Circulating immune complexes are present in the sera of patients with active disease. Different assay techniques, however, are required to detect complexes of different sizes, and there is controversy about how closely the level of soluble circulating immune complexes correlates with disease activity.

4. Antierythrocyte antibodies–These antibodies belong to the IgG, IgA, and IgM classes and can be detected by the direct Coombs test. The prevalence of these antibodies among SLE patients ranges from 10 to 65%. Hemolytic anemia does occasionally occur and, when present, is associated with a complement-fixing warm antierythrocyte antibody.

5. Circulating anticoagulants, antiphospholipids, and antiplatelet antibodies–Antiphospholipid antibodies develop in 10–15% of patients with SLE. These antibodies are often associated with a false-positive Venereal Disease Research Laboratory (VDRL) test and possess activity against cardiolipin. Some antiphospholipid antibodies have anticoagulant activity. Although these anticoagulants prolong the partial thromboplastin and prothrombin times, hemorrhagic complications are rare. Paradoxic thrombotic states may develop owing to actions of antiphospholipid antibodies on platelets, vascular endothelial cells, or erythrocytes. Patients with antiphospholipid antibodies are at increased risk for thrombotic events, and women with these antibodies are subject to recurrent spontaneous abortions. Specific antifactor VIII antibodies have also been described. These antibodies are potent anticoagulants and may be associated with bleeding. Antiplatelet antibodies are found in 75–80% of patients with SLE. These antibodies inhibit neither clot retraction nor thromboplastin generation in normal blood. They probably induce thrombocytopenia by direct effects on platelet surface membrane.

6. False-positive serologic test for syphilis–A false-positive VDRL test is seen in 10–20% of patients with SLE. The serologic test for syphilis can be considered an autoimmune reaction, because the antigen is a phospholipid present in many human organs (see item 5).

7. Rheumatoid factors–Almost 30% of patients with SLE have a positive latex fixation test for rheumatoid factors.

8. Anticytoplasmic antibodies–Numerous anticytoplasmic antibodies (antimitochondrial, antiribosomal, antilysosomal) have been found in patients with SLE. These antibodies are not organ- or species-specific. Antiribosomal antibodies are found in the sera of 25–50% of patients. The major antigenic determinant is ribosomal RNA. Antimitochondrial antibodies are more common in other diseases (eg, primary biliary cirrhosis) than in SLE.

C. Tissue Immunofluorescence

1. Kidneys–Irregular or granular accumulation of immunoglobulin and complement occurs along the glomerular basement membrane and in the mesangium in patients with lupus nephritis. On electron microscopy, these deposits are seen in subepithelial, subendothelial, and mesangial sites.

2. Skin–Almost 90% of patients with SLE have immunoglobulin and complement deposition in the dermal–epidermal junction of skin that is *not* involved with an active lupus rash. The immunoglobulins are IgG or IgM and appear as a brightly staining homogeneous or granular band. Patients with discoid lupus erythematosus show deposition of immunoglobulin and complement only in involved skin.

Differential Diagnosis

The diagnosis of SLE in patients with classic multisystem involvement and a positive ANA test is not difficult. The onset of the disease can be vague and insidious, however, and can therefore present a perplexing diagnostic problem. The polyarthritis of SLE is often similar to that seen in viral infections, infective endocarditis, mixed connective tissue disease, rheumatoid arthritis, and rheumatic fever. When Raynaud's phenomenon is the predominant complaint, progressive systemic sclerosis should be considered. SLE can present with a myositis similar to that of polymyositis–dermatomyositis. The clinical constellation of arthritis, alopecia, and a positive VDRL may denote secondary syphilis. Felty's syndrome (thrombocytopenia, leukopenia, splenomegaly in patients with rheumatoid arthritis) can simulate SLE. Takayasu's disease should be considered in a young woman who presents with arthralgias, fever, and asymmetric pulses. Some patients with discoid lupus erythematosus may develop leukopenia, thrombocytopenia, hypergammaglobulinemia, a positive ANA, and an elevated sedimentation rate. Ten percent of patients with discoid lupus erythematosus have mild systemic symptoms. The frequent presence of anti-ds-RNA in discoid lupus erythematosus suggests that SLE and discoid lupus erythematosus are part of a single disease spectrum.

Treatment

The efficacy of the drugs used in the treatment of SLE is difficult to evaluate, since spontaneous remissions do occur. There are few controlled studies, because it is difficult to withhold therapy in the face of the life-threatening disease that can develop in fulminant SLE. Depending on the severity of the disease, no treatment, minimal treatment (nonsteroidal anti-inflammatory drugs, antimalarials), or intensive treatment (corticosteroids, cytotoxic drugs) may be required.

When arthritis is the predominant symptom and other organ systems are not significantly involved, high-dose aspirin or another fast-acting nonsteroidal anti-inflammatory drug may suffice to relieve symptoms. When the skin or mucosa is predominantly involved, antimalarials (hydroxychloroquine or chloroquine) and topical corticosteroids are very beneficial. Because high-dosage antimalarial therapy may be associated with irreversible retinal toxicity, these drugs should be used judiciously and in as low doses as can be effective.

Systemic corticosteroids used to treat severe SLE can suppress disease activity and prolong life. The mode of action is unknown, but the immunosuppressive and anti-inflammatory properties of these agents presumably play a significant role in their therapeutic efficacy. High-dosage corticosteroid treatment (eg, prednisone, 1 mg/kg/d orally) decreases immunoglobulin levels and autoantibody titers and suppresses immune responses. This treatment is recommended in acute fulminant lupus, acute lupus nephritis, acute central nervous system lupus, acute autoimmune hemolytic anemia, and thrombocytopenic purpura. One or more courses of "pulse" therapy (ie, 15 mg/kg/d intravenously for 3 days) may be effective in patients with recalcitrant disease. The course of corticosteroid therapy should be monitored by the clinical response and meticulous follow-up of laboratory and immunologic parameters, such as complete blood count, platelet count, urinalysis, anti-ds-DNA titer, and complement levels.

If the clinical and immunologic status of the patient fails to improve or if serious side effects of corticosteroid therapy develop, immunosuppressive therapy with cytotoxic agents, such as cyclophosphamide, chlorambucil, or azathioprine is indicated. Intravenous "pulse" therapy with cyclophosphamide is a practical and effective means of treating lupus nephritis. Because of serious complications (cancer, marrow suppression, infection, and liver and gastrointestinal toxicity), immunosuppressive agents should be used with discretion.

Complications & Prognosis

SLE may run a very mild course confined to one or a few organs, or it may be a fulminant fatal disease. Renal failure and central nervous system lupus were the leading causes of death until the corticosteroids and cytotoxic agents came into widespread use. Since then, the complications of therapy, including atherosclerosis, infection, and cancer, have become common causes of death. The 5-year survival rate of patients with SLE has markedly improved over the past decade and now approaches 80–90%.

RHEUMATOID ARTHRITIS

Major Immunologic Features

- Monomeric and pentameric IgM, IgA, and IgG rheumatoid factors exist in serum and synovial fluid.
- Vasculitis and synovitis are present.

General Considerations

Rheumatoid arthritis is a chronic, recurrent, systemic inflammatory disease primarily involving the joints. It affects 1–3% of people in the USA, with a female-to-male ratio of 3:1. Constitutional symptoms include malaise, fever, and weight loss. The disease characteristically begins in the small joints of the hands and feet and progresses in a centripetal and symmetric fashion. Elderly patients may present with more proximal large-joint involvement. Deformities are common. Extra-articular manifestations include vasculitis, atrophy of the skin and muscle, subcutaneous nodules, lymphadenopathy, splenomegaly, and leukopenia.

Immunologic Pathogenesis

The cause of rheumatoid arthritis is unknown. Approximately 70% of patients with rheumatoid arthritis carry the HLA-DR4 haplotype. This haplotype has several different variants. Certain HLA-DR alleles determine both susceptibility to and severity of the disease. It is possible that these and perhaps other genetic determinants impart susceptibility to an unidentified environmental factor, such as a virus, that initiates the disease process. Although no virus particles have ever been identified, theoretically an antigenic stimulus leads to the appearance of an abnormal IgG that results in the production of rheumatoid factors and the eventual development of rheumatoid disease (Fig 33–2).

Whatever the primary stimulus, synovial lymphocytes produce IgG, monomeric IgM, and pentameric IgM anti-immunoglobulins (ie, rheumatoid factors). The presence of IgG aggregates or IgG–rheumatoid factor complexes could activate the complement system and lead to a number of inflammatory phenomena, including histamine release, the production of factors chemotactic for polymorphonuclear neutrophils (PMN) and mononuclear cells, and membrane damage with cell lysis (see Chapter 11). There is a marked influx of leukocytes into the synovial space. Prostaglandins and leukotrienes produced by inflammatory cells are thought to play a major role in mediation of the inflammatory process. In addition, lysosomal enzymes released into the synovial space by leukocytes further amplify the inflammatory and proliferative response of the synovium. The mononuclear infiltrate characteristically seen within the synovium includes perivascular collections of CD4 cells and interstitial collections of CD8 cells, B lymphocytes, lymphoblasts, plasma cells, and macrophages. The immunologic interaction of these cells leads to the liberation of cytokines responsible for the accumulation of macrophages within the inflammatory synovium. The various inflammatory cells in the joint produce proteinases and collagenases that damage cartilage and articular supporting structures.

Rheumatoid factors may play a role in the causation of extra-articular disease. Patients with rheumatoid vasculitis have high titers of monomeric and pentameric

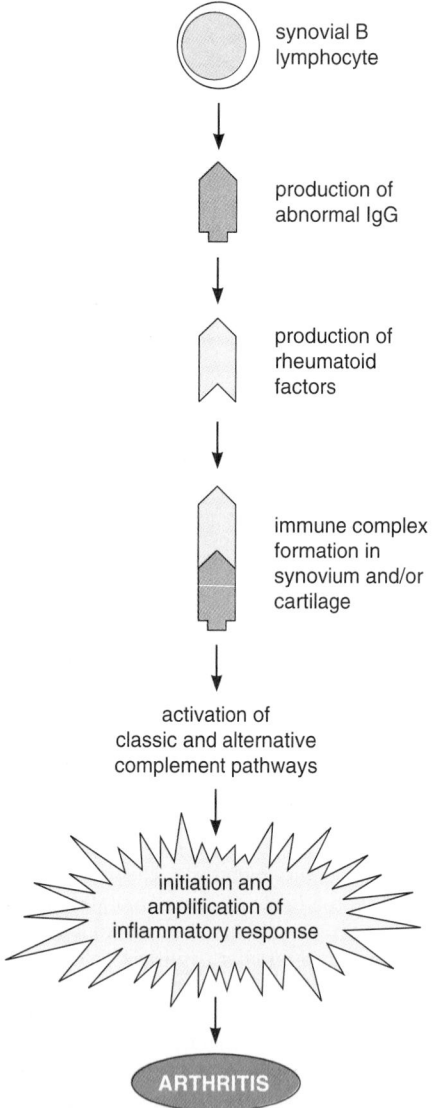

Figure 33–2. Hypothetical immunopathogenesis in rheumatoid arthritis.

synovial B lymphocyte

↓

production of abnormal IgG

↓

production of rheumatoid factors

↓

immune complex formation in synovium and/or cartilage

↓

activation of classic and alternative complement pathways

↓

initiation and amplification of inflammatory response

↓

ARTHRITIS

IgM, IgA, and IgG rheumatoid factors. Antigen–antibody complexes infused into experimental animals in the presence of IgM rheumatoid factor induce necrotizing vasculitis. Theoretically, immune complexes initiate vascular inflammation by the activation of complement. Pulmonary involvement is associated with the deposition of 11S and 15S protein complexes containing aggregates of IgG in the walls of pulmonary vessels and alveoli. 19S IgM rheumatoid factor has also been detected in arterioles and alveolar walls adjacent to cavitary nodules. Rheumatoid factors probably do not initiate the inflammatory process in rheumatoid disease, but they might perpetuate and amplify that process.

Clinical Features
A. Symptoms and Signs:

1. Onset–The usual age at onset is 20–40 years. In most cases the disease presents with joint manifestations; however, some patients first develop extra-articular manifestations, including fatigue, weakness, weight loss, mild fever, and anorexia.

2. Articular manifestations–Patients experience stiffness and joint pain, which are generally worse in the morning and improve throughout the day. These symptoms are accompanied by signs of articular inflammation, including swelling, warmth, erythema, and tenderness on palpation. The arthritis is symmetric, involving the small joints of the hands and feet (ie, the proximal interphalangeals, metacarpophalangeals, wrists, and subtalars). Large joints (knees, hips, elbows, ankles, shoulders) commonly become involved later in the course of the disease, although in some patients large-joint involvement predominates. The cervical spine may be involved; the thoracic and lumbosacral spine is usually spared.

Periarticular inflammation is common, with tendonitis and tenosynovitis resulting in weakening of tendons, ligaments, and supporting structures. Joint pain leads to muscle spasm, limitation of motion, and, in advanced cases, muscle contractions and ankylosis with permanent joint deformity. The most characteristic deformities in the hand are ulnar deviation of the fingers, the "boutonnière" deformity (flexion of the proximal interphalangeal joints and hyperextension of the distal interphalangeal joints resulting from volar slippage of the lateral bands of the superficial extensor tendons), and the "swan neck" deformity (hyperextension of the proximal interphalangeal joints and flexion of the distal interphalangeal joints resulting from contactures of intrinsic muscles of the hand).

3. Extra-articular manifestations–From 20 to 25% of patients (particularly those with severe disease) have subcutaneous or subperiosteal nodules, so-called rheumatoid nodules. Rheumatoid nodules consist of an irregularly shaped central zone of fibrinoid necrosis surrounded by a margin of large mononuclear cells with an outer zone of granulation tissue containing plasma cells and lymphocytes. They are thought to be a late stage in the evolution of a vasculitic process. Mature nodules are firm, nontender, round or oval masses that can be movable or fixed. They frequently develop over boney prominences, most commonly the olecranon process and proximal ulna. Rheumatoid nodules may also be found in the myocardium, pericardium, heart valves, pleura, lungs, sclera, dura mater, spleen, larynx, and synovial tissues.

Lung involvement includes pleurisy, interstitial lymphocytic pneumonitis or fibrosis, and Caplan's syndrome (development of large nodules in the lung parenchyma of patients with rheumatoid arthritis who also have pneumoconiosis). The manifestations of rheumatoid cardiac disease include pericarditis, myocarditis, valvular insufficiency, and conduction disturbances.

Several types of vasculitis occur in rheumatoid arthritis. The most common is a small-vessel obliterative vasculitis that leads to peripheral neuropathy. Less common is a subacute cutaneous arteriolitis associated with ischemic ulceration of the skin. The rarest form of rheumatoid vasculitis is a necrotizing vasculitis of medium and large vessels indistinguishable from polyarteritis nodosa. The major neurologic abnormalities in rheumatoid arthritis involve peripheral nerves. In addition to the peripheral neuropathy associated with vasculitis, a number of entrapment syndromes occur due to impingement by periarticular inflammatory tissue or amyloid on nerves passing through tight fascial planes. The carpal tunnel syndrome is a well-known complication of wrist disease; however, entrapment can also occur at the elbow, knee, and ankle. Destruction of the transverse ligament of the odontoid can result in atlantoaxial subluxation with cord or nerve root impingement.

Sjögren's syndrome (keratoconjunctivitis sicca and xerostomia) occurs in up to 30% of patients. Myositis with lymphocytic infiltration of involved muscle is rare. Ocular involvement ranges from benign inflammation of the surface of the sclera (episcleritis) to severe inflammation of the sclera, with nodule formation. Scleronodular disease can lead to weakening and thinning of the sclera (scleromalacia). A catastrophic but rare complication of scleromalacia is perforation of the eye with extrusion of vitreous (scleromalacia perforans).

4. Felty's syndrome–Felty's syndrome is the association of rheumatoid arthritis, splenomegaly, and neutropenia. Possible mechanisms of the hematologic abnormalities seen in these patients include anti-stem cell antibodies, antigranulocyte antibodies, and splenic sequestration of immune complex-coated polymorphonuclear leukocytes. The syndrome almost always develops in patients with high rheumatoid factor titers and rheumatoid nodules, although the arthritis itself is frequently inactive. Other features of hypersplenism and lymphadenopathy may also be present. These patients are at increased risk of developing bacterial infections.

B. Laboratory Findings: A normochromic, normocytic anemia and thrombocytosis are common among patients with active disease. The sedimentation rate is elevated, and the degree of elevation correlates roughly with disease activity.

The synovial fluid is more inflammatory than that seen in degenerative osteoarthritis or SLE. The leukocyte count is usually 5000–20,000/μL (occassionally higher than 50,000/μL). Two thirds of the cells are PMN that discharge lysosomal enzymes into the synovial fluid, presumably leading to depolymerization of synovial hyaluronate, decreased viscosity, and a poor mucin clot. The glucose level may be low or normal.

The rheumatoid pleural effusion is an exudate containing fewer than 5000 mononuclear or polymorphonuclear leukocytes per microliter. Protein exceeds 3 g/dL, and glucose is often reduced below 20 mg/dL. Rheumatoid factors can be detected, and complement levels are usually low.

C. X-Ray Findings: The first detectable x-ray abnormalities are soft tissue swelling and juxta-articular demineralization. The destruction of articular cartilage leads to joint space narrowing. Bony erosions develop at the junction of the synovial membrane and the bone just adjacent to articular cartilage. Destruction of the cartilage and laxity of ligaments lead to maladjustment and subluxation of articular surfaces. Spondylitis is usually limited to the cervical spine and may lead to osteoporosis, joint space narrowing, erosions, and, finally, subluxation of the involved articulations.

Immunologic Diagnosis

The most important serologic finding is the elevated rheumatoid factor titer, present in over 75% of patients. Rheumatoid factors are immunoglobulins with specificity for the Fc fragment of IgG. Most laboratory techniques detect pentameric IgM rheumatoid factor, but rheumatoid factor properties are also seen in monomeric IgM, IgG, and IgA. Pentameric IgM rheumatoid factor may combine with IgG molecules to form a soluble circulating high-molecular-weight immunoglobulin complex in the serum.

In rheumatoid arthritis, serum protein electrophoresis may show increased α_2-globulin, polyclonal hypergammaglobulinemia, and hypoalbuminemia. Cryoprecipitates composed of immunoglobulins are often seen in rheumatoid vasculitis. Serum complement levels are usually normal but may be low in the presence of active vasculitis. Many patients have antinuclear antibodies.

Several tests are available in the laboratory to detect rheumatoid factors. The latex fixation test is a commonly used method for detection of rheumatoid factor. Aggregated γ-globulin (Cohn's fraction II) is adsorbed onto latex particles, which then agglutinate in the presence of rheumatoid factors. The latex fixation test is not specific but is very sensitive, resulting in a high incidence of false-positive results. The sensitized sheep erythrocyte test (Rose-Waaler test) depends on specific antibody binding and is more specific than the latex fixation assay. Sheep erythrocytes are coated with rabbit antibody against sheep erythrocytes. The sensitized sheep erythrocytes then agglutinate in the presence of rheumatoid factor. Other techniques, capable of detecting rheumatoid factors of all classes, include indirect immunofluorescence, ELISA, and laser nephelometry.

It is important to emphasize that a negative rheumatoid factor by routine laboratory procedures does not exclude the diagnosis of rheumatoid arthritis. Approximately 20% of patients with otherwise typical rheumatoid arthritis are seronegative. Some of these patients may have IgG, IgA or monomeric IgM rheumatoid factors. Conversely, rheumatoid factors are not unique to rheumatoid arthritis. Rheumatoid factors are also present in patients with SLE (30%), in a high percentage (90%) of patients with Sjögren's syndrome, and less often in patients with scleroderma or polymyositis. Positive agglutination reactions with the latex test also occur in patients with a number of chronic inflammatory conditions, including chronic active hepatitis, kala-azar, sarcoidosis, neoplasia, and syphilis. The sensitized sheep erythrocyte test is usually negative in these conditions. In some chronic infectious diseases, such as leprosy and tuberculosis, both the latex and the sensitized sheep erythrocyte tests may be positive. In subacute bacterial endocarditis, both tests may be positive during active disease and revert to negative as patients improve. The transient appearance of rheumatoid factor has been noted following vaccinations in military recruits. Epidemiologic studies have shown that a small number of normal people also have rheumatoid factors. A large proportion of the elderly have a positive latex test, though the sensitized sheep erythrocyte test is generally negative.

Differential Diagnosis

In the patient with classic articular changes, bony erosions of the small joints of the hands and feet, and positive rheumatoid factors, the diagnosis of rheumatoid arthritis is not difficult. Early in the disease, or when extra-articular manifestations dominate the clinical picture, other rheumatic diseases (including SLE, Reiter's syndrome, gout, psoriatic arthritis, degenerative osteoarthritis, and the peripheral arthritis of chronic inflammatory bowel disease) or infectious processes may mimic rheumatoid arthritis. Patients with SLE can be distinguished by their characteristic skin lesions, renal disease, and diagnostic serologic abnormalities. Reiter's syndrome occurs predominantly in young men, generally affects joints of the lower extremity in an asymmetric fashion, and is often associated with urethritis and conjunctivitis. Gouty arthritis is usually an acute monoarthritis with negatively birefringent sodium urate crystals present within the white cells of inflammatory synovial fluid. Psoriatic arthritis is usually asymmetric and often involves distal interphalangeal joints. Degenerative arthritis is characterized by Heberden's nodes, lack of symmetric joint involvement, and involvement of the distal interphalangeal joints. The peripheral arthritis of bowel disease usually occurs in large weight-bearing joints and is often associated with bowel symptoms. The polyarthritis associated with rubella vaccination, parvovirus infection, hepatitis A, sarcoidosis, and infectious mononucleosis can mimic early rheumatoid arthritis.

Treatment

A. Physical Therapy: A rational program of physical therapy is vital in the treatment of patients with rheumatoid arthritis. Such a program should consist of an appropriate balance of rest and exercise and the judicious use of heat or cold therapy. The patient may require complete or intermittent bedrest on a regular basis to combat inflammation or fatigue. In addition, specific joints may have to be put at rest through the use of braces, splints, or crutches. An exercise program emphasizing active range-of-motion movements helps to maintain strength and mobility. Heat or cold is valuable in alleviating muscle spasm, stiffness, and pain. Many patients need a hot shower or bath to loosen up in the morning, and others cannot perform their exercises adequately without prior heat treatment. Heating pads or paraffin baths are often used to apply heat to specific joints. In some patients ice massage is more effective than heat. Physical and occupational therapists provide valuable help in devising an appropriate physical therapy program.

B. Drug Treatment:

1. Nonsteroidal anti-inflammatory drugs (NSAIDs)–NSAIDs (Table 33–2) may provide symptomatic benefit to patients with rheumatoid arthritis. Although their exact mechanism of action is uncertain, they effectively inhibit the production of prostaglandins, thereby reducing inflammation. These agents are associated with numerous side effects. Gastric distress is common but can be partly alleviated by using antacids, histamine H_2 receptor blockers, sucralfate, or misoprostol (prostaglandin E_1) and by encouraging patients to take their drugs with meals. Although any of these modalities may alleviate gastrointestinal symptoms in the individual patient, only misoprostol has been shown to decrease gastritis and gastric ulcer formation in patients on nonsteroidal anti-inflammatory drugs. Microscopic blood loss from the gastrointestinal tract is common but is not an indication for stopping NSAID therapy. Since NSAIDs do decrease platelet adhesiveness, their use should be avoided in patients about to have surgery, those with a bleeding diathesis, or those receiving coumarin anticoagulants. Combining two or more nonsteroidal anti-inflammatory agents provides little or no additional benefit over maximum

Table 33–2. Nonsteroidal anti-inflammatory drugs (NSAIDs).

Carboxylic acid derivatives	Salicylates: aspirin, salsalate, diflunisal, choline magnesium trisalicylate. Propionic acids: ibuprofen, naproxan, fenoprofen, flurbiprofen, ketoprofen, oxaprozin. Pyranocarboxylic acids: etodolac. Aromatic acetic acids: indomethacin, sulindac, tolmetin. Phenylacetic acids: diclofenac. Fenamic acids: meclofenamate sodium.
Enolic acid derivatives	Pyrazolones: phenylbutazone, oxyphenbutazone. Oxicams: piroxicam.
Nonacidic NSAIDs	Naphthylalkanone: nabumetone.

doses of single agents and may increase gastrointestinal toxicity.

2. Antimalarial Drugs–Many rheumatologists advocate the use of antimalarial drugs for prolonged periods in patients with severe disease. Their mechanism of action is unclear, but they appear to affect monocyte function. The antimalarial drugs act slowly, often requiring 1–6 months of treatment for maximum therapeutic benefit. The preparation most often used is hydroxychloroquine, 200–600 mg/d. Toxic side effects include skin rashes, nausea and vomiting, myopathy, and both corneal and retinal damage. Eye toxicity is rare at the low doses used in rheumatoid arthritis, but patients should have ophthalmologic examinations every 6–12 months while on antimalarial therapy.

3. Gold salt therapy–Although associated with a high incidence of toxic side effects, parenteral gold salt therapy is of significant benefit to some patients. Gold shots have to be administered every week for up to 20 weeks and then monthly for as long as the patient has active disease. Toxic side effects occur in 40% of patients and include dermatitis, photosensitivity, stomatitis, thrombocytopenia, agranulocytosis, hepatitis, aplastic anemia, peripheral neuropathy, nephritis with nephrotic syndrome, ulcerative enterocolitis, pneumonitis, and keratitis.

An oral gold salt preparation, auranofin, is available. Most side effects, although similar to those of parenteral gold salt preparations, may occur less frequently. Diarrhea, however, is more common. The usual dose is 3 mg twice daily. As with parenteral gold preparations, it may take 3–6 months to achieve therapeutic benefit.

4. Penicillamine–Penicillamine has been used in the treatment of rheumatoid arthritis. Like gold, penicillamine is a slow-acting nonsteroidal anti-inflammatory agent, and it may take up to 6 months for a therapeutic response to become apparent. The toxic side effects of penicillamine can be severe. They include rash, loss of sense of taste, nausea and vomiting, anorexia, proteinuria, agranulocytosis, aplastic anemia, and thrombocytopenia. Less commonly, myasthenia, myositis, Goodpasture's syndrome, pemphigus, bronchiolitis, and a lupus-like syndrome may be seen.

5. Sulfasalazine–Sulfasalazine was developed as a treatment for rheumatoid arthritis over 40 years ago. The mode of action is unknown but may be related to the pharmacologic actions of its two constituent components, sulfapyridine and 5-aminosalicylate. The anti-inflammatory dose is 2–3 g/d. It takes 6–12 weeks for the clinical benefits of the drug to become apparent, and approximately two thirds of patients derive some benefit from sulfasalazine therapy. Side effects include anorexia, nausea and vomiting, pruritus, rash, urticaria, anemia, leukopenia, and thrombocytopenia.

6. Corticosteroids–Intermittent intra-articular injection of corticosteroids is useful for the patient with only a few symptomatic joints. Relief may last for months. Low-dose systemic corticosteroids may be indicated in patients who do not respond to other anti-inflammatory therapy. The usual dose is 5–10 mg of prednisone daily. Withdrawal from corticosteroids should be gradual, since clinical exacerbation of arthritis or steroid withdrawal syndrome may occur. Long-term systemic corticosteroid treatment results in hyperadrenocorticism and disruption of the pituitary–adrenal axis. Manifestations of corticosteroid toxicity include weight gain, moon facies, ecchymoses, hirsutism, diabetes mellitus, hypertension, osteoporosis, avascular necrosis of bone, cataracts, myopathy, mental disturbances, activation of tuberculosis, and predisposition to infections.

7. Immunosuppressive agents–The antimetabolite methotrexate can produce dramatic improvement in patients with severe disease. Methotrexate has largely replaced gold and penicillamine in the treatment of rheumatoid arthritis. Side effects include marrow suppression, liver toxicity, oral ulcers, and teratogenesis. Alkylating agents (eg, chlorambucil, cyclophosphamide) purine analogs (eg, mercaptopurine, azathioprine) and cyclosporin have also been used in the treatment of rheumatoid arthritis. These drugs are associated with major toxic side effects, however, including an increased incidence of neoplasms and infection. They should, therefore, be used with great caution.

C. Orthopedic Surgery: Surgery to correct or compensate for joint damage is often an essential part of the general management of rheumatoid arthritis. Arthroplasty is employed to relieve pain and to maintain or improve joint motion. Arthrodesis can be used to correct deformity and alleviate pain, but it results in loss of motion. Early synovectomy might prevent joint damage or tendon rupture and decreases pain and inflammation in a given joint, but the synovium often grows back and symptoms may return.

Complications & Prognosis

Several clinical patterns of rheumatoid arthritis are apparent. Spontaneous remission may occur, usually within 2 years after the onset of the disease. Some patients have brief episodes of acute arthritis with longer periods of low-grade activity or remission. Rare patients have sustained progression of active disease resulting in deformity and death. The development of classic disease within 1 year of the onset of symptoms, an age of less than 30 years at onset of disease, and the presence of rheumatoid nodules and high titers of rheumatoid factor are unfavorable prognostic factors.

Follow-up of patients after 10–15 years shows that 50% are stationary or improved, 70% are capable of full-time employment, and 10% are completely incapacitated. Death from vasculitis or atlantoaxial subluxation is rare. Fatalities are more often associated with sepsis or the complications of therapy.

JUVENILE ARTHRITIS

Major Immunologic Features
- Overt or "hidden" rheumatoid factors exist.
- Antinuclear antibodies may occur.

General Considerations

Juvenile arthritis consists of a group of disorders that occur in individuals under 16 years of age. The incidence of the disease peaks in boys at age 2 and again at age 9, whereas in girls it peaks between 1 and 3 years of age. Juvenile arthritis may present as a systemic illness (Still's disease), as a seronegative pauci- or polyarthritis, or as a seropositive polyarthritis identical to adult rheumatoid arthritis. The outlook for girls with pauciarticular disease is excellent, whereas boys with pauciarticular disease may eventually develop ankylosing spondylitis. Although upper respiratory infections and trauma have both been implicated as precipitating factors, the roles of infection, trauma, and heredity in the pathogenesis of the disease are unclear.

Immunologic Pathogenesis

The basic immunopathogenic mechanisms in juvenile arthritis are unknown. Both humoral and cellular defects occur in these patients, however. Diffuse hypergammaglobulinemia, involving IgG, IgA, and IgM, is present. Rheumatoid factors of all immunoglobulin classes have been detected. Approximately 10% of children with juvenile arthritis have a positive latex fixation test for IgM rheumatoid factor. The sera from some patients with negative latex fixation tests may actually contain IgM rheumatoid factors. Two major theories have been offered in an attempt to explain the presence of these "hidden" rheumatoid factors in juvenile arthritis. First, IgM rheumatoid factor may bind avidly to native IgG in the patient's serum and therefore may not be able to bind IgG coating the latex particles. Second, an abnormal IgG may be present that preferentially binds IgM, thereby blocking latex fixation. Cold-reacting (4 °C) pentameric IgM rheumatoid factors (cryoglobulins) are associated with severe disease.

Serum components of both the classic and alternative (properdin) complement systems are elevated, although this elevation is less in patients who have rheumatoid factors or severe disease. Elevation of serum complement may reflect a secondary overcompensation in response to increased consumption, or a general increase in protein synthesis. Studies of the metabolism of complement actually demonstrate hypercatabolism. The depression of complement in synovial fluid is probably secondary to complement activation by immune complexes, similar to that seen in rheumatoid arthritis.

Studies suggest that patients with juvenile arthritis possess certain HLA tissue types with greater than expected frequencies. Thus, patients with early-onset pauciarticular disease tend to be HLA-DR5- or HLA-DR8-positive, whereas those with late-onset pauciarticular disease tend to be HLA-B27-positive. Patients with rheumatoid factor-positive polyarticular disease tend to be HLA-D4-positive, and those with systemic disease tend to be HLA-DR5-positive.

Clinical Features

A. Symptoms and Signs:

1. Onset–

a. Twenty percent of children, usually under age 4, present with high, spiking fever, an evanescent rash, polyserositis, hepatosplenomegaly, and lymphadenopathy (Still's disease).

b. Forty percent of patients present with polyarthritis (more than four joints involved during the first 6 months of illness), sometimes accompanied by low-grade fever and malaise. In 25% of this group, the onset is in late childhood and is associated with rheumatoid factor.

c. Forty percent of patients present with pauciarticular (involvement of four or fewer joints) disease and few systemic manifestations. Slightly more than 50% of these patients are young girls with antinuclear antibodies, who are particularly likely to develop iridocyclitis.

2. Joint manifestations–
Even in the presence of severe arthritis, young children may not complain of pain but may instead limit the use of an extremity. The knees, wrists, ankles, and neck are common sites of initial involvement. Early involvement of the hip is extremely rare in young children with pauciarticular disease. Older children occasionally develop symmetric involvement in the small joints of the hands (metacarpophalangeal, proximal interphalangeal, and distal interphalangeal) similar to that seen in adults. In seronegative patients, the metacarpophalangeal joints may be spared. With severe hand involvement, children are more likely to develop radial rather than ulnar deviation. Involvement of the feet may lead to hallux valgus or to "hammer toe" deformity. Achillobursitis and achillotendinitis may cause tender, swollen heels. Older boys with pauciarticular disease may develop ankylosing spondylitis during the third decade of life.

3. Systemic manifestations–
Fever, often with a high evening spike, is characteristic of Still's disease. Anorexia, weight loss, and malaise are common. Most children with Still's disease develop an evanescent, salmon-colored maculopapular rash that coincides with periods of high fever. Occasional patients manifest cardiac involvement. Pericarditis occurs commonly but rarely leads to dysfunction or constriction. Myocarditis is an unusual manifestation of the cardiac disease, but, when present, can lead to heart failure. Acute pneumonitis or pleuritis sometimes occur, but chronic lung disease is rare.

Iridocyclitis occurs most commonly in young girls with pauciarticular disease and can precede articular involvement. It typically runs an insidious course and often persists even when joint disease becomes quiescent. Iridocyclitis is best monitored by frequent slit lamp examinations, at least through puberty.

Lymphadenopathy and hepatosplenomegaly are associated with severe systemic disease and are uncommon in patients with chiefly articular manifestations.

Subcutaneous nodules occur in children with polyarticular disease, usually in association with a positive test for rheumatoid factors.

Rarely, Still's disease occurs in adults. Characteristic manifestations include high spiking fevers, evanescent rash, arthritis, and elevated leukocyte count and hepatic enzyme levels.

4. Complications–The major complication of juvenile arthritis is impairment of growth and development secondary to early epiphyseal closure. This is particularly common in the mandible, causing micrognathia, and in the metacarpals and metatarsals, leading to abnormally small fingers and toes. The extent of growth impairment usually correlates positively with the severity and duration of disease but may also reflect the growth-inhibiting effects of steroids. Children in whom arthritis begins before age 5 occasionally undergo increased growth of an affected extremity. Vasculitis and encephalitis are sometimes observed in patients with juvenile arthritis. Secondary amyloidosis occurs rarely.

B. Laboratory Findings: Mild leukocytosis (15,000–20,000/μL) is the rule, but some patients develop leukopenia. A normochromic microcytic anemia, an elevated erythrocyte sedimentation rate, and an abnormal C-reactive protein occur commonly. Because an elevated ASO titer is so frequently encountered, this test cannot be used to differentiate juvenile arthritis from rheumatic fever. Positive tests for rheumatoid factors occur in older children with polyarticular disease, whereas antinuclear antibodies are found both in patients with polyarticular disease and in young patients with pauciarticular disease. A positive ANA almost never occurs in Still's disease. Serum protein electrophoresis shows an increase in acute-phase reactants (α-globulins) and a polyclonal increase of γ-globulin. The synovial fluid in active juvenile rheumatoid arthritis is exudative, with a leukocyte count of 5000–20,000/μL (mostly neutrophils), a poor mucin clot, and decreased glucose compared with serum glucose. Mononuclear cells may predominate in the synovial fluid of patients with pauciarticular disease.

C. X-Ray Findings: Radiographic changes early in the disease include juxta-articular demineralization, periosteal bone accretion, premature closure of the epiphyses, cervical zygapophyseal fusion (particularly at C2–3), osseous overgrowth of the interphalangeal joints, and erosion and narrowing of the joint space. Carpal arthritis with ankylosis is seen as a late manifestation of Still's disease.

Immunologic Diagnosis

Currently, the diagnosis of juvenile arthritis is based on clinical criteria. Although certain abnormalities of immunoglobulins, complement, and cellular immunity are compatible with the diagnosis of juvenile arthritis, no specific immunologic test is diagnostic.

Differential Diagnosis

The diagnosis of juvenile arthritis is extremely difficult, since the disease can present with nonspecific constitutional signs and symptoms in the absence of arthritis. Other causes of fever, particularly infections and cancer, must be considered. Leukemia can present in childhood with fever, lymphadenopathy, and joint pains. Rheumatic fever closely resembles juvenile arthritis, particularly early in the disease, but the patient with juvenile arthritis tends to have higher spiking fevers, lymphadenopathy and hepatosplenomegaly in the absence of carditis, and a more refractory, long-lasting arthritis. Patients with rheumatic fever are more likely to have evidence of recent streptococcal infection, including elevated titers of antihyaluronidase, antistreptokinase, and antistreptodornase antibodies. In addition, patients with rheumatic fever tend to have a less intense leukocytosis and respond more dramatically to low doses of aspirin. An expanding skin lesion followed in weeks or months by arthritis suggests the diagnosis of Lyme disease, an inflammatory arthropathy caused by the spirochete *Borrelia burgdorferi*. Rheumatic diseases that may begin in childhood, such as SLE or dermatomyositis, can be differentiated by their different clinical course, different organ system involvement, and characteristic serologic abnormalities.

When juvenile arthritis presents as a monoarticular arthritis, examination of synovial fluid is of paramount importance in excluding infection.

Treatment

The major goals of therapy are to relieve pain, prevent contractures and deformities, and promote normal physical and emotional development. These goals are best achieved by a comprehensive program of physical, medical, and, when necessary, surgical therapy.

A. Physical Therapy: Exercise promotes muscle strength, encourages growth, and prevents deformity. The goal in children is to maintain mobility. The tricycle is always preferable to the wheelchair! As in the treatment of adult rheumatoid arthritis, rest can be an important part of physical therapy. Complete rest is indicated during severe exacerbations and may be necessary for short afternoon periods on a routine basis. Specific joints can be put at rest by the use of splints, collars, and braces that support the joint and help prevent deformity. Judicious use of heat decreases pain and muscle spasm and is particularly useful before exercising.

B. Drug Treatment:

1. Aspirin–The disease responds to aspirin at a dosage level of 90–130 mg/kg/d given in four to six divided doses. Tinnitus and decreased hearing are poor indicators of aspirin toxicity in children. Irritability, drowsiness, or intermittent periods of hyperpnea are early signs of salicylate intoxication. Therefore, it is essential to monitor blood salicylate levels during aspirin therapy. Acidosis and ketosis may develop in infants. Respiratory alkalosis, due to primary stimulation of the respiratory center, occurs in older children. Many of the newer NSAIDs are new approved for use in children.

2. Remittive agents–Children with refractory arthritis may benefit from injectable or oral gold, antimalarials, penicillamine, or methotrexate.

3. Corticosteroids–Intra-articular corticosteroid injections are useful in pauciarticular disease. Systemic corticosteroids are reserved for patients with myocarditis, vasculitis, refractory iridocyclitis, or Still's disease that is unresponsive to aspirin therapy. Patients with iridocyclitis may require prolonged corticosteroid therapy. In children, the major toxic effects of corticosteroid therapy include subcapsular cataract formation, vertebral osteoporosis and collapse, infection, premature skeletal maturation with diminished growth, and pseudotumor cerebri with intracranial hypertension.

C. Surgical Treatment: The aims of surgery in juvenile arthritis are to relieve pain and maintain or improve joint function. Synovectomy may diminish pain due to chronic synovitis, but long-term effectiveness is questionable. Synovectomy for severe extensor tenosynovitis of the hand may prevent tendon rupture. Tendon release procedures help relieve joint contractures. Hip replacement is of benefit in selected cases but should be delayed as long as possible, since in some children hip cartilage may regenerate with continued weight-bearing.

Complications & Prognosis

Seventy percent of patients experience a spontaneous and permanent remission by adulthood. Patients with Still's disease tend to have several recurrences per year. Patients presenting with oligoarthritic disease, particularly if they are female, tend to remain oligoarthritic, and those presenting with polyarthritis remain polyarthritic. Rarely, the disease persists into adulthood. This usually occurs in children with symmetric polyarthritis similar to that seen in adults. Sometimes a patient with juvenile arthritis in apparent remission develops rheumatoid arthritis as an adult. In an occasional unfortunate case, the disease is relentless and crippling. Small-joint involvement, positive serum rheumatoid factor, and onset in later childhood all portend a poor prognosis.

SJÖGREN'S SYNDROME

Major Immunologic Features

■ Lymphocytes and plasma cells infiltrate involved tissues.
■ There are rheumatoid factors and antinuclear antibodies.
■ There are autoantibodies against salivary duct antigens.

General Considerations

Sjögren's syndrome is a chronic inflammatory disease of unknown cause characterized by diminished lacrimal and salivary gland secretion resulting in keratoconjunctivitis sicca and xerostomia. There is dryness of the eyes, mouth, nose, trachea, bronchi, vagina, and skin. In half of patients, the disease occurs as a primary pathologic entity (primary Sjögren's syndrome). In the other half, it occurs in association with rheumatoid arthritis or other connective tissue disorders. Ninety percent of patients with Sjögren's syndrome are female. Although the mean age at onset is 50 years, the disease does occur in children.

Immunologic Pathogenesis

Patients with Sjögren's syndrome may have an abnormal immunologic response to one or more unidentified antigens, perhaps viral antigens or virus-altered autoantigens. This abnormal response is characterized by excessive B cell and plasma cell activity, manifested by polyclonal hypergammaglobulinemia and the production of rheumatoid factors, antinuclear antibodies, cryoglobulins, and antisalivary duct antibodies. Immunofluorescence studies have shown both B and T helper lymphocytes and plasma cells infiltrating involved tissues. Large quantities of IgM and IgG are synthesized by these infiltrating lymphocytes. In patients with coexisting macroglobulinemia, monoclonal IgM may be synthesized in the salivary glands. Excessive B-cell activity could be due either to a primary B-cell defect or to defective T-lymphocyte regulation. There is evidence of decreased suppressor T-cell function in patients with Sjögren's syndrome.

Pathology

Histologically, there is lymphocytic infiltrate in exocrine glands of the respiratory, gastrointestinal, and vaginal tracts as well as glands of the ocular and oral mucosa. Histologic demonstration of lymphocytic infiltration in a biopsy specimen taken from the minor labial salivary glands is the most specific and sensitive single diagnostic test for Sjögren's syndrome.

Clinical Features

A. Symptoms and Signs:

1. Oral–Dryness of the mouth is usually the most distressing symptom and is often associated with burning discomfort and difficulty in chewing and swallowing dry foods. Parotid salivary flow is less than the normal 5 mL/10 minutes/gland. Polyuria and nocturia develop as the patient drinks increasing amounts of water in an effort to relieve oral symptoms. The oral mucous membranes are dry and erythematous, and the tongue becomes fissured and ulcerated. Severe dental caries is often present. Half of patients have intermittent parotid gland enlargement. The parotid gland in Sjögren's syndrome is firm, in contrast to the soft parotid enlargement characteristic of diabetes mellitus or alcohol abuse. Glossitis and angular cheilitis are manifestations of oral candidiasis in Sjögren's syndrome.

2. Ocular–The major ocular finding is keratoconjunctivitis sicca. Symptoms include burning, itching, decreased tearing, ocular accumulation of thick mucoid material during the night, photophobia, pain, and a "gritty" or "sandy" sensation in the eyes. Decreased tearing is demonstrated by diminished flow of tears down a strip of filter paper inserted into the lower palpebral fissure (Schirmer's test). Rose bengal or fluorescein reveals punctate staining of the conjunctiva and cornea. Tear break-up time is shortened. Severe ocular involvement may lead to ulceration, vascularization with opacification, or perforation of the cornea.

3. Miscellaneous–Dryness of the nose, posterior oropharynx, larynx, and respiratory tract may lead to epistaxis, dysphonia, recurrent otitis media, tracheobronchitis, or pneumonia. Dryness of the vagina may cause dyspareunia. Active synovitis is a common finding, particularly in patients who also have rheumatoid arthritis. Twenty percent of patients with primary Sjögren's syndrome complain of Raynaud's phenomenon. Ten percent of patients have extraglandular lymphocytic infiltrates, particularly in the kidneys, lungs, lymph nodes, and muscles. A few such patients develop lymphoma.

B. Laboratory Findings: Anemia, leukopenia, and an elevated erythrocyte sedimentation rate are common features. Secretory sialography with radiopaque dye demonstrates glandular disorganization. Salivary scintigraphy with technetium Tc99m pertechnetate reveals decreased parotid secretory function.

Immunologic Diagnosis

No immunologic test is diagnostic for Sjögren's syndrome; however, a myriad of nonspecific immunologic abnormalities occur in these patients.

A. Humoral Abnormalities: Hypergammaglobulinemia is seen in half of patients. Although serum protein electrophoresis usually shows a polyclonal hypergammaglobulinemia, occasional patients develop a monoclonal IgM paraproteinemia, usually of the kappa type. Patients who develop lymphoma sometimes become severely hypogammaglobulinemic and show disappearance of autoantibodies. Rheumatoid factors can be detected in 90% of patients with Sjögren's syndrome. ANA in a speckled or homogeneous pattern is present in 70% of patients. Many of these antinuclear antibodies are directed against acid-extractable nuclear antigens. Antibodies against one such antigen, termed SS-B, are relatively specific for patients with primary Sjögren's syndrome. Antibodies against a second acid-extractable nuclear antigen, SS-A, may be found in Sjögren's syndrome alone or in Sjögren's syndrome associated with SLE. Patients with Sjögren's syndrome and rheumatoid arthritis have neither anti-SS-A nor anti-SS-B antibodies. Autoantibodies against salivary duct antigens have been detected in 50% of patients with Sjögren's syndrome associated with rheumatoid arthritis.

B. Cellular Abnormalities: Thirty percent of patients with Sjögren's syndrome have decreased lymphocyte responses to mitogenic stimulation. A few patients also have decreased numbers of circulating T lymphocytes in the peripheral blood (see the section Immunologic Pathogenesis).

C. HLA Associations: HLA typing studies suggest a genetic predisposition to the development of Sjögren's syndrome. The prevalence of HLA-B8, -DR3, -DR2, and, most markedly, -DRw52 is significantly increased in patients with primary Sjögren's syndrome. HLA-DR3, -DQ1, and -DQ2, but not -DRw52, are associated with polyclonal hypergammaglobulinemia and high titers of anti-SSA antibodies.

Differential Diagnosis

The diagnosis of Sjögren's syndrome can be made on the basis of two of the three classic manifestations of xerostomia, keratoconjunctivitis sicca, and rheumatoid arthritis. The varied and multisystemic nature of the disease, however, may obscure the diagnosis. Other causes of bilateral parotid swelling include nutritional deficiencies, endocrine disorders, sarcoidosis, drug reactions, infections (including human immunodeficiency virus [HIV]), amyloid, and obesity. Parotid gland cancer must always be considered in a patient with unilateral parotid swelling.

Treatment

A. Symptomatic Measures:

1. Oral–Patients must be urged to maintain fastidious oral hygiene, with regular use of fluoride toothpaste and mouthwashes and with regular dental examinations. Frequent sips of water and the use of sugarless gum or candy to stimulate salivary secretion are sometimes helpful in relieving xerostomia. Pilocarpine is sometimes useful in cases that don't respond to conservative measures. Many patients find aerosolized preparations of artificial saliva helpful. A bedroom humidifier helps decrease nocturnal xerostomia and nasal dryness. The most effective treatment for oral candidiasis in Sjögren's syndrome is the oral use of nystatin lozenges.

2. Ocular–Artificial tears alleviate ocular signs and symptoms. Shielded glasses offer protection against the drying effects of wind. Therapy for refractory ocular complications includes mucolytic agents, punctal occlusion, soft contact lenses, and partial tarsorrhaphy.

3. Other–Dryness of the skin can be treated with moisturizing skin creams or oils. Vaginal and nasal dryness is often relieved with sterile, water-miscible lubricants.

B. Systemic Measures: Sjögren's syndrome can usually be controlled with symptomatic therapy. Nonsteroidal anti-inflammatory drugs are useful in the treatment of the nonerosive arthritis of Sjögren's syndrome. Corticosteroids or immunosuppressive agents may be required in treating patients with severe or life-threatening disease, such as lymphoma, Waldenström's macroglobulinemia, or massive lymphocytic infiltration of vital organs.

Complications & Prognosis

In the vast majority of patients, significant lymphoproliferation is confined to salivary, lacrimal, and other mucosal glandular tissue, resulting in a benign chronic course of xerostomia and xerophthalmia. Rarely, patients develop significant extraglandular lymphoid infiltration or neoplasia.

Splenomegaly, leukopenia, and vasculitis with leg ulcers may occur. Hypergammaglobulinemic purpura, often associated with renal tubular acidosis, has been described and may be a presenting complaint. Five percent of patients with Sjögren's syndrome develop chronic autoimmune thyroiditis. Other associations include primary biliary cirrhosis, chronic active hepatitis, gastric achlorhydria, pancreatitis, renal and pulmonary lymphocytic infiltration, cryoglobulinemia with glomerulonephritis, hyperviscosity syndrome, and adult celiac disease. Neuromuscular complications include polymyositis, peripheral or cranial (particularly trigeminal) neuropathy, and cerebral vasculitis. Rarely, patients with Sjögren's syndrome develop lymphoma, immunoblastic sarcoma, or Waldenström's macroglobulinemia.

PROGRESSIVE SYSTEMIC SCLEROSIS (SCLERODERMA)

Major Immunologic Features

- Antinuclear antibodies with a speckled or nucleolar pattern occur frequently.
- Anticentromere antibodies occur in 75% of patients.
- Antibodies against topoisomerase 1 (Scl-70) may occur.

General Considerations

Scleroderma is a disease of unknown cause characterized by abnormally increased collagen deposition in the skin. The course is usually slowly progressive and chronically disabling, but it can be rapidly progressive and fatal because of involvement of internal organs. It commonly begins in the third or fourth decade of life, but children are occassionally affected. The prevalence of the disease is one case per 100,000 in the population. Women are affected twice as often as men. There is no racial predisposition. Scleroderma has been categorized based on the nature and extent of end-organ involvement. Patients with severe, widespread involvement have progressive systemic sclerosis. Morphea and localized scleroderma are forms of disease limited to the skin. Limited scleroderma (ie, CREST syndrome) is a form of scleroderma defined by *c*alcinosis, *R*aynaud's phenomenon, *e*sophogeal dysfunction, and *t*elangiectasias.

Immunologic Pathogenesis

The association of progressive systemic sclerosis with Sjögren's syndrome and, less often, with thyroiditis or primary biliary cirrhosis—and the serologic abnormalities seen in the majority of cases (presence of ANA, rheumatoid factors, polyclonal hypergammaglobulinemia)—are suggestive of an immunologic aberration in these patients. At present, there is scanty evidence for a humoral mechanism in the pathogenesis of the disease, although a serum factor toxic to vascular endothelium has been identified. Humoral factors may stimulate increased collagen production by fibroblasts. Immunoglobulins have not been found at the dermal–epidermal junction in scleroderma, although examination of the fibrinoid lesions seen in the walls of renal arterioles has revealed the presence of immunoglobulins and complement. T cells and macrophages may injure vascular endothelium, leading to activation of fibroblasts and subsequent fibrosis.

Breast implants containing silicone have been implicated as a cause of scleroderma and other rheumatic diseases. Silicone, a polymer of silicon oxide, could be immunogenic or function as an adjuvant; however, no good study has conclusively linked silicone to a rheumatic illness.

Pathology

Biopsy of clinically involved skin reveals thinning of the epidermis with loss of the rete pegs, atrophy of the dermal appendages, hyalinization and fibrosis of arterioles, and a striking increase of compact collagen fibers in the reticular dermis.

Synovial findings range from an acute lymphocytic infiltration to diffuse fibrosis with relatively little inflammation.

The histologic changes in muscles include interstitial and perivascular inflammatory infiltration followed by fibrosis and myofibrillar necrosis, atrophy, and degeneration.

In patients with renal involvement, the histologic appearance of the kidney is similar to that of malignant hypertensive nephropathy, with intimal proliferation of the interlobular arteries and fibrinoid changes in the intima and media of more distal interlobular arteries and of afferent arterioles.

There is increased collagen deposition in the lamina propria, submucosa, and muscularis of the gastrointestinal tract. Small-vessel changes similar to those that occur in the skin may also result. With loss of normal smooth muscle, the large bowel is subject to development of the characteristic wide-mouthed diverticula and to infiltration of air into the wall of the intestine (pneumatosis cystoides intestinalis).

Clinical Features

A. Symptoms and Signs:

1. Onset–Raynaud's phenomenon heralds the onset of the disease in at least 90% of patients. It may precede the other manifestations by many years. Scleroderma frequently begins with skin changes, but in one third of patients polyarthralgias and polyarthritis are the first manifestations. Initial visceral involvement without skin changes is very unusual.

2. Skin abnormalities–There are three stages in the clinical evolution of scleroderma. In the edematous phase, symmetric nonpitting edema is present in the hands and, rarely, in the feet. The edema can progress to the forearms, arms, upper anterior chest, abdomen, back, and face. In the sclerotic phase, the skin is tight, smooth, and waxy and seems bound down to underlying structures. Skin folds and wrinkles disappear. The hands are involved in most patients, with painful, slowly healing ulcerations of the fingertips in half of those cases. The face appears stretched and masklike, with thin lips and a "pinched" nose. Pigmentary changes and telangiectases are frequent at this stage. The skin changes may stabilize for prolonged periods and then either progress to the third (atrophic) stage or soften and return to normal. It should be emphasized that not all patients pass through all the stages. Subcutaneous calcifications, usually in the fingertips (calcinosis circumscripta), occur more often in women than in men. The calcifications vary in size from tiny deposits to large masses and may develop over bony prominences throughout the body.

3. Joints and muscles–Articular complaints are very common and may begin at any time during the course of the disease. The arthralgias, stiffness, and frank arthritis seen in progressive systemic sclerosis may be difficult to distinguish from those of rheumatoid arthritis, particularly in the early stages of the disease. Involved joints include the metacarpophalangeals, proximal interphalangeals, wrists, elbows, knees, ankles, and small joints of the feet. Flexion contractures caused by changes in the skin or joints are common. Muscle involvement is usually mild but may be clinically indistinguishable from that of polymyositis, with muscle weakness, tenderness, and pain of proximal muscles of the upper and lower extremities.

4. Lungs–The lungs are frequently involved in progressive systemic sclerosis, either clinically or at autopsy. A low diffusion capacity is the earliest evidence of interstitial fibrosis, preceding alterations in ventilation or clinical and radiologic evidence of disease. Dyspnea on exertion is the most frequently reported symptom. Orthopnea, paroxysmal nocturnal dyspnea, chronic cough, hemoptysis, chest pain, and hoarseness are also manifestations of pulmonary involvement. Pleurisy (with associated pleural friction rub) can also occur. Interstitial fibrosis is the major pulmonary manifestation of progressive systemic sclerosis and may occur early in patients with truncal involvement. Pulmonary hypertension, which can best be detected by echocardiography, is more likely to be seen in limited scleroderma. Patients with diffuse pulmonary involvement have intimal proliferation of small and medium-sized pulmonary arteries and arterioles and may have an intense bronchiolar epithelial proliferation.

5. Heart–Because of the frequency of pulmonary fibrosis, cor pulmonale is the most common cardiac finding. Myocardial fibrosis, leading to resistant left-sided heart failure, carries a poor prognosis. Cardiac arrhythmias and conduction disturbances are common manifestations of myocardial fibrosis. Pericarditis is usually asymptomatic and is found incidentally at autopsy. Although 40% of patients have pericardial effusion, tamponade is extremely rare.

6. Kidneys–Renal involvement is an uncommon but life-threatening development in patients with diffuse disease. Although renal insufficiency may follow an indolent course, it frequently presents as rapidly progressive oliguric renal failure with or without malignant hypertension.

7. Gastrointestinal tract–The gastrointestinal tract is commonly affected. The esophagus is the most frequent site of involvement, with dysphagia or symptoms of reflux esophagitis occurring in 80% of patients. Gastric and small bowel involvement presents with cramping, bloating, and diarrhea alternating with constipation. Hypomotility of the gastrointestinal tract with bacterial overgrowth may result in malabsorption. Colonic scleroderma is associated with chronic constipation.

8. Sjögren's syndrome–Sicca syndrome is seen in 5–7% of patients.

9. Mixed connective tissue disease–Mixed connective tissue disease is a syndrome with features of scleroderma, rheumatoid arthritis, SLE, and polymyositis–dermatomyositis. The manifestations of the disease include arthritis, Raynaud's phenomenon, scleroderma of the fingers, muscle weakness and tenderness, interstitial lung disease, and a skin rash resembling either dermatomyositis or SLE. These patients have a high-titer speckled pattern of ANA and antibody to the ribonuclease-sensitive component of extractable nuclear antigen (eg, RNP). Renal disease is unusual in these patients. The disease appears to respond to moderate doses of corticosteroids.

B. Laboratory Findings: The normochromic normocytic anemia of chronic inflammatory disease is occasionally seen in progressive systemic sclerosis. Microangiopathic anemia can also occur. An elevated erythrocyte sedimentation rate and polyclonal hypergammaglobulinemia are common. A positive speckled or nucleolar pattern ANA is frequently encountered.

C. X-Ray Findings:

1. Bones–Thickening of the periarticular soft tissues and juxta-articular osteoporosis are seen in involved joints. Absorption of the terminal phalanges is often associated with soft tissue atrophy and subcutaneous calcinosis.

2. Chest–Characteristically, a diffuse increase in interstitial markings is seen in the lower lung fields of patients with moderate to severe pulmonary involvement. "Honeycombing," nodular densities, and disseminated pulmonary calcifications may also occur.

3. Gastrointestinal tract–Upper gastrointestinal series often reveal decreased or absent esophageal peristaltic activity, even in patients without symptoms of dysphagia. Long-standing disease leads to marked dilation of the lower two thirds of the esophagus. Gastrointestinal reflux is present in the majority of cases, and ulcers or strictures of the lower esophagus due to peptic esophagitis are commonplace. With gastrointestinal involvement, barium is often retained in the second and third portions of the duodenum. Intestinal loops become dilated and atonic, with irregular flocculation and hypersegmentation.

The barium enema may reveal large, wide-mouthed diverticular along the antimesenteric border of the colon.

4. Renal arteriography–Marked changes are seen on renal arteriography in patients with scleroderma kidney. Irregular arterial narrowing, tortuosity of the interlobular arterioles, persistence of the arterial phase, and absence of a nephrogram phase are typical findings.

Immunologic Diagnosis

Polyclonal hypergammaglobulinemia is a frequent serologic abnormality in progressive systemic sclerosis. The fluorescent ANA test shows a speckled or nucleolar pattern in 70% of cases. Anticentromere antibodies occur commonly in patients with limited scleroderma. Antibodies to topoisomerase 1 (Scl-70) typically are seen in patients with diffuse disease.

Differential Diagnosis

When classic skin changes and Raynaud's phenomenon are associated with characteristic visceral complaints, the diagnosis is obvious. In patients presenting with visceral or arthritic complaints and no skin changes, the diagnosis is difficult. In many cases, only the presence or absence of antibodies to RNP makes it possible to differentiate scleroderma from mixed connective tissue disease. Patients with eosinophilic fasciitis present with marked thickening of the skin similar to that seen in the edematous phase of scleroderma. In eosinophilic fasciitis, however, Raynaud's phenome-

non and visceral involvement are rare and fibrosis and inflammatory cell infiltration are seen in the deep facial layers, whereas in scleroderma the fibrosis occurs predominantly in the dermis. The differential diagnosis also includes scleromyxedema, polyvinyl chloride toxicity, L-tryptophan-induced eosinophilia myalgia syndrome, toxic oil syndrome, carcinoid syndrome, phenylketonuria, porphyria cutanea tarda, amyloidosis, Werner's syndrome, and progeria.

Treatment

There is no cure for progressive systemic sclerosis. Sympathectomy has resulted in only transient relief of vascular symptoms, but vasodilating agents, particularly calcium channel blockers, have provided relief for patients with severe Raynaud's phenomenon. Corticosteroids have no effect on the visceral progression of the disease, though they are beneficial in scleroderma with myositis and in mixed connective tissue disease. Colchicine has limited efficacy in treatment of the cutaneous manifestations of the disease. Penicillamine is often effective in the treatment of cutaneous scleroderma, and evidence suggests that it may be of benefit in slowing the progression of visceral disease.

Patients should avoid exposure to cold and should wear gloves to protect their hands. Tobacco should be avoided. Skin ulcers require careful antiseptic care. Cor pulmonale and left-sided heart failure may be treated with diuretics and digitalization (treatment with digitalis), although the response is often poor. Antibiotics may be beneficial in decreasing intestinal bacterial overgrowth that leads to malabsorption.

Hypertensive crisis in renal disease associated with progressive systemic sclerosis is very difficult to control even with potent hypotensive agents. Angiotensin-converting enzyme inhibitors may be of benefit in treating the renal disease associated with scleroderma. The arthritis can usually be controlled with aspirin and other fast-acting nonsteroidal anti-inflammatory drugs. Skin lubricants can alleviate dryness and cracking.

Complications & Prognosis

Spontaneous remissions occur, but the usual course of the disease is one of relentless progression from dermal to visceral involvement. Involvement of the heart, lungs, or kidneys is associated with a high mortality rate. Aspiration pneumonia resulting from esophageal dysfunction is a complication in advanced disease.

Although the prognosis for any given patient is extremely variable, the overall 5-year survival rate for progressive systemic sclerosis is approximately 40%.

POLYMYOSITIS–DERMATOMYOSITIS

Major Immunologic Features

■ There is lymphocytic and plasma cell infiltration of involved muscle.

- Antibodies to the nuclear antigens Jo-1, PM-Scl, Mi-2, and RNP are present.
- Antibodies to the cytoplasmic antigen, SRP, are characteristic.

General Considerations

Polymyositis–dermatomyositis is an acute or chronic inflammatory disease of muscle and skin that may occur at any age. Women are affected twice as commonly as men. There is no racial preponderance. The prevalence of the disease is one per 200,000 population.

Polymyositis–dermatomyositis can be subclassified into 6 categories: (1) idiopathic polymyositis, (2) idiopathic dermatomyositis, (3) polymyositis–dermatomyositis associated with cancer, (4) childhood polymyositis–dermatomyositis, (5) polymyositis–dermatomyositis associated with other rheumatic diseases (Sjögren's syndrome, SLE, progressive systemic sclerosis, mixed connective tissue disease), and (6) inclusion body myositis.

Immunologic Pathogenesis

Although the precise pathogenetic mechanisms are unknown, evidence suggests that autoimmunity plays a role. Experimental polymyositis has been induced in rats and guinea pigs by the injection of allogeneic muscle tissue in Freund's complete adjuvant. Polymyositis–dermatomyositis may coexist with other autoimmune diseases.

A. Humoral Factors: Polyclonal hypergammaglobulinemia is common in patients with polymyositis–dermatomyositis, and rheumatoid factors and antinuclear antibodies occur in 20% of cases. In children, focal deposits of complement, IgG, and IgM have been seen in vessel walls of involved skin and muscle. Some patients with polymyositis–dermatomyositis produce nonspecific antibodies against skeletal muscle.

B. Cellular Factors: Cellular immunity may play a role in the pathogenesis of polymyositis–dermatomyositis. Lymphocytes from patients with polymyositis–dermatomyositis, after incubation with normal autologous muscle, produce a lymphokine that is toxic to monolayers of human fetal muscle cells. The lymphocytes in the muscle infiltrate of patients with polymyositis–dermatomyositis produce this lympho-

toxin on simple incubation of involved muscle. Thus, the lymphocytes of patients with polymyositis–dermatomyositis may respond to their own muscle antigens as if they were foreign (Fig 33–3). It is not known whether this is a primary defect in antigen recognition by the lymphocytes or whether these muscle antigens are cross-reactive with an unidentified foreign antigen. Polymyositis has been induced in rats and guinea pigs by the transfer of sensitized lymphoid cells.

Pathology

Biopsy of involved muscles is diagnostic in only 50–80% of cases. Therefore, a normal muscle biopsy does not rule out the diagnosis of polymyositis–dermatomyositis in a patient with a characteristic clinical picture, muscle enzyme elevations, and an abnormal electromyogram. The histologic findings in acute and subacute polymyositis–dermatomyositis include (1) focal or extensive primary degeneration of muscle fibers, (2) signs of muscle regeneration (fiber basophilia, central nuclei), (3) necrosis of muscle fibers, and (4) a focal or diffuse lymphocytic infiltration. Patients with inclusion body myositis have evidence of nuclear inclusion bodies on light and electron micrography. Chronic myositis leads to a marked variation in the cross-sectional diameter of muscle fibers and a variable degree of interstitial fibrosis.

Clinical Features

A. Symptoms and Signs:

1. Onset–Although the symptoms may begin abruptly, the onset of the disease is usually insidious.

2. Muscle involvement–The commonest manifestation is weakness of involved striated muscle. The proximal muscles of the extremities are most often affected, usually progressing from the lower to the upper limbs. The distal musculature is involved in only 25% of patients. Weakness of the cervical muscles with inability to raise the head and weakness of the posterior pharyngeal muscles with dysphagia and dysphonia are also seen. Facial and extraocular muscle involvement is unusual. Muscle pain, tenderness, and edema also occur.

3. Skin involvement–The characteristic rash of dermatomyositis, present in approximately 40% of

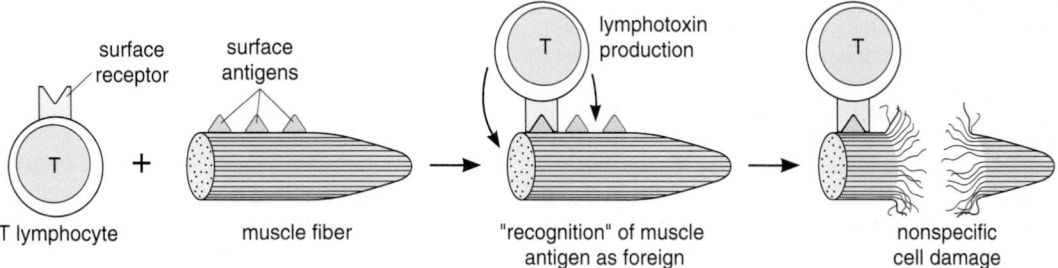

Figure 33–3. Defective "recognition" in polymyositis.

patients, consists of raised, smooth or scaling, dusky red plaques over bony prominences of the hands, elbows, knees, and ankles. An erythematous telangiectatic rash may appear over the face and sun-exposed areas. Less commonly seen is the pathognomonic "heliotrope" rash (a dusky, lilac suffusion of the upper eyelids). One fourth of patients have various dermatologic manifestations ranging from skin thickening to scaling eruptions to erythroderma.

4. Cancer–Some patients with polymyositis–dermatomyositis are found to have a concomitant malignant tumor. In patients older than 40 years, the association between polymyositis–dermatomyositis and cancer appears to be more common. Removal of the tumor may result in a dramatic improvement in the polymyositis–dermatomyositis.

5. Miscellaneous features–A mild transitory arthritis is not unusual. Sjögren's syndrome occurs in 5–7% of cases. In children, vasculitis may result in gastrointestinal ulceration with abdominal pain, hematemesis, and melena. Patients with severe muscle disease are particularly susceptible to the development of interstitial pneumonia and pulmonary fibrosis. Raynaud's phenomenon occurs occasionally.

B. Laboratory Findings: An elevated erythrocyte sedimentation rate and a mild anemia are very common. Half of patients have elevated α_2- and γ-globulins on serum protein electrophoresis. Myoglobinemia and myoglobinuria are often seen. Up to 20% of patients with acute polymyositis have nonspecific T-wave abnormalities on the ECG.

1. Muscle enzymes–When muscle cells are injured, a number of muscle enzymes, including glutamic-oxaloacetic transaminase, creatine phosphokinase, and aldolase, are released into the blood. The serum enzyme elevation reflects the severity of muscle damage as well as the amount of muscle mass involved.

2. Urinary creatine–Creatine is normally produced in the liver and transported via the circulatory system to the musculature. After attaching to receptor sites on the muscle cell surface, it is carried into the cell, where it is converted to creatinine. Polymyositis–dermatomyositis and other myopathies lead to a decrease in the number of cell surface receptors, causing an increase in circulating creatine that is quickly cleared by the kidneys. An increase in the urine creatine concentration is the most sensitive laboratory test for muscle damage and is an indicator of disease activity. It is the first detectable laboratory abnormality in relapse of disease.

3. Electromyography–When involved muscles are examined, 70–80% of patients demonstrate myopathic changes on electromyography. These changes are nonspecific but can point to the diagnosis of myositis. They include (1) spontaneous "sawtooth" fibrillatory potentials and irritability on insertion of the test needle; (2) complex polyphasic potentials, often of short duration and low amplitude; and (3) salvos of repetitive high-frequency action potentials (pseudomyotonia).

Immunologic Diagnosis

The diagnosis must be based on the nonimmunologic clinical and laboratory data already discussed. Antibodies to the nuclear antigen histidyl-sRNA synthetase (Jo-1), however, occur in a substantial number of patients with polymyositis, particularly those with pulmonary involvement. Patients with dermatomyositis have antibodies to the nuclear antigen Mi-2. Those with acute-onset polymyositis may have antibodies to a cytoplasmic antigen, signal recognition protein (SRP). Antibodies to PM-Scl (a nucleolar antigen) are more common in patients with polymyositis and scleroderma. Anti-RNP antibodies occur most frequently in patients with myositis as a component of mixed connective tissue disease.

Differential Diagnosis

At least three of the following criteria must be present for a definite diagnosis of polymyositis: (1) weakness of the shoulder or pelvic girdle musculature, (2) biopsy evidence of myositis, (3) elevation of muscle enzymes, and (4) electromyographic findings of myopathy. Typical skin changes must also be present for a definite diagnosis of dermatomyositis. A number of diseases can affect muscles and lead to clinical and laboratory abnormalities that are identical to those seen in polymyositis–dermatomyositis. The diagnostic criteria outlined previously cannot be strictly applied in patients with infection (including HIV), sarcoidosis, muscular dystrophy, SLE, progressive systemic sclerosis, mixed connective tissue disease, drug-induced myopathy (alcohol, clofibrate), rhabdomyolysis, and various metabolic and endocrine disorders (McArdle's syndrome, hyperthyroidism, myxedema, acid maltase deficiency, carnitine palmityl transferase deficiency, and adenosine monophosphate [AMP] deaminase deficiency). In addition, various neuropathies and muscular dystrophies can mimic inflammatory myopathy. A diligent search for occult cancers should be made in any patient who develops polymyositis–dermatomyositis as an adult.

Treatment

A. Corticosteroids: Prednisone, 60–80 mg orally daily, usually decreases muscle inflammation and improves strength. The dose is tapered slowly, with clinical and laboratory monitoring. Assessment of muscle strength and determination of serum enzyme levels are helpful indicators of disease activity. Some patients require chronic prednisone therapy (5–20 mg daily) to control the disease.

B. Cytotoxic Agents: Methotrexate and azathioprine have each been used with success in patients who do not respond to corticosteroids or who develop severe complications of corticosteroid therapy.

Complications & Prognosis

Polymyositis–dermatomyositis is a chronic disease characterized by spontaneous remissions and exacerbations. Most patients respond to corticosteroid therapy. Patients with severe muscle atrophy show little response to either corticosteroid or other immunosuppressive therapy. When the disease is associated with cancer, the prognosis depends on the response to tumor therapy.

BEHÇET'S DISEASE

Behçet's disease is a chronic recurrent inflammatory disease affecting adults of both sexes. The major manifestations of the disease are aphthous stomatitis, iritis, and genital ulcers. Other findings include vasculitis (particularly of the skin), pulmonary artery aneurysms, arthritis, meningomyelitis, enterocolitis, erythema nodosum, thrombophlebitis, and epididymitis. The differential diagnosis includes viral (herpes simplex) or chlamydial (inclusion conjunctivitis, lymphogranuloma venereum) infections, Reiter's syndrome, inflammatory bowel disease, Stevens-Johnson syndrome, oral pemphigus, and SLE. A pustular lesion appearing after needle puncture of the skin is highly suggestive of Behçet's disease.

Genetic and environmental factors probably play a role in pathogenesis. Some studies show an increased prevalence of HLA-B5 and HLA-B51 in Behçet's disease. There is also evidence suggesting that a virus may play a role in disease causation. Antibodies against various human mucosal antigens have been detected, and indirect immunofluorescence has demonstrated vascular deposition of immunoglobulins as well as circulating anticytoplasmic antibodies. There is a decrease in circulating helper T lymphocytes and an increase in gamma-delta T cells and natural killer cells. Furthermore, lymphocytes and plasma cells are prominent in the perivascular infiltrate of Behçet's vasculitis. Amyloidosis may develop in some patients.

Local corticosteroids are useful in the treatment of mild ocular and oral disease. Systemic corticosteroids are helpful in the treatment of systemic manifestations, but chlorambucil is thought to be the most useful agent for treating severe ocular or central nervous system disease. Unproved remedies include whole-blood transfusions, transfer factor, levamisole, colchicine, cyclosporin, and thalidomide.

ANKYLOSING SPONDYLITIS

Ankylosing spondylitis is a chronic progressive inflammatory disorder involving the sacroiliac joints, spine, and large peripheral joints. Ninety percent of cases occur in males, with the usual age at onset being the second or third decade of life.

The disease begins with the insidious onset of low back pain and stiffness, usually worse in the morning. Manifestations include pain on compression of the sacroiliac joints and spasm of the paravertebral muscles. Findings in advanced disease include ankylosis of the sacroiliac joints and spine, with loss of lumbar lordosis, marked dorsocervical kyphosis, and decreased chest expansion. Peripheral arthritis, when present, usually involves the shoulder or hips. Twenty-five percent of patients also have iritis or iridocyclitis. Carditis with or without aortitis occurs in 10% of patients, and a few patients develop insufficiency of the aortic valves. Rare complications include pericarditis and pulmonary fibrosis.

Patients with ankylosing spondylitis are seronegative for rheumatoid factors and ANA, but an elevated erythrocyte sedimentation rate and a mild anemia are common during active disease. Electrocardiographic abnormalities, such as atrioventricular block, left or right bundle branch block, and left ventricular hypertrophy reflect cardiac involvement. X-rays of the sacroiliac joints reveal osteoporosis and erosions early in the disease and sclerosis with fusion in advanced disease. Calcification of the anterior longitudinal ligament of the spine and squaring of the vertebrae are seen on lateral x-rays of the spine. Ossification of the outer margins of the intervertebral disk (syndesmophyte formation) may lead to fusion of the spine.

The proliferative synovitis in these patients is similar pathologically to that of rheumatoid arthritis. In advanced disease the characteristic skeletal change is ossification of the sacroiliac joints and interspinous and capsular ligaments. Pathologic cardiac findings include focal inflammation and fibrous thickening of the aortic wall and the base of the valve cusps.

The physical findings in patients with severe osteoarthritis of the spine may resemble those of patients with end-stage ankylosing spondylitis. Degenerative osteoarthritis, however, begins much later in life, does not extensively involve the sacroiliac joints, and is characterized radiographically by osteophytes rather than syndesmophytes. The differentiation of ankylosing spondylitis from other diseases associated with sacroiliitis and spondylitis, such as psoriatic arthritis, Reiter's syndrome, regional enteritis, and ulcerative colitis, depends on the presence or absence of the clinical and radiologic characteristics of those diseases. The flowing ossification of the spine that occurs in patients with diffuse idiopathic skeletal hyperostosis (DISH) typically involves only one side of the vertebral bodies and spares the annulus fibrosis.

The basic pathogenesis of ankylosing spondylitis is unknown. There is a strong genetic predisposition to ankylosing spondylitis. Several members of the same family are often involved, and twin concordance for ankylosing spondylitis has been described. Furthermore, 90% of white patients with ankylosing spondylitis have HLA-B27, compared with about 8% in the white US population.

The treatment of ankylosing spondylitis consists of giving anti-inflammatory agents to decrease acute inflammation and relieve pain and of instituting physical therapy to maintain muscle strength and flexibility. Therapy is designed to maintain a position of function even if ossification and ankylosis progress. Posturing exercises (lying flat for periods during the day, sleeping without a pillow, breathing exercises), the judicious use of local heat, and job modification are all part of a rational physical therapy program. Total hip replacement may offer considerable relief to patients with ankylosis of the hips, although recurrent ankylosis is sometimes a problem.

REITER'S SYNDROME

Reiter's syndrome is clinically defined as a triad consisting of arthritis, urethritis, and conjunctivitis. The arthritis, however, is frequently accompanied by only one of the other characteristic manifestations. Although Reiter's syndrome usually affects men, it may also occur in women and children. The arthritis tends to be asymmetric, and polyarticular, involving primarily joints of the lower extremity. Fever, malaise, and weight loss occur commonly with episodes of acute arthritis. Frequently the urethritis is asymptomatic. The conjunctivitis is mild, but 20–50% of patients develop iritis. Balanitis circinata, painless oral ulcerations, and keratoderma blennorrhagicum (thick keratotic lesions of the palms and soles) are mucocutaneus manifestations. Complications include spondylitis and carditis. The manifestations of Reiter's syndrome appear to be more severe in patients with AIDS.

Most patients have a mild leukocytosis. The urethral discharge is purulent, but smear and culture are negative for *Neisseria gonorrhoeae*. Synovial fluid is sterile, with a leukocyte count of 2000–50,000/μL, mostly PMN. The classic radiographic finding is fluffy periosteal proliferation of the heels, ankles, metatarsals, phalanges, knees, and elbows. Bony erosions may be seen in severe cases but rarely, if ever, occur in upper extremities.

Major diseases in the differential diagnosis include gonococcal arthritis, psoriatic arthritis, ankylosing spondylitis, Lyme arthritis, and the arthritis of inflammatory bowel disease. Patients with psoriatic arthritis occasionally develop urethritis or conjunctivitis. The differentiation of psoriatic arthritis and Reiter's syndrome is difficult to make on the basis of the skin lesion, since keratoderma blennorrhagicum is histologically indistinguishable from pustular psoriasis. Reiter's syndrome can be differentiated from ankylosing spondylitis by the presence of the urethritis and conjunctivitis, the prominent involvement of distal joints, and the presence of asymmetric radiologic changes in the sacroiliac joints and spine.

In Reiter's syndrome, the arthritis is thought to be an immunologic response to infection elsewhere in the body. Predisposing infectious agents include shigellae, salmonellae, gonococci, mycoplasmas, chlamydiae, yersiniae, and campylobacters. Eighty percent of patients with Reiter's syndrome have HLA-B27. It is not known whether this antigenic marker imparts an increased susceptibility to environmental or infectious agents or is associated with an unusual immune response gene.

NSAIDs or slow-acting antirheumatic drugs like sulfasalazine may be used to control acute inflammation. Immunosuppressive drugs, such as methotrexate or azathioprine, may be necessary in treatment of patients with recalcitrant disease. Although the acute attack usually subsides in a few months, recurrences are common and some patients develop a chronic deforming arthritis.

PSORIATIC ARTHRITIS

Psoriatic arthritis is a chronic, recurrent, asymmetric, erosive polyarthritis that occurs in about 25% of patients with psoriasis. The onset of the arthritis may be acute or insidious and is usually preceded by skin disease. It characteristically involves the distal interphalangeal joints of the fingers and toes and may involve the hips, sacroiliac joints, and spine. Distal interphalangeal joint disease is frequently accompanied by nail pitting or onycholysis secondary to psoriasis of the nail matrix or nail bed. Constitutional signs and symptoms, such as fever and fatigue, may occur. Severe erosive disease may lead to marked deformity of the hands and feet (arthritis mutilans), and marked vertebral involvement can result in ankylosis of the spine.

An elevated erythrocyte sedimentation rate and a mild anemia are common. Hyperuricemia is occasionally seen in patients with severe skin disease. Serum immunoglobulin levels are normal, and rheumatoid factor is absent. Synovial fluid examination reveals a leukocyte count of 5000–40,000/μL, mostly PMN. Characteristic x-ray findings include "pencil cup" erosions, fluffy periosteal proliferation, and bony ankylosis of peripheral joints. Sacroiliac changes, including erosions, sclerosis, and ankylosis similar to that in Reiter's syndrome, occur in 10–30% of patients.

The major diseases that must be differentiated from psoriatic arthritis include rheumatoid arthritis, ankylosing spondylitis, and Reiter's syndrome. Psoriatic arthritis is differentiated from rheumatoid arthritis by the absence of rheumatoid factor and subcutaneous nodules, the involvement of distal interphalangeals, the characteristic x-ray findings of psoriatic arthritis, and the presence of psoriasis. The involvement of distal interphalangeals and differences in the radiologic appearance of the spine help differentiate psoriatic arthritis from ankylosing spondylitis. The differentiation of psoriatic arthritis from Reiter's syndrome is particularly difficult, because both diseases are associated with HLA-B27 and involve the sacroiliac joints and spine and because keratoderma blennorrhagicum is histologically indistinguishable from pustular psoriasis. A helpful clinical distinction is the greater likelihood of upper extremity involvement in psoriatic arthritis.

The cause of psoriasis and psoriatic arthritis is unknown. Genetic factors appear to play a role in disease causation. Psoriasis and rheumatic diseases are found in family members of approximately 15% of patients. Patients with psoriasis and peripheral arthritis have an increased prevalence of haplotypes HLA-DR4, DR7, B13, B17, B38 and B39. Forty-five percent of patients with psoriasis and spondylitis have HLA-B27. Evidence for an immunopathogenesis in psoriatic arthritis includes the presence of antibodies directed against skin antigens and of activated T cells in skin and synovium.

Skin and arthritic manifestations require therapy. Topical corticosteroids, coal tar and ultraviolet light, or immunosuppressive drugs can be used to treat the skin disease. Treatment of arthritis is similar to that of rheumatoid arthritis.

RELAPSING POLYCHONDRITIS

Relapsing polychondritis is a rare disease characterized by recurrent episodes of inflammatory necrosis involving cartilaginous tissues of the ears, nose, upper respiratory tract, and peripheral joints. It may occur alone or in association with other diseases such as RA, SLE, systemic vasculitis, or malignancy. Relapsing polychondritis begins abruptly with swollen, painful, erythematous lesions of the nose or ears, usually associated with fever. Destruction of supporting cartilaginous tissues leaves patients with characteristic "floppy ear" and "saddle nose" deformities and can lead to collapse of the trachea. The commonest cause of death in these patients is airway obstruction. Recurrent episcleritis, anterior inflammatory ocular disease, auditory and vestibular defects, systemic vasculitis, necrotizing glomerulitis, vasculitis, and arthritis are other manifestations of relapsing polychondritis. Aortic insufficiency due to destruction and dilatation of the aortic valve ring occurs rarely.

Laboratory abnormalities include an elevated erythrocyte sedimentation rate, increased serum immunoglobulins, a false-positive VDRL, and mild anemia. Pathologic examination reveals infiltration of the cartilage–connective tissue interface with lymphocytes, plasma cells, and PMN. As the lesion evolves, the cartilage loses its basophilic stippling and stains more acidophilic. Eventually, the cartilage becomes completely replaced by fibrous tissue.

The pathogenesis of this disease is unknown; however, there is some evidence that autoimmune phenomena play a role. Immunofluorescence has revealed the presence of immune complexes at the fibrocartilaginous junction. Antibodies to human cartilage and to type II collagen are frequently present but also occur in other rheumatic diseases. Electron microscopy reveals electron-dense deposits of lysosomal origin in involved cartilage. In some patients with relapsing polychondritis, cartilage antigen induces lymphocyte activation and lymphocyte production of migration inhibitory factor (MIF).

Corticosteroids, dapsone, colchicine, nonsteroidal anti-inflammatory drugs, and cytotoxic agents have been used with success in the treatment of relapsing polychondritis.

RELAPSING PANNICULITIS
(Weber-Christian Disease)

Relapsing panniculitis is a rare syndrome characterized by recurrent episodes of discrete nodular inflammation and nonsuppurative necrosis of subcutaneous fat. Most patients are women. Painful, erythematous nodules usually appear over the lower extremities but may involve the face, trunk, and upper limbs and progress to local atrophy and fibrosis. Occasionally, they may undergo necrosis, with the discharge of a fatty fluid. Constitutional signs, including fever, usually accompany an acute episode. Histologically, one sees edema, mononuclear cell infiltration, fat necrosis, perivascular inflammatory cuffing, and endothelial proliferation. The differential diagnosis includes superficial thrombophlebitis, polyarteritis nodosa, necrotizing vasculitis, erythema induratum, erythema nodosum, and factitious disease.

The cause of relapsing panniculitis is not known, and, in fact, the syndrome may be simply a nonspecific response to any one of a number of inciting factors, including trauma, cold, exposure to toxic chemicals, and infection. It has been seen in patients with SLE, rheumatoid arthritis, diabetes mellitus, sarcoidosis, tuberculosis, withdrawal from corticosteroid therapy, acute and chronic pancreatitis, pancreatic carcinoma, and α_1-antitrypsin deficiency. An autoimmune mechanism is suggested by the presence of hypocomplementemia, circulating immune complexes, and the association of relapsing panniculitis with several autoimmune diseases. The only autoantibodies demonstrated to date are circulating leukoagglutinins.

Acute episodes respond to corticosteroid therapy. Prostaglandin inhibitors, antimalarial drugs, and immunosuppressive drugs have been used to treat severe disease.

HEREDITARY COMPLEMENT DEFICIENCIES
& COLLAGEN VASCULAR DISEASES

Complement deficiency occurs in approximately one in a million normal adults and is associated with various rheumatoid diseases. C2 deficiency is the most common hereditary complement deficiency (see Chapters 11 and 25).

Deficiencies of C1r, C1s, C2, C4, C5, C6, C7, C8, and C1 esterase have all been associated with lupus-like syndromes. Hereditary complement deficiency could lead to an increased susceptibility to infectious agents, which may then stimulate the autoimmunity. Lack of complement could impair clearance of immune complexes. Alternatively, a neighboring gene predisposing to autoimmune phenomena could be inherited along with the defective gene for complement production.

HYPOGAMMAGLOBULINEMIA & ARTHRITIS

Hypogammaglobulinemia is an acquired or congenital disorder that may involve all or any one of the specific classes of immunoglobulin (see Chapter 21). Hypogammaglobulinemia is associated with infec-

tions, chronic inflammatory bowel disease, sarcoidosis, SLE, scleroderma, Sjögren's syndrome, polymyositis–dermatomyositis, and cancer. Patients with classic adult and juvenile rheumatoid arthritis may develop hypogammaglobulinemia.

Hypogammaglobulinemia patients may develop a seronegative, symmetric arthritis, with morning stiffness, occasional nodule formation, and radiographic evidence of demineralization and joint space narrowing. Bony erosions are rarely seen. Biopsy of the synovium reveals chronic inflammatory changes without plasma cells. Despite the reduction of serum immunoglobulins, immunoglobulin may be detected in the inflammatory synovial fluid. Total hemolytic complement is commonly depressed in the synovial fluid, suggesting immune complex formation.

The mono- or pauciarticular arthritis seen in hypogammaglobulinemia may be caused by mycoplasma, ureaplasma, or enterovirus infection.

Hypogammaglobulinemic arthritis may improve after the administration of gamma globulin.

REFERENCES

SYSTEMIC LUPUS ERYTHEMATOSUS
Boumpas DT et al: Systemic lupus erythematosus: Emerging concepts. Part 1: Renal, neuropsychiatric, cardiovascular, pulmonary, and hematologic disease. *Ann Int Med* 1995;**122**:940.

Boumpas DT et al: Systemic lupus erythematosus: Emerging concepts. Part 2: Dermatologic and joint disease, the antiphospholipid antibody syndrome, pregnancy and hormonal therapy, morbidity and mortality, and pathogenesis. *Ann Int Med* 1995;**123**:42.

Budman D, Steinberg A: Hematologic aspects of systemic lupus erythematosus: Current comments. *Ann Intern Med* 1977;**86**:220.

Dubois EL: Antimalarials in the management of discoid and systemic lupus erythematosus. *Semin Arthritis Rheum* 1978;**8**:35.

Fessler BJ, Boumpas DT: Severe major organ involvement in systemic lupus erythematosus. Diagnosis and management. *Rheum Dis Clin North Am* 1995;**21**:81.

Fritzler MJ: Antinuclear antibodies in the investigation of rheumatic diseases. *Bull Rheum Dis* 1985;**35**(6):1.

Haupt H et al: The lung in systemic lupus erythematosus: Analysis of the pathologic changes in 120 patients. *Am J Med* 1981;**71**:791.

Mandell BF: Cardiovascular involvement in systemic lupus erythematosus. *Semin Arthritis Rheum* 1987;**17**:126.

McCluskey R: The value of renal biopsy in lupus nephritis. *Arthritis Rheum* 1982;**25**:867.

McCune WJ, Golbus J: Neuropsychiatric lupus. *Rheum Dis Clin North Am* 1988;**14**:149.

Meyer O: A critical appraisal of the classification criteria for systemic lupus erythematosus. *Clin Exper Rheumatol* 1994;**12**(suppl 11):41.

Steinberg A et al: Systemic lupus erythematosus: Insights from animal models. *Ann Intern Med* 1984;**100**:714.

Tan EM et al: 1982 Revised criteria for the classification of systemic lupus erythematosus. *Arthritis Rheum* 1982; **25**:1271.

Ward MM et al: Causes of death in systemic lupus erythematosus. Long-term followup of an inception cohort. *Arthritis Rheum* 1995;**38**:1492.

RHEUMATOID ARTHRITIS
Alarcón GS: Epidemiology of rheumatoid arthritis. *Rheum Dis Clin North Am* 1995;**21**:589.

Albani S et al: Genetic and environmental factors in the immune pathogenesis of rheumatoid arthritis. *Rheum Dis Clin North Am* 1992;**18**:729.

Arnett FC et al: The American Rheumatism Association 1987 revised criteria for the classification of rheumatoid arthritis. *Arthritis Rheum* 1988;**31**:315.

Hurd ER: Extra-articular manifestations of rheumatoid arthritis. *Semin Arthritis Rheum* 1979;**8**:151.

Kremer JM et al: Methotrexate for rheumatoid arthritis. Suggested guidelines for monitoring liver toxicity. *Arth Rheum* 1994;**37**:316.

Nepom GT, Nepom BS: Prediction of susceptibility to rheumatoid arthritis by human leukocyte antigen typing. *Rheum Dis Clin North Am* 1992;**18**:785.

Pincus T et al: Quantitative analysis of hand radiographs in rheumatoid arthritis: Time course of radiographic changes, relation to joint examination measures, and comparison of different scoring methods. *J Rheumatol* 1995;**22**:1983.

Vollertsen RS, Conn DL: Vasculitis associated with rheumatoid arthritis. *Rheum Dis Clin North Am* 1990;**16**:445.

JUVENILE ARTHRITIS
Cassidy JT et al: The development of classification criteria for children with juvenile rheumatoid arthritis. *Bull Rheum Dis* 1989;**38**:1.

De Inocencio J et al: Can genetic markers contribute to the classification of juvenile rheumatoid arthritis? *J Rheumatol* 1993;**20:**12.

Giannini EH et al: Comparative efficacy and safety of advanced drug therapy in children with juvenile rheumatoid arthritis. *Semin Arthritis Rheum* 1993;**23:**34.

Lawrence JM: Autoantibody studies in juvenile rheumatoid arthritis. *Semin Arthritis Rheum* 1993;**22:**265.

Singsen BH: Rheumatic diseases of childhood. *Rheum Dis Clin North Am* 1990;**16:**581.

SJÖGREN'S SYNDROME

Daniels TE, Fox PC: Salivary and oral components of Sjögren's syndrome. *Rheum Dis Clin North Am* 1992;**18:**571.

Daniels TE, Whitcher JP: Association of patterns of labial salivary gland inflammation with keratoconjunctivitis sicca. Analysis of 618 patients with suspected Sjögren's syndrome. *Arthritis Rheum* 1994;**37:**869.

Fox RI, Saito I: Criteria for diagnosis of Sjögren's syndrome. *Rheum Dis Clin North Am* 1994;**20:**391.

Price E, Venables PJW: The etiopathogenesis of Sjögren's syndrome. *Semin Arth Rheum* 1995;**25:**117.

Talal N: Sjögren's syndrome: Historical overview and clinical spectrum of disease. *Rheum Dis Clin North Am* 1992;**18:**507.

PROGRESSIVE SYSTEMIC SCLEROSIS

Barnett A et al: A survival study of patients with scleroderma over 30 years (1953–1983): The value of a simple cutaneous classification in the early stages of disease. *J Rheumatol* 1988;**15:**276.

Nimelstein S et al: Mixed connective tissue disease: A subsequent evaluation of the original 25 patients. *Medicine* 1980;**59:**239.

Rocco V, Hurd E: Scleroderma and sclerodermalike disorders. *Semin Arthritis Rheum* 1986;**16:**22.

Rothfield NF: Autoantibodies in scleroderma. *Rheum Dis Clin North Am* 1992;**18:**483.

Steen VD: Systemic sclerosis. *Rheum Dis Clin North Am* 1990;**16:**641.

Subcommittee for Scleroderma Criteria of the American Rheumatism Association Diagnostic and Therapeutic Criteria Committee: Preliminary criteria for the classification of systemic sclerosis (scleroderma). *Arthritis Rheum* 1980;**23:**581.

POLYMYOSITIS–DERMATOMYOSITIS

Hochberg M et al: Adult onset polymyositis/dermatomyositis: An analysis of clinical and laboratory features and survival in 76 patients with a review of the literature. *Semin Arthritis Rheum* 1986;**15:**168.

Miller FW: Classification and prognosis of inflammatory muscle disease. *Rheum Dis Clin North Am* 1994;**20:**811.

Oddis CV: Therapy of inflammatory myopathy. *Rheum Dis Clin North Am* 1994;**20:**899.

Targoff IN: Immune manifestations of inflammatory muscle disease. *Rheum Dis Clin North Am* 1994;**20:**857.

BEHÇETS DISEASE

James D: "Silk route disease" (Behçet's disease) *West J Med* 1988;**148:**433.

O'Duffy J: Vasculitis in Behçet's disease. *Rheum Dis Clin North Am* 1990;**16:**423.

Shimizu T et al: Behçet's disease (Behçet's syndrome). *Semin Arthritis Rheum* 1979;**8:**223.

ANKYLOSING SPONDYLITIS

Calin A et al: Ankylosing spondylitis—an analytical review of 1500 patients: The changing pattern of disease. *J Rheumatol* 1988;**15:**1234.

Gran JT, Husby G: The epidemiology of ankylosing spondylitis. *Semin Arthritis Rheum* 1993;**22:**319.

Khan MA: An overview of clinical spectrum and heterogeneity of spondyloarthropathies. *Rheum Dis Clin North Am* 1992;**18:**1.

REITER'S SYNDROME

Aho K et al: Reactive arthritis. *Clin Rheum Dis* 1985;**11:**25.

Calin A, Fries J: An "experimental" epidemic of Reiter's syndrome revisited: Follow-up evidence on genetic and environmental factors. *Ann Intern Med* 1976;**84:**564.

Hughes RA, Keat AC: Reiter's syndrome: A current view. *Semin Arthritis Rheum* 1994;**24:**190.

PSORIATIC ARTHRITIS

Gladman D: Psoriatic arthritis. Recent advances in pathogenesis and treatment. *Rheum Dis Clin North Am* 1992;**18:**247.

POLYCHONDRITIS

McAdam LP et al: Relapsing polychondritis. Prospective study of 23 patients and a review of the literature. *Medicine* 1976;**55:**193.

Michet CJ et al: Relapsing polychondritis. Survival and predictive role of early disease manifestations. *Ann Intern Med* 1986;**104:**74.

PANNICULITIS

Panush R et al: Weber-Christian disease: Analysis of 15 cases and review of the literature. *Medicine* 1985;**64:**181.

HEREDITARY COMPLEMENT DEFICIENCY

Atkinson JA: Complement deficiency. Predisposing factor to autoimmune syndrome. *Am J Med* 1988;**85**(suppl 6a):45.

Frank M: Complement in the pathophysiology of human disease. *N Engl J Med* 1987;**316:**1525.

Moulds JM et al: Genetics of the complement system and rheumatic diseases *Rheum Dis Clin North Am* 1992;**18:**893.

HYPOGAMMAGLOBULINEMIA & ARTHRITIS

Lee AH et al: Hypogammaglobulinemia and rheumatic disease. *Semin Arthritis Rheum* 1993;**22:**252.

Puéchal X et al: Ureaplasma urealyticum destructive septic polyarthritis revealing a common variable immunodeficiency. *Arthritis Rheum* 1995;**38:**1524.

Sneller MC et al: New insights into common variable immunodeficiency. *Ann Intern Med* 1993;**118:**720.

Endocrine Diseases

James R. Baker, Jr., MD

In the more than 40 years since the first demonstration of the immune basis for thyroiditis, autoimmune disease has been identified as a major cause of dysfunction of all endocrine organs. It is now apparent that such diverse disorders as idiopathic Addison's disease, insulin-dependent diabetes mellitus (IDDM), and the polyglandular endocrinopathy syndromes all have an autoimmune pathogenesis. Although primary therapy for these disorders remains the replacement of hormones deficient as a result of the destruction of endocrine organs, research is now being conducted into the genesis of the autoimmune process itself. It is hoped that through this research treatments could be developed to forestall the autoimmune process before the gland is destroyed, thereby allowing normal endocrine function to continue.

MECHANISM OF DEVELOPMENT OF AUTOIMMUNE ENDOCRINE DISEASE

Endocrine disease has become a favored model for the study of autoimmune pathogenesis. Two possible factors in the development of human autoimmunity have been identified specifically through the study of endocrine disorders. The first is the discovery of aberrant expression of class II human leukocyte antigens (HLA) (see Chapter 6), on the surface of target cells in autoimmune disease (Fig 34–1). It is postulated that autoimmunity begins with an inflammatory process, possibly of infectious origin, in an endocrine organ. The inflammatory cells in the gland produce interferon gamma and other cytokines, which induce the aberrant de novo expression of class II HLA molecules on endocrine cell membranes. After expression of class II major histocompatibility complex (MHC) molecules, endocrine cells may function as antigen-presenting cells for their own cellular proteins, which are recognized by autoreactive T and B cells. This leads to enzymatic and oxidative destruction of endocrine cells, which further releases cellular proteins for processing by antigen-presenting cells, propagating the autoimmune response. Either abnormalities in the presentation of antigen owing to allogenic specificities in class II MHC or inappropriate recognition of the class II HLA-antigen complex as a result of their inherited differences in the T-cell antigen recep-

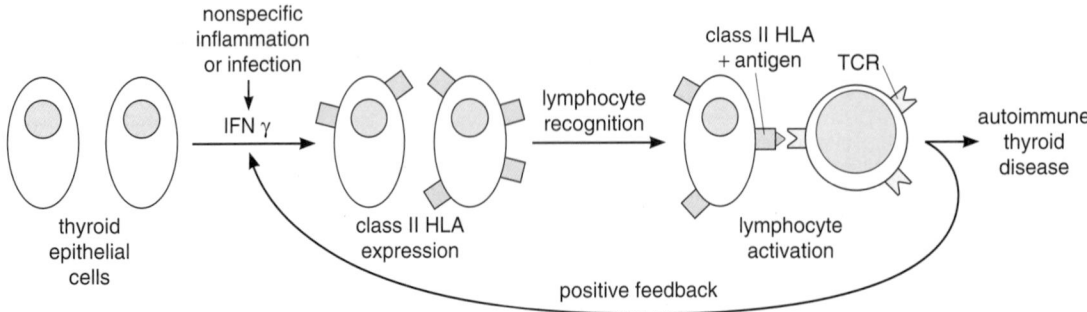

Figure 34–1. Initiation of autoimmunity through class II HLA expression. The expression of class II HLA results in lymphocyte activation, which causes the production of more lymphokines. These cause feedback stimulation of HLA expression and produce cytotoxic cells, which can destroy epithelial cells.

tor structure can then cause these autoantigens to be recognized as foreign in a genetically susceptible host.

Another potentially important factor in the genesis of autoimmunity is antigen cross-reactivity. The mechanism by which an immune response to a pathogen or an environmental or dietary protein might lead to a cross-reactive response to an autoantigen is not fully understood. However, several examples are now documented for Graves' disease and IDDM (Fig 34–2), and it is apparent that this cross-reactivity may occur at either the T- or B-cell level.

ORGAN-SPECIFIC AUTOANTIBODIES

The presence of organ-specific autoantibodies is often used as an adjunct to the diagnosis and occasionally the management of some autoimmune disorders. Table 34–1, showing the relative sensitivity and specificity of autoantibodies in different diseases, should be referred to during study of this chapter.

Organ-specific antibodies are defined by several methods, including their binding to tissue as determined by immunohistologic staining and the binding of specific proteins, lipids, carbohydrates, and hormones in immunoassays. In addition, autoantibody

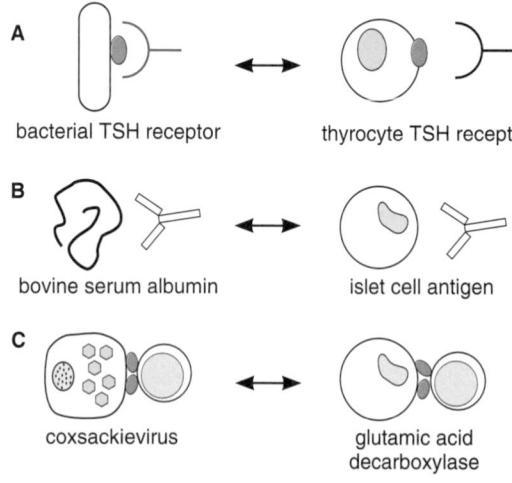

Figure 34–2. Proposed examples of molecular mimicry in the pathogenesis of autoimmune endocrine disease. **A:** Cross-reactive antibodies to bacterial thyroid-stimulating hormone (TSH) receptors and thyroid cell TSH receptors in Graves' disease. **B:** Cross-reactivity of antibodies to bovine serum albumin and an islet antigen in IDDM. **C:** Cross-recognition of coxsackievirus peptides and glutamic acid decarboxylase (GAD).

Table 34–1. Specificity and sensitivity of autoantibodies.

Autoantigen–Autoantibody	Associated Autoimmune Disease	Percentage of Patients Having Autoantibody (Sensitivity)	Specificity for Disorder
Thyroid peroxidase (microsomal antigen)	Hashimoto's thyroiditis	80–95	High
	Graves' disease	50–80	Low
	Subacute thyroiditis	30–50	Moderate
	Idiopathic hypothyroidism	50–80	Moderate
Thyroglobulin	Hashimoto's thyroiditis	40–70	Moderate
	Graves' disease	20–40	Low
	Subacute thyroiditis	10–30	Moderate
	Idiopathic hypothyroidism	10–30	Low
Thyroid-stimulating immunoglobulin (TSI)	Graves' disease	50–90	High
	Hashimoto's thyroiditis	10–20	Low
	Idiopathic hypothyroidism	0–5	ND[1]
Thyroid growth-stimulating immuno-globulin (TGSI)	Graves' disease	20–50	Moderate
	Hashimoto's thyroiditis	0–5	ND
	Idiopathic hypothyroidism	0–5	ND
Thyrotropin binding-inhibitory immuno-globulin (TBI)	Graves' disease	50–80	High
	Hashimoto's thyroiditis	5–10	Low
	Idiopathic hypothyroidism	10–20	Moderate
Anti-islet cell antibodies	IDDM	35–80	High
Glutamic acid decarboxylase	IDDM	50–80	High
Anti-insulin antibodies	IDDM	20–60	Low
	Insulin resistance	0–2	High
Antibodies to insulin receptors	IDDM	5–10	Low
	Type B insulin resistance	90–100	High
Antibodies to adrenal cortex	Addison's disease	30–60	High
21-Hydroxylase	Addison's disease	60–80	High

[1] ND, not determined.

activity is characterized by the inhibition of hormone binding to receptor or through physiologic alterations of organ and cells in vitro. There are difficulties, however, in the use of these autoantibodies in diagnosis and evaluation of autoimmune diseases. There are often inconsistencies in the way many of the bioassays are conducted, leading to variability in sensitivity of autoantibody results. Also, in immunoassays for antibodies to ill-defined antigens, differences in the antigen preparation can cause variable results.

Often, even well-characterized autoantibodies are not specific for an associated autoimmune disorder. This raises concern about the pathogenic role of the autoantibody in the autoimmune disorder. A good example of this is the presence of antithyroglobulin antibodies in healthy relatives of patients with autoimmune thyroid disease and in some healthy elderly individuals. In contrast, some antibodies found in only a small proportion of patients with autoimmune disease, such as insulin receptor antibodies, correlate well with disease activity in those patients (see Table 34–1). Thus, it is always important to evaluate autoantibody findings in the context of the patient's clinical situation.

THYROID AUTOIMMUNE DISEASES

CHRONIC THYROIDITIS (Hashimoto's Thyroiditis)

Major Immunologic Features
- There is lymphocytic infiltration of the thyroid gland.
- Antibodies to thyroid antigens are present.
- There is cellular sensitization to thyroid antigens.

General Considerations
Hashimoto's thyroiditis is an inflammatory disorder of unknown etiology, which results in progressive destruction of the thyroid gland. It is found most commonly in the middle-aged and elderly, but it also occurs in other age groups, including children in whom it may cause goiter. Females make up the vast majority, about 85%, of patients. Although it is distributed throughout the world without racial or ethnic restriction, it occurs more commonly in families in which another member has an autoimmune thyroid disease. It is observed in conjunction with Graves' disease in a form of autoimmune-overlap syndrome. In addition, it is associated with other autoimmune disorders, such as systemic lupus erythematosus (SLE), chronic active hepatitis, dermatitis herpetiformis, and scleroderma. Although no formal mode of inheritance is recognized, there have been reported associations with several class II HLA antigens, including DR4 and DR5. These associations, however, are not consistent among different ethnic populations.

Pathology
The hallmark of Hashimoto's thyroiditis is lymphocytic infiltration that almost completely replaces the normal glandular architecture of the thyroid (Fig 34–3). Plasma cells and macrophages abound, whereas scattered through this infiltrate are dying thyroid cells with acidophilic granules called Askenasze cells. Formations of germinal centers often give the impression that the thyroid gland is being converted into a lymph node. Lymphocytes infiltrating the thyroid are mainly B cells and CD4 T cells, although CD8 cytotoxic T cells have been cloned from Hashimoto's glands.

Clinical Features
Hashimoto's thyroiditis is primarily associated with symptoms of altered thyroid function. Early in the course of the disease euthyroidism is usually the case but clinical hyperthyroidism may arise due to the inflammatory breakdown of thyroid follicles with release of thyroid hormones. In contrast, late in the disease hypothyroidism often occurs because of progressive destruction of the thyroid gland. The most common eventual outcome of Hashimoto's disease is hypothyroidism.

A consistent physical sign seen in Hashimoto's disease is an enlarged thyroid gland. The goiter is often large and "rubbery" and may feel nodular, similar to its condition in other goitrous diseases. Often, lymph nodes surrounding the gland become enlarged. Rarely, patients show symptoms of generalized vasculitis with urticaria and nephritis, and this has been associated with the presence of circulating immune complexes.

Generally, laboratory findings are not helpful in making the diagnosis and relate primarily to the thyroid status of the patient. Patients with hyperthyroidism are differentiated from those with Graves' disease by the demonstration of patchy or decreased uptake on a radioiodine scan of the thyroid.

Immunologic Diagnosis
The hallmark of the diagnosis of Hashimoto's disease is the presence of circulating autoantibodies to thyroglobulin and thyroid microsomal antigen (now known to be the enzyme thyroid peroxidase). These antibodies were first detected by immunofluorescence (Fig 34–4), but they are now measured by agglutination assays or ELISA (see Chapter 14). They are present in the serum of more than 90% of Hashimoto's disease patients, with antimicrosomal antibodies being more common and of higher titer than antithyroglobulin antibodies. In patients without serum antibodies, autoantibody production may be localized to the intrathyroidal lymphocytes and plasma cells. Of interest, the immune responses to both thyroglobulin and thyroid peroxidase are heterogeneous, with several areas of each molecule conferring immunogenicity.

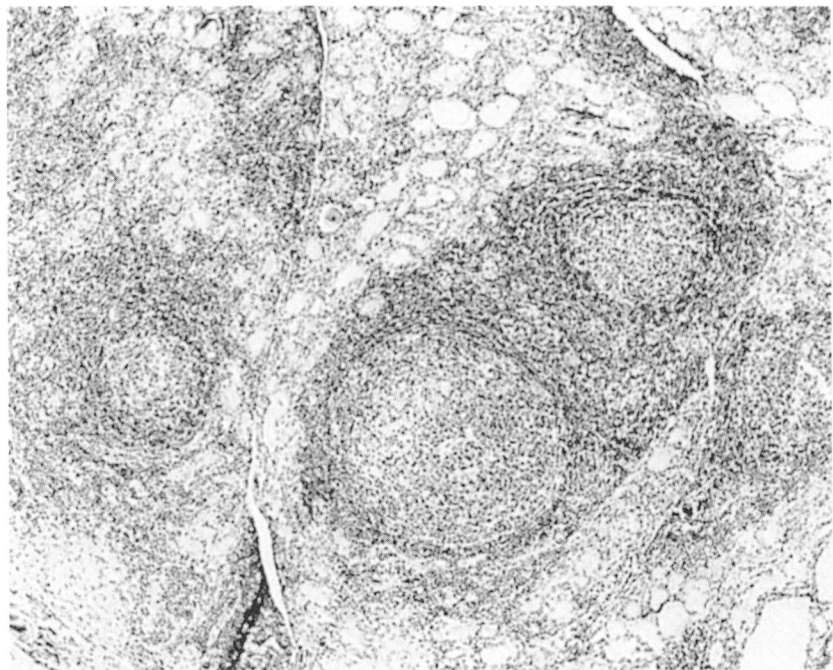

Figure 34–3. Pathology of Hashimoto's thyroiditis. Note the germinal centers and the lack of normal thyroid architecture. (Original magnification ×100.)

Other thyroid antibodies are often present in Hashimoto's disease patients, including antibodies that displace thyroid-stimulating hormone (TSH) from its receptor on thyroid cells and others that stimulate thyroid cells to produce hormones. Other important thyroid antigens stimulate the production of autoantibodies, since multiple unidentified protein bands are recognized by sera from patients with Hashimoto's thyroiditis in Western blots of thyroid membranes. In addition, lymphocytes of these patients proliferate in response to thyroid antigens.

Differential Diagnosis

One must differentiate Hashimoto's disease from other forms of goiter. This is usually done by using clinical criteria with the help of antithyroid antibody titers. On occasion, the rapid enlargement of one lobe of the thyroid gland is confused with thyroid cancer or thyroid lymphoma, which are observed with an increased incidence in Hashimoto's glands. In these cases, needle biopsy of the nodule may be helpful, whereas computed tomograms or magnetic resonance images of the neck can be used to evaluate cervical adenopathy.

Treatment

Treatment of Hashimoto's disease usually consists of thyroid hormone replacement for hypothyroidism. If the patient has a symptomatic goiter, doses of thyroid hormone that suppress TSH secretion can often decrease the size of the gland. Rarely, thyroidectomy is necessary for an unusually large or painful gland.

Prognosis

The prognosis of Hashimoto's disease is excellent, but serial thyroid function tests, especially TSH levels, are necessary to monitor the requirement for thyroid hormone replacement.

TRANSIENT THYROIDITIS SYNDROMES

Major Immunologic Features

- There is giant-cell infiltration of the thyroid.
- There is transient production of antithyroid antibodies.

General Considerations

Several heterogeneous, self-limited thyroiditis syndromes have been described that have in common a transient immune activity against the thyroid. The two most common are subacute (de Quervain's) thyroiditis and postpartum thyroiditis. Subacute thyroiditis is possibly caused by a viral infection of the thyroid gland. It has a seasonal and geographic distribution common to infections with mumps virus, coxsackievirus, and echo virus. Patients with this disorder usually have an acute phase of thyroiditis in which the gland may be painful and antithyroid antibodies may be present. At this time, patients are thyrotoxic, with an elevated serum T4 and decreased radioiodine uptake. Progressive euthyroid and hypothyroid periods of 4–8 weeks may follow before thyroid functions finally normalize.

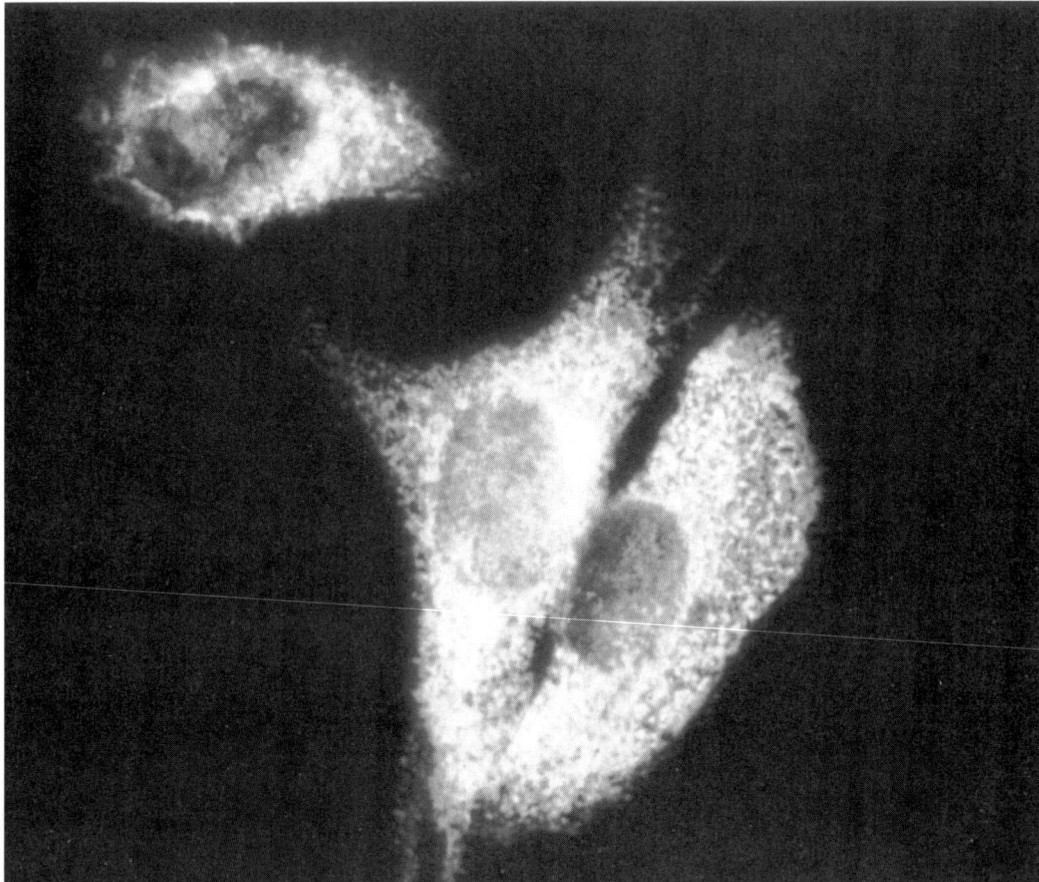

Figure 34–4. Immunofluorescent staining of a cultured human thyroid cell by antithyroglobulin antibodies showing the distribution of the antigen. (Original magnification ×400.) (Courtesy of Donald Sellitti.)

Similar in clinical course, postpartum thyroiditis is a common disorder that usually presents within 3 months of delivery. Patients may experience either hypothyroidism or hyperthyroidism, and a significant percentage develop chronic thyroid dysfunction. Of interest, patients who have this disorder often have recurrent courses with subsequent pregnancies.

Postpartum thyroiditis occurs in about 5–8% of pregnant women and, unlike subacute thyroiditis, is not thought to be related to a viral infection of the thyroid. Supporting this are the presence of antithyroid antibodies preceding the onset of clinical disease and an association with HLA-DR3 and -DR5 haplotypes.

Pathology

Although the lymphocytic infiltrate seen in subacute thyroiditis is similar to that in Hashimoto's disease, two findings in subacute thyroiditis are distinctive. First, giant cells with a small center of thyroid colloid can be seen (this is known as colloidophagy) and the follicular infiltration tends to progress to form granulomas. These findings are not seen in postpartum thyroiditis, however.

Clinical Features

Subacute thyroiditis and postpartum disease have in common the clinical presentation of rapidly enlarging thyroid gland and signs of thyroid dysfunction. Subacute thyroiditis has a much more acute course than postpartum disease and is more commonly associated with pain and tenderness in the area of the gland. Postpartum thyroiditis and other types of transient thyroiditis without pain or other symptoms are sometimes termed "silent" thyroiditis.

Subacute thyroiditis is also accompanied by an elevated erythrocyte sedimentation rate. Both syndromes can cause "low-uptake" toxicosis, in that they can produce elevated serum levels of thyroid hormones in the face of low to normal levels of radioactive iodine uptake.

Immunologic Diagnosis

Antibodies to thyroglobulin and thyroid microsomes (peroxidase enzyme) are present acutely in both syndromes; however, they tend to be transient and of low titer in subacute thyroiditis. Thyroid-stimulating antibodies have also been demonstrated in a few patients with postpartum disease.

Treatment & Prognosis

In most cases thyroid function returns to normal within several months in both disorders. Patients with subacute thyroiditis who have especially painful glands may be treated with anti-inflammatory drugs. Postpartum patients who are clinically hypothyroid can benefit from thyroid hormone replacement. This finding offers a means for monitoring patients for eventual therapy with thyroid hormone or antithyroid drugs.

GRAVES' DISEASE

Major Immunologic Features

- Antibodies against thyroid antigens are present that stimulate thyroid cell function and displace TSH binding.
- There is class II HLA expression on the surface of thyroid cells.
- There is associated autoimmune ophthalmopathy and dermopathy.

General Considerations

Graves' disease is an autoimmune disorder of unknown etiology, which presents as thyrotoxicosis with a diffuse goiter. It is unique among autoimmune disorders since it is probably mediated by autoantibodies that actually stimulate thyroid cellular activity. In addition, patients with Graves' disease often have associated phenomena of ophthalmopathy and a proliferative dermopathy, which appear to be autoimmune in nature. The endocrine, skin, and eye disorders are most commonly seen in combination. They can exist separately, however, and often have different clinical courses even when they coexist in the same patient.

Graves' disease is most common in the third and fourth decades of life and has a marked female predominance of 7:1. Unlike Hashimoto's disease, it rarely occurs in children but is often seen in individuals past the fifth decade of life. It is a relatively common disorder, occurring in 0.1–0.5% of the general population.

Graves' disease was among the first autoimmune disorders noted to have an association with HLA haplotypes. There is a strong association with DR3 and several DQβ and a DQα genotype in whites and with Bw35 and Bw46 in Asians. Also, the disease tends to occur in families and is linked with HLA and Gm haplotypes in affected kindred. The disease seem to be associated with a type of generalized "autoimmune susceptibility" in some families, since other family members often have autoimmune disorders such as Hashimoto's disease and antibodies to gastric parietal cells and intrinsic factor.

Pathology

Thyroid glands from patients with Graves' disease present as a uniformly enlarged and diffuse goiter. Microscopic analysis reveals small thyroid follicles with hyperplastic epithelium, but little colloid. Although there is often a lymphocytic and plasma cell infiltrate, it is much less intense and does not have the associated destruction of normal tissue seen in Hashimoto's disease. These findings resolve in patients treated with antithyroid drugs.

Immunofluorescence analysis indicates that a high proportion of thyroid cells express HLA-DR antigens on their surface. In addition, analysis of the lymphocyte subsets in the gland reveals both CD4 and CD8 T and B cells.

Clinical Features

Graves' disease typically presents with diffuse goiter and thyrotoxicosis. The signs of hyperthyroidism are heat intolerance, hand tremor, nervousness, irritability, warm moist skin, weight loss, muscle reflex changes, hyperdynamic cardiovascular status with tachycardia, hyperdefecation, and changes in mental status. The exception to this is in the elderly, in whom apathetic hyperthyroidism may present with tachycardia as the sole clinical manifestation. Patients with accompanying ophthalmopathy may have proptosis, lid lag, and a characteristic "stare." Dermopathy usually presents as a swelling in the pretibial area (myxedema), and in the feet, face, or hands.

Laboratory findings are those of hyperthyroidism, with elevated levels of total and free T3 and T4. TSH levels in this disease are low or undetectable because the stimulation of the thyroid gland is exogenous rather than from the pituitary axis and the elevated levels of the thyroid hormones cause a feedback inhibition of pituitary TSH secretion.

The thyroid gland in patients with Graves' disease always shows an increased uptake of radioactive iodine. A diffuse homogeneous uptake on a radio isotopic scan of the thyroid is almost pathognomonic of Graves' disease.

Immunologic Diagnosis

The immunologic diagnosis of Graves' disease rests on the identification of antithyroid antibodies with the ability to alter thyroid cell function. These antibodies tend to fall into three categories (Fig 34–5): (1) antibodies that stimulate the production of cyclic adenosine monophosphate (cAMP) (thyroid-stimulating immunoglobulins [TSI]), (2) antibodies causing proliferation of thyroid cells as measured by the incorporation of [³H]thymidine into their DNA (thyroid growth-stimulating immunoglobulins [TGSI]), and (3) antibodies that displace the binding of TSH from its receptor (thyroid-binding inhibitory immunoglobulins [TBI]). Although these antibodies have been found in several other disorders, especially Hashimoto's thyroiditis, their presence in the appropriate clinical

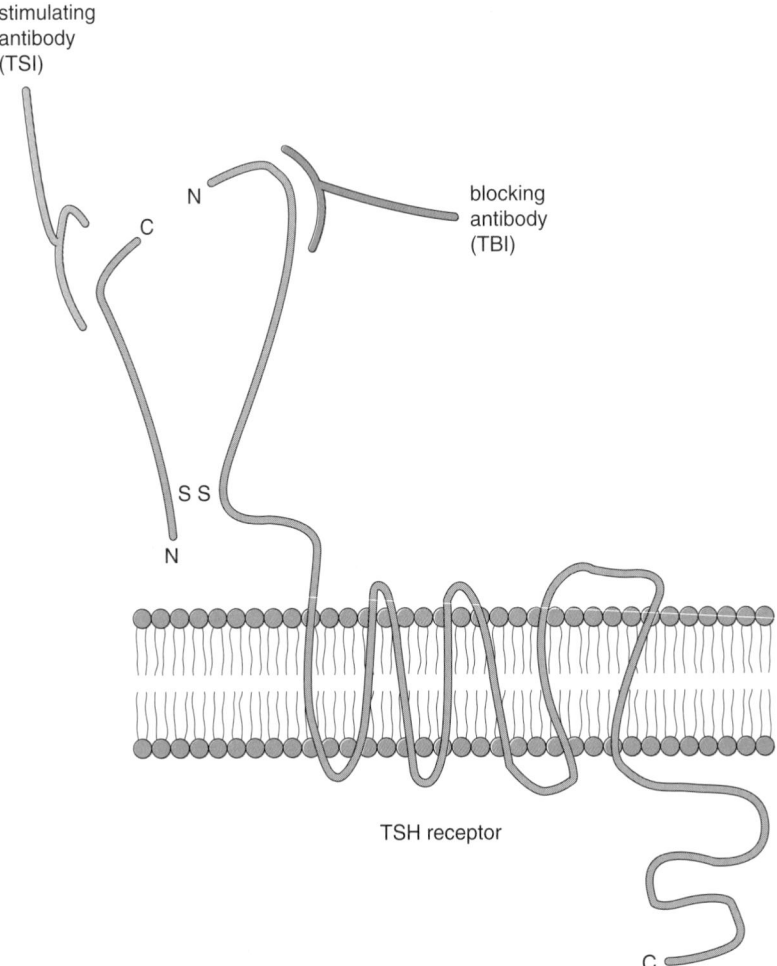

stimulating
antibody
(TSI)

N

C

blocking
antibody
(TBI)

S S

N

TSH receptor

C

Figure 34–5. TSH receptor structure and antibody binding sites. The TSH receptor is a major antigen in autoimmune thyroid disease. It appears that the autoantibodies bind to different sites on the external domain of the receptor and mediate stimulation of the receptor (in Graves' disease) or inhibition of receptor activation by TSH (atrophic thyroiditis).

setting is virtually pathognomonic of Graves' disease. In addition, monitoring the function of these antibodies may, in some cases, correlate with the clinical course of the disease and its response to antithyroid drugs.

Initial efforts to measure the activity of TSI involved injecting IgG fractions from patients with Graves' disease into animals and measuring thyroid activity. This test has been replaced by the Fisher rat thyroid line 5 (FRTL-5). These cells are grown in culture with IgG from patients with Graves' disease, and the effect on cell function (either the production of cAMP or the incorporation of [^{3}H]thymidine) is measured. The ability of the IgG to displace TSH from its receptor is still measured as described more than 15 years ago. The test involves the incubation of IgG with porcine thyroid membranes and radiolabeled TSH. The amount of TSH bound to the membrane is then calculated and compared with the amount bound in the presence of control IgG or unlabeled TSH. This

results in a "percent displacement" of radiolabeled TSH, which gives a relative activity of the IgG.

Recently, studies with recombinant TSH receptor protein have tried to identify specific sites in the receptor bound by autoantibodies. These studies are inconclusive but suggest that there are several sites in the external domain of the receptor to which autoantibodies bind. No specific biologic activity, however, has been uniquely associated with autoantibodies to a particular epitope. This suggests that the autoantibody response to the TSH receptor in Graves' disease is complex and heterogeneous.

Differential Diagnosis

The differential diagnosis of Graves' disease involves exclusion of other thyroid disorders manifesting hyperthyroidism, such as Hashimoto's disease, pituitary tumors, or thyroid adenomas. Most of these can be ruled out by determining that the thyroid gland has a diffuse increase in iodine uptake. The presence of ophthalmopathy and dermopathy also supports the diagnosis of Graves' disease.

Treatment

The initial treatment of Graves' disease involves the inhibition of symptomatic beta-adrenergic hyperstimulation with beta-adrenergic blocking agents. Therapy with drugs to inhibit thyroid cell function is also given soon after diagnosis. These drugs, propylthiouracil and methimazole, offer several advantages in the treatment of Graves' disease. They not only inhibit the production of thyroid hormones, relieving hyperthyroidism, but also decrease the size and vascularity of the goiter, making it more amenable to definitive therapy with surgery or radioactive iodine. Of interest, these drugs may also interrupt the perpetuation of the underlying autoimmune process, possibly through the resolution of the hyperthyroidism, as thyroid hormones appear to have nonspecific immunostimulatory activities in vitro.

Recently, it has been shown that administering suppressive doses of thyroid hormone in conjunction with antithyroid drugs may lead to long-term remission of Graves' disease. The mechanism of this effect is unknown but may be the result of suppression of thyrocyte autoantigen expression.

Definitive therapy for Graves' disease involves the destruction of the thyroid gland, either by ^{131}I or by complete surgical removal of the gland. Although personal preference and experience often dictate which therapy is used, surgery has been the therapy of choice in women of childbearing age because of the potential risks of radiation to the gonads and fetus. Recent studies do not show risk to the ovaries, however, and radioiodine is becoming increasingly popular in premenopausal women once pregnancy is ruled out.

Prognosis & Complications

The prognosis for most patients is very good once their thyroid function is controlled. The most serious problems in Graves' disease often come from the associated ophthalmopathy and dermopathy, which in some cases do not respond to treatments that normalize thyroid function. Treatment with corticosteroids provides relief in some cases, but occasionally the ophthalmopathy progresses to a point that vision is threatened. At that point, radiotherapy or surgical decompression of the orbit is often required. More aggressive treatment protocols with immunosuppressive drugs such as cyclosporine have shown some success in reversing the autoimmune process in these patients.

PRIMARY HYPOTHYROIDISM

Major Immunologic Features
■ There is lymphocytic infiltration of the thyroid gland.

■ Antithyroid antibodies can be present.

General Considerations

Primary hypothyroidism, or thyroid atrophy, is the most common cause of hypothyroidism (other than iatrogenic ablation) in adults. Much like the other autoimmune thyroid diseases, it is more common in women than men and occurs most often from age 40 to 60 years. The atrophy probably results from asymptomatic or unrecognized thyroiditis with resulting progressive destruction of the gland. However, some data suggest that some of these cases are related to antibodies which block TSH binding to its receptor, thereby inhibiting the trophic effect of the hormone. Thyroid atrophy also occurs as part of the polyglandular syndromes (see later section).

Pathology

The thyroid is markedly atrophic and often fibrotic. In some cases residual lymphocytic infiltration occurs.

Clinical Features

Although most patients demonstrate the usual findings of hypothyroidism and a small, impalpable thyroid gland, some present with palpable fibrosis in the area of the thyroid gland. Laboratory findings include elevated TSH levels with low (or low normal) levels of circulating thyroid hormones. TSH response to thyrotropin-releasing hormone (TRH) administration is often exaggerated, indicating an increased state of activation of the pituitary axis.

Immunologic Diagnosis

Antithyroid antibodies are found in a high proportion of patients (>80%), but they are not necessary for the diagnosis. No other specific immunologic tests are available.

Treatment & Prognosis

Treatment consists of thyroid hormone replacement. Most patients do well with this therapy. Replacement is required throughout the rest of the patient's life, however.

DISORDERS OF THE ENDOCRINE PANCREAS

INSULIN-DEPENDENT DIABETES MELLITUS (IDDM or Type I Diabetes)

Major Immunologic Features
■ There is monocytic and lymphocytic infiltration of the islets of Langerhans.
■ There are antibodies against multiple antigens of islet beta cells.

- There is HLA-DR expression on the beta cells.
- There is some evidence for partial responses to immunosuppressive therapy.

General Considerations

IDDM is a disorder in which the destruction of the insulin-producing beta cells of the pancreatic islets of Langerhans results in a deficiency of insulin. This is in contrast to the defect in type II diabetes mellitus, in which resistance of target organs to the effects of insulin is present. Although IDDM has only recently been associated with an immune pathogenesis, it is now clear that there is an autoimmune cause in essentially all patients with this disorder. The postulated sequence of events leading to islet cell destruction is similar to the scheme outlined in Figure 34–1. After an initiating event such as a viral infection, an inflammatory response to beta cells of the islets results. This inflammation is characterized by HLA-DR expression on the beta cells and lymphocytic infiltration of the islets. Subsequently, either a persistent stimulation of the immune system or a defect in immune regulation allows the propagation of the autoimmune response in a genetically predisposed individual. This causes destruction of the beta cells and leads to insulin deficiency.

The hypothesis that a viral infection is the initial insult leading to the development of IDDM in humans is unproven. There is, however, much evidence in favor of this hypothesis, including reports of the development of IDDM following infections with viruses, such as mumps virus, cytomegalovirus, influenza virus, and rubella virus, as well as a direct relationship between viral infection and diabetes in experimental animals. Mumps virus, coxsackievirus types B3 and B4, and reovirus type 3 can infect and destroy human islet cells in vitro. In addition, evidence now suggests amino acid sequence similarities between coxsackievirus proteins and the islet cell autoantigen, glutamic acid decarboxylase. As yet, however, there is no direct causal link between the common occurrence of infections with these viruses and the rare event of developing autoimmune diabetes mellitus. It seems that the heterogeneous genetic susceptibility to development of autoimmunity is what has made identification of a specific environmental cause difficult.

Epidemiologic studies support the concept of a genetic susceptibility to develop IDDM. Seen almost entirely in individuals under the age of 30 years, it has a peak age of onset between 10 and 14 years. It occurs predominantly in whites and has a prevalence of approximately 0.25% in both the USA and Europe. Unlike most other autoimmune disorders, males are more commonly affected than females, by a small margin. The incidence of this disorder has increased slightly over the past 50 years. There are also seasonal fluctuations.

The genetics of type I diabetes mellitus have come under intense study recently. It is well documented that more than 90% of patients have HLA-DR3, -DR4, or both and that there is a negative association with HLA-DR2. An additive risk occurs when both HLA-DR3 and -DR4 are present. Few individuals who have the HLA-DR3 and -DR4 haplotypes develop IDDM, however. This paradox may be partially explained by the association of the MHC antigens with particular DQβ genotypes. It has been noted that unique substitutions of amino acids at critical positions in this DQβ chain may be related to susceptibility to diabetes. One substitution (an uncharged amino acid for Asp at position 57) was noted in animals genetically susceptible to diabetes. Although this substitution does not perfectly identify humans at risk for this disease, it does indicate the potential importance of MHC antigens in diabetes.

Pathology

Patients show evidence of lymphocytic infiltration in the pancreatic islets even before evidence of glucose intolerance is noted. This inflammatory lesion progresses to cause specific destruction of the beta cells with atrophy and scarring of the islets. The other endocrine cells in the islets usually remain functional.

Immunofluorescence staining of the islet inflammation reveals several interesting findings. First, there is HLA-DR expression on the beta cells, as well as on the infiltrating lymphocytes. The majority of these lymphocytes stain positively with monoclonal antibodies for CD8, indicating a cytotoxic–suppressor phenotype. Antibody-producing cells are also seen, and antibody and complement components are present on the surface of the beta cells.

Clinical Features

The signs and symptoms are well known and are beyond the scope of this chapter. Unlike type II disease, there is a true insulin deficiency in type I diabetes mellitus, which leaves the patient prone to greater fluctuations in blood glucose concentration and to subsequent ketosis.

The laboratory diagnosis still rests on the documentation of elevated blood glucose concentrations. A fasting blood glucose level greater than 140 mg/dL in the appropriate clinical setting is diagnostic for diabetes. If the fasting glucose concentration is normal, the use of a glucose tolerance test may be helpful, but this is controversial. The level of hemoglobin A1c is helpful primarily in monitoring the ongoing control of blood glucose concentrations in patients on therapy.

Immunologic Diagnosis

Presently, no immunologic test is useful clinically. Antibodies to both islet cell cytoplasm and membranes can be identified by using immunofluorescence; however, these antibodies are not helpful in determining whether a susceptible individual will develop the disease. In the future, genetic analysis of HLA polymorphism or antibodies against a specific pancreatic antigen may serve this purpose. In this regard, the recent description that antibodies to glutamic acid decarboxylase precede the development of clinical glucose intolerance may suggest that the immune response to this enzyme will be a useful marker to monitor.

Treatment

Treatment of diabetes requires normalization of blood glucose concentrations by using oral hypoglycemic drugs or insulin injections. Most patients with IDDM require insulin, and the availability of human insulin may allow better therapy for some patients with insulin antibodies. Segmental pancreas or islet cell transplantation may offer a more physiologic form of insulin replacement in the future.

There have now been many trials of immunosuppressive therapy to attempt to reverse the inflammatory process that causes islet cell destruction (see Fig 34–5). Although most of these trials were started a short time after the development of glucose intolerance, there have been some (Table 34–2) successful increases in C peptide levels and clinical improvement in blood glucose control, obviating a need for insulin injections. All of these drugs have potentially severe toxicity, which has prevented their use in most diabetics.

ADRENAL INSUFFICIENCY
(Addison's Disease)

Major Immunologic Features

- Circulating antibodies against adrenal cells are present.
- Complement is fixed on the surface of adrenal cells.
- It is associated with other autoimmune diseases.

General Considerations

Since the decline of tuberculosis, idiopathic Addison's disease is the most common form of adrenal insufficiency, accounting for 70–80% of all cases. The prevalence is relatively low, only 40–50 cases per million, and it tends to affect young individuals in their third or fourth decade. The female-to-

Table 34–2. Immunotherapy trials in type I diabetes mellitus.

Drug	C Peptide Increase Period	Insulin Therapy-Free Period
Prednisone	24 months	Transient
Interferon alpha	None	None
Prednisone, antithymocyte globulin, and azathioprine	12 months	3–26 months
Cyclosporine	>12 months	12 months (25% of subjects)

male ratio is lower than that seen in other autoimmune disorders, only 1.8:1. It can present as an isolated disorder or in combination with other autoimmune diseases. It is most commonly seen as part of a polyglandular syndrome (see later discussion), which accounts for up to 40% of the cases of this disease. The disease is associated with HLA-DR 3/4 in a manner similar to type I diabetes mellitus, except when part of a polyglandular syndrome.

Pathology

Grossly, adrenal glands from patients with idiopathic Addison's disease show progressive scarring and atrophy. Microscopic examination often reveals a lymphocytic infiltrate early in the course of the disease, and immunofluorescence shows antibody and complement fixed to cortical cells.

Clinical Features

Idiopathic Addison's disease is usually slowly progressive, with the development of clinical manifestations such as salt wasting, hypotension, anorexia, malaise, and hyperpigmetation occurring so gradually that they can easily be undetected. Serum levels of adrenocorticotropic hormone (ACTH) are often elevated long before clinical disease develops. The finding of small, noncalcified adrenal glands on x-ray or computed tomography of the abdomen helps to differentiate this disorder from adrenal insufficiency secondary to carcinoma (primary or metastatic) and tuberculosis. The laboratory diagnosis rests on the lack of a cortisol (and possibly aldosterone) response to ACTH administration.

Immunologic Diagnosis

Serum antibodies against adrenal cortical cells are demonstrable by immunofluorescence in up to 80% of cases.

Treatment

Treatment consists of corticosteroid hormone replacement and, when needed, replacement of mineralocorticoid hormones. No trials of immunosuppressive therapy have been published.

LYMPHOCYTIC ADENOHYPOPHYSITIS

Lymphocytic adenohypophysitis is a rare disorder characterized by the rapid development of hypopituitarism without evidence of pituitary adenoma. It occurs most often in women during or after pregnancy. Although the incidence of this disorder is unknown, the finding of antibodies against pituitary cells in 18% of patients with Sheehan's syndrome suggests that at least some of these patients may have had an autoimmune basis for their hypopituitarism. It also occurs as part of a polyglandular syndrome (as discussed in a later section), in which it has been associated with isolated deficiencies of gonadotropic hormones.

PREMATURE OVARIAN FAILURE

Evidence is accumulating that some individuals may have an autoimmune basis for premature gonadal failure. There have been several cases in which autoimmune oophoritis is associated with other autoimmune endocrine diseases, especially adrenal insufficiency. This is especially true in polyglandular syndromes.

IDIOPATHIC HYPOPARATHYROIDISM

This is another uncommon disorder seen primarily in polyglandular autoimmune syndromes. Although antibodies against parathyroid tissue commonly occur in the polyglandular syndromes, their presence does not correlate with overt hypoparathyroidism. It has been reported that antibodies from patients with this disorder cause complement-mediated cytolysis of parathyroid cells, suggesting that a subset of antibodies may have pathogenic significance.

AUTOIMMUNE POLYGLANDULAR SYNDROMES

Major Immunologic Features
- There are circulating antibodies against multiple endocrine organs.
- There is evidence of HLA-DR expression on affected cells.
- There is genetic susceptibility to autoimmunity.

General Considerations
Polyglandular syndromes are groupings of multiple endocrine dysfunctions of autoimmune origin in a genetically susceptible individual. There were initially many versions of these syndromes identified by multiple eponyms; however, recently a classification scheme for these disorders has been developed (Table 34–3).

A. Type I Syndrome: The type I syndrome is a disorder that occurs in childhood, usually before the age of 10 years, with a slight female predominance. It was previously known as mucocutaneous candidiasis endocrinopathy. The most common association is between candidiasis and hypoparathyroidism (>70% of cases), but 40–70% of patients also go on to develop adrenal insufficiency. With the exception of gonadal failure, which occurs in approximately 40% of patients, the other autoimmune endocrine disorders are less common in the type I syndrome. There is, however, an association with chronic active hepatitis (10–15% of cases), alopecia areata, malabsorption, and pernicious anemia.

Table 34–3. Classification of polyglandular syndromes.

Syndrome	Major Criteria	Minor Criteria
Type I	Candidiasis Adrenal failure Hypoparathyroidism	Gonadal failure Alopecia Malabsorption Chronic hepatitis
Type II	Adrenal failure Thyroid disease IDDM	Gonadal failure Vitiligo Nonendocrine autoimmune disease
Type III[1]	Thyroid disease	a. IDDM b. Gastric disease c. Nonendocrine autoimmune disease

[1] Type III is composed of thyroid disease plus only one of a, b, or c.

The pathogenesis of this disorder is unknown, but the problems with chronic fungal infection suggest a defect in cell-mediated immunity. Autoantibodies against cells from most affected organs are also seen in a large percentage of patients.

Although type I polyglandular syndrome occurs sporadically, it is more commonly seen as a familial disorder with inheritance suggestive of an autosomal-recessive trait. It has not, however, been associated with a particular HLA haplotype.

B. Type II Syndrome: Type II polyglandular syndrome was originally known as Schmidt's syndrome. It tends to occur most often between the ages of 20 and 30 years and has a 2:1 female predominance. It is a rare disorder, with a prevalence of 20 per million. It is characterized by the presence of a second, autoimmune disorder (usually diabetes or thyroid disease or both) with idiopathic Addison's disease. Gonadal failure occurs in a smaller percentage of cases, and nonendocrine autoimmune disorders have been occasionally noted.

Although at least half the cases of type II polyglandular syndrome are familial, the mode of inheritance is unknown. Both autosomal-dominant and -recessive patterns have been suggested, and there is also a high frequency of HLA-DR3 in these patients. Autoantibodies against cells of the affected organs are present in the majority of patients, and there have also been reports of alterations in cell-mediated immunity.

C. Type III Syndrome: Type III polyglandular syndrome is the least well characterized but probably the most common of the disorders. It is defined by the presence of autoimmune thyroid disease with another autoimmune disorder. This syndrome comprises at least three clinical entities. The first is the association of diabetes mellitus with autoimmune thyroid disease. The second is the association of autoimmunity against gastric components such as parietal cells or intrinsic factor in association with autoimmune thyroid disease. The association of any other organ-specific autoimmune disorder, such as myasthenia gravis, with autoimmune thyroid disease constitutes the third component. Patients with type III polyglandular syndrome, by definition, do not have Addison's disease.

The cause of type III polyglandular syndrome is unclear, but it tends to primarily involve female patients (7:1 female predominance) who have HLA-DR3-associated autoimmune disease. Again, organ-specific autoantibodies are present in the sera of patients with this disorder.

D. Other Considerations: The pathology, symptoms, and treatment of patients with the polyglandular syndromes are the same as for the individual autoimmune disorders, with a few important exceptions. Patients with type I polyglandular syndrome should have their candidiasis treated with ketoconazole. This not only provides symptomatic relief but also may help resolve some of the defects in cell-mediated immunity. In addition, all patients with the polyglandular syndromes should be monitored for the development of other autoimmune disorders associated with their syndrome. This prevents the possibility of missing disorders such as Addison's disease, which may develop later in the course of the syndrome.

REFERENCES

GENERAL

Bach JF: Antireceptor or antihormone autoimmunity and its relationship with the idiotype network. *Adv Nephrol* 1987;**16**:25.

Bigazzi PE: Autoimmunity in diabetes mellitus and polyendocrine syndromes: Current concepts of pathogenesis and etiology. *Immunol Ser* 1990;**52**:295.

Boehm BO, Farid NR: Molecular aspects of endocrine autoimmunity. *Clin Invest Med* 1993;**71**(1):79.

Patrick CC: Organ-specific autoimmune diseases. *Immunol Ser* 1990;**50**:435.

Pujol-Borrell R et al: Inappropriate major histocompatibility complex class II expression by thyroid follicular cells in thyroid autoimmune disease and by pancreatic beta cells in type I diabetes. *Mol Biol Med* 1986;**3**:159.

Zouali M et al: Autoimmune diseases—at the molecular level. *Immunol Today* 1993;**14**(10):473.

THYROID DISEASES

Baker JR Jr et al: Seronegative Hashimoto thyroiditis with thyroid autoantibody production localized to the thyroid. *Ann Intern Med* 1988;**108**:26.

Burman KD, Baker JR Jr: Immune mechanisms in Graves' disease. *Endocr Rev* 1985;**6**:183.

Kosugi S et al: Use of thyrotropin receptor (TSHR) mutants to detect stimulating TSHR antibodies in hypothyroid patients with idiopathic myxedema, who have blocking TSHR antibodies [see comments]. *J Clin Endocrinol Metab* 1993;**77**(1):19.

Mooij P, Drexhage HA: Autoimmune thyroid disease. *Clin Lab Med* 1993;**13**(3):683.

Nagayama Y, Rapoport B: The thyrotropin receptor 25 years after its discovery: New insight after its molecular cloning. *Mol Endocrinol* 1992;**6**(2):145.

Perros P, Kendall-Taylor P: Thyroid-associated ophthalmopathy: Pathogenesis and clinical management. *Baillieres Clin Endocrinol Metab* 1995;**9**(1):115.

Sundbeck G et al: Prevalence of serum antithyroid peroxidase antibodies in 85-year-old women and men. *Clin Chem* 1995;**41**(5):707.

Weetman AP, McGregor AM: Autoimmune thyroid disease: Developments in our understanding. *Endocr Rev* 1984;**5**:309.

INSULIN-DEPENDENT DIABETES MELLITUS

Atkinson MA, Maclaren NK: The pathogenesis of insulin-dependent diabetes mellitus. *N Engl J Med* 1994;**331**(21):1428.

Baekkeskov S et al: Identification of the 64K autoantigen in insulin-dependent diabetes as the GABA-synthesizing enzyme glutamic acid decarboxylase. *Nature* 1990;**347**:151.

Baekkeskov S et al: The glutamate decarboxylase and 38kd autoantigens in type 1 diabetes: Aspects of structure and epitope recognition. *Autoimmunity* 1993;**15**(suppl):24.

Baisch JM et al: Analysis of HLA-DQ genotypes and susceptibility in insulin-dependent diabetes mellitus. *N Engl J Med* 1990;**322**:1836.

Bonifacio E et al: Islet autoantibody markers in IDDM: Risk assessment strategies yielding high sensitivity. *Diabetologia* 1995;**38**(7):816.

Gottsater A et al: Glutamate decarboxylase antibody levels predict rate of beta-cell decline in adult-onset diabetes. *Diabetes Res Clin Pract* 1995;**27**(2):133.

Karjalainen J et al: A bovine albumin peptide as a possible trigger of insulin-dependent diabetes mellitus. *N Engl J Med* 1992;**327**:302.

Lernmark A: Molecular biology of IDDM. *Diabetologia* 1994;**37**(suppl 2):S73.

Riley WJ et al: A prospective study of the development of diabetes in relatives of patients with insulin-dependent diabetes. *N Engl J Med* 1990;**323**:1167.

ADDISON'S DISEASE

Betterle C et al: Complement-fixing adrenal autoantibodies as a marker for predicting onset of idiopathic Addison's disease. *Lancet* 1983;**1**:1238.

Falorni A et al: High diagnostic accuracy for idiopathic Addison's disease with a sensitive radiobinding assay for autoantibodies against recombinant human 21-hydroxylase. *J Clin Endocrinol Metab* 1995;**80**(9):2752.

Latinne D et al: Addison's disease: Immunological aspects. *Tissue Antigens* 1987;**30**:23.

Vita JA et al: Clinical clues to the cause of Addison's disease. *Am J Med* 1985;**78**:461.

Weetman AP et al: HLA associations with autoimmune Addison's disease. *Tissue Antigens* 1991;**38**:31.

Winqvist O et al: 21-Hydroxylase, a major autoantigen in idiopathic Addison's disease. *Lancet* 1992;**339**:1559.

LYMPHOCYTIC ADENOHYPOPHYSITIS & HYPOPARATHYROIDISM

Brandi ML et al: Antibodies cytotoxic to bovine parathyroid cells in autoimmune hypoparathyroidism. *Proc Natl Acad Sci USA* 1986;**83**:8366.

Guay AT et al: Lymphocytic hypophysitis in a man. *J Clin Endocrinol Metab* 1987;**64:**631.

Homberg JC: Hypoparathyroidism, ovarian insufficiency and adrenal insufficiency of autoimmune origin. *Rev Prat* 1986;**36:**3505.

McDermott MW et al: Lymphocytic adenohypophysitis. *Can J Neurol Sci* 1988;**15:**38.

AUTOIMMUNE OVARIAN FAILURE

Moncayo R, Moncayo HE: The association of autoantibodies directed against ovarian antigens in human disease: A clinical review. *J Intern Med* 1993;**234**(4):371.

POLYGLANDULAR SYNDROMES

Ahonen P: Autoimmune polyendocrinopathy candidosis ectodermal dystrophy (APECED): Autosomal recessive inheritance. *Clin Genet* 1985;**27:**535.

Appleboom TM, Flowers FP: Ketoconazole in the treatment of chronic mucocutaneous candidiasis secondary to autoimmune polyendocrinopathy candidiasis syndrome. *Cutis* 1982;**30:**71.

Brun JM: Juvenile autoimmune polyendocrinopathy. *Horm Res* 1982;**16:**308.

Leshin M: Polyglandular autoimmune syndromes. *Am J Med Sci* 1985;**290:**77.

Neufeld M et al: Autoimmune polyglandular syndromes. *Pediatr Ann* 1980;**9:**154.

Hematologic Diseases

35

J. Vivian Wells, MD, FRACP, FRCPA, & James P. Isbister, FRACP, FRCPA

Many areas in hematology are significantly affected by immunologic processes. An important group of disorders—the autoimmune hemolytic anemias, autoimmune neutropenias, and immune thrombocytopenias—are characterized by immunologic destruction of circulating blood cells. Even hematopoietic precursor cells in the bone marrow may be affected by immunologic mechanisms, as seen in pure erythrocyte aplasia and some cases of aplastic anemia. Another large group of hematologic disorders—the plasma cell dyscrasias, lymphatic leukemias, and lymphomas—represent abnormal proliferations of primary cells of the immune system (see Chapter 46).

This chapter is devoted primarily to hematologic disorders in which immunologic cells or mechanisms play a major role. The chapter discusses immunologic disorders of leukocytes, erythrocytes, and coagulation.

LEUKOCYTE DISORDERS

LEUKOPENIA

Leukopenia is defined as a reduction in the number of circulating leukocytes below 4000/μL. Granulocytopenia may be caused either by decreased granulocyte production by the bone marrow or by increased granulocyte utilization or destruction. Decreased granulocyte production occurs in aplastic anemia, leukemia, and other diseases marked by bone marrow infiltration; many drugs also cause leukopenia by this mechanism. Increased granulocyte use or destruction occurs in hypersplenism, autoimmune neutropenia, and some forms of drug-induced leukopenia. The major causes of leukopenia are listed in Table 35–1.

Table 35–1. The major causes of leukopenia.

Infections
Viral—rubella
Bacterial—typhoid fever, miliary tuberculosis, brucellosis
Rickettsial
Therapy
Ionizing radiation
Cytotoxic drugs
Drugs
Selective neutropenia
Agranulocytosis
Aplastic anemia
Hematologic diseases
Megaloblastic anemia
Acute leukemia
Myelodysplasia
Aplastic anemia
Multiple myeloma
Paroxysmal nocturnal hemoglobinuria
Leukoerythroblastic anemia
Metastatic carcinoma
Autoimmune neutropenia
Hypersplenism
SLE
Felty's syndrome
Chronic idiopathic neutropenia
Cyclic neutropenia
Miscellaneous
Anaphylaxis
Hypopituitarism

Abbreviations: SLE = systemic lupus erythematosus.

1. AUTOIMMUNE NEUTROPENIA

Autoimmune neutropenia may occur as an isolated disorder or secondary to an autoimmune disease. These patients may be asymptomatic or may have recurrent infections. Antigranulocyte antibodies have been detected by a variety of procedures, including the utilization of anti-immunoglobulin antisera with fluorescence or antiglobulin consumption techniques, functional assays, and cytotoxicity assays. The presence of leukoagglutinins does not correlate well with leukopenia. Bone marrow function is relatively normal in autoimmune neutropenia, with myeloid hyperplasia and a shift to the left in maturation, or maturation arrest, presumably in response to increased peripheral granulocyte destruction. The autoantibody may also suppress bone marrow myeloid cell growth in vitro and in vivo.

Autoimmune neutropenia may also be seen in systemic lupus erythematosus (SLE), Felty's syndrome (rheumatoid arthritis, splenomegaly, and severe neutropenia), and other autoimmune disorders. Immune neutropenia in these disorders may be caused by adsorption of immune complexes onto the neutrophil membrane with premature cell destruction rather than by an antibody directed at specific neutrophil antigens. Some patients with Felty's syndrome also appear to have depressed granulocyte production by the bone marrow, probably also on an immunologic basis.

2. CYCLIC NEUTROPENIA

These patients have a 3- to 6-week cycle, which includes a period of neutropenia lasting 4–10 days. Patients may be asymptomatic, but many show a pattern of recurrent fever, pharyngitis, recurrent aphthous stomatitis, lymphadenopathy, and infections during the period of neutropenia. The treatment of choice for symptomatic patients is granulocyte colony-stimulating factor (G-CSF; see section on management of neutropenia).

3. DRUG-INDUCED IMMUNE NEUTROPENIA

Although most drugs produce neutropenia by bone marrow suppression, some may cause neutropenia by the attachment of drug–antibody immune complexes to the surface of the granulocytes, with premature cell destruction. This "innocent-bystander" mechanism is known to occur in drug-induced immune hemolytic anemia and thrombocytopenia. Cephalothin causes granulocytopenia in approximately 0.1% of patients given the drug, probably by this mechanism.

4. AGRANULOCYTOSIS

Agranulocytosis is characterized by the total absence of granulocytes and granulocyte precursors from the peripheral blood and bone marrow. This most often results from exposure of the patient to certain drugs, such as aminopyrine, dipyrone, and phenylbutazone. Patients with agranulocytosis usually present with infections—often serious, life-threatening ones. Prior to the antibiotic era, agranulocytosis was almost invariably fatal. Patients now usually recover with intensive antibiotic treatment and granulocyte transfusions when necessary. Unlike

drug-induced aplastic anemia, agranulocytosis usually resolves spontaneously within a few days to a few weeks after discontinuing the offending drug.

Although antigranulocyte antibodies or leukocyte drug-dependent antibodies generally have not been demonstrated in agranulocytosis, there is circumstantial evidence that immunologic damage to peripheral blood and bone marrow granulocytic cells is the mechanism of cell destruction, at least in some cases. Such patients often develop agranulocytosis after taking the responsible drug for weeks or months. If they recover from the agranulocytosis after the drug is discontinued and later are rechallenged with a small test dose of the same drug, acute agranulocytosis occurs immediately, associated with the acute onset of fever, chills, and hypocomplementemia.

5. MANAGEMENT OF NEUTROPENIA

The first step in the management of neutropenia is identification of any underlying disease or drugs that may be responsible for the neutropenia.

The offending drug should be withdrawn, unless it is "essential" treatment, such as antitumor cytotoxic chemotherapy, antiretroviral therapy in human immunodeficiency virus (HIV)-infected patients, or recombinant interferon alfa in hairy cell leukemia. Underlying diseases such as SLE should be treated appropriately, and generally no specific treatment is required for the neutropenia, which tends to resolve as the underlying disease goes into remission or is controlled. On occasion, patients with autoimmune neutropenia have required treatment with corticosteroids, immunosuppressive drugs, or splenectomy.

The major advance in the management of cytopenias has been the therapeutic use of cytokines along with hemolymphopoietic growth factors.

Cytokines are bioactive cell secretions, which function as hormones for immune and other cells. The growth factors function as growth regulators, and more than 20 such factors have been identified and their genes cloned, including erythropoietin, the colony-stimulating factors, and the interleukins (IL). A few are now used in clinical practice (see Chapter 10), but their use is still restricted in many ways. Many ongoing clinical trials are assessing the role of cytokines in treating various diseases. Table 35–2 lists the major cytokines currently in clinical use or suggested for further studies.

For the management of neutropenia, cytokine therapy has been used in the following clinical settings:

1. Chronic neutropenia/cyclic neutropenia: G-CSF is now the treatment of choice.

2. Autoimmune neutropenia: G-CSF is considered for symptomatic patients not responding to corticosteroid therapy.

3. Drug-associated neutropenia: GM-CSF has been used in HIV-infected patients who developed

Table 35–2. Cytokines/hemolymphopoietic growth factors with clinical applications.

Cytokine	Major Biologic Effects	Clinical Applications[1]
Erythropoietin.	Erythrocyte production.	Anemia of end-stage renal disease. Zidovudine anemia in AIDS patients.
Granulocyte colony-stimulating factor (G-CSF).	Granulocyte lineage and differentiation. Early myeloid stem cell action. Neutrophil phagocytosis increase. Release of neutrophils from bone marrow.	Neutropenia. Aplastic anemia. Transplantation.
Granulocyte–monocyte colony-stimulating factor (GM-CSF).	Granulocyte, macrophage, and megakaryocyte proliferation and differentiation. Enhancement of neutrophil functions.	Neutropenia. Aplastic anemia. Transplantation.
Colony-stimulating factor-1 (CSF-1).	Macrophage–monocyte proliferation and differentiation (lesser for granulocytes). Stimulation of macrophage activities.	Neutropenia. (Cancer).
Interleukin-2 (IL-2).	Growth induction for T cells. Activation of cytotoxic T cells. Enhancement of NK function.	(AIDS). (Cancer).
Interleukin-3 (IL-3).	Stimulatin of proliferation and differentiation of granulocyte, macrophage, mast cell, megakaryocyte, early myeloid stem cell, and T- and B-cell lineages.	Neutropenia. Aplastic anemia. Transplantation.
Interleukin-6 (IL-6).	Stimulation of B-cell differentiation and IgG secretion. Synergy with IL-3 for stimulation of early myeloid stem cells. Stimulation of platelet production.	(Aplastic anemia). (Transplantation).

[1] Items in parentheses indicate conditions that have been tested but not proven.

significant neutropenia after treatment with the anti-retroviral agent zidovudine. Its role in this setting is still unproven.

4. Neutropenia associated with hairy cell leukemia: G-CSF is effective in this setting.

5. Cytotoxic chemotherapy: Neutropenia is virtually inevitable following full-dose multidrug cytotoxic therapy. Several trials have studied G-CSF and GM-CSF to determine whether they prevent or modify the severity of the neutropenia and permit complete treatment courses at full dosage. Encouraging but variable results have been reported, but it is likely that a combination of cytokines will prove to be the best approach.

6. Transplantation: There are two possible uses in transplantation medicine. The first is to use cytokines to increase the neutrophil count in patients who have neutropenia after transplantation. The second is to use the cytokines in nonneutropenic patients to mobilize stem cells from bone marrow to the periphery for collection, cryopreservation and, autografting.

7. Aplastic anemia: GM-CSF, G-CSF, and interleukin-3 (IL-3) have all produced increases in neutrophil counts in such patients, but only while the drug is continued and with no effect on red cell and platelet counts. Their current use in this setting is therefore limited, mainly to supporting patients pending bone marrow transplantation for severe aplastic anemia.

The side effects of G-CSF are few, mainly axial bone pain during intravenous (but not subcutaneous) therapy and splenomegaly with long-term treatment. GM-CSF has a wider range of side effects, including fever and, at higher doses, capillary leak (fluid retention) syndrome, pericarditis, and pleuritis.

It is clear that cytokine/growth factor therapy will increase in the future, especially with the development of combination therapy for multilineage effects (eg, IL-3 and G-CSF or GM-CSF).

ERYTHROCYTE DISORDERS

The erythrocyte disorders in which immune processes play an important role are the immune hemolytic anemias, paroxysmal nocturnal hemoglobinuria, and aplastic anemia and related disorders.

IMMUNE HEMOLYTIC ANEMIAS

The immune hemolytic disorders are classified in Table 35–3. The classification is based on the behavioral characteristics of antibodies involved and whether there is a demonstrable underlying disease. The clinical picture may be one of an acute self-limiting hemolytic disorder but is more often chronic.

Table 35–3. Classification of immune hemolytic anemias.

Autoimmune hemolytic anemias
A. Warm antibody types
  1. Idiopathic warm autoimmune hemolytic anemia (AIHA)
  2. Secondary warm autoimmune hemolytic anemias
    a. SLE and other autoimmune disorders
    b. Chronic lymphocytic leukemia, lymphomas, etc
    c. Hepatitis and other viral infections
B. Cold antibody types
  1. Idiopathic cold agglutinin syndrome
  2. Secondary cold agglutinin syndrome
    a. *Mycoplasma pneumoniae* infection; infectious mononucleosis and other viral infections
    b. Chronic lymphocytic leukemia, lymphomas, etc
  3. Paroxysmal cold hemoglobinuria
    a. Idiopathic
    b. Syphilis, viral infections
Drug-induced immune hemolytic anemias
  1. Drug absorption mechanism
  2. Membrane modification mechanism
  3. Immune complex mechanism
Partial list of drugs:

Aminosalicylic acid (PAS)	Methyldopa
Antihistamines	Penicillin
Carbromal	Phenacetin
Cephalothin	Pyramidon
Chlorinated hydrocarbons	Quinidine
Chlorpromazine	Quinine
Dipyrone	Rifampin
Insulin	Stibophen
Isoniazid	Sulfonamides
Levodopa	Sulfonylureas
Mefenamic acid	Tetracyclines
Melphalan	

Alloantibody-induced immune hemolytic anemias
A. Hemolytic transfusion reactions
B. Hemolytic disease of the newborn
C. Allograft-associated anemias

Since identification of the type of antibody is essential to correct diagnosis in patients with suspected immune hemolytic anemia, the immunologic laboratory investigation of such patients is discussed before the individual diseases.

Immunologic Laboratory Investigations

There are two groups of immunologic tests used to investigate patients with suspected immune hemolytic anemias: (1) tests to detect and characterize antibodies involved in the hemolytic process, and (2) tests to aid in diagnosis of possible underlying disease processes. Tests that define underlying disorders include detection of anti-DNA antibodies and antinuclear antibody (ANA) in SLE, rheumatoid factors in rheumatoid arthritis, and monoclonal B cells in chronic lymphocytic leukemia.

The serologic tests used to characterize antibodies in serum and on erythrocytes are basic blood-banking procedures, with the addition of monospecific antisera to identify specific proteins on erythrocytes and titration techniques to precisely quantitate antibody activity. Laboratory evaluation of such patients addresses a series of questions:

1. Are the erythrocytes of the patient coated with immunoglobulin, complement components, or both?
2. How heavily are the erythrocytes sensitized?
3. What antibodies are eluted from the erythrocytes?
4. What antibodies are present in the serum?

Routine screening is performed by means of the direct antiglobulin (Coombs') test by tube or slide agglutination (see Chapter 16) using antisera with broad specificity. Subsequent evaluation requires testing the red cells with dilutions of monospecific antisera, especially antisera to IgG and C3. The autoantibody is examined at different temperatures to see whether the temperature of maximal activity identifies it as a "warm" or "cold" antibody.

False-negative and false-positive results can be obtained in direct antiglobulin tests. Approximately 20% of all patients with immune hemolytic anemias have a negative or only weakly positive direct antiglobulin test unless the antiserum contains adequate titers of antibodies to complement components, especially C3. A positive direct antiglobulin test may be seen in situations other than autoantibodies on erythrocytes and does not necessarily mean autoimmune hemolytic anemia. Causes of such reactions include: (1) antibody formation against drugs rather than intrinsic erythrocyte antigens (see section on drug-induced hemolytic anemia); (2) damage to the erythrocyte membrane due to infection or cephalosporins, leading to nonimmunologic binding of proteins; (3) in vitro complement sensitization of erythrocytes by low-titer cold antibodies (present in many normal individuals) in clotted blood samples stored at 4 °C prior to separation; (4) delayed transfusion reactions; and (5) unknown mechanisms. The above-mentioned reactions are generally weak and can be differentiated by clinical and detailed serologic studies.

Serologic investigations of the patient's serum and erythrocyte eluates should then answer another series of questions: (1) Are antibodies present? (2) Do they act as agglutinins, hemolysins, or incomplete antibodies? (3) What is their thermal range of activity? (4) What is their specificity?

The patient's serum is tested both undiluted and with fresh added complement against untreated and enzyme-treated pools of erythrocytes. Enzyme treatment enhances the sensitivity of the Ii system or abolishes activity in the case of the Pr system. The tests are run at both 37 and 20 °C and examined after 1 hour for agglutination and lysis. Cold agglutinin titration at 4 °C is also performed. Erythrocyte eluate is similarly tested.

Specialized tests may be performed to detect antibodies to drugs (eg, penicillin) in cases of drug-induced immune hemolytic anemia.

The specificity of the antibodies is tested at different temperatures with a panel of erythrocytes of different Rh genotypes and with cells of different types in the Ii blood group system.

The results of the serologic investigations are then correlated with clinical and other laboratory investigations to establish a definitive diagnosis.

1. WARM AUTOIMMUNE HEMOLYTIC ANEMIA

Major Immunologic Features
- There is a positive direct antiglobulin (Coombs') test.
- Associated lymphoreticular cancer or autoimmune disease may be present.
- Splenomegaly is common.

General Considerations
Warm antibody autoimmune hemolytic anemia is the most common type of immune hemolytic anemia. It may be either idiopathic or secondary to chronic lymphocytic leukemia, lymphomas, SLE, or other autoimmune disorders or infections (see Table 35–3). The idiopathic form may follow overt or subclinical viral infection.

Clinical Features
A. Symptoms and Signs: Patients usually present with symptoms of anemia and hemolysis. There may also be manifestations of an underlying disease, such as lymphadenopathy, hepatosplenomegaly, or manifestations of autoimmune disease.

B. Laboratory Findings: Normochromic normocytic or slightly macrocytic anemia is usually present; spherocytosis is common, and nucleated erythrocytes may occasionally be found in the peripheral blood. Leukocytosis and thrombocytosis are often present, but occasionally (especially in SLE) leukopenia and thrombocytopenia are seen. A moderate to marked reticulocytosis usually occurs. The bone marrow shows marked erythroid hyperplasia with plentiful iron stores. The serum level of indirect (unconjugated) bilirubin increases. Stool and urinary urobilinogen may be greatly increased. Transfused blood has a shortened survival time.

Immunologic Diagnosis
The results of the serologic tests discussed earlier are summarized in Table 35–4. The most common pattern is IgG and complement on erythrocytes, with IgG in the eluate. The eluate generally has no activity if the erythrocytes are sensitized only with complement.

Warm hemolysins active against enzyme-treated erythrocytes occur in 24% of sera, but warm serum agglutinins or hemolysins against untreated erythrocytes are rare. The indirect antiglobulin test (see Chapter 16) is positive at 37 °C in approximately 50–60% of patients' sera tested with untreated erythrocytes but in 90% of serum samples tested with en-

zyme-treated erythrocytes. This warm antibody is usually IgG but rarely may be IgM, IgA, or both.

The specificity of antibodies in warm antibody autoimmune hemolytic anemia is very complex, but the main specificity is directed against determinants in the Rh complex.

Differential Diagnosis
Congenital nonspherocytic hemolytic anemia, hereditary spherocytosis, and hemoglobinopathies can usually be differentiated by the family history, routine hematologic tests, hemoglobin electrophoresis, and a negative direct antiglobulin test.

Treatment
A. General Measures: Treatment of the primary disease is necessary. Blood transfusions may be necessary for life-threatening anemia but should be avoided when possible, since the transfused cells are rapidly destroyed. Careful serologic studies are needed to minimize the risks of serious hemolytic transfusion reactions, and successful crossmatching can be difficult or impossible in this situation. Alloantibodies are common and are difficult to detect.

B. Specific Measures: Hemolysis can be controlled with high doses of corticosteroids in most patients (40–120 mg of prednisone per day). The steroids are fairly rapidly tapered and then slowly reduced until the clinical state, hemoglobin level, and reticulocyte count indicate the appropriate maintenance dose. Occasionally it is possible to gradually withdraw steroids completely. Regular monitoring is necessary since relapses often occur.

Monitoring generally includes serologic studies, such as direct and indirect antiglobulin tests, and these may show improvement with reduced amounts of IgG and complement on erythrocytes and lower antibody titers or a negative antibody test. There is no consistent correlation between clinical response and serologic tests; however, prednisone often induces clinical remissions in patients with warm antibody autoimmune hemolytic anemia despite persistently positive direct antiglobulin tests.

If prednisone therapy fails or if unacceptable side effects occur, splenectomy is usually performed. Splenectomy is the treatment of choice if hemolysis persists after 2–3 months of corticosteroids and 60% respond to this procedure. ^{51}Cr-labeled erythrocyte survival studies can be used to identify abnormal splenic erythrocyte sequestration prior to splenectomy; however, clinical remissions may occur after splenectomy even when abnormal splenic sequestration cannot be documented. Continued significant hemolysis or late relapse sometimes occurs after splenectomy and requires therapy with steroids with or without other immunosuppressive agents.

Other immunosuppressive drugs include oral azathioprine, cyclophosphamide at low dosage, or cyclosporine.

Table 35–4. Summary of serologic findings in patients with autoimmune hemolytic anemia.

Disease Group	Erythrocytes			Serum		
	Direct Antiglobulin Test		Eluate	Immunoglobulin Type	Serologic Characteristics	Specificity
Warm antibody type	IgG 30% IgG + complement 50% Complement 20%		IgG IgG No activity	IgG (rarely also IgA or IgM)	Positive indirect antiglobulin test 50%. Agglutination of enzyme-treated erythrocytes 90%. Hemolysis of enzyme-treated erythrocytes 24%. Agglutination of untreated erythrocytes (20 ˚C) 20%. Agglutination or hemolysis of untreated erythrocytes (37 ˚C). Very rare.	Rh system (often with a "nonspecific" component).
Cold agglutinin syndrome	Complement		No activity	IgM (rarely IgA)	High-titer cold agglutinin (usually 1:1000 at 4 ˚C) up to 32 ˚C; monoclonal IgM in chronic disease.	Anti-I usually (can be anti-i or anti-Pr).
Paroxysmal cold hemoglobinuria (very rare)	Complement		No activity	IgG	Potent hemolysin also agglutinates normal cells. Biphasic (usually sensitizes cells in cold up to 15 ˚C and hemolyzes them at 37 ˚C).	Anti-P blood group.

Source: Modified, with permission, from Petz LD, Garratty G: Laboratory correlations in immune hemolytic anemias. In: *Laboratory Diagnosis of Immunologic Disorders.* Vyas GN et al (editors). Grune & Stratton, 1975, p. 139.

Prognosis

The prognosis of idiopathic warm antibody autoimmune hemolytic anemia is fairly good; however, relapses are not infrequent, and death sometimes occurs. The prognosis of secondary warm autoimmune hemolytic anemia is determined by the underlying disease (eg, SLE or lymphoma).

2. COLD AGGLUTININ SYNDROMES

These diseases may be primary or may be secondary to infection or lymphoma (see Table 35–3). The infections include mycoplasmal pneumonia and infectious mononucleosis and other viral infections.

The clinical features are often those of the underlying disease. Cold-reactive symptoms such as Raynaud's phenomenon, livedo reticularis, or vascular purpura are seen in some patients. Hemolysis is generally mild but occasionally severe, especially in cases secondary to lymphoreticular cancer. The onset may be acute in cases secondary to infection. The idiopathic form is generally gradual in onset and runs a chronic and usually benign course in older patients.

These diseases usually are characterized by very high serum titers of agglutinating IgM antibodies that react optimally in the cold. These patients have cold agglutinin titers in the thousands or millions, whereas normal individuals may have low-titer IgM cold agglutinins, and patients with chronic parasitic infections and most patients with *Ancylostoma* infection have titers up to 1:500. The presence of hemolysis is determined by the thermal range of the cold agglutinin. The high-titer, narrow-thermal-range antibodies

cause acral ischemic symptoms. Some, however, may have a low titer but a thermal range reacting up to 37 °C. The specificity of the IgM is generally anti-I in the Ii system, but occasionally it is anti-i or anti-Pr (see Table 35–4). In chronic idiopathic cases or cases associated with lymphoreticular malignancy, the cold agglutinin is generally a monoclonal IgM-κ paraprotein. The direct antiglobulin test is always positive using antiserum to C3.

Treatment consists of keeping the patient warm and waiting for spontaneous resolution in acute cases. Chronic cases sometimes respond to chlorambucil or cyclophosphamide in low doses. Corticosteroids and splenectomy are probably not helpful, unless an underlying lymphoma is present.

The prognosis is generally good except for patients with severe underlying disease such as malignant lymphoma.

3. DRUG-INDUCED IMMUNE HEMOLYTIC ANEMIA

Many cases of immune hemolytic anemia have been reported in association with drug administration; the most common examples are included in Table 35–3. There are three stages in the investigation of a patient with suspected drug-induced hemolytic anemia: a history of intake of the drug, confirmation of hemolysis, and serologic tests. Detailed serologic tests are necessary, since different drugs produce hemolysis by different mechanisms. The immunopathologic mechanisms and clinical and laboratory features are summarized in Table 35–5. The mechanisms are

Table 35–5. Summary of immunopathologic mechanisms and clinical and laboratory features in drug-induced immune hemolytic disorders.

Mechanism	Drugs	Clinical Findings	Serologic Evaluation	
			Direct Antigiobulin Test	Antibody Characterization
Immune complex formation (drug + antidrug antibody)	Quinine, quinidine, phenacetin	History of small doses of drugs. Acute intravascular hemolysis and renal failure. Thrombocytopenia occasionally found.	Complement (IgG) occasionally also present).	Drug + patient's serum + enzyme-treated erythrocytes → Hemolysis, agglutination, or sensitization. Antibody often complement-fixing IgM. Eluate generally nonreactive.
Drug adsorption to erythrocyte membrane (combination with high-titer serum antibodies to drug)	Penicillins, cephalosporins	History of large doses of drugs. Other allergic features may be absent. Usually subacute extravascular hemolysis.	IgG (strongly positive if hemolysis occurs). Rarely, weak complement sensitization also present.	Drug-coated erythrocytes + serum → Agglutinaton or sensitization (rarely hemolysis). High-titer antibody. Eluate reacts only with antibiotic-coated erythrocytes.
Membrane modification (non-immunologic adsorption of proteins to erythrocytes)	Cephalosporins	Hemolytic anemia rare.	Positive with reagents with antibodies to a variety of serum proteins.	Drug-coated erythrocytes + serum → Sensitization to antiglobulin antisera in low titer.
Unknown	Methyldopa	Gradual onset of hemolytic anemia. Common.	IgG (strongly positive if hemolysis occurs).	Antibody sensitizes normal erythrocytes without drug. Antibody in serum and eluate identical to warm antibody. No in vitro tests demonstrate relationship to drug.

Source: Adapted, with permission, from Garratty G, Petz LD: Drug-induced immune hemolytic anemia. *Am J Med* 1975;**58:**398.

classified as immune complex formation, hapten adsorption, nonspecific adsorption, and other, unknown mechanisms.

1. Immune-complex formation: Circulating preformed immune complexes between the drug and antibody to the drug sensitize the erythrocyte ("innocent-bystander" phenomenon). Quinine in low doses is a typical example. There is great variability in clinical features and serologic findings.

2. Drug (hapten) adsorption: The drug acts as a hapten in that it is bound to the erythrocyte membrane and stimulates the production of a high titer of antidrug antibodies.

3. Nonspecific adsorption: The drug affects the erythrocytes so that various nonimmunologic proteins are adsorbed onto erythrocytes and give a positive Coombs' test. This does not result generally in marked hemolysis.

4. Unknown mechanisms: This type is exemplified by the positive Coombs' test that develops within 3 months in 20% of patients treated with methyldopa. The IgG that coats erythrocytes in these patients does not have antibody activity against the drug, and the drug is not required in in vitro tests.

The hemolysis may be acute and severe, but only rarely is blood transfusion required. The main treatment is to stop the offending drug and monitor the patient to be sure the hemolysis disappears. The prognosis is therefore excellent.

4. PAROXYSMAL COLD HEMOGLOBINURIA

This rare disease may be transient or chronic and constitutes 10% of the cold autoimmune hemolytic anemias. It may occur as a primary idiopathic disease or secondary to syphilis or viral infection. It is characterized clinically by signs of hemolysis and hemoglobinuria following local or general exposure to cold. Symptoms may include combinations of fatigue; pallor; aching and pain in the back, legs, or abdomen; chills and fever; and the passing of dark brown urine. The symptoms may appear from within a few minutes to a few hours after exposure to cold.

The disease is characterized by the presence of the classic biphasic Donath-Landsteiner antibody. This polyclonal IgG antibody sensitizes erythrocytes in the cold (usually below 15 °C), so that complement components are detected on the erythrocytes by the direct antiglobulin test after rewarming. Heavily sensitized cells are hemolyzed when warmed to 37 °C. The antibody has specificity for the P antigen.

Acute attacks are treated symptomatically, and postinfectious cases generally resolve spontaneously, but transfusion is often necessary.

5. HEMOLYTIC DISEASE OF THE NEWBORN

Immunologic Pathogenesis

During pregnancy, very small amounts of fetal blood leak into the maternal circulation, especially during the last trimester but usually does not trigger antibody formation in the mother. During delivery, when the placenta is detached, bleeding of cord blood into the mother's circulation can elicit an immune response to fetal erythrocyte alloantigens.

Hemolytic disease of the newborn results from the mother's antibodies crossing the placenta and destroying fetal erythrocytes. This leads to hemolytic anemia and hydrops in the newborn infant. Hyperbilirubinemia occurs as a postnatal complication.

The first child is seldom affected by the hemolytic disease, but the chances for alloimmunization increase with each incompatible pregnancy. The primary stimulus for immunization can also be a previous blood transfusion or abortion.

Formation of Rh antibodies is the most common form of alloimmunization to give rise to clinically important disease. Antibodies to blood groups A and B (see Chapter 16) may also cause hemolysis of fetal cells if IgG maternal antibodies cross the placenta. In these cases, the mother usually belongs to group O and the baby to group A. In fact, ABO immunization during pregnancy occurs more often than Rh immunization, but it seldom results in serious problems. If the fetus secretes soluble A or B substances, the maternal antibodies become neutralized before they cause damage to erythrocytes, since A or B substances are also present on other tissues, including the placental endothelium.

Clinical Features

The most frequent signs in the newborn are anemia and rapidly developing jaundice, usually within the first 24 hours (in contrast to the physiologic icterus that occurs later). The infant's response to the anemia is marked reticulocytosis and erythroblastosis. As bilirubin accumulates in the plasma, it may cross the blood–brain barrier and cause damage to the nervous system (kernicterus). Severe alloimmunization causes fetal hydrops, and the fetus may die in utero. In these cases, if the father is homozygous for the relevant blood group, the prognosis is very poor for future babies.

Immunologic Diagnosis

Since the cause of the disease is antibody on erythrocyte membrane, the direct Coombs' test is usually positive. In ABO incompatibility, it is often negative. The reason for this is somewhat unclear, but the relatively small amount of IgG antibody and the adsorption by other tissues may result in so few antibody molecules on the erythrocyte surface that the conventional Coombs' method is not able to detect them. Thus, a negative direct Coombs' test does not rule out an immunologic cause for neonatal icterus. If antibodies are not found in the mother's serum, however, immune hemolysis is unlikely.

Alloimmunization should be detected during pregnancy. In many countries, all Rh-negative women are screened for the presence of blood group antibodies during pregnancy. As the number of D immunizations decreases, the relative proportion of immunizations to other blood groups has increased. Consequently, antibody screening should not be restricted to Rh-negative women. No reliable screening test is available for ABO disease, although several assays for detection of clinically important IgG anti-A or anti-B have been used.

When unexpected antibodies are found in the mother's serum, the father's blood groups should be determined. If the father is negative for the relevant blood group, there is no risk; if he is heterozygous, the baby has only a 50% chance of being affected. Increasing antibody titer or a history of previously ill children increases suspicion that the fetus can be affected, and amniocentesis is done to determine the concentration of bile pigments and possibly antibodies in the amniotic fluid. With these procedures and with ultrasound examination, the presence and seriousness of the hemolytic disease can be assessed. Detectable amounts of antibodies sometimes develop in the serum so late in the pregnancy that they remain unnoticed until the time of delivery. Alloimmunization should always be suspected if the bilirubin level starts rising rapidly in an anemic newborn infant.

Treatment & Prevention

Treatment is started during the last trimester of pregnancy if amniocentesis and antibody determinations indicate that the fetus has serious disease. Compatible blood is injected into the abdominal cavity of the fetus and is rapidly absorbed into the circulation. Direct intravascular transfusion may be achieved by fetoscopy as early as 18 weeks, but only in specialized centers. The blood should be free of viable leukocytes to avoid the risk of subsequent graft-versus-host disease. Intrauterine transfusions may help the fetus to survive until mature enough to live outside the uterus. The last weeks of pregnancy are the most critical time for the fetus. Careful monitoring of clinical data by the obstetrician and neonatologist may prompt a decision to deliver the affected baby prior to term.

Immediately after delivery, the infant's blood group is determined and the cord cells are tested by the direct Coombs' technique. If the baby is affected, exchange transfusions are usually needed, although in mild cases phototherapy with ultraviolet light or close supervision of bilirubin levels may be sufficient.

Women who have antibodies to the fetal erythrocytes should deliver in hospitals experienced in exchange transfusion. Despite modern advances in the treatment of hemolytic disease of the newborn, the mortality rate in severe intrauterine cases remains high.

Over 90% of Rh-negative women having Rh-positive offspring do not form anti-D antibodies. The immunization of the rest can be prevented by giving the mother 100 μg of concentrated anti-D (Rh$_o$) immunoglobulin within 72 hours of delivery if she does not have any preexisting anti-D antibodies. Since it is not possible to predict who will make antibodies, all Rh-negative women with an Rh-positive baby must be given prophylaxis. Since Rh antigens are detectable in an embryo a few weeks after conception, anti-D immunoglobulin should also be given to Rh-negative women who have aborted.

The mechanism of inhibition of antibody synthesis is unclear, but rapid destruction and clearance of Rh-positive cells from the circulation seem to play a role. In experimental conditions, Rh-positive cells coated with blood group antibodies other than anti-D are quickly destroyed and anti-D antibodies are not formed. Mothers with anti-A or anti-B antibodies reacting with fetal cells produce Rh antibodies less often than in ABO-compatible pregnancies.

Systematically applied anti-D prophylaxis has reduced the number of immunized women from about 7–8% to a little over 1% if measured by the number of Rh-negative women with antibodies after two consecutive Rh-positive babies. Several reasons have been suggested for the few failures: immunization early during the pregnancy (not starting at the time of delivery); abnormally large volume of fetal blood leaking into the maternal circulation with insufficient anti-D immunoglobulin; and unusual sensitivity of the maternal immune system to the antigen D.

PAROXYSMAL NOCTURNAL HEMOGLOBINURIA

Paroxysmal nocturnal hemoglobinuria (PNH) is a rare acquired disease that can occur in adults as a chronic hemolytic anemia with acute exacerbations. It may follow other hematologic disorders such as idiopathic or drug-induced bone marrow aplasia and may terminate in acute myelogenous leukemia. The intravascular hemolysis causes intermittent hemoglobinemia and hemoglobinuria. This activity fluctuates throughout the day, but the classic nocturnal timing of hemoglobinuria is seen in only 25% of cases. Venous thrombosis is a recognized complication.

The diagnosis is suggested by the findings of intermittent or chronic intravascular hemolysis, iron deficiency, hemosiderinuria, a low leukocyte alkaline phosphatase value, and frequently pancytopenia. The diagnosis of PNH is confirmed by any of the following tests: the acid hemolysis (Ham) test, the sugar water test, and the inulin test. These tests detect the abnormal clones with the two presently known abnormalities in PNH: the exquisite sensitivity of PNH erythrocytes to complement lysis and the abnormally low acetylcholinesterase activity in the erythrocyte membrane.

In PNH there is deficient synthesis by hematopoietic cells of the glycosyl-phosphatidylinositol molecules that anchor proteins to the cell membrane. Complement-mediated hemolysis is a prominent feature of the disease due to deficient cell surface expression of decay-accelerating factor (DAF), CD55, and CD59, which protect blood cells from the action of complement. DAF operates at the level of C3/C5 activation. DAF does not have a central role in controlling hemolysis of erythrocytes, but it regulates the deposition of C3 on nucleated cells. PNH arises from a mutant hemopoietic clone and this explains the association with several other blood disorders such as aplastic anemia and leukemia.

The end result is that cells from such patients are more easily destroyed by complement than are normal cells. Patients' cells are lysed by approximately 4% of the amount of complement required to lyse normal erythrocytes.

Treatment is mainly symptomatic but otherwise unsatisfactory. Transfusions are often required, and reactions are not infrequent. Androgens may be useful if there is underlying bone marrow hypoplasia. Corticosteroids and splenectomy are probably not useful. Rarely, bone marrow transplantation may be possible.

APLASTIC ANEMIA & RELATED DISORDERS

Some cases of aplastic anemia and related disorders may be immunologic in origin.

Pure Erythrocyte Aplasia

This rare form of anemia is characterized by a marked reduction or absence of bone marrow erythroblasts and blood reticulocytes, with normal granulopoiesis and thrombopoiesis. It occurs as an acquired disorder in adults, either in an idiopathic form or associated with thymoma (in 30–50% of cases), lymphoma, other tumors, or certain drugs. Patients usually present with progressive anemia requiring transfusion support. Bone marrow examination confirms the diagnosis. Thymoma is present in a small number of patients. Other immunologic abnormalities, such as hypogammaglobulinemia, monoclonal gammopathy, autoimmune hemolytic anemia, myasthenia gravis, and features of SLE may be seen in patients with pure erythrocyte aplasia.

Many patients with pure erythrocyte aplasia, with or without thymoma, have serum IgG antibodies that fix complement and are cytotoxic for bone marrow erythroblasts. This IgG antibody in plasma from patients with pure erythrocyte aplasia suppresses in vitro erythropoiesis by normal bone marrow.

Patients with pure erythrocyte aplasia usually require total erythrocyte transfusion support. Patients with thymomas should have these tumors removed, which produces a remission in about 30% of these patients. Patients with idiopathic pure erythrocyte aplasia and those who do not respond to thymectomy should be treated with intravenous gamma globulin (IVGG) if they do not have parvovirus infection, since some patients respond well to IVGG. If not, the next step is immunosuppressive drugs. Corticosteroids are usually used first, but few patients respond, and most are subsequently treated with cyclophosphamide plus prednisone. This combination produces remissions in 30–50% of patients, but relapses may occur when drugs are discontinued. Splenectomy has also been advocated for refractory pure erythrocyte aplasia, as has plasma exchange.

Diamond-Blackfan Syndrome

This disorder, also known as congenital hypoplastic anemia, represents the congenital form of pure erythrocyte aplasia seen in infants. Anemia is usually noted in the first year of life but may occur later. This syndrome must be distinguished from transient erythroblastopenia of infancy and childhood, which is a less serious, self-limited disorder.

The clinical features of this syndrome vary, and, although it is familial, no single genetic mode of transmission has been confirmed.

The abnormality appears to be mainly in early erythroid stem cells since erythropoietin is normal. Recent studies have suggested that responses may be obtained with GM-CSF and IL-3, and a reduction in transfusion requirements is obtained with these agents.

Aplastic Anemia

Aplastic anemia is defined as pancytopenia due to bone marrow aplasia. Patients with severe aplastic anemia have no hematopoietic precursor cells present in their bone marrow and must be supported with erythrocyte and platelet transfusions and antibiotics.

In the past, aplastic anemia was usually associated with exposure to toxic drugs or chemicals (benzene, chloramphenicol, arsenicals, gold, anticonvulsants, etc). Recent series, however, indicate that most patients have no such exposure and no other associated illness, so that they are classified as having idiopathic aplastic anemia. Such patients should be tested for HIV infection.

Lymphocytes from the bone marrow of about one third of patients with aplastic anemia suppress the growth of or kill granulocyte colonies from normal bone marrow in vitro. When these abnormal suppressor lymphocytes are separated from the marrow granulocytic stem cells or killed with a specific cytotoxic antilymphocyte serum, increased granulocyte colony formation occurs. Other investigators found that peripheral blood lymphocytes from patients with aplastic anemia may suppress erythropoiesis of normal bone marrow when cultured in vitro.

Problems in management exist with continuing transfusion support; even with optimal supportive care, severe aplastic anemia rarely undergoes spontaneous remission, and there is a 75–90% mortality rate. Trials have confirmed the efficacy of antilymphocyte globulin (ALG) in selected patients, with response in approximately 50% of patients. Treatment with high doses of androgens may benefit some patients, but few patients with severe aplasia respond. Treatment with GM-CSF, G-CSF, IL-3, or CSF-1 is only a short-term measure. Bone marrow transplantation produces long-term remissions in 50–80% of patients with severe aplastic anemia, and early bone marrow transplantation is currently considered the treatment of choice for patients with a histocompatibly matched donor.

Aplastic anemia, therefore, may result from different defects involving the stem cells, the hematopoietic environment, cytokines/hemolymphopoietic growth factors, or suppressor cells. Characterization of the nature of the defects would permit more rational management of aplastic anemia, since those cases with evidence of increased suppressor cell activity would be considered for treatment with immunosuppressive drugs or antithymocyte globulin (ATG) and those with obvious stem cell defects would be considered for early bone marrow transplantation.

PLATELET DISORDERS

Thrombocytopenia may be caused by decreased platelet production, increased platelet destruction, or abnormal platelet pooling. Immunologic thrombocytopenias, the subject of this section, are caused by increased platelet destruction, usually following platelet sensitization with antibody. Thrombocytopenias from decreased platelet production (aplastic anemia, leukemias, etc) have already been discussed with regard to immunologic features. Thrombocytopenia due to abnormal platelet pooling in an enlarged spleen (hypersplenism) is generally not associated with immunologic abnormalities.

Immunologic Mechanisms of Platelet Destruction

Several immunologic mechanisms of platelet damage leading to thrombocytopenia have been described. Platelet autoantibodies sensitize circulating platelets in idiopathic thrombocytopenic purpura and related disorders, leading to premature destruction of these cells in the spleen and generally involving Fc receptors on macrophages and other parts of the monocyte–machrophage system (see following section). Platelet alloantibodies may develop after multiple transfusions with blood products, or maternal sensitization can occur during pregnancies. Such platelet alloantibodies are becoming a major problem in long-term platelet support for patients with bone marrow failure. Alloantibodies may cause shortened platelet survival after transfusion or produce immediate platelet lysis with severe fever and chill reactions. Shortened platelet survival appears to be mediated by noncomplement-dependent IgG or IgM antibodies similar to autoantibodies seen in idiopathic thrombocytopenic purpura and platelet lysis by complement-dependent cytotoxic antibodies. These alloantibodies are directed primarily at human leukocyte antigens (HLA), but non-HLA platelet antigens may also be involved. Alloantibody-dependent lymphocyte-mediated cytotoxicity has also been described in some patients.

The classification of platelet-specific antigens has continued to pose problems. The antigens of the five human platelet antigen (HPA) systems are inherited in an autosomal-codominant manner. The clinically relevant platelet alloantigens have their origins in single amino acid substitutions within the polypeptide chain of the glycoprotein (GP) that bears the alloantigenic epitope. The original platelet antigen system was based on the name of the patients, but this has resulted in major problems with nomenclature. The new classification system, based on internationally agreed-on platelet antigen numbers, has not been universally accepted.

Other immunologic mechanisms of platelet destruction include development of antibodies to drugs or other antigenic substances (haptens) absorbed to the platelet membrane and adsorption of preformed antigen–antibody complexes onto the platelet membrane, with rapid removal of these sensitized cells from the circulation (innocent-bystander phenomenon). The reactions are often complement-dependent. These mechanisms occur in drug-induced immune thrombocytopenia, in some infections, especially HIV, and in autoimmune disorders such as SLE. It has been suggested that cell-mediated immunity, that is, lymphocyte activation, may alone be able to cause platelet damage and thrombocytopenia. Lymphocyte activation has been observed in response to autologous platelets in some patients with idiopathic thrombocytopenic purpura. Whether this represents a true cellular immune response or whether the lymphocytes are reacting to immune complexes or otherwise altered platelets remains uncertain. Finally, it is known that bacterial endotoxin can cause thrombocytopenia directly, usually involving activation of the complement system. Antibodies are not required for this reaction.

Table 35–6. Classification of immune thrombocytopenias.

Idiopathic (autoimmune) thrombocytopenic purpura (ITP)

Secondary autoimmune thrombocytopenias
  Systemic lupus erythematosus (SLE) and other autoimmune disorders
  Chronic lymphocytic leukemia, lymphomas, some nonlymphoid malignancies
  Human immunodeficiency virus (HIV) infection
  Infectious mononucleosis and some other infections

Drug-induced immune thrombocytopenias (partial list of drugs)

Acetazolamide	Imipramine
Allymid	Meprobamate
Aminosalicylic acid (PAS)	Methyldopa
Antazoline	Novobiocin
Apronalide	Phenolphthalein
Aspirin	Phenytoin
Carbamazepine	Quinidine
Cephalothin	Quinine
Chlorthiazide	Rifampin
Digitoxin	Spironolactone
Factor VIII concentrate	Stibophen
Heparin	Sulfamethazine
Hydrochlorothiazide	Thioguanine

Posttransfusion purpura

Thrombotic thrombocytopenic purpura (TTP)

Neonatal immune thrombocytopenias
  Due to autoantibodies (ITP)
  Due to alloantibodies (maternal sensitization)

Due to alloantibodies (destruction of transfused platelets)
  Sensitization from previous transfusions
  Maternal sensitization during pregnancies

Table 35–6 shows a classification of immunologic thrombocytopenias that are discussed in more detail in the following section.

IDIOPATHIC THROMBOCYTOPENIC PURPURA

Major Immunologic Features

- Antiplatelet antibodies are demonstrable on platelets and in serum.
- Platelet survival is shortened.
- There is a therapeutic response to prednisone and splenectomy.

General Considerations

Idiopathic thrombocytopenic purpura is an autoimmune disorder characterized by increased platelet destruction by antiplatelet autoantibody. IgG autoantibodies sensitize the circulating platelets, leading to accelerated removal of these cells by the macrophages of the spleen and at times of the liver and other components of the monocyte–macrophage system. Although there is a compensatory increase in platelet production by the bone marrow (total platelet turnover may be 10–20 times the normal rate), thrombocytopenia occurs, and, depending on the severity, gives rise to the two typical clinical features of the disease: purpura and bleeding.

Idiopathic thrombocytopenic purpura most often occurs in otherwise healthy children and young adults. Childhood idiopathic thrombocytopenic purpura often occurs within a few weeks following a viral infection, suggesting possible cross-immunization between viral and platelet antigens, or adsorption of immune complexes, or a hapten mechanism. Adult idiopathic thrombocytopenic purpura is less often associated with a preceding infection. An identical form of autoimmune thrombocytopenia can also be associated with SLE, chronic lymphocytic leukemia, lymphomas, nonlymphoid cancers, infectious mononucleosis, and other viral and bacterial infections. Certain drugs can also cause immune thrombocytopenia, and these can produce a clinical picture that is indistinguishable from idiopathic thrombocytopenic purpura.

Although adult and childhood idiopathic thrombocytopenic purpura appear to have similar basic pathophysiologic features, there are significant differences in their course and therefore their treatment. The features of idiopathic thrombocytopenic purpura in children and adults are compared in Table 35–7. Most children have spontaneous remissions within a few weeks to a few months, and splenectomy is rarely necessary. Adult patients, on the other hand, rarely have spontaneous remissions and usually require splenectomy within the first few months after diagnosis. HIV-associated immune thrombocytopenic purpura is recognized more frequently in patients with HIV who have not yet had an AIDS-defining disease.

Immunologic Diagnosis

W. Harrington and coworkers first showed in 1951 that the plasma from patients with idiopathic thrombocytopenic purpura caused thrombocytopenia when transfused into normal human recipients. Techniques to detect antiplatelet antibodies are shown in Table 35–8. Immunoinjury techniques (platelet factor 3 release, ^{14}C-serotonin release) detect antiplatelet antibodies in the serum of 60–70% of adult patients with idiopathic thrombocytopenic purpura. Other methods to show positive results in almost all patients with idiopathic thrombocytopenic purpura include methods to detect platelet–autoantibody complexes by lymphocyte activation or ingestion by granulocytes, or

Table 35–7. Idiopathic thrombocytopenic purpura in children and adults.

Parameter	Children	Adults
Peak age incidence (yr)	2–6	20–30
Sex incidence (M:F)	1:1	1:3
Clinical onset	Acute	Gradual
Antecedent infection	Common	Uncommon
Average duration of disease	1 mo	Months to years
Spontaneous remission	90%	10–20%
Presenting platelet count	$<20 \times 10^9$ L	$(30–50) \times 10^9$ L

Table 35–8. Tests for platelet autoantibodies in idiopathic thrombocytopenic purpura (ITP).

Method	Percent Positive
Standard immunologic tests (agglutination, complement fixation, etc)	0
Transfusion of plasma from patients with ITP into normal donors	63–75
Platelet factor 3 release	65–70
^{14}C-serotonin release	60
Lymphocyte activation by autologous platelets	70
Lymphocyte activation by platelet-antibody immune complexes	90+
Phagocytosis of platelet-antibody immune complexes by granulocytes	90+
Measurement of platelet-associated IgG by competitive binding assays	90+
Radiolabeled Coombs antiglobulin test	90+
Fluorescein-labeled Coombs antiglobulin	90+
Enzyme-linked immunosorbent assay (ELISA)	90+

competitive binding assays or antiglobulin tests for the measurement of antiplatelet antibodies on the platelet surface.

Platelet Kinetics

^{51}Cr-platelet kinetic studies show that all patients with idiopathic thrombocytopenic purpura and other types of autoimmune thrombocytopenia have markedly shortened platelet survival times ($t_{1/2}$ 0.1–30 hours; normal $t_{1/2}$ 100–120 hours) and have normal or only slightly subnormal platelet recoveries at t_0 (40–80%; normal 60–80%). About 75% of patients have splenic platelet sequestration, and 25% have both splenic and hepatic sequestration. Patients with thrombocytopenia due to an enlarged splenic platelet pool can be easily distinguished from patients with autoimmune thrombocytopenia by these kinetic methods. Both groups had an 85–90% complete remission rate at 2 years' follow-up postsplenectomy.

Clinical Features

A. Symptoms and Signs: The onset may be acute, with sudden development of petechiae; ecchymoses; epistaxis; and gingival, gastrointestinal, or genitourinary tract bleeding. More commonly, the disease is gradual in onset and chronic in course. Often, however, chronic idiopathic thrombocytopenic purpura is slowly progressive or suddenly becomes acute.

B. Laboratory Findings: The platelet count is usually less than 20,000–30,000/μL in acute cases and 30,000–100,000/μL in chronic cases. There may be moderate anemia due to blood loss and iron deficiency. The leukocyte count is normal or slightly increased but may be low in SLE. Platelets are often larger than normal on peripheral blood smear, and no immature leukocytes are present. The bone marrow shows normal or increased numbers of megakaryocytes and is otherwise normal. The megakaryocytes may be normal or immature in appearance but at times are larger than normal with increased numbers of nuclei.

Differential Diagnosis

All causes of thrombocytopenia must be considered when evaluating a patient with suspected idiopathic thrombocytopenic purpura (Table 35–9). Patients with idiopathic thrombocytopenic purpura characteristically feel and look well, and all physical and laboratory findings are normal except for thrombocytopenia and the associated purpura and possible bleeding. Patients with "consumptive" thrombocytopenias, on the other hand, tend to be acutely ill, often with fever and evidence of multisystem disease, especially renal disease. These patients generally have microangiopathic hemolytic anemia, the fragmented erythrocytes being a critical diagnostic finding on the peripheral blood smear. Abnormalities of clotting function are also often present. Patients with acute leukemia, aplastic anemia, and other serious bone marrow disorders are also often acutely ill, and bone marrow examination is diagnostic. Patients with hypersplenism sufficient to cause thrombocytopenia usually have an easily palpable spleen; hypersplenism alone rarely causes a platelet count of less than 50,000/µL.

Secondary causes of autoimmune thrombocytopenia, such as HIV infection and SLE, must be ruled out by appropriate laboratory tests. If a patient with apparent idiopathic thrombocytopenic purpura has been taking any suspicious drugs, the possibility of drug-induced thrombocytopenia must be considered. In some areas, HIV-associated disease is now the most common cause of thrombocytopenic purpura, especially in males between 20 and 50 years of age. Testing for antibodies to HIV is an essential part of the assessment of idiopathic thrombocytopenic purpura.

Treatment

Treatment of patients with idiopathic thrombocytopenic purpura is based mainly on clinical features and progress.

If the patient is asymptomatic and the platelet count remains over 30,000/µL, observation is the preferred approach.

Children with mild or moderately severe idiopathic thrombocytopenic purpura should be observed without therapy. In children who require active treatment, IVGG is the treatment of choice. A 5-day course of 400 mg/kg/d is given. Responses occur in 75% in 1–4 days, but many patients respond for only a short time, and repeat courses may be necessary.

Splenectomy is the treatment of choice for adult patients with idiopathic thrombocytopenic purpura who have persistent symptomatic thrombocytopenia. Corticosteroids (prednisone, 1–2 mg/kg/d) usually increase the platelet count temporarily but do not alter the course of the underlying disease, and most patients relapse when steroid use is tapered or discontinued. Adults rarely have spontaneous remissions, and splenectomy is therefore usually necessary within the first few months after diagnosis. Large doses of steroids over long periods should be avoided in these patients, since 75–90% will have prolonged complete remissions following splenectomy. Immunosuppressive therapy with cytotoxic drugs should generally not be used until the patient has had the benefit of splenectomy; this is particularly true for younger patients, since these drugs may cause serious late adverse effects.

Vincristine seems to be a valuable agent in treating patients with autoimmune thrombocytopenia who do not respond to splenectomy, who relapse after an initial response to splenectomy, or in whom the risk of splenectomy is unacceptable. A significant increase in platelet count occurs in 70–80% of patients with refractory autoimmune thrombocytopenia treated with vincristine. Vincristine appears to be more effective, less toxic, and better tolerated than cyclophosphamide or other standard immunosuppressive drugs. IVGG may be used as a short-term measure in adults prior to splenectomy, if corticosteroid therapy has failed to maintain a satisfactory platelet count at an acceptable dose. IVGG is also used in patients with HIV-associated immune thrombocytopenic purpura, prior to splenectomy, where one would prefer not to use long-term immunosuppressive and cytotoxic therapy. Zidovudine (AZT) is effective in raising platelet counts in patients with HIV-associated immune thrombocytopenic purpura.

Corticosteroids may be given when severe thrombocytopenia and bleeding occur in children, although the platelet count does not respond as consistently to steroids in children as in adults. Splenectomy should be considered in children only when severe

Table 35–9. Differential diagnosis of thrombocytopenic purpuras.

Thrombocytopenias due to increased platelet destruction
  Immune thrombocytopenias
    Idiopathic thrombocytopenic purpura
    Secondary autoimmune thrombocytopenias
    Drug-induced immune thrombocytopenias
    Posttransfusion purpura
    Neonatal immune thrombocytopenias
    Thrombocytopenia due to use of factor VIII concentrate
    HIV infection
  Consumptive thrombocytopenias
    Thrombotic thrombocytopenic purpura
    Hemolytic–uremic syndrome
    Disseminated intravascular coagulation
    Vasculitis
    Sepsis
  Hypersplenism
Thrombocytopenias due to decreased platelet production
  Bone marrow suppression by drugs, alcohol, toxins, infections
  Aplastic anemia
  Leukemias and other bone marrow cancers
  Megaloblastic anemia
  Refractory anemias, preleukemia, hematopoietic dysplasia

thrombocytopenia persists for 3–6 months, since most children will have had a spontaneous remission by that time. The postsplenectomy state is much more likely to predispose young children to serious or overwhelming infection than in adults. Immunosuppressive drugs should generally not be used in children.

DRUG-INDUCED IMMUNE THROMBOCYTOPENIAS

The principal drugs that may cause immune thrombocytopenic purpura are listed in Table 35–6. The best studied example was the sedative apronalide (Sedormid) (no longer in use); the drugs most commonly used in clinical practice that can produce immune thrombocytopenic purpura are sulfonamides, thiazide diuretics, chlorpropamide, quinidine, heparin, and gold. A syndrome resembling acute drug-induced immune thrombocytopenia has also been observed in heroin addicts. Further reports have confirmed the increasing frequency of the heparin-induced thrombosis thrombocytopenia syndrome. This unusual combination includes clinical features of hemorrhagic tendencies due to development of thrombocytopenia in patients treated with heparin for thrombosis. It appears that the heparin-dependent IgG-class antibody induces thromboxane synthesis and aggregation of the platelets.

There is a variable period of sensitization after initial exposure to the drug, but subsequent drug reexposure is rapidly followed by thrombocytopenia. Patients therefore usually give a history of having taken the drug in the past for at least several weeks if this is their first exposure. A very small plasma concentration of the drug and very small amounts of antibody may induce severe thrombocytopenia. The drug itself generally shows only weak and reversible binding to the platelet; the thrombocytopenia in most cases appears to be caused by adsorption of the drug–antibody complexes to the platelet membrane with complement activation.

Treatment consists mainly of withdrawal of the offending drug (or all drugs) and monitoring for return of normal platelet counts, generally within 7–10 days. Thrombocytopenia may persist if the drug is excreted slowly. When a patient who is taking a number of suspicious drugs is first seen, it is often impossible to tell whether the patient has drug-induced immune thrombocytopenia or idiopathic thrombocytopenic purpura. In vitro tests can now be used in some centers to confirm drug–antibody reactions involving platelets. In vivo drug challenges of sensitized patients for confirmation of drug-induced immune thrombocytopenia should be avoided, since they are too hazardous.

POSTTRANSFUSION PURPURA

There are two types of posttransfusion purpura. The first is due to dilution and occurs during massive blood replacement, as in the treatment of hemorrhage and shock. Further bleeding from the dilutional thrombocytopenia may complicate clinical management. The second type, which is due to alloantibodies, is an acute severe thrombocytopenic state appearing about 1 week after transfusion of a blood product. It occurs almost exclusively in women. It is mediated by an alloantibody, usually directed against the platelet Pl^{A1} antigen. Platelets both with and without the Pl^{A1} antigen are destroyed.

The diagnosis is suspected when acute thrombocytopenia occurs 7–10 days after blood transfusion. Coagulation studies are normal, and the bone marrow shows abundant megakaryocytes. The anti-Pl^{A1} antibody is detected in the plasma.

Gradual recovery from posttransfusion purpura usually occurs in 1–6 weeks. Corticosteroids do not appear to alter the course of the disease. Massive exchange transfusions have been associated with more rapid recovery, but severe transfusion reactions often occur. Aggressive plasma exchange has also been shown to be effective without the risks of severe transfusion reactions.

NEONATAL ALLOIMMUNE THROMBOCYTOPENIA

Neonatal alloimmune thrombocytopenia (NAIT) is a rare syndrome, occurring in approximately 1 in 5000 newborn infants as a result of maternal alloimmunization against a platelet-specific antigen on fetal platelets for which the mother is antigen-negative. The syndrome is characterized by an isolated, transient, severe thrombocytopenia due to platelet destruction by maternal IgG alloantibody that has crossed the placenta. It may result in serious intrauterine, neonatal, or perinatal immune thrombocytopenia, which may cause extensive hemostatic failure, especially intracerebral hemorrhage. It is now possible to establish immune thrombocytopenia, allowing for the cause of appropriate treatment and eventually the care of future pregnancies. Treatment in utero of fetomaternal alloimmunization has altered the natural course of fetal thrombocytopenia, assisting in the management of pregnancies at risk.

NAIT should be suspected in neonates with otherwise unexplained isolated thrombocytopenia and confirmed with demonstration of a platelet antibody in the mother's serum. The typical presentation for an infant with NAIT is dramatic petechiae, purpura, and extreme thrombocytopenia in an otherwise healthy infant. There is significant risk of serious, life-threatening hemorrhage. There is no significant obstetric history in the mother, the maternal platelet count is normal, and there is no present or past history of immune thrombocytopenia (ITP). If the mother or infant have other perinatal or hematologic problems, alternative diagnosis need to be considered to explain the thrombocytopenia, including maternal autoimmune or drug induced, preeclampsia hemolysis-elevated liver enzymes low platelet count syndrome (HELLP), sepsis, congenital viral infections, congenital bone marrow hypoplasia, osteopetrosis, prematurity, and birth asphyxia. Babies of first pregnancies are affected in about half the cases.

Treatment is dictated by the presence of bleeding and the degree of thrombocytopenia. Infants who are bleeding or severely thrombocytopenic should receive a platelet transfusion compatible with the mother's serum. Washed and irradiated maternal platelets are suitable. A single platelet transfusion is usually adequate. High-dose intravenous IgG (IVIG) can serve as an alternative form of treatment if compatible platelets cannot be procured. Pregnancies known to be at risk for NAIT should be monitored with ultrasound examinations from about the twentieth week of gestation. Fetal blood sampling for platelet count and allotype should be considered around 20 weeks. This should be performed at a center experienced in percutaneous umbilical cord blood sampling (PUBS) and capable of preparing maternal platelets for transfusion. The importance of cooperative care among the obstetrician, hematologist, and neonatologist cannot be overemphasized. Accurate assessment of the past obstetric and transfusion history is important. Before the next pregnancy or early in subsequent pregnancies, the the father's platelets should be phenotyped to determine if all subsequent infants will have the target antigen.

THROMBOTIC THROMBOCYTOPENIC PURPURA

Thrombotic thrombocytopenic purpura (TTP) is a rare potentially fulminant and life-threatening disorder characterized by platelet microthrombi in small vessels resulting in organ dysfunction and a microangiopathy. Coagulation activation is not a prominent feature. The clinical syndrome is manifest by the pentad of thrombocytopenia, microangiopathic hemolytic anemia, fever, renal dysfunction, and neurologic abnormalities. Abdominal symptoms, hepatic dysfunction, and pulmonary abnormalities may also occur. With the clinical features and a microangiopathic blood smear with thrombocytopenia the diagnosis is relatively easy. The acute form of the condition can be fulminant and life-threatening and in the past was rapidly fatal in the majority of patients.

The pathophysiology of this syndrome is enigmatic and the mechanisms may not be the same in individual cases, and there could be a final common pathway for a variety of initiating causes. Pathologically, there appears to be an abnormal interaction between the vascular endothelium and platelets, but the primary event remains undertain. In some cases there may be circulating platelet-aggregating factors or abnormalities in high-molecular-weight von Willebrand factor (vWF) multimers that mediate the platelet aggregation.

There is a primary idiopathic form that usually has an acute presentation and probably has an underlying autoimmune mechanism. This form may be associated with a variety of prodromal infections (viral—CMV, HIV, herpes—and bacterial) and typically may occur in the third trimester of pregnancy. Bacterial cytotoxins, produced by *Shigella dysenteriae* I and certain *Escherichia coli* serotypes, have been related to TTP and hemolytic–uremic syndrome (HUS) probably in initiating damage to vascular endothelial cells, possibly via cytokine mechanisms. TTP may be associated with various drugs (cytotoxic agents), toxins, and bites. Chemotherapy-associated TTP/HUS may be associated with a range of cytotoxic medications, especially mithromycin. Pathogenesis may be related to drug toxicity on endothelial cells in the kidney microvasculature or the formation of soluble circulating platelet aggregators, such as immune complexes, autoantibodies, or abnormal amounts of large-molecular-weight vWF multimers from stimulated endothelial cells. Severe microangiopathy resembling TTP has also been reported as a complication of acute graft-versus-host disease in patients receiving cyclosporine, prophylaxis following allogeneic bone marrow transplantation. It is hypothesized that cytokines may induce the endothelial damage.

In the past TTP was fatal in 90% of patients, but dramatic improvement in its outcome has occurred over the past two decades with the development of effective therapy. Plasma infusion or exchange have become the cornerstones of the treatment of TTP. Cryoprecipitate-poor plasma (depleted in vWF) may offer advantages over whole fresh-frozen plasma. It is now possible to achieve remissions in the majority of patients, and cures are now common, but unfortunately up to half the patients relapse. The clinical course at relapse is usually milder than the disease at presentation, and less aggressive therapy may be needed. Patients resistant to this approach may respond to alternative therapy, including high-dose intravenous immunoglobulin, dextran, platelet inhibitory drugs, corticosteroids, vincristine, or splenectomy.

HEMOLYTIC–UREMIC SYNDROME

This syndrome has many similarities to TTP, but renal involvement is the hallmark in association with microangiopathic hemolytic anemia and thrombocytopenia. It usually occurs in children, related to bacterial or viral infections. It may rarely be seen in adults, in whom the disease is commonly drug-related and may take a more chronic and serious course. Quinine-associated hemolytic–uremic syndrome has been recently described and probably occurs more often than is recognized. It is important to recognize this syndrome in order to avoid further quinine exposure. The prognosis and approach to management of HUS is similar to that for TTP.

QUININE-INDUCED IMMUNE THROMBOCYTOPENIA WITH HEMOLYTIC–UREMIC SYNDROME

Quinine-induced immune thrombocytopenia with HUS is a recently defined clinical entity. The disease is characterized by the onset of chills, sweating, nausea and vomiting, abdominal pain, oliguria, and petechial rash following quinine exposure. Anemia, severe thrombocytopenia, increased serum lactate dehydrogenase levels, and azotemia are noted. Quinine-dependent platelet-reactive antibodies can usually be identified. Patients are treated with plasma exchange (range 1–12 procedures) and may also require hemodialysis. All survive without residual abnormality. Adult patients presenting with HUS should routinely be asked about exposure to quinine in the form of medication or beverages. The mechanism of renal failure is unclear but may be due to drug-induced antibodies reactive with endothelial cells leading to margination of granulocytes in renal glomeruli. Quinine-induced HUS has a better prognosis than other forms of adult HUS.

COAGULATION DISORDERS

HEMOPHILIA & VON WILLEBRAND'S DISEASE

Classic hemophilia and von Willebrand's disease (vWD) are both congenital bleeding disorders caused by abnormalities of the factor VIII molecule complex. Hemophilia is an X-linked disorder characterized by severe deficiency of factor VIII procoagulant activity (VIII:C), which is measured in clotting assays. Von Willebrand's disease is an autosomally inherited disorder also characterized by a deficiency of VIII:C, but it is also associated with defective platelet function, resulting in a prolonged bleeding time. The abnormal platelet function in von Willebrand's disease is due to a deficiency of factor VIII-related protein (VIIIR), which is also known as von Willebrand factor (vWF). vWF activity is measured by testing the ability of plasma to support platelet agglutination by the antibiotic ristocetin or ristocetin cofactor (VIIIR:RC) activity.

Von Willebrand's disease is the commonest congenital bleeding disorder and is due to quantitative or qualitative defects of von Willebrand factor (the pivotal protein in platelet adhesion) and thrombus formation at sites of vascular injury. Molecular defects in vWF and its receptors are responsible for the heterogeneity of the disease. Recently the disease was classified into four groups based on specific pathophysiologic features and therapy for the prevention and treatment of bleeding episodes.

Quantitative Deficiency
- Partial: Type I (75–80%)
- Total: Type III (rare <5%)

Qualitative Defects: Type II
- Type IIA: Platelet function is impaired, and high-molecular-weight (HMW) multimers are absent.
- Type IIB: Affinity vWF for platelet GPIb is associated with thrombocytopenia.
- Type IIM: Platelet-dependent function is impaired, HMW multimers=N, GPIb affinity occurs.
- Type IIN: FVIII affinity to platelets leads to increased VIII clearance.

Acquired vWD has been described in association with autoimmune disorders, monoclonal gammopathies, and chronic lymphoproliferative and myeloproliferative diseases. Possible mechanisms include autoantibodies against the vWF, abnormal adsorption of vWF to tumor cells, and increased plasma clearance of vWF.

The gene for factor VIII is located near the tip of the long arm of the X chromosome (Xq2.9/Ter). The large gene has approximately 186 kb with 27 exons. Defects in the hemophilia A gene include point mutations and partial deletions, so there is heterogeneity in defective factor VIII molecules.

Heterogeneous antibodies made to purified factor VIII are able to detect antigenic determinants on VIIIR (VIIIR:Ag). VIIIR:Ag has been found to be normal in patients with classic hemophilia, indicating that these patients have a normal amount of the basic factor VIII molecule but that they lack the portion of the molecule necessary for normal procoagulant activity. The heterologous antibodies therefore appear to recognize antigenic determinants distinct from the functional site responsible for procoagulant activity. Patients with von Willebrand's disease, on the other hand, have reduced levels of both VIII:C and VIIIR:Ag, indicating a true deficiency of factor VIII complex molecules. Measurement of VIII:C and VIIIR:Ag can therefore be used to differentiate between classic hemophilia and von Willebrand's disease and in most cases can differentiate between female carriers of hemophilia (heterozygotes) and normal individuals. Measurement of ristocetin cofactor (VIIIR:RC) can also be used to identify patients with von Willebrand's disease. Studies with antibodies have helped to clarify the relationships of the factor VIII complex.

Prenatal diagnosis is now possible for hemophilia A with a chorionic villus biopsy and restriction fragment length polymorphism methods or a polymerase chain reaction (PCR) assay.

Human antibodies to factor VIII, unlike heterologous antibodies, are usually directed at antigenic determinants at the functional procoagulant site of factor VII (VIII:CAg), and these antibodies are capable of blocking factor VIII clotting activity. These antibodies sometimes develop in patients with severe hemophilia after they have been transfused with factor VIII-containing blood products and sometimes develop spontaneously in otherwise healthy individuals. When present in high titer, they cause a severe hemorrhagic disorder that is difficult to correct with factor VIII transfusions, since the transfused factor VIII is simply inactivated by the factor VIII antibodies (see next section).

Most hemophiliacs treated in the early 1980s with factor VIII concentrate have developed AIDS, and AIDS is now the most common cause of death in hemophiliacs. Centers switched from treating the hemophiliac with factor VIII concentrate from large donor pools back to using cryoprecipitate from a single donor. Infectivity can be abolished by heating the preparation.

Recombinant engineered factor VIII is now available to overcome problems with supply, purity, and cross-infection.

CIRCULATING INHIBITORS OF COAGULATION

Abnormal bleeding is occasionally due to circulating inhibitors that block one or more plasma coagulation factors. These inhibitors, also called endogenous circulating anticoagulants, have in most cases been shown to be IgG antibodies. Inhibitors against factor VIII and against the prothrombin activator complex ("lupus inhibitor") occur most often, but inhibitors directed against factors V, IX, XIII, and vWF have also been reported. There are rare reports of human monoclonal proteins (especially IgM) with antibody activity directed against clotting components, for example factor VIII, phospholipid. Inhibitors may appear abruptly and be associated with life-threatening hemorrhage or may be chronic and associated with little or no bleeding.

Factor VIII inhibitors develop in 15% of patients with classic hemophilia after they have been transfused with factor VIII-containing blood products; genetic factors sppear to determine which patients develop inhibitors. Factor VIII inhibitors also occasionally occur spontaneously in women postpartum, in patients with autoimmune disorders such as SLE, and in older patients without demonstrable underlying disease. Rarely, the paraprotein in a monoclonal gammopathy has specific inhibitor activity against factor VIII or other clotting factors.

High-titer factor VIII inhibitors (antibodies) often cause serious bleeding and require aggressive treatment. Patients with serious bleeding can be given several times the calculated amount of factor VIII to saturate the inhibitor, provided the inhibitor titer is not too high. When bleeding cannot be stopped, even after giving large amounts of factor VIII, activated prothrombin complex concentrates should be given, since these often stop the bleeding by providing activated clotting factors that bypass the factor VIII step. If this is unsuccessful, aggressive large-volume plasma exchange can be used to remove the inhibitor.

Combination therapy with factor VIII, cyclophosphamide, vincristine, and prednisone (CVP) is highly effective in the eradication of factor VIII inhibitors in nonhemophiliacs, but not in hemophiliacs.

ANTICARDIOLIPIN ANTIBODY SYNDROME

Major Immunologic Features

- Anticardiolipin antibodies (IgG or IgM class) are present.
- Ninety percent of patients with lupus anticoagulants also have anticardiolipin antibody.
- Eleven percent of anticardiolipin antibodies cross-react with heparin and heparan sulfate.
- There is frequent association with SLE.

General Considerations

Anticardiolipin antibody syndrome comprises a clinical diagnosis of arterial or venous thrombosis, thrombocytopenia, or recurrent fetal loss and a laboratory results of positive tests for IgG-class or IgM-class anticardiolipin antibodies or lupus anticoagulants on at least two occasions 12 weeks apart.

The female-to-male ratio is 2:1, and smoking, hyperlipidemia, and hypertension are risk factors.

The condition is primary if associated autoimmune disease (especially SLE) has been excluded. There are no clear differences in major features or treatment of primary or secondary anticardiolipin antibody syndrome.

Immunologic Pathogenesis

The cause of the production of these antibodies is not known, but frequently an infection precedes the development and detection of the various antibodies. In some cases the antiphospholipid antibodies appear to follow the use of drugs, such as procainamide, hydralazine, chlorpromazine, quinidine, isoniazide, methyldopa.

Cross-reactivity between these antibodies and natural body components may account for some features. Thus, 11% of anticardiolipin antibodies cross-react with the glycosaminoglycans heparin and heparan sulfate, and thereby impair the heparin-dependent antithrombin III inhibition of thrombin. Other proposed mechanisms by which anticardiolipin antibodies promote thrombosis include platelet activation, inhibition of prostacyclin production, interference with protein C, and initiation of vascular injury.

Clinical Features

A. Symptoms and Signs:

1. Venous Thrombosis: This may occur in up to 50% of patients (especially younger patients) and included deep venous thrombosis, venous thromboembolism, and thrombosis at unusual sites.

2. Arterial Ischaemic and Infarct Syndromes: These may take various forms and occur in up to 50% of patients and include stroke, transient ischemic attacks, multi-infarct dementia, migraine headaches; myocardial infarction; vasculitic rashes and arthralgias in 50%; digital infarcts or skin necrosis; pulmonary hypertension; retinal artery or venous occlusion, amaurosis fugax; splenic infarction or hyposplenism; adrenal infarction and hemorrhage; and livedo reticularis and multiple ischemic cerebrovascular lesions (Sneddon's syndrome).

3. Recurrent Fetal Loss: This may occur in up to 35% of female patients. IgG or IgM anticardiolipin antibodies occur in 2% of women with one or two fetal losses, 9% of women with two losses and 10% of women with three or more. Anticardiolipin antibodies may occur with severe preeclampsia late in the second or early in the third trimester.

4. Cardiac Abnormalities: Valvular insufficiency or stenosis may result from verrucous endocardial lesions or Libman-Sacks endocarditis. There is a strong association with anticardiolipin antibodies in patients with SLE.

5. Autoimmune Hemolytic Anemia: Anticardiolipin antibodies may have a direct role in the production of hemolytic anemia in some patients with SLE by acting as autoantibodies to red blood cells.

6. Drug-Induced ACLAS: This syndrome may appear following drug treatment, and many patients show features of SLE. The drugs include procainamide, hydralazine, chlorpromazine, quinidine, isoniazide, and methyldopa. More frequently, patients treated with drugs who develop autoantibodies are asymptomatic. These antibodies include anticardiolipin (especially IgM class), lupus anticoagulants, and ANA and DNA antibodies.

7. Association with Infections: It is uncommon to find the clinical features of ACLAS although it is common for anticardiolipin antibodies and lupus antioagulants to develop with an infection and disappear with resolution of the infection. Infections include syphilis; Lyme disease; and viral infections due to adenovirus, rubella, chickenpox, and HIV.

B. Laboratory Findings

1. Thrombocytopenia: Thrombcytopenia occurs in 30–50%, especially in patients with SLE.

2. Anticardiolipin Antibody: Cofactor (β_2-glycoprotein)-dependent anticardiolipin antibodies have been associated with autoimmune disease and the presence of clinical manifestations of the syndrome. This is in contrast to cofactor-independent anticardiolipin antibodies in which the association is with infectious diseases and drug-induced anticardiolipin antibodies.

Lupus anticoagulant activity is demonstrated on two occasions, 12 weeks apart, in 50% of patients. Antiphospholipid antibodies that prolong the phospholipid-dependent coagulation assays. Not all reagents in clotting assays are equally sensitive to lupus anticoagulant. The combination of anticardiolipin antibody and β_2-glycoprotein is essential for binding to cardiolipin and lupus anticoagulant activity. Low β_2-glycoprotein levels (<50 mg/L) may result in false-negative lupus anticoagulant tests.

3. Other Serology: ANA is present in 50% in low titer 1/40–1/160. Antibodies to single-stranded DNA are frequent. Occasionally the Coombs' direct antiglobulin test is positive with associated autoimmune hemolytic anemia. Antibodies to double-stranded DNA and ENA are negative.

Treatment

Treatment of the clinical features of anticardiolipin antibody syndrome remains controversial and is often unsatisfactory. This is partly because of the multifactorial nature of the syndrome, partly because definition of the syndrome is still developing, and partly because of the marked clinical variability.

If SLE is associated with the syndrome, then treatment of the underlying SLE is a priority (see Chapter 00). With mild thrombotic symptoms, aspirin is the most common first-line drug therapy. With more severe thrombotic features, more aggressive anticoagulant treatment is given, with varying claims for its efficacy. Corticosteroid therapy is often used now in women with the syndrome who experience recurrent early fetal loss to attempt to achieve a viable fetus.

REFERENCES

LEUKOPENIAS

Christie DJ: Specificity of drug-induced immune cytopenias. *Transf Med Rev* 1993;**7**:230.

Hartman KR: Anti-neutrophil antibodies of the immunoglobulin M class in autoimmune neutropenia. *Am J Med Sci* 1994;**308**:102.

Levine JD et al: Recombinant human granulocyte–macrophage colony-stimulating-factor ameliorates zidovudine-induced neutropenia in patients with acquired immunodeficiency syndrome (AIDS)/AIDS-related complex. *Blood* 1991;**78**:3148.

Martino R et al: Combined autoimmune cytopenias. *Haematologica* 1995;**80**:305.

Martino R et al: Successful treatment of chronic autoimmune neutropenia with cyclosporine A. *Haematologica* 1994;**79**:66.

Postiglione K et al: Immune mediated agranulocytosis and anemia associated with thymoma. *Am J Hematol* 1995;**49**:336.

Robinson BE, Quesenberry PJ: Hematopoietic growth factors: Overview and clinical applications. *Am J Med Sci* 1990;**300**:163, 237, 311. (Three parts.)

Shastri KA, Logue GL: Autoimmune neutropenia. *Blood* 1993;**81**:1984.

Shulman NR, Reid DM: Mechanisms of drug-induced immunologically mediated cytopenias. *Transf Med Rev* 1993;**7**:215.

Stroneck DF: Drug-induced immune neutropenia. *Transf Med Rev* 1993;**7**:268.

Verhoef G, Boogaerts M: In vivo administration of granulocyte–macrophage colony-stimulating factor enhances neutrophil function in patients with myelodysplastic syndromes. *Br J Haematol* 1991;**79**:177.

ERYTHROCYTE DISORDERS

Beal RW, Isbister JP: *Blood Component Therapy in Clinical Practice.* Blackwell, 1985.

Bourantas K: High-dose recombinant human erythropoietin and low-dose corticosteroids for treatment of anemia in paroxysmal nocturnal hemoglobinuria. *Acta Haematol* 1994;**91**:62.

Contreras MC: Antenatal tests in the diagnosis and assessment of severity of haemolytic disease (hd) of the fetus and newborn (hdn). *Vox Sang* 1994;**67**(suppl 3):207.

Gilsanz F et al: Acquired pure red cell aplasia. A study of six cases. *Ann Hematol* 1995;**71**:181.

Griscelli-Bennaceur A et al: Aplastic anemia and paroxysmal nocturnal hemoglobinuria: Search for a pathogenetic link. *Blood* 1995;**85**:1354.

Jefferies LC: Transfusion therapy in autoimmune hemolytic anemia. *Hematol Oncol Clin North Am* 1994;**8**:1087.

Korbling M et al: Allogeneic blood stem cell transplantation: Peripheralization and yield of donor-derived primitive hematopoietic progenitor cells (CD34+ Thy-1dim) and lymphoid subsets, and possible predictors of engraftment and graft-versus-host disease. *Blood* 1995;**86**:2842.

Mahbub B et al: Decay-accelerating factor-deficient erythrocytes during the long-term clinical course of patients with paroxysmal nocturnal hemoglobinuria. *Acta Haematol* 1995;**93**:91.

Nakakuma H et al: Paroxysmal nocturnal hemoglobinuria clone in bone marrow of patients with pancytopenia. *Blood* 1995;**85**:1371.

Narayanan MN et al: Long term follow-up of aplastic anemia. *Br J Haematol* 1994;**86**:837.

Noble AL et al: Predicting the severity of haemolytic disease of the newborn: An assessment of the clinical usefulness of the chemiluminescence test. *Br J Haematol* 1995;**90**:718.

Petz LD: Drug-induced autoimmune hemolytic anemia. *Transf Med Rev* 1993;**7**:242.

Rosse WF, Ware RE: The molecular basis of paroxysmal nocturnal hemoglobinuria. *Blood* 1995;**86**:3277.

Zon LI: Developmental biology of hematopoiesis. *Blood* 1995;**86**:2876.

PLATELET DISORDERS

Blanchette VS et al: Role of intravenous immunoglobulin G in autoimmune hematologic disorders. *Semin Hematol* 1992;**29**(suppl 2):72.

Goldman M et al: Neonatal alloimmune thrombocytopenia. *Transf Med Rev* 1994;**8**:123.

Gottschall JL et al: Quinine-induced immune thrombocytopenia with hemolytic uremic syndrome: Clinical and serological findings in nine patients and review of literature. *Am J Hematol* 1994;**47**:283.

Imbach WF: Immune thrombocytopenia in children. The immune character of destructive thrombocytopenia and the treatment of bleeding. *Semin Thromb Hemost* 1995;**21**:305.

Kaplan C et al: Management of fetal and neonatal alloimmune thrombocytopenia. *Vox Sang* 1994;**67**(suppl 3):85.

Linares M et al: Chronic idiopathic thrombocytopenic purpura in the elderly. *Acta Haematol* 1995;**93**:80.

McFarand JG: Laboratory investigation of drug-induced immune thrombocytopenias. *Transf Med Rev* 1993;**7**:275.

Panzer S et al: Maternal alloimmunization against fetal platelet antigens: A prospective study. *Br J Haematol* 1995;**90**:655.

Reiner A et al: Pulse cyclophosphamide therapy for refractory autoimmune thrombocytopenic purpura. *Blood* 1995;**85**:351.

Rutherford CJ, Frenkel ER: Thrombocytopenia. Issues in diagnosis and therapy. *Med Clin North Am* 1994;**78**:555.

Stasi R et al: Long-term observation of 208 adults with chronic idiopathic thrombocytopenic purpura. *Am J Med* 1995;**98**:436.

Taub JW et al: Characterization of autoantibodies against the platelet glycoprotein antigens IIb/IIIa in childhood idiopathic thrombocytopenic purpura. *Am J Hematol* 1995;**48**:104.

Udom-Rice I, Bussel JB: Fetal and neonatal thrombocytopenia. *Blood Rev* 1995;**9**:57.

COAGULATION DISORDERS

Aledort L: Inhibitors in hemophilia patients. Current status and management. *Am J Hematol* 1994;**47**:208.

Ames PRJ et al: Antiphospholipid antibodies, haemostatic variables and thrombosis—A survey of 144 patients. *Thromb Haemost* 1995;**73**:768.

Antonarakis SE: Molecular genetics of coagulation factor VIII gene and hemophilia A. *Thromb Haemost* 1995;**74**:322.

Baker WF Jr, Bick RL: Antiphospholipid antibodies in coronary artery disease. A review. *Semin Thromb Hemost* 1994;**20**:27.

Bick RL, Baker WF Jr: The antiphospholipid and thrombosis syndromes. *Med Clin North Am* 1994;**78**:667.

Evatt BL: AIDS and hemophilia-current issues. *Thromb Haemost* 1995;**74**:36.

Furie B et al: A practical guide to the evaluation and treatment of hemophilia. *Blood* 1994;**84**:3.

Ginsberg JS et al: Antiphospholipid antibodies and venous thromboembolism. *Blood* 1995;**86**:3685.

Harris EN, Pierangeli SS: Anticardiolipin and lupus anticoagulant testing and significance. *J Clin Immunoassay* 1994;**17**:108.

Hinton RC: Neurological syndromes associated with antiphospholipid antibodies. *Semin Thromb Hemost* 1994;**20**:46.

Hoyer LW, Scandella D: Factor VIII inhibitors: Structure and function in autoantibody and hemophilia A patients. *Semin Hematol* 1994;**31**(suppl 4):1.

Kampe CE: Clinical syndromes associated with lupus anticoagulants. *Semin Thromb Hemost* 1994;**20**:16.

Khamashta MA et al: The management of thrombosis in the antiphospholipid-antibody syndrome. *N Engl J Med* 1995;**332**:993.

Lethagen S: Desmopressin (DDAVP) and hemostasis. *Ann Hematol* 1994;**69**:173.

Ludlam CA et al: Treatment of acquired hemophilia. *Semin Hematol* 1994;**31**(suppl 4):16.

Lusher JM: Response to 1-deamino-8-D-arginine vaso-pressin in von Willebrand disease. *Haemostasis* 1994;**24**:276.

Lynch A et al: Antiphospholipid antibodies in predicting adverse pregnancy outcome: A prospective study. *Ann Intern Med* 1994;**120**:470.

Ordi-Ros J et al: Clinical and therapeutic aspects associated to phospholipid binding antibodies (lupus anticoagulant and anticardiolipin antibodies). *Haemostasis* 1994;**24**:165.

Rick ME: Diagnosis and management of von Willebrand's syndrome. *Med Clin North Am* 1994;**78**:609.

Ruggeri ZM: Pathogenesis and classification of von Willebrand disease. *Haemostasis* 1994;**24**:265.

Sadler JE et al: Molecular mechanism and classification of von Willebrand disease. *Thromb Haemost* 1995;**74**:161.

Schwartz RS et al: A prospective study of treatment of acquired (autoimmune) factor VIII inhibitors with high-dose intravenous gammaglobulin. *Blood* 1995;**86**:797.

Thompson AR: Progress towards gene therapy for the hemophilias. *Thromb Haemost* 1995;**74**:36.

Cardiac & Vascular Diseases

36

Thomas R. Cupps, MD

CARDIAC DISEASES

A variety of immunologic diseases probably involve cardiac tissues without causing any clinically relevant effects; nevertheless, there are several recognized syndromes characterized by clinically significant immune-mediated damage of the pericardium, myocardium, and endocardium.

PERICARDIAL DISEASES

Relapsing Pericarditis
This is a disease of unknown cause, characterized by chronic recurrent episodes of pericardial inflammation. Other disease processes associated with pericarditis, including infection, neoplasm, and collagen vascular disease, should be actively excluded. Chest pain and shortness of breath with or without pericardial effusion make up the characteristic pattern during an episode of pericarditis. Complications including pericardial tamponade, hemopericardium, and constrictive pericarditis have been reported. Nonsteroidal anti-inflammatory drugs, such as aspirin and ibuprofen, constitute the initial form of treatment. Some patients with relapsing pericarditis develop a chronic pattern, which requires treatment with corticosteroids. A subset of these patients may become corticosteroid-dependent, requiring a brief course of more aggressive immunosuppressive treatment. Pericardiectomy may be considered in patients who cannot be successfully treated medically.

An immunologic pathogenesis for this disease is presumed, largely on the basis of histopathology, which includes infiltration by acute and chronic inflammatory cells and fibrin deposition.

Postinfarction Syndrome & Postpericardiotomy Syndrome
Pericardial inflammation also occurs following damage to cardiac tissue after myocardial infarction,

cardiac surgery, or trauma. **Postinfarction (Dressler's) syndrome** is characterized by chest pain, profound malaise, fever, pericardial inflammation and effusion, leukocytosis with or without pleural effusion, pulmonary infiltrates, arthralgia, or transient arthritis that develops 2–3 weeks following surgical or traumatic opening of the pericardium. The presence of myocyte antibodies detected by immunofluorescence and rising titers of antiviral antibodies suggests that these syndromes may be associated with a concurrent or reactivated viral illness triggering the immunologic response that produces the characteristic clinical syndrome. Increasing titers of antibodies to coxsackie virus type B, cytomegalovirus, and adenovirus occur frequently. The response is therefore not limited to a particular type of virus. The postinfarction syndrome occurs in 3% or fewer of patients with myocardial infarction and is very rare in patients receiving thrombolytic therapy. The presence of a pericardial friction rub during the first several days after infarction increases the likelihood of developing the syndrome. The **postpericardiotomy syndrome** occurs in approximately 25% of patients following surgical intervention or blunt trauma to the heart. Rare complications include pericardial tamponade and restrictive pericarditis. Nonsteroidal anti-inflammatory drugs suppress the clinical symptoms in most cases. A brief course of corticosteroid therapy may be required in the more severe cases. These syndromes generally run a self-limited course lasting several weeks to several months.

MYOCARDIAL DISEASES

Autoimmune Myocarditis
This is a rare disease characterized by an aberrant immune response that damages myocardial tissue and is generally seen as part of a systemic autoimmune syndrome. Autoimmune myocarditis is associated most commonly with polymyositis–dermatomyositis and systemic lupus erythematosus (SLE) and less

commonly with rheumatoid arthritis, scleroderma, mixed connective tissue disease, and sarcoidosis. Little is known about the etiology of autoimmune myocarditis. The presence of mononuclear cell infiltrates in the myocardium and the association with immunologically mediated diseases suggest an autoimmune pathogenesis. Autoimmune myocarditis may present with signs and symptoms of congestive heart failure, arrhythmias, or conduction abnormalities. Chest pain from an associated pericarditis may also be present. Findings on chest radiograph, echocardiogram, and electrocardiogram may reflect diffuse myocardial dysfunction and rhythm or conduction abnormalities. Other laboratory studies may suggest the diagnosis of an associated autoimmune disease. There is an increased occurrence of the antiribonucleoprotein (RNP) autoantibody in patients with SLE who develop autoimmune myocarditis. Autoimmune myocarditis generally responds rapidly and dramatically to corticosteroid therapy. The outlook is generally favorable, with the patient's prognosis being determined by the underlying disease.

Autoimmune myocarditis is differentiated clinically from viral myocarditis by its association with SLE, rheumatoid arthritis, myositis, and, less commonly, scleroderma. Favorable response to immunosuppressive and anti-inflammatory treatment is also a distinguishing feature. The histopathology of mononuclear cell infiltration in autoimmune and viral pericarditis is identical, however.

Dilated Cardiomyopathy

A subset of patients with dilated cardiomyopathy may have a component of myocarditis. This disease is associated with low cardiac output and ejection fraction, in contrast to the hypertrophic and restrictive forms of cardiomyopathy. Transvenous endomyocardial biopsy studies in patients with nonischemic dilated cardiomyopathy demonstrate a 15–25% prevalence of myocarditis. The clinical presentation, including signs and symptoms associated with congestive heart failure and disturbances in rhythm and conduction is similar whether or not myocarditis is present. Treatment with immunosuppressive drugs including corticosteroids may result in a short-term improvement in myocardial function but does not appear to alter the long-term prognosis. The prolonged use of immunosuppressive therapy does not produce sustained clinical benefit in patients with inflammatory dilated cardiomyopathy. Treatment is directed at the underlying congestive heart failure. The prognosis is guarded and is associated with the cardiac functional status. Selected patients may be considered for cardiac transplantation.

ENDOMYOCARDIAL DISEASES

The association of eosinophilia with endomyocardial fibrosis is recognized in a number of clinical syndromes, including **tropical endomyocardial fibrosis, Löffler's endomyocardial disease, eosinophilic leukemia,** and the **hypereosinophilic syndrome.** It has been suggested that these clinical entities may represent a spectrum of a single disease process. Morphologic abnormalities of eosinophils include decreased numbers of crystalloid granules, vacuolation, and hypersegmentation. Presumably, aberrant tissue invasion and inappropriate degranulation of the eosinophils result in the endomyocardial pathology, which involves both ventricles. Three stages of the disease are recognized: (1) an acute stage with infiltration of eosinophils and myocytolysis; (2) an intermediate thrombotic stage, in which a thickened endocardium is covered by thrombus; and (3) a fibrotic stage, in which dense fibrosis occurs in the endocardium and myocardium. An immunologic pathogenesis is presumed because of the eosinophilia. In these conditions there is a marked tendency for clot formation with fibrosis on resolution of the clots, and it is possible that the eosinophilia is secondary to this process.

The clinical presentation is that of a restrictive cardiomyopathy with a pattern of biventricular involvement. Emboli from intraventricular thrombi may be a prominent clinical component of the disease. Therapy is directed at the management of the cardiac dysfunction and thromboembolic complications. Treatment with prednisone and hydroxyurea may benefit patients with hypereosinophilic syndrome. Surgical intervention (endomyocardiectomy, thrombectomy, or valve replacement) may benefit carefully selected patients. Despite therapeutic intervention, the prognosis remains guarded.

VASCULAR DISEASES: THE VASCULITIDES

Vasculitis is defined as a clinicopathologic process characterized by inflammation and necrosis of blood vessels. The clinical spectrum ranges from a primary disease involving blood vessels exclusively to an involvement of vessels as a relatively insignificant component of another systemic disease. Because vasculitis can potentially involve any blood vessel, a complex and often confusing array of clinical syndromes results (Table 36–1). The vasculitides are a heterogeneous group of clinical syndromes, and therefore no single cause explains the pathophysiology of all of the inflammatory vessel diseases. The best characterized mechanism is **immune complex-mediated vasculitis.** The elements necessary for the expression of this process include (1) soluble immune complexes larger than 19S formed in slight antigen excess, (2) increased vascular permeability with passive deposition of complexes in the vessel wall, (3) activation of complement with subsequent attraction of polymorphonuclear neu-

Table 36–1. Classification of the vasculitides.

Systemic necrotizing vasculitis
 Polyarteritis nodosa.
 Allergic angiitis and granulomatosis.
 Overlap syndromes (ie, overlap angiitis, microscopic polyarteritis nodosa).
 Associated diseases (connective tissue diseases, hepatitis B, hepatitis C virus, essential mixed cryoglobulinemia, cytomegalovirus infection, hairy cell leukemia).

Small-vessel (hypersensitivity) vasculitis
 Henoch-Schönlein purpura.
 Serum sickness.
 Other drug-related vasculitides.
 Vasculitis associated with food, foreign protein, or other exogenous antigens.
 Vasculitis associated with a systemic disease (Table 36–2).
 Hypocomplementemic urticarial vasculitis.
 Congenital deficiencies of the complement system.
 Erythema elevatum diutinum.

Behçet's disease

Wegener's granulomatosis

Arteritis of larger arteries
 Giant cell (temporal) arteritis
 Takayasu's arteritis
 Large-artery arteritis-complicating diseases, such as ankylosing spondylitis, Reiter's syndrome, and relapsing polychondritis
 Aortitis-associated syphilis

Thromboangiitis obliterans (Buerger's disease)

Isolated angiitis of the central nervous system

Mucocutaneous lymph node syndrome (Kawasaki disease)

Miscellaneous vasculitis syndromes

trophils (PMN) to the site of immune complex deposition, and (4) release of inflammatory mediators and disruption of vascular integrity.

Studies of the mononuclear cell profiles in temporal artery biopsies suggest an important role for CD4 T cells in the pathogenesis of giant-cell arteritis. A small percentage of the infiltrating CD4 T cells show a pattern of activation, including recent activation through the T-cell receptor (TCR), IL-2R expression, and the production of interferon gamma (IFNγ). Analysis of the TCR expression demonstrates the following pattern: (1) only a small percentage of the CD4 T cells are clonally expanded, (2) clonally expanded CD4 T cells with identical TCR patterns can be identified in anatomically distinct lesions from the same biopsy, and (3) the clonally expanded T cells at the site of disease are enriched relative to the peripheral blood compartment. These observations provide compelling indirect evidence that a localized, antigen-driven T-cell immune response is important in the pathogenesis of giant-cell arteritis.

Other potential mechanisms are less well established. Aberrant regulation of T-cell, B-cell, monocyte, fixed tissue macrophage, and endothelial cell function may be important in some of the vasculitides. In addi-

tion, soluble cytokines and the expression of cell surface adhesion molecules on leukocytes and blood vessels may play a role in the expression of vasculitis.

SMALL-VESSEL (HYPERSENSITIVITY) VASCULITIS

Major Immunologic Features
- Small vessels undergo inflammation.
- It is an immune complex-mediated process.

General Considerations
Small-vessel vasculitis, which includes a heterogenous group of clinical syndromes, is characterized by inflammation of arterioles, capillaries, and venules. The most commonly involved vessel is the venule, producing a venulitis. Skin involvement is characteristic of small-vessel vasculitis, although any organ system can be affected. Immune complex deposition is an important mechanism in at least a subset of cases of small-vessel vasculitis. A variety of agents have been suggested as causal factors in hypersensitivity vasculitis; these include (1) microorganisms (bacteria, mycobacteria, viruses, and parasites), (2) foreign proteins (animal serum and monoclonal antibodies), (3) chemicals (insecticides, herbicides, and petroleum products), and (4) drugs (antibiotics, antihypertensives, antiarrhythmics, nonsteroidal anti-inflammatory drugs, antirheumatic drugs, and others). The chemicals and drugs are presumed to function as haptens, binding covalently to unknown host carrier molecules and thereby eliciting an immune response. Small-vessel vasculitis can also occur in association with a wide variety of systemic diseases. It most commonly occurs in the fifth decade of life, with a slight female predominance.

Pathology
The most common histologic pattern is a neutrophilic leukocyte infiltrate of the postcapillary venules with leukocytoclasis (presence of nuclear debris), fibrinoid necrosis, endothelial swelling, and disruption of vascular integrity (Fig 36–1). Patterns of mixed acute and chronic inflammatory infiltrates, as well as a chronic infiltrate composed predominantly of lymphocytes, are also recognized.

Clinical Features
A nonblanching palpable purpuric lesion (**palpable purpura**) is characteristic. Other associated skin findings include papular, petechial, and ulcerative lesions. The lesions tend to recur in crops varying in number from a few to more than 100. Each crop resolves over 2–4 weeks. The lesions have a symmetric distribution and are most often found in dependent areas, particularly the distal lower extremities. Vasculitis produces pain, a burning sensation, or dependent edema in up to 40% of patients. Evidence of joint, kidney, lung, gastrointestinal, or peripheral nervous system involvement is present in the minority of cases.

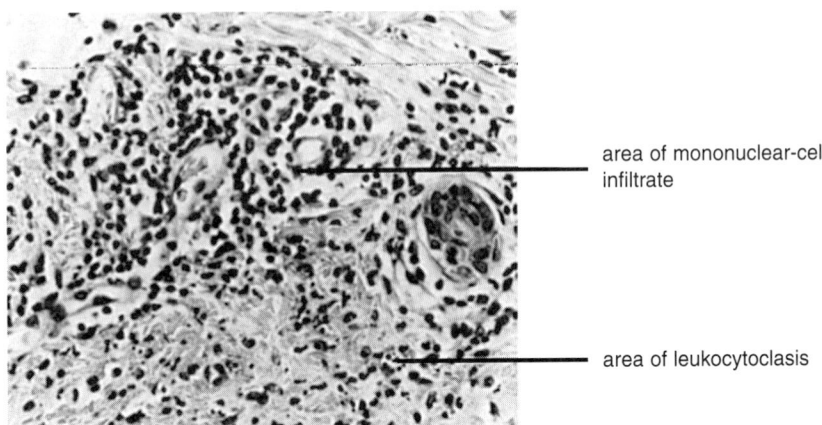

area of mononuclear-cell infiltrate

area of leukocytoclasis

Figure 36–1. Skin biopsy specimen from a patient with hypersensitivity vasculitis. A venulitis with a mixed cellular infiltrate is seen. A mononuclear cell infiltrate around a venule is present in one area of the specimen, but a neutrophil infiltrate with early leukocytoclasis (presence of nuclear debris) is seen in an adjacent area. Hematoxylin and eosin stain. (Original magnification ×330.) (Reproduced, with permission, from Cupps TR, Fauci AS: The vasculitides. In: *Major Problems in Internal Medicine.* Vol 21. Smith LH [editor]. WB Saunders, 1981.)

Immunologic Diagnosis

No specific laboratory test is diagnostic for small-vessel vasculitis. The following tests may or may not be abnormal: sedimentation rate, cryoglobulins, immune complexes, rheumatoid factor, and serum complement levels. A biopsy of a newly developing skin lesion should establish the diagnosis.

Differential Diagnosis

Once the diagnosis of small-vessel vasculitis is established, the patient should be evaluated for evidence of visceral involvement or an associated underlying disease process.

Treatment

Treatment should be directed at eliminating any inciting agent or treating any underlying systemic disease. A brief course of corticosteroid therapy or period of bedrest may expedite the resolution of an acute flare. Lengthy regimens of high-dose or split-dose daily corticosteroid treatment should be avoided. Analgesics may be required for symptomatic relief.

Complications & Prognosis

With rare exceptions, small-vessel vasculitis does not progress to life-threatening complications. The disease may be self-limited or, less commonly, develop a chronic recurrent pattern.

SYNDROMES ASSOCIATED WITH SMALL-VESSEL VASCULITIS

Several subgroups of hypersensitivity vasculitis have distinctive clinicopathologic patterns and are considered separate syndromes. In clinical practice these subsets may overlap. In this section the unique features of Henoch-Schönlein purpura, Behçet's disease, urticarial vasculitis, and small-vessel vasculitis associated with systemic disease processes are reviewed.

1. HENOCH-SCHÖNLEIN PURPURA

This syndrome, a distinctive subset of the small-vessel vasculitides, is characterized by normal platelet count, purpuric skin lesions, arthralgias, colicky abdominal pain with bleeding, and renal disease. It is the systemic form of small-vessel vasculitis. Deposition of IgA-containing immune complexes with activation of the alternative complement pathway may be an important pathophysiologic mechanism. The majority of patients have symptoms of an upper respiratory tract infection prior to the onset of their disease. Other suspected causes, including drugs (antibiotics and thiazides), foods (milk, fish, eggs, rice, nuts, beans, and others), and immunizations may appear to precipitate the disease clinically. There is a slight male predominance. The peak age of onset is between the ages of 4 and 7 years, although the disease does occur in adults. The disease has a seasonal variation, with the peak incidence reported in spring.

A. Histopathology: The histopathology is a diffuse leukocytoclastic vasculitis involving small vessels of any involved organ system. In the bowel, hemorrhage may occur in the submucosal surface or subserosal areas. The kidneys show focal or diffuse glomerulonephritis.

B. Clinical Manifestation: The clinical manifestation varies with age. In children, symptoms localized to skin, gut, and joints predominate. In adults, the disease presents predominantly with skin findings, whereas initial complaints related to the gastrointestinal tract or joints are present in fewer than one quarter of patients. The cutaneous lesion of Henoch-Schönlein purpura evolves through the following phases: (1) an initial small urticarial lesion that may be pruritic; (2) a pink maculopapular spot that develops over several hours; (3) maturation of this spot to a raised, darkened lesion; (4) progression the following day to a 0.5–2 cm maculopapular lesion that, in some cases, may become a confluent patch; and (5) final resolution in 2 weeks without scarring. Arthralgias without synovitis tend to follow a migratory pattern involving most commonly the large joints of the lower extremities. Abdominal symptoms, including colicky pain, nausea, vomiting, and blood loss, are present in the majority of patients. Life-threatening gastrointestinal tract problems, such as major bleeding, bowel perforation, or intussusception, are present in fewer than 5% of patients. The most common form of intussusception is ileoileal. The mean age of patients with this complication is 6 years, although intussusception has been reported in young adults. Clinically, the diagnosis of intussusception is suggested in a patient with a worsening clinical course, an unchanging abdominal mass, bright-red rectal bleeding, and the clinical pattern of complete bowel obstruction. Kidney involvement is characteristically very mild, although a few patients may develop progressive renal failure. Radiographic studies of the bowel may be useful in diagnosing an intussusception.

IgA-containing immune complexes may be present. These complexes, however, are not pathognomonic and are not detected by C1q assay, although the Raji cell assay may be positive. A skin biopsy establishes the vasculitic nature of the process, and immunofluorescence showing IgA deposition in vessel walls further supports the diagnosis of Henoch-Schönlein purpura.

C. Differential Diagnosis: The differential diagnosis for a patient presenting with rash, abdominal pain, and joint symptoms includes, in part, inflammatory bowel disease, *Yersinia* enterocolitis, meningococcemia, Rocky Mountain spotted fever, rheumatic fever, and viral infections.

D. Prognosis and Therapy: The disease usually resolves spontaneously after one or more recurrent episodes; consequently, the prognosis of even untreated patients is excellent. Therapy consists of supportive care and symptomatic relief. Timely surgical intervention may be required for the rare patients with life-threatening bowel complications. In the small number of patients with renal involvement with progressive functional impairment, corticosteroid therapy may be required.

2. BEHÇET'S DISEASE

Behçet's disease is characterized by recurrent episodes of oral ulcers, eye lesions, genital ulcers, thrombophlebitis, and other cutaneous lesions. The characteristic pathologic lesion is a venulitis, although vessels of any size in any organ system can be affected.

The primary lesion is a **small-vessel vasculitis,** presumably reflecting an antibody- or T cell-mediated response, although no antigenic epitope has yet been identified as a cause. Serum complement levels are normal, but circulating immune complexes may be present. There are studies showing complement deposition in lesions, but it is not known whether this is a primary or secondary event.

The oral lesions begin as raised erythematous areas with progression to shallow, punched-out lesions with yellow necrotic bases. These are discussed further in Chapter 35. The genital ulcers have similar appearance and follow a similar time course. Ocular involvement is most frequently observed in the anterior chamber, with iridocyclitis and hypopyon, which generally resolve without long-term complications. Involvement of the posterior structures is less frequent, but recurrent episodes over several years may lead to impaired vision. Renal, cardiovascular, and gastrointestinal tract involvement occurs in a minority of patients. In the absence of central nervous system or bowel involvement, the prognosis is good. No drug is uniformly successful in the treatment of Behçet's disease, but favorable results have been reported with indomethacin, colchicine, levamisole, and corticosteroids. Azathioprine in combination with corticosteroids is effective in the treatment of ocular manifestations of Behçet's disease. The need for early aggressive therapy of central nervous system disease has been emphasized.

3. HYPOCOMPLEMENTEMIC URTICARIAL VASCULITIS

This disease is a clinicopathologic entity characterized by a reduction of the early complement components in serum, persistent urticaria, and a pattern of leukocytoclastic vasculitis. Characteristically, there is a selective depression of the C1q component of complement because of the binding of C1q by IgG molecules through the F(ab)$'_2$—not Fc—portion of the molecule. The clearance of C1q is increased. The primary clinical feature of this disease is a persistent urticarial eruption, with lesions lasting a day or longer. Additional findings may include angioedema with occasional laryngeal involvement, joint symptoms, abdominal distress, neurologic abnormalities, and glomerulonephritis. The characteristic complement profile is a **depressed C1q level** with near-normal C1r and C1s levels. Other complement components, including C2, C3, and C4, may be depressed. The alternative pathway complement components are normal. Diseases such as SLE, urticaria–angioedema, and inherited partial C3 deficiency may present with a similar clinical pattern. Antihistamines, anti-inflammatory

Table 36–2. Systemic diseases associated with small-vessel vasculitis.

Systemic vasculitides
Systemic necrotizing vasculitis of the polyarteritis nodosa group (particularly the Churg-Strauss syndrome and overlap syndromes, including microscopic polyarteritis nodosa), Wegener's granulomatosis, Behçet's disease, Henoch-Schönlein purpura.

Collagen vascular diseases
SLE, rheumatoid arthritis, Sjögren's syndrome, dermatomyositis, scleroderma, rheumatic fever, sarcoidosis, C2 deficiency, essential mixed cryoglobulinemia.

Neoplasms
Lymphoproliferative neoplasms, carcinoma.

Infections
Bacterial (endocarditis), viral, mycobacterial, rickettsial.

Miscellaneous syndromes
Chronic active hepatitis, inflammatory bowel disease, primary biliary cirrhosis, retroperitoneal fibrosis.
Goodpasture's syndrome, relapsing polychondritis, α-antitrypsin deficiency, celiac disease, and others

drugs (indomethacin), and immunosuppressive drugs have been tried, but their therapeutic efficacy has not been established.

4. SMALL-VESSEL VASCULITIS ASSOCIATED WITH SYSTEMIC DISEASES

Small-vessel vasculitis occurs in association with a wide variety of systemic diseases (Table 36–2). It generally resolves when the underlying disease process is adequately treated.

SYSTEMIC NECROTIZING VASCULITIS

Systemic necrotizing vasculitis is a category that includes polyarteritis nodosa, allergic angiitis and granulomatosis (Churg-Strauss syndrome), and overlap syndromes, including microscopic polyarteritis nodosa. These diseases have in common a multisystem necrotizing vasculitis.

1. POLYARTERITIS NODOSA

Major Immunologic Features
■ There is necrotizing vasculitis of small- and medium-sized muscular arteries.
■ Pulmonary involvement is uncommon.

General Considerations
Classic polyarteritis nodosa is a necrotizing vasculitis of small and medium-sized muscular arteries. Involvement of renal and visceral arteries with sparing of the pulmonary circulation is characteristic. Immune complex deposition in involved arteries is considered to

be the relevant pathophysiologic mechanism. In patients with polyarteritis nodosa in association with chronic hepatitis B virus infection, hepatitis B surface antigen, IgM, and complement components can be demonstrated in early vasculitic lesions. With more than 1000 cases reported, polyarteritis nodosa is considered an uncommon but not rare disease. The male-to-female ratio is 2.5:1. The mean age at onset is 45 years, although the disease occurs at both extremes of age.

Pathology
Involvement of the kidneys, heart, abdominal organs, and nervous system (both central and peripheral nervous systems) is characteristic. With the exception of the bronchial arteries, the pulmonary vessels are uninvolved. The vasculitic lesions are **segmental** and have a predilection for branching and bifurcating points of small- and medium-sized muscular arteries (Fig 36–2). Arterioles, venules, and veins are characteristically spared, and granuloma formation is rare. Destruction of the media and internal elastic lamina with **aneurysm formation** is characteristic. Endothelial proliferation, vessel wall degeneration with fibrinoid necrosis, thrombosis, ischemia, and infarction are present to various degrees. Lesions at all stages of evolution, including (1) the degenerative stage, (2) the acute inflammatory stage, (3) the chronic inflammatory stage, and (4) healing with scarring, may be present at any given time. Renal pathology includes the presence of vasculitis, hypertensive changes, and glomerulonephritis.

Immunologic Pathogenesis
Polyarteritis nodosa is associated with various infections, especially hepatitis B but also tuberculosis,

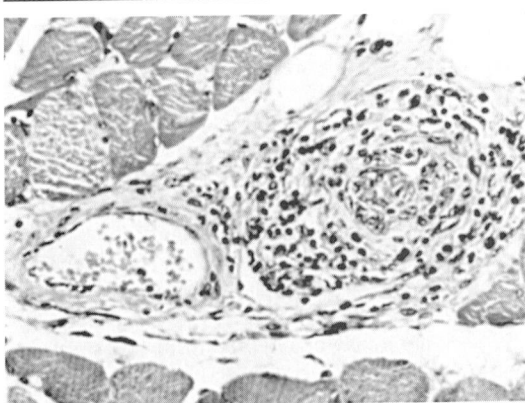

Figure 36–2. Muscle biopsy from a patient with classic polyarteritis nodosa. A necrotizing vasculitis of a small, muscular artery with a predominantly mononuclear cell infiltrate is seen. The adjacent vein is not involved. Hematoxylin and eosin stain. (Original magnification ×330.) (Reproduced, with permission, from Cupps TR, Fauci AS: The vasculitides. In: *Major Problems in Internal Medicine.* Vol 21. Smith LH [editor]. WB Saunders, 1981).

streptococcal infections, and otitis media. Evidence for an exogenous antigen causing the vasculitis is strongest when hepatitis B virus is present. The surface antigen of the virus is present at higher concentrations in plasma than are other viral antigens. It is found in immune complexes, and it can also be detected in tissues. Immune complexes containing IgM antibody could bind to the surface antigen nonspecifically, so definite proof that the vasculitis is caused by a viral antigen–antibody immune complex is lacking.

Clinical Features

Nonspecific signs and symptoms are common at the presentation of polyarteritis nodosa; these include weakness, abdominal pain, leg pain, neurologic symptoms, fever, and cough. The nonspecific nature of the presentation and the relatively uncommon occurrence of polyarteritis nodosa may contribute to the difficulty in establishing the diagnosis. Kidney involvement is common but tends to be asymptomatic. Arthritis, arthralgia, or myalgia occurs in more than half of the patients, as does hypertension. Diffuse renal vasculitis with secondary hyperreninemia appears to be an important cause of hypertension in patients with polyarteritis nodosa. The peripheral nervous system is involved in half of the cases. Several patterns of involvement are recognized. Mixed motor–sensory involvement with a pattern of mononeuritis multiplex suggests the diagnosis of vasculitis. There is clinical evidence for abdominal involvement in 45% of patients. Nausea, vomiting, and abdominal pain, which may suggest pancreatitis, are present. Less common manifestations of gastrointestinal tract disease include "intestinal angina" (postprandial abdominal pain, anorexia, and weight loss), malabsorption, and steatorrhea. Although rare, bowel infarction is a life-threatening complication, which requires rapid diagnosis and prompt surgical intervention.

Skin involvement is present in 40% of patients. The most common pattern is a maculopapular rash. In addition, subcutaneous painful nodules or livedo reticularis (a red to blue net-like mottling of the skin) can be seen. Clinical involvement of the heart is present in one third of patients. Cardiac disease may be secondary to the hypertension, coronary vasculitis, or pericarditis. Central nervous system involvement, including stroke, altered mental status, and seizures, can be seen in one quarter of patients. At autopsy there are changes secondary to hypertension as well as active vasculitis. Similarly, retinal vessel involvement from hypertension and vasculitis is recognized in patients with polyarteritis nodosa.

Abnormal laboratory studies include elevated erythrocyte sedimentation rate, leukocytosis, anemia, thrombocytosis, and cellular casts in the urinary sediment, indicating glomerular disease. Angiographic evaluation is important in establishing the diagnosis (Fig 36–3). Two abnormalities suggest the diagnosis of polyarteritis nodosa: (1) aneurysms (vascular

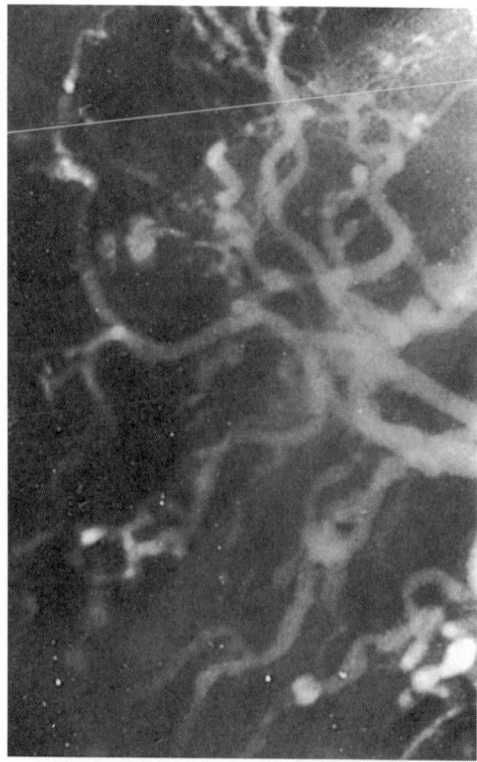

Figure 36–3. Hepatic angiogram from a patient with classic polyarteritis nodosa. Multiple saccular aneurysms and areas of symmetric narrowing are seen.

dilatation with a circular appearance), and (2) changes in vessel caliber (these tend to have an asymmetric pattern). The aneurysms in a given individual tend to be similar in size, ranging most commonly between 1 and 5 mm. Angiography establishes the diagnosis of polyarteritis nodosa in approximately 80% of cases; consequently, a negative study does not totally exclude the diagnosis.

Immunologic Diagnosis

There may be immune complexes, cryoglobulins, rheumatoid factors, and reduced level of complement components. Antineutrophil cytoplasmic antibodies with a perinuclear pattern (p-ANCA) and specificity for myeloperoxidase are seen in some patients. The histologic diagnosis of systemic necrotizing vasculitis can be established from a variety of tissue sites. Biopsy specimens taken from symptomatic sites such as skeletal muscle or nerves have a higher diagnostic yield than those from asymptomatic sites.

Differential Diagnosis

Because the initial signs and symptoms of polyarteritis nodosa are nonspecific, vasculitis should be considered in all patients with an undiagnosed systemic illness. At initial presentation many patients with polyarteritis nodosa are believed to have a neoplasm, infection, or other collagen vascular disease. The presence of an abnormal urinary sediment, recent onset of hypertension, or mononeuritis multiplex suggests the diagnostic possibility of vasculitis. A number of diseases occur in association with polyarteritis nodosa, including infections (hepatitis B virus infection, acute otitis media, endocarditis, and streptococcal infection), collagen vascular diseases (SLE, rheumatoid arthritis, Sjögren's syndrome, and others), and neoplasms (hairy cell leukemia).

Treatment

Although corticosteroids alone are generally recommended in the less fulminant cases of polyarteritis nodosa, cyclophosphamide is the treatment of choice in severe progressive polyarteritis nodosa. The drug is started at 2 mg/kg as a single daily oral dose, with monitoring of the leukocyte count to avoid a total leukocyte count of less than 3000 cells/mm^3. Prednisone (60 mg orally per day) is also started during the induction period of 10–14 days. After this induction period, a taper to an alternate-day schedule is initiated. The taper to alternate-day prednisone administration is generally completed in 2–3 months.

Complications & Prognosis

Cyclophosphamide induces long-term clinical remission of systemic necrotizing vasculitis, including cases that have been refractory to other treatment modalities. Meticulous control of hypertension is needed for several reasons. One reason is the potential for accelerated atherosclerosis in arteries damaged by the necrotizing vasculitis. Another major reason is that kidneys initially damaged by vasculitis or glomerulonephritis should be protected from the additional insult of poorly controlled blood pressure. Angiotensin-converting enzyme inhibitors may be particularly effective in this clinical setting.

2. ALLERGIC ANGIITIS & GRANULOMATOSIS (Churg-Strauss Syndrome)

Major Immunologic Features

- There is vasculitis of blood vessels of various type and sizes (including small- and medium-sized muscular arteries).
- Pulmonary involvement is common.

General Considerations

Allergic angiitis and granulomatosis is a rare disease characterized by a granulomatous vasculitis of multiple organ systems. Although vascular lesions identical to the pattern seen in polyarteritis nodosa may be present, this disease is unique for the following findings: (1) frequency of involvement of pulmonary vessels, (2) vasculitis of blood vessels of various types and sizes (small- and medium-sized muscular arteries, veins, and small vessels), (3) intravascular and extravascular granuloma formation, (4) eosinophilic tissue infiltrates, and (5) association with severe asthma and peripheral eosinophilia. The pathophysiology of this syndrome appears to be similar to the pattern described for polyarteritis nodosa. There is a slight male predominance, and the mean age at the onset of disease is 44 years. In one series of patients with systemic necrotizing vasculitis, approximately 30% of patients had a clinical pattern of allergic angiitis and granulomatosis.

Pathology

In autopsy studies, the frequent involvement of the spleen and pulmonary vessels with sparing of central nervous system contrasts with the pattern seen in polyarteritis nodosa. In addition to the pattern of arteritis seen in polyarteritis nodosa, involvement of smaller vessels is commonly seen. **Eosinophils and granulomata** are seen in and around the vascular infiltrates. The veins are involved in approximately half of the patients, and small-vessel vasculitis is seen in the purpuric skin lesions.

Clinical Features

The clinical manifestation of allergic angiitis and granulomatosis is similar to the pattern seen in polyarteritis nodosa, except for the high frequency of pulmonary signs and symptoms. Asthma and transient pulmonary infiltrates are frequently noted. Symptoms related to the lungs generally precede the diagnosis of systemic vasculitis by 2 years, although the range is from 0 to 30 years. A short duration of pulmonary symptoms has been associated with a poorer prognosis. Peripheral blood eosinophilia is seen in 85% of cases at some point in the course of the disease.

Immunologic Diagnosis

Elevation of IgE has been reported in allergic angiitis and granulomatosis. The p-ANCA test is positive in some patients. In addition to the peripheral biopsy sites described for polyarteritis nodosa, an open-lung biopsy may be useful to establish the diagnosis of necrotizing vasculitis.

Differential Diagnosis

In addition to the differential diagnosis discussed for polyarteritis nodosa, the diagnosis of allergic angiitis and granulomatosis should be considered in patients with bronchospasm and pulmonary infiltrates.

Treatment, Complications, & Prognosis

Treatment and prognosis are similar to those of polyarteritis nodosa. The bronchospasm may persist after successful treatment for the systemic vasculitis, and specific treatment of asthma may be required.

3. OVERLAP SYNDROMES

There are patients who share clinical and pathologic features characteristic of both polyarteritis nodosa and allergic angiitis and granulomatosis, as well as other vasculitic syndromes, but do not fit precisely into these strictly defined diagnostic categories. The presence of an overlap syndrome emphasizes that there is a continuum of disease manifestations in patients with systemic necrotizing vasculitis. The approach to the patients with overlap syndromes is similar to the one described for other systemic necrotizing vasculitides.

WEGENER'S GRANULOMATOSIS

Major Immunologic Features

- This is a necrotizing granulomatous vasculitis.
- There is focal segmental glomerulonephritis.
- There are antineutrophil cytoplasmic autoantibodies.

General Considerations

Wegener's granulomatosis is a clinicopathologic complex of a necrotizing, granulomatous vasculitis of the upper and lower respiratory tracts, glomerulonephritis, and variable degrees of small-vessel vasculitis. The cause is unknown. Because of the predominant involvement of the upper and lower respiratory tracts in this disease, it has been suggested that an infectious agent or an inhaled antigen may trigger an aberrant immune response. However, no such antigen or infectious agent has been identified as yet. A potential role for the antineutrophil cytoplasmic antibodies with a diffuse cytoplasmic pattern (c-ANCA) in the pathogenesis of Wegener's granulomatosis has been suggested. There is a slight male predominance. The majority of cases begin in the fourth or fifth decade of life, although the disease has been described at both extremes of age.

Pathology

Wegener's granulomatosis is characterized by **fibrinoid necrosis** of predominantly small arteries and veins, with early infiltration of neutrophils followed by mononuclear cells. This is followed by healing with fibrosis. The vasculitis lesions occur at all stages of evolution. **Granulomata** are well-formed with plentiful multinucleated giant cells. Renal involvement is characterized by a focal segmental glomerulonephritis. Crescent formation can be seen in the more severe cases. Renal vasculitis or granuloma formation is less frequent.

Clinical Features

The most common presenting complaints (present in 85% of patients) involve the **upper respiratory tract** and include sinusitis, nasal obstruction, otitis, hearing loss, and oropharyngeal symptoms. Lower respiratory tract symptoms occur in 35% of patients; these include cough, sputum production, dyspnea, pleuritic chest pain, and, less commonly, hemoptysis. Other presenting complaints include arthralgias, weight loss, and weakness. Wegener's granulomatosis can involve any organ system, but the lungs are involved in virtually all patients. Lung disease may be asymptomatic, but it can be seen radiographically. In addition to the presenting symptoms of cough and dyspnea, massive pulmonary hemorrhage can occur but it is rare. There is evidence of **sinus** involvement in 95% of patients; this can be complicated by a superimposed bacterial infection. Inflammatory lesions may involve any site in the upper airways. Destruction of the nasal septum results in the saddle nose deformity (Fig 36–4). A persistent sore throat is a frequent complaint. Shallow oral ulcerations with sharp margins occur.

Renal involvement is generally asymptomatic but can be documented in 80% of cases. Functional impairment may progress very rapidly in the absence of appropriate treatment. In contrast to patients with systemic necrotizing vasculitis, renal vascular hypertension is not a significant clinical problem. **Joint** symptoms are present in more than half of the patients, but a deforming arthritis is not characteristically seen.

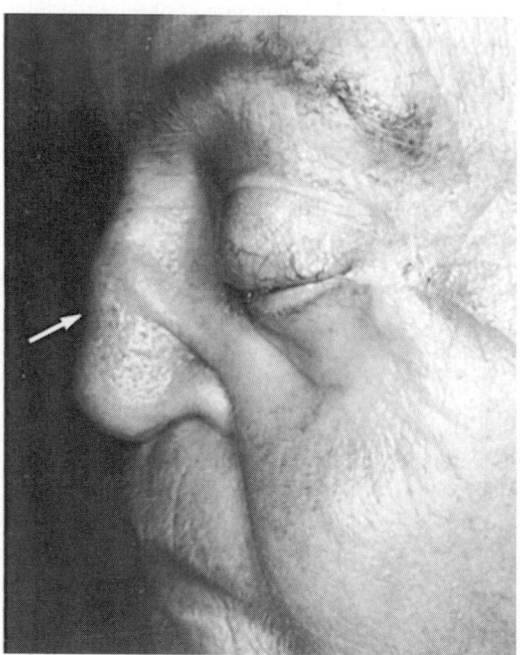

Figure 36–4. The saddle nose deformity of Wegener's granulomatosis (arrow) results from inflammation, scarring, and loss of height of the cartilaginous portion of the bridge of the nose. The bony portion (os nasale) is uninvolved. Note also the proptosis of the eye secondary to retroorbital inflammation.

Skin involvement, including ulceration, vesicles, petechiae, and subcutaneous nodules, occurs in almost half of the patients. The **eyes** are involved in 40% of patients. The most common abnormalities are proptosis secondary to a retroorbital inflammatory mass and inflammation of the anterior ocular structures (ie, conjunctivitis, episcleritis, scleritis, and corneoscleral ulceration). Vasculitis of the vessels in the optic nerve or retina occurs in 10% of cases. **Cardiac** involvement is reported in one quarter of patients. The most common abnormality is pericarditis, but inflammation of other structures, including the endocardium, the myocardium, and the coronary vessels, has been reported. The **nervous system** is involved in one quarter of patients. Different patterns of peripheral nerve involvement, including mononeuritis multiplex, are noted. Involvement of the central nervous system is less common but is a well-recognized complication.

Laboratory studies show leukocytosis, thrombocytosis, elevated sedimentation rate, and presence of C-reactive protein. An abnormal urinary sediment is present in 80% of patients. Hematuria, with or without cellular casts, and proteinuria make up the most common pattern. The most common pattern seen on a chest radiograph is multiple, nodular, bilateral cavitary infiltrates, although virtually any pattern has been described. Computed tomography of the chest may be more sensitive for identifying subtle lung lesions. Computed tomography of the orbits may be useful in diagnosing and monitoring retroorbital eye involvement.

Immunologic Diagnosis

Polyclonal elevations of IgG and IgA with normal levels of IgM is the characteristic pattern seen in active Wegener's granulomatosis. Elevation is variable. Circulating immune complexes can be detected in some patients. The c-ANCA directed against proteinase 3 is present in most patients with active systemic disease. In some patients, the c-ANCA titer reflects disease activity, and a rising titer may precede clinical recurrence in a subset of patients. A definitive diagnosis of Wegener's granulomatosis is made by seeing the histologic pattern of granulomatous necrotizing vasculitis on a biopsy specimen. Open-lung biopsy has the highest diagnostic yield. Tissue taken from other sites has an approximately 10% yield in demonstrating the diagnostic pattern. Renal tissue provides a histologic pattern that is consistent with the diagnosis of Wegener's granulomatosis.

Differential Diagnosis

Wegener's granulomatosis is included in the differential diagnosis of patients with chronic sinusitis or otitis media. Diseases that are associated with a pulmonary renal syndrome (SLE, Goodpasture's syndrome, thrombotic thrombocytopenia purpura, etc) may be confused with Wegener's granulomatosis during the initial phases.

Treatment

Cyclophosphamide at 2 mg/kg orally as a single daily dose is the most effective form of treatment. After the initial induction period the total leukocyte count is monitored to adjust the dose of cyclophosphamide. Care should be taken to avoid lowering the leukocyte count below 3000 cells/mm^3. In addition, oral prednisone at 1 mg/kg/d is used. After 2 weeks of daily prednisone, a taper to an alternate-day regimen of prednisone is initiated; the taper is completed after 2–3 months. Treatment should continue until the patient is free of disease for 1 year before the drugs are discontinued; withdrawal should be gradual. Weekly oral methotrexate up to a maximum dose of 20–25 mg/wk in combination with prednisone as outlined earlier may also be effective in selected patients with Wegener's granulomatosis. The efficacy of methotrexate in the setting of progressive renal disease is not established.

Complications & Prognosis

Treatment with cyclophosphamide and prednisone results in marked improvement in 90% of patients and in a complete remission in 75%. The occurrence of relapse following discontinuation of therapy may approach 50%. Late relapses, years after successful induction, have been reported. Sinus damage by the disease may predispose to recurrent episodes of bacterial sinusitis. Obstruction from scarring of large airways can be seen in patients with severe endobronchial disease. The most common obstructed site is the subglottic region.

The potential toxicities from oral cyclophosphamide administration are significant and include hemorrhagic cystitis, bladder fibrosis, and neoplasia. The estimated prevalence of bladder transitional-cell carcinoma after the first exposure to cyclophosphamide is 5% at 10 years and 15% at 15 years. A history of nonglomerular microscopic hematuria, a total accumulated dose exceeding 100 g of cyclophosphamide, and a duration of therapy greater than 2.7 years are associated with the development of bladder carcinoma. Long-term follow-up monitoring for the development of delayed drug-associated toxicities is warranted in patients who have received oral cyclophosphamide.

GIANT-CELL ARTERITIS

Major Immunologic Features

- This is a granulomatous panarteritis.
- It affects the elderly.
- Headache is common, but presenting symptoms are nonspecific.
- It is associated with polymyalgia rheumatica.

General Considerations

Giant-cell arteritis (temporal arteritis) is a systemic panarteritis affecting any medium-sized or large artery. The disease predominantly affects the elderly, with clinical signs and symptoms resulting from vasculitis in branches of the carotid artery. There is a slight female predominance, and the average age at onset of the disease is 70 years. More than 95% of cases occur in patients older than 50 years. The age-specific incidence (new cases per 100,000 population per year) increases with age, rising from 1.7 in the sixth decade to 55.5 for patients older than 80 years.

Pathology

The disease is characterized by a panarteritis consisting of mononuclear cells. The dominant infiltrating cell type is the CD4 lymphocyte. A small subset of CD4 T cells shows a pattern of activation through the TCR, expression of IL-2R on the cell surface, production of IFNγ and clonal expansion. Activated macrophages producing interleukin (IL)-1 and IL-6 are also present in inflammatory lesions. In the fully developed arteritis lesion, the major site of involvement is the media, with smooth muscle necrosis and disruption of the internal elastic membrane. The inflammatory lesions have a segmental pattern.

Clinical Features

The presenting signs and symptoms of giant-cell arteritis have a nonspecific pattern. The most frequent presenting complaints of headache, malaise, and fatigue are common symptoms in an older population. Less common presenting problems include jaw or extremity claudication, fever, arthralgias, chronic sore throat, and tender scalp nodules. **Headache** is the most common manifestation. The pain has a continuous, boring quality with intermittent exacerbations. Although the pain is most commonly located over the distribution of the **temporal artery,** radiation to the neck, face, jaw, or tongue occurs. Although abnormalities along the course of the temporal artery, including tenderness, absent pulse, and nodules, are seen in half of the patients (Fig 36–5), these findings appear later in the course of disease. Other findings include hair loss, erythema, and necrosis along the course of the temporal artery. **Eye problems,** including visual impairment, blindness, amaurosis fugax, and diplopia, occur in more than one third of patients. Although giant-cell arteritis may present with sudden blindness, the majority of patients have other symptoms for an average of 3.5 months prior to developing visual impairment. Because the loss of vision is the result of ischemic optic neuritis in the majority of cases, the funduscopic examination may be normal for several days after the onset of blindness.

Jaw claudication (pain brought on by chewing or talking and relieved by rest) occurs in one third of patients and suggests the diagnosis of giant-cell arteritis. **Polymyalgia rheumatica,** a syndrome characterized by proximal muscle pain, periarticular pain, and morning stiffness, occurs in approximately half of the patients with giant-cell arteritis. Conversely, up to 50% of

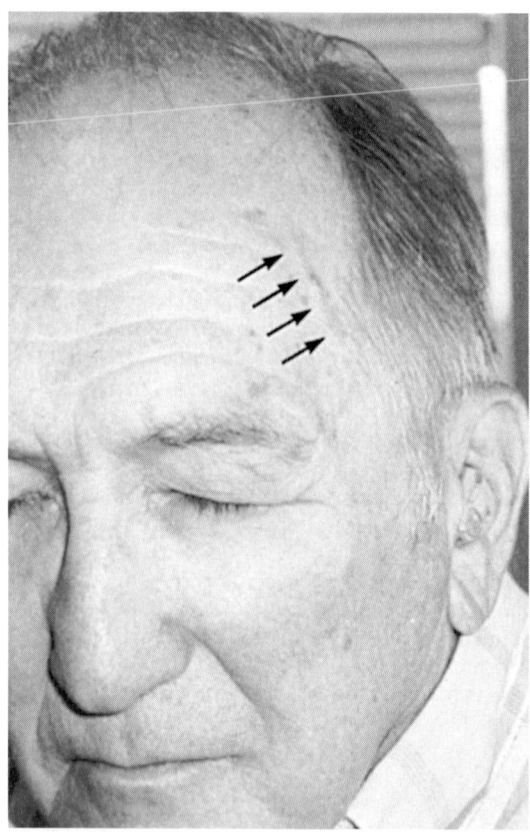

Figure 36–5. Giant-cell arteritis involving the temporal artery (arrows) is shown. The temporal artery was swollen and tender. Biopsy of the contralateral temporal artery demonstrated the characteristic granulomatous panarteritis. The swelling and tenderness resolved following treatment with corticosteroids. (Courtesy of S. Ray Mitchell, Georgetown University Medical School, Washington, D.C.)

patients presenting with symptoms of polymyalgia rheumatica may have a positive temporal artery biopsy.

Laboratory abnormalities include a normochromic, normocytic anemia, elevated alkaline phosphatase, and mild elevation of hepatic transaminases.

Immunologic Diagnosis

The sedimentation rate, total IgG, and acute-phase reactants are characteristically elevated. The diagnosis is established by finding the characteristic panarteritis on a temporal artery biopsy. Because of the segmental nature of the inflammation, the need for generous biopsy specimens and serial sectioning has been emphasized.

Differential Diagnosis

Because of the nonspecific nature of the majority of presenting symptoms, giant-cell arteritis can be confused with a wide variety of disease processes, including neoplasia, chronic infection, abnormal thyroid function, and other connective tissue diseases.

Treatment

Prednisone at 40–60 mg/d orally is the initial treatment. As manifestations of the disease are suppressed, an attempt should be made to taper the dose of the drug. Although some patients may be adequately treated with 6 months of therapy, most require a more prolonged course of 1–2 years or longer. Prednisone should be tapered to the minimum effective dose, generally in the range of 7.5–10 mg/d. The use of weekly oral methotrexate as a steroid-sparing agent is currently under investigation.

Complications & Prognosis

Corticosteroids are effective in suppressing the symptoms of giant-cell arteritis and preventing visual impairment. In general, visual impairment is not reversible once present.

Problems with thoracic aortic aneurysm or dissection may be seen as a remote complication, generally following successful therapeutic intervention for the inflammatory phase of the disease. Complications from the prolonged use of corticosteroids in an elderly population is a potential source of morbidity as well.

TAKAYASU'S ARTERITIS

Major Immunologic Features

■ There is inflammation and stenosis of large and intermediate-sized arteries.
■ There is frequent involvement of the aortic arch.

General Considerations

Takayasu's arteritis is characterized by inflammation and stenosis of large and intermediate-sized arteries with frequent involvement of the aortic arch and its branches. There is a marked female predominance (about 9:1). The onset of symptoms presents at a median age of 25 years. Although originally recognized in Asian women, Takayasu's arteritis has a worldwide distribution.

Pathology

Takayasu's arteritis is characterized by a panarteritis of large elastic arteries, with infiltration of all layers of the artery wall by mononuclear cells and giant cells. Other findings include intimal proliferation, fibrosis, disruption of elastic lamina, and vascularization of the media. Aneurysms, dissection, and hemorrhage are less common. In descending order of frequency, the following arteries are involved: subclavian artery (85%), descending aorta (58%), renal artery (56%), carotid artery (43%), ascending aorta (30%), abdominal aorta (20%), vertebral artery (17%), iliac artery (16%), innominate artery (15%), and pulmonary artery (15%).

Clinical Features

Although historically reported to present in three phases (prepulseless inflammation, followed by painful, ischemic arteries and ending in a "burned-out" occlusive phase), the clinical manifestation of Takayasu's arteritis is quite varied. Approximately 20% of patients present with monophasic, apparently self-limited disease. An additional 33% present with systemic symptoms, including malaise, fever, night sweats, and arthralgias. Less common manifestations include skin nodules similar to erythema nodosum, arthritis, episcleritis, and iritis. Symptoms during the occlusive phase reflect ischemia of the involved organ systems. Signs of vascular insufficiency are present in almost all patients. The pulse of the radial, ulnar, and carotid arteries is decreased or absent in 98% of patients. Bruits can be detected in 86% of patients. Symptoms of claudication or pain over the distribution of an artery occur in approximately one third of patients. Central hypertension is present in half of the cases. Blood pressure determinations of the lower extremities more reliably reflect the true central blood pressure in the presence of severe aortic arch involvement. Sixty percent of patients experience difficulty in looking up, resulting in the characteristic "face-down" position. Patients assume this position to avoid transient decreases in visual acuity and narrowing of visual fields caused by a further decrement of compromised blood flow to the central nervous system. Ischemic changes to the retina and anterior structures of the eye are seen in a minority of patients. Cardiac symptoms are present in one third of patients. Palpitations and congestive heart failure (right- and left-sided failure) secondary to hypertension are the most common manifestations. Less commonly, cardiac ischemia (secondary to coronary arteritis), aortic insufficiency, myocarditis, and pericarditis have been reported. Routine blood tests may show a mild anemia and leukocytosis.

Immunologic Diagnosis

The erythrocyte sedimentation rate is generally elevated but is not a reliable indicator of disease activity. IgG, IgA, and IgM may be elevated, but the rheumatoid factor and antinuclear antibodies are generally negative. **Arteriography** is important in the diagnosis and management of Takayasu's arteritis (Fig 36–6). Arteriographic abnormalities include symmetric narrowing to complete occlusion of large arteries with collateralization of flow. Less commonly aneurysms, including both saccular and fusiform patterns, can be seen. Other noninvasive tests to measure blood flow may be useful for serial follow-up evaluations.

Differential Diagnosis

Other causes of aortitis, including syphilis, mycotic aneurysm, rheumatic fever, Reiter's syndrome, and ankylosing spondylitis, should be excluded. Vascular occlusion secondary to emboli can also mimic Takayasu's arteritis.

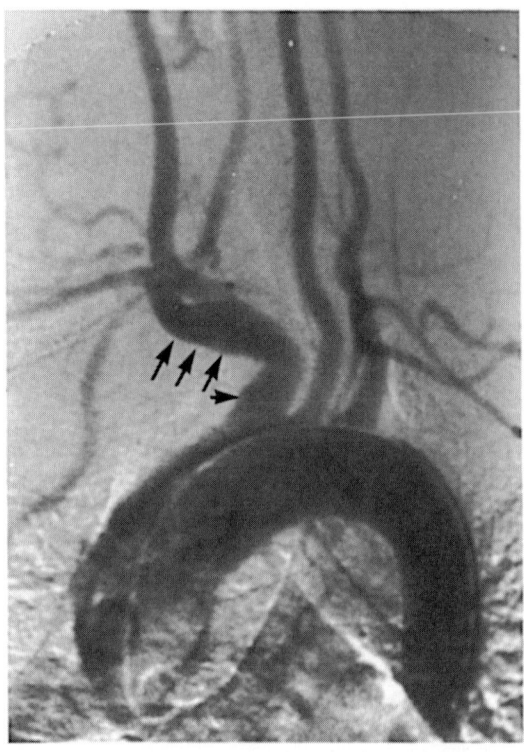

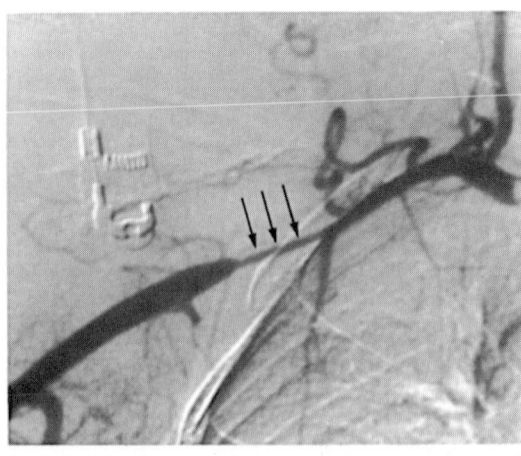

Figure 36–6. ***A:*** Angiographic findings in Takayasu's arteritis include saccular aneurysm of the brachiocephalic and common carotid arteries (arrows), ***B:*** a prolonged segment of symmetric narrowing of the subclavian and axillary arteries (arrows) producing a "string sign," and ***C:*** complete occlusion of the major aortic arch vessel (large arrow) with blood flow to the head established through collateral vessels (thin arrow).

Treatment

Patients with self-limited monophasic disease do not require treatment with immunosuppressive agents. Glucocorticoids are the initial form of treatment of patients with active disease. Oral prednisone can be started at a dose of 1 mg/kg/d with a goal of tapering to an alternate-day regimen within a 6-month period. Patients who develop reactivation of the disease when tapered to an alternate-day regimen or those who develop recurrent disease after a year of glucocorticoid therapy should be treated with weekly oral methotrexate starting at a dose of 15 mg/week with 2.5-mg incremental increases up to a total dose of 25 mg/week. Patients whose disease progresses despite the use of methotrexate and glucocorticoids may respond to the use of cytotoxic agents, such as azathioprine or cyclophosphamide. Remote relapse of disease may be seen after successful induction of remission. A subset of patients may benefit from a chronic low-dose immunosuppressive regimen. Percutaneous transluminal angioplasty may be useful in selected patients, although the incidence of restenosis is significant. Vascular surgery, if required, should be performed during periods of disease inactivity.

Complications & Prognosis

In two large series a 10% mortality rate was noted. The most common cause of death was congestive heart failure, and the second most common was myocardial infarction. Less common causes of death were renal failure and central nervous system hemorrhage.

THROMBOANGIITIS OBLITERANS (Buerger's Disease)

This syndrome is characterized by inflammatory occlusive vascular disease of the intermediate to small arteries and veins of the extremities. Three histopathologic phases of the disease are recognized: (1) neutrophil infiltrate of the vessel wall associated with microabscesses and thrombosis, (2) a subacute phase with mononuclear cell and giant-cell infiltrates, and (3) a chronic phase with fibrosis and recanalization of the thrombus. Although the disease predominantly affects males younger than 40 years of age with a significant smoking history, an increasing incidence among women has been noted. The most common presenting symptoms are lower extremity claudication or migratory thrombophlebitis. Less than 5% of patients present with upper extremity problems. During the course of the disease the majority of patients develop Raynaud's syndrome, and upper extremity involvement is seen in 90% of cases. Systemic symptoms are characteristically absent. Protection of ischemic tissue and cessation of tobacco use are imperative. Carefully selected patients may benefit from surgical intervention. Morbidity from tissue loss may be great, but survival is not affected.

Circulating immune complexes have been reported by some investigators but not others. There are no diagnostic immunologic tests. It is not known whether tobacco has a toxic or immunologic effect in this disease. The possibility of an immune pathogenesis, however, is raised by the close resemblance of the histopathology in the early phase of the disease with that of a hyperacute graft rejection.

OTHER VASCULITIC SYNDROMES

1. ISOLATED ANGIITIS OF THE CENTRAL NERVOUS SYSTEM

This is a distinct clinicopathologic entity characterized by vasculitis restricted to the vessels of the central nervous system. The arteriole is the most commonly affected vessel, although any size of vessel can be affected. The disease generally presents with a pattern of higher cortical dysfunction or severe headache and progresses to a pattern of multifocal neurologic deficits. Immunosuppressive therapy is successful in inducing long-term clinical remissions.

2. ERYTHEMA NODOSUM

This is a clinical syndrome characterized by recurrent crops of painful nodular lesions (Fig 36–7) and is generally associated with infection (mycobacterial, fungal, or bacterial) or with sarcoidosis. The histopathology is characterized by acute and chronic inflammation of the dermis and subcutaneous tissue including a vasculitic component.

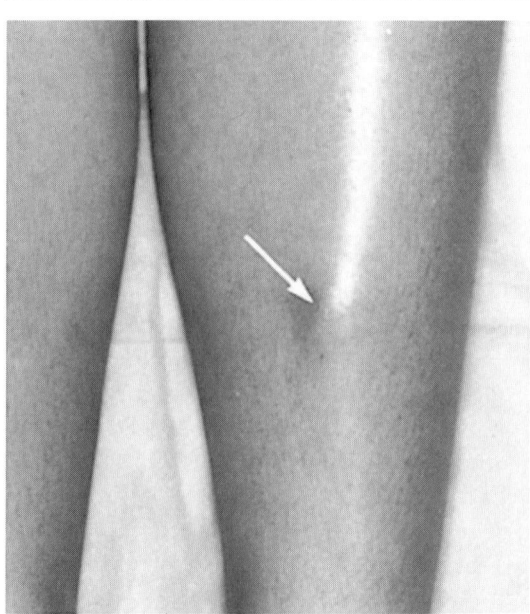

Figure 36–7. Erythema nodosum. A 2–3 cm raised, red nodule in the characteristic pretibial distribution is shown (arrow).

REFERENCES

GENERAL

American College of Rheumatology Subcommittee on Classification of Vasculitis: The American College of Rheumatology 1990 criteria for the classification of vasculitis. *Arthritis Rheum* 1990;**33**:1065.

Churg A, Churg J (editors): *Systemic Vasculitides.* Igaku-Shoin, 1991.

Cupps TR, Fauci AS: The vasculitides. In: *Major Problems in Internal Medicine.* Vol 21. Smith LH (editor). WB Saunders, 1981.

Hunder GG (guest editor): Vasculitis. In: *Rheum Dis Clin North Am* 1995;**21:** Entire issue.

Jennette JC et al: Nomenclature of systemic vasculitides: Proposal of an international conference. *Arthritis Rheum* 1994;**37**:187.

Schlant RC, Alexander RW (editors): *Hurst's the Heart: Arteries and Veins,* 8th ed. McGraw Hill, 1994.

PERICARDIAL DISEASE

Gregoratos G: Pericardial involvement in acute myocardial infarction. *Cardiol Clin* 1990;**8**:601.

Khan AH: The postcardiac injury syndromes. *Clin Cardiol* 1992;**15**:67.

Marcolongo R et al: Immunosuppressive therapy prevents recurrent pericarditis. *J Am Coll Cardiol* 1995;**26**:1276.

MYOCARDIAL DISEASE

Brown CA, O'Connell JB: Myocarditis and idiopathic dilated cardiomyopathy. *Am J Med* 1995;**99**:309.

Grogan M et al: Long-term outcome of patients with biopsy-proved myocarditis: Comparison with idiopathic dilated cardiomyopathy. *J Am Coll Cardiol* 1995;**26**:80.

Mason JW et al: A clinical trial of immunosuppressive therapy for myocarditis. The Myocarditis Treatment Trial Investigators. *N Engl J Med* 1995;**333**:269.

ENDOMYOCARDIAL DISEASE

Felice PV et al: Endomyocardial disease and eosinophilia. *Angiology* 1993;**44**:869.

Chusid MJ et al: The hypereosinophilic syndrome: Analysis of fourteen cases with review of the literature. *Medicine* 1975;**54**:1.

SMALL-VESSEL VASCULITIS

Cupps TR, Fauci AS: Cutaneous vasculitis. In: *Current Therapy in Allergy and Immunology 1983–1984.* Lichtenstein LM, Fauci AS (editors). BC Decker, 1983, p 136.

Gibson LE: Cutaneous vasculitis: Approach to diagnosis and systemic associations. *Mayo Clin Proc* 1990;**65**:221.

Ilan Y, Naparstek Y: Schönlein-Henoch syndrome in adults and children. *Semin Arthritis Rheum* 1991;**21**(2):103.

Wisnieski JJ et al: Hypocomplementemic urticarial vasculitis syndrome: Clinical and serologic findings in 18 patients. *Medicine* 1995;**74**:24.

Yazici H et al: A controlled trial of azathioprine in Behçet's syndrome. *N Engl J Med* 1990;**322**:322.

SYSTEMIC NECROTIZING VASCULITIS

Falk RJ and The Glomerular Disease Collaborative Network: Clinical course of anti-neutrophil cytoplasmic autoantibody-associated glomerulonephritis and systemic vasculitis. *Ann Intern Med* 1990;**113**:656.

Fauci AS et al: Cyclophosphamide therapy of severe systemic necrotizing vasculitis. *N Engl J Med* 1979; **301**:235.

Guillevin L et al: Prognostic factors in polyarteritis nodosa and Churg-Strauss syndrome. *Medicine* 1996;**75**:17.

WEGENER'S GRANULOMATOSIS

Hoffman GS et al: Wegener granulomatosis: An analysis of 158 patients. *Ann Intern Med* 1992;**116**:488.

Nolle B et al: Anticytoplasmic autoantibodies: Their immunodiagnostic value in Wegener granulomatosis. *Ann Intern Med* 1989;**111**:28.

Sneller MC et al: An analysis of forty-two Wegener's granulomatosis patients with methotrexate and prednisone. *Arthritis Rheum* 1995;**38**:608.

Talar-Williams C et al: Cyclophosphamide-induced cystitis and bladder cancer in patients with Wegener granulomatosis. *Ann Intern Med* 1996;**124**:477.

TEMPORAL ARTERITIS

Evans JM et al: Increased incidence of aortic aneurysm and dissection in giant cell (temporal) arteritis. A population-based study. *Ann Intern Med* 1995;**122**:502.

Machado EB et al: Trends in incidence and clinical presentation of temporal arteritis in Olmsted Country, Minnesota. *Arthritis Rheum* 1988;**31**:745.

Weyand CM, Coronzy JJ: Giant cell arteritis as an antigen-driven disease. *Rheum Dis Clin North Am* 1995;**21**:1027.

TAKAYASU'S ARTERITIS

Hoffman GS et al: Treatment of glucocorticoid-resistant or relapsing Takayasu arteritis with methotrexate. *Arthritis Rheum* 1994;**37**:578.

Kerr GS et al: Takayasu Arteritis. *Ann Intern Med* 1994;**120**:919.

THROMBOANGIITIS OBLITERANS

Lie JT: Thromboangiitis obliterans (Buerger's disease) in women. *Medicine* 1986;**65**:65.

OTHER SYNDROMES

Cupps TR et al: Isolated angiitis of the central nervous system: Prospective diagnostic and therapeutic experience. *Am J Med* 1983;**74**:97.

37

Gastrointestinal, Hepatobiliary, & Orodental Diseases

Stephen P. James, MD, Warren Strober, MD, & John S. Greenspan, BDS, PhD, FRCPath

As reviewed in Chapter 13, the gastrointestinal tract is normally a site of intense immunologic activity. The gastrointestinal lumen contains a complex mixture of harmless (and necessary) microbial flora, potential pathogens, and large quantities of complex macromolecules capable of eliciting immune responses. The mucosal immune system has evolved mechanisms to downregulate immune responses to harmless flora and food antigens while eliciting protective responses to pathogens. The diseases reviewed in this chapter are thought to be the result of aberrations of the mucosal immune response to harmless exogenous antigens or autoantigens, resulting in inappropriate injury to the host, or diseases such as hepatitis in which the immunologic host response to a pathologic agent is an important component of the disease process.

GASTROINTESTINAL DISEASES

Stephen P. James, MD, & Warren Strober, MD

GLUTEN-SENSITIVE ENTEROPATHY (Celiac Disease)

Major Immunologic Features

- Hypersensitivity to cereal grain proteins (gliadins).
- Antigliadin antibodies are present.
- The lamina propria is infiltrated with lymphocytes and plasma cells, associated with villous atrophy.
- Strong HLA association exists.
- Association with dermatitis herpetiformis exists.

General Considerations

Gluten-sensitive enteropathy (celiac sprue, nontropical sprue) is a disease of the small intestine that is characterized by villous atrophy and malabsorption.

It is caused by hypersensitivity to cereal grain storage proteins (gluten or gliadin, both alcohol-soluble wheat proteins) found in wheat, barley, and rye. The disease is most common in caucasians and occurs only occasionally in African blacks and not in Asians. It is either limited to the intestine or associated with a vesicular skin disease, dermatitis herpetiformis.

Pathology

The inflammatory lesions are restricted primarily to the small-intestinal mucosa, with the most severe changes being in the area most often in contact with ingested gluten, the proximal small intestine. Gliadin challenge studies show that the disease begins with subepithelial edema and thickening of the basement membrane followed by an influx of inflammatory cells. The latter initially consists of polymorphonuclear leukocytes, but these are soon replaced by lymphocytes and plasma cells. Although IgA plasma cells increase in number and continue to predominate, there is a disproportionate increase in IgG plasma cells; in contrast, few if any IgE plasma cells appear. These inflammatory changes are accompanied by shortening and eventual flattening of the villi and lengthening of the crypts; the latter is indicative of a marked increase in epithelial cell turnover (Fig 37–1). When dermatitis herpetiformis is present, the intestinal lesions are similar to (but usually milder than) those when it is absent, and the skin lesions consist of subepidermal collections of inflammatory cells near areas of fluid accumulation. A characteristic feature of the skin lesions is the presence of granular deposits of IgA and complement in both lesional and normal skin.

Immunologic Pathogenesis

Gluten-sensitive enteropathy is most probably due to a specific immunologic hyperreactivity to peptides derived from certain grains that leads to activation of lymphocytes in the mucosa. Consistent with this hypothesis, patients have antibody responses to gliadin

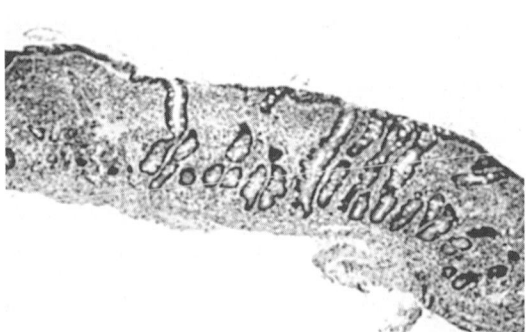

Figure 37–1. Gluten-sensitive enteropathy. Jejunal biopsy specimen shows complete loss of villi, elongation of crypts, and lymphocytic infiltrate in a severe case.

that are quantitatively and qualitatively distinct from those found in the other gastrointestinal tract diseases. They also have gliadin-specific T-cell-mediated responses that are not seen in controls. Further evidence of an immunologic origin comes from organ culture studies that show that gliadin is not toxic by itself but instead requires the participation of an endogenous effector mechanism. In addition, 80–90% of patients both with and without dermatitis herpetiformis have HLA-DQ antigens encoded by DQA1*0501 and DQB1*0201 in *cis* or *trans*. Most of the remaining patients have DQA1*0301 and DQB1*0302. This finding suggests that particular immune response genes are necessary for the inappropriate antigliadin immune responses that are presumably causing the disease. Although these HLA phenotypes are necessary for the disease, they are not sufficient since the majority of individuals with these genes do not have celiac disease.

Clinical Features

In gluten-sensitive enteropathy alone, the clinical course is dominated by gastrointestinal tract symptoms and malabsorption, whereas when dermatitis herpetiformis is present the course is dominated by a vesicular skin eruption and the intestinal symptoms are usually absent. The intestinal symptoms of gluten-sensitive enteropathy are highly variable and consist of weight loss, diarrhea, symptoms due to nutritional deficiencies, and growth failure in children. When dermatitis herpetiformis is present, the skin disease consists of a vesicular, intensely pruritic skin eruption on extensor and exposed surfaces. Typical laboratory findings in gluten-sensitive enteropathy include evidence of malabsorption: increased fecal fat, abnormal D-xylose absorption, vitamin deficiencies, anemia, and, in severe cases, biochemical evidence of osteomalacia and abnormal coagulation due to vitamin K deficiency. Intestinal contrast studies during active disease show dilatation and thickening of the proxi-

mal small bowel. The intestinal biopsy is the most important specific diagnostic test, particularly in association with gluten challenge studies.

Immunologic Diagnosis

The diagnosis of gluten-sensitive enteropathy is established by demonstrating villous atrophy in the small-bowel biopsy, which resolves with removal of gluten from the diet and which reappears with gluten challenge. Antigliadin antibodies are present in active disease, but their presence is not entirely specific, unless they are present in high titers and are of the IgA class. Antiendomyseal antibodies are also relatively specific for celiac disease.

Differential Diagnosis

The differential diagnosis includes all intestinal diseases causing malabsorption. Small-bowel biopsy showing villous atrophy and inflammation, however, considerably narrows the diagnostic possibilities to gluten-sensitive enteropathy, tropical sprue, hypogammaglobulinemia, and some forms of intestinal lymphoma.

Treatment

Treatment consists of lifelong elimination of gluten-containing foods from the diet. It is recommended that such treatment be instituted even in patients with mild disease because a major complication of gluten-sensitive enteropathy is an increased prevalence of small-bowel carcinoma and lymphoma, and it is thought that reduction of chronic inflammation by gluten restriction may diminish the risk of this complication. Nutritional supplements should be instituted as needed in patients with active disease. Very severe disease, particularly associated with severe villous atrophy and small-bowel ulceration, may respond to corticosteroids. When dermatitis herpetiformis is present, both the intestinal and skin lesions can also be treated with a gluten-free diet. More usually, however, diaminodiphenylsulfone (dapsone), an anti-inflammatory drug that provides good control of the skin lesions, is used.

Complications & Prognosis

Unrecognized and untreated gluten-sensitive enteropathy may lead to severe debility and death, but following treatment, patients usually return to normal health and have a normal life expectancy. As noted above, the incidence of intestinal carcinoma and lymphoma is increased. Recently it has been shown that intestinal lymphoma is most often a CD8 T-cell lymphoma. Patients with long-standing intestinal changes may be relatively unresponsive to a gluten-free diet and may require corticosteroid therapy. Rarely, patients develop villous atrophy associated with severe intestinal ulceration (ulcerative iliojejunitis), a syndrome that in some instances becomes life-threatening.

NONGLUTEN (NONGLIADIN) FOOD HYPERSENSITIVITY

Major Immunologic Features
- IgE-mediated hypersensitivity or gluten-sensitive enteropathy-like hypersensitivities are present.
- Ill-defined mucosal abnormalities marked by eosinophilic infiltration or villous atrophy of the mucosa occur.

General Considerations

Several conditions marked by hypersensitivity to food substances other than gluten (gliadin) also occur. These include IgE-mediated food allergy localized to the gastrointestinal tract, usually associated with non-gastrointestinal allergic symptoms. The causative food substance in this case can induce an increase in mucosal IgE plasma cells and mast cell degranulation, which may lead to a severe protein-losing enteropathy. Treatment consists of eliminating the offending food from the diet (see Chapter 27).

A second type of hypersensitivity is due to food substances that induce a clinical picture nearly identical to that in gluten-sensitive enteropathy: villous atrophy and malabsorption developing days to weeks after exposure to the causative substance. This condition is more or less limited to young children and is most frequently caused by cow's milk protein; however, soy, egg, and wheat proteins have also been implicated. It frequently occurs after a gastrointestinal infection and resolves spontaneously after the age of 3 years. It may be due to immaturity of the mucosal immune system and hence an inability to develop immunologic tolerance to food antigens.

Finally, there is an ill-defined group of gastrointestinal tract hypersensitivity states marked by either eosinophilic infiltration of the bowel or villous atrophy and not definitely associated with a causative food or other agent. In some cases these conditions may be due to a self-perpetuating inflammation that was initiated by an inappropriate immune response, whereas in other cases it may be due to an autoimmune process.

CROHN'S DISEASE

Major Immunologic Feature
- Transmural granulomatous inflammation of the bowel wall is present.
- Extraintestinal inflammation of the skin, eyes, joints, and liver can occur.

General Considerations

Crohn's disease (regional ileitis, granulomatous ileitis, or colitis) is a syndrome of unknown origin characterized by transmural inflammation of any portion of the bowel wall. It occurs worldwide, but is most common in persons of European origin. The prevalence ranges from 10 to 70 per 100,000, and it is much more common in industrialized countries. There is a slight female predominance. The disorder can begin at any age, but most typically begins between 15 and 30 years of age. There is a familial aggregation of cases but no clear mode of inheritance.

Pathology

Crohn's disease may involve any part of the alimentary tract from the mouth to the anus, although most patients fall into one of the typical patterns of the disease, having predominant involvement of the ileocolic, small-intestinal, or colonic–anorectal regions. The gross pathology of Crohn's disease is characterized by transmural inflammation of the bowel wall, often in a discontinuous fashion, with ulceration, strictures, and fistulae being typical findings. The histopathologic findings are those of a discontinuous granulomatous inflammatory process (true granulomas are found in about 60% of surgically resected specimens) (Fig 37–2), crypt abscesses, fissures, and aphthous ulcers. The inflammatory infiltrate is mixed, consisting of lymphocytes (both T and B cells), plasma cells, macrophages, and neutrophils. There is a disproportionate increase in IgM- and IgG-secreting plasma cells compared with IgA-secreting cells, but the latter are also increased. The number of T cells is increased, but a normal proportion of CD4 and CD8 cells is maintained.

Crohn's disease (like ulcerative colitis, see later section) is found primarily in industrialized countries, suggesting that one or more environmental factors are important in pathogenesis; however, no such factors have yet been identified. Infection with *Mycobacterium paratuberculosis* species has been suggested as a cause, but recent evidence makes it more likely that this organism is a commensal that does not have an etiologic role. Early childhood infection has also been implicated. Because of the failure to identify a specific causative infectious microorganism, it has been suggested that the disease has a primary immunologic basis. One leading possibility in this regard is that the

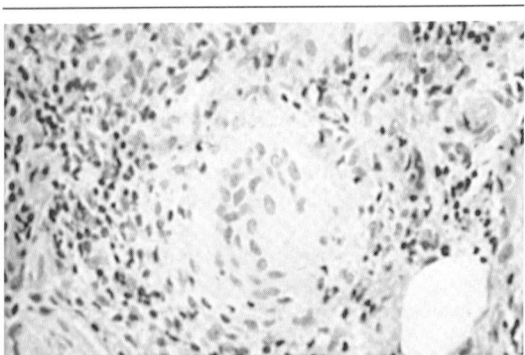

Figure 37–2. Crohn's disease. Rectal biopsy specimen shows mucosal granuloma.

mucosal inflammation in Crohn's disease is the result of abnormality of mucosal T-cell regulation, which leads to an inappropriate mucosal immune response to ubiquitous intestinal antigens (see Chapter 13). In support of this concept are the facts that (1) the inflammatory lesion in Crohn's disease begins as a follicular collection of lymphocytes that resembles a normal (if inappropriate) immune response; (2) patients manifest excessive responses to oral antigen challenge; and (3) several immunoregulatory defects have been identified, including the presence of circulating suppressor T cells and abnormal lymphokine secretory patterns in the mucosa. These data are not conclusive, however, and additional work is needed to establish an immunologic origin.

Clinical Features

Typical symptoms include abdominal pain, anorexia, weight loss, fever, diarrhea, perianal discomfort and discharge, and extraintestinal symptoms involving the skin, eyes, and joints. The manifestations vary somewhat according to the predominant pattern of intestinal involvement. Extraintestinal manifestations are not unusual and include arthritis, erythema nodosum, pyoderma gangrenosum, aphthous mouth ulcers, uveitis, anemia, urinary calculi, and sclerosing cholangitis. Typical laboratory abnormalities include anemia (chronic disease, iron deficiency, vitamin B_{12} deficiency, folate deficiency), leukocytosis, thrombocytosis, elevation of the erythrocyte sedimentation rate, hypoalbuminemia, electrolyte abnormalities (in severe diarrhea), and presence of occult blood in the stool. Many radiographic abnormalities may be present in small-bowel and colon contrast studies. These include aphthous ulceration, linear ulceration, edema, and thickening of the bowel wall (Fig 37–3), as well as strictures, fissures, fistulae, and mass lesions (inflammatory mass or abscess); the chronic inflammation also may lead to a characteristic "cobblestone" pattern. When the areas involved are accessible, endoscopy provides a direct method of evaluating disease activity and permits collection of biopsy material for pathologic confirmation as well as screening for colon carcinoma.

Immunologic Diagnosis

Multiple abnormalities of immune function have been described, but none has diagnostic specificity.

Differential Diagnosis

Diseases sometimes having an appearance similar to Crohn's disease are appendicitis, diverticulitis, intestinal neoplasia, and intestinal infections (*M tuberculosis, Chlamydia, Yersinia enterocolitica, Campylobacter jejuni, Entamoeba histolytica, Cryptosporidium,* herpes simplex virus, cytomegalovirus, *Salmonella,* and *Shigella*). A combination of stool cultures, intestinal biopsies, and clinical follow-up are usually sufficient to exclude these possibilities.

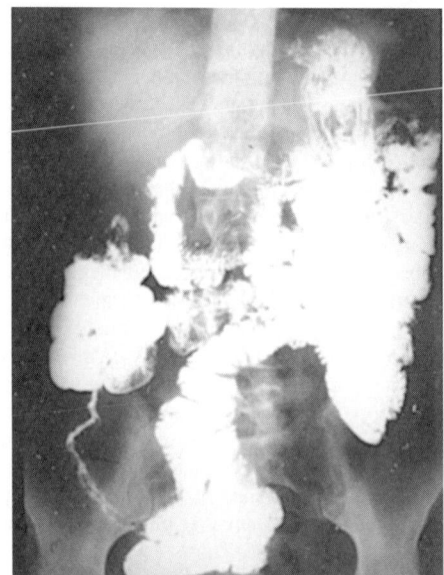

Figure 37–3. Crohn's disease. Small-bowel barium contrast x-ray shows marked narrowing of the terminal ileum as a result of transmural inflammation.

Treatment

The anti-inflammatory drug sulfasalazine and newer 5-aminosalicylic acid (5-ASA) agents are useful in treating mildly active colonic Crohn's disease and is commonly used in an attempt to maintain remission of disease. Metronidazole and ciprofloxacin are similar in efficacy to sulfasalazine and appear to be particularly useful for treating perianal disease. In more severe active disease, corticosteroids are effective in treating acute exacerbations and possibly in maintaining remission in some patients. There is no evidence, however, that corticosteroids prevent the progression of subclinical disease. Azathioprine and 6-mercaptopurine are used as steroid-sparing drugs in patients who require chronic corticosteroids and are not amenable to surgical therapy; in addition, it has been suggested but not proved that these drugs may have a role in long-term prophylaxis. There may be a long delay in the onset of action of these drugs (6 months) when used in conventional doses. Weekly, low-dose oral methotrexate is effective in some patients. Antidiarrheal drugs provide symptomatic relief in some patients. Dietary management with elemental diets or total parenteral nutrition is useful for improving the nutritional status of patients and in inducing symptomatic improvement of acute disease, but diet alone does not induce sustained clinical remissions. Antibiotics are used in treating secondary small-bowel bacterial overgrowth and in treatment of pyogenic complications. Cyclosporin has largely been abandoned due to toxicity and lack of efficacy. Finally, surgical treatment is necessary when the disease is not controlled medically and when various complications occur (see following paragraph).

Complications & Prognosis

Patients typically have recurrent episodes of active disease with periods of intervening quiescence. They often have low-grade symptoms, however, even during periods of apparent disease inactivity, and the disease has high social and economic costs. Approximately two thirds of patients require surgery at some time during their life for diseases not treatable with tolerable doses of steroids or for complications such as obstruction, abscess, fistula, hemorrhage, or megacolon. The disease is clearly not curable by surgical resection, however, and recurs at a rate approaching 90% in very long-term follow-up. The mortality rate of Crohn's disease is approximately twice that in the general age-matched population, although most mortality occurs early in the course of the disease and there is only a small increase in mortality in patients with long-standing disease. The incidence of intestinal carcinoma is increased, but the frequency is much lower than that associated with ulcerative colitis.

ULCERATIVE COLITIS

Major Immunologic Features

■ Colonic mucosa is chronically inflamed, with ulceration of the epithelial layer.
■ Anticolon antibodies are present.
■ ANCA is present in subgroups of patients.
■ Extraintestinal manifestations occur in joints, skin, liver, and eyes.

General Considerations

Idiopathic ulcerative colitis is a disease of unknown origin characterized by chronic inflammation of the colonic mucosa. As with Crohn's disease, ulcerative colitis is found primarily in industrialized nations, although it does occur worldwide. The prevalence ranges from 37 to 80 per 100,000 with a slight female predominance. It is more prevalent in Ashkenazi Jewish populations. There are two peaks of incidence: one in the third decade and one in the fifth decade. There is a significant familial association but no clear pattern of inheritance.

Pathology

Ulcerative colitis, in contrast to Crohn's disease, is limited to the colon and involves mainly the superficial layers of the bowel. In addition, the inflammation is continuous and is not associated with granulomas. Typically, the disease is found in the distal colon and rectosigmoid area, but it extends proximally to involve the entire colon in more severe cases. Gross pathologic findings include edema, increased mucosal friability, and frank ulceration. Histologic features are crypt abscesses consisting of accumulations of polymorphonuclear cells adjacent to crypts, necrosis of the epithelium, and surrounding accumulations of chronic inflammatory cells (Fig 37–4). Over time,

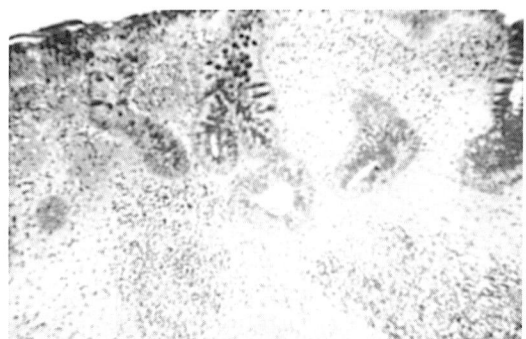

Figure 37–4. Ulcerative colitis. Rectal biopsy specimen shows distortion of crypts and lymphoid aggregates.

there is distortion of the crypt architecture. Finally, in long-standing disease, epithelial cell dysplasia and colonic carcinoma may be found.

As in Crohn's disease, the immunopathogenesis is uncertain. Autoantibodies reactive with mucin-associated antigens or with colonic epithelial cell antigens have been identified in patients. These antibodies have in some cases been demonstrated to cross-react with bacterial cell wall antigens and have been identified in relatives of patients. Other studies have shown that lymphocytes from patients with ulcerative colitis can be cytotoxic for colonic epithelial cells; although not completely proven, this is probably due to arming of Fc receptor-bearing cytotoxic cells with antiepithelial cell antibodies. These findings suggest that primary immunologic mechanisms, possibly involving an autoimmune component, are the basis of the disease. Overall, the disease mechanism appears to be similar but not identical to that underlying Crohn's disease.

Clinical Features

The clinical features are highly variable. The onset may be insidious or abrupt. Symptoms include diarrhea, tenesmus, and relapsing rectal bleeding. With fulminant involvement of the entire colon, toxic megacolon, a life-threatening emergency, may occur. Extraintestinal manifestations include arthritis, pyoderma gangrenosum, uveitis, and erythema nodosum. As mentioned earlier, colonic dysplasia and carcinoma may ensue in long-standing disease. Typical laboratory abnormalities include anemia (chronic disease, iron deficiency), leukocytosis, thrombocytosis, elevation of the erythrocyte sedimentation rate, electrolyte abnormalities (in severe diarrhea), and the presence of occult blood in stool. A barium enema study may demonstrate ulcerations and, in more severe disease, pseudopolyps. In chronic disease the colon may be shortened, narrowed, and tubular. Colonoscopy is useful for direct assessment of the degree and extent of inflammation, for biopsy confirmation of the diagnosis, and for screening for dysplasia and carcinoma.

Immunologic Diagnosis

No immunologic test is specific for the disease. Anticolon epithelial cell antibodies have been identified in research laboratories, but they have not been shown to be of diagnostic utility. Antineutrophil cytoplasmic antibodies (ANCA) have been identified in subgroups of patients, but their presence does not correlate with disease activity and is not specific for ulcerative colitis.

Differential Diagnosis

The differential diagnosis is similar to that listed in the previous section for Crohn's disease, with the addition of ischemic colitis, radiation-induced enteritis, and pseudomembranous colitis. It is occasionally difficult to distinguish between Crohn's disease of the colon and ulcerative colitis. Such differentiation is usually based on the fact that Crohn's disease, but not ulcerative colitis, is a discontinuous lesion and is associated with granulomatous inflammation.

Treatment

As in the case of Crohn's disease, sulfasalazine and related salicylate-containing drugs are effective in mild cases and corticosteroid drugs are effective in severe cases. Sulfasalazine is used to maintain remission, although with variable results. Topical administration of either salicylates or corticosteroids is effective in some patients, particularly those with disease limited to distal bowel, and is associated with decreased side effects compared with systemic use. Supportive measures such as administration of iron and antidiarrheal agents are sometimes indicated. Azathioprine, 6-mercaptopurine, and methotrexate are sometimes used in refractory corticosteroid-dependent cases. Patients with severe colitis have been rescued from imminent colectomy with parenteral cyclosporin.

Complications & Prognosis

Ulcerative colitis patients usually respond to medical therapy and enjoy a reasonable quality of life without surgical intervention. Patients with severe intractable disease or with megacolon, however, may require colectomy. In contrast to Crohn's disease, surgery completely eliminates the disease. In patients who have the disease for longer than two decades, the incidence of colon carcinoma increases significantly, and so patients should receive periodic screening examinations. Whether the presence of colonic dysplasia is an indication for prophylactic colectomy is controversial.

ALPHA HEAVY-CHAIN DISEASE

Major Immunologic Features

- The small intestine is infiltrated with malignant, α-chain-producing B cells.
- α-Heavy chain protein is present in serum.

General Considerations

The immunoproliferative small-intestinal diseases (IPSID) consist of a rare group of premalignant or malignant lymphomas that are limited mostly to the small bowel. The pathognomonic feature is infiltration of the bowel by aberrant B cells, which produce α-heavy chains in 70% of patients. The diseases are usually found in underdeveloped countries, especially in the Middle East, and generally in young patients of low socioeconomic status. It has been suggested that the disease begins as a response to excessive antigenic stimulation as a result of infectious agents in the setting of malnutrition, since it may respond initially to antibiotic administration. The diffuse infiltration of the intestine is associated with villous flattening and malabsorption. Mucosal ulceration and small-bowel obstruction may occur with progression. The diagnosis is established by intestinal biopsy and the presence of α-heavy chain in the serum of intestinal secretions. Early stages may respond to prolonged antibiotic therapy, whereas advanced stages may respond to combined chemotherapy.

PERNICIOUS ANEMIA

Major Immunologic Features

- Antiparietal cell antibodies are present.
- Anti-intrinsic factor antibodies are present.

General Considerations

Pernicious anemia is an autoimmune disease in which progressive destruction of the gastric fundic glands takes place, leading to atrophic gastritis, achlorhydria, loss of production of intrinsic factor, and vitamin B_{12} malabsorption. The disease presents insidiously with megaloblastic anemia and rarely with neurologic complications due to vitamin B_{12} deficiency. Recognition and treatment of the disease prior to onset of neurologic symptoms is important to prevent irreversible neurologic damage. There is an increased familial incidence and an association with other autoimmune diseases, particularly those involving the thyroid and adrenal glands. Other associations include vitiligo, hypoparathyroidism, and common variable hypogammaglobulinemia. Most patients with pernicious anemia have antiparietal cell antibodies, and the majority have anti-intrinsic factor antibodies. The fact that such antibodies are found with increased frequency in unaffected family members as well as in patients with other autoimmune diseases suggests that (1) the disease has a genetic component and (2) these antibodies do not cause disease by themselves. This fact, as well as other data, suggests that the disease is caused primarily by T-cell-mediated immune damage to the stomach. Routine laboratory abnormalities in pernicious anemia include the presence of megaloblastic anemia, vitamin B_{12} deficiency, and increased serum gastrin. The diagnosis is confirmed by the demonstration of achlorhydria and an abnormal Schilling test, which corrects with addition of intrinsic factor. Treatment consists of vitamin B_{12} replacement. Patients with pernicious anemia have an increased incidence of gastric polyps and gastric carcinoma, and therefore attention to gastric symptoms and screening for occult blood in the stool are indicated.

WHIPPLE'S DISEASE

Major Immunologic Features
- Massive infiltration of the lamina propria occurs with periodic acid-Schiff-positive macrophages.
- Secondary T-cell abnormalities are present.

General Considerations
Whipple's disease is a rare infectious disease caused by the bacterium *Tropheryma whippelii,* which has not yet been cultured. Characteristic features include abdominal pain, diarrhea, weight loss, and a variety of central nervous system manifestations. The diagnosis is established by intestinal biopsy, which discloses free-lying bacteria and the characteristic presence of large numbers of macrophages containing bacterial cell wall debris (periodic acid-Schiff-positive material) in the lamina propria. The infection is not limited to the gastrointestinal tract and can involve the heart, lungs, serosal surfaces, joints, and central nervous system. In the gastrointestinal tract, the cell infiltration leads to "clubbed" villi, lymphatic obstruction, malabsorption, and protein-losing enteropathy. These patients suffer progressive inanition. In addition, when lymphatic obstruction is severe, they may lose lymphocytes into the gastrointestinal tract, become lymphopenic, and develop a secondary T-cell immunodeficiency. The cause of the disease is unclear, but it may be due to an inability to respond immunologically to particular bacterial antigens. In any case, the disease frequently responds to antibiotic therapy.

HEPATOBILIARY DISEASES

Stephen P. James, MD, & Warren Strober, MD

Several diseases of the liver and biliary tract have important immunologic features in pathogenesis. These include acute viral hepatitis (Table 37–1), chronic hepatitis, and primary sclerosing cholangitis.

HEPATITIS A

Major Immunologic Feature
- Antibodies to HAV occur (IgG antibodies are long-lived).

General Considerations
Hepatitis A is an acute liver infection caused by a small RNA picornavirus (hepatitis A virus, HAV). The virus may cause dramatic epidemics or appear sporadically. Transmission is virtually always by the fecal–oral route. During acute viral hepatitis, there is ballooning and acidophilic degeneration of hepatocytes and portal and periportal infiltration with mononuclear cells. In severe disease, there may be massive necrosis of the liver. HAV particles may be identified in the cytoplasm of infected hepatocytes. Young children with hepatitis A may be asymptomatic, whereas adults usually have nausea, vomiting, dark urine, abdominal pain, and fatigue. Hepatomegaly, abdominal tenderness, and jaundice are typical findings in symptomatic patients. HAV is one of the causes of fulminant hepatitis, which is associated with hepatic encephalopathy and a high mortality rate. Although a relapsing course may rarely occur, the disease usually resolves completely. Typical laboratory features include striking elevations of the serum aminotransferases.

It is thought that the mechanism of liver injury in hepatitis A is not due to the virus itself but rather to the immune response to viral antigens present on the surface of the hepatocytes. In this regard, cytolytic CD8 T cells, which specifically kill hepatitis A-infected target cells, have been shown to be present in the liver in hepatitis A patients. It is thought that variability in the outcome of acute hepatitis A infection (ie, mild versus fulminant disease) might be due in part to genetically controlled differences in the magnitude of the immune response to the virus.

Immunologic Diagnosis
The diagnosis is confirmed by the presence of IgM anti-HAV antibodies. IgG antibodies are long-lived and may persist for the life of the host, and their presence signifies immunity to infection.

Differential Diagnosis
The differential diagnosis of acute hepatocellular necrosis includes acute viral hepatitis from other viruses; toxic hepatitis due to drugs, chemicals, or physical agents; acute fatty liver associated with pregnancy; acute reactivation of chronic hepatitis; fulminant Wilson's disease; and Reye's syndrome.

Treatment
Hepatitis A usually resolves quickly, and there is no evidence of a long-lasting carrier state. Treatment is supportive. Vaccination is recommended for individuals at increased risk of exposure to hepatitis A.

HEPATITIS B

Major Immunologic Features
- In acute hepatitis HBsAg, HBeAg, and IgM anti-HBc are present in serum.

Table 37–1. Viral and serologic characteristics of hepatitis.

Type	Viral Markers Antigen	Characteristics	Serologic Markers Antibody	Characteristics
Hepatitis A	HAAg (hepatitis A antigen)	Found in stool during incubation and transiently during acute symptomatic phase.	IgG anti-HAV IgM anti-HAV	Acute hepatitis. Long-lived antibody found during convalescence.
Hepatitis B	HBsAg (hepatitis B surface antigen)	Viral coat; present in acute and chronic phase.	Anti-HBe	Found during convalescence.
	HBcAg	Core antigen found in nuclei of infected hepatocytes.	IgM anti-HBc IgG anti-HBc	Acute hepatitis. High titer in chronic hepatitis.
	HBeAg	Virus-encoded protein of unknown function; marker of active viral replication.	Anti-HBe	Found after resolution of active replication.
	DNA polymerase (HBV DNA)	Found in serum during active replication.		
Hepatitis D	Delta antigen	Found primarily in hepatocyte nuclei and occasionally in serum during active infection.	Antidelta	High titer in chronic infection.
	HBV markers	Requires coinfection with HBV.		
Hepatitis C	HCV recombinant antigens	HCV mRNA in serum	Anti-HCV	Acute and chronic hepatitis.
Hepatitis E			Anti-HEV	Acute and chronic hepatitis.

- In acute hepatitis (convalescent phase) IgG anti-HBs is present in serum.
- In chronic hepatitis (active viral replication phase) HBV DNA, DNA polymerase, HBsAg, HBeAg, and high-titer IgG anti-HBc are present in serum.
- In chronic hepatitis (viral integration phase) HBsAg, anti-HBc, and anti-HBe are present in serum.
- HBV is not cytopathic; immune mechanisms are thought to cause hepatocyte necrosis.

General Considerations

Hepatitis B virus (HBV) infection is a double-stranded DNA virus of worldwide distribution. The mode of transmission is parenteral or maternal–infant. Individuals at risk for infection include recipients of blood or blood products, drug addicts, dialysis patients, male homosexuals, some health care workers, and infants born to HBV-infected mothers. The risk of chronic infection is higher in infants, immunosuppressed patients, patients with lymphoid cancer, and children with Down syndrome. Infection has many possible outcomes, including an acute asymptomatic infection or symptomatic hepatitis, a chronic carrier state with or without development of chronic or progressive live disease, fulminant hepatitis, and hepatocellular carcinoma. Other syndromes associated with HBV include polyarteritis nodosa, aplastic anemia, glomerulonephritis, and essential mixed cryoglobulinemia.

Pathology

The histologic features of acute HBV infection include ballooning and eosinophilic degeneration of he-patocytes, the presence of focal areas of necrosis of hepatocytes, and lymphocytic infiltration of the parenchyma and portal areas. In more severe cases, extensive areas of necrosis of hepatocytes may be present in central and midzones, which may lead to collapse of the reticulin framework, giving the pattern of "bridging necrosis." In chronic HBV infection, the pathologic findings are variable. In chronic carriers who are clinically well, there may be variable degrees of hepatic inflammation ranging from scattered focal areas of hepatocyte necrosis and lymphocyte infiltration of portal tracts to more severe inflammation, resulting in disruption of the limiting plate between the portal tract and the parenchyma. The latter features are known as piecemeal necrosis. In addition, "ground-glass" hepatocytes, which contain large amounts of hepatitis B surface antigen (HBsAg), may be visible in hematoxylin-eosin-stained sections. Chronic type B hepatitis may progress to cirrhosis and hepatocellular carcinoma. Specific antibody staining for HBsAg or hepatitis B core antigen (HBcAg) in acute hepatitis B shows little detectable viral antigen in the liver. In chronic hepatitis, large amounts of HBsAg and (if viral replication is active) HBcAg may be found in hepatocytes.

There is no evidence that HBV is cytopathic, and thus it is thought that hepatocyte injury is mediated by the immune response against the virus. In this regard, evidence has been presented that lymphocytes derived from the liver or circulation of patients with hepatitis B infection are cytotoxic for autologous hepatocytes, but the specificity and mechanism of this cytotoxicity have not yet been completely defined.

Clinical Features

The symptoms of hepatitis B infection are highly variable. As many as half the cases of acute infection are anicteric, and patients have no symptoms or mild nonspecific symptoms of a viral illness. Symptoms already described for acute hepatitis A may occur in typical symptomatic cases. Acute hepatitis B is occasionally preceded by a serum sickness-like syndrome. Approximately 5–10% of patients develop chronic infection (lasting more than 6 months). They often have had a mild or asymptomatic acute infection. During the phase of active viral replication, nonspecific symptoms or symptoms of acute viral hepatitis may be present. With progressive chronic hepatitis, symptoms attributable to cirrhosis or hepatic decompensation may supervene.

Physical findings in acute hepatitis B infection are few. Icterus may be present, the liver may be enlarged and mildly tender, and splenomegaly is sometimes present. In chronic hepatitis B infection, there are often no physical abnormalities until chronic liver damage occurs; at that point, findings common to other chronic liver diseases are seen.

Laboratory findings of acute hepatitis B are similar to those of hepatitis A. In chronic hepatitis B, the serum aminotransferase levels are highly variable and may be normal. If significant liver damage is present, however, hypoalbuminemia and prolongation of the prothrombin time may occur.

Immunologic Diagnosis

Serum immunologic findings in hepatitis B infection are variable, depending on the length and clinical outcome of the infection (Fig 37–5). During acute infection, both HBsAg and IgM anti-HBc are present; in addition, HBV, DNA, and a viral protein anti-

gen known as HBeAg make a transient appearance. With resolution of the acute infection, HBsAg disappears (usually after 1–6 months) and anti-HBsAg appears and persists for years. In chronic infection, the serum findings are variable and depend on the stage of the natural history of the infection. HBsAg is often present in very high titers, as is anti-HBc, but anti-HBs is absent. During the period of active viral replication, HBeAg, DNA polymerase, and HBV DNA are also present. Patients with asymptomatic chronic infection may have episodes of acute reactivation that correlate with the appearance of markers of active viral replication. Eventually, evidence of viral replication may disappear, and there is seroconversion to anti-HBe positivity.

Differential Diagnosis

The serologic diagnosis of acute and chronic hepatitis B infection is usually definitive. In the setting of chronic hepatitis B infection, an apparent relapse should prompt a search for other possible causes of liver disease, including superimposed delta hepatitis (see next major section) or drug-induced hepatotoxicity.

Treatment

Acute hepatitis B usually resolves completely, and supportive care is needed only for severe hepatitis. Interferon alpha therapy may induce remission in some patients with chronic hepatitis. Liver transplantation may save patients with fulminant hepatitis.

Prevention

Screening of blood products for hepatitis B virus has nearly eliminated blood products as a mode of transmission. Individuals at high risk of acquiring hepatitis B should be immunized with HBsAg vac-

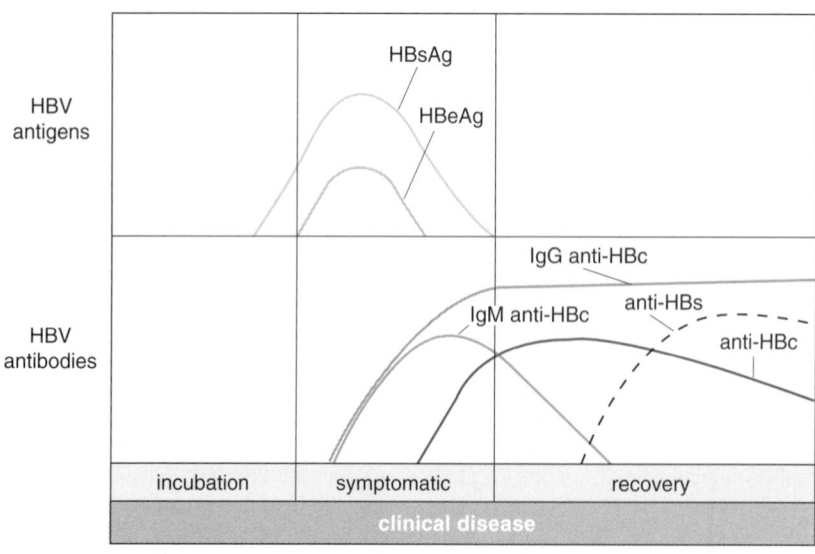

Figure 37–5. Hepatitis B antigens and antibody titers during the course of an acute hepatitis B infection.

cine, which is safe and confers long-lasting immunity in most individuals.

HEPATITIS D
(Delta Hepatitis)

Major Immunologic Features
- Defective virus requiring the presence of HBV infection (hepatitis B markers present in serum) causes this infection.
- Antidelta antibody is present in serum.

General Considerations
Hepatitis D is caused by a small defective (ie, unable to replicate in the absence of another virus) RNA virus (delta agent), which requires the presence of HBV for replication and production of infectious particles. The virus may be associated with acute or fulminant hepatitis due to coinfection with HBV, or it may cause a superimposed acute or chronic hepatitis in patients with chronic hepatitis B infection. The virus is found worldwide and has caused epidemics with high mortality rates. Transmission is primarily parenteral. Since inflammation is not a prominent feature, it is thought that the virus is directly cytopathic. Diagnosis is established by the presence of serum antidelta antibody and consistent clinical features. There is no effective specific treatment; however, it may be prevented by immunization for hepatitis B, since this prevents the hepatitis B infection necessary for hepatitis D virus replication.

HEPATITIS C
(Non-A, Non-B Hepatitis)

Major Immunologic Features
- Acute and chronic hepatitis similar to hepatitis B is the mode of presentation.
- There is a specific immunoassay for antibody to viral protein.
- Hepatitis C viral RNA is present in serum.

General Considerations
Shortly after the development of serologic tests for hepatitis B, it became clear that a significant proportion of patients with acute and chronic posttransfusion hepatitis did not have hepatitis B. A substantial literature subsequently evolved concerning this form of hepatitis, named non-A, and non-B. Hepatitis C virus was not identified until 1989, when Choo and coworkers isolated a cDNA clone from the blood of a patient with non-A, non-B hepatitis and showed that patients with non-A, non-B hepatitis have serum antibodies reactive with synthetic proteins derived from the cDNA sequence. This led quickly to the routine screening of blood donors with an antibody assay, even before complete isolation of the virus.

Hepatitis C virus is an RNA virus that is a member of the Flavivirus group, which includes dengue and yellow fever viruses. Recent work has shown considerable heterogeneity of hepatitis C virus sequences, and these differences may cause differences in their pathogenicity. The distribution of the virus is worldwide and its frequency in blood donors is relatively uniform, ranging from 0.3 to 1.5%. The major known mode of transmission of the virus is by blood, and thus the risk groups for this viral infection include patients who have had blood transfusion, hemodialysis patients, recipients of blood products, intravenous drug abusers, and health care workers. A significant proportion of cases of sporadic, community-acquired hepatitis C virus infection are not associated with any known risk, and in these patients the mode of transmission is unknown. Unlike hepatitis B, vertical transmission from mother to infant does not occur at a significant frequency, probably because patients with chronic hepatitis C virus infection have very low levels of viremia. Furthermore, the risk of sexual transmission appears to be low. Screening of blood donors by using an assay that detects multiple different hepatitis C antigens has greatly diminished the risk of transmission of this disease by blood transfusion. Since antibody-positivity does not appear immediately after infection, however, antibody screening cannot completely eliminate the risk of transmission by blood transfusion. The only definitive test for hepatitis C viremia is based on reverse transcription and polymerase chain reaction (PCR) amplification of viral sequences.

Liver disease caused by hepatitis C virus has many similarities to hepatitis B. The infection frequently has an onset with a typical, acute hepatitis-like illness as described earlier. Other presentations are possible, including fulminant hepatitis and subclinical infection. Chronic infection with chronic hepatitis is a common sequela of hepatitis C infection, occurring in about one half of patients. The illness may be characterized by marked fluctuation in the serum transaminase levels. Progression to significant fibrosis and cirrhosis is also relatively common, occurring in about 10% of patients overall. It is now clear that some patients who had been classified as having autoimmune hepatitis in the past have evidence of hepatitis C virus infection (see later section). Furthermore, many patients previously classified as having cryptogenic cirrhosis have evidence of hepatitis C virus infection. As with hepatitis B, there is a significant association of hepatocellular carcinoma with cirrhosis due to hepatitis C virus infection. Other syndromes are also associated with this infection, such as mixed cryoglobulinemia with glomerulonephritis.

Randomized controlled trials have demonstrated that some patients with chronic hepatitis C virus infection have beneficial response to long-term (26 weeks) treatment with interferon alpha. Because of the great expense, toxicity, and relatively low response rate, this therapy is generally limited to patients with evidence of significant disease activity. About one half of patients have a beneficial response as indicated by a marked fall in transaminase levels and disappearance of viral RNA from serum; however, only about 10–20% of patients have a sustained remission.

HEPATITIS E

Antihepatitis E antibody is present in serum. Hepatitis E virus is an RNA virus that is a major cause of acute hepatitis resembling hepatitis A. The virus is a major cause of both sporadic and epidemic hepatitis in developing countries and is transmitted by the fecal–oral route. To date the only cases found in the United States have been found in travelers from areas where the infection is endemic. Hepatitis E has clinical features very similar to those of hepatitis A. It does not cause chronic hepatitis and is not associated with hepatocellular carcinoma. One interesting aspect of the disease that has not been explained is that there is a high fatality rate in pregnant women. Hepatitis E virus infection is associated with the appearance of serum antibodies that can be detected by enzyme-linked immunosorbent assay (ELISA). Hepatitis E viral RNA has been detected in stool by PCR assays. Preliminary studies have indicated that animals exposed to hepatitis E virus develop protective immunity, suggesting that the development of an effective vaccine is feasible.

AUTOIMMUNE CHRONIC ACTIVE HEPATITIS

Major Immunologic Features

- Antinuclear antibodies and autoantibodies are present to smooth muscle and liver membranes.
- Polyclonal hypergammaglobulinemia occurs.
- HLA-B8/DR3 association exists.
- Destruction of hepatocytes is associated with portal infiltration of lymphocytes.

General Considerations

Autoimmune hepatitis is a rare form of chronic hepatitis of unknown cause and is associated with various autoimmune phenomena. The disease usually affects women and is more common in individuals of northern European descent. The great majority of cases are sporadic. Of interest, there is a significant association with HLA-B8/DR3 as well as an association with the Gm allotype of IgG, termed "ax." For unknown reasons the incidence of the disease has been declining.

Pathology

The major histologic finding in the liver, one not specific to this disease and mentioned before in rela-

tion to hepatitis B infection, is piecemeal necrosis, in which there is necrosis of hepatocytes in the periportal region, disruption of the limiting plate of the portal tract, and local infiltration of lymphoid cells (Fig 37–6). The degree of piecemeal necrosis is variable, but in some patients it may lead to bridging necrosis and cirrhosis. The lymphoid cells infiltrating lesions of autoimmune hepatitis consist of plasma cells and CD4-positive T cells. There are immunoglobulin deposits on hepatocytes.

The mechanism of liver damage in autoimmune hepatitis is unknown. Although autoantibodies against the liver have been shown to be present, it is not clear that they play a role in liver damage. Lymphocyte-mediated killing of autologous hepatocytes has been demonstrated in vitro; however, the specificity and mechanism of this killing are uncertain.

Clinical Features

Typical symptoms of autoimmune hepatitis include easy fatigability, jaundice, dark urine, abdominal pain, anorexia, myalgia, delayed menarche, and amenorrhea. Late in the disease, symptoms attributable to progressive chronic liver disease may supervene. Abnormal physical findings include hepatomegaly, jaundice, splenomegaly, spider nevi, and cushingoid features. Common laboratory findings include elevation of serum aminotransferase levels and hypergammaglobulinemia.

Immunologic Diagnosis

There are no serologic features that are diagnostic of the disease. Polyclonal hypergammaglobulinemia is typically found, however, and autoantibodies are common, particularly antinuclear antibodies and smooth muscle antibodies. In addition, antibodies against liver membrane antigens are present. Antimitochondrial antibodies are usually absent and, when present, are found in low titer. Serologic markers of hepatitis viruses are absent. The presence of HLA-B8 supports the diagnosis.

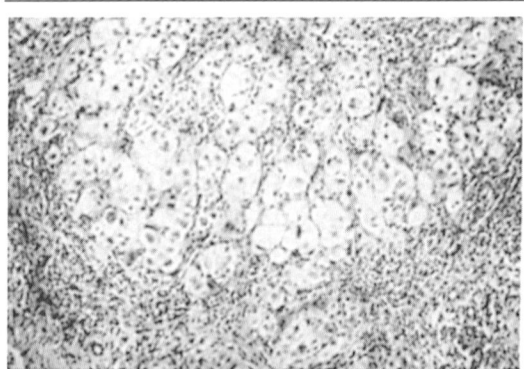

Figure 37–6. Chronic HBV infection. Liver biopsy specimen shows ballooning of hepatocytes and piecemeal necrosis typical of chronic active hepatitis.

Differential Diagnosis

Since there are no specific diagnostic tests, viral hepatitis and drug- or chemical-induced liver injury must be excluded as well as rare liver diseases such as Wilson's disease and other metabolic liver diseases such as α_1-antitrypsin deficiency. Primary biliary cirrhosis may have features that overlap those of autoimmune hepatitis, but this disease is associated with the presence of antimitochondrial antibodies (see later discussion). Primary sclerosing cholangitis is occasionally misdiagnosed as autoimmune hepatitis, but this disease is associated with characteristic radiographic abnormalities of the biliary system.

Treatment

Unlike those with viral hepatitis, patients with severe autoimmune hepatitis respond favorably to corticosteroid treatment. This therapy may prevent or retard the development of cirrhosis and may improve survival.

PRIMARY BILIARY CIRRHOSIS

Major Immunologic Features

- Associated autoimmune syndromes are frequent.
- The titer of antimitochondrial antibodies is high in most patients.
- Serum IgM with abnormal properties is elevated.
- There is lymphocytic infiltration and destruction of intrahepatic bile ducts.

General Considerations

Primary biliary cirrhosis is a chronic disease of unknown cause, primarily affecting middle-aged women. It is characterized by chronic intrahepatic cholestasis due to chronic inflammation and necrosis of intrahepatic bile ducts and progresses insidiously to biliary cirrhosis. Although syndromes resembling primary biliary cirrhosis may follow ingestion of drugs such as chlorpromazine or contraceptive steroids, no toxic or infectious agent has been identified. It has been suggested that primary biliary cirrhosis is an autoimmune disease because of the frequent association of other autoimmune syndromes, the presence of autoantibodies, and histologic features of the disease. Its prevalence has been estimated to be 2.3–14.4 per 100,000. The distribution of the disease is worldwide, without predilection for any racial or ethnic groups. The usual age at diagnosis is in the fifth and sixth decades, but age at onset varies widely from the third to the ninth decade. Ninety percent of patients are female. Familial aggregation has been reported but is rare; however, although there is no known HLA association, the incidence of immunologic abnormalities has been reported to be increased in family members.

Pathology

The histologic abnormalities in the liver have been divided into four stages, although they overlap, and more than one stage may be found in biopsies from the same patient. The earliest changes (stage I) are most specific and consist of localized areas of infiltration of intrahepatic bile ducts with lymphocytes and necrosis of biliary epithelial cells; these lesions may have granulomas in close proximity (Fig 37–7). In stage II there is proliferation of bile ductules, prominent infiltration of portal areas with lymphoid cells, and early portal fibrosis. Stage III is characterized by reduction of the inflammatory changes, paucity of bile ducts in the portal triads, and increased portal fibrosis. In stage IV, fibrosis is prominent in biliary cirrhosis and a marked increase in hepatic copper is found. Thus, the pathologic process is characterized by slowly progressive, spotty destruction of bile ducts, with associated inflammation and fibrosis and, ultimately, cirrhosis. Hepatocellular necrosis is not a prominent feature, although there are occasional cases of primary biliary cirrhosis/chronic active hepatitis overlap syndromes with piecemeal necrosis. Immunofluorescence shows predominantly IgM plasma cells in portal triads and deposition of IgM. CD4 T cells predominate in portal triads, but CD8 T cells have been observed in close proximity to damaged epithelial cells. HLA-DR antigen expression is increased on biliary epithelial cells, a finding associated with autoimmunity (see Chapter 32).

Although the mechanisms of liver injury in this disease are unknown, the presence of associated autoimmune syndromes and other features suggests that primary biliary cirrhosis is an autoimmune disease. Patients frequently have circulating immune complex–like materials, abnormalities of the complement cascade, and nearly always antimitochondrial antibodies. These antibodies have different specificities, the most prevalent being against the E2 component of pyruvate dehydrogenase, which is present on the inner mitochondrial membrane. In recent years, ample evidence of immunoregulator abnormalities have been found, and it is thought that these underlie the autoimmunity.

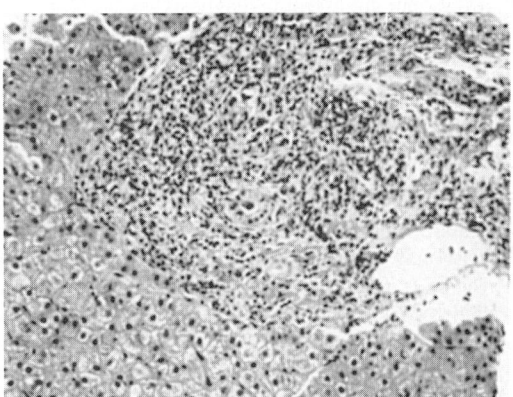

Figure 37–7. Primary biliary cirrhosis. Percutaneous liver biopsy specimen shows bile duct surrounded by dense lymphoid infiltrate typical of stage I disease.

Clinical Features

The onset of symptoms is typically insidious, and as many as half of all patients are asymptomatic at diagnosis. Typical symptoms include pruritus, fatigue, increased skin pigmentation, arthralgias, and dryness of the mouth and eyes. Jaundice and gastrointestinal bleeding from varices are uncommon presentations. There may be no abnormalities on physical examination. Typical findings that occur with disease progression include hepatomegaly, splenomegaly, skin hyperpigmentation, excoriations, xanthomata, xanthelasma, spider telangiectasia, and, late in the disease, deep jaundice, petechiae, purpura, and signs of hepatic decompensation. In addition, symptoms or signs of the many associated autoimmune syndromes may be present. The most common include keratoconjunctivitis sicca, arthritis, hypothyroidism, scleroderma (CREST variant), Raynaud's phenomenon, and pulmonary alveolitis.

Common laboratory abnormalities include elevation of serum alkaline phosphatase and γ-glutamyl transpeptidase. Total bilirubin is normal early in the disease but increases progressively as the disease advances. Hypercholesterolemia is also common. Nonspecific laboratory changes of hepatic decompensation are found late in the disease. Cholangiography is normal early in the course of the disease but may reveal distortion of bile ducts due to cirrhosis late in the disease.

Immunologic Diagnosis

The nearly pathognomonic immunologic feature of primary biliary cirrhosis is the presence in high titer of nonspecies-specific, nonorgan-specific antibodies against the inner-membrane components of mitochondria. Antimitochondrial antibodies are found in other autoimmune syndromes but only in low titer. Less than 10% of primary biliary cirrhosis patients lack these antibodies. Many other autoantibodies are commonly found in patients but are not useful in diagnosis. Other immunologic abnormalities, such as circulating immune complex-like materials, complement abnormalities, and abnormalities of lymphocyte function, are not useful in diagnosis.

Differential Diagnosis

Chronic cholestasis may follow the administration of drugs such as chlorpromazine, but this does not lead to progressive loss of bile ducts, and it resolves following withdrawal of the drug. Hepatic sarcoidosis may closely mimic primary biliary cirrhosis, but mitochondrial antibodies are absent. Graft-versus-host disease may be found in patients with primary biliary cirrhosis, but in the former disease the basement membrane around bile ducts remains intact. Hepatic allograft rejection may also be associated with nonsuppurative destructive cholangitis.

Treatment

Medical treatment includes supportive treatment such as anion exchange resins to relieve pruritus and administration of lipid-soluble vitamins for nutritional deficiencies. Attempts to suppress the primary inflammatory process have been disappointing. Corticosteroids are considered to be contraindicated because of their tendency in uncontrolled studies to exacerbate metabolic bone disease, complicating the disease. Azathioprine and colchicine may improve survival marginally. D-Penicillamine does not increase survival and is associated with severe side effects. Cyclosporin has been used on an investigational basis but has not yet been proved to be efficacious. Treatment with ursodeoxycholic acid has been associated with improved clinical findings and chance of survival in some patients. The only treatment for end-stage disease is hepatic transplantation.

Complications & Prognosis

Progressive disease is often associated with metabolic bone disease and may lead to chronic hepatic decompensation. Survival from the time of diagnosis is highly variable; asymptomatic patients may have a normal life span. For symptomatic patients, survival from diagnosis is about 12 years. Patients with end-stage disease may be excellent candidates for transplantation, and the long-term prognosis in patients who survive the procedure is good.

PRIMARY SCLEROSING CHOLANGITIS

Major Immunologic Features

- Chronic inflammation and fibrosis of intrahepatic and extrahepatic bile ducts are present.
- Association with inflammatory bowel disease is common.

General Considerations

Primary sclerosing cholangitis is a disease of unknown origin characterized by inflammation and fibrosis of both intrahepatic and extrahepatic bile ducts. The disease occurs primarily in young men but may be found in children and older adults. It is often associated with chronic inflammatory bowel disease (usually ulcerative colitis). It is usually progressive and leads to biliary cirrhosis. In addition, it has a significant association with cholangiocarcinoma.

The symptoms are similar to those of other chronic cholestatic diseases and include fatigue, pruritus, hyperpigmentation, xanthelasma, and jaundice. Patients may have fever and abdominal pain associated with superimposed acute bacterial cholangitis. Symptoms of underlying inflammatory bowel disease may be prominent, mild, or absent. Extrahepatic manifestations (other than inflammatory bowel disease) are unusual. Laboratory findings are generally similar to those in primary biliary cirrhosis; however, it is distinct from the latter disease in that antimitochondrial antibodies are absent.

The most important laboratory test is cholangiography, which demonstrates tortuosity and areas of dilatation and stricture of either intrahepatic bile ducts, extrahepatic bile ducts, or both.

The liver biopsy is usually abnormal but is often not diagnostic; in fact, the abnormalities occasionally resemble those in primary biliary cirrhosis or autoimmune hepatitis. A characteristic feature that does occur is a fibrous–obliterative process in which segments of bile ducts are replaced by solid cords of connective tissue, leading to an "onion skin" appearance. The differential diagnosis includes biliary stricture secondary to stones, surgery, or neoplasia. Like primary biliary cirrhosis, treatment is supportive (eg, antibiotics for cholangitis), and the underlying disease has proved resistant to treatment with anti-inflammatory agents. Patients with localized areas of high-grade obstruction in large bile ducts may benefit from palliative surgical procedures to relieve obstruction. Patients with advanced diseases who have not had prior surgery may be excellent candidates for hepatic transplantation.

ORODENTAL DISEASES

John S. Greenspan, BDS, PhD, FRCPath

The mouth is the portal of entry for a variety of antigens, including numerous microorganisms, into the alimentary and respiratory systems. Normally, these antigens do not cause disease and are flushed away with swallowed saliva into the distal parts of the alimentary tract. The mucosal barrier, continual desquamation of oral epithelium, toothbrushing, and other forms of mouth cleaning mechanically protect the mouth. Immunologic defense mechanisms, particularly secretory IgA antibodies, probably prevent adherence of microorganisms to mucosal and tooth surfaces by aggregating them and possibly rendering them more susceptible to phagocytosis.

Several of the most important oral diseases, including caries, the common forms of gingival and periodontal disease, oral herpes simplex virus infections, candidal infections, and the oral manifestations of primary and secondary immunodeficiency, especially AIDS, are due to an imbalance between oral organisms and the host response. This imbalance results from **hypersensitivity, immunologic deficiency,** or **direct tissue damage** regardless of the status of the host response, as in the case of dental caries and chronic inflammatory periodontal disease.

Another group of oral diseases in which immunologic factors have been implicated are those in which oral tissues are a target for **autoimmune reactions.** Manifestations may be confined to the mouth or may involve other systemic organs. Many are mucocutaneous diseases, several are rheumatoid diseases, and others involve mainly the gastrointestinal tract. The role of **tumor immune mechanisms** in oral homeostasis and the part that defects in these mechanisms play in the cause and pathogenesis of oral precancerous lesions and mucosal malignancy constitute a growing field of interest. Tumor immune mechanisms are probably important but must be considered in the context of other factors, including oncogenic viruses and chemical carcinogens.

LOCAL ORAL DISEASES INVOLVING IMMUNOLOGIC MECHANISMS

1. INFLAMMATORY PERIODONTAL DISEASES: GINGIVITIS & PERIODONTITIS

Major Immunologic Features

- Bacterial dental plaque induces inflammation of tissues immediately surrounding the teeth.
- The local responses of the host are not effective in eliminating the bacteria, which continue to adhere to the tooth surfaces. Humoral and cellular immunity are both involved in these responses.
- Local responses include complement activation, infiltration of leukocytes, release of lysosomal enzymes and cytokines, and production of a serous gingival crevicular exudate.
- Inflammatory agents from the bacteria and immunopathologic reactions of the host result in gingivitis and periodontitis.

General Considerations

Inflammation of the supporting tissues of the teeth produces one of the most common forms of human diseases. Depending on its severity, the destructive process may involve both the gingiva (**gingivitis**) and the periodontal ligament and alveolar bone surrounding and supporting the teeth (**periodontitis**). Periodontitis may involve both the direct cytotoxic and proteolytic effects of dental plaque and the indirect pathologic consequences of the host immune response to the continued presence of bacterial plaque microorganisms (Fig 37–8).

Dental plaque consists of a mass of bacteria that adheres tenaciously to the tooth surfaces. In gingivitis, the plaque generates inflammation of the gingival tissue without affecting the underlying periodontal ligament and bone. In periodontitis, attachment between the gingiva and the involved teeth is lost, subgingival bacterial plaque forms on the root surfaces, and bone loss is clinically apparent (Figs 37–9 and 37–10). Elimination of the plaque usually stops the inflammatory process. In children with poor oral hygiene, gingivitis is common but periodontitis is rare.

The microflora of the dental plaque is complex, comprising many different strains of bacteria including gram-positive rods and cocci and gram-negative rods, cocci, and filamentous forms. In general, the healthy gingival crevice contains only a few gram-positive

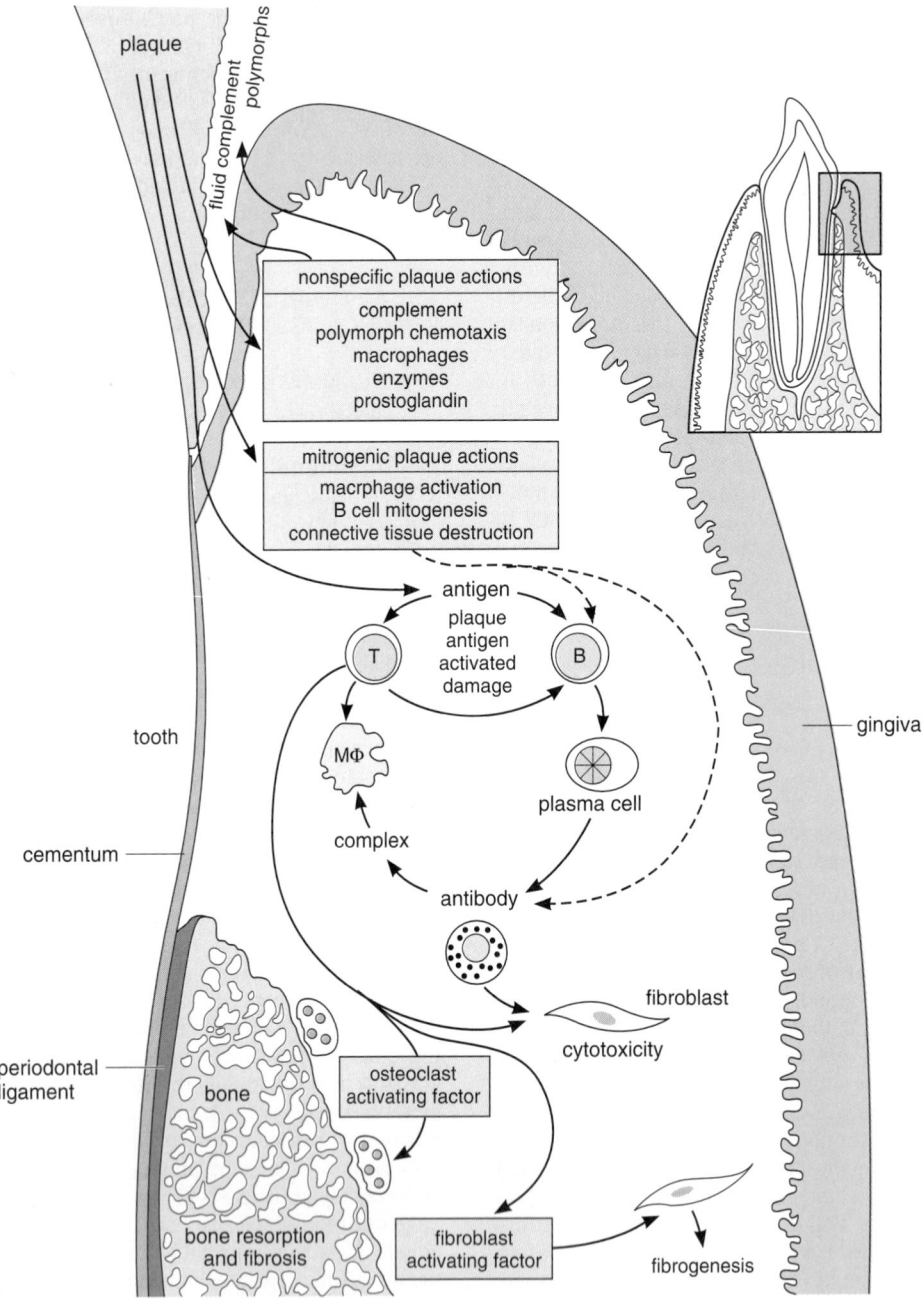

Figure 37–8. The pathogenesis of periodontal disease.

streptococcal and facultative *Actinomyces* species. As gingivitis develops, many more gram-negative organisms are found, including *Fusobacterium nucleatum, Bacteroides intermedius,* and *Haemophilus* species. Many motile rods and spirochetes are also seen. In advanced adult periodontitis, the organisms usually cultured are predominantly gram-negative anaerobic rods, such as *Bacteroides gingivalis, B intermedius,* and *F nucleatum.* Furthermore, phase-contrast examination shows that as many as 50% of organisms from such lesions are motile rods and spirochetes. There is some indirect evidence for a relationship between particular forms of periodontal disease and specific microorganisms. Thus, elevated levels and increased frequency of serum antibodies to *Actinobacillus actinomycetemcomitans, Capnocytophaga* spp, and *Eikenella corrodens* are found in localized juvenile periodontitis (rapidly progressive periodontitis) (see section 2).

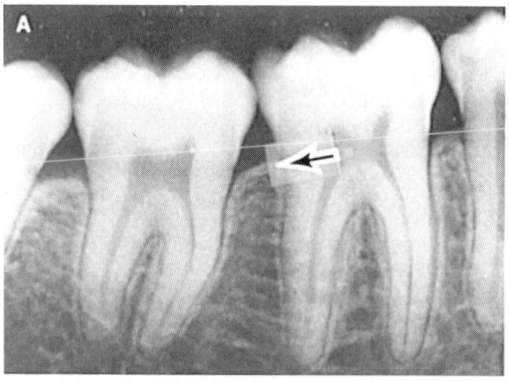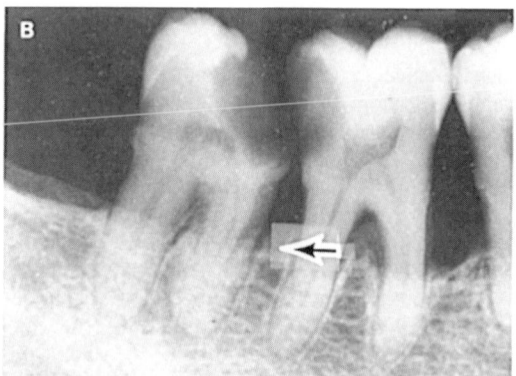

Figure 37–9. *A:* Radiographs of the lower molars of a 25-year-old man with a normal periodontium and *B:* a 45-year-old man with advanced periodontitis and severe dental caries. In the patient with periodontitis, more than half of the supporting alveolar bone has been destroyed (arrows). (Courtesy of GC Armitage.)

Immunologic Pathogenesis

A delicate balance exists between dental plaque organisms and the host response. In healthy individuals, the immunologic response provides a well-regulated specific defense against infiltration by plaque substances. The tissue-destructive mechanisms thought to be involved in periodontal disease include direct effects of plaque bacteria, polymorphonuclear-induced damage, neutrophil complement-mediated damage initiated by both antibody and the alternative pathway, and cell-mediated damage.

Clinically apparent gingivitis is probably the result of an exaggerated response to bacterial plaque. Individuals with mild gingivitis have, in addition to a continued polymorphonuclear infiltration, a gingival influx of a few T lymphocytes. Those with prolonged severe gingivitis and severe periodontitis, however, have an influx composed mainly of B lymphocytes and plasma cells, with resulting IgG antibody production. Most noteworthy in severe periodontal disease is the extremely low proportion of gingival plasma cells committed to IgG2 production, while serum levels of the other IgG subclasses are normal. The proportions of antibodies of IgG3, IgG1, or IgG4 subclasses with specific antibody activity for plaque antigens in the gingival tissues are unknown. This unusual local IgG subclass response may indicate a degree of nonspecific activation of B lymphocytes arriving in the inflamed area, possibly caused by a variety of mechanisms involving bacterial mitogens and proteinases. The bacteria may also activate the alternative complement pathway. Associated with gingivitis is the generation of a serum exudate known as **crevicular fluid,** which flows from around the teeth and contacts the dental plaque. This exudate, like serum, contains functional complement components as well as low levels of specific antibodies to the various plaque antigens.

The onset of flow of crevicular fluid is an important stage in the progression of periodontal disease. Crevicular fluid complement is rapidly activated by a

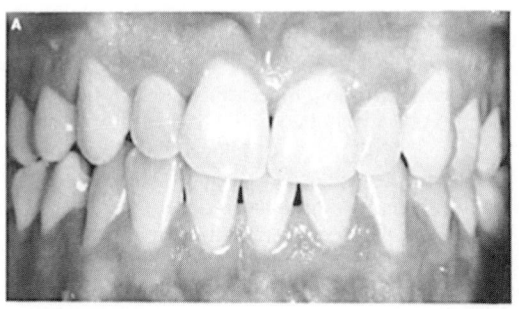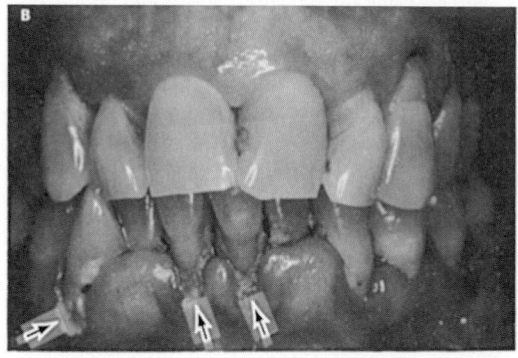

Figure 37–10. *A:* Clinical appearance of the anterior teeth and periodontal tissues of a 22-year-old man with healthy gingiva and *B:* a 48-year-old man with advanced periodontitis. Note the heavy deposits of plaque and calculus (arrows) in the patient with periodontitis. Marked gingival inflammation is particularly noticeable around the lower anterior teeth. Most teeth have either pocket formation or extensive gingival recession. (Courtesy of GC Armitage.)

combination of effects. These include activation of the classic pathway by IgG and IgM antibodies to subgingival plaque antigens; activation of the alternative complement pathway by endotoxins and peptidoglycan from gram-negative and gram-positive microorganisms, respectively; and activation of complement components by host and bacterial proteolytic enzymes. Complement activation results first in the release of C3a and C5a, which cause additional edema and increase crevicular fluid flow, and subsequently in chemotactic attraction of polymorphonuclear leukocytes. Other chemotactic factors are produced directly by the plaque microorganisms. The release of proteolytic enzymes with collagenase and trypsin-like activities by host cells is believed to damage tissue and activate additional complement components and subsequent release of prostaglandin E. In vitro, prostaglandin E can induce bone resorption through its effect on osteoclasts.

Cell-mediated immunity may also play a role in the progression of periodontal disease. In some studies, individuals with periodontal disease generally exhibit increased peripheral blood T-lymphocyte reactivity to plaque antigens. Yet, for reasons unknown, in severe gingivitis and severe periodontitis the local T-cell response to the plaque is conspicuously small. Bone destruction in periodontal disease may be mediated by lymphokines, including osteoclast-activating factor, as well as by parathyroid hormone and prostaglandins. Individuals with reduced immunologic capacity, notably primary immunodeficiency and immunodeficiency secondary to treatment associated with kidney transplantation, do not have more gingival and periodontal disease than do normal controls. Severe periodontal disease is seen in association with HIV infection, however.

Immunologic Diagnosis

Lymphocytes from individuals with periodontal disease are more responsive to dental plaque antigens in vitro than are lymphocytes from normal individuals, but no clear relationships have been found between disease severity and serum or salivary antibody levels. At present, immunologic tests are not generally useful in the diagnosis of gingivitis and periodontitis. Most individuals with inflammatory periodontitis have gingivitis, but the clinical symptoms of the latter may be masked by fibrosis.

Treatment

Although gingivitis and periodontitis are apparently caused by dental bacterial plaque, there is a reluctance to treat this disease with antibiotics because elimination of one group of organisms by antibiotics may lead to the emergence of antibiotic-resistant strains. Some clinicians, however, use local application of tetracycline depending on the severity of the periodontal disease. Treatment may range from simply good routine oral hygiene to periodontal surgery.

Reduction of plaque accumulation to an absolute minimum is essential for the arrest of gingivitis or the reduction of periodontal ligament destruction and bone loss. Topical antibacterial agents, notably chlorhexidine, are valuable for this purpose.

2. JUVENILE PERIODONTITIS

In a small percentage of the population, periodontal bone loss occurs very rapidly, sometimes within 2–5 years. In this condition—juvenile periodontitis, formerly known simply as periodontitis—conventional periodontal treatment is ineffective. There is a characteristic gram-negative anaerobic flora, different from that in the more slowly progressive form of periodontitis. Short-term antibiotics are probably useful in these cases, but there is no evidence that the results of such treatment are permanent. Several reports suggest that defects in granulocyte or monocyte function may be involved.

RECURRENT APHTHOUS ULCERATION
(Aphthous Stomatitis)

Major Immunologic Features

- Lymphocyte infiltration is present at the earliest stage of the lesion.
- Circulating antibodies to oral mucous membranes are present in some patients and may cross-react with oral organisms.
- Cellular immunity to the same antigens is reported.
- Circulating immune complexes are found in some patients.
- There is association with HLA-B12.
- Response to topical or systemic corticosteroids is favorable.

General Considerations

After caries and chronic periodontal disease, oral ulceration probably represents the most common lesion of the mouth. Although oral ulcers can be due to a large number of diseases, the most common form is **recurrent aphthous ulceration (RAU)** (aphthous stomatitis) (Fig 37–11). Recurrent oral ulcers usually occur alone but may be a local manifestation of **Behçet's disease** when accompanied by uveitis, genital ulcers, and perhaps lesions of other systems. Estimates of the prevalence of recurrent oral ulceration vary, but probably 20% of the population experiences it. The condition may recur only once or twice a year or may be so frequent that a new set of ulcers overlaps a previous group. There is slight evidence of a familial incidence. Severe RAU can be seen in association with HIV infection. Emotional, hematologic, and nutritional factors may play a causative role, and

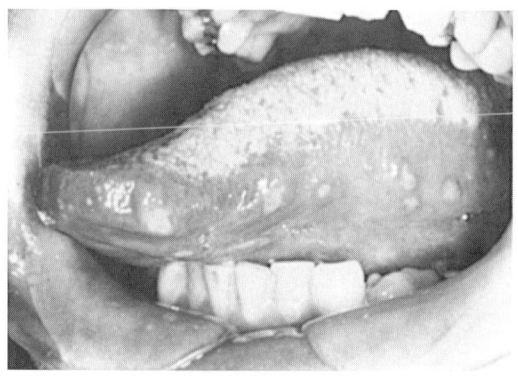

Figure 37–11. Recurrent aphthous ulcers.

an association has been suggested with changes in the hormone status during the menstrual cycle. Extensive searches for specific bacterial or viral causes have been unsuccessful. A possible role for herpes simplex virus type I has again been raised by the observation that part of the herpes simplex virus genome is present and transcribed in peripheral blood mononuclear cells of patients with recurrent aphthae and Behçet's disease. Additional evidence also indicates a possible role for *Streptococcus sanguis,* since this organism has been cultured from the ulcers and patients exhibit delayed hypersensitivity reactions to the organism and significant inhibition of leukocyte migration by antigens of this organism in vitro. The organism is a common commensal, however. One study has shown reduced lymphocyte transformation to *S sanguis* in patients compared with controls. A likely role for bacterial or viral agents in this disease is that of cross-reacting antigens, which elicit host responses to autologous oral mucous membrane antigens.

Immunologic Pathogenesis

Patients have a raised level of **circulating antibody** to a saline extract of fetal oral mucous membrane. Slightly raised levels of the same antibody have been found in other ulcerative conditions but in lower titers. The antibodies are of the agglutinating and complement-fusing types, suggesting that antibody cytotoxicity might be involved in the tissue destruction. Some studies, however, show poor correlation between the level of antimucous membrane antibody and clinical features of the disease. In addition, two other mechanisms could explain the presence of circulating autoantibodies of this type. The antibodies may cross-react with antigens of an organism present in the mouth, such as *S sanguis* or a virus, and oral mucous membrane epithelial cells. Alternatively, the antibodies may be a response to exposed tissue antigens from chronic ulcerations that had previously been protected from the immune system. Attempts to show that patient serum containing significant titers of this anti-

body has a direct cytotoxic effect against oral epithelial cells have been unsuccessful. Thus, it is unlikely that a cytotoxic antioral mucosal antibody is directly involved in the pathogenesis.

Interest in the role of **cellular immunity** in the pathogenesis of recurrent aphthous ulceration was aroused by the observation that the earliest histologic changes involve the presence of an infiltrate of lymphocytes. Other cells do not appear until a later stage. Furthermore, patients with recurrent oral ulceration have peripheral blood lymphocytes that are sensitized to oral mucous membrane antigen. These two observations support the hypothesis that a cell-mediated hypersensitivity mechanism might be involved in the pathogenesis of the lesion. Lymphocytes from some patients with recurrent aphthous ulceration are cytotoxic to oral epithelial cells. The antigen eliciting the cytotoxic reaction has not been identified. It might be one or more epithelial cell surface autoantigens, determinants cross-reacting with an infecting organism or organisms, or food or microbial antigens attached to oral epithelial cell surfaces or even by a hapten. Increased antibody-dependent cell-mediated cytotoxicity has been found, but the identity of the population of lymphocytes involved in these reactions is also unknown. Increased production of tumor necrosis factor (TNF) by peripheral blood lymphocytes of patients with RAU has been observed. There is at present no acceptable hypothesis linking oral mucous membrane autoantigens and effector mechanisms, although transient defects in immunoregulation have been postulated.

Patients with Behçet's disease and recurrent oral ulceration show elevated levels of serum C9 and of circulating soluble immune complexes. IgG and C3 have also been demonstrated in the basement membrane zone of the lesions. It is not clear whether these observations are clues to the immunologic pathogenesis of the disease or represent epiphenomena. There is also some evidence for an increased incidence of HLA-B12 in recurrent oral ulceration.

Treatment & Prognosis

Effective treatment depends on identification of any underlying systemic disease. In such cases, treatment of the systemic condition usually leads to cure of the oral ulceration. For the remaining group, uncomplicated by known systemic disease, several treatment forms are available. They are the use of topical corticosteroids, antibiotics, and immunostimulants. The most effective topical corticosteroids available are 0.1% triamcinolone in Orabase, 2.5-mg tablets of hydrocortisone sodium succinate, and 0.025% fluocinonide in Orabase. Some cases of major aphthous ulceration are sufficiently severe to warrant the use of systemic prednisone. Tetracycline mouth rinses have been used with some success in the herpetiform variety of recurrent aphthous ulceration. The treatment of Behçet's disease is discussed in Chapters 33 and 36.

ACQUIRED IMMUNODEFICIENCY SYNDROME

The oral mucosa is particularly hospitable to **opportunistic pathogens.** Thus, primary and recurrent herpes simplex virus, varicella-zoster virus, and several fungi, notably *Candida* species, are frequent features of primary cellular immunodeficiency syndromes (see Chapters 22 and 53). The same conditions, as well as a number of others, are seen in patients whose immune systems are compromised by chemotherapy, those receiving bone marrow transplants, patients with leukemia or lymphoma, and those with clinical expressions of HIV-induced immunosuppression.

The oral features of acquired immunodeficiency syndrome (AIDS) include Kaposi's sarcoma, non-Hodgkin's lymphoma, and severe oral candidiasis (Fig 37–12), as well as persistent herpesvirus lesions (herpes simplex virus and varicella-zoster virus). Other conditions seen in AIDS and other HIV disease include severe periodontal disease, oral warts, and the recently described lesion known as **oral hairy leukoplakia.**

Hairy leukoplakia (Fig 37–13) is seen on the tongue in HIV-immunosuppressed patients. Ninety-nine percent of patients are HIV antibody-positive, and the majority of those tested carry the virus in blood lymphocytes. This lesion has characteristic histopathologic features suggestive of human papillomavirus, further evidence for the presence of which is provided by antigen staining. No human papillomavirus DNA is found by hybridization techniques, however. Instead, clear evidence for the presence of Epstein-Barr virus (EBV) comes from immunocytochemistry with monoclonal antibodies, from electron microscopic morphology, and from DNA studies with EBV probes. Southern blot hybridization provides evidence for the presence of EBV DNA in complete linear virion form and in very high copy number. At the time of diagnosis of hairy leukoplakia, about 20% of patients have AIDS, but a very large number of those

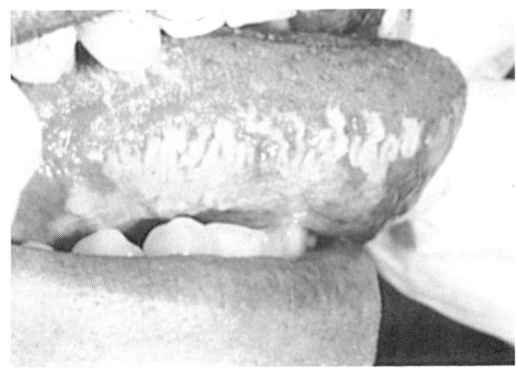

Figure 37–13. Hairy leukoplakia in an HIV-positive man.

who are AIDS-free when first seen subsequently develop AIDS, with mean conversion rates at 48% at 16 months and 83% at 30 months, mostly with *Pneumocystis carinii* pneumonia.

Oral hairy leukoplakia is a significant indicator of HIV-induced immunosuppression and is highly predictive of the subsequent development of AIDS, although rare cases are seen in HIV-negative people, mostly in association with other forms of secondary immunodeficiency. It appears to be one of only two oral lesions specifically associated with HIV infection. It is the first form of oral leukoplakia consistently associated with a virus or viruses. The mechanism whereby HIV favors oral opportunistic infection presumably involves viral elimination of helper T cells and thus the loss of cell-mediated immunity to herpesviruses and fungi as well as to other organisms. Other mechanisms may also mediate the immune defect, however, including loss of Langerhans' cells or their functions as well as polymorphonuclear cell and macrophage aberrations.

ORAL CANDIDIASIS

Major Immunologic Features
- There are many associated immunologic defects.
- It is the most significant oral indication of an underlying immunodeficiency.
- It is a prominent feature of HIV-induced immunodeficiency.

General Considerations

Oral candidiasis is the most common oral fungal disease. It may occur in acute or chronic form at any age. The disease may be a sign of life-threatening systemic disease or may be confined to a small part of the oral mucous membrane and have no general significance. *Candida* species are frequent oral commensals, and it has not yet been established whether candidiasis is predominantly of endogenous or exogenous origin.

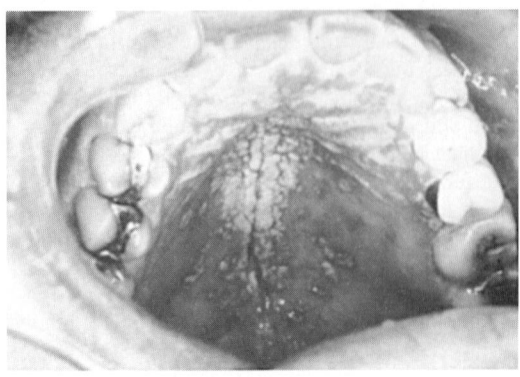

Figure 37–12. Pseudomembranous candidiasis in an HIV-positive man.

Immunologic Pathogenesis

The immunologic features of generalized candidiasis are discussed in Chapters 22 and 50. A wide range of **immunologic defects** have been found, including defects in cytotoxicity to *Candida*, reduced lymphokine production, failure of anticandidal antibody response of one or more classes, generalized cytotoxicity defects, failure of lymphocyte activation to candidal antigen, absence of the delayed hypersensitivity skin test to *Candida* or to many antigens, and presence of an abnormal suppressor T-cell population. Immunologic defects alone do not explain the pathogenesis of candidiasis, however. High glucose levels in diabetics and low levels of serum iron transferrin and blood folate are also important factors. Granulocyte defects have been shown in some patients, as have defects in leukocyte myeloperoxidase. A few patients have been described in whom antibody production to *Candida* and other antigens was enhanced while cellular immune function was depressed.

Immunologic Diagnosis

The diagnosis of pseudomembranous candidiasis **(thrush)** is based on the clinical appearance and history. The immunologic approach is directed toward establishing the nature of the immunologic defect, if any. Although immunologic investigation of patients with oral candidiasis is still predominantly a research tool, it is likely that subtypes of patients will be identified and that specific immunologic treatment will be directed toward the correction of localized defects in cell-mediated immunity. The differential diagnosis of candidal leukoplakia from other white oral lesions involves smear, culture, and biopsy.

Treatment & Prognosis

Treatment of localized oral candidiasis consists of elimination of predisposing factors, when known, and administration of topical antifungal therapy. This may be prolonged in the treatment of chronic oral candidiasis. Systemic therapy is used in cases that are resistant to local measures and in generalized mucocutaneous candidiasis.

REFERENCES

GENERAL

James SP: The immune system. In: *Bockus' Gastroenterology,* Haubrich W et al (editors). WB Saunders, 1995, p 3345.

Schiff L, Schiff ER: *Diseases of the Liver.* JB Lippincott, 1993.

Sleisenger M et al: *Gastrointestinal Diseases.* WB Saunders, 1993.

GASTROINTESTINAL DISEASES

Celiac Disease

Fry L: Dermatitis herpetiformis. *Baillieres Clin Gastroenterol* 1995;**9**(2):371.

Goggins M, Kelleher D: Celiac disease and other nutrient related injuries to the gastrointestinal tract. *Am J Gastroenterol* 1994;**89**(8 suppl):S2.

Inflammatory Bowel Disease

Peppercorn MA: Inflammatory Bowel Disease. *Gastroenterol Clin N Am* 1995;**24**:1–738, Entire issue.

Intestinal Lymphoma

Isaacson PG: Gastrointestinal lymphoma. *Hum Pathol* 1994;**25**:1020.

Pernicious Anemia

Pruthi RK, Tefferi A: Pernicious anemia revisited. *Mayo Clin Proc* 1994;**69**:144.

LIVER DISEASES

Viral Hepatitis

Choo QL et al: Isolation of a cDNA clone derived from a blood-borne non-A, non-B viral hepatitis genome. *Science* 1989;**244**:359.

Carreno V et al: Hepatitis delta virus infection: Molecular biology and treatment. *Dig Dis* 1994;**12**:265.

Conjeevaram HS et al: Predictors of a sustained beneficial response to interferon alfa therapy in chronic hepatitis C. *Hepatology* 1995;**22**:1326.

Katkov WN, Dienstag JL: Hepatitis vaccines. *Gastroenterol Clin North Am* 1995;**24**:147.

Martin P, Friedman LS: Viral Hepatitis. *Gastroenterol Clin N Am* 1994;**23**:619. Entire issue.

Primary Biliary Cirrhosis

Laurin JM, Lindor KD: Primary biliary cirrhosis. *Dig Dis* 1994;**12**(6):331.

Autoimmune Hepatitis

Czaja AJ, Manns MP: The validity and importance of subtypes in autoimmune hepatitis: A point of view. *Am J Gastroenterol* 1995;**90**(8):1206.

Donaldson P et al: The molecular genetics of autoimmune liver disease. *Hepatology* 1994;**20**:225.

Primary Sclerosing Cholangitis

Lee YM, Kaplan MM: Primary sclerosing cholangitis. *N Engl J Med* 1995;**332**:924.

ORODENTAL DISEASES

Periodontal Disease

Boughman JA et al: Early onset periodontal disease: A genetics perspective. *Oral Biol Med* 1990;**1**:89.

Genco RJ: Host responses in periodontal diseases: Current concepts. *J Periodontol* 1992;**63**:338.

Page RC: The role of inflammatory mediators in the pathogenesis of periodontal disease. *J Periodont Res* 1991; **26**:230.

Ranney RR: Immunologic mechanisms of pathogenesis in periodontal diseases: An assessment. *J Periodont Res* 1991;**26**:243.

Socransky SS, Haffajee AD: Microbial mechanisms in the pathogenesis of destructive periodontal diseases: A critical assessment. *J Periodont Res* 1991;**26**:195.

Stiehm ER: New and old immunodeficiencies. *Pediatr Res* 1992;**33**(suppl):S2.

Williams RC: Periodontal disease. *N Engl J Med* 1990; **322**:373.

Recurrent Aphthous Ulcers

MacPhail LA et al: Recurrent aphthous ulcers in association with HIV infection: Diagnosis and treatment. *Oral Surg Oral Med Oral Pathol* 1992;**73**:283.

Nolan A et al: Recurrent aphthous ulceration: Vitamin B1, B2, and B6 status and response to replacement therapy. *J Oral Pathol Med* 1991;**20**:389.

Taylor LJ et al: Increased production of tumour necrosis factor by peripheral blood leukocytes in patients with recurrent oral aphthous ulceration. *J Oral Pathol Med* 1992;**21**:21.

Verdickt GM et al: Expression of the CD54 (ICAM-1) and CD11a (LFA-1) adhesion molecules in oral mucosal inflammation. *J Oral Pathol Med* 1992;**21**:65.

AIDS & Candidiasis

Agabian N: Candidiasis and HIV infection. In: *Oral Manifestations of HIV Infection.* Greenspan JS, Greenspan D (editors). Quintessence, 1995.

Greenspan D et al: *AIDS and the Mouth: Diagnosis and Management of Oral Lesions.* Munksgaard, 1990.

Katz MH et al: Progression to AIDS in HIV-infected homosexual and bisexual men with hairy leukoplakia and oral candidiasis. *AIDS* 1992;**6**:95.

Miyasaki SH et al: The identification and tracking of *Candida albicans* isolates from oral lesions in HIV-seropositive individuals. *J Acquired Immune Defic Syndr* 1992;**5**:1039.

Greenspan D, Greenspan JS: HIV-related oral disease. *Lancet.* In press.

Renal Diseases

38

Curtis B. Wilson, MD, Lili Feng, MD, & David M. Ward, MB, ChB, FRCP

Immunologically induced glomerulonephritis and tubulointerstitial nephritis are estimated to be responsible for at least 25% of instances of end-stage renal failure and its consequent mortality, morbidity, and expense. Nephritogenic antibody–antigen reactions most often lead directly or indirectly to glomerular or tubular immune deposits. The subsequent activation of humoral and cellular mediator systems produces foci of inflammation (Table 38–1). In addition, experimental antibody reactions with glomerular cell antigens can lead to immune deposit formation as seen with epithelial cell antigens in the Heymann nephritis model of membranous glomerulonephritis. Alternatively, antibody reactions with mesangial cell Thy-1 antigens lead to complement-dependent mesangial cell lysis followed by mesangial proliferation. Human counterparts of these mechanisms are being sought. Immune activation of mediator systems, such as complement or as postulated to occur in vasculitic injury associated with antineutrophil cytoplasmic antibodies (ANCA), must also be considered.

Immune deposits develop when nephritogenic antibodies react directly with antigens in the kidney. In humans, the major nephritogenic structural antigens are in the glomerular basement membrane (GBM). Antibodies may also react with nonrenal, often exogenous, antigens that have been "trapped" in the GBM by physiologic, immunologic, or physicochemical mechanisms such as the reaction of cationic molecules with the polyanionic glomerular capillary wall.

The most common nephritogenic mechanisms of glomerular immune deposit formation involve soluble antigens that, in the presence of circulating antibody, can lead to deposits through a continuum of circulating immune complex accumulation to in situ immune complex formation. In addition, once a glomerular immune deposit has formed, interaction of additional antigen, antibody, or immune complex material from the circulation can be a major factor in increasing the deposit or, in cases of extreme antigen excess, actually dissolving it. The key to shifting the continuum from circulating immune complex accumulation to in situ immune complex formation is the characteristics of the antigen, antibody, or immune complex that allow a physicochemical or otherwise selective interaction with the glomerulus, such as charge interaction. The in situ immune complex formation and "trapped" antigen mechanisms are similar, with the latter usually implying fixation of a soluble antigen prior to the presence of circulating antibody.

In renal biopsy tissue, antibodies reactive with the GBM have a characteristic linear configuration by immunofluorescence microscopy. In contrast, a granular pattern is much more common and can be due either to the accumulation of immune complexes or to antibodies directly reactive with fixed glomerular antigens that are distributed irregularly.

In glomerulonephritis, humoral mechanisms appear to dominate, and there is much less evidence for a contribution by cellular immunity. A cellular immune response has been recognized in some forms of human glomerulonephritis. Sometimes T cells can be identified in nephritic glomeruli, and a role for T cells in some forms of experimental glomerulonephritis has been shown by cell transfer studies.

The glomerular (or tubular) injury caused by antibody reactions results in large part from the action of immunologic mediator systems. The most extensively studied of these are complement and neutrophils, representing the humoral and cellular mediator groups, respectively. Complement activation generates biologically active fragments that initiate vasoconstriction, platelet aggregation, immune adherence, opsonization, histamine release, and leukocyte chemotaxis. Complement products also can serve to solubilize immune-complex material and may affect handling of complexes via erythrocyte CR1 receptors. C5b–9, the membrane attack complex (MAC), is found in human glomerular immune deposits, and manipulative studies in experimental models indicate its contribution to injury in some situations. In addition to the chemotaxins, C3a and C5a, the MAC may

Table 38–1. Immunopathogenesis of humorally mediated renal disease classified by the solubility of the antigen.

Solubility	Mechanism	Antigen	Condition
Insoluble or tissue-fixed antigens	Antibodies react with structural components of the kidney.	GBM	Glomerulonephritis.
		TBM	Tubulointerstitial nephritis.
		Other glomerular wall antigens.	Experimental glomerulonephritis.
		Cell surface antigens.	Experimental glomerulonephritis, tubulointerstitial nephritis.
	Antibodies react with antigens trapped or "planted" in the glomerulus.	Mesangial accumulations, immune-complex components, lectins, cationic materials; possibly bacterial antigens, DNA.	Experimental glomerulonephritis. May contribute to human glomerulonephritis as well.
Soluble antigens	Antibodies react with antigens in the vascular compartment to form circulating immune complexes, which accumulate in glomeruli by active or passive mechanisms.	Exogenous antigens: drugs, products of infectious agents, etc.	Glomerulonephritis, tubulointerstitial nephritis, vasculitis.
		Endogenous antigens; nuclear antigens, tumor antigens, etc.	
	Antibodies react with antigens in the extravascular fluid near the site of antigen release.	Tubular antigens.	Experimental tubulointerstitial nephritis.

promote leukocyte adhesion by increasing expression of P-selectin (CD62). The MAC can also enhance eicosanoid production as well as interleukin-1 (IL-1) and tumor necrosis factor (TNF), which in turn activate a cascade of cytokines, including the chemokines monocyte chemoattractant protein-1 (MCP-1) and IL-8. Other humoral mediators include the coagulation proteins. Coagulation can be induced by glomerular tissue factor, procoagulant activity of infiltrating macrophages, and platelet aggregation. The anticoagulant protein C with its cofactor protein S and activator thrombomodulin are found in the kidney along with protein C inhibitor. Abnormalities in fibrinolysis may occur in glomerular injury related to enhanced expression of plasminogen activator inhibitor-1, which inhibits the action of urokinase and tissue plasminogen activator. Fibrinolytic therapy may be beneficial in some models.

Recruitment of neutrophils includes chemotaxis by complement, platelet-activating factor (PAF), thrombin, and the actions of platelet-derived growth factor (PDGF), IL-1, and TNF. Molecules from the chemokine family, such as IL-1, are also strong neutrophil chemoattractants. Molecules that promote neutrophil adhesion include P-selectin, E-selectin, and intracellular adhesion molecule-1 (ICAM-1), with its corresponding β_2-integrin (CD11a or CD11b/CD18). Neutrophils, as well as macrophages (which are also attracted to the site of injury), produce reactive oxygen species, nitric oxide, bioactive lipids, cytokines including IL-1 and TNF, proteinases, and growth factors. Platelets can also contribute factors including thrombospondin, thromboxane, PDGF, and platelet factor 4. PAF released from many cells associated with the inflammatory response has spasmogenic and vascular permeability properties.

Glomerular cells themselves can produce numerous mediator and adhesion molecules involved in the local inflammatory process. These include IL-1, IL-6, IL-8, TNF, MCP-1, PAF, colony-stimulating factor, endothelin, proteinases, and eicosanoids. The glomerular cells are also involved in the resolution of the injury, which, unfortunately, is often complicated by sclerosis and loss of function. The evolution of sclerosis is multifactorial and includes hemodynamic factors, lipid accumulation, and growth factor production. The growth factors, PDGF and transforming growth factor β, can lead to excessive production of extracellular matrix components, including various collagens, proteoglycans, and laminin. Insufficiency or inhibition of proteinases responsible for degrading and remodeling the excess matrix may also contribute.

ANTIGLOMERULAR BASEMENT MEMBRANE ANTIBODY-INDUCED GLOMERULONEPHRITIS

Major Immunologic Features

- Linear deposition of immunoglobulin and often of C3 occurs along the GBM.
- Anti-GBM antibodies are usually detectable in serum by radioimmunoassay (RIA), less often by indirect immunofluorescence techniques.

General Considerations

Anti-GBM antibodies can produce glomerulonephritis, Goodpasture's syndrome (glomerulonephritis and pulmonary hemorrhage), and, occasionally, idiopathic pulmonary hemosiderosis. The pathogenicity of these antibodies was demonstrated (1) by transfer to subhuman primates by using anti-GBM antibodies recovered from the serum of or eluted from the kidneys of affected patients and (2) by the observation of recurrence of anti-GBM antibody disease in renal transplants inadvertently placed in patients with residual circulating anti-GBM antibodies.

The nephritogenic GBM antigens appear to be in the noncollagenous carboxyl extension of the type IV procollagen molecule, a region termed NC1. This region of the type IV molecule is involved in intermolecular joining. The NC1 region of the α3 chain of type IV collagen carries a major reactive GBM epitope. In a recent large study, all patients detected with anti-GBM antibody with our radioimmunoassay had reactivity with α3(IV) NC1, with 15% having an additional reactivity with α1(IV) NC1 and 3% with α4(IV) NC1.

Of interest, anti-GBM antibodies do not react with the GBM from affected individuals in some kindreds of patients with hereditary nephritis (Alport's syndrome), a condition with GBM abnormalities. Transplantation of a normal kidney to such an individual lacking the reactive antigen may induce nephritogenic anti-GBM antibodies in the recipient. The genetic abnormalities of the α5 chain of type IV collagen associated with the different kindreds of Alport's syndrome and observed morphologic defects in GBM, characterized by structure, are being defined. An added defect in α6(IV) is found in patients with Alport's syndrome and diffuse leiomyomatosis.

Little is known about the events responsible for the induction of spontaneous anti-GBM antibodies in humans. There is a suggested genetic association with HLA-DR2. Materials cross-reactive with the GBM have been identified in the urine of animals and humans. Mercuric chloride administered to rats produces a transient anti-GBM antibody response. Both hydrocarbon solvent inhalation and influenza A2 virus infections have been temporally associated with anti-GBM antibody production and Goodpasture's syndrome in a few patients. The duration of the anti-GBM antibody response is self-limited, suggesting that the immunologic stimulus is also transient. Most affected individuals have only a single episode, although two or more episodes have been reported.

Less than 5% of human glomerulonephritis is caused by anti-GBM antibodies. There is a bimodal age distribution. Anti-GBM antibody-associated Goodpasture's syndrome is most commonly identified in males in the second to fourth decades of life; however, either sex can be involved, and children under 5 and adults over 70 can be affected. A second grouping of cases occurs in patients older than 50 years. Glomerulonephritis alone is more common in this group, and there is a female predominance.

Pathology

The renal pathology induced by anti-GBM antibodies is related to quantitative and temporal factors of antibody binding. Lesions may vary from mild focal proliferative glomerulonephritis to diffuse proliferative necrotizing glomerulonephritis with crescent formation. The latter is more common, however, and may progress to glomerular destruction and hyalinization. The anti-GBM antibody deposits are not visualized by electron microscopy, in contrast to the electron-dense deposits of immune complexes. Tubulointerstitial nephritis in patients with anti-GBM antibody disease is caused by concomitant antitubular basement membrane (TBM) antibodies. The pulmonary pathology of Goodpasture's syndrome is intra-alveolar hemorrhage with hemosiderin-laden macrophages in alveoli and sputum.

Clinical Features

Half to two thirds (depending on age and sex) of patients with anti-GBM antibody glomerulonephritis also have pulmonary hemorrhage and often respiratory impairment. This condition is referred to as Goodpasture's syndrome. The first symptoms may be either renal or pulmonary, occurring nearly simultaneously or separated by as much as 1 year. Episodes of pulmonary hemorrhage may occur at any time during anti-GBM antibody production. Alteration in the accessibility of the alveolar basement membrane antigen by such factors as fluid overload, toxin exposure (smoking, hydrocarbons), or infection may facilitate the binding of anti-GBM antibodies and precipitate the episodes of lung injury. In many patients, particularly those with Goodpasture's syndrome, influenza-like symptoms precede the onset of renal or pulmonary symptoms. Arthritis is an early complaint in fewer than 10% of patients, and central nervous system involvement may occur infrequently. Overall, about 75% of patients develop renal failure, necessitating dialysis, although the outlook is improving somewhat as a result of early diagnosis and more aggressive treatment. Milder forms of disease account for fewer than 10% of cases. Clinical presentations confined to the lung are rare. Nephrotic syndrome is unusual in anti-GBM antibody glomerulonephritis.

Immunologic Diagnosis

The diagnosis of anti-GBM antibody disease can be established by finding at least two of the following: (1) linear deposits of immunoglobulins along the GBM by immunofluorescence, (2) elution of anti-GBM antibody from renal tissue, and (3) detection of circulating anti-GBM antibody. By immunofluorescence, anti-GBM antibodies appear as linear deposits of IgG and infrequently IgA or IgM along the GBM (Fig 38–1). Linear deposits of IgG are present along the TBM in about 70% of patients and may also be found along the alveolar basement membranes in some patients with pulmonary involvement; however, lung tissue is not as useful for detection of antibody as is kidney. Irregular glomerular IgM deposits may also be present. The linear glomerular deposits of im-

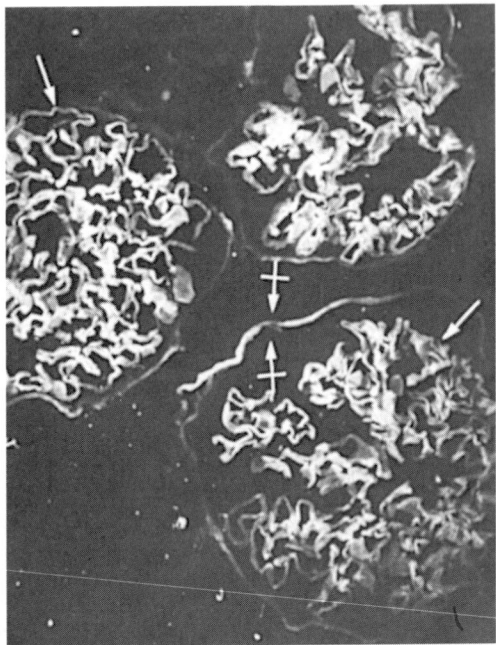

Figure 38–1. Smooth linear deposits of IgG (arrows) representing anti-GBM antibodies are seen outlining the GBM of three glomeruli from a young man with Goodpasture's syndrome. The antibody also had reactivity with Bowman's capsule (opposed hatched arrows). (Original magnification ×160.)

munoglobulins are accompanied by linear or irregular deposits of C3 in about two thirds of kidneys from patients with linear IgG deposits. Fibrin may be striking in areas of extracapillary proliferation and crescent formation. When C3 is present, it is usually accompanied by deposits of other components of the classic complement pathway. Nonimmunologic linear accumulations of IgG are sometimes found in kidneys from patients with diabetes mellitus, in kidneys perfused in preparation for transplantation, and in some normal kidneys. These must be distinguished from linear anti-GBM antibody deposits; the latter can be eluted from the renal tissue.

Circulating anti-GBM antibodies are usually detected by indirect immunofluorescence or by assays using immunopurified human GBM antigens or other type IV collagen NC1 fractions. It is important clinically to understand the specificity and reliability of the particular test chosen. Almost all patients with confirmed anti-GBM antibody deposits have circulating anti-GBM antibodies detected by RIA with immunopurified GBM antigen in serum obtained early in the course of the disease.

Differential Diagnosis

Although anti-GBM antibodies are the classic cause of Goodpasture's syndrome and an important

cause of crescentic glomerulonephritis, these clinical presentations are more commonly due to other immunologic mechanisms. "Pulmonary–renal" syndrome may also be related to immune-complex deposition, as in systemic lupus erythematosus (SLE), and to similar lesions with no or minimal immune deposits frequently associated with ANCA, as in Wegener's granulomatosis or polyarteritis (see later discussion). Crescentic glomerulonephritis in the absence of pulmonary involvement has a similar spectrum of pathogeneses.

Treatment

There is no immunologically specific treatment. High-dose corticosteroids are generally helpful in the management of acute pulmonary hemorrhage in patients with anti-GBM antibody-associated Goodpasture's syndrome. To hasten the disappearance of antibodies, repeated and intensive plasmapheresis, in conjunction with immunosuppression, is usually performed. This appears useful if the combined therapy is instituted before irreversible renal damage has taken place, although data from controlled trials are limited.

Complications & Prognosis

The mean duration of the anti-GBM antibody response measured by sensitive RIA is about 15 months; it ranges from a few weeks to 5 years. Immunosuppression and plasmapheresis hasten the disappearance of the anti-GBM antibody. Nephrectomy has no immediate effect on the levels of circulating anti-GBM antibody but may speed its eventual disappearance. The ultimate outcome is influenced by the severity of disease at the initiation of therapy. Initial improvement is not sustained in all patients, so that long-term follow-up is needed. Circulating anti-GBM antibodies can transfer glomerulonephritis to a transplanted kidney, so transplantation should be postponed until circulating anti-GBM antibodies are absent or greatly reduced. Posttransplant immunosuppression may help suppress the recrudescence of the anti-GBM antibody response.

IMMUNE-COMPLEX GLOMERULONEPHRITIS

Major Immunologic Features

- Granular deposits of immunoglobulins and complement occur in glomeruli.
- Circulating immune complexes are most easily detectable in the nephritis of systemic lupus erythematosus and some systemic infections.

General Considerations

The demonstration by immunofluorescence of granular deposits of immunoglobulins in the glomerulus can usually be interpreted as evidence of immune complex-mediated glomerulonephritis. It must be kept in mind that the direct reaction of antibody with irregularly distributed fixed or "planted" antigens, as noted earlier, could be confused with immune-complex deposits by immunofluorescence; this stresses the need for identification of the antigen–antibody systems involved.

The glomerulus seems to be a uniquely susceptible site for immune-complex accumulation; this is probably related in part to its function as a filter with a fenestrated endothelial lining. Several factors may influence the tissue localization of immune complexes in terms of (1) the characteristics and quantity of immune complexes reaching the glomerulus and (2) local factors within the glomerulus itself. A number of factors influence the delivery of immune complexes to the glomerulus, including the blood flow or its alteration and the systemic clearance of immune complexes by the mononuclear phagocytic system. It has been demonstrated, for example, that patients with autoimmune disease and tissue deposition of immune complexes have defective Fc receptor-mediated phagocytic clearance, and complement receptor handling of immune complexes may also be altered.

The size of the circulating immune complex, which, in turn, is determined by the relative antigen–antibody ratio, the size, valence, and nature of the antigen, and the antibody class and affinity, also influence the fate of the immune complex. Great antigen excess produces small immune complexes that are not particularly nephritogenic. Great antibody excess produces large, often insoluble immune complexes, which are rapidly removed from the circulation by the mononuclear phagocytic system and are not available for vascular localization. Experimentally, large complexes in antibody excess that are delivered to the circulation leading to the kidney localize in vessels and mesangial areas but are rapidly removed, in contrast to those formed during a period when the antigen–antibody ratio is more closely balanced.

Local factors that affect immune-complex deposition in the glomerulus include permeability and electric charge of the glomerular capillary wall and the composition of the immune complex. Vasoactive substances released as part of the immune response may enhance vascular permeability and immune-complex localization. The physicochemical properties of the antigen, antibody, and resultant immune complex have a bearing on their affinity for the highly charged glomerular capillary wall. Interchange with circulating antigens and antibodies appears to be particularly important. The size and composition of the immune complex are subject to modification with shifts in the relative concentration of either antigen or antibody. Once localization has begun, antigen, antibody, or immune complexes can interact at the site. The interchange of immune-complex components is influenced by such factors as the location, degree of inflammation, affinity of the antibody reaction, and physicochemical factors. Immune-complex cross-linking via secondary immune reactions with rheumatoid factors or anti-idiotypic antibodies could alter free interchange between the primary immune-complex reactants. Complement activation can solubilize the immune complex and could contribute to immune-complex lability.

Granular immunoglobulin or complement deposits (or both) appear to be responsible for more than 75% of cases of human glomerulonephritis of various histologic types, clinical courses, and demographic presentation (Table 38–2).

The granular deposits may represent immune complexes that accumulate from the circulation or that form in situ in the glomeruli as well as possibly representing reactions with irregularly distributed glomerular antigens, native or trapped. Experimental studies suggest that charge-related immune deposits may favor a subepithelial location, such as in acute poststreptococcal nephritis and in membranous glomerulonephritis, as described later on.

Immunogenetic factors may influence susceptibility to immune-complex disease with increasing numbers of associations between the HLA-DR system and glomerulonephritis being recognized (see Table 38–2). It is not known how the actual gene products are involved in the generation of the disease. The ever-increasing number of antigen–antibody systems identified in immune-complex glomerulonephritis in humans can be divided into exogenous (or foreign) and endogenous (or self) antigens (Table 38–3). In most cases of presumed human immune-complex glomerulonephritis, however, the causative antigen–antibody systems are unknown, and screening for antigens is difficult.

Pathology

Primary immune-complex glomerulonephritis (ie, glomerulonephritis in patients without identifiable systemic disease) is usually classified histologically (see Table 38–2). The secondary forms of glomerulonephritis (principally those associated with systemic diseases such as SLE, essential mixed cryoglobulinemia, Henoch-Schönlein purpura, and subacute infective endocarditis) are often of a proliferative type, although other histologic variants (noted earlier) occur. The main histologic patterns are described in Table 38–2 and Figure 38–2. The immune-complex deposits are visualized as electron-dense deposits by electron microscopy and may appear in subepithelial, subendothelial, intramembranous, and mesangial locations (see Table 38–2).

Clinical Features

Since immune-complex accumulation in glomeruli can induce all histologic forms of glomerulonephritis, the clinical features vary widely depending on the type and severity of glomerulonephritis (see Table 38–2). Proteinuria is almost always present and may be mild, moderate, or severe. Nephrotic syndrome occurs when

Table 38–2. Morphologic, immunopathologic, serologic, and clinical features of the major histologic classifications of immune-complex glomerulonephritis.

Morphology of Glomeruli	Immunofluorescence of Glomeruli (Granular Pattern)	Immunology Laboratory Findings (Serology)	Clinical Presentation and Features
Glomerulonephritis types **Diffuse proliferative glomerulonephritis, including poststreptococcal glomerulonephritis** Diffuse hypercellularity, electron-dense deposits in the mesangia or along GBM. Poststreptococcal form: subepithelial "humps" by electron microscopy.	IgG and C3 scattered along GBM. Variable IgA and IgM. In poststreptococcal form, C3 may be present when immunoglobulin is minimal or absent.	Nonpoststreptococcal forms: usually no abnormalities. Decreased C3, C4, and C1q, or presence of immune complex suggests underlying disease (eg, SLE or chronic infection). Poststreptococcal form: increased antistreptolysin O titer, decreased C3 (usually normal C4). Immune complexes and cryoglobulins may be present.	Nonpoststreptococcal forms: microscopic hematuria and/or proteinuria, gross hematuria, hypertension. Onset and course variable. May progress to renal failure. Poststreptococcal form: acute nephritic syndrome, usually resolves, especially in children. Prevalence variable depending on serotype of streptococcus.
Diffuse proliferative crescent-forming glomerulonephritis Diffuse hypercellularity with extracapillary crescents. Electron microscopy as above.	Heavy fibrinogen-related antigen in areas of crescents. Immunoglobulin and complement as above.	Secondary forms: features of underlying disease as above. Idiopathic form: complement is normal or reduced. Variable immune-complex and cryoglobulin detection.	Rapidly progressive renal failure, even anuric or oliguric from onset. Microscopic or gross hematuria, erythrocyte casts in urine, proteinuria, nephrotic syndrome unusual. Uncommon; more common above age 50.
Focal proliferative glomerulonephritis, including mesangial IgA nephropathy Focal and segmental mesangial hypercellularity, with electron-dense deposits.	IgA often prominent, with or without C3 and IgG, sometimes IgM, in mesangial pattern (often segmental).	Variable increased serum IgA. Often immune complex of IgA class (less reactivity in usual immune-complex assays). IgA-fibronectin complexes often present in serum. Some association with HLA-Bw35 and -DR4.	Microscopic hematuria and/or proteinuria. Recurrent gross hematuria, may accompany intercurrent respiratory infections. Occasionally progresses to renal failure. Prevalent in young adults.
Membranous glomerulonephritis Thickening of GBM, little or no hypercellularity. Subepithelial spikes by silver stains, diffuse subepithelial electron-dense deposits.	IgG and C3 diffusely along the GBM. IgA and IgM unusual in idiopathic form.	Usually no abnormality in idiopathic form. (SLE form described below.)	Proteinuria, often nephrotic syndrome. Slow progression in one third of cases. In older patients, may rarely be related to neoplasm. Common in adults; unusual before age 15.
Membranoproliferative glomerulonephritis Mesangial proliferation with interposition between endothelium and thickened GBM. At least two variants by electron microscopy: type I (subendothelial deposits) and type II (intramembranous dense deposits).	Type I: Heavy C3, some IgG along GBM; occasional IgA or IgM. Type II: Heavy C3 along GBM. Immunoglobulin deposits uncommon.	Persistent low C3 in most type I and all type II. C4 usually normal. Nephritic factor often present, especially in type II.	Proteinuria, microscopic or gross hematuria, often nephrotic syndrome, often hypertension. Usually progresses over several years to renal failure. Type I is somewhat uncommon. Type II is rare. Type II can be associated with partial lipodystrophy.

(continued)

Table 38–2. Morphologic, immunopathologic, serologic, and clinical features of the major histologic classifications of immune-complex glomerulonephritis. *(continued)*

Morphology of Glomeruli	Immunofluorescence of Glomeruli (Granular Pattern)	Immunology Laboratory Findings (Serology)	Clinical Presentation and Features
End-stage (chronic) glomerulonephritis Hyalinized glomeruli, extensive tubulointerstitial destruction. Electron microscopy occasionally detects features of original disease process.	Variable IgG, IgA, IgM, and C3 in least damaged glomeruli. C3 may persist in absence of immuno-globulin deposits.	Abnormalities typical of original disease occasionally persist.	Renal failure, often hypertension, variable degree of proteinuria and/or hematuria. End stage of many morphologic forms of glomerulonephritis.
Systemic diseases with glomerulonephritis **Systemic lupus erythematosus** Classified into mesangial only, membranous glomerulonephritis, diffuse proliferative glomerulonephritis, and focal proliferative glomerulonephritis. Resemble lesions listed above. Some transitions from one type to another.	IgG, IgA, IgM (typically all three) and C3 (also C4 and C1q). Patterns of glomerular deposition in accord with morphologic type. Often prominent tubulo-interstitial immune deposits.	ANA positive. Decreased C3, C4, and C1q; increased anti-DNA; circulating immune complexes, with or without cryoglobulins, especially in diffuse proliferative type; often fluctuating with changes in disease activity and can be normalized by immunosuppressive treatment.	Only mild urinary abnormalities with minimal mesangial lesions. Proteinuria and microscopic hematuria, nephrotic syndrome in others; 10–50% progression to end-stage renal failure by 5 years, depending on morphologic type. Rapidly progressive course when crescentic glomerulonephritis. Lupus nephritis affects half or more of all patients with SLE.
Essential mixed cryoglobulinemia Usually proliferative glomerulonephritis (diffuse, occasionally focal or membranoproliferative).	IgG, IgM, C3 diffusely along the GBM; sometimes massive deposits in capillary lumens. Fibrinogen-related antigen variable.	Decreased C4, cryoglobulins (especially IgM$_K$-IgG), rheumatoid factor.	Proteinuria, microscopic hematuria, acute nephritic episodes, hypertension, episodes of purpura. Progresses slowly to renal failure. Rare disease; affects females more than males.
Henoch-Schönlein purpura Focal or diffuse proliferative glomerulonephritis, sometimes crescentic.	IgA prominent, usually with IgG and C3, with or without IgM. Fibrinogen-related antigen frequently prominent.-	Variable increased serum IgA. Often immune complex of IgA class (less reactivity in usual immune-complex assays). Some association with HLA-Bw35.	Microscopic hematuria, proteinuria, nephrotic syndrome, acute nephritic syndrome. Generally favorable outcome, but some cases progress to end-stage renal failure. Nephritis occurs in more than half of patients with Henoch-Schönlein purpura.

Abbreviations: GBM = glomerular basement membrane; SLE = systemic lupus erythematosus.

urinary protein loss exceeds the body's capacity to completely replace it, after which serum oncotic pressure decreases and edema develops along with other disturbances in salt and water balance. Nephrotic syndrome most frequently accompanies membranous glomerulonephritis. Hematuria is more common in patients with proliferative or membranoproliferative histologic findings. The presence of erythrocyte casts in the urinary sediment suggests an acute phase of glomerular inflammation. Acute nephritic syndrome frequently accompanies diffuse proliferative and membranoproliferative glomerulonephritis. It is characterized by hematuria, proteinuria, edema, hypertension, and a reduced glomerular filtration rate. Hypertension can be present from the outset of any of these diseases or may appear later if the nephritis progresses. The syndrome of rapidly progressive glomerulonephritis resembles that of acute glomerulonephritis except for the rapid progression (within weeks or a few months) toward end-stage renal failure.

Renal failure and chronic glomerulonephritis may follow any form of immune-complex glomerular injury, usually related to the particular histologic type (see Table 38–2).

Table 38–3. Antigen–antibody systems known to cause or strongly suspected of causing immune-complex glomerulonephritis in humans.

Antigens	Clinical Condition
Exogenous or foreign antigens	
Iatrogenic agents	
Drugs, toxoids, foreign serum	Serum sickness, heroin nephropathy (?), gold nephropathy (?), etc.
Infectious agents	
Bacterial: Nephritogenic streptococci, *Staphylococcus albus* and *S aureus, Corynebacterium bovis,* enterococci, *Streptococcus pneumoniae, Propionibacterium acnes, Klebsiella pneumoniae, Yersinia enterocolitica, Treponema pallidum, Salmonella typhi, Mycoplasma pneumoniae.*	Poststreptococcal glomerulonephritis, infected ventriculo-atrial shunts, endocarditis, pneumonia, yersiniasis, syphilis, typhoid fever, pneumonia.
Parasitic: Plasmodium malariae, P falciparum, Schistosoma mansoni, Echinococcus granulosus, Toxoplasma gondii.	Malaria, schistosomiasis, toxoplasmosis, hydatid disease.
Viral: Hepatitis virus, retrovirus-related antigen, measles virus, Epstein-Barr virus, cytomegalovirus.	Hepatitis, leukemia, subacute sclerosing panencephalitis, Burkitt's lymphoma, cytomegalovirus infection.
Fungal: Candida albicans.	Candidiasis.
Perhaps others as yet undetermined.	Endocarditis, leprosy, kala-azar, dengue, mumps, varicella, infectious mononucleosis, Guillain-Barré syndrome, AIDS (?)
Endogenous or self antigens	
Nuclear antigens	SLE.
Immunoglobulin	Cryoglobulinemia.
Tumor antigens	Neoplasms.
Thyroglobulin	Thyroiditis.

Abbreviations: AIDS = acquired immunodeficiency syndrome; SLE = systemic lupus erythematosus.

Immunologic Pathogenesis

The presumptive diagnosis of immune-complex glomerulonephritis is based on the finding in renal biopsy of granular deposits of immunoglobulin, usually accompanied by complement, in the glomeruli. IgG is the most common, with IgA or IgM occasionally predominating (see Table 38–2). The glomerular immune deposits may diffusely involve all capillary loops in membranous or diffuse proliferative glomerulonephritis (Fig 38–3A). In focal glomerulonephritis the deposits tend to involve only segments of the glomerular capillary wall or mesangium, but they may be more widespread than expected from the focal nature of the histologic change, and in some patients the immune deposit is confined to the mesangium (see Fig 38–3B).

Predominant IgA deposits are seen in patients with focal glomerulonephritis. The association has been so striking that the term "mesangial IgA nephropathy" has been coined to denote the condition. Circulating IgA-containing immune complexes can be detected in IgA nephropathy, and the rapidity with which hematuria follows an infectious episode suggests that the immune complexes may be formed during antibody excess, possibly with preformed antibody to a common infectious microorganism in the oropharynx. The large, antibody-excess complexes would preferentially accumulate in the mesangium. Fifty percent of patients have raised serum IgA levels and evidence of abnormal regulation of IgA production in vitro, suggesting a primary immune abnormality. Many patients also have demonstrable circulating aggregates of IgA and fibronectin. Alternative explanations for the IgA accumulation include IgA multimers and antimesangial antibodies. Occasionally, patients with similar clinical courses have predominantly IgM mesangial deposits.

Mesangial deposition of IgA, usually in a more diffuse pattern with C3 and fibrin, occurs in Henoch-Schönlein purpura. This is a systemic disease typified by arteriolar and venular lesions causing skin purpura, arthralgias, abdominal pain, intestinal hemorrhage, and often a proliferative glomerulonephritis that rarely progresses to end-stage renal failure. It has been suggested that the disease may be triggered by infectious agents or drugs presented at mucosal surfaces and eliciting abnormal IgA responses. The role of food allergy is controversial.

Acute poststreptococcal glomerulonephritis is characterized by acute inflammatory changes due to immune deposits in a subepithelial location. These contain large amounts of C3 and smaller amounts of IgG. A streptococcal antigen that becomes trapped at this site is implicated; one proposed candidate is a streptococcal protein that may directly activate the alternative complement pathway.

Membranous glomerulonephritis often has nearly continuous granular IgG and C3 deposits (see Fig 38–3), seen as electron-dense deposits along the subepithelial aspect of the GBM by electron microscopy. Experimentally, cationic antigen can lead to such deposits; however, native bovine serum albumin, which is weakly anionic, causes similar deposits in serum sickness protocols. The search for an antigen–antibody system similar to the glomerular epithelial cell antigen of the Heymann nephritis model of membranous nephritis in rats is ongoing.

In SLE, the immune deposits may be widespread, involving glomeruli and, in 70% of instances, extraglomerular renal tissues as well. Indeed, granular deposits of immunoglobulin and complement in TBM or peritubular capillaries should suggest the diagnosis of

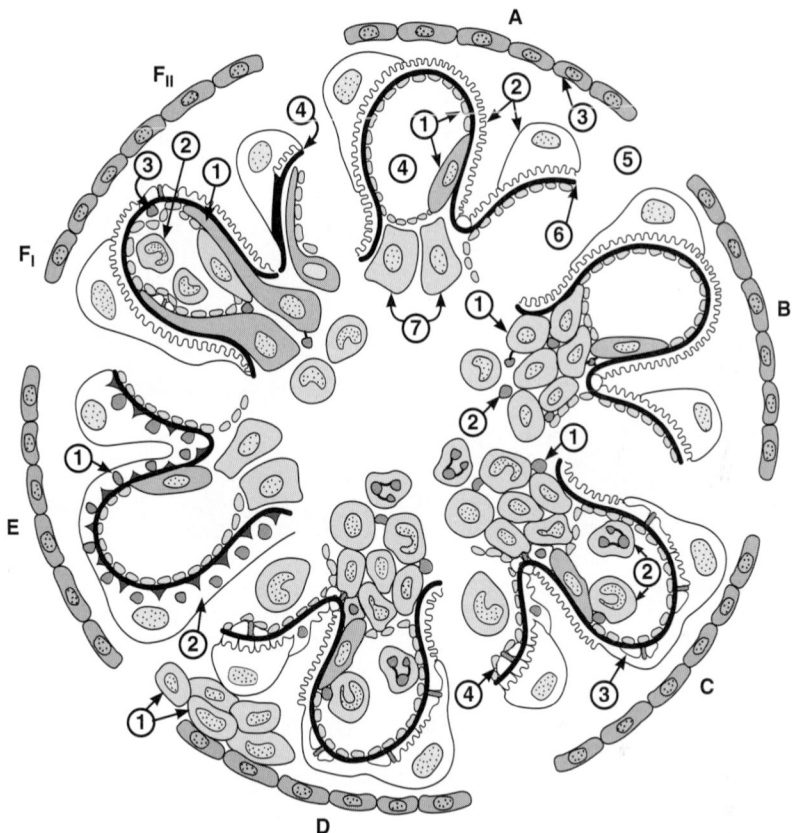

Figure 38–2. Major histologic forms of presumed immune-complex glomerulonephritis. ***A:** Normal glomerular anatomy.* 1, Glomerular endothelial cells, with fenestrated endothelium; 2, glomerular epithelial cells with specialized foot processes; 3, parietal epithelium lining Bowman's capsule; 4, glomerular capillary lumen; 5, urinary space; 6, glomerular basement membrane (GBM); 7, the glomerular mesangium, composed predominantly of smooth muscle-like mesangial cells and occasional mononuclear phagocytes. ***B:** Focal proliferative glomerulonephritis.* The lesion is characterized by focal (some glomeruli) and segmental (portions of glomeruli) mesangial hypercellularity (1). Immune deposits of immunoglobulin and C3 (2) are found in the mesangial area. IgA deposits predominate in IgA nephropathy. ***C:** Diffuse proliferative glomerulonephritis.* Extensive and widespread hypercellularity is present with infiltration of polymorphonuclear and mononuclear inflammatory cells (2). Immune deposits of immunoglobulin and C3 may be found in mesangial (1), subepithelial (3), or subendothelial (4) locations. In post-streptococcal proliferative glomerulonephritis, the subepithelial deposits have a characteristic hump-like appearance in electron microscopy. ***D:** Diffuse proliferative glomerulonephritis with crescent formation.* In addition to the features of diffuse proliferative glomerulonephritis, macrophages and parietal epithelial cells accumulate in Bowman's space (1) in response to fibrin deposits, which accumulate in this area when severe glomerular capillary wall damage has occurred. The inflammation may be sufficiently intense to cause necrosis in the glomerular tuft. ***E:** Membranous glomerulonephritis.* This is typified by marked thickening of the GBM, the accumulation of immunoglobulin and C3 immune deposits in a subepithelial position (1), and a lack of glomerular hypercellularity. With time, GBM extensions or "spikes" (2) develop between the immune deposits and eventually engulf them. ***F_I/F_{II}:** Membranoproliferative glomerulonephritis.* Interposition of mesangial cells between the endothelium and the GBM (1) produces a "tram-track" appearance of the glomerular capillary wall. Mesangial hypercellularity and inflammatory cells are present (2). In type I, immune deposits of immunoglobulin and C3 are present predominantly in subendothelial positions (3). In type II, also called dense-deposit disease, the GBM is thickened and abnormally electron dense (4). Heavy C3 deposits are seen in the GBM and mesangial areas with little or no immunoglobulin.

SLE. IgA and C1q deposits are prominent in kidneys of patients with SLE.

Immunologic Diagnosis

It is helpful to identify antigen–antibody systems in individuals with suspected immune-complex glomerulonephritis. Serologic tests for common infectious etiologies should include streptococcal antibodies, hepatitis B antigen, hepatitis C antibodies, and human immunodeficiency virus (HIV) antibody. Antinuclear and anti-DNA antibodies should be sought, since SLE glomerulonephritis can occur without other overt organ involvement. The presence of ANCA, rheumatoid factors, or cryoglobulins may provide additional insight into the pathogenic process. In most cases, however, serum antibody testing is unrevealing.

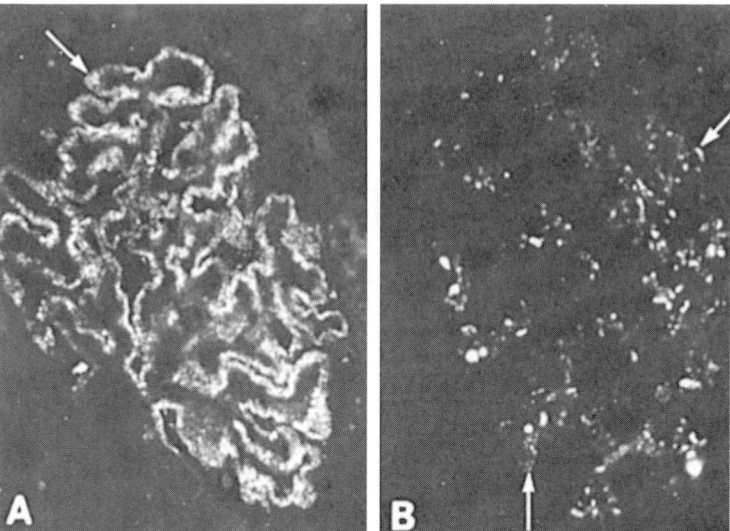

Figure 38–3. Granular deposits of IgG are seen in the glomeruli of patients with immune complex-induced glomerulonephritis. **A:** Heavy diffuse deposits (arrow) are present in a patient with membranous glomerulonephritis and nephrotic syndrome. **B:** Focal granular deposits (arrows), largely confined to the mesangium, are present in a patient with focal proliferative glomerulonephritis and mild proteinuria. (Original magnification ×250.)

Serum complement levels may be helpful (see Table 38–2). C3, C4, and total hemolytic complement (CH_{50}) are normal in the majority of cases of glomerulonephritis, but when abnormalities occur, they are of considerable diagnostic importance. Hypocomplementemia occurs frequently in certain forms of immune-complex glomerulonephritis, especially SLE, essential mixed cryoglobulinemia, and infection-associated glomerulonephritis (poststreptococcal, endocarditis, infected ventriculoatrial shunts, etc).

Hypocomplementemia is also common in membranoproliferative glomerulonephritis, a group of diseases incorporating at least two varieties of nephritis with differing pathogenetic mechanisms: type I and type II membranoproliferative glomerulonephritis. Type I is an etiologically heterogeneous group with granular immune-complex deposits. Type II, or dense-deposit disease, is identified by electron-dense transformation of the GBM, in which chemical analysis of the GBM suggests an increase in sialic acid-rich GBM glycoproteins, rather than the accumulation of a nonbasement membrane component.

A serum factor, termed nephritic factor, capable of activating the alternative complement pathway is present in many patients with membranoproliferative glomerulonephritis, particularly type II. Nephritic factor has been shown to be an immunoglobulin with immunoconglutinin properties, capable of reacting with activated components of the alternative complement pathway, specifically the bimolecular complex of C3b and activated factor B, stabilizing its C3 convertase activity.

An increasingly prevalent secondary cause of type I membranoproliferative glomerulonephritis is infec-

tion with the hepatitis C virus, and such patients often have hypocomplementemia, rheumatoid factor, and mixed cryoglobulinemia. In contrast, hepatitis B infection may be associated with membranous glomerulonephritis and polyarteritis nodosa.

Several sensitive methods for the detection of circulating immune complexes are available (see Chapter 14). In general, the immune-complex assays are positive when large amounts of circulating immune complexes are present in patients with SLE and with glomerulonephritis associated with other systemic immune-complex diseases.

Differential Diagnosis

The simultaneous presence of proteinuria (more than 1 g daily) and urinary casts almost invariably indicates a glomerular disease. The differential diagnosis is extensive and includes familial renal disease, hypertension, SLE, streptococcal infection, viral hepatitis, rheumatoid arthritis, and cryoglobulinemia.

Treatment

The most commonly used drugs are corticosteroids, cyclophosphamide, and azathioprine, and occasionally other "immunosuppressive" therapy used singly or in combination. Primary (idiopathic) membranous glomerulonephritis may respond somewhat to corticosteroids or regimens including chlorambucil, but the benefit is uncertain and the toxicity is of concern.

The subset of patients who do show marked reduction in proteinuria during a six-month course of such treatment may obtain lasting remission, or if they relapse they are likely to respond again to repeat therapy. Primary proliferative and membranoproliferative forms are usually quite unresponsive to immunosuppressive therapy. In contrast, patients with SLE nephritis often show considerable benefit from corticosteroid therapy, and in severe cases with diffuse proliferative histology, the addition of cyclophosphamide or azathioprine is often appropriate.

High-dose pulse methylprednisolone infusions (eg, 1000 mg daily for 3 days) can be used as initial treatment for acute flares of lupus nephritis. Idiopathic diffuse crescentic glomerulonephritis can be treated in the same way initially but usually also requires further corticosteroids, cyclophosphamide, or plasmapheresis. Whereas the anti-GBM type of crescentic glomerulonephritis responds poorly once renal failure is established, immune-complex types and those associated with ANCA antibodies may still respond.

Ideally, management of immune-complex glomerulonephritis should either eradicate the source of antigen or inhibit production of the specific antibody. These approaches stress the need for identification of the antigen–antibody systems in each patient.

That the course of established poststreptococcal glomerulonephritis is not influenced by appropriate antibiotics may simply reflect the self-limiting nature of the disease. In contrast, the proliferative immune-complex glomerulonephritis that often insidiously complicates subacute bacterial endocarditis responds to protracted antibacterial therapy. Similarly, removal of antigen by treating *Treponema pallidum* infection has been beneficial to individuals with syphilitic immune-complex glomerulonephritis, as has removal of malignant tissue in immune-complex glomerulonephritis associated with neoplasia. The use of plasmapheresis and of specific immunoadsorbents to remove circulating antibodies, antigens, or immune complexes is under investigation.

Complications & Prognosis

The prognosis is extremely variable, depending on the histologic form of glomerulonephritis (see Table 38–2). Generally, diffuse proliferative forms have worse prognoses than focal proliferative or nonproliferative forms. An exception is diffuse proliferative postinfectious glomerulonephritis, which usually remits in 90% of cases. Complications include progressive loss of glomerular filtration leading to renal failure and the eventual need for dialysis or kidney transplantation. Hypertension may occur with any form of immune-complex glomerulonephritis and is occasionally severe. Proteinuria of the degree found in the nephrotic syndrome may cause hypoalbuminemia (leading to edema or anasarca), depletion of the serum IgG level, and disturbed balance of coagulation factors manifesting as venous thrombosis, pulmonary embolism, or renal vein thrombosis.

Recurrence of some of the forms of glomerulonephritis in kidney transplants has been reported, especially with focal mesangial IgA nephropathy and type II membranoproliferative glomerulonephritis.

Because recurrence is infrequent in the former and slow in the latter, however, transplantation is not contraindicated.

TUBULOINTERSTITIAL NEPHRITIS

Major Immunologic Features

- There are extensive interstitial mononuclear cell infiltrates, predominantly T cells.
- In anti-TBM tubulointerstitial nephritis, linear deposits of immunoglobulin usually accompanied by complement are found along the TBM; circulating anti-TBM antibody may be detected.
- In immune-complex tubulointerstitial nephritis, granular deposits of immunoglobulin and complement are found in the TBM, interstitium, or peritubular capillaries; circulating immune complexes may be detected.
- In presumed cell-mediated tubulointerstitial nephritis, there is no detectable immunoglobulin along the TBM, and no anti-TBM antibody or immune complex is detected in the circulation.

Immune processes that lead to tubulointerstitial nephritis are similar to those described earlier for the glomerulus. These include anti-TBM antibodies, immune complexes, and cell-mediated immunity. Immune tubulointerstitial nephritis can accompany glomerulonephritis or occur as an independent event. Experimental models of anti-TBM antibody- and immune complex-induced tubulointerstitial nephritis have been developed, and similar processes have been identified in humans. Evidence exists that sensitized cells may transfer or contribute to tubulointerstitial nephritis in experimental models. Despite the conspicuous infiltration of interstitial mononuclear cells, including T cells, the pathogenetic role of cell-mediated immunity, other than in renal allografts, is not well established in humans.

General Considerations

Anti-TBM antibodies occur in about 70% of patients with anti-GBM glomerulonephritis and correlate with greater degrees of interstitial inflammation. Anti-TBM antibodies are occasionally found in drug-induced tubulointerstitial nephritis, in tubulointerstitial nephritis associated with immune complex-induced glomerulonephritis, in renal allografts, and rarely in primary tubulointerstitial nephritis.

In immune-complex tubulointerstitial nephritis, granular deposits of immunoglobulin and complement are found along the TBM, interstitium, or peritubular capillaries. These deposits are present in 50–70% of patients with SLE nephritis and infrequently in those with cryoglobulinemia, Sjögren's syndrome, membranoproliferative and rapidly progressing glomerulonephritis, and primary idiopathic tubulointerstitial nephritis. Tubulointerstitial immu-

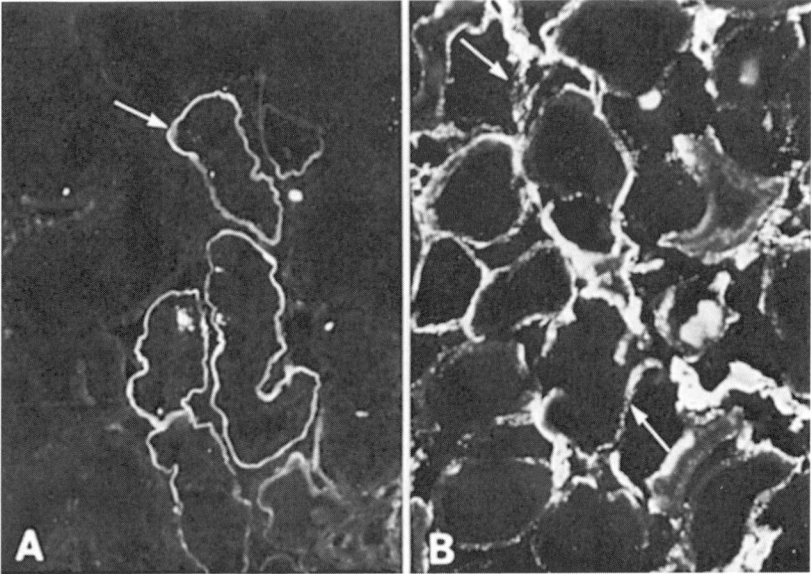

Figure 38–4. *A:* Linear deposits of IgG (arrow) are present along the TBM of focal renal tubules in the renal biopsy of a patient with anti-GBM glomerulonephritis. *B:* Diffuse granular deposits of IgG (arrows) are seen along the TBM of most renal tubules in the renal biopsy of a patient with SLE and immune-complex glomerulonephritis. (Original magnification ×250.)

noglobulin deposits may be present in the absence of glomerular immune-complex deposits and have occasionally been found in patients with SLE.

Mononuclear interstitial infiltrates without anti-TBM antibodies or immune complexes are the most common form of tubulointerstitial nephritis in humans. Frequently, the disease appears to be a hypersensitivity reaction to drugs, which may include a wide range of antibiotics, nonsteroidal anti-inflammatory drugs, and diuretics. Other situations in which mononuclear interstitial infiltrates may be prominent include acute allograft rejection, anti-GBM glomerulonephritis, pyelonephritis, sarcoidosis, Sjögren's syndrome, chronic active hepatitis, and idiopathic interstitial nephritis.

Pathology

Depending on the duration, underlying causes, and severity of disease, renal pathology varies from focal to diffuse mononuclear interstitial infiltrates composed primarily of T lymphocytes and macrophages. Tubular lesions may range from minimal degeneration of the tubular epithelium to necrosis and atrophy. Neutrophils may be associated with necrotic tubules. As the inflammation advances, interstitial fibrosis and thickened TBM develop. Eosinophils may be prominent in drug hypersensitivity. The glomerulus is not involved unless there is an associated glomerulonephritis.

Clinical Features

The clinical course is usually that of renal functional impairment without urinary findings suggestive of glomerular disease. When anti-TBM antibody- and

immune complex-induced tubulointerstitial nephritis is associated with glomerulonephritis, the features of the glomerulonephritis usually predominate. Evidence of tubular dysfunction manifesting as complete or partial Fanconi's syndrome may occur. When anti-TBM antibodies occur in transplant recipients, their effects may be indistinguishable from those of cell-mediated immune rejection.

Drug-induced tubulointerstitial nephritis usually presents acutely with fever, rash, hematuria, azotemia, and eosinophilia associated with a course of drug therapy. Other features, such as pyuria, eosinophiluria, mild proteinuria, flank pain, and arthralgia, may also be present, together with an elevated serum IgE level. Progressive renal failure is the general rule unless the offending drug is discontinued.

Immunologic Diagnosis

To distinguish the immune mechanism responsible for the mononuclear infiltrate characteristic of tubulointerstitial nephritis, renal biopsy for immunopathologic studies is needed and should include determination of the phenotypes of the infiltrating cells. Linear deposits of immunoglobulin and complement are found along the TBM (Fig 38–4A) in anti-TBM antibody-associated tubulointerstitial nephritis. As in anti-GBM antibody disease, the specificity should be confirmed by elution studies or detection of circulating anti-TBM antibodies. Rarely, anti-TBM antibodies have been found in drug-induced tubulointerstitial nephritis in which the drug or its metabolites can be detected bound to the TBM.

In immune-complex disease, the tubules, vessels,

and interstitium should be carefully examined for immunofluorescent deposits of immunoglobulin (see Fig 38–4B) and complement, which are often focal and less intense than are glomerular deposits. Prominent or widespread tubulointerstitial immunoglobulin deposits suggest SLE.

In presumed cell-mediated tubulointerstitial nephritis, no immunoglobulin deposits are found. T lymphocytes are the predominant cells, although a few B cells are also present. Monoclonal antibodies directed to T-cell subsets identify both CD4 (helper/inducer) and CD8 (suppressor/cytotoxic) cells. The proportion of CD4 to CD8 cells, however, appears to vary depending on the underlying cause of disease. CD8 cells are the predominant phenotype found in drug-induced cases, whereas either CD4 or CD8 cells may be the major cells found in renal allograft rejection. The patient's reactivity to the drug can be tested by antibody measurement and lymphocyte proliferation (see Chapter 15).

Treatment

Tubulointerstitial nephritis associated with glomerulonephritis is treated as outlined in the previous sections. In cases of drug-induced tubulointerstitial nephritis, the offending drug should be discontinued immediately and replaced as needed with a structurally unrelated alternative drug. Corticosteroids may aid in quicker resolution of drug-induced tubulointerstitial nephritis.

MINIMAL-CHANGE NEPHROPATHY

General Considerations

Minimal-change nephropathy is the most common cause of nephrotic syndrome in children; however, it causes less than 10% of adult cases. No clear epidemiologic factor has been established. Abnormal T-cell function or T-cell products have been suggested as possible etiologic factors.

Pathology

Typically, no abnormalities are detected by light microscopy, and no immunoglobulin deposits are found by immunofluorescence. By electron microscopy, there is a diffuse effacement of the epithelial cell foot processes.

Clinical Features

Patients have nephrotic edema and selective proteinuria with no impairment of renal function, no hypertension, rare microscopic hematuria, and no hypocomplementemia; however, hypoproteinemia may be marked. The disease follows a naturally remitting and relapsing course. Repeated relapses in childhood are often followed by permanent remission in adolescence.

Treatment

Minimal-change nephropathy is particularly corticosteroid-sensitive, so that a rapid remission, in 2–8 weeks, on steroid therapy is considered diagnostic in children. In adults, more prolonged therapy is usually needed. Relapses occur, and may require repeated courses of corticosteroids. For patients with frequent relapses, adjunctive treatment should be considered. This usually consists of oral cyclophosphamide or chlorambucil, in low dosage, for no more than 8–10 weeks. Cyclosporine is also now recognized as useful, but, unlike the alkylating agents, it rarely induces lasting remissions.

FOCAL GLOMERULOSCLEROSIS

General Considerations

Focal glomerulosclerosis is another common cause of nephrotic syndrome in children and young adults. It is usually an idiopathic disease; however, a similar disease may develop in heroin abusers and in some patients with AIDS. Focal glomerulosclerosis may be difficult to distinguish from minimal-change nephropathy early in the course of the two diseases.

Pathology

The glomerular lesion is that of segmented hyalinosis and sclerosis. IgM, C3, and fibrin are present in small quantities in the hyalinized segments of glomeruli, although their immunopathogenic significance is unclear. AIDS nephropathy cases may have distinctive additional features, such as tubuloreticular structures on electron microscopy of the glomeruli and microcyst formation in the renal tubulointerstitial regions.

Clinical Features

Nephrotic syndrome is common and may be associated with hypertension and microscopic hematuria and then progressive impairment of renal function. A large percentage of cases reach end-stage renal failure within 10 years. Patients with heroin or AIDS nephropathy typically progress even more quickly.

Treatment

Most focal glomerulosclerosis is corticosteroid-resistant, and there is little evidence that any other specific treatment alters the natural history of progression to renal failure. A trial of treatment, however, may be worthwhile because those few who do respond by significantly reducing proteinuria also improve their long-term prognosis. Cyclophosphamide and cyclosporine have also been used with some claims of success, although cyclosporine may exacerbate the renal interstitial fibrosis that accompanies this disease. Angiotensin-converting enzyme inhibitors may reduce the rate of glomerular sclerosis and are particularly important in hypertensive patients.

Transplantation is not contraindicated, despite slow and inconsistent recurrence of the same histologic lesion in the transplant.

VASCULITIS

General Considerations

The vasculitides are syndromes with a spectrum of clinicopathologic features with the essential common component of vasculitis, an inflammatory reaction in vessel walls, leading to ischemia of the supplied tissues. Increasing evidence points to an immunologic pathogenesis of the vascular lesions, particularly the deposition of circulating immune complexes triggering the inflammatory process through humoral and cellular mediators. Several vasculitides involve the renal vessels and glomeruli. Of these, Henoch-Schönlein purpura has already been discussed. Polyarteritis nodosa, Wegener's granulomatosis, and some cases of crescentic glomerulonephritis without overt vasculitis are increasingly being recognized as a group of closely related entities in which a substantial subset of patients have circulating ANCA. In addition to being useful markers for the diagnosis and classification of these diseases, there is evidence that ANCA are directly involved in the pathogenesis of the vasculitic lesions.

Pathology

Vasculitis is diagnosed by the presence of segmental vasculitic lesions, with a perivascular inflammatory infiltrate, fibrinoid necrosis, and, in the extreme, aneurysm formation. The lesion may have evidence of coagulation, luminal obliteration, and downstream ischemia.

Polyarteritis nodosa is a necrotizing vasculitis of small and medium-sized muscular arteries with arteriolar and glomerular lesions (often segmental and focal), glomerular necrosis, and proliferative and crescentic glomerulonephritis. Lesions may be present at all stages of development. Wegener's granulomatosis is a necrotizing granulomatous angiitis involving arteries and veins. The renal lesion consists of a proliferative necrotizing glomerulonephritis with crescent formation and granulomatous angiitis.

Clinical Features

Polyarteritis nodosa is a multisystemic disease, and its prognosis is influenced by the degree of kidney involvement. Renovascular hypertension occurs in more than 50% of the cases, and end-stage renal failure is the common cause of death. Wegener's granulomatosis occurs equally in both sexes and often involves the upper respiratory tract, the lungs, and the kidneys.

Immunologic Diagnosis

The diagnosis is based on a combination of renal biopsy and other biopsy studies, angiographic demonstration of vasculitis or vascular aneurysms, and serologic tests for ANCA. ANCA are of various types with different specificities, and two major categories predominate. Those with cytoplasmic staining (c-ANCA) are often specific for proteinase-3 and are common in patients with Wegener's granulomatosis. ANCA, whose staining is perinuclear in alcohol-fixed targets (p-ANCA), are often specific for myeloperoxidase and are common in patients with disease limited to the kidneys. There is a considerable overlap, however, of antibody specificities and clinical syndromes; for instance, rapidly progressive glomerulonephritis is a common feature of both specificities, and alveolar capillaritis with lung hemorrhage may occur with either. Immunofluorescence microscopy of renal biopsy specimens in ANCA-positive cases typically reveals no or scant immune deposits, leading to the description "pauci-immune" to differentiate this from the more abundant immunoglobulin and complement deposits seen in "immune-complex" lesions.

Treatment

Therapy with corticosteroids and cyclophosphamide has been shown to be effective in Wegener's granulomatosis, even when acute renal failure is already advanced. This therapy may be less effective in polyarteritis nodosa, and plasmapheresis therapy has been recommended in resistant cases. ANCA-positive crescentic glomerulonephritis in the absence of systemic vasculitis appears also to respond to treatment with corticosteroids and cyclophosphamide. For cases of polyarteritis nodosa associated with hepatitis B virus, trials of antiviral agents associated with plasmapheresis have shown promise.

REFERENCES

GENERAL

Couser WG: Pathogenesis of glomerulonephritis. *Kidney Int* 1993;**44**(suppl 42):S19.

Couser WG: New insights into mechanisms of immune glomerular injury. *West J Med* 1994;**160**:440.

Main IW, Atkins RC: The role of T-cells in inflammatory kidney disease. *Curr Opin Nephrol Hyperten* 1995; **4**:354.

Makker SP: Mediators of immune glomerular injury. *Am J Nephrol* 1993;**13**:324.

O'Meara YM et al: The nephritogenic immune response. *Curr Opin Nephrol Hyperten* 1994;**3**:318.

Wilson CB: Renal response to immunologic glomerular injury. In: *The Kidney*, 5th ed. Vol 2. Brenner BM (editor). WB Saunders, 1996, p 1253.

Wilson CB, Tang WW: Immunological renal diseases. In: *Samter's Immunological Diseases,* 5th ed. Frank MM et al (editors). Little, Brown, 1994, p 1033.

ANTIGLOMERULAR BASEMENT MEMBRANE ANTIBODY-INDUCED GLOMERULONEPHRITIS

Glassock RJ et al: Primary glomerular diseases. In: *The Kidney,* 5th ed. Vol 2. Brenner BM (editor). WB Saunders, 1996, p 1392.

Kashgarian M, Sterzel RB: The pathobiology of the mesangium. *Kidney Int* 1992;**41:**524.

Wilson CB: Autoimmune renal disease. In: *The Molecular Pathology of Autoimmune Diseases.* Bona C et al (editors). Harwood Academic, 1993, p 673.

IMMUNE COMPLEX GLOMERULONEPHRITIS

Adler SG et al: Secondary glomerular diseases. In: *The Kidney,* 5th ed. Vol 2. Brenner BM (editor). WB Saunders, 1996, p 1498.

Emancipator SN: IgA nephropathy: Morphologic expression and pathogenesis. *Am J Kidney Dis* 1994 **23:**451.

TUBULOINTERSTITIAL NEPHRITIS

Meeus F et al: Cellular immunity in interstitial nephropathy. *Ren Fail* 1993;**15:**325.

Neilson EG: The nephritogenic T lymphocyte response in interstitial nephritis. *Semin Nephrol* 1993;**13:** 496.

VASCULITIS

Jennette JC, Falk RJ: Update on the pathobiology of vasculitis. *Monogr Pathol* 1995;**37:**156.

39 Immune-Mediated Dermatologic Diseases

Neil J. Korman, MD, PhD, Sanford M. Goldstein, MD, & Bruce U. Wintroub, MD

A large and growing number of skin diseases are autoimmune in nature and are characterized by the presence of skin blisters. These autoimmune blistering skin diseases are among the most intriguing, well-characterized, and potentially serious skin diseases known.

Until approximately 45 years ago, the diagnosis of blistering diseases was based solely on the clinical presentation, morphology, lesion distribution, and occasionally therapeutic trials. Although these clinical clues are very important in developing a working diagnosis, absolute diagnosis requires the use of laboratory methods, including histologic, immunopathologic, immunochemical, and ultrastructural studies. It has become increasingly clear that the autoantibodies found in these autoimmune blistering diseases bind to specific structures within the skin (Figs 39–1 and 39–2). Thus, the discovery of these autoantibodies has revolutionized the understanding and classification of these diseases. Furthermore, these autoantibodies, which may also be found bound to the skin as well as circulating in the blood, serve as important diagnostic markers. On a more basic level, the existence of these antibodies has allowed us to identify and characterize several important proteins in the skin that are thought to play an important role in cell adhesion.

The major routine techniques used to diagnose immune-mediated blistering diseases are histology and direct and indirect immunofluorescence. The most accurate diagnostic features for routine histology are obtained from skin biopsy samples taken from early lesions, including inflamed skin or small vesicles. Direct immunofluorescence, a technique that enables the determination of antibodies bound to the skin, should be performed on perilesional unaffected skin. Indirect immunofluorescence, a technique that probes for the presence of circulating antibodies directed against molecules found in the skin, is also frequently indicated in the diagnostic evaluation of patients with autoimmune blistering diseases.

BULLOUS PEMPHIGOID

Major Immunologic Features
- There is linear deposition of IgG and C3 at the dermal–epidermal junction.
- Circulating IgG binds to bullous pemphigoid antigens in the lamina lucida of the dermal–epidermal junction.

General Considerations
A. Definition: Bullous pemphigoid is characterized by tense, often pruritic blisters located on the flexor surfaces of the extremities, axilla, groin, and lower abdomen. There is characteristic deposition of IgG or C3 or both at the dermal–epidermal junction, without which the diagnosis is in question.

B. Etiology: In vivo and in vitro models suggest that the binding of IgG to bullous pemphigoid antigens (named for the disease) at the lamina lucida of the dermal–epidermal junction is an initiating event in the disease. Autoantibodies in bullous pemphigoid recognize two distinct keratinocyte hemidesmosomal proteins named BP 230 (BPAG1) and BP 180 (BPAG2), which were recently cloned. BP 230 is a cytoplasmic protein, whereas BP 180 is a transmembrane protein, whose clinically relevant epitopes map to a short region between an extracellular collagenous domain and the transmembrane domain. BP 230 and BP 180 map to chromosome 6 and 10, respectively. The primary stimulus for production of the autoantibody is unknown. The disease has been passively transferred to animals by injection of patient antibody. Immunohistochemical studies also demonstrate activation of the complement cascade through the classic and alternative complement pathways. Antibody and complement, in addition to mast cell activation in situ, appear to direct the influx of inflammatory cells, including eosinophils, into the area. The release of mediators from inflammatory cells, including proteolytic enzymes, may contribute to the characteristic separa-

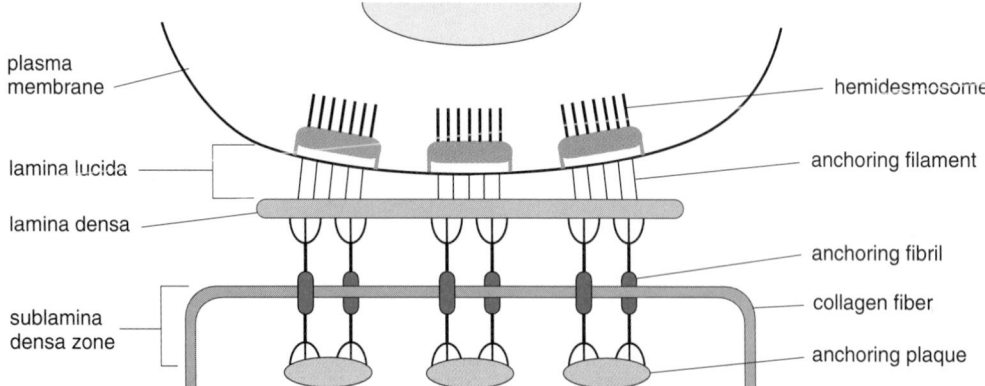

Figure 39–1. Schematic of epithelial basement membrane zone indicates major regions and structures. The lamina lucida is the electron-lucent region just below the keratinocyte plasma membrane and just above the electron-dense lamina densa. Skin incubated in 1 mol/L NaCl splits through the lamina lucida. (Reproduced and modified, with permission, from Gammon WR et al: Immunofluorescence on split skin for the detection and differentiation of basement membrane zone autoantibodies. *J Am Acad Dermatol* 1992;**27**:79.)

tion of the epidermis from the dermis. The typical distribution of lesions on the body surface may be correlated with the regional distribution and concentration of the bullous pemphigoid antigen at those sites.

C. Prevalence: Bullous pemphigoid is an uncommon but not rare disease. There is no sex or race predominance. Although the disease has been occasionally identified in children, it is primarily a disease of individuals 60 years of age or older. There are no known patterns of inheritance, and no HLA associations have been found.

Pathology

Biopsy specimens (3–4 mm in diameter) are obtained from the edge of a fresh blister and should also contain perilesional skin. A subepidermal bulla is seen with inflammatory infiltrate that may be eosinophil-rich (Fig 39–3). The epidermis is intact and not necrotic. A biopsy performed on older lesions may give the false appearance of an intraepidermal blister if the epidermis has begun to regenerate. The dermal infiltrate varies depending on whether the base of the clinical lesion is grossly inflamed or normal,

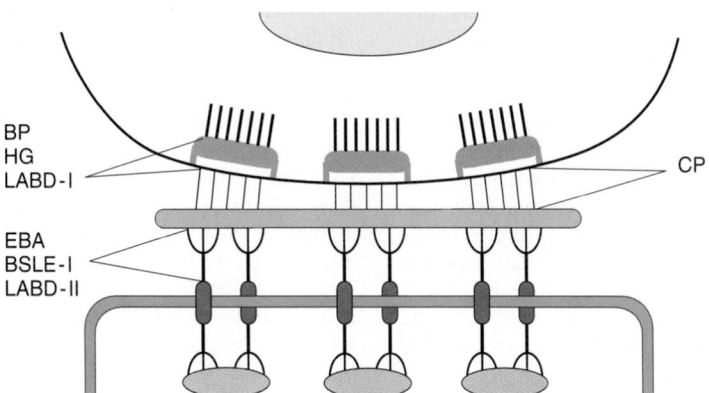

Figure 39–2. Schematic of the epithelial basement membrane zone shows ultrastructural binding sites of BMZ autoantibodies. BP, bullous pemphigoid; BSLE-I, bullous systemic lupus erythematosus type I; CP, cicatricial pemphigoid; EBA, epidermolysis bullosa acquisita; LABD, linear IgA bullous disease. (Reproduced and modified, with permission, from Gammon WR et al: Immunofluorescence on split skin for the detection and differentiation of basement membrane zone autoantibodies. *J Am Acad Dermatol* 1992;**27**:79.)

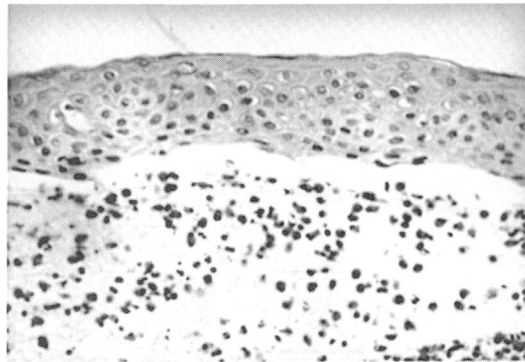

Figure 39–3. Histopathology of bullous pemphigoid. Note the full thickness of epidermis that makes up the blister roof. (Courtesy of Philip LeBoit.)

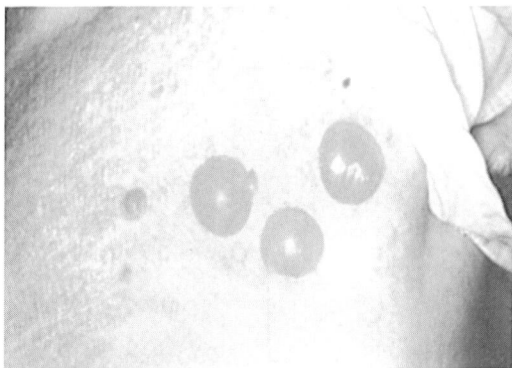

A

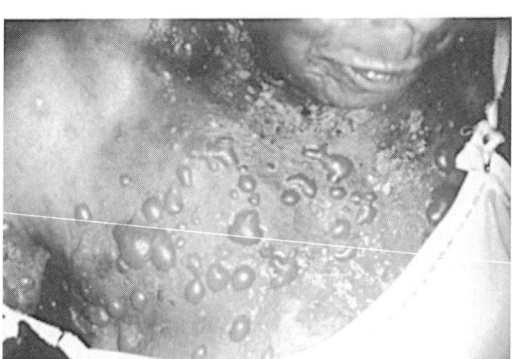

B

Figure 39–4. *A:* Tense blisters on a red base on the back of a patient with bullous pemphigoid. *B:* Multiple blisters on the chest of a patient. (Courtesy of Richard Odom.)

the former being characterized by an infiltrate in the papillary dermis similar to that seen in the blister cavity.

Clinical Features

A. Signs and Symptoms: The classic lesion of bullous pemphigoid is a tense blister with a diameter of 1 cm or more, appearing on a normal or erythematous base (Fig 39–4). The tenseness of the blisters in bullous diseases usually correlates with the thickness of the blister roof, which in bullous pemphigoid is full-thickness epidermis (see Fig 39–3). The lesions may be very pruritic, but this is variable. Bullae are distributed over the extremities and trunk as noted earlier and may rupture and then heal. Smaller blisters, called vesicles, are sometimes seen in a clinical variant called vesicular pemphigoid. Blisters may remain localized to areas such as the lower legs in a variant termed localized pemphigoid. Frequently, elderly patients present with urticarial lesions. This presentation is known as urticarial pemphigoid and precedes the eruption of blisters. Recognizing the existence of these clinical variants allows the physician to obtain appropriate skin biopsy specimens for routine stains and direct immunofluorescence. Blisters may be found in the oral cavity in up to one third of patients and, rarely, on other mucous membranes, including the esophagus, vagina, and anus.

B. Laboratory Findings: Peripheral eosinophilia and elevated serum IgE were present in 50 and 70% of patients, respectively, in one series. These tests are not routinely ordered, but one study did demonstrate a correlation between disease activity and eosinophil counts.

Immunologic Diagnosis

Punch biopsy specimens for immunofluorescence studies should be processed the same day and stored in liquid nitrogen or in a special holding medium. Direct immunofluorescence studies performed on normal appearing or erythematous nonbullous perile-

sional skin reveal linear basement membrane zone deposits of IgG (Fig 39–5) and the third component of complement in the majority of patients, but similar findings can be observed in epidermolysis bullosa acquisita, cicatricial pemphigoid, herpes gestationis, and bullous eruption of systemic lupus erythematosus. The sera of approximately 70% of patients with bullous pemphigoid have circulating IgG antibodies that bind to the basement membrane. Similar findings may also be observed in patients with epidermolysis bullosa acquisita. The amount of these circulating antibodies has no correlation with the degree of disease activity. In order to distinguish bullous pemphigoid from conditions such as epidermolysis bullosa acquisita, special studies, such as indirect immunofluorescence using salt-split skin, are necessary. In this technique, normal human skin is treated with 1.0 M sodium chloride solution for 3 days. This causes a split to occur within the epidermal basement membrane such that most bullous pemphigoid antibodies bind only to the epidermal side, but all epidermolysis bullosa acquisita antibodies bind solely to the dermal side of split skin.

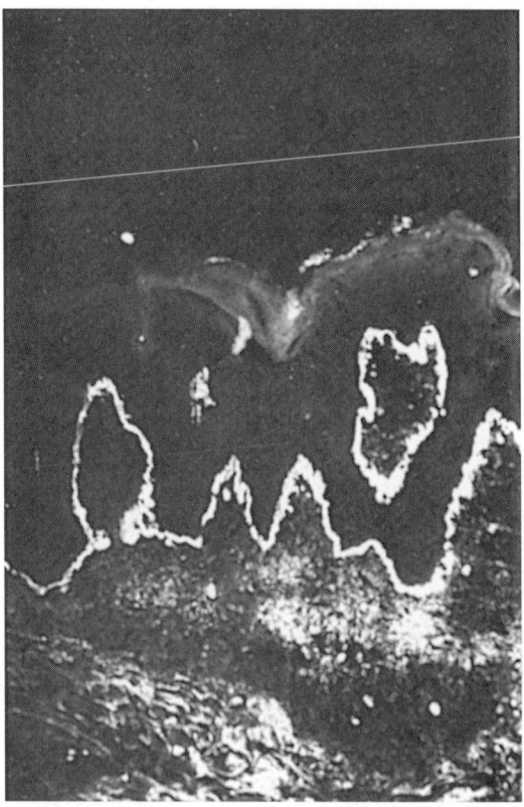

Figure 39–5. Linear deposition of IgG and C3 on direct immunofluorescence of lesional skin. (Courtesy of Richard Odom.)

Differential Diagnosis

The differential diagnosis includes several diseases characterized by blistering. These may be definitively separated from bullous pemphigoid, most often on the basis of immunofluorescence tests and histopathology and less often by clinical features and natural course. In elderly patients with tense blisters, the presence of a subepidermal blister on light microscopy and the linear basement membrane zone deposition of IgG or C3 (or both) on direct immunofluorescence is very suggestive of the diagnosis. However, indirect immunofluorescence studies demonstrating the presence of a circulating IgG antibody that binds to the roof of salt-split skin are required to absolutely confirm the diagnosis of bullous pemphigoid. The same clinical, histologic, and immunologic features in a young woman who is pregnant or taking oral contraceptive drugs, however, strongly suggests the diagnosis of herpes gestationis. Another diagnostic possibility is a bullous drug eruption, which may be similar histologically but has negative immunofluorescence studies. Bullous erythema multiforme often shows a few "target," or "bull's eye," lesions with central blisters and has distinct histologic and usually negative or nonspecific immunofluorescence findings. Other blistering diseases, such as cicatricial pemphigoid, dermatitis herpetiformis, pemphigus vulgaris, epidermolysis bullosa acquisita, and porphyria cutanea tarda, are distinguished from bullous pemphigoid on clinical grounds and laboratory findings.

Treatment

Patients with localized disease can often be successfully treated with high-potency topical steroids. Patients with mild generalized disease are usually successfully treated with low-dose prednisone (approximately 0.5 mg/kg/day, in a single morning dose). Patients with more severe disease should be treated with moderate-dose prednisone (0.75–1.25 mg/kg/day, in a single morning dose). As the disease comes under control, prednisone should be tapered to an alternate-day regimen to minimize steroid side effects. Patients with contraindications to systemic therapy may be treated with dapsone, a combination of tetracycline and nicotinamide, or immunosuppressive agents, particularly azathioprine. The combination of tetracycline and nicotinamide works nicely in younger patients with contraindications to systemic corticosteroids. Older patients with generalized disease, who have contraindications to systemic corticosteroids, can be treated with azathioprine alone (1.0–1.5 mg/kg/day) with excellent results. These patients generally respond within 2–6 months after treatment initiation. Subsequent flares of disease respond well to reinstitution of azathioprine. Older patients with bullous pemphigoid who have severe disease can often be successfully treated with the combination of moderate-dose prednisone along with azathioprine. As the disease comes under control, the prednisone is tapered to alternate days, as described earlier. Other options to be considered in patients with the most progressive disease that is uncontrollable with this combination therapy include the combination of moderate- to high-dose prednisone along with cyclophosphamide or chlorambucil, as well as pulse steroids and plasmapheresis.

Prognosis

Bullous pemphigoid is usually a self-limited disease with a benign, if sometimes prolonged, course. Factors predictive of prognosis have been difficult to identify. Fatal complications may arise in the oldest and most debilitated of patients. The key to successful management is adequate control of the disease while avoiding the complications of systemic corticosteroids. Patients with bullous pemphigoid were thought to have an increased prevalence of internal cancers, but data from several series have refuted this impression. It is possible, but unproven, that patients with negative indirect immunufluorescence tests ("seronegative") may be at increased risk for neoplasia. Because the disease typically affects older adults, concurrent internal cancers may be expected. A thorough history and physical examination is therefore indicated in every case.

CICATRICIAL PEMPHIGOID

Major Immunologic Feature
■ There is linear deposition of IgG and C3 at the submucosal–epithelial junction.

Cicatricial pemphigoid is a chronic subepidermal blistering disease involving primarily mucosal surfaces, including, in decreasing order of frequency, the oropharynx and nasopharynx, conjunctiva, larynx, genitalia, and esophagus. Morbidity and mortality are caused by the scarring that results from recurrent lesions. Cutaneous involvement occurs in only about one fourth of patients with cicatricial pemphigoid. The major criteria for differentiating between bullous pemphigoid and cicatricial pemphigoid is the prominent scarring secondary to blistering that is seen in cicatricial pemphigoid. In bullous pemphigoid, lesions are largely found on the skin, whereas in cicatricial pemphigoid lesions are largely found on the mucosa. Clinical features should therefore be used to differentiate between these two entities. The diagnosis of cicatricial pemphigoid is based on three criteria: (1) scarring mucosal blisters or erosions; (2) subepithelial blister with intact basal cell and variable inflammatory cell infiltrate; and (3) direct immunofluorescence of perilesional epithelium revealing linear deposits of IgG and C3 along the basement membrane. Although early reports indicated that routine indirect immunofluorescence (IIF) studies for circulating antibodies in cicatricial pemphigoid are often negative, recent studies demonstrate that the use of salt-split human skin increases the frequency of detection of both IgG and IgA circulating autoantibodies.

Recent studies, using sophisticated immunopathologic and immunochemical techniques, have demonstrated the presence of several distinct subgroups of patients that fit within the cicatricial pemphigoid phenotype. The first group includes patients with antiepiligrin cicatricial pemphigoid. These patients are immunochemically distinct in that they have circulating IgG autoantibodies that bind to the dermal side of salt-split skin and recognize epiligrin, now known as laminin 5, but they lack distinguishing clinical features that separate them from other cicatricial pemphigoid variants. The other three major groups that form the cicatricial pemphigoid spectrum have recently been delineated in a large study of 123 patients with immune-mediated subepithelial blistering diseases who were categorized on the basis of clinical and immunopathologic features. The first of these distinct groups of patients have pure ocular disease in the absence of skin, oral, or other mucous membrane disease. These patients rarely have circulating IgG antibodies and have negative serologic reactivity to BP antigens or other defined basement membrane zone antigens. The second group consists of patients who have oral mucosal disease (with or without other mucosal lesions) along with skin lesions and have circulating IgG antibodies and serologic reactivity to bullous pemphigoid antigens, which occur at the same frequency as patients with bullous pemphigoid. These patients have been classified as having anti-BP antigen mucosal pemphigoid. The third and final group of patients is itself a heterogeneous one that includes patients who have oral mucosal disease (along with ocular and other mucous membrane lesions) in the absence of any skin lesions, and patients with oral disease alone.

Cicatricial pemphigoid is a chronic disease, and treatment regimens should be dictated by the organs involved. Patients with involvement limited to the nasopharynx or oropharynx should be treated with topical or intralesional steroids, short bursts of oral corticosteroids, or dapsone. If the eyes, esophagus, or larynx become involved, then the anticipated morbidity can be severe, including blindness and asphyxiation, and aggressive therapy with systemic corticosteroids and immunosuppressive agents is warranted. Cyclophosphamide has been most effective in the treatment of patients with severe involvement, and the majority go into clinical remission after an 18- to 24-month course.

HERPES GESTATIONIS

Major Immunologic Features
■ The third component of complement is always and IgG is occasionally linearly deposited along the dermal–epidermal junction of a perilesional skin biopsy.
■ Frequently there are circulating IgG antibodies that avidly bind complement.

General Considerations
A. Definition: Herpes gestationis is characterized by extremely pruritic vesicles and bullae appearing during pregnancy. *Herpes* refers to the Greek word meaning "to creep," but this disease has no association with herpes simplex virus or varicella-zoster virus.

B. Etiology: The cause is unknown. The primary stimulus for antibody production is not known, but the antigen is the same BP 180 (BPAG2) epidermal basement membrane hemidesmosomal protein that is one of the target antigens in bullous pemphigoid. The onset of herpes gestationis appears to require placental tissue, choriocarcinoma, or hydatidiform moles; recurrences may be caused by exogenous estrogen alone. Antibodies bound to placental tissue in these patients are not cross-reactive with the skin. The antibody also reacts with the amnion epithelial basement membrane of second-trimester and full-term placentas, although the significance of this finding is unclear. Fixation of complement and activation of the classic complement pathway may be involved in the blistering seen clinically.

C. Prevalence: Herpes gestationis is rare, ranging from 1:3000–1:10,000 births in early studies to 1:50,000 births in recent series. There have been few reports of herpes gestationis occurring in blacks, which may reflect the lower frequency of HLA-DR4 in this population. Between 61 and 83% of patients have the HLA-DR3 haplotype, and 45% have both HLA-DR3 and DR4, compared with 3% of women in the general population. The HLA type, however, does not correlate with duration, severity, or recurrence of disease or with antibody titer. Abnormal regulation of anti-HLA idiotype antibodies during pregnancy was demonstrated in one patient, but the prevalence and significance in this defect in immune regulation are not known.

Pathology

The classic picture on light microscopy of a subepidermal bulla with eosinophils in the blister cavity is seen in only a minority of cases. The papillary dermis shows edema and a mixed perivascular lymphohistiocytic infiltrate with eosinophils. Spongiosis (edema between epidermal cells), with or without eosinophils, liquefactive degeneration, or necrosis in the epidermis may be present. Eosinophils are an important histologic feature when present (Fig 39–6A).

Clinical Features

A. Signs and Symptoms: The onset is usually in the second or third trimester; in 20% of cases it occurs in the first few days postpartum. Intense pruritus accompanies and at times precedes the eruption, which often begins around the umbilicus or on the extremities as hive-like plaques, blisters, or rings of vesicles at the edges of hive-like plaques (Figs 39–6B and 39–6C). The disease may worsen at delivery. It tends to recur with subsequent pregnancies and lasts for weeks to months postpartum, occasionally flaring with ovulation, menstruation, or use of oral contraceptives. Lactation may shorten the natural course of untreated postpartum skin disease. Barring secondary bacterial infection, the blisters heal without scarring.

B. Laboratory Findings: Routine investigations are not clinically useful. Peripheral eosinophilia may occur, with an elevated erythrocyte sedimentation rate. Serum complement concentrations are usually normal.

Immunologic Diagnosis

A skin biopsy specimen obtained at the edge of a fresh blister for direct immunofluorescence testing reveals linear deposition of C3 at the epidermal basement membrane zone in virtually all cases. IgG is also found in 25% of biopsy specimens. Routine indirect immunofluorescence studies are usually negative, but the complement fixation assay is positive in about 50% of cases. When positive, the IIF pattern is identical to that seen in bullous pemphigoid.

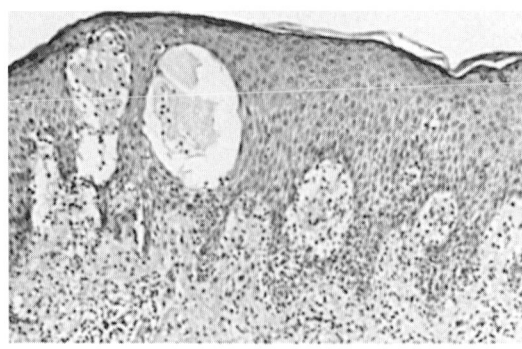

A

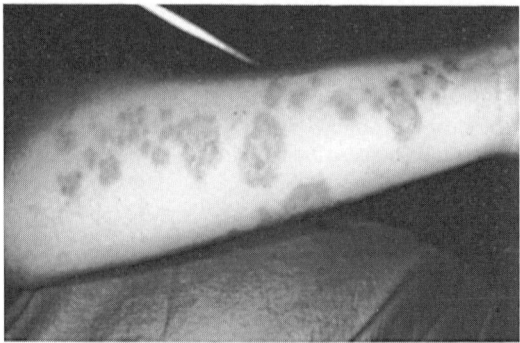

B

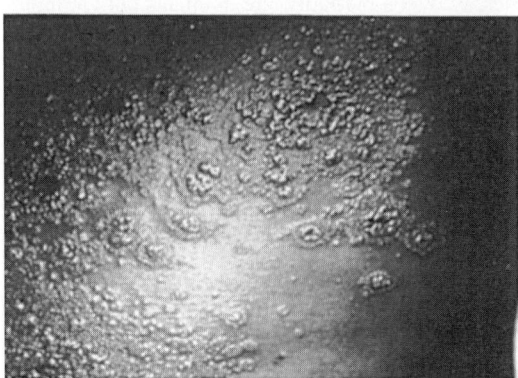

C

Figure 39–6. A: Histopathology of herpes gestationis showing early subepidermal blister formation. The teardrop-shaped vesicle at the left is characteristic of early herpes gestationis. (Courtesy of Philip LeBoit.) **B:** Hive-like and ringed lesions with vesicular edges on the arm of a patient with herpes gestationis. (Courtesy of Richard Odom.) **C:** Rings of vesicles at the edges of plaques in herpes gestationis. (Courtesy of Richard Odom.)

Differential Diagnosis

The onset of pruritic, hive-like plaques with tense blisters in a pregnant woman requires punch biopsy specimens for light and immunofluorescence microscopy to confirm the diagnosis. The greatest confusion may exist in cases of herpes gestationis prior to the appearance of blisters, and one must rule out disorders causing pruritus and those causing hive-like rashes. There are reports of a large number of poorly defined pruritic cutaneous syndromes in pregnant women. One should also rule out atopic dermatitis, scabies, and dry skin. Hive-like or edematous plaques may be caused by pruritic urticarial papules and plaques of pregnancy (which, unlike herpes gestationis, typically spares the umbilicus), urticaria, and erythema multiforme, but these may be ruled out by skin biopsy.

Treatment and Prognosis

Treatment should be undertaken in consultation with the patient's obstetrician. Prednisone at 40–60 mg/day controls the disease in most cases within a week, but higher or divided doses may be necessary in the event of a poor response. The steroid therapy is then slowly tapered over several weeks to a maintenance dose. Some patients improve spontaneously in the third trimester, but the condition flares at delivery. Cytotoxic immunosuppressive agents should be avoided during pregnancy. Antihistamines have little, if any, effectiveness.

Herpes gestationis often recurs in subsequent pregnancies and it may appear earlier. Skin lesions in infants are uncommon and usually are transient, requiring no therapy. Although early studies suggested an increased fetal mortality rate in infants born to mothers with herpes gestationis, subsequent studies have not supported this finding. Several studies do suggest an increased incidence of low-birth-weight and premature infants in herpes gestationis. It is therefore prudent that these patients be cared for jointly by a dermatologist and an obstetrician and delivery be performed in a facility that has a neonatal intensive care unit.

EPIDERMOLYSIS BULLOSA ACQUISITA

Major Immunologic Features

■ IgG and, less frequently, IgA, IgM, C3, C1q, C4, factor B, and properdin are linearly deposited at the basement membrane zone in the sublaminar densa zone.

General Considerations

Epidermolysis bullosa acquisita is a blistering disease marked by skin fragility. It occurs on noninflamed skin over the distal extremities and heals with scarring. Immunoelectron microscopy detects linear immunoglobulin deposits in the sublaminar dense zone of the dermal–epidermal junction. These may also be seen by immunofluorescence microscopy on the dermal side of skin separated at the dermal–epidermal junction after incubation in NaCl.

The cause is unknown. The epidermolysis bullosa acquisita antigen is the globular carboxy terminus of type VII procollagen, which is also synthesized by epidermal cells and fibroblasts in culture. Aggregates of type VII collagen form the anchoring fibrils that bind the epidermis and dermis together. Passive transfer experiments with human epidermolysis bullosa acquisita antibody in animals have not been successful. In vitro organ culture models of the disease indicate that epidermolysis bullosa acquisita antibody fixes complement and directs an influx of leukocytes into the skin, resulting in epidermal–dermal separation.

Pathology

A subepidermal blister is characteristic of epidermolysis bullosa acquisita. Other features, especially the dermal infiltrate, are variable and correlate with clinical characteristics. Noninflammatory lesions may resemble porphyria cutanea tarda. Inflammatory lesions resemble bullous pemphigoid but with a greater predominance of neutrophils.

Clinical Features

A. Signs and Symptoms: Epidermolysis bullosa acquisita is a disease of adult onset with two distinct presentations. The "classic presentation" involves acral skin fragility and blisters, which heal with scarring and milia. Alternatively, almost half of all patients have widespread vesicles and bullae on red or inflamed bases; these are associated with pruritus, erosions, and erythematous plaques. These lesions may be accentuated in skin folds and flexural areas. This second presentation resembles bullous pemphigoid. Patients may also have combinations of both presentations during the evolution of their disease. Some patients also have nail changes, oral lesions, or a scarring process in the scalp, leading to hair loss. Epidermolysis bullosa acquisita may be significantly associated with inflammatory bowel disease, particularly Crohn's disease. Individual patients have been reported to have other systemic diseases, such as thyroiditis, systemic lupus erythematosus (SLE), diabetes mellitus, or rheumatoid arthritis, but these associations are unclear.

B. Laboratory Findings: Routine tests are generally normal. Twenty-four-hour urine porphyrin levels are normal.

Immunologic Diagnosis

Direct immunofluorescence examination of perilesional skin demonstrates a broad linear band of IgG, C3, and, occasionally, other immune deposits at the dermal–epidermal junction. Immune deposits are also found in several other conditions, especially bullous pemphigoid, so these findings are not pathognomonic for epidermolysis bullosa acquisita. Twenty-five to 50% of patients have positive indirect immunofluorescence of the basement membrane zone below stratified squamous epithelium, but the autoantibodies do not cross-react with the lungs and kidneys. When skin that has been split between the epidermis and dermis by incubation in a solution high in salt is used as the substrate for indirect immunofluorescence tests, a characteristic staining of the sera on the dermal side helps define epidermolysis bullosa acquisita. In the absence of positive indirect immunofluorescence, immunoelectron microscopy localizes the immune deposits to the sublaminar densa fibrillar zone.

Differential Diagnosis

Family history and immunofluorescence testing help to rule out hereditary forms of epidermolysis bullosa. Noninflammatory lesions may be clinically and histologically confused with those of porphyria cutanea tarda, but determination of 24-hour urinary porphyrin excretion and the finding of immune deposits in dermal vessels should be diagnostic of porphyria cutanea tarda. Bullous pemphigoid may be similar clinically and histologically to one presentation of epidermolysis bullosa acquisita. However, immunoelectron microscopy, indirect immunofluorescence on split-skin substrates, the presence or absence of scarring and milia, and the response to treatment aid in distinguishing between the two diseases. The bullous eruption of SLE may be very difficult to distinguish from epidermolysis bullosa acquisita by clinical and histologic features, immunofluorescence testing, and by Western immunoblot analysis of patient sera against epidermolysis bullosa acquisita antigen. Patients with bullous SLE, however, are said to respond more readily to dapsone, have less skin fragility, heal without scars and milia, and have a more granular staining pattern at the dermal–epidermal junction on direct immunofluorescence than patients with epidermolysis bullosa acquisita.

Treatment

Treatment is difficult, since patients respond poorly to topical and systemic corticosteroid therapy, even with the addition of dapsone and various immunosuppressive drugs. Initial studies with cyclosporin A have been promising. Other therapies, including colchicine and even plasmapheresis, occasionally prove beneficial. Careful and gentle local measures to promote skin cleanliness, control infections, and minimize trauma are important.

Complications and Prognosis

Epidermolysis bullosa acquisita is a chronic, nonremitting disease with great morbidity secondary to pain, scarring, and, ultimately, disfiguring skin lesions.

DERMATITIS HERPETIFORMIS

Major Immunologic Features
■ Granular deposits of IgA and complement components are found at the dermal–epidermal junction

in dermal papillae in lesional and normal-appearing skin.
■ There is a critical sensitivity to dietary gluten.

General Considerations

Dermatitis herpetiformis is characterized by pruritic grouped papules, papulovesicles, and vesicles and the granular deposition of IgA in dermal papillae at the dermal–epidermal junction. The cause is unknown. The stimuli for production of IgA antibodies found on the skin, the antigen(s) to which they are bound, and cellular and biochemical causes of the clinical disease remain to be determined. The IgA antibody does not react with gluten or gliadin and may be found in clinically normal-appearing skin. It is presumed that the primary stimulus for the disease occurs in the gastrointestinal tract. Patients with dermatitis herpetiformis also have circulating IgA antiendomysial antibodies. In 21 patients on a gluten-free diet and 80 controls not on the diet, who all had bullous and other dermatologic or noncutaneous diseases, the sensitivity and specificity of these antibodies for dermatitis herpetiformis were 90 and 96%, respectively.

Prevalence estimates range from 10 to 39 persons per 100,000 in Scandinavia, but the rate is much lower in Japan. The rate may relate to the frequency of HLA types. Between 80 and 95% of patients with granular deposits of IgA in normal skin have the HLA-B8 haplotype, and up to 95% have HLA-DR3. More than 90% of patients may express the HLA antigen Dqw2. The strongest HLA associations on a molecular level are with HLA-DQB1*0201 and HLA-DQA1*0501 and HLA-DRB1*0301, as seen with gluten-sensitive enteropathy. The association with HLA-DP antigens is less strong than with HLA-DQw2 or HLA-DR3. HLA-B8 is also associated with "ordinary" gluten-sensitive enteropathy without skin lesions (see Chapter 37).

Pathology

The skin lesions optimal for biopsy are early papules or fresh, unbroken vesicles for light microscopy. Neutrophils are seen at the dermal papillary tips in early lesions that may evolve into subepidermal blisters. Eosinophils and a mild perivascular lymphohistiocytic infiltrate may be seen. Older vesicles and crusted lesions may yield nondiagnostic findings. For direct immunofluorescence tests, biopsy of normal-appearing perilesional skin is recommended.

Clinical Features

Grouped red papules, hive-like plaques, and vesicles are symmetrically distributed on the elbows and knees, upper back, buttocks, and posterior neck and scalp (Fig 39–7). This distribution may be quite helpful to the diagnosis. The lesions are extremely pruritic or may burn or sting. When excoriated, they leave crusted areas.

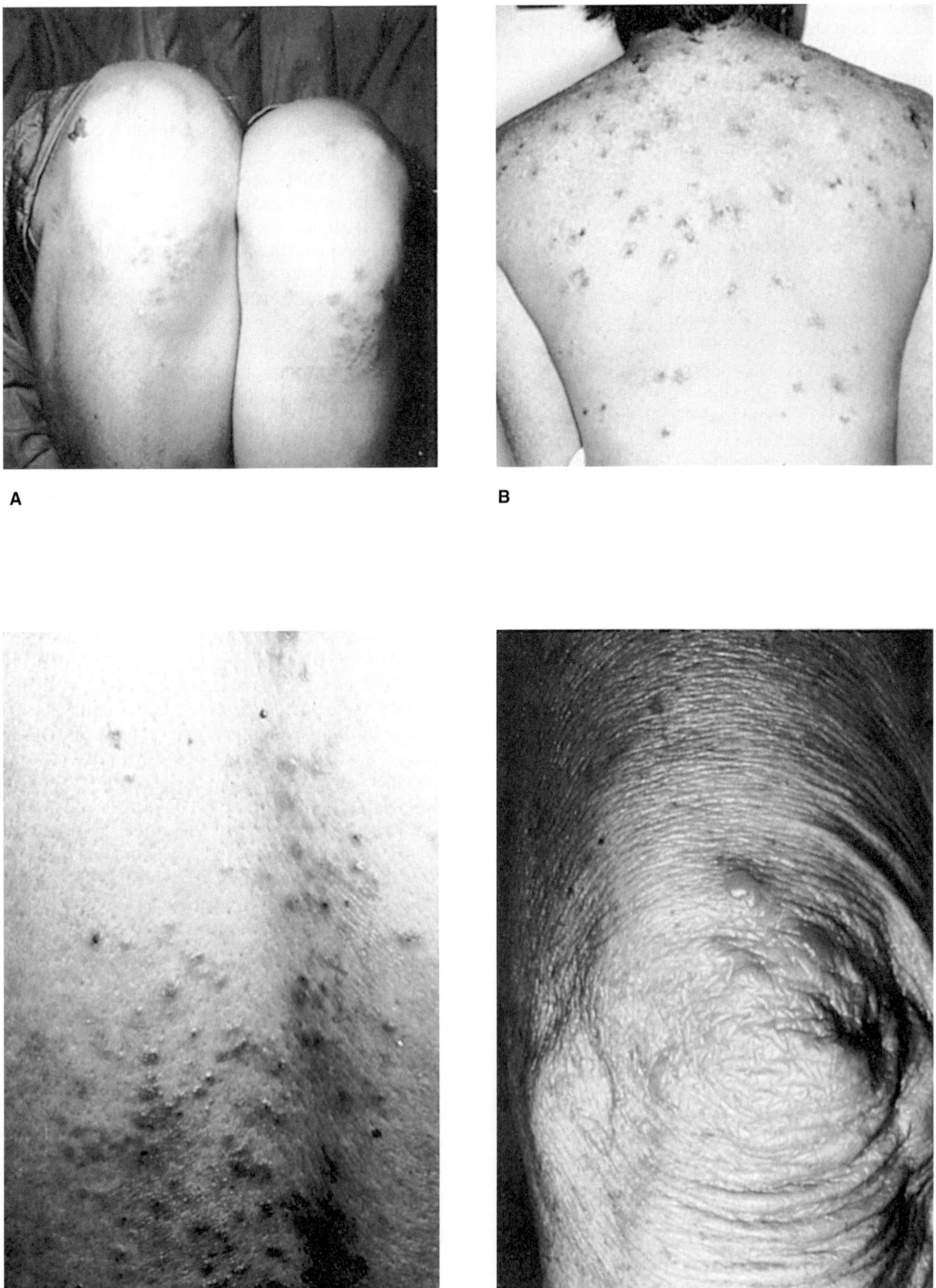

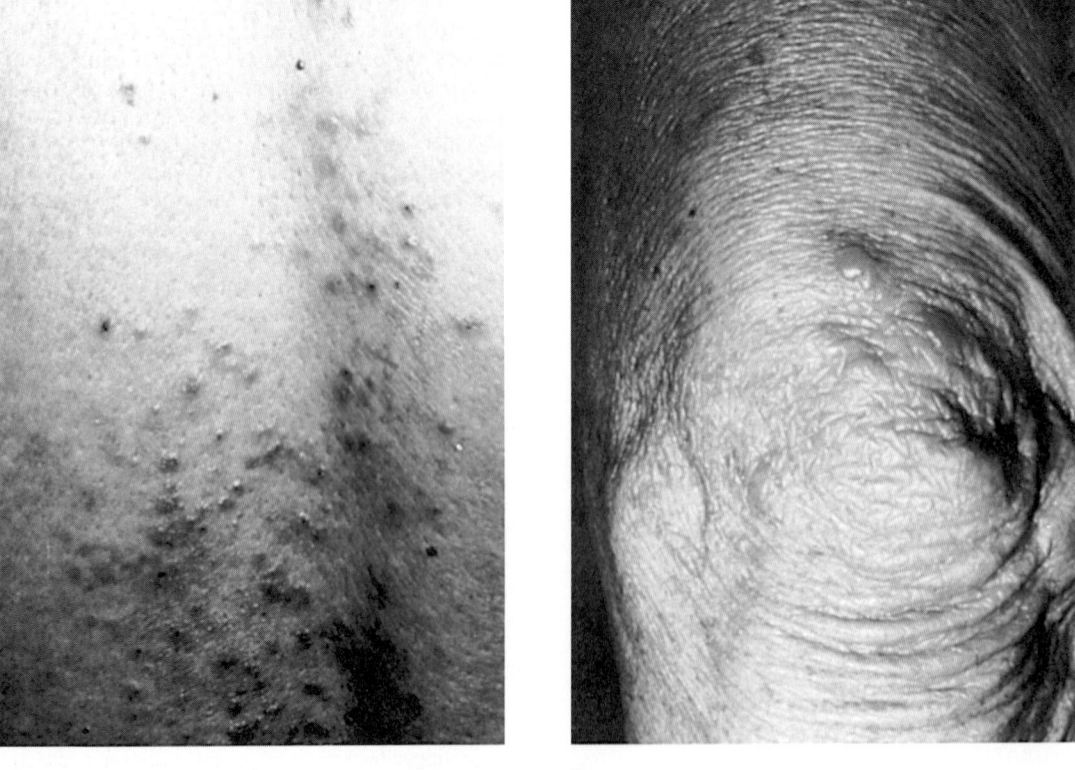

Figure 39–7. Dermatitis herpetiformis. **A** and **B:** Typical distribution of lesions on knees and upper back. (Courtesy of Richard Odom.) **C:** Papular lesions on the mid-back. (Courtesy of John Reeves.) **D:** Close-up view of papulovesicular lesions on elbow. (Courtesy of John Reeves.)

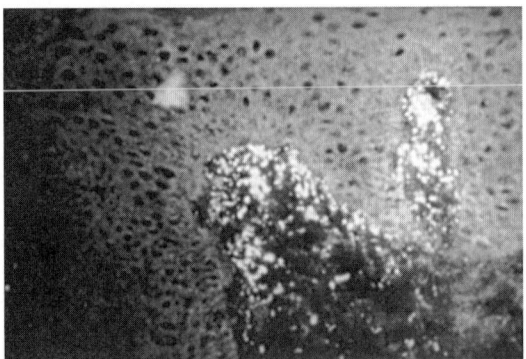

Figure 39–8. Direct immunofluorescence of perilesional skin demonstrates IgA deposition in dermal papillae in dermatitis herpetiformis. (Courtesy of Richard Odom.)

There are no diagnostic laboratory findings. Endoscopy with biopsy or radiographic studies may detect signs seen in gluten-sensitive enteropathy, but this is neither clinically useful nor necessary for diagnosis or management. Thyroid abnormalities, including hyperthyroidism and hypothyroidism, occur more frequently in patients with dermatitis herpetiformis.

Immunologic Diagnosis

A biopsy of normal-appearing perilesional skin reveals granular deposits of polyclonal IgA along dermal papillae in all patients, and this defines the disease (Fig 39–8). IgA may not always be found in lesional skin. C3 may also be found.

Differential Diagnosis

Vesicles may be seen in a variety of diseases, including varicella, herpes simplex, and herpes zoster. Cytologic smears and cultures, as well as their nongrouped or asymmetric distribution of lesions, distinguish these diseases from dermatitis herpetiformis. A clinically similar disease with different HLA associations, called linear IgA disease, is characterized by linear deposits of IgA in or below the lamina lucida of the basement membrane zone. Direct immunofluorescence can also rule out diseases such as bullous pemphigoid, herpes gestationis, and chronic bullous disease of childhood, all of which are usually clinically distinguishable as well.

Treatment

Strict avoidance of dietary gluten may control the disease entirely after 1–4 years or may lower the dosage of sulfones required. Although gluten may not be the only dietary factor that plays a role in this disease, gluten avoidance by some patients has been shown to lead to a clearing of skin IgA deposits after more than a decade of dietary treatment. It is difficult to follow such a diet. Less than total avoidance may be helpful but is not as effective. It may also be best

to restrict gluten in the diet before initiating sulfone therapy. Most patients can completely control their skin disease by treatment with 100–200 mg per day of dapsone. A glucose-6-phosphate dehydrogenase (G6PD) level must be determined for all patients prior to therapy with dapsone. Hemolysis may occur at high dapsone doses even in patients with normal G6PD levels. Patients on dapsone must be monitored for hemolysis and methemoglobinemia, as well as hepatic, renal, and neurologic complications of therapy.

Prognosis and Associated Diseases

Dermatitis herpetiformis is a chronic disease unless dietary avoidance of gluten is maintained. Even after the lesions clear, reintroduction of gluten rapidly results in disease exacerbation. Lesions heal without scarring, although pigmentary changes may remain. There are reported associations of dermatitis herpetiformis with antigastric parietal cell antibodies, gastric hypochlorhydria or achlorhydria, antithyroid antibodies, IgA nephropathy, and possibly, gastrointestinal lymphoma.

LINEAR IGA BULLOUS DERMATOSIS

Major Immunologic Feature

■ There are linear basement membrane zone deposits of IgA.

A subset of patients (10%) with vesicles and bullae appear to have a disease that falls between bullous pemphigoid and dermatitis herpetiformis. Like patients with bullous pemphigoid, they have larger bullae than are seen in dermatitis herpetiformis, as well as linear deposits of immunoglobulin, usually IgA but sometimes IgG and C3 as well. Unlike patients with bullous pemphigoid, these patients respond to sulfones but not to corticosteroids, and deposits are at and below the lamina lucida. Other patients have small vesicles like those of dermatitis herpetiformis, but occasionally without the marked symmetry of dermatitis herpetiformis. Unlike dermatitis herpetiformis, however, the histopathology of linear IgA bullous dermatosis shows a linear band-like infiltrate of polymorphonuclear neutrophils at the dermal–epidermal junction, in addition to papillary neutrophil microabscesses and linear deposits of IgA at the dermal–epidermal junction, in and below the lamina lucida. Patients present with vesicles and bullae that may clinically resemble bullous pemphigoid or dermatitis herpetiformis, or both. Oral lesions and ulcers may be minor findings or, rarely, the major manifestation of the disease. Direct immunofluorescence is positive for linear deposits of IgA and occasionally other immunoglobulins at and below the lamina lucida. Indirect immunofluorescence may be positive in some cases. In this disease there is a lower prevalence of HLA-B8 than in dermatitis herpetiformis. The patients do not have jejunal changes of gluten-sensitive enteropathy, they lack the antiendomysium antibodies seen in dermatitis herpetiformis and gluten-sensitive enteropathy, they do not benefit from a gluten-free diet, they respond to sulfones, and their disease tends to have a chronic course. The antigen that binds the IgA is a 97-kd molecule named LAD-1.

PEMPHIGUS VULGARIS & PEMPHIGUS FOLIACEOUS

Major Immunologic Features
- IgG is deposited on the epidermal cell surface.
- Circulating IgG antibody binds to the cell surface of stratified squamous epithelium.

General Considerations
Pemphigus vulgaris and pemphigus foliaceous are described together because they are blistering diseases characterized by acantholysis and the deposition of cell surface autoantibodies. They may be distinguished clinically, histologically, and immunologically.

Pemphigus vulgaris and pemphigus foliaceous are characterized by widespread blistering and denudation of skin and mucous membranes. They have a distinctive histologic picture demonstrating acantholysis (loss of cohesion) of epidermal cells and a typical pattern on direct immunofluorescence tests. The lesion is superficial in pemphigus foliaceous and deeper in pemphigus vulgaris.

A. Etiology: A large body of clinical and experimental evidence demonstrates that pemphigus autoantibodies are pathogenic. The clinical evidence includes the observations that circulating antibody titers correlate with disease activity in many patients and that treatment with plasmapheresis has induced short term remissions in some patients. Furthermore, the occurrence of neonatal pemphigus vulgaris, with spontaneous resolution of the disease by several months of age, demonstrates that maternal pemphigus IgG can cross the placenta and cause disease. Organ culture studies convincingly demonstrate that treatment of skin with pemphigus vulgaris or pemphigus foliaceous IgG leads to epidermal acantholysis (in the suprabasilar and granular layer, respectively). These studies also reveal that pemphigus antibody alone, without complement or inflammatory cells, is sufficient to induce acantholysis. It has been shown in this system that treatment with pemphigus IgG leads to the release of a proteinase, thought to be plasminogen activator, which mediates acantholysis. Finally, when either pemphigus foliaceous or pemphigus vulgaris IgG antibodies are injected into neonatal mice, these animals develop the clinical, histologic, and immunopathologic features of the corresponding subtype of pemphigus.

Recent studies have concentrated on characterizing the keratinocyte cell surface molecules to which pemphigus autoantibodies bind. This work has demonstrated that patients with pemphigus vulgaris have circulating autoantibodies directed against a 130-kd cadherin, pemphigus vulgaris antigen, a desmosomal protein that is bound to plakoglobin, an 85-kd molecule of desmosomes and adherens junctions. Patients with pemphigus foliaceous have circulating autoantibodies directed against desmoglein, a 160-kd desmosomal protein, which is also bound to plakoglobin. These findings establish that patients with pemphigus have circulating autoantibodies directed against molecular complexes that contain adhering junction molecules. Although the exact sequence of events that occurs after pemphigus antibody binds to the epidermal cell surface is not known, there is evidence to support a role for proteolytic enzymes and complement activation. Based on the evidence that pemphigus autoantibodies bind to cell adhesion junction molecules, it must also be considered that pemphigus autoantibodies could directly interfere with assembly or function of cell adhesion junctions and, thereby, lead to blister formation.

B. Epidemiology: Pemphigus vulgaris occurs predominantly but not exclusively in persons of Jewish or Mediterranean ancestry. It may occur in all age groups, with an incidence of 0.5–3.2 cases per 100,000 per year, but it is more common in the fourth and fifth decades and is rare after age 60. The familial occurrence of pemphigus has been reported in 25 families.

C. Genetics: HLA-A10 was first identified as being more commonly represented among patients with pemphigus vulgaris than in the general population. More recently it has been shown that 95% of pemphigus vulgaris patients are positive for HLA-DR4/DQw3 or HLA-DRw6/DQw1, and it is thought that pemphigus may segregate with DQ alleles. In a series of 13 DQw1-positive patients with pemphigus vulgaris, all were identified as positive for an allele designated $PV6_b$ versus 1 of 13 DR/DQ-matches controls. This allele differs from the normal DQ_b allele in codon 57, where asparagine replaces valine or serine.

Pathology
Skin biopsy shows a suprabasal intraepidermal blister with loss of cohesion of keratinocytes (acantholysis) in pemphigus vulgaris (Fig 39–9). Pemphigus foliaceous demonstrates a superficial subcorneal or subgranular acantholytic blister.

Clinical Features
Pemphigus vulgaris is characterized by blisters that most commonly affect the scalp, chest, umbilicus, and body folds (Fig 39–10). In contrast to the lesions of bullous pemphigoid, these blisters are flaccid and fragile because the epidermal split occurs within the epidermis, resulting in a thinner roof (see Fig 39–9). Lesions may easily rupture, and in some cases only crusts and no blisters are seen. Oral lesions may be the initial or, uncommonly, the only presentation of the disease. Nikolsky's sign (sloughing of the epidermis after lateral pressure with a cotton applicator or tongue

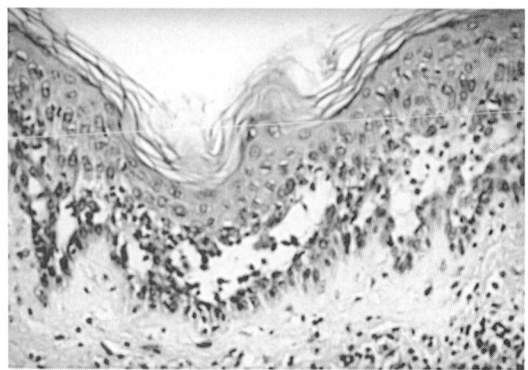

Figure 39–9. Histopathology of pemphigus vulgaris demonstrates intraepidermal blister formation with loss of cohesion of keratinocytes (acantholysis). (Courtesy of Philip LeBoit.)

blade) is positive in involved skin. Pemphigus foliaceous, with its more superficial histologic process of blistering, may show only scaly, crusted, and superficial erosions without frank blisters. Oral lesions are rarely seen in pemphigus foliaceous. Routine laboratory tests are not helpful in diagnosis or management.

Immunologic Diagnosis

In virtually all patients, direct immunofluorescence reveals the deposition of IgG. In 50% of patients, complement components (mostly C3) deposit on the epidermal cell surface, forming a honeycomb pattern (Fig 39–11). Between 80 and 90% of patients also have circulating IgG that stains the cell surface of stratified squamous epithelium in target substrates such as monkey esophagus or human skin. Although it has been reported that pemphigus foliaceous sera stain the more superficial layers of the epidermis compared with pemphigus vulgaris sera, this seldom is seen in practice.

Differential Diagnosis

Several diseases may be confused with pemphigus vulgaris. The diagnosis depends on clinical suspicion when the patient presents with blisters and crusting with appropriate immunofluorescence on biopsy. Oral lesions may be confused with aphthous ulcers or oral erythema multiforme. Scalp lesions may appear similar to impetigo. Occasionally pemphigus vulgaris resembles other pemphigus variants, including pemphigus foliaceous and pemphigus erythematosus, but light microscopy is helpful in this situation. Other blistering eruptions (see earlier discussion) are readily distinguished by clinical appearance (size, grouping, distribution, and tenseness of blisters), histopathology, and immunofluorescence pattern. Since pemphigus vulgaris and pemphigus foliaceous may be somewhat confused with widespread dermatitis or impetigo, the persistence of disease in spite of empirical treatment of a patient for these other diseases without a biopsy often delays the correct diagnosis.

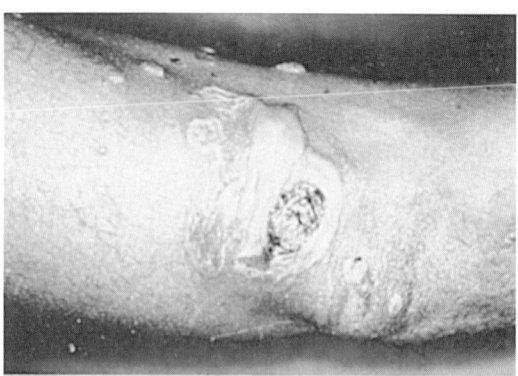

A

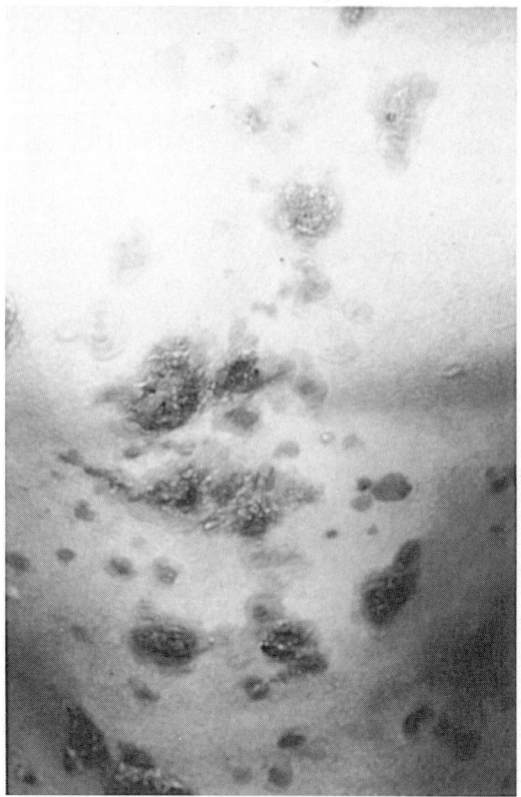

B

Figure 39–10. *A:* Flaccid blister on the elbow of a patient with pemphigus vulgaris (compare with the tense blister in bullous pemphigoid in Fig 39–4). *B:* Crusted and bullous lesions on the chest of a patient with pemphigus vulgaris. (Courtesy of Richard Odom.)

Treatment

All patients with pemphigus vulgaris require systemic therapy with glucocorticosteroids to clear the circulating antibodies. Pemphigus foliaceous patients tend to have a more benign course, can often be

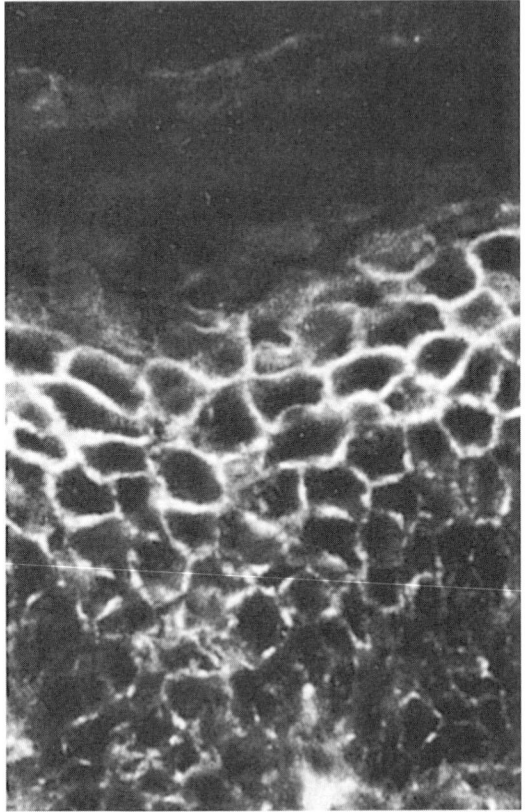

Figure 39–11. Direct immunofluorescence pattern of IgG deposition in pemphigus vulgaris. The immunoglobulins and complement components are deposited in intercellular regions in the epidermis forming a honeycomb pattern. (Courtesy of Denny Tuffanelli.)

treated with lower dosages of glucocorticosteroids, and occasionally respond to topical steroid therapy alone. Patients with pemphigus are generally treated with prednisone at 1–2 mg/kg/day in a single morning dosage, depending on disease severity, with tapering toward an alternate-day dosage within a 1–3 month period as the disease allows. Short- and long-term toxicities of prednisone are numerous and include gastrointestinal bleeding, diabetes mellitus, cataracts, osteoporosis, increased risk of infection, and central nervous system changes. Every effort should therefore be made to minimize the dosage of systemic glucocorticosteroids and to switch to alternate-day dosing as soon as is feasible.

Immunosuppressive drugs, most commonly cyclophosphamide and azathioprine, are used, particularly in pemphigus vulgaris, for their steroid-sparing effects. Cyclophosphamide appears to be the more effective of the two but it has numerous toxicities, including bone marrow suppression, hemorrhagic cystitis, bladder fibrosis, sterility, alopecia, and an increased risk of malignancy. The major toxicities of azathioprine include bone marrow suppression, hepatotoxicity, and increased risk of malignancy. Monitoring of patients treated with these immunosuppressive agents should include frequent blood counts, urinalyses, and liver function testing. Other therapies used in specific settings but with lower success rates as steroid-sparing agents in pemphigus, include dapsone, the combination of tetracycline and niacinamide, hydroxychloroquine, gold, and cyclosporine. Patients with the most severe disease may be treated with the combination of systemic glucocorticosteroids, immunosuppressive drugs and plasmapheresis.

Prognosis and Associated Diseases

Several factors have been shown to predict the clinical outcome of patients with pemphigus. The age of the patient is very important, with elderly patients having a worse prognosis. One large study found that the average age of pemphigus patients dying within 3 months of the initiation of therapy was 75 years as compared with 55 years for those surviving the first 3 months of therapy. The extent of disease activity is another important factor, because patients with generalized disease have an increased mortality rate. Disease progression prior to the onset of therapy correlates with prognosis because patients with minimal disease activity for prolonged periods do better than patients whose disease rapidly progresses after short periods without therapy. Furthermore, several studies demonstrate that the majority of patients who die from their pemphigus do so within the first few years of their disease.

Although the dose of glucocorticosteroids necessary to control disease has been cited as an important prognostic factor, complications of systemic steroid therapy make it difficult to separate disease-related from treatment-related morbidity and mortality. Before glucocorticosteroids became available, the mortality rate from pemphigus ranged from 60 to 90%. With the current use of systemic corticosteroids and immunosuppressive agents the mortality rate has fallen to the 5–10% range.

Pemphigus may occur in association with myasthenia gravis or thymoma or rarely with other autoimmune diseases. Although pemphigus is generally considered to be idiopathic, certain medications, including penicillamine and captopril, may occasionally lead to a drug-related pemphigus.

PARANEOPLASTIC PEMPHIGUS

Major Immunologic Features

- Cell surface deposits of IgG and C3 occur along with occasional granular basement membrane deposits of C3 on direct immunofluorescence.
- Circulating IgG antibodies are present that bind to cell surface of skin and mucosa in a typical pemphigus pattern but in addition bind to simple, columnar, and transitional epithelia.

Paraneoplastic pemphigus is an autoimmune disease that has features reminiscent of both pemphigus vulgaris and erythema multiforme. Patients with this disease have an underlying malignancy that is usually lymphoreticular in origin. The disease is characterized by ocular and oral blisters and erosions along with generalized skin lesions that may resemble toxic epidermal necrolysis, lichen planus, bullous pemphigoid, or erythema multiforme. Paraneoplastic pemphigus is rapidly progressive leading to death in most patients who have an associated malignant neoplasm (such as lymphoma) but may resolve in patients after surgical removal of an associated benign neoplasm, such as a thymoma. Histologic features of both pemphigus vulgaris (suprabasilar acantholysis) and erythema multiforme (basal keratinocyte necrosis and lymphocyte infiltrate) may be seen. Immunofluorescence studies show the presence of circulating and tissue-bound IgG antibodies in paraneoplastic pemphigus that bind to the cell surface of stratified squamous epithelia in a pattern indistinguishable from pemphigus antibodies. These circulating IgG antibodies also recognize the cell surface of simple columnar and transitional epithelia such as colon, small bowel, liver, lung, and bladder, in contrast to pemphigus IgG antibodies, which recognize only the cell surface of stratified squamous epithelia. In addition, there may also be IgG antibodies that bind to the basement membrane. The circulating antibodies in paraneoplastic pemphigus recognize a complex of epidermal proteins that include 250- and 210-kd proteins (desmoplakin I and II),

the 230-kd bullous pemphigoid antigen and as yet uncharacterized 190- and 170-kd proteins. Although the etiology of this severe mucocutaneous disease is poorly understood, it is thought that it may result from the combination of both a cellular and humoral immune response to tumor antigens that have some overlapping reactivity to normal components of skin and other epithelia.

The syndrome of paraneoplastic pemphigus must be considered in patients with severe mucocutaneous disease reminiscent of pemphigus who present with atypical features. These patients may not have a known neoplasm at the time of presentation. If there is sufficient suspicion for the diagnosis of paraneoplastic pemphigus, then a search for an occult neoplasm is warranted. This entails extensive laboratory and diagnostic investigation because these patients may have associated tumors that are difficult to diagnose, including rare entities such as retroperitoneal sarcoma, thymoma, and Waldenström's macroglobulinemia, along with more commonly recognized tumors such as Hodgkin's lymphoma and chronic lymphocytic leukemia. Most patients are treated very aggressively with high-dose glucocorticosteroids and immunosuppressive drugs, often with poor results. The best treatment for patients who have an associated benign tumor is surgical removal of the tumor. Unfortunately, the majority of patients with paraneoplastic pemphigus have associated malignant tumors, and there are no known effective therapies. These patients present exceedingly difficult treatment problems.

REFERENCES

BULLOUS PEMPHIGOID

Ahmed AR et al: Bullous pemphigoid: Clinical and immunologic follow-up after successful therapy. *Arch Dermatol* 1977;**113:**1043.

Berk MA, Lorincz AL: The treatment of bullous pemphigoid with tetracycline and niacinamide. *Arch Dermatol* 1986;**122:**670.

Dubertret L et al: Cellular events leading to blister formation in bullous pemphigoid. *Br J Dermatol* 1980;**104:**615.

Giudice GJ et al: Cloning and primary structural analysis of the bullous pemphigoid autoantigen BP 180. *J Invest Dermatol* 1992;**99:**243.

Hadi SM et al: Clinical, histological, and immunological studies in 50 patients with bullous pemphigoid. *Dermatologica* 1988;**176:**6.

Jordon RE et al: Basement membrane zone antibodies in bullous pemphigoid. *JAMA* 1967;**200:**751.

Korman NJ: Bullous pemphigoid. *Dermatol Clin* 1993; **11:**483.

Mueller S et al: A 230 kd basic protein is the major bullous pemphigoid antigen. *J Invest Dermatol* 1989;**92:**33.

Stanley JR: A specific antigen–antibody interaction triggers the cellular pathophysiology of bullous pemphigoid. *Br J Dermatol* 1985;**113**(suppl 28):67.

Venecie PY et al: Bullous pemphigoid and malignancy:

Relationship to indirect immunofluorescence findings. *Acta Derm Venereol* (Stockh) 1984;**64:**316.

Venning VA, Wojnarowska F: Lack of predictive factors for the clinical course of bullous pemphigoid. *J Am Acad Dermatol* 1992;**26:**585.

Wintroub BU et al: Morphologic and functional evidence for release of mast cell products in bullous pemphigoid. *N Engl J Med* 1978;**298:**417.

CICATRICIAL PEMPHIGOID

Domloge-Hultsch N et al: Anti-epiligrin cicatricial pemphigoid. A subepithelial bullous disorder. *Arch Dermatol* 1994;**130:**1521.

Chan LS et al: Immune-mediated subepithelial blistering diseases of mucous membranes. *Arch Dermatol* 1993;**129:**448.

Foster CS: Cicatricial pemphigoid. *Trans Am Ophthalmol Soc* 1986;**84:**527.

Mutasim DF et al: Cicatricial pemphigoid. *Dermatol Clin* 1993;**11:**499.

HERPES GESTATIONIS

Holmes RC, Black MM: The specific dermatoses of pregnancy. *J Am Acad Dermatol* 1983;**8:**405.

Jordon RE et al: The immunopathology of herpes gestationis: Immunofluorescence studies and characterization of "HG factor." *J Clin Invest* 1976;**57**:1426.

Katz SI et al: Herpes gestationis: immunopathology and characterization of the HG factor. *J Clin Invest* 1976;**57**:1434.

Lawley TJ et al: Pruritic urticarial papules and plaques of pregnancy. *JAMA* 1979;**241**:1696.

Morrison LH et al: Herpes gestationis autoantibodies recognize a 180-kd human epidermal antigen. *J Clin Invest* 1988;**81**:2023.

Shornick JK et al: Herpes gestationis: Clinical and histologic features of twenty-eight cases. *J Am Acad Dermatol* 1983;**8**:214.

EPIDERMOLYSIS BULLOSA ACQUISITA

Briggaman RA et al: Epidermolysis bullosa acquisita of the immunopathological type (dermolytic pemphigoid). *J Invest Dermatol* 1985;**85**(suppl):79.

Crow LL et al: Clearing of epidermolysis bullosa acquisita on cyclosporine. *J Am Acad Dermatol* 1988;**19**:937.

Gammon WR et al: Epidermolysis bullosa acquisita—A pemphigoid-like disease. *J Am Acad Dermatol* 1984;**11**:820.

Gammon WR et al: Direct immunofluorescence studies of sodium chloride-separated skin in the differential diagnosis of bullous pemphigoid and epidermolysis bullosa acquisita. *J Am Acad Dermatol* 1990;**22**:664.

Woodley DT et al: Review and update of epidermolysis bullosa. *Semin Dermatol* 1988;**7**:111.

DERMATITIS HERPETIFORMIS

Fronek Z et al: Molecular analysis of HLA-DP and DQ genes associated with dermatitis herpetiformis. *J Invest Dermatol* 1991;**97**:799.

Fry L: Fine points in the management of dermatitis herpetiformis. *Semin Dermatol* 1988;**7**:206.

Hall RP: The pathogenesis of dermatitis herpetiformis: Recent advances. *J Am Acad Dermatol* 1987;**16**:1129.

Kadunce DP et al: The effect of an essential diet with and without gluten on disease activity in dermatitis herpetiformis. *J Invest Dermatol* 1991;**97**:175.

Katz SI et al: HLA-B8 and dermatitis herpetiformis in patients with IgA deposits in skin. *Arch Dermatol* 1977;**113**:155.

Mazzola G et al: Immunoglobulin and HLA-DP genes contribute to the susceptibility to juvenile dermatitis herpetiformis. *Eur J Immunogenet* 1992;**19**:129.

Otley CC et al: DNA sequence analysis and restriction fragment length polymorphism (RFLP) typing of the HLA-Dqw2 alleles associated with dermatitis herpetiformis. *J Invest Dermatol* 1991;**97**:318.

Peters MS, McEvory MT: IgA antiendomysial antibodies in dermatitis herpetiformis. *J Am Acad Dermatol* 1989;**21**:1225.

LINEAR IgA DISEASE

Haftek M et al: Immunogold localization of the 97-kd antigen of linear IgA bullous dermatosis detected with patients sera. *J Invest Dermatol* 1994;**103**:656.

Webster GF et al: Cicatrizing conjunctivitis as a predominant manifestation of linear IgA bullous dermatosis. *J Am Acad Dermatol* 1994;**30**:355.

Zone JJ et al: Identification of the cutaneous basement membrane zone antigen and isolation of antibody in linear immunoglobulin A bullous dermatosis. *J Clin Invest* 1990;**85**:812.

PEMPHIGUS

Ahmed AR et al: Pemphigus-current concepts. *Ann Intern Med* 1980;**92**:396.

Amagai M et al: Autoantibodies against a novel epithelial cadherin in pemphigus vulgaris, a disease of cell adhesion. *Cell* 1991;**67**:869.

Anhalt GJ et al: Induction of pemphigus in neonatal mice by passive transfer of IgG from patients with the disease. *N Engl J Med* 1982;**306**:1189.

Beutner EH, Jordon RE: Demonstration of skin antibodies in sera of pemphigus vulgaris patients by indirect immunofluorescent staining. *Proc Soc Exp Bio Med* 1964;**117**:505.

Bystryn JC: Adjuvant therapy of pemphigus. *Arch Dermatol* 1984;**120**:941.

Fellner MJ et al: Successful use of cyclophosphamide and prednisone for initial treatment of pemphigus vulgaris. *Arch Dermatol* 1978;**114**:889.

Judd KP, Lever WF: Correlation of antibodies in skin and serum with disease severity in pemphigus. *Arch Dermatol* 1979;**115**:428.

Korman N: Pemphigus. *J Acad Dermatol* 1988;**18**:1219.

Korman NJ et al: Demonstration of an adhering-junction molecule (plakoglobin) in the autoantigens of pemphigus foliaceus and pemphigus vulgaris. *N Engl J Med* 1989;**321**:631.

Krain LS: Pemphigus. Epidemiologic and survival characteristics of 59 patients, 1955–1973. *Arch Dermatol* 1974;**110**:862.

Lever WF: Pemphigus. *Medicine* 1953;**32**:Entire issue.

Lever WF, Schaumberg-Lever G: Immunosuppressants and prednisone in pemphigus vulgaris. Therapeutic results obtained in 63 patients between 1961 and 1975. *Arch Dermatol* 1977;**113**:1236.

Lever WF, White H: Treatment of pemphigus with corticosteroids. Results obtained in 46 patients over a period of 11 years. *Arch Dermatol* 1963;**87**:12.

PARANEOPLASTIC PEMPHIGUS

Anhalt GJ et al: Paraneoplastic pemphigus. *N Engl J Med* 1990;**323**:1729.

Camisa C et al: Paraneoplastic pemphigus: A report of three cases including one long-term survivor. *J Am Acad Dermatol* 1992;**27**:547.

Fullerton SH et al: Paraneoplastic pemphigus with autoantibody deposition in bronchial epithelium after autologous bone marrow transplantation. *JAMA* 1992;**267**:1500.

Joly P et al: Overlapping distribution of autoantibody specificities in paraneoplastic pemphigus and pemphigus vulgaris. *J Invest Dermatol* 1994;**103**:65.

Mehregan DR et al: Paraneoplastic pemphigus: A subset of patients with pemphigus and neoplasia. *J Cut Pathol* 1993;**20**:203.

Neurologic Diseases

40

Hillel S. Panitch, MD, Paul S. Fishman, MD, PhD, & Christopher T. Bever, Jr., MD

The role of immunologic mechanisms in diseases of the nervous system is the focus of increasing interest, and there have recently been major advances in the study of several of these conditions. In acute disseminated encephalomyelitis and acute inflammatory demyelinating polyneuropathy (Guillain-Barré syndrome), the host response to an infectious agent may trigger a direct autoaggressive assault on the nervous system. The pathogenesis of multiple sclerosis is less clear, but immunogenetic studies, defects of immunoregulation, and responses to immunomodulatory therapy strongly suggest that the immune system is involved in the pathogenesis of the disease. In myasthenia gravis, an antibody response directed against the acetylcholine receptor directly inhibits neuromuscular transmission. In other conditions, such as the paraneoplastic syndromes, amyotrophic lateral sclerosis, and certain chronic neuropathies, abnormal immune responses are known to occur; however, their significance is uncertain. Among the most surprising recent developments in this area has been the realization that conditions not previously suspected of being immunologically based, such as some forms of epilepsy and stroke, do in fact have autoimmune features. In degenerative conditions such as Alzheimer's disease, the role of the immune system in pathogenesis is almost entirely conjectural.

DEMYELINATING DISEASES

The commonly accepted pathologic criteria for a demyelinating disease are destruction of myelin sheaths of nerve fibers with relative sparing of neurons and axons. Lesions are frequently perivascular in location and are accompanied by mononuclear inflammatory infiltrates, suggesting that immunologic mechanisms participate in their pathogenesis.

MULTIPLE SCLEROSIS

Major Immunologic Features
- There is inflammatory demyelination in central nervous system white matter.
- There are alterations in immunoregulatory T-cell function and cytokine production.
- There are oligoclonal immunoglobulins in cerebrospinal fluid.
- It responds to immunosuppressive and immunomodulating agents.

General Considerations
Multiple sclerosis is a chronic relapsing disease in which signs and symptoms of central nervous system involvement are separated both in time and in location. Is is by far the most common and clinically important of the demyelinating diseases. Epidemiologic studies have uncovered important clues about multiple sclerosis, but the cause remains unknown. In high-risk areas the prevalence is 50–100 per 100,000 population, whereas in low-risk areas, such as Africa and Japan, the rate is less than 5 per 100,000. Individuals who migrate from high-risk to low-risk areas, or vice versa, after age 15 carry with them their native risk of acquiring the disease. The peak onset is at age 30, with few cases before age 15 or after age 55, suggesting that some critical event in determining the risk of acquiring multiple sclerosis occurs in adolescence. The risk of disease in a first-degree relative is 10–50 times higher than the risk in the general population, and the concordance rate in identical twins is approximately 30%, indicating a strong genetic component. Localized outbreaks of multiple sclerosis have been described, however, most notably in the Faroe Islands, where the temporal clustering of cases suggests a transmissible cause. Studies of histocompatibility antigens have shown significant associations with HLA-DR2 and HLA-DQw1, which may be closely linked to a multiple sclerosis susceptibility gene.

Viruses have been implicated as possible etiologic agents by the presence of specific antibodies in spinal fluid, identification of viral DNA or RNA in brain tissue or mononuclear cells, and, in some cases, actual viral isolation. None of these observations has been consistently confirmed. It is more likely that certain epitopes of viral proteins resemble myelin antigens sufficiently to initiate an autoimmune response, a process known as molecular mimicry.

Numerous immunoregulatory defects have been identified, perhaps the best documented being abnormal suppressor T-cell function in acute attacks and in the chronic progressive phase. Although decreases in the CD8 T-cell subset are not consistently found, the defect may reside in a loss of CD4 suppressor/inducer cells or in a relative deficiency of T_H2 cells that secrete suppressive cytokines such as IL-4 and IL-10. In addition, there are excessive numbers of activated T cells of the T_H1 phenotype, that secrete proinflammatory cytokines, such as interferon gamma and IL-2, in the blood and cerebrospinal fluid. Increased levels of adhesion molecules such as soluble intercellular adhesion molecule-1 (ICAM-1) are also found in active disease. Monocytes and macrophages play important roles in multiple sclerosis as well, related in part to their sensitivity to interferon gamma, which induces the class II major histocompatibility complex (MHC) surface molecules essential for antigen presentation to T cells (Fig 40–1). Activated macrophages are prevalent in multiple sclerosis plaques, where they release proteinases and cytokines leading to demyelination (see Fig 40–1). The importance of interferon gamma as an immune activator was emphasized by a clinical trial in which patients treated with interferon gamma developed acute exacerbations. Minor viral infections often precipitate attacks; this effect may be mediated by interferon gamma or other cytokines. Within the central nervous system, interferon gamma induces class II antigens on astrocytes and microglia, enabling them to present antigens to T cells and to propagate the disease process. Although the specific antigen in question is unknown, it is likely to be a structural component of myelin such as myelin basic protein, proteolipid protein, or myelin oligodendrocyte glycoprotein. The autoimmune theory of multiple sclerosis is strengthened by its response to immunosuppressive drugs such as corticosteroids. Interferons alpha and beta, which inhibit the synthesis of interferon gamma and reverse some of its immunostimulatory effects, also seem to be effective in preventing exacerbations.

Pathology

The lesions of multiple sclerosis are confined to the central nervous system and primarily involve the white matter of the cerebrum, cerebellum, brain stem, and spinal cord. In the early stages they consist of perivascular infiltrates of T lymphocytes and macrophages. In older lesions, macrophage-mediated demyelination is further advanced and large numbers of

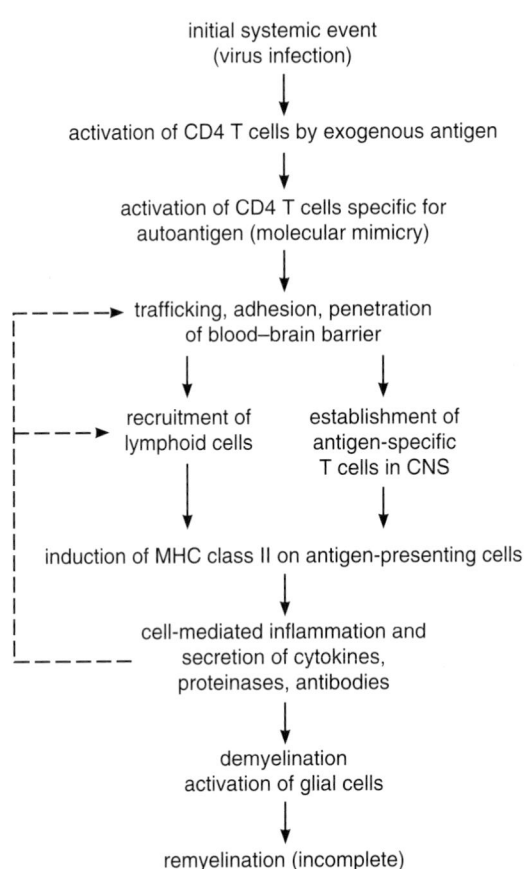

Figure 40–1. Postulated mechanism of disease induction and progression in multiple sclerosis. Solid lines and arrows indicate inflammatory-demyelinating pathways. Dashed lines and arrows indicate suppressive-regulatory pathways. Activated T cells enter the central nervous system and secrete interferon gamma and other proinflammatory cytokines which induce MHC class II molecules on macrophages, microglia, and perhaps other antigen-presenting cells. Activated macrophages, T cells, and B cells secrete cytokines, proteinases, and antibodies that may all play roles in an autoimmune attack on myelin antigens. At the same time, a regulatory process involving suppressor T cells and regulatory cytokines is initiated, which eventually slows or terminates the disease process.

reactive astrocytes are seen. These lesions, or plaques, appear to be of different ages and correlate with the appearance of clinical signs and symptoms at different times during the illness. Plasma cells within the plaques secrete oligoclonal IgG into the extracellular and cerebrospinal fluid. Activation of glial cells may, in some cases, lead to abortive attempts at remyelination. The similarities between the lesions of multiple sclerosis and the inflammatory demyelination seen in experimental allergic encephalomyelitis (particularly the relapsing form) suggest that cellular immune mechanisms are involved in the pathogenesis of multiple sclerosis.

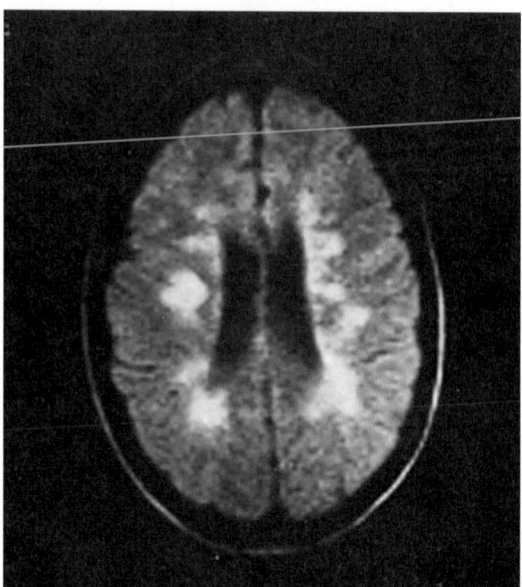

Figure 40–2. Magnetic resonance image of the brain of a multiple sclerosis patient, showing lesions (irregular white areas) in the white matter surrounding the lateral ventricles.

CSF electrophoresis

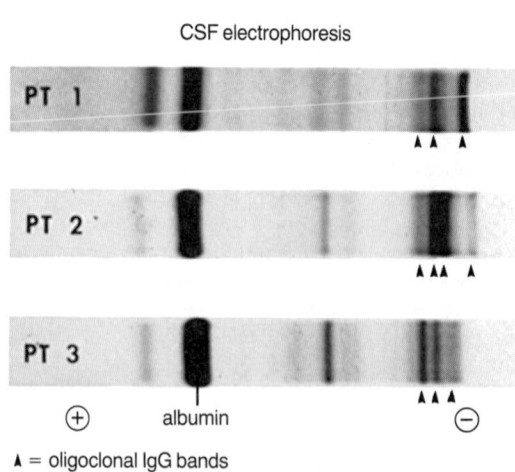

⏶ = oligoclonal IgG bands

Figure 40–3. Oligoclonal bands in cerebrospinal fluid (CSF) specimen from a patient with subacute sclerosing parencephalitis. Cerebrospinal fluid electrophoresis pattern in agarose gel demonstrates the phenomenon of oligoclonal banding. In the gamma region (to the right), several dark, distinct bands are noted for all these patients. Similar abnormalities are noted in CSF specimens from multiple sclerosis patients.

Clinical Features

Because multiple sclerosis plaques tend to involve many areas of the central nervous system, the symptoms and signs are extremely varied. The most common manifestations are motor weakness, paresthesias, impairment of visual acuity, and diplopia. Ataxia, urinary bladder dysfunction, impotence, spasticity, and mild to moderate cognitive impairment are also common. Symptoms may occur rapidly as acute exacerbations that develop over a few days and persist for days to weeks with gradual recovery, or more slowly in the chronic progressive form of the disease. Exacerbations occur at varying intervals and tend to subside with less complete recovery of function and increasing disability as the disease progresses. Visual, auditory, and somatosensory evoked potentials are often abnormal and assist in diagnosis. The most important recent diagnostic advance, however, has been the introduction of magnetic resonance imaging (MRI), which provides striking visualization of plaques in the cerebral white matter (Fig 40–2).

Immunologic Diagnosis

Despite the many immunologic abnormalities already described, there is no single diagnostic test for multiple sclerosis. Oligoclonal IgG bands are detectable in cerebrospinal fluid by electrophoresis or isoelectric focusing in more than 90% of patients (Fig 40–3). An elevated IgG index (ratio of cerebrospinal fluid to serum IgG corrected for albumin concentration in each compartment) indicates local IgG synthesis, but this can be found in other inflammatory dis-

eases of the nervous system. Myelin basic protein may be detected by radioimmunoassay in the cerebrospinal fluid, but it is largely a reflection of myelin damage and can be seen in other conditions such as head trauma and stroke. Other immunologic findings such as HLA haplotypes, abnormal CD4/CD8 T-cell ratios, reduced suppressor cell activity, activated T cells, and increased levels of tumor necrosis factor alpha or other cytokines in blood and cerebrospinal fluid are not specific or consistent enough to be useful in diagnosis.

Differential Diagnosis

Acute episodes of multiple sclerosis must be differentiated from structural lesions of the central nervous system such as brain and spinal cord tumors or from vascular malformations. A host of other medical conditions may produce signs, symptoms, spinal fluid findings, and, in some cases, MRIs that mimic those of multiple sclerosis, and they must be excluded by appropriate testing. These diseases include neurosyphilis, sarcoidosis, systemic lupus erythematosus, Sjögren's syndrome, vitamin B_{12} deficiency, and Lyme disease. Spinal and cerebellar disorders such as Friedreich's ataxia and olivopontocerebellar degeneration can mimic multiple sclerosis but tend to be familial, chronically progressive, and associated with normal spinal fluid. Finally, tropical spastic paraparesis or HTLV-I–associated myelopathy should be considered in patients with slowly progressive paraparesis. The diagnosis of HTLV-I–associated myelopathy may be made if antibody to HTLV-I is present.

Treatment

High doses of intravenous methylprednisolone given for 5–7 days have become the mainstay of therapy for severe acute exacerbations and may shorten their duration, particularly when optic neuritis is present; however, the long-term benefits of such therapy are uncertain. For less severe attacks, oral prednisone may be used, although it should not be given in the presence of acute optic neuritis, as it may precipitate subsequent relapses. Intensive immunosuppression with cyclophosphamide was initially reported to arrest progression in some patients, but other studies have shown no benefit, and the use of this drug in multiple sclerosis remains controversial. Other suppressive agents, in particular methotrexate and azathioprine, are sometimes used as well. A study of cyclosporine in patients with chronic progressive disease showed a statistically significant effect on outcome, but was associated with unacceptable side effects of hypertension and nephrotoxicity.

The most striking advance in the therapy of multiple sclerosis in over 20 years occurred in 1993, with the publication of a multicenter, double-blind, placebo-controlled study showing that large doses of recombinant interferon beta-1b, given by subcutaneous injection every other day, significantly reduced exacerbation rates and the appearance of new or enlarging lesions on MRI scans in patients with relapsing-remitting disease. In a follow-up report, the effect persisted for up to 5 years, but in about one third of patients neutralizing antibodies to interferon beta-1b developed and were associated with some loss of therapeutic efficacy. Since its approval by the Food and Drug Administration, over 40,000 multiple sclerosis patients have been treated with interferon beta-1b, and it is now an established form of therapy in clinical practice. In an article published in 1996, a slightly different molecule, recombinant interferon beta-1a, was also shown to be safe and effective in a large well-controlled trial in patients with early relapsing-remitting multiple sclerosis. In addition to reducing the relapse rate and appearance of new lesions on MRI scans, interferon beta-1a had a modest, but significant, effect on slowing progression of disability, perhaps conferring a therapeutic advantage over interferon beta-1b. Copolymer-1, a synthetic polypeptide that inhibits experimental allergic encephalomyelitis in animals, was highly effective in preventing exacerbations of multiple sclerosis in a pilot study, and these results were recently confirmed in a larger multicenter, randomized, placebo-controlled trial. Copolymer-1 was as effective as either of the interferon beta products in reducing relapse rates and also had a significant effect on disease progression. As with interferon beta-1a, its place in clinical practice remains to be established.

The status of other immunomodulators in multiple sclerosis therapy is still experimental. Targeted immunotherapy with monoclonal antibodies directed against CD4 T cells seemed promising on the basis of preclinical studies, but recent controlled trials in patients have been disappointing. Other experimental approaches include induction of oral tolerance to myelin antigens, monoclonal antibodies to adhesion molecules, and vaccines made from antigen-specific T cells or from T-cell receptor peptides specific for immunodominant epitopes of myelin antigens. These have all been effective in preventing or suppressing experimental allergic encephalomyelitis; however, it remains to be seen which, if any, of these modalities will survive testing in rigorously controlled clinical trials in multiple sclerosis.

Complications & Prognosis

The prognosis of multiple sclerosis is difficult to predict because of its extremely variable nature. Benign cases in which patients function normally or with little neurologic deficit are not uncommon, while fulminant cases of acute multiple sclerosis can result in severe disability or death within a few years. Most patients fall between these extremes and continue to have exacerbations and remissions, or chronic progression, for many years. Despite substantial evidence for defective immunoregulation, patients with multiple sclerosis do not have increased susceptibility to other autoimmune disorders, infections, or neoplasms.

ACUTE DISSEMINATED ENCEPHALOMYELITIS

Major Immunologic Features

- It follows infectious diseases or immunizations.
- Inflammatory demyelination occurs in central nervous system white matter.
- There is cellular immunity to myelin basic protein and other myelin antigens.

General Considerations

Although acute disseminated encephalomyelitis is uncommon, it is important because of the widespread practice of vaccination for prevention of infectious diseases and its potential for leaving patients severely disabled. The onset of clinical illness occurs several days to weeks following vaccination; in the case of natural viral infections, such as measles, rubella, varicella, mumps, and influenza, it can occur concomitantly with the illness (parainfectious) or after the acute phase (postinfectious). Except for measles, in which the incidence of acute disseminated encephalomyelitis is well defined and constant at 1:1000, reliable figures are not available; however, they are all much lower than the prevalence following measles. The argument favoring an immunologic pathogenesis of this disorder is based on its similarity to experimental allergic encephalomyelitis, in which animals are immunized with extracts of brain tissue or specific myelin proteins, resulting in an autoimmune response to myelin antigens mediated by T lymphocytes.

Pathology

Acute disseminated encephalomyelitis is marked by perivascular mononuclear cell infiltrates in which matter throughout the brain and spinal cord; polymorphonuclear leukocytes and microhemorrhages are seen in the most acute form of the disease. As the lesions age, they become sclerotic, with proliferation of astrocytes and formation of glial scars. The lesions are pathologically all of the same age, reflecting the monophasic nature of the illness.

Clinical Features

Systemic symptoms of fever, malaise, headache, myalgia, nausea, and vomiting generally precede neurologic symptoms by 24–48 hours. Neurologic symptoms and signs develop rapidly thereafter and include pain, paresthesias, motor weakness, spasticity, incoordination, dysarthria, dysphagia, and respiratory distress. Seizures may occur in severe cases and in the acute hemorrhagic form, and widespread brain lesions can lead to stupor and coma. A more restricted form of the same pathologic process may be confined to the spinal cord as acute transverse myelitis.

Immunologic Diagnosis

Cellular immunity to myelin basic protein can sometimes be demonstrated in acute disseminated encephalomyelitis by measuring the activation in vitro of peripheral blood or spinal fluid lymphocytes during the acute phase of the illness. Cerebrospinal fluid is usually abnormal, with moderate pleocytosis, elevated levels of IgG, and oligoclonal IgG bands on electrophoresis, similar to those found in multiple sclerosis.

Differential Diagnosis

Acute multiple sclerosis can be difficult to distinguish from acute disseminated encephalomyelitis. Fever and a preceding viral illness or vaccination favor the latter diagnosis. The vasculitis of systemic lupus erythematosus can affect the central nervous system, but neurologic symptoms generally accompany the systemic illness and tend to be more focal than in acute disseminated encephalomyelitis. Primary infections of the nervous system with herpes simplex virus or the arboviruses tend to involve gray as well as white matter, and they produce neuronal dysfunction such as seizures, stupor, and coma early in the illness. Direct isolation of viruses from cerebrospinal fluid and increasing serum antibody titers are helpful in differentiating viral encephalitides from acute disseminated encephalomyelitis. The subacute encephalitis of acquired immunodeficiency syndrome (AIDS) develops more slowly and is not usually associated with focal neurologic deficits. Toxoplasmosis of the central nervous system may be distinguished serologically. Magnetic resonance imaging may be useful in diagnosis and in distinguishing this conditions from multiple sclerosis; however, a diagnostic

brain biopsy is sometimes necessary to exclude a treatable central nervous system infection.

Treatment

Although the course is unpredictable, high doses of corticosteroids given intravenously may be of value in treatment. The successful prevention of experimental allergic encephalomyelitis with immunosuppressive and immunomodulating agents offers hope that similar treatment may inhibit the attack of sensitized T lymphocytes on the nervous system in acute disseminated encephalomyelitis. A few cases have been treated successfully with plasmapheresis, suggesting that antibodies or other soluble factors may be involved.

Complications & Prognosis

The mortality rate varies but may be as high as 25%, with the highest rates reported in association with measles. Neurologic sequelae persist in 25–40% of survivors. The occasional occurrence of relapses blurs the distinction between this condition and multiple sclerosis in about 5% of cases.

ACUTE INFLAMMATORY DEMYELINATING POLYNEUROPATHY (Guillain-Barré Syndrome)

Major Immunologic Features

- It commonly follows acute viral infections or enteric infection with *Campylobacter jejuni*.
- There is inflammatory demyelination of peripheral nerves.
- There is cellular and humoral immunity to peripheral nerve antigens.

General Considerations

Acute inflammatory demyelinating polyneuropathy, like acute disseminated encephalomyelitis, frequently follows an infectious illness. Upper respiratory infections, exanthems, vaccinations, and viral illnesses such as infectious mononucleosis and hepatitis often precede acute inflammatory demyelinating polyneuropathy by 1–3 weeks. Serological evidence of infection with the enteric bacterium *C jejuni* occurs in 15–45% of patients. Increasing numbers of cases have also been reported in patients with AIDS. The disease affects all age groups and is not related to sex, race, or genetic background. The annual incidence is approximately 2 per 100,000.

Pathology

Acute inflammatory demyelinating polyneuropathy is a multifocal demyelinating disease of the peripheral nervous system characterized by perivascular mononuclear cell infiltrates with segmental demyelination in the areas of inflammation. In areas of most severe involvement, axonal destruction and wallerian degeneration occur. In cases associated with *C jejuni*, especially those reported recently from northern China, the lesions are more suggestive of a primary immune attack on motor and sensory axons rather than on myelin.

Clinical Features

The onset is characterized by rapidly progressive weakness first of the lower extremities, then of the upper extremities, and finally of the facial, pharyngeal, and respiratory musculature. Weakness and paralysis are frequently preceded by paresthesias and numbness of the limbs, but objective sensory loss is mild and transient. The tendon reflexes are decreased or lost early in the illness, and nerve conduction in affected limbs in moderately to markedly slowed. Cerebrospinal fluid protein is increased in all cases but usually not during the first few days of the illness. The cerebrospinal fluid cell count is normal, except when the disease occurs in association with AIDS. The usual clinical course is one of rapid evolution of symptoms over 3 days to 3 weeks with improvement and return to normal function over 6–9 months. Other patterns, however, such as a more gradual onset, a prolonged period of complete paralysis, recovery with severe residual deficits, and a relapsing course have also been described.

Immunologic Diagnosis

In patients tested early in the course of their illness, high titers of complement-fixing antimyelin antibody of the IgM class have been detected. Clearance of this antibody from the serum often correlates with clinical improvement. Other antinerve and antimyelin antibodies have also been found, but it is not yet certain whether these are pathogenic or reflect reactions secondary to nerve tissue destruction. IgM and IgG antibodies to the membrane glycolipids GM1 and GD1b are often found in patients with evidence of *Campylobacter* infection, suggesting that molecular mimicry between bacterial and peripheral nerve antigens may underlie the pathogenesis of the disease in such patients. Spontaneously transformed circulating lymphocytes have been described, as well as lymphocytes that respond to peripheral-nerve myelin proteins by proliferation or cytokine production. However, most evidence now favors a primary role for humoral immune responses in the pathogenesis of the disease.

Differential Diagnosis

Neuropathies associated with porphyria or heavy-metal poisoning can be excluded by appropriate blood or urine tests. Acute transverse myelitis or early spinal cord compression may resemble acute inflammatory demyelinating polyneuropathy, but increased reflexes and spasticity occur days to weeks after initial flaccidity, usually with bowel and bladder involvement. Vasculitides such as polyarteritis nodosa can produce peripheral neuropathies, but these tend to present with asymmetric multifocal involvement. Acute myasthenia gravis may resemble acute inflammatory demyelinating polyneuropathy but is more likely to be associated with oculomotor weakness and generally responds to anticholinesterase drugs. Botulism and tick paralysis, uncommon diseases causing subacute generalized weakness through the effect of their associated toxins on the neuromuscular junction, can usually be distinguished by the clinical history and by neurophysiologic testing.

Treatment

Plasmapheresis, especially if begun as early as possible, is effective in shortening the course of the illness (Fig 40–4). Therapy with high doses of intravenous immunoglobulin is as effective as plasmapheresis and is now generally accepted as an alternative treatment, although its mechanism of action is very poorly understood. Intensive supportive care, including respiratory assistance, must be given as required. Corticosteroids tend to prolong the duration of illness and are therefore contraindicated, except in some cases of recurrent polyneuropathy.

Complications & Prognosis

Modern methods for assisting and maintaining respiration have resulted in a marked decrease in the mortality rate of acute inflammatory demyelinating polyneuropathy, which currently ranges from 1 to 5%. However, residual neurologic deficits, caused by irreversible axonal disruption and wallerian degeneration, occur in as many as 50% of patients. Cases associated with *C jejuni* infection and axonal degeneration tend to be more severe than others and have a higher mortality rate. Respiratory muscle and pharyngeal weakness favor the development of infections, which may be life-threatening, and associated autonomic neuropathy may produce vasomotor instability and cardiac arrhythmias, resulting in sudden death despite adequate respiratory care.

CHRONIC DEMYELINATING POLYNEUROPATHIES

These are uncommon disorders that resemble acute inflammatory demyelinating polyneuropathy pathologically and physiologically but follow a more indolent and frequently relapsing course. Clinical manifestations include variable degrees of extremity weakness and sensory symptoms. Nerve conduction studies show profound slowing with conduction block. Cerebrospinal fluid protein is characteristically increased; deposits of immunoglobulin may be found in peripheral nerves; and complement-fixing antibody to myelin may be detected, suggesting an immune system-mediated process. Patients frequently respond to plasma exchange, intravenous immunoglobulin, long-term corticosteroid treatment (particularly in the

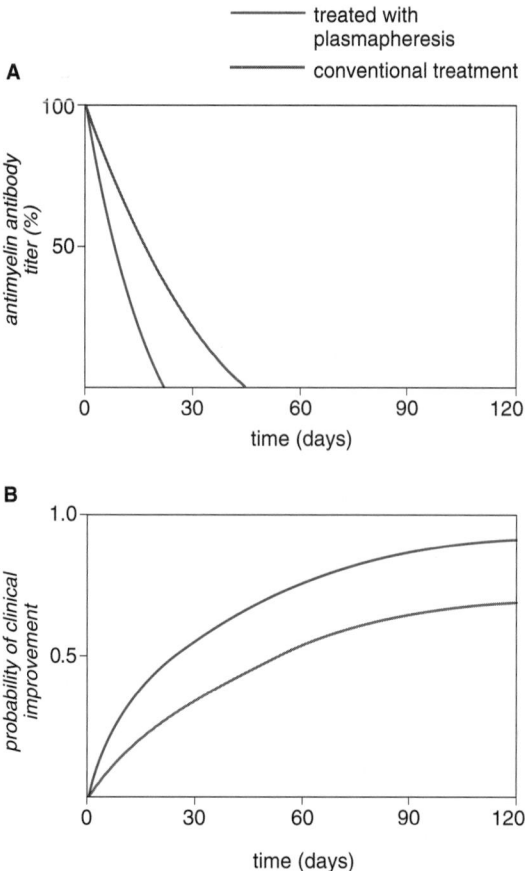

Figure 40–4. ***A:*** Effect of plasmapheresis on antimyelin antibody, and ***B:*** clinical recovery in acute inflammatory demyelinating polyneuropathy (AIDP). Titers decline faster and recovery is more rapid and more nearly complete with plasma exchange, especially when performed during the first week of illness. (Panel A adapted from data provided by CL Koski; panel B adapted from Guillain-Barré Syndrome Study Group Clinical Trial, *Neurology* 1985;**35**:1096.)

relapsing type), or treatment with other immunosuppressive drugs.

Patients with multiple myeloma, Waldenström's macroglobulinemia, and primary systemic amyloidosis sometimes develop peripheral neuropathies in which the pathologic pattern is primarily axonal degeneration with secondary demyelination. The pathogenesis of those conditions has been largely unexplored. In patients with benign monoclonal gammopathy and peripheral neuropathy, however, the circulating paraproteins, usually of the IgM isotype, are monoclonal antibodies directed against the myelin-associated glycoprotein or other glycoprotein and glycolipid components of peripheral nerves. Evidence that these antibodies actually initiate demyelination is inconclusive. Nevertheless, plasma exchange and immunosuppression have produced remissions with reversal of conduction block and disappearance of the paraprotein from the serum in some cases. The role of immune cells has not been determined, although mononuclear cell infiltrates are often present in demyelinated areas of peripheral nerve, and secretion of

the IgM paraprotein is under T-cell control. Another group of neurologic disorders, including a multifocal motor neuropathy with conduction block, has recently been described in association with high titers of circulating antibody to GM_1 ganglioside. They respond to treatment with various combinations of plasma exchange, intravenous immunoglobulin, and cyclophosphamide. Not only are these disorders immunologically interesting in their own right, they also may serve as models for other more common immune-mediated diseases of the peripheral and central nervous systems.

DISORDERS OF NEUROMUSCULAR TRANSMISSION

Myasthenia gravis and the myasthenic (Lambert-Eaton) syndrome are the neurologic diseases for which an autoimmune pathogenesis is best established.

MYASTHENIA GRAVIS

Major Immunologic Features
- It is commonly associated with thymic hyperplasia or thymoma.
- Pathogenic autoantibodies are directed against the acetylcholine receptor.
- It is often associated with other autoantibodies and autoimmune diseases.

General Considerations
Myasthenia gravis is a disease of unknown cause in which there is muscle weakness due to a disorder of neuromuscular transmission. The frequent occurrence of myasthenia gravis with thymomas, thymic hyperplasia, autoantibodies, and other autoimmune diseases strongly suggests that the immune system is involved in its pathogenesis. Antiacetylcholine receptor antibody, which binds at the postsynaptic membrane of the neuromuscular junction, interrupts transmission by increasing endocytosis of acetylcholine receptors and forms immune complexes that bind complement, causing further destruction of the postsynaptic membrane (Fig 40–5). The prevalence of myasthenia gravis is 2–10 per 100,000. It occurs at all ages, but different subgroups are recognized. In patients with thymoma, in whom the onset is usually after age 40, there is no sex or HLA antigen association; in patients without thymoma and with onset before age 40, there is a female preponderance and association with HLA-A1, -B8, and -DR3; in patients without thymoma and with onset after age 40, there is a male preponderance and association with HLA-A3, -B7, and -DR2.

Pathology
Scattered aggregates of lymphocytes are observed in the muscles. At the neuromuscular junction there is widening of the synaptic cleft and a marked abnormality of the postsynaptic membrane, with sparse, shallow postsynaptic folds. Eighty percent of patients have hyperplasia of lymphoid follicles with active germinal centers in the medulla of the thymus, whereas 10% have a thymoma (a locally invasive thymic neoplasm), and in the remaining 10% the thymus appears normal.

Clinical Features
Skeletal muscles are normal at rest but become increasingly weak with repetitive use. Weakness is often first noted in the extraocular muscles as diplopia or ptosis, whereas pharyngeal and facial weakness results in dysphagia and dysarthria. Skeletal muscle weakness is more often proximal than distal and causes difficulty in climbing stairs, rising from chairs, combing the hair, or even holding up the head. When respiratory muscles are weak, ventilatory assistance is sometimes necessary. Exacerbations can occur spontaneously but are often related to intercurrent infections, surgery, or emotional stress and may result in

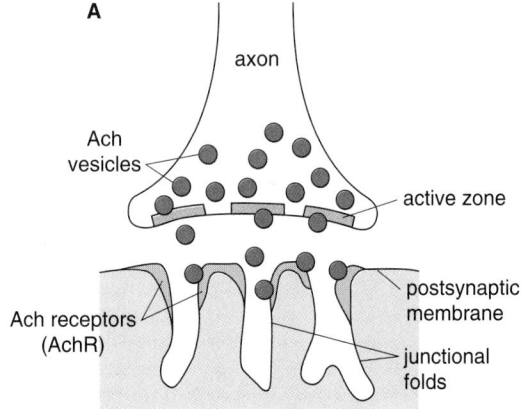

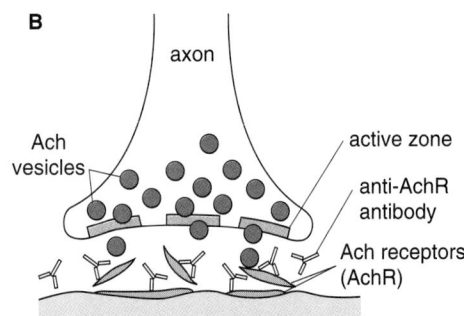

Figure 40–5. *A:* Normal, and *B:* myasthenic neuromuscular junctions. At the normal junction, acetylcholine (Ach) is released from the nerve terminal and taken up by receptors on the complex folded postsynaptic membrane. In myasthenia gravis, antiacetylcholine receptor (AchR) antibodies and immune complexes induce complement-mediated destruction of the membrane, with loss of normal folds and receptor sites.

myasthenic crisis with severe bulbar and respiratory weakness. Except for muscle weakness and depressed reflexes, the neurologic examination is normal. Intravenous injection of edrophonium, a short-acting anticholinesterase, is useful in diagnosis, as it produces dramatic transient improvement of weakness by prolonging the availability of acetylcholine at the postsynaptic receptor.

Immunologic Diagnosis
Antiacetylcholine receptor antibodies are found in 90% of myasthenia gravis patients and occasionally in thymoma patients without muscle weakness, but they may be absent in patients with purely ocular myasthenia. As they are found in no other neuromuscular disease, their presence in the appropriate clinical setting is diagnostic. Antistriated muscle antibodies are often detected in patients with an associated thymoma, but their pathogenic significance is unknown.

Differential Diagnosis

Myasthenia gravis can be differentiated from other myopathies on the basis of its response to anticholinesterase drugs. The various forms of periodic paralysis do not show the oculomotor involvement of myasthenia. The myasthenic (Lambert-Eaton) syndrome usually associated with small-cell carcinoma of the lung can be differentiated by electrodiagnostic studies and by lack of response to anticholinesterase agents. Botulism and tick paralysis can be diagnosed on the basis of the clinical history and electrophysiologic testing.

Treatment

Anticholinesterase drugs such as pyridostigmine and neostigmine were, for many years, the mainstays of long-term therapy. Thymectomy is beneficial in the majority of cases, and all patients with myasthenia gravis except those with nondisabling ocular myasthenia should be considered for thymectomy. Dramatic improvement also occurs in severely ill patients treated with plasmapheresis, which removes antiacetylcholine receptor antibodies from the circulation. Plasmapheresis is most effective when combined with corticosteroids and other immunosuppressive drugs to diminish the rapid increase in antireceptor antibody that follows plasma exchange. As in the autoimmune neuropathies, intravenous immunoglobulin is an effective, and less expensive, alternative to plasmapheresis. Chronic treatment with low-dose azathioprine is frequently used for maintenance therapy.

Complications & Prognosis

The course of myasthenia gravis prior to the availability of modern intensive respiratory care was one of remission in 25% of cases and chronic persistent weakness in 75% of patients, with a 20–30% mortality rate. Improvement or complete remission within 5 years can now be expected in up to 90% of patients undergoing thymectomy supplemented by the other treatment modalities. Potential hazards for the myasthenic patient include myasthenic crisis with respiratory impairment, cholinergic crisis with weakness caused by overdosage of anticholinesterase drugs, pulmonary infections resulting from respiratory insufficiency and pharyngeal weakness, and lowered resistance to invading organisms as a result of immunosuppressive therapy.

MYASTHENIC SYNDROME

This condition, also known as Lambert-Eaton syndrome, superficially resembles myasthenia gravis, but commonly spares ocular and bulbar muscles, affects proximal limb muscles, and is characterized by increasing strength with repeated muscle contraction. This phenomenon is reflected electrophysiologically in increased amplitude of motor unit action potentials evoked by rapid repetitive nerve stimulation. Approximately 50% of cases occur as a remote effect of small-cell carcinoma of the lung. Patients have circulating IgG antibodies to presynaptic voltage-sensitive calcium channels, located in portions of the membrane known as active zones, that are important in releasing acetylcholine at nerve terminals. The antibodies are thought to be directed at tumor antigens and to cross-react with determinants on calcium channels. The disease can be experimentally transmitted to mice with serum IgG from affected patients, and sometimes responds to treatment with plasmapheresis and immunosuppressive drugs. Symptoms respond poorly to cholinesterase inhibitors but do respond to guanidine hydrochloride, which increases intracellular calcium, and to aminopyridines, which prolong the duration of presynaptic action potentials.

IMMUNOLOGIC ABNORMALITIES IN OTHER NEUROLOGIC DISEASES

Immunologic findings have been described in several neurodegenerative diseases. Autoimmune mechanisms have been most clearly implicated in a group of nervous system disorders associated with systemic cancer, known as paraneoplastic syndromes. The significance of immunologic abnormalities in amyotrophic lateral sclerosis and Alzheimer's disease remains speculative. Recently, other neurologic conditions have been linked to antibodies directed against neurotransmitter receptors and synthetic enzymes. Autoantibodies have also been implicated in the pathogenesis of some cases of stroke.

PARANEOPLASTIC CEREBELLAR DEGENERATION

This is the best described syndrome of neural degeneration occurring as an indirect effect of systemic cancer. Patients develop gait instability or ataxia and gross incoordination of their arms. If untreated, the condition can progress to disabling incoordination and unintelligible speech in a few months. Although such degeneration has been described in patients with a variety of cancers, it is strongly associated with carcinomas of the lung and ovary. In patients who present with nervous system disease, an occult tumor may be discovered only after prolonged investigation. Two features dominate the pathology of this condition: extensive loss of Purkinje cells (the major output neuron of the cerebellum) and proliferation of microglial cells. A patchy lymphocytic infiltrate may also be seen. Many patients have serum antibodies that bind to human cerebellum tissue slices. These antibodies are usually polyclonal IgG. Autoantibodies against three different nervous system antigens have been identified. Each is associated with a particular type of malignancy and a distinguishable clinical syndrome. Patients with antibodies against the cytoplasmic antigen termed Yo usually are women with ovarian or breast cancer and have the typical subacute cerebellar degeneration just described. Yo is highly expressed by both normal cerebellar neurons and ovarian cancer cells. An antinuclear antigen called Hu is strongly associated with small-cell carcinoma of the lung. Patients with this antibody frequently develop neuropathy and encephalopathy as well as cerebellar ataxia. Another neuronal nuclear antigen, called Ri, has been found in a few women with breast cancer together with an unusual syndrome of ataxia, myoclonus, and opsoclonus (irregular jerking eye movements). Paraneoplastic cerebellar degeneration without specific antineuronal antibodies is sometimes associated with lymphoma. In antibody-mediated paraneoplastic disease, antibodies raised as a natural immune defense against tumor cells cross-react with a normal tissue component. This early immune response to cancer cells may account for the association of paraneoplastic syndromes with otherwise occult malignancies. The presence of these antibodies in the serum of a patient with one of these clinical syndromes should raise strong suspicion of an occult cancer. The antibodies are usually detectable in the cerebrospinal fluid as well as the serum, and they seem to be produced by clones of lymphocytes residing within the central nervous system. Intrathecal production of the pathogenic antibody may explain the poor remission rate of this condition with either treatment of the malignancy or systemic immunosuppression.

LIMBIC ENCEPHALITIS

Limbic encephalitis is an unusual syndrome characterized by impairment of short-term memory and behavioral disturbances, as well as psychiatric symptoms of delusions and hallucinations. The syndrome usually develops over days to weeks, and may occur either as a paraneoplastic syndrome or without any underlying cause. When associated with small-cell carcinoma of the lung, it is usually part of the more generalized anti-Hu antibody syndrome along with sensorimotor neuropathy. Imaging studies frequently show nonspecific evidence of inflammation such as areas of increased signal or contrast enhancement on MRI scans of the brain. Inflammatory changes in the cerebrospinal fluid are also commonly found. Although a rare syndrome, there have been several reports of recovery after oncologic and immunosuppressive treatment.

AMYOTROPHIC LATERAL SCLEROSIS

Amyotrophic lateral sclerosis causes progressive weakness, atrophy, and fasciculations due to degener-

ation of motor neurons of the spinal cord. Most patients also show degeneration of corticospinal upper motor neurons, resulting in spasticity, hyperreflexia, and poor control of voluntary movement. The disease progresses inexorably to death, usually within 3–5 years. Survival is poorest in patients who have wasting and weakness of the muscles of the pharynx, chest, and diaphragm, leading to aspiration pneumonia and respiratory failure. Commonly known as Lou Gehrig's disease, amyotrophic lateral sclerosis typically affects males after age 40. Although pathologic examination reveals neuronal loss and glial proliferation without inflammatory cells, an immunologic basis has been proposed for a subgroup of patients with a monoclonal IgM paraproteinemia. Recent work has identified the possible target antigens as glycolipids known as gangliosides, which are normal neural membrane components. Autoantibodies against other neuronal membrane and structural components such as neurofilaments have also been detected. Immunoglobulins have been localized to motor neurons in tissue from patients with amyotrophic lateral sclerosis, but the significance of this observation is unclear since other plasma proteins can enter motor neurons by similar nonspecific mechanisms. Antibodies directed against calcium channels, similar to those found in the Lambert-Eaton myasthenic syndrome, have also been detected in serum from amyotrophic lateral sclerosis patients and appear to be cytotoxic. Several immunosuppressive agents have been tested in patients with amyotrophic lateral sclerosis without altering the course of the disease. Another condition with very similar clinical manifestations does appear to have an autoimmune basis. Multifocal motor neuropathy with conduction block causes progressive weakness, muscle wasting, and motor fasciculations without sensory loss, and usually requires electrophysiologic studies to distinguish it from amyotrophic lateral sclerosis. Although autoantibodies are variably present, many patients respond to immunosuppressive therapy.

ALZHEIMER'S DISEASE

Alzheimer's disease was originally described as a presenile dementia. It is now clear that the same pathology occurs in patients older than 65 years and that it is the commonest cause of senile dementia. Memory and abstract reasoning are affected early in the course of the disease, which eventually renders patients unable to care for themselves and makes Alzheimer's disease the single largest reason for nursing-home care. The disease is defined by its pathologic changes. Large neurons, particularly in the cortex and hippocampus, develop cytoplasmic filamentous abnormalities called "neurofibrillary tangles." Clusters of degenerating nerve terminals mixed with deposits of an amyloid-type protein form senile plaques, the other pathologic hallmark of Alzheimer's disease. The presence of amyloid protein in Alzheimer's disease was previously thought to suggest an immune-mediated process, since immunoglobulins can form amyloid deposits. The amyloid of Alzheimer's disease has now been characterized and is composed primarily of an abnormal cleavage product of a transmembrane protein, the A4 fragment of β amyloid. Although this fragment may be derived from the brain, it is found in the circulation as well. The role of the immune system in the pathogenesis of Alzheimer's disease is currently unclear. Although inflammation is usually not seen, activation of macrophage-equivalent microglial cells has been described. Immunogenic antigens, as well as complement components, have been detected in or near senile plaques. Some investigators believe that amyloid deposition stimulates production of cytokines, which may potentiate the neurotoxicity of the amyloid protein. Use of nonsteroidal anti-inflammatory drugs has been associated with a reduced risk of Alzheimer's disease, and clinical trials of those agents are currently underway.

CENTRAL NERVOUS SYSTEM DISEASES WITH AUTOIMMUNE FEATURES

Rasmussen's encephalitis and "stiff-man" syndrome are two rare neurologic diseases that have recently been proposed as possible autoimmune conditions. Rasmussen's encephalitis presents as a progressive syndrome of unilateral cerebral dysfunction in children, manifested by hemiparesis and intractable seizures. Active inflammation with perivascular infiltration and neuronal destruction are seen on pathologic specimens, usually taken from patients undergoing surgical hemispherectomy in an attempt to control their seizures. Recently, an animal model of this condition has been described, based on sensitization to a portion of the neuronal membrane receptor for the excitatory neurotransmitter glutamate. Not only do immunized animals have a similar clinicopathologic syndrome, but IgG from those animals and from some affected patients with antiglutamate receptor antibodies can induce hyperexcitability in neuronal cultures. Some patients have improved with plasma exchange. Stiff-man syndrome is a condition characterized by excessive muscular contraction leading to progressive rigidity with spontaneous muscle spasms. The excessive muscular contraction results from hyperactivity of spinal motor neurons similar to that seen in clinical tetanus. Stiff-man syndrome is suspected of having an autoimmune basis because it is usually associated with such other autoimmune disorders as thyroiditis, insulin-dependent diabetes mellitus, pernicious anemia, and myasthenia gravis. Antibodies against a component of the enzyme glutamic acid decarboxylase have been detected in the serum and cerebrospinal fluid in up to 60% of patients. Glutamic acid decarboxylase is the enzyme controlling the synthesis of the major inhibitory neurotransmitter γ-aminobutyric acid. Improvement in symptoms has been observed after immunosuppressive therapy, including plasma exchange, corticosteroids, or intravenous immunoglobulin.

IMMUNOLOGICAL FEATURES OF STROKE

In the past several years, it has become clear that some patients with atypical cerebrovascular disease have circulating antibodies to phospholipids, which are major constituents of all cell membranes. The first such antibody to be implicated in stroke was the so-called lupus anticoagulant, which is neither a true anticoagulant, nor always associated with systemic lupus, but probably accounts for some of the thrombotic disorders seen in that disease. The most common antiphospholipid antibodies in stroke patients are the anticardiolipin antibodies, also responsible for positive (or false-positive) serologic tests for syphilis. Patients with stroke associated with antiphospholipid antibodies are typically young women with previous histories of deep venous thrombosis, spontaneous abortion, or thrombocytopenia; but without the common stroke risk factors of hypertension, diabetes, hyperlipidemia, or smoking. Antiphospholipid antibodies are usually of the IgG isotype and are detected by enzymatic immunoassays that are widely available in clinical laboratories. They should be sought in all stroke patients under the age of 45, especially those with a history of previous thrombotic disorders. The mechanism of antiphospholipid antibody activity is unclear, but several possibilities have been investigated, including activation of clotting factors, binding to platelets or endothelial cell membranes, and inhibition of serum proteins known as S and C, that normally inhibit coagulation or promote fibrinolysis. Therapy currently consists of anticoagulation with antiplatelet agents, heparin, or warfarin. Studies of corticosteroids, immunosuppressants, plasma exchange, and intravenous immunoglobulin infusions have been limited and largely unsuccessful to date; however, further clinical testing is needed.

REFERENCES

MULTIPLE SCLEROSIS

Beck RW et al: The effect of corticosteroids for acute optic neuritis on the subsequent development of multiple sclerosis. *N Engl J Med* 1993;**239:**1764.

IFNB Multiple Sclerosis Study Group and University of British Columbia MS/MRI Analysis Group: Interferon beta-1b in the treatment of multiple sclerosis: Final outcome of the randomized controlled trial. *Neurology* 1995;**45:**1277.

Jacobs LD et al: Intramuscular interferon beta-1a for disease progression in relapsing multiple sclerosis. *Ann Neurol* 1996;**39:**285.

Johnson KP et al: Copolymer 1 reduces relapse rate and improves disability in relapsing-remitting multiple sclerosis: Results of a phase III multicenter, double-blind, placebo-controlled trial. *Neurology* 1996;**45:**1268.

Owens T, Sriram S: The immunology of multiple sclerosis and its animal model, experimental allergic encephalomyelitis. *Neurol Clin* 1995;**13:**51.

Weiner HL et al: Therapy for multiple sclerosis. *Neurol Clin* 1995;**13:**173.

Weinstock-Gutmann B et al: The interferons: Biological effects, mechanisms of action, and use in multiple sclerosis. *Ann Neurol* 1995;**37:**7.

ACUTE DISSEMINATED ENCEPHALOMYELITIS

Johnson RT et al: Postinfectious encephalomyelitis. *Semin Neurol* 1985;**5:**180.

Kanter DS et al: Plasmapheresis in fulminant acute disseminated encephalomyelitis. *Neurology* 1995;**45:**824.

Kesselring J et al: Acute disseminated encephalomyelitis. MRI findings and the distinction from multiple sclerosis. *Brain* 1990;**113:**291.

ACUTE & CHRONIC INFLAMMATORY DEMYELINATING POLYNEUROPATHIES

Griffin JW et al: Pathology of the motor-sensory axonal Guillain-Barré syndrome. *Ann Neurol* 1996;**39:**17.

Latov N: Pathogenesis and therapy of neuropathies associated with monoclonal gammopathies. *Ann Neurol* 1995;**37**(S1):S32.

Ropper AH: The Guillain-Barré syndrome. *N Engl J Med* 1992;**326:**1130.

van der Meché FGA et al: Guillain-Barré syndrome and chronic inflammatory demyelinating polyneuropathy: Immune mechanisms and update on current therapies. *Ann Neurol* 1995;**37**(S1):S14.

Vriesendorp FJ et al: Serum antibodies to GM1, GD1b, peripheral nerve myelin, and *Campylobacter jejuni* in patients with Guillain-Barré syndrome and controls: Correlation and prognosis. *Ann Neurol* 1993;**34:**130.

MYASTHENIA GRAVIS & MYASTHENIC SYNDROME

Drachman DB: Myasthenia gravis. *N Engl J Med* 1994;**330:**1797.

Sanders DB: Lambert-Eaton myasthenic syndrome: Clinical diagnosis, immune-mediated mechanisms, and update on therapies. *Ann Neurol* 1995;**37**(S1):S63.

Watson DF, Lisak RP: Myasthenia gravis: An overview. In: *Handbook of myasthenia gravis and myasthenic syndromes.* Lisak RP (editor). Marcel Dekker, 1994, p 1.

PARANEOPLASTIC SYNDROMES

Anderson NE et al: Paraneoplastic cerebellar degeneration: Clinical-immunological correlations. *Ann Neurol* 1988;**24:**599.

Bakheit AM et al: Paraneoplastic limbic encephalitis: Clinico-pathological correlations. *J Neurol Neurosurg Psychiatry* 1990;**53:**1084.

Dropcho EJ: Autoimmune central nervous system paraneoplastic disorders: Mechanisms, diagnosis, and therapeutic options. *Ann Neurol* 1995;**37**(S1):S102.

Graus F et al: Plasmapheresis and antineoplastic treatment in CNS paraneoplastic syndrome with antineuronal antibodies. *Neurology* 1992;**42:**536.

AMYOTROPHIC LATERAL SCLEROSIS

Appel SH et al: Autoimmunity as an etiologic factor in sporadic amyotrophic lateral sclerosis. *Adv Neurol* 1995;**68:**47.

Rowland LP: Amyotrophic lateral sclerosis and autoimmunity. *N Engl J Med* 1992;**327:**1752.

Tan E et al: Immunosuppressive treatment of motor neuron syndromes: Attempts to distinguish a treatable disorder. *Arch Neurol* 1994;**51:**194.

ALZHEIMER'S DISEASE

McGeer PL et al: Immune system response in Alzheimer's disease. *Can J Neurol Sci* 1989;**16:**516.

Rich JB et al: Non-steroidal anti-inflammatory drugs in Alzheimer's disease. *Neurology* 1995;**45:**51.

Yankner BA et al: Beta-amyloid and the pathogenesis of Alzheimer's disease. *N Engl J Med* 1991;**325:**1894.

OTHER DISEASES OF THE CENTRAL NERVOUS SYSTEM WITH AUTOIMMUNE FEATURES

Amato AA et al: Treatment of stiff-man syndrome with intravenous immunoglobulin. *Neurology* 1994;**44:**1652.

Brey RL: Antiphospholipid antibodies and cerebral ischemia in young people. *Neurology* 1990;**40:**1190.

Hart YM et al: Medical treatment of Rasmussen's syndrome (chronic encephalitis and epilepsy): Effect of high-dose steroids or immunoglobulin in 19 patients. *Neurology* 1994;**44:**1030.

Feldman E, Levine SR: Cerebrovascular disease with antiphospholipid antibodies: Immune mechanisms, significance, and therapeutic options. *Ann Neurol* 1995;**37**(S1):S114.

Rogers SW et al: Autoantibodies to glutamate receptor 3 in Rasmussen's encephalitis. *Science* 1991;**265:**648.

Solimena M et al: Autoantibodies to GABA-ergic neurons and pancreatic beta cells in stiff-man syndrome. *N Engl J Med* 1990;**322:**1555.

Eye Diseases

41

Mitchell H. Friedlaender, MD, & G. Richard O'Connor, MD

The eye is frequently considered to be a special target of immunologic disease processes, but proof of the causative role of these processes is lacking for all but a few disorders. In this sense, the immunopathology of the eye is much less clearly delineated than that of the kidney, the testis, or the thyroid gland. Because the eye is a highly vascularized organ and because the rather labile vessels of the conjunctiva are embedded in a nearly transparent medium, inflammatory eye disorders are more obvious (and often more painful) than those of such other organs as the thyroid or the kidney. The iris, ciliary body, and choroid are the most highly vascularized tissues of the eye. The similarity of the vascular supply of the uvea to that of the kidney and the choroid plexus of the brain has given rise to justified speculation concerning the selection of these three tissues, among others, as targets of immune complex diseases (eg, serum sickness).

Immunologic diseases of the eye can be grossly divided into two major categories: antibody-mediated and cell-mediated diseases. As is the case in other organs, there is ample opportunity for the interaction of these two systems in the eye.

ANTIBODY-MEDIATED DISEASES

Before it can be concluded that a disease of the eye is antibody-dependent, the following criteria must be satisfied: (1) There must be evidence of specific antibody in the patient's serum or plasma cells. (2) The antigen must be identified and, if feasible, characterized. (3) The same antigen must be shown to produce an immunologic response in the eye of an experimental animal, and the pathologic changes produced in the experimental animal must be similar to those observed in the human disease. (4) It must be possible to produce similar lesions in animals passively sensitized with serum from an affected animal on challenge with the specific antigen.

Unless all of the above criteria are satisfied, the disease may be thought of as *possibly* antibody-dependent. In such circumstances, the disease can be regarded as antibody-mediated if only one of the following criteria is met: (1) antibody to an antigen is present in higher quantities in the ocular fluids than in the serum (after adjustments have been made for the total amounts of immunoglobulins in each fluid); (2) abnormal accumulations of plasma cells are present in the ocular lesion; (3) abnormal accumulations of immunoglobulins are present at the site of the disease; (4) complement is fixed by immunoglobulins at the site of the disease; (5) an accumulation of eosinophils is present at the site of the disease; or (6) the ocular disease is associated with an inflammatory disease elsewhere in the body for which antibody dependency has been proved or strongly suggested.

VERNAL CONJUNCTIVITIS & ATOPIC KERATOCONJUNCTIVITIS

These two diseases belong to the group of atopic-like disorders. Both are characterized by itching and lacrimation of the eyes but are more chronic than hay fever conjunctivitis. Furthermore, both ultimately result in structural modifications of the lids and conjunctiva. The immunologic basis for these diseases is not delineated.

Vernal conjunctivitis characteristically affects children and adolescents; the incidence decreases sharply after the second decade of life. Like hay fever conjunctivitis, vernal conjunctivitis occurs only in the warm months of the year. Most of its victims live in hot, dry climates. The disease characteristically produces giant ("cobblestone") papillae of the tarsal conjunctiva (Fig 41–1).

Atopic keratoconjunctivitis affects individuals of all ages and has no specific seasonal incidence. The

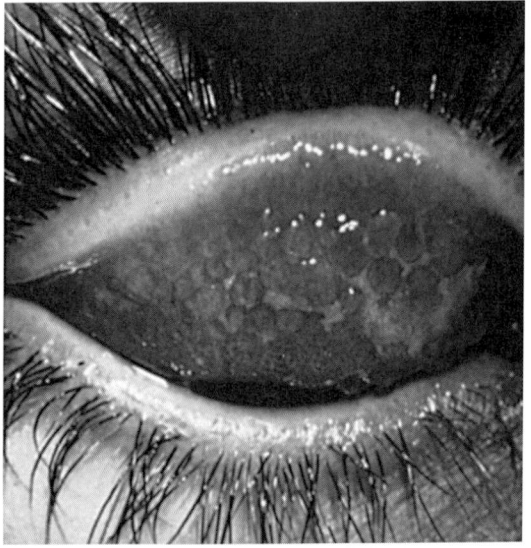

Figure 41–1. Giant papillae ("cobblestone") in the tarsal conjunctiva of a patient with vernal conjunctivitis.

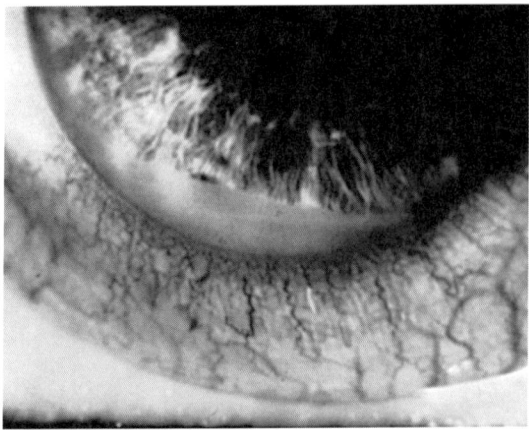

Figure 41–2. Acute iridocyclitis in a patient with ankylosing spondylitis. Note the fibrin clot in the anterior chamber.

skin of the lids has a characteristic dry, scaly appearance. The conjunctiva is pale and boggy. Both the conjunctiva and the cornea may develop scarring in the later stages of the disease. Atopic cataract has also been described. Staphylococcal blepharitis, manifested by scales and crusts on the lids, commonly complicates this disease.

RHEUMATOID DISEASES AFFECTING THE EYE

The diseases in this category vary greatly in their clinical manifestations depending on the specific disease entity and the age of the patient. Uveitis and scleritis are the principal ocular manifestations of the rheumatoid diseases. **Juvenile rheumatoid arthritis** affects females more frequently than males and is commonly accompanied by iridocyclitis of one or both eyes. The onset is often insidious, the patient having few or no complaints and the eye remaining white. Extensive synechia formation, cataract, and secondary glaucoma may be far advanced before the parents notice that anything is wrong. The arthritis generally affects only one joint (eg, a knee) in cases with ocular involvement.

Ankylosing spondylitis affects males more frequently than females, and the onset is in the second to sixth decades. It may be accompanied by iridocyclitis of acute onset, often with fibrin in the anterior chamber (Fig 41–2). Pain, redness, and photophobia are the initial complaints, and synechia formation is common. Over 90% of patients with ankylosing spondylitis and over 50% of all iridocyclitis patients express the HLA-B27 allele.

Rheumatoid arthritis of adult onset may be accompanied by acute scleritis or episcleritis (Fig 41–3). The ciliary body and choroid, lying adjacent to the sclera, are often involved secondarily with the inflammation. Rarely, serous detachment of the retina results. The onset is usually in the third to fifth decade, and women are affected more frequently than men. The sclera may become thin and may even perforate.

Reiter's disease affects men more frequently than women. The first attack of ocular inflammation usually consists of a self-limited papillary conjunctivitis. It follows, at a highly variable interval, the onset of nonspecific urethritis and the appearance of inflammation in one or more of the weight-bearing joints. Subsequent attacks of ocular inflammation may consist of acute iridocyclitis of one or both eyes, occasionally with hypopyon (Fig 41–4). Over 90% of patients with Reiter's disease express the HLA-B27 allele.

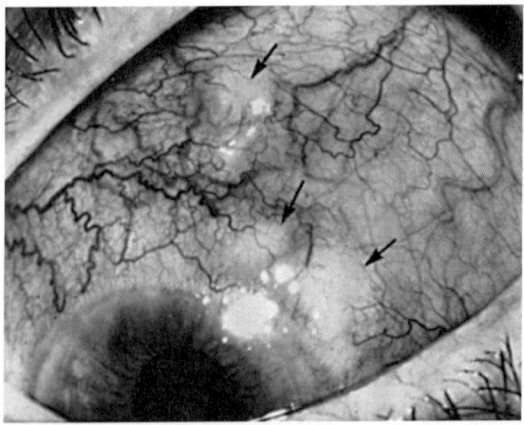

Figure 41–3. Scleral nodules in a patient with rheumatoid arthritis. (Courtesy of S Kimura.)

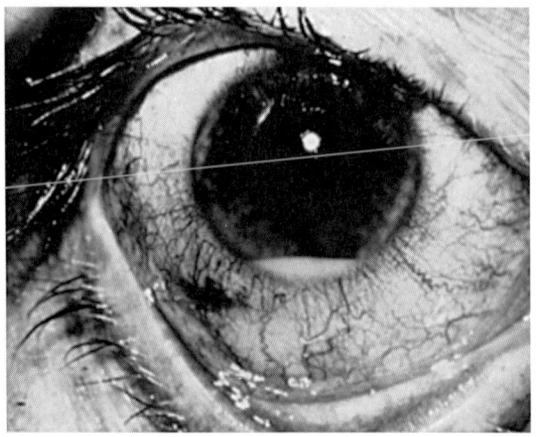

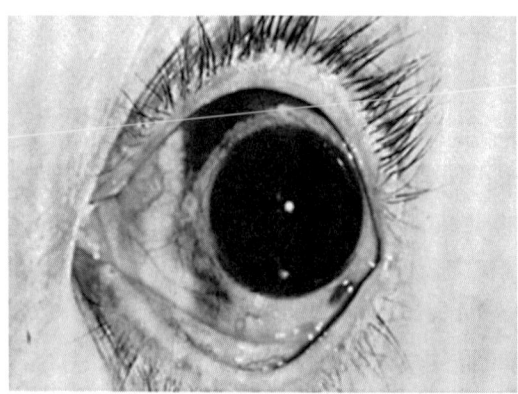

Figure 41–5. Scleral thinning in a patient with rheumatoid arthritis. Note the dark color of the underlying uvea.

Figure 41–4. Acute iridocyclitis with hypopyon in a patient with Reiter's disease.

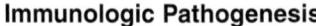

Immunologic Pathogenesis

Rheumatoid factor, an IgM autoantibody directed against the patient's own IgG, probably plays a major role in the pathogenesis of certain clinical manifestations of rheumatoid arthritis. The union of IgM antibody with IgG is followed by fixation of complement at the tissue site and the attraction of leukocytes and platelets to this area. An occlusive vasculitis resulting from this train of events is thought to be the cause of rheumatoid nodule formation in the sclera as well as elsewhere in the body. The occlusion of vessels supplying nutrients to the sclera is thought to be responsible for the "melting away" of the scleral collagen that is so characteristic of rheumatoid arthritis (Fig 41–5).

Although this explanation may suffice for rheumatoid arthritis, patients with the ocular complications of juvenile rheumatoid arthritis, ankylosing spondylitis, and Reiter's syndrome usually have negative tests for rheumatoid factor, so other explanations must be sought.

Outside the eyeball itself, the lacrimal gland has been shown to be under attack by circulating antibodies. Destruction of acinar cells within the gland and invasion of the lacrimal gland (as well as the salivary glands) by mononuclear cells result in decreased tear secretion. The combination of dry eyes (keratoconjunctivitis sicca), dry mouth (xerostomia), and rheumatoid arthritis (or other connective tissue disease) is known as Sjögren's syndrome (see Chapter 33).

A growing body of evidence indicates that the immunogenetic background of certain patients accounts for the expression of their ocular inflammatory disease in specific ways. Analysis of the HLA antigen system shows that the incidence of HLA-B27 is significantly greater in patients with ankylosing spondylitis and Reiter's syndrome than could be expected by chance alone. It is not known how this molecule controls specific inflammatory responses.

Immunologic Diagnosis

Rheumatoid factor can be detected in the serum by a number of standard tests involving the agglutination of IgG-coated erythrocytes or latex particles. Unfortunately, the test for rheumatoid factor is not positive in the majority of isolated rheumatoid afflictions of the eye.

The HLA types of individuals suspected of having ankylosing spondylitis and related diseases can be determined by standard cytotoxicity tests with specific antisera. These tests are generally done in tissue-typing centers where HLA typing for organ transplantation necessitates such studies. X-ray of the sacroiliac area is a valuable screening procedure that may show evidence of spondylitis prior to the onset of low back pain in patients with the characteristic form of iridocyclitis.

Treatment

Patients with uveitis associated with rheumatoid disease respond well to local instillations of corticosteroid drops (eg, dexamethasone 0.1%) or ointments. Orally administered corticosteroids must occasionally be resorted to for brief periods. Aspirin given orally in divided doses with meals is thought to reduce the frequency and blunt the severity of recurrent attacks. Atropine drops 1% are useful for the relief of photophobia during the acute attacks. Shorter acting mydriatics such as phenylephrine 10% should be used in the subacute stages to prevent synechia formation. Corticosteroid-resistant cases, especially those causing progressive erosion of the sclera, have been treated successfully with immunosuppressive drugs such as chlorambucil. Hydroxychloroquine, an antimalarial drug, has been useful in the treatment of Sjögren's syndrome and other collagen-vascular diseases. Eye examinations at 6–12-month intervals are recommended, since deposits in the cornea and retina have been reported with high-dose hydroxychloroquine therapy.

OTHER ANTIBODY-MEDIATED DISEASES

The following antibody-mediated diseases are infrequently seen by the practicing ophthalmologist.

Systemic lupus erythematosus (SLE), associated with the presence of circulating antibodies to DNA, produces an occlusive vasculitis of the nerve fiber layer of the retina. Such infarcts result in cytoid bodies, or "cotton-wool" spots, in the retina (Fig 41–6).

Pemphigus vulgaris produces painful intraepithelial bullae of the conjunctiva. It is associated with the presence of circulating antibodies to an intercellular antigen located between the deeper cells of the conjunctival epithelium.

Cicatricial pemphigoid is characterized by subepithelial bullae of the conjunctiva. In the chronic stages of this disease, cicatricial contraction of the conjunctiva may result in severe scarring of the cornea, dryness of the eyes, and, ultimately, blindness. Pemphigoid is associated with local deposits of tissue antibodies directed against one or more antigens located in the basement membrane of the epithelium.

Lens-induced uveitis is a rare condition that may be associated with circulating antibodies to lens proteins. It is seen in individuals whose lens capsules have become permeable to these proteins as a result of trauma or other disease. Interest in this field dates back to 1903, when P. Uhlenhuth first demonstrated the organ-specific nature of antibodies to the lens. R. Witmer showed in 1962 that antibody to lens tissue may be produced by lymphoid cells of the ciliary body.

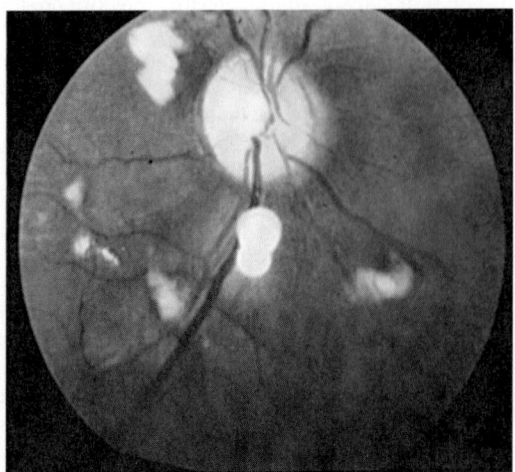

Figure 41–6. Cotton-wool spots in the retina of a patient with SLE.

CELL-MEDIATED DISEASES

This group of diseases appears to be associated with T-cell-mediated immunity (delayed hypersensitivity). Various structures of the eye are invaded by mononuclear cells, principally lymphocytes and macrophages, in response to one or more chronic antigenic stimuli. In chronic infections, such as tuberculosis, leprosy, toxoplasmosis, and herpes simplex, the antigenic stimulus has clearly been identified as an infectious agent in the ocular tissue. Such infections are often associated with delayed skin test reactivity following the intradermal injection of an extract of the organism.

More intriguing but less well understood are the granulomatous diseases of the eye for which no infectious cause has been found. Such diseases are thought to represent cell-mediated, possibly autoimmune processes, but their origin remains obscure.

OCULAR SARCOIDOSIS

Ocular sarcoidosis is characterized by a panuveitis with occasional inflammatory involvement of the optic nerve and retinal blood vessels. It often presents as iridocyclitis of insidious onset. Less frequently, it occurs as acute iridocyclitis, with pain, photophobia, and redness of the eye. Large precipitates resembling drops of solidified mutton fat are seen on the corneal endothelium. The anterior chamber contains a good deal of protein and numerous cells, mostly lymphocytes. Nodules are often seen on the iris, both at the pupillary margin and in the substance of the iris stroma. The latter are often vascularized. Synechiae are commonly encountered, particularly in patients with dark skin. Severe cases ultimately involve the posterior segment of the eye. Coarse clumps of cells ("snowballs") are seen in the vitreous, and exudates resembling candle drippings may be seen along the course of the retinal vessels. Patchy infiltrations of the choroid or optic nerve may also be seen.

Infiltrations of the lacrimal gland and of the conjunctiva have been noted on occasion. When the latter are present, the diagnosis can easily be confirmed by biopsy of the small opaque nodules.

Immunologic Pathogenesis

Although many infectious or allergic causes of sarcoidosis have been suggested, none has been confirmed. Noncaseating granulomas are seen in the uvea, optic nerve, and adnexal structures of the eye as well as elsewhere in the body. The presence of macrophages and giant cells suggests that particulate matter is being phagocytized, but this material has not been identified.

Patients with sarcoidosis are usually anergic to extracts of the common microbial antigens such as those of mumps, *Trichophyton, Candida,* and *Mycobacterium tuberculosis.* As in other lymphoproliferative disorders, such as Hodgkin's disease and chronic lymphocytic leukemia, suppression of T-cell immunity impairs normal delayed hypersensitivity responses to common antigens. Meanwhile, circulating immunoglobulins are usually detectable in the serum at higher than normal levels.

Immunologic Diagnosis

The diagnosis is largely inferential. Negative skin tests to a battery of antigens to which the patient is known to have been exposed are highly suggestive, and the same is true of the elevation of serum immunoglobulins. Biopsy of a conjunctival nodule or scalene lymph node may provide positive histologic evidence of the disease. X-rays of the chest reveal hilar adenopathy in many cases. Elevated levels of serum lysozyme or serum angiotensin-converting enzyme may be detected. A gallium scan, using gallium-67, may be useful in detecting clinically inapparent lesions.

Treatment

Sarcoid lesions of the eye respond well to corticosteroid therapy. Frequent instillations of prednisolone acetate 1% eye drops generally bring the anterior uveitis under control. Atropine drops should be prescribed in the acute phase of the disease for the relief of pain and photophobia; short-acting pupillary dilators such as phenylephrine should be given later to prevent synechia formation. Systemic corticosteroids are sometimes necessary to control severe attacks of anterior uveitis and are always necessary for the control of retinal vasculitis and optic neuritis. The latter condition often accompanies cerebral involvement and carries a grave prognosis.

SYMPATHETIC OPHTHALMIA & VOGT-KOYANAGI-HARADA SYNDROME

These two disorders are discussed together because they have certain common clinical features. Both are thought to represent autoimmune phenomena affecting pigmented structures of the eye and skin, and both may give rise to meningeal symptoms.

Clinical Features

Sympathetic ophthalmia is an inflammation in the second eye after the other has been damaged by penetrating injury. In most cases, some portion of the uvea of the injured eye has been exposed to the atmosphere for at least 1 hour. The uninjured, or "sympathizing," eye develops minor signs of anterior uveitis after a period ranging from 2 weeks to several years. Floating spots and loss of the power of accommodation are among the earliest symptoms. The disease may progress to severe iridocyclitis with pain

and photophobia. Usually, however, the eye remains relatively quiet and painless while the inflammatory disease spreads around the entire uvea. Despite the presence of panuveitis, the retina usually remains uninvolved except for perivascular cuffing of the retinal vessels with inflammatory cells. Papilledema and secondary glaucoma may occur. The disease may be accompanied by vitiligo (patchy depigmentation of the skin) and poliosis (whitening) of the eyelashes.

Vogt-Koyanagi-Harada syndrome consists of inflammation of the uvea of one or both eyes characterized by acute iridocyclitis, patchy choroiditis, and serous detachment of the retina. It usually begins with an acute febrile episode with headaches, dysacusis, and occasionally vertigo. Patchy loss or whitening of the scalp hair is described in the first few months of the disease. Vitiligo and poliosis are commonly present but are not essential for the diagnosis. Although the initial iridocyclitis may subside quickly, the course of the posterior disease is often indolent, with long-standing serous detachment of the retina and significant visual impairment.

Immunologic Pathogenesis

In both sympathetic ophthalmia and Vogt-Koyanagi-Harada syndrome, delayed hypersensitivity to melanin-containing structures is thought to occur. Although a viral cause has been suggested for both disorders, there is no convincing evidence of an infectious origin. It is postulated that some insult, infectious or otherwise, alters the pigmented structures of the eye, skin, and hair in such a way as to provoke delayed hypersensitivity responses to them. Soluble materials from the outer segments of the photoreceptor layer of the retina have recently been incriminated as possible autoantigens. Patients with Vogt-Koyanagi-Harada syndrome are usually Asians, which suggests an immunogenetic predisposition to the disease.

Histologic sections of the traumatized eye from a patient with sympathetic ophthalmia may show uniform infiltration of most of the uvea by lymphocytes, epithelioid cells, and giant cells. The overlying retina is characteristically intact, but nests of epithelioid cells may protrude through the pigment epithelium of the retina, giving rise to **Dalen-Fuchs nodules.** The inflammation may destroy the architecture of the entire uvea, leaving an atrophic, shrunken globe.

Immunologic Diagnosis

Skin tests with soluble extracts of human or bovine uveal tissue are said to elicit delayed hypersensitivity responses in these patients. Several investigators have recently shown that cultured lymphocytes from patients with these two diseases undergo transformation to lymphoblasts in vitro when extracts of uvea or rod outer segments are added to the culture medium. Circulating antibodies to uveal antigens have been found in patients with these diseases, but such antibodies are to be found in any patient with long-standing uveitis, including those suffering from several infectious entities. The spinal fluid of patients with Vogt-Koyanagi-Harada syndrome may show increased numbers of mononuclear cells and elevated protein in the early stages.

Treatment

Mild cases of sympathetic ophthalmia may be treated satisfactorily with locally applied corticosteroid drops and pupillary dilators. The more severe or progressive cases require systemic corticosteroids, often in high doses, for months or years. An alternate-day regimen of oral corticosteroids is recommended for such patients to minimize adrenal suppression. The same applies to the treatment of patients with Vogt-Koyanagi-Harada syndrome. Occasionally, patients with long-standing progressive disease become resistant to corticosteroids or cannot take additional corticosteroid medication because of pathologic fractures, mental changes, or other reasons. Such patients may become candidates for immunosuppressive therapy. Chlorambucil and cyclophosphamide have been used successfully for both conditions. More recently, cyclosporin has shown promise in the treatment of corticosteroid-resistant uveitis.

OTHER CELL-MEDIATED DISEASES

Giant-cell arteritis (temporal arteritis) (see Chapter 36) may have disastrous effects on the eyes, particularly in elderly individuals. The condition is manifested by pain in the temples and orbit, blurred vision, and scotomas. Examination of the fundus may reveal extensive occlusive retinal vasculitis and choroidal infarcts. Atrophy of the optic nerve head is a frequent complication. Such patients have an elevated erythrocyte sedimentation rate. Biopsy of the temporal artery reveals extensive infiltration of the vessel wall with giant cells and mononuclear cells.

Polyarteritis nodosa (see Chapter 36) can affect both the anterior and posterior segments of the eye. The corneas of such patients may show peripheral thinning and cellular infiltration. The retinal vessels reveal extensive necrotizing inflammation characterized by eosinophil, plasma cell, and lymphocyte infiltration.

Behçet's disease (see Chapters 33 and 36) has an uncertain place in the classification of immunologic disorders. It is characterized by recurrent iridocyclitis with hypopyon and occlusive vasculitis of the retinal vessels. Although it has many of the features of a delayed hypersensitivity disease, dramatic alterations of serum complement levels at the very beginning of an attack suggest an immune complex disorder. Furthermore, high levels of circulating immune complexes have recently been detected in patients with this disease. Most patients with eye symptoms are positive for HLA-B5 (subtype B51).

Contact dermatitis (see Chapter 30) of the eyelids represents a significant though minor disease caused by delayed hypersensitivity. Atropine, perfumed cosmetics, materials contained in plastic spectacle frames, and other locally applied agents may act as the sensitizing hapten. The lower lid is more extensively involved than the upper lid when the sensitizing agent is applied in drop form. Periorbital involvement with erythematous, vesicular, pruritic lesions of the skin is characteristic.

Phlyctenular keratoconjunctivitis (Fig 41–7) represents a delayed hypersensitivity response to certain microbial antigens, principally those of *M tuberculosis*. It is characterized by acute pain and photophobia in the affected eye, and perforation of the peripheral cornea has been known to result. The disease responds rapidly to locally applied corticosteroids. Since the advent of chemotherapy for pulmonary tuberculosis, phlyctenulosis is much less of a problem than it was 30 years ago. It is still encountered occasionally, however, particularly among Native Americans and Inuit peoples. Rarely, other pathogens such as *Staphylococcus aureus* and *Coccidioides immitis* have been implicated in phlyctenular disease.

Acquired immunodeficiency syndrome (AIDS) (see Chapter 53) is commonly associated with ocular disorders, seen mainly in homosexual men, intravenous drug abusers, and hemophiliacs. Cotton-wool exudates are the most common ocular sign. They have the same appearance as those seen in SLE (see Fig 41–6), but it is not known whether the cotton-wool spots of AIDS have the same pathogenesis. As is the case with SLE, patients suffering from AIDS may have elevated levels of serum immune complexes.

In addition to cotton-wool spots, AIDS patients may develop Kaposi's sarcoma of the conjunctiva or lids as well as chorioretinitis associated with any one

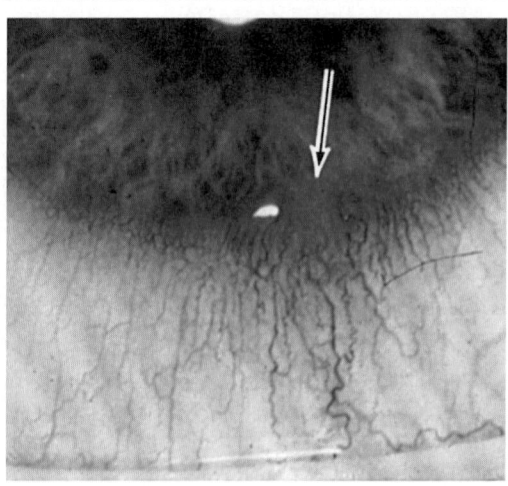

Figure 41–7. Phlyctenule (arrow) at the margin of the cornea. (Courtesy of P Thygeson.)

of a number of different opportunistic pathogens such as cytomegalovirus, *Cryptococcus, Toxoplasma,* or *Candida.* These patients have a fundamental disorder of cell-mediated immunity reflected in reduced levels of CD4 cells and chronic infection by HIV. These patients often die of systemic opportunistic infections such as *Pneumocystis carinii* pneumonia or toxoplasmal encephalitis. Since cotton-wool spots are an early sign of AIDS, the ophthalmologist may be the first physician to alert the patient to the existence of this serious disorder.

CORNEAL GRAFT REACTIONS

General Considerations

Blindness due to opacity or distortion of the central portion of the cornea is a remediable disease (Fig 41–8). If all other structures of the eye are intact, a patient whose vision is impaired solely by corneal opacity can expect great improvement from a graft of clear cornea into the stroma, and a single-layered endothelium. Although the surface epithelium may be sloughed and later replaced by the recipient's epithelium, certain elements of the stroma and all of the donor's endothelium remain in place for the rest of the patient's life. This has been firmly established by sex chromosome markers in corneal cells when donor and recipient were of opposite sexes. The endothelium must remain healthy for the cornea to remain transparent, and an energy-dependent pump mechanism is required to keep the cornea from swelling with water.

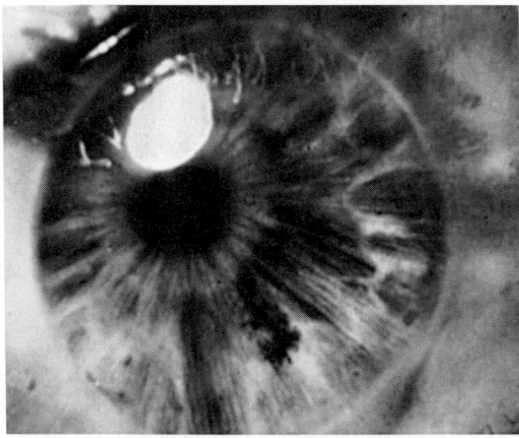

Figure 41–8. A cornea severely scarred by chronic atopic keratoconjunctivitis into which a central graft of clear cornea has been placed. Note how distinctly the iris landmarks are seen through the transparent graft.

Since the recipient's endothelium is in most cases diseased, the central corneal endothelium must be replaced by healthy donor tissue.

A number of foreign elements exist in corneal grafts that might stimulate the immune system of the host to reject this tissue. In addition to those already mentioned, the corneal stroma is regularly perfused with IgG and serum albumin from the donor, although none—or only small amounts—of the other blood proteins are present. Although these serum proteins of donor origin rapidly diffuse into the recipient stroma, these substances are theoretically immunogenic.

Although the ABO blood antigens have been shown to have no relationship to corneal graft rejection, the HLA antigen system probably plays a significant role in graft reactions. HLA incompatibility between donor and recipient has been shown by several authors to be significant in determining graft survival, particularly when the corneal bed is vascularized. It is known that most cells of the body possess these HLA antigens, including the endothelial cells of the corneal graft as well as certain stromal cells (keratocytes). The epithelium has been shown by J. Hall and others to possess a non-HLA antigen that diffuses into the anterior third of the stroma. Thus, although much foreign antigen may be eliminated by purposeful removal of the epithelium at the time of grafting, that amount of antigen which has already diffused into the stroma is automatically carried over into the recipient. Such antigens may be leached out by soaking the donor cornea in tissue culture for several weeks prior to engraftment.

Immunologic Pathogenesis

Both antibody and cellular mechanisms have been implicated in corneal graft reactions. It is likely that early graft rejections (within 2 weeks) are cell-mediated reactions. Cytotoxic lymphocytes have been found in the limbal area and stroma of affected individuals, and phase microscopy in vivo has revealed an actual attack on the grafted endothelial cells by these lymphocytes. Such lymphocytes generally move inward from the periphery of the cornea, making what is known as a "rejection line" as they move centrally. The donor cornea becomes edematous as the endothelium becomes compromised by an accumulation of lymphoid cells.

Late rejection of a corneal graft may occur several weeks to many months after implantation of donor tissue into the recipient eye. Such reactions may be antibody-mediated, since cytotoxic antibodies have been isolated from the serum of patients with a history of disease in this area. Trauma, including chemical burns, is one of the most common causes of central corneal opacity. Others include scars from herpetic keratitis, endothelial cell dysfunction with chronic corneal edema (Fuchs' dystrophy), keratoconus, and opacities from previous graft failures. All of these conditions represent indications for penetrating corneal grafts, provided the patient's eye is no longer inflamed and the opacity has been allowed maximal time to undergo spontaneous resolution (usually 6–12 months). It is estimated that approximately 10,000 corneal grafts are performed in the USA annually. Of these, about 90% can be expected to produce a beneficial result.

The cornea was one of the first human tissues to be successfully grafted. The fact that recipients of corneal grafts generally tolerate them well can be attributed to (1) the absence of blood vessels or lymphatics in the normal cornea and (2) the lack of presensitization to tissue-specific antigens in most recipients. Reactions to corneal grafts do occur, however, particularly in individuals whose own corneas have been damaged by previous inflammatory disease. Such corneas may have developed both lymphatics and blood vessels, providing afferent and efferent channels for immunologic reactions in the engrafted cornea.

Although attempts have been made to transplant corneas from other species into human eyes (xenografts), particularly in countries where human material is not available for religious reasons, most corneal grafts have been taken from human eyes (allografts). Except in the case of identical twins, such grafts always represent the implantation of foreign tissue into a donor site; thus, the chance for a graft rejection due to an immune response to foreign antigens is virtually always present.

The cornea is a three-layered structure composed of a surface epithelium, an oligocellular stroma, and a single endothelial layer of cells. Each layer can undergo single or multiple graft reactions in vascularized corneal beds. Graft reactions can be cell-mediated or antibody-mediated. These antibody reactions are complement-dependent and attract polymorphonuclear leukocytes, which may form dense rings in the cornea at the sites of maximum deposition of immune complexes. In experimental animals, similar reactions have been produced by corneal xenografts, but the intensity of the reaction can be markedly reduced either by decomplementing the animal or by reducing its leukocyte population through mechlorethamine therapy.

Treatment

The mainstay of the treatment of corneal graft reactions is corticosteroid therapy. This medication is generally given in the form of frequently applied eye drops (eg, prednisolone acetate 1%, hourly) until the clinical signs abate. These clinical signs consist of conjunctival hyperemia in the perilimbal region, a cloudy cornea, cells and protein in the anterior chamber, and keratic precipitates on the corneal endothelium. The earlier that treatment is applied, the more effective it is likely to be. Neglected cases may require systemic or periocular corticosteroids in addition to local eye drop therapy. Occasionally, vascularization and opacification of the cornea occur so rapidly that corticosteroid therapy is useless, but even the most hopeless-appearing graft reactions have occasionally been reversed by corticosteroid therapy. Topical corticosteroids are often used once or twice a day as prophylaxis against transplant rejection. More recently, topical cyclosporin eye drops have been used.

Patients known to have rejected many previous corneal grafts are treated somewhat differently, particularly if disease affects their only remaining eye. An attempt is made to find a close HLA match between donor and recipient. Pretreatment of the recipient with immunosuppressive agents such as azathioprine has also been resorted to in some cases. Although HLA testing of the recipient and the potential donor is indicated in cases of repeated corneal graft failure or in cases of severe corneal vascularization, such testing is not necessary or practicable in most cases requiring keratoplasty.

REFERENCES

Dugel PU, Rao NA: Ocular infections in acquired immunodeficiency syndrome. *Int Ophthalmol Clin* 1993; **33:**103.

Friedlaender MH (editor): Ocular allergy. *Int Ophthalmol Clin* 1988;**28:**261.

Friedlaender MH: *Allergy and Immunology of the Eye,* 2nd ed. Raven, 1993.

Friedlaender MH: New and evolving ocular infections. *Int Ophthalmol Clin* 1993;**33:**1–193. Entire issue.

Gold DH: Systemic associations of ocular disease. *Int Ophthalmol Clin* 1991;**31:**1–184. Entire issue.

Mannis MJ et al: *Eye and Skin Disease.* Lippincott-Raven, 1996.

Michelson JB, Nozik RA: *Surgical Treatment of Ocular Inflammatory Disease.* Lippincott, 1988.

O'Connor GR, Chandler JW (editors): *Advances in Immunology and Immunopathology of the Eye.* Masson, 1985.

Smith R, Nozik R: *Uveitis: A Clinical Approach to Diagnosis and Management.* Williams & Wilkins, 1983.

Smolin G, O'Connor GR: *Ocular Immunology.* Little, Brown, 1986.

Tabbara KF: Posterior uveitis. Part 1. *Int Ophthalmol Clin* 1995;**35:**1–138. Entire issue.

Tabbara KF: Posterior uveitis. Part 2. *Int Ophthalmol Clin* 1995;**35:**1–152. Entire issue.

Tabbara KF, Hyndiuk RA: *Infections of the Eye.* Little, Brown, 1996.

Respiratory Diseases

42

John F. Fieselmann, MD, & Hal B. Richerson, MD

Respiratory diseases of putative disordered immune regulation include those caused by exaggerated inflammation to exogenous antigen (hypersensitivity or allergic response), immune response to self-antigen (autoimmunity), or the failure to mount a protective immune response to a harmful agent (immunodeficiency). **Hypersensitivity responses** to known antigens include hypersensitivity pneumonitis, allergic asthma (atopic and occupational), some examples of eosinophilic pneumonias (parasitic, drug-induced, and allergic bronchopulmonary aspergillosis), and other manifestations of drug-induced lung diseases. Most respiratory diseases attributed to disordered immune regulation are of unknown etiology, but their pathology appears to involve immunologic mechanisms. Examples include collagen-vascular diseases, granulomatous diseases, vasculitis syndromes, and idiopathic interstitial fibrosis. Respiratory diseases associated with **primary** or **secondary immunodeficiency** are caused by infectious agents: viral, bacterial, fungal, or parasitic.

The lung must cope with antigens, including infectious organisms, that reach it by way of inspired air, aspiration, and the circulation. The pulmonary immune system normally mounts a protective effector response against harmful agents and ignores those that are harmless. Protection is helped by nonspecific clearance mechanisms involving alveolar macrophages, ciliary action, secretions, and cough. In general, the combination of specific (immunologic) and nonspecific mechanisms protects the lung very well. Why the system fails and how it leads to disease in some individuals is not well understood for many of the conditions included in this chapter.

Several respiratory diseases of disordered immune regulation are fully discussed elsewhere in this volume. For completeness, they are mentioned at the end of this chapter with reference to the chapters where they are treated in full.

DRUG-INDUCED RESPIRATORY DISEASES

Drugs cause adverse pulmonary effects by several different mechanisms, although details of pathogenesis are lacking in most cases. Potential mechanisms include hypersensitivity, direct toxicity, production of free oxygen radicals, stimulation of collagen synthesis, and lipidosis induction. This section primarily considers reactions involving proven or suspected immunologic mechanisms. Lists of common drugs are provided in Table 42–1.

Immunologic Mechanisms

Drug-induced hypersensitivity reactions involving the lungs may be associated with one or more types of immunologic response that damage host tissue. In the Gell and Coombs classification system, hypersensitivity responses may involve IgE antibodies (type I), cellular cytotoxicity (type II), antigen–antibody complexes (type III), or T-cell-mediated hypersensitivity (type IV). Except for wheal-and-flare (immediate-type) skin tests in type I hypersensitivity, documentation of drug allergy by in vivo or in vitro testing has not been clinically useful. In the following section, selected drugs are discussed to illustrate prototypic manifestations of adverse pulmonary reactions.

Airway Involvement

Bronchospasm and cough are the most common symptoms of airway dysfunction. Asthma may be caused by drugs eliciting IgE-mediated systemic anaphylaxis. This is commonly seen in response to beta-lactam antibiotics, foreign proteins, and exogenous hormones. Latex from surgical gloves or catheters is an increasing problem. Inhalation of psyllium (eg, Metamucil) dusts may induce asthma in a sensitized individual administering or otherwise handling the drug.

Table 42–1. Drug-induced respiratory diseases that may involve immunologic mechanisms.

Structure Affected or Disease Induced	Drug	Major Pulmonary Manifestations	Suspected Mechanism
Airways	ACE inhibitors Aspirin and other NSAIDs Sulfites Cisplatin, L-asparaginase D-Penicillamine Psyllium (inhaled)	Cough, asthma (rare) Asthma Bronchospasm Bronchospasm Bronchiolitis obliterans Asthma	Unknown Unknown Unknown Unknown Hypersensitivity IgE-mediated

Parenchyma	Anti-infectious agents
	  Isoniazid
	  Nitrofurantoin
	  p-Aminosalicylic acid
	  Penicillin
	  Sulfonamides
		Pulmonary infiltrates	Hypersensitivity

	Chemotherapeutic agents
	  Azathioprine
	  Methotrexate
	  Procarbazine
		Pulmonary infiltrates	Hypersensitivity

	Chemotherapeutic agents
	  Azathioprine
	  Bleomycin
	  Busulfan
	  Chlorambucil
	  Cyclophosphamide
	  Melphalan
	  Mitomycin
	  Nitrosureas
		Pulmonary fibrosis/pneumonitis	Unknown
			
			Oxidants?
			Toxic metabolites?
			Toxic metabolites?
			Toxic metabolites?
			Toxic metabolites?
			Toxic metabolites?
			Oxidants?

	Miscellaneous agents
	  Carbamazepine
	  Cromolyn
	  Gold salts
	  NSAIDs
		Pulmonary infiltrates	Hypersensitivity

	Miscellaneous agents
	  Amiodarone
	  Diphenylhydantoin
	  D-Penicillamine
	  Fluoxetine
	  Methysergide
	  Nitrofurantoin
		Pulmonary fibrosis/pneumonitis	Toxic lipidosis?
			Free oxygen radicals?

Pleura	Chemotherapeutic agents
	  Bleomycin, busulfan, methotrexate
	    mitomicin, procarbazine
	  Methysergide, ergonovine
	  Bromocryptine
	  Nitrofurantoin
		Pleurisy and effusion	Unknown

Mediastinum	Diphenylhydantoin	Pseudolymphoma with adenopathy	Hypersensitivity
Lupus syndrome	Diphenylhydantoin Hydralazine Isoniazid Procainamide	Infiltrates, pleuritis, effusion	Hypersensitivity
Pseudo-Goodpasture's syndrome	D-Penicillamine	Pulmonary hemorrhage	Unknown

Abbreviations: ACE, angiotensin-converting enzyme; NSAID, nonsteroidal anti-inflammatory drug.

Aspirin and other nonsteroidal anti-inflammatory agents can cause sudden, severe bronchospasm. No evidence exists that IgE antibodies play a role; rather, shunting of the arachidonic pathway toward lipoxygenase products (leukotrienes C_4, D_4, and E_4) has been suggested as a possible mechanism. Asthma can also be provoked by the direct pharmacologic effects of drugs such as beta-adrenergic blockers or an idiosyncratic effect of drugs such as angiotensin-converting enzyme (ACE) inhibitors.

Parenchymal Involvement

Parenchymal involvement induced by drugs includes diffuse, discrete, or interstitial infiltrates that may be associated with eosinophilia or with fibrosis. Chest computed tomography (CT) has been reported to be helpful in the diagnosis and monitoring of pulmonary damage in patients receiving potentially toxic drugs. **Nitrofurantoin** may cause acute or, less commonly, chronic pulmonary disease. The acute form usually has a sudden onset of fever, cough, dyspnea, and occasionally pleurisy within 7–10 days of beginning medication. Crackles and wheezes may be heard, and eosinophilia is found in 20–30% of patients. Chest x-rays show an interstitial, alveolar, or mixed pattern most prominent at the bases (Fig 42–1). Patients usually improve rapidly after the drug is withdrawn. The uncommon chronic form begins after months to years of nitrofurantoin use and is manifested by an insidious onset of dyspnea on exertion, bibasilar crackles, and diffuse interstitial pneumonitis or fibrosis. Some resolution typically occurs on discontinuation of the drug, but the fibrosis may progress. Studies suggest an immunologic pathogenesis in the acute form and cumulative toxicity, perhaps from oxygen radicals, in the chronic form. **Amiodarone** pneumonitis occurs in 4–6% of patients taking this antiarrhythmic agent and results in death in about 25% of those affected. The risk of this complication is dose- and duration-related and is manifested by dyspnea and cough with x-ray findings of interstitial and alveolar infiltrates. Although hypersensitivity may play a role, the condition is associated with lipid accumulation in lung cells (lipidosis), which may be the cause of the inflammatory response. Withdrawing the drug early in the course of pulmonary involvement results in resolution in most patients. **Chemotherapeutic agents,** especially methotrexate, carmustine (N,N'-bis(2-chloroethyl)-N-nitrosourea [BCNU], and bleomycin, are well known to cause ad-

verse pulmonary responses. Methotrexate generates pulmonary complications in about 8% of patients, but there appears to be a threshold dose requirement of 20 mg/week. The time interval before onset of symptoms may vary from days to years. The acute syndrome of fever, cough, dyspnea, and bilateral pulmonary infiltrates progresses over 1–2 weeks and then regresses whether or not methotrexate therapy is stopped. Acute lymphocytic leukemia of childhood seems to be a specific risk factor for the acute syndrome, and it results in death in 10% of those affected. BCNU, especially in higher doses, has been reported to cause pulmonary fibrosis in 20–30% of patients. The mechanism of injury is probably oxidant toxicity rather than an immunologic one. Bleomycin produces both acute and chronic pulmonary injury with inflammatory infiltrates and fibrosis. The chronic, but not the acute, form is dose-dependent, occurring in about 15% of patients receiving total doses that exceed 450 mg. Older age, previous irradiation, and oxygen therapy increase the risk. The chest x-ray most commonly shows lower lobe linear or nodular densities.

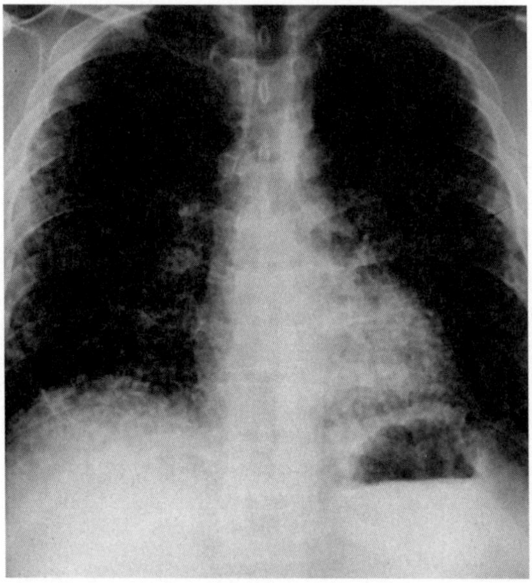

Gold salts produce pneumonitis in fewer than 1% of patients; this condition occurs 1–26 months after institution of therapy. Eosinophilia and lymphokine production provide evidence favoring types I and IV hypersensitivity responses. **Sulfasalazine** has been reported to cause pulmonary infiltrates, eosinophilia, fibrosis, and bronchiolitis obliterans after months or years of therapy. Hypersensitivity is the most likely mechanism.

Pleura

Drugs causing inflammation of the pleura with or without other lung structures are listed in Table 42–1. Pleuritis may also occur as a part of the lupus syndrome.

Mediastinum

Diphenylhydantoin may cause a pseudolymphoma affecting mediastinal as well as peripheral lymph nodes.

Lupus Syndrome

Procainamide and **hydralazine** are the most common agents that cause drug-induced systemic lupus erythematosus with pulmonary manifestations of pneumonitis or pleural effusions. **Isoniazid, D-penicillamine,** and **diphenylhydantoin** are less frequent lupus inducers. Features of the syndrome suggest hypersensitivity mechanisms that may involve an adjuvant effect or alteration of DNA nucleoproteins and subsequent autoantibody production.

Pseudo-Goodpasture's Syndrome

D-Penicillamine in high doses occasionally causes pseudo-Goodpasture's syndrome with abrupt onset of dyspnea, cough, hemoptysis, and hematuria, followed by increasing respiratory distress and renal failure. Intra-alveolar hemorrhage and fibrosis are seen his-

Figure 42–1. Chest x-ray of a patient with drug-induced lung disease secondary to nitrofurantoin showing nodular and linear interstitial infiltrates in the periphery and at the bases.

tologically. In contrast to Goodpasture's syndrome, antibasement membrane antibodies are not found.

EOSINOPHILIC PNEUMONIAS

Peripheral blood eosinophilia is commonly associated with atopic diseases, parasitic infestations, and some allergic drug reactions. There are many less common causes. When eosinophilia is present together with pulmonary infiltrates, however, the diagnostic possibilities are more limited and constitute the eosinophilic pneumonias or pulmonary infiltrates with eosinophilia (PIE) syndromes (Table 42–2). Although the etiology is usually unknown, hypersensitivity is suspected because similar syndromes result from hypersensitivity to known agents. Affected patients usually have peripheral blood eosinophilia over 10% or 500 eosinophils/mm³, but some have eosinophilic pulmonary infiltrates without peripheral eosinophilia.

Many eosinophilic pneumonias are associated with asthma, and the presence or absence of asthma is useful in the differential diagnosis (see Table 42–2).

Asthma essentially always occurs in and usually predates the onset of allergic bronchopulmonary aspergillosus (ABPA) and allergic granulomatosis of Churg and Strauss, and it is often associated with Carrington's chronic eosinophilic pneumonia. The pa-

tient is always atopic in ABPA (with demonstrable IgE antibodies to *Aspergillus fumigatus*), often atopic in allergic granulomatosis of Churg-Strauss, but not atopic in Carrington's chronic eosinophilic pneumonia.

ABPA is fully discussed in Chapter 29.

Chronic Idiopathic Eosinophilic Pneumonia

This disease is often called Carrington's chronic eosinophilic pneumonia. Clinical manifestations include fever, night sweats, weight loss, and progressive dyspnea. Most patients are white women with a history of recent-onset nonatopic asthma. The classic x-ray shows widespread shadows in a peripheral distribution (Figs 42–2 and 42–3), described as the "photographic negative" of that produced by pulmonary edema, although localized nonsegmental transient or migratory infiltrates are also found. Chest computed tomography may reveal predominant peripheral airspace consolidation even when the x-ray does not. Glucocorticoid therapy produces prompt remission of this potentially fatal disease, but relapses are common after discontinuation of treatment.

Allergic Granulomatosis of Churg and Strauss

This disease typically begins with upper respiratory symptoms of rhinitis and sinusitis followed by asthma

Table 42–2. Eosinophilic pneumonias.

Disease Entity	Association with Asthma	Comments
Allergic bronchopulmonary aspergillosis	Essentially always (extrinsic asthma)	Complication of atopic asthma with evidence of IgE and IgG antibodies to *Aspergillus fumigatus.*
Chronic idiopathic eosinophilic pneumonia (Carrington's)	Frequent (intrinsic asthma)	Subacute to chronic symptoms of cough, fever, dyspnea, sweats, and weight loss; classically peripheral infiltrates on radiogram.
Allergic granulomatosis (Churg-Strauss syndrome)	Essentially always	Multisystem vasculitis with fever, malaise, weight loss, pulmonary infiltrates, peripheral neuropathy, arthralgias, myalgias.
Acute simple idiopathic pulmonary eosinophilia (Löffler's syndrome)	Occasional	Migratory or transient infiltrates on chest x-ray and minimal or no symptoms.
Acute eosinophilic pneumonia	None	Recently described noninfectious eosinophilic pneumonia with rapid progressive respiratory failure.
Eosinophilia–myalgia syndrome	None	Caused by dietary supplements of tryptophan (L-tryptophan); sometimes associated with pulmonary infiltrates.
Drug-induced eosinophilic pneumonia	None	Penicillins, sulfonamides, nitrofurantoin, isoniazid, and many others (see Table 42–3).
Parasite-induced eosinophilic pneumonia (including visceral larva migrans and tropical pulmonary eosinophilia)	Occasional	*Ascaris, Trichinella, Strongyloides, Dirofilaria, Wuchereria, Toxocara,* and others (see Table 42–3).
Hypereosinophilic syndrome	None	Eosinophilia >1500/mm³ for 6 months or more; characteristic organ involvement; absence of secondary cause.

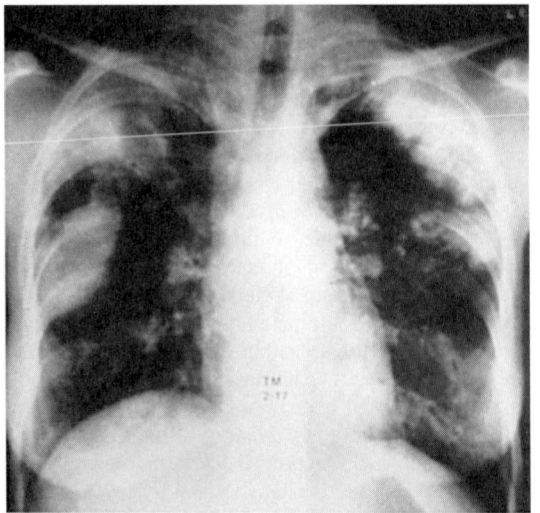

A

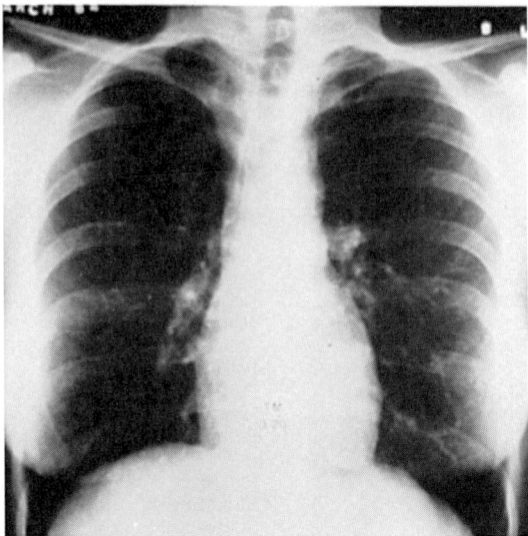

B

Figure 42–2. Chest x-ray of a patient with chronic idiopathic (Carrington's) eosinophilic pneumonia, **A:** showing peripheral distribution of infiltrates during the active phase of the disease and **B:** resolution of the lesions within days of starting glucocorticoid therapy.

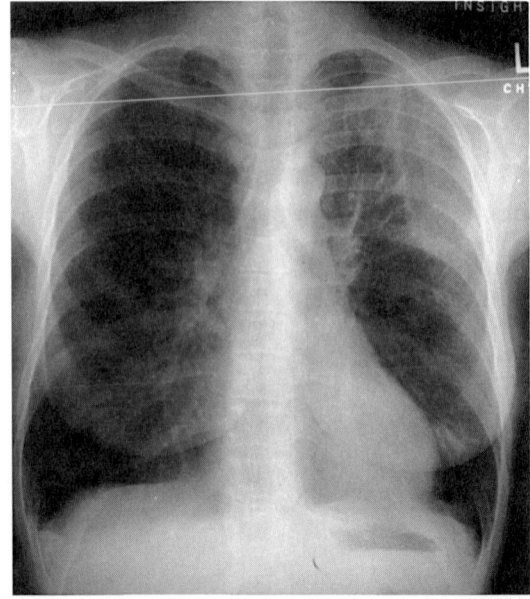

A

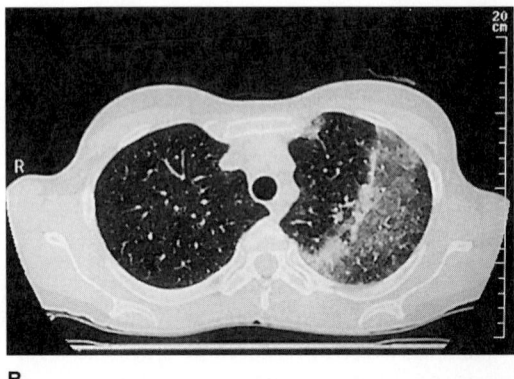

B

Figure 42–3. **A:** Chest x-ray of a 52-year-old woman during third exacerbation of chronic eosinophilic pneumonia, interpreted as showing a vague opacity overlying the peripheral margin of the left upper hemithorax and stranded opacities radiating out from the left heart border. **B:** High-resolution chest computed tomography taken on patient shown in **A** on the same day, with demonstration of confluent "ground-glass" densities in the left upper lobe. Note the rather distinct demarcation of the involved peripheral portion of the left upper lobe in this axial slice. Scattered areas of abnormal ground-glass density throughout both lungs were also seen.

and marked peripheral blood eosinophilia, with concurrent or subsequent pulmonary infiltrates. This is followed by evidence of a systemic vasculitis that may involve the heart, skin, and peripheral nerves. The kidneys are spared or only mildly involved. Mononeuritis multiplex is common, but polyneuropathy also occurs. Treatment requires glucocorticoids in this previously fatal disease; in resistant cases, immunosuppressants such as cyclophosphamide or azathioprine are needed.

Simple Idiopathic Pulmonary Eosinophilia (Löffler's Syndrome)

This is the name that has been applied to a self-limited, relatively mild illness with transient or migratory pulmonary infiltrates and peripheral eosinophilia regardless of etiology. Current usage arguably applies the term Löffler's syndrome to simple pulmonary eosinophilia of unknown cause; similar manifestations due to drugs or parasites are better classified under specific etiology.

The condition is expected to resolve within a month, so the patient with minimal symptoms does not require treatment.

Acute Eosinophilic Pneumonia

This is an acute form of eosinophilic lung disease considered to be distinct from previously described syndromes. It was first reported by two groups in 1989. Specific features include (1) acute febrile illness, (2) severe hypoxemia, (3) diffuse infiltrates on the chest x-ray, (4) over 25% eosinophils in bronchoalveolar lavage fluid, (5) no pulmonary or systemic infection, (6) no history of asthma or atopic illness, (7) prompt response to glucocorticoid therapy, and (8) complete resolution with no sequelae. Distinctive features are the rapid development of severe dyspnea and hypoxemia (PO_2 46–58 mm Hg) within a few days of onset of an acute febrile illness in a previously healthy subject. Lung biopsy has shown diffuse alveolar edema, intra-alveolar and interstitial eosinophils, and no vasculitis.

Eosinophilia–Myalgia Syndrome

This syndrome is included here because it may present with pulmonary infiltrates and peripheral blood eosinophilia. The most notable clinical features are severe disabling myalgias, muscle weakness, skin rash, and soft tissue induration resembling scleroderma. This syndrome is associated with the ingestion of L-tryptophan (containing one or more contaminants) used in large doses as a dietary supplement.

Drug-Induced Eosinophilic Pneumonias

Pulmonary diseases induced by drugs and involving suspected immunologic mechanisms were described earlier. Drugs most commonly incriminated in eosinophilic pneumonia are listed in Table 42–3. Nitrofurantoin may produce acute or chronic eosinophilic pneumonia, whereas most incriminated drugs produce acute syndromes beginning within a month of the institution of therapy. Treatment involves withdrawal of the drug with or without glucocorticoid therapy.

Parasite-Induced Eosinophilic Pneumonias

Eosinophilia is characteristic of all invasive helminthic infestations. Those that remain localized to the intestinal tract and cause minimal inflammatory lesions produce little if any eosinophilia; examples include oxyuriasis (pinworm) and trichuriasis (whipworm). Encystment of larval forms may be followed by disappearance of eosinophilia. Protozoan infestations (malaria, amebiasis, giardiasis, toxoplasmosis, leishmaniasis, trypanosomiasis) are not usually accompanied by eosinophilia. Thus, parasite-induced

eosinophilic pneumonias are limited to tissue-invasive stages of helminthic parasites trafficking through the lung. Documented examples are listed in Table 42–3.

Visceral larva migrans most commonly affects young children and is caused by infection with the dog and cat ascarids, *Toxocara canis* and *T cati,* respectively; the raccoon ascarid *Bayliascaris procyonsis,* hookworm, and *Strongyloides stercoralis* are occasionally responsible. Clinical manifestations are due to free migration of larvae in the liver, lungs, brain, eyes, heart, and skeletal muscles, causing inflammation, eosinophilia, and, eventually, granuloma formation. Patients are often asymptomatic but may present with fever, hepatomegaly, splenomegaly, skin rash, and recurrent pneumonia.

Tropical pulmonary eosinophilia is associated with microfilarial infection (*Wuchereria bancrofti* and *Brugia malayi*) and is characterized by fever, weight loss, fatigue, dyspnea, wheezing, and cough, which are usually worse at night. The disease is seen mainly in India, Southeast Asia, and South Pacific islands. Treatment with diethylcarbamazine is usually successful, but progressive fibrosis has been reported following inadequate eradication of the organisms.

Table 42–3. Eosinophilic pneumonias secondary to drugs and parasites.

Drugs	
Ampicillin	Minocycline
Aspirin	Naproxen
Arsenicals	Nickel
Beclomethasone	Nitrofurantoin
Bleomycin	Aminosalicylic acid
Carbamazepine	Penicillamine
Chlorpromazine	Penicillin
Chlorpropamide	Phenothiazine
Clofibrate	Propylthiourasil
Crack cocaine	Phenylbutazone
Cromolyn	Piroxicam
Diclofenac	Streptomycin
Dilantin	Sulfasalazine
Gold salts	Sulfonamide
Hydralazine	Tetracycline
Imipramine	Thiazide
Mephenesin	Tolazamide
Methotrexate	Tricyclic antidepressants
Methylphenidate	

Parasites
Ancylostoma brasiliense (hookworm)
Ancylostoma duodenale (hookworm)
Ascaris species (roundworm)
Brugia malayi
Dirofilaria immitis (dog heartworm)
Fasciola hepatica (liver fluke)
Necator americanus (hookworm)
Schistosoma species (blood flukes)
Strongyloides stercoralis
Taenia saginata (beef tapeworm)
Toxocara canis (dog roundworm)
Toxocara cati (cat heartworm)
Trichinella spiralis
Trichuris trichiura (whipworm)
Wuchereria bancrofti

Hypereosinophilic Syndrome

Diagnostic criteria for this idiopathic condition include (1) persistent eosinophilia greater than 1500 eosinophils/mm^3 for longer than 6 months; (2) lack of other known causes of eosinophilia; (3) systemic involvement of the heart, liver, spleen, central nervous system, or lungs. Fever, weight loss, and anemia are common. The heart is frequently involved, with tricuspid valve abnormalities and biventricular restrictive and obliterative cardiomyopathy. Treatment is aimed at lowering the eosinophil count. Some patients progress with morphologic, cytologic, and karyotypic features of eosinophilic leukemia.

OCCUPATIONAL AND ENVIRONMENTAL LUNG DISEASES

Indoor air quality has become an increasingly important issue for workplace and home environments. For the most part, immune-mediated occupational and environmental diseases involving the lung are either asthma (Chapter 27) or hypersensitivity pneumonitis (Chapter 30). The environmental antigens associated with these disorders make up long and growing lists.

In addition to asthma and hypersensitivity pneumonitis, environmental exposures may result in nonimmunologic disorders, such as the organic dust toxic syndrome (discussed in a later section) or the sick building syndrome.

The **sick building syndrome** has symptoms of cough, irritation of the nose or throat, headache, fatigue, and difficulty concentrating. Investigations of outbreaks of these and other symptoms reported by workers in modern office buildings determine a specific cause, such as accumulation of toxic gases or contaminated humidification systems, in only about 25% of cases. Inadequate ventilation with outdoor air has also been reported.

SARCOIDOSIS

Major Immunologic Features

- T-cell-mediated hypersensitivity to various skin test antigens is lost (anergy).
- T lymphocytes are activated, with cytokine release at foci of disease.
- There is CD4 lymphocytic alveolitis from a proliferation of local lymphocytes and chemotaxis of blood T lymphocytes.
- There is granuloma formation.
- Polyclonal gammopathy is found.

General Considerations

Sarcoidosis is a multisystem granulomatous disease of unknown origin; it occurs most commonly in young adults. There appears to be a higher prevalence of this disease in the black population. It is character-

ized by a lymphocytic alveolitis or noncaseating granulomas (or both) involving multiple systems. Pulmonary manifestations occur in more than 90% of patients. Cutaneous, ocular, or hepatic manifestations are also common.

Immunologic Pathogenesis

The assumed inciting antigen of this disorder is unknown. Once the antigen is processed by monocytes or macrophages, however, a well-described cascade of immune-mediated events begins. The macrophage initially presents antigen to antigen-specific T lymphocytes, becomes activated, and produces interleukin-1. This in turn activates the CD4 lymphocyte to release interleukin-2, which results in the presence of a large number of T cells at the site of disease through two mechanisms: (1) chemotaxis (the attraction of T cells from the circulation to sites of granuloma formation) and (2) mitogenesis (the stimulation of T cells to proliferate at sites of granuloma formation). This compartmentalization of inflammatory cells in sites of disease results in peripheral blood lymphocytopenia and a CD4 lymphocyte-rich alveolitis. The activated T cells found at the periphery of the granuloma play an important role in the pathogenesis of this disorder by releasing a number of lymphokines. One of these, a monocyte chemotactic factor, attracts monocytes that are essential building blocks of the granuloma. Most components of the granuloma (macrophages, epithelioid cells, and multinucleated giant cells) are derived from blood monocytes. Other lymphokines activate macrophages and inhibit macrophage migration.

Activated T cells at sites of granuloma formation are probably responsible for the polyclonal gammopathy sometimes found in sarcoid. T-cell/B-cell interactions release B-cell growth factor and B-cell differentiation factor, which nonspecifically activate B cells to differentiate into immunoglobulin-secreting plasma cells.

Clinical Features

Textbook descriptions of acute sarcoidosis include fever, erythema nodosum, iritis, and polyarthritis. More often, however, patients note the insidious onset of fatigue, weight loss, malaise, weakness, anorexia, fever, sweats, nonproductive cough, and progressive exertional dyspnea. Patients may also be asymptomatic, diagnosed only by the presence of an abnormality on a routine chest x-ray. (Fig 42–4; Table 42–4). Pulmonary function studies may be normal or may reveal evidence of a restrictive lung disease characterized by loss of lung volume, decreased diffusing capacity, and exercise-induced hypoxemia. Up to 40% of patients have an obstructive ventilatory defect secondary to airway involvement.

Diagnosis

The diagnosis can be established by the following criteria: (1) a compatible clinical picture; (2) his-

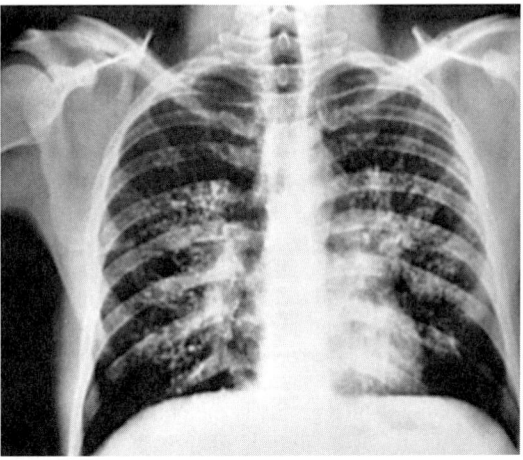

Figure 42–4. Chest x-ray of a patient with sarcoidosis (type II) showing bilateral hilar and parenchymal fibronodular infiltrates.

tologic evidence of a systemic granulomatous disease compatible with sarcoidosis; and (3) no evidence of exposure to an agent that is known to cause granulomatous disease. The disorder is also frequently associated with a peripheral-blood T lymphocytopenia, anergy to a panel of skin tests for cellular immunity, hypergammaglobulinemia, circulating immune complexes, increased serum angiotensin-converting enzyme activity, and increased numbers of macrophages and CD4 T cells in bronchoalveolar lavage fluid. These findings suggest but are not specific for sarcoidosis. The Kveim test, a cutaneous hypersensitivity test formerly used to diagnose sarcoidosis, is largely of historical interest owing to the unavailability of the antigen and to the availability of other diagnostic tests.

Differential Diagnosis

Sarcoidosis must be differentiated from a variety of granulomatous diseases, including various infectious diseases (particularly tuberculosis, nontuberculous mycobacterial infection, fungal infection), hypersensitivity pneumonitis, berylliosis, drug reactions, and neoplasms such as lymphomas. Type III sarcoidosis must also be distinguished from the large number of other interstitial lung disorders.

Treatment & Prognosis

The overall prognosis is favorable, with the likelihood of spontaneous remission somewhat linked to

Table 42–4. Chest radiography in sarcoidosis.

Type	Description
0	Normal.
I	Bilateral hilar adenopathy alone.
II	Hilar adenopathy and parenchymal abnormalities.
III	Parenchymal abnormalities without hilar adenopathy.

the stage of the disease. Patients with a type 0 or I chest x-ray have a very good prognosis with a greater than 80% chance of spontaneous remission, whereas those with type II or III chest x-ray have a less favorable prognosis. Treatment with corticosteroids is normally reserved for symptomatic pulmonary disease; systemic involvement of the eyes, myocardium, and central nervous system; disfiguring skin lesions; and hypercalcemia.

IDIOPATHIC PULMONARY FIBROSIS

Major Immunologic Features
- Immune complexes can be found in the blood and in the lungs.
- Immune complexes may stimulate macrophages to release neutrophilic chemoattractants, oxidants, and growth signals for mesenchymal cells.
- T cells may direct lung B cells to produce "autoimmune" antibodies and mediate cellular immune processes directed against lung parenchymal cells.

General Considerations

Although there is a rare familial form of the disease, idiopathic pulmonary fibrosis is, for the most part, an interstitial lung disease of unknown origin. Therefore, known causes of pulmonary fibrosis must be excluded prior to making this diagnosis. These include exposure to environmental inorganic dusts or toxic fumes; a history of underlying conditions such as sarcoidosis, eosinophilic granuloma, and collagen vascular disease; and pulmonary fibrosis secondary to lung infections, chronic aspiration, and drugs. Although some patients respond to treatment with corticosteroid or cytotoxic drug therapy, the prognosis, in general, is poor.

Immunologic Pathogenesis

The trigger of this disorder is still unknown. It is known, however, that **immune complexes** are present in serum and in the lungs in the early, active phase of the disease. Although these immune complexes may trigger an inflammatory process in the lungs by activating the complement cascade, there is no evidence to date that this process actually occurs in the lungs. Immune complexes in the lungs, however, stimulate **alveolar macrophages** to release various factors that may play a role in the pathogenesis of this disorder. One such factor released by alveolar macrophages is leukotriene B_4 (LTB_4), a lipid chemotactic factor that attracts neutrophils and eosinophils. The alveolar macrophages also release oxidants, which injure the pulmonary epithelium, and a variety of growth factors for fibroblasts, which increase the numbers of fibroblasts in the lungs and hence leads to the deposition of collagen. These observations are consistent with the pathologic features of the disease: increased numbers of polymorphonuclear leukocytes and generalized fibrosis of the lung parenchyma. New data suggest a complex but poorly defined relationship between these cellular components, their potential to release a variety of potent inflammatory mediators, and cellular receptors that modify these responses.

Clinical Features

Although patients at any age can be affected by this disease, the average age at diagnosis is 60 years. The disease has an insidious onset, with patients often noting symptoms for weeks to months before seeking medical attention. The usual presenting symptoms are progressive dyspnea on exertion and a nonproductive cough. Constitutional symptoms such as fatigue, weight loss, malaise, and arthralgias are not uncommon. Physical examination reveals dry bibasilar crackles ("Velcro rales"). In advanced cases, one may find clubbing, cyanosis, and evidence of cor pulmonale. The chest x-ray shows interstitial fibrosis predominantly in the basilar areas of the lungs. Honeycombing may occur in later stages. A chest CT may show focal or diffuse "ground glass" infiltrates or increased interstitial markings which are more prominent in the bases and periphery. A peripheral honeycomb pattern is fre-

quently observed (Fig 45–5). Pulmonary function testing shows a restrictive defect with decreases in lung volumes and diffusing capacity. Arterial blood gases show normal or decreased oxygen tension, which may fall significantly with exertion.

Diagnosis

Because this is a diagnosis of exclusion, no definitive or specific confirmatory tests exist. Serologic abnormalities may include positive tests for antinuclear antibodies or rheumatoid factor, increased amounts of immunoglobulins, and circulating immune complexes. Various immunologic tests are used primarily to exclude the presence of other interstitial lung disorders. Pathologic abnormalities often reveal wide variability among patients. Even when several biopsy specimens are taken from an individual patient, pathologic heterogeneity is not uncommon, suggesting that lung injury occurs at different rates. The histologic pattern varies from an acute alveolitis to an acellular stage with marked distortion of lung architecture and fibrosis. Bronchoscopy with biopsy and lavage is often used to exclude other causes of chronic interstitial lung disease. Bronchoalveolar lavage reveals increased numbers of alveolar macrophages and

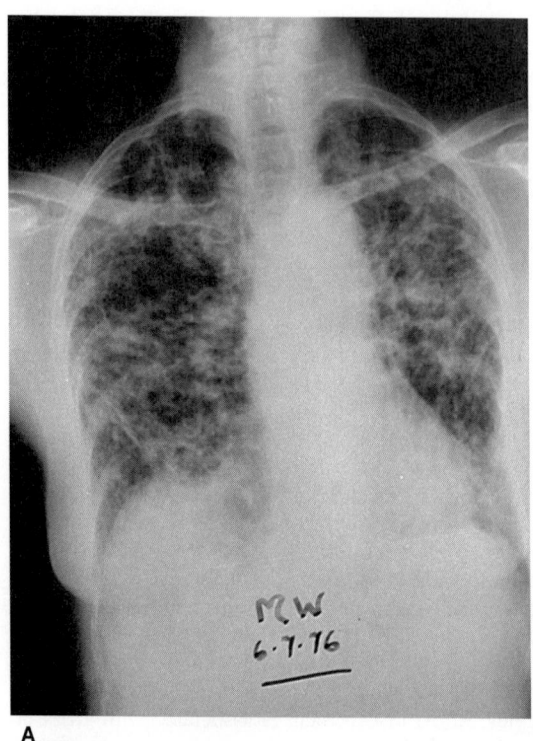

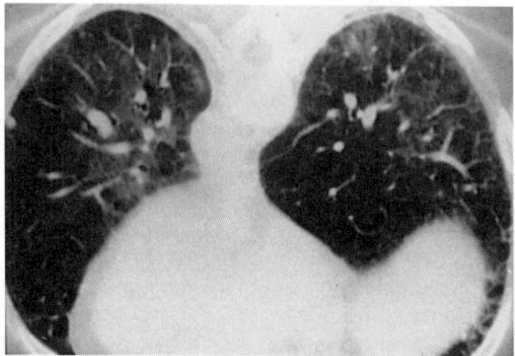

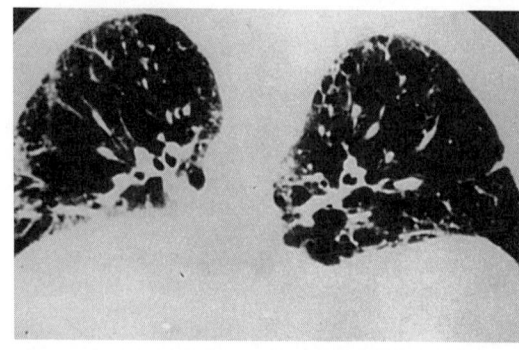

A

B

C

Figure 42–5. Radiographic evaluation of patients with idiopathic pulmonary fibrosis. **A:** Chest x-ray shows diffuse, bilateral interstitial infiltrates. Chest CT examples show the spectrum and heterogeneity of this process. **B:** An alveolar filling process is noted, and **C:** a more chronic, fibrotic process with honeycombing.

Table 42–5. Differential diagnosis of idiopathic pulmonary fibrosis.

Aspiration pneumonia
Collagen vascular diseases
Drugs (antibiotics and chemotherapy)
Eosinophilic lung syndromes
Histiocytosis X
Hypersensitivity pneumonitis
Infections (mycobacterial, viral, or fungal)
Lymphocytic interstitial diseases
Noxious gases (eg, oxides of nitrogen)
Pneumoconioses
Radiation
Sarcoidosis

polymorphonuclear leukocytes; the most characteristic feature is an increased percentage of both neutrophils and eosinophils. Since the histology of bronchoscopically obtained specimens is often nonspecific, an open or transthoracic thoracoscopic lung biopsy is usually necessary to exclude other disorders (eg, granulomatous infections, sarcoidosis, or bronchiolitis with obstructive pneumonia) and select the patients most likely to respond to treatment.

Differential Diagnosis

The differential diagnosis includes a large number of interstitial lung diseases of both known and unknown origin (Table 42–5). The principal considerations, however, include sarcoidosis, hypersensitivity pneumonitis, interstitial lung disease associated with collagen vascular diseases, and interstitial lung disease associated with certain inorganic dust exposures.

Treatment & Prognosis

Therapy is directed at suppressing active inflammation (alveolitis) and thus preventing further loss of function. High doses of corticosteroids may result in improvement and stabilization of pulmonary functions in approximately 20% of patients. Cytotoxic drugs have also been reported to benefit some patients. Unfortunately, despite treatment with corticosteroids or cytotoxic drugs, there is only a 50% survival at 5 years. This high mortality is secondary to progressive respiratory failure, infections related to treatment, pulmonary emboli, lung cancer, right heart failure, and the complications of prolonged immunosuppressive therapy. Most recently, there has been some enthusiasm for single-lung transplantation in patients who respond poorly to medical trials.

GOODPASTURE'S SYNDROME

Major Immunologic Features

- This syndrome is a type II cytotoxic antibody-mediated process.
- It is associated with circulating antiglomerular basement membrane (anti-GBM) antibodies.
- There are linear deposits of immunoglobulin

(principally IgG) and complement (C3) along the basement membrane of renal glomeruli, renal tubules, and pulmonary alveoli.

General Considerations

Goodpasture's syndrome, a disease of unknown origin, is characterized by the triad of pulmonary hemorrhage, glomerulonephritis, and circulating antibody to basement membrane antigens. Intrapulmonary hemorrhage may be insignificant or may be severe and life-threatening, often preceding renal involvement by 1–12 months. Renal involvement is commonly rapidly progressive, with oliguric renal failure occurring within weeks to months of the clinical onset of the disease. Without early treatment, permanent renal failure is the rule.

Immunologic Pathogenesis

In more than 90% of cases, circulating anti-GBM antibodies can be demonstrated early in the course of the disease. These antibodies are directed against renal tubular, renal glomerular, and pulmonary alveolar basement membranes. Immunofluorescence techniques can demonstrate that these tissues contain antibody deposited in a characteristic linear pattern, often accompanied by C3 deposition (see Fig 38–1). In a type II cytotoxic hypersensitivity reaction, antibody bound to basement membrane activates the complement cascade, resulting in the generation of chemotactic factors for various inflammatory cells. The inflammatory cells subsequently destroy the renal tubular, renal glomerular, and pulmonary alveolar basement membranes via the release of various reactive oxygen species and proteolytic enzymes. In addition, a host of other noncomplement mediators of inflammation are also activated. Recent studies demonstrate that the membrane antigenic site is the noncollagenous domain of the alpha 3 chain of type IV collagen.

Clinical Features

Goodpasture's syndrome occurs predominantly in young males, often following a viral infection. Pulmonary manifestations include pulmonary hemorrhage with or without hemoptysis, dyspnea, weakness, fatigue, and cough. Recurrent pulmonary hemorrhage may result in iron deficiency anemia. The chest x-ray typically reveals bilateral opacities that radiate from the hilum involving predominantly the middle and lower lobes in a confluent or acinar pattern. The pattern may change in intensity depending on the degree of intra-alveolar hemorrhage (see Fig 42–6). Bronchoalveolar lavage produces hemosiderin-laden macrophages with or without erythrocytes. Renal involvement is associated with gross or microscopic hematuria and variable amounts of proteinuria, a decreased 24-hour urine creatinine clearance, and an increase in blood urea and serum creatinine levels.

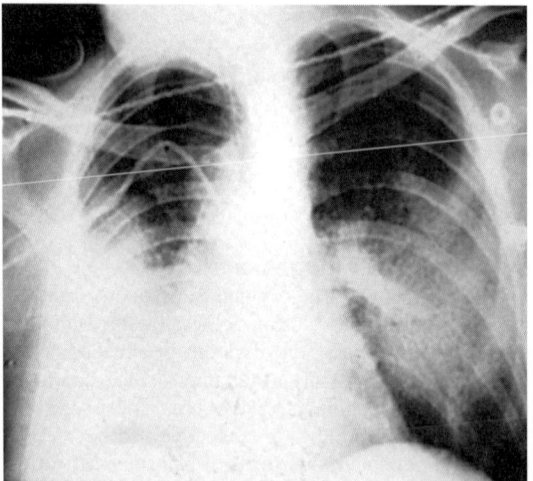

Figure 42–6. Chest x-ray of a patient with Goodpasture's syndrome, showing extensive bilateral pulmonary filtrates typical of intra-alveolar hemorrhage.

Differential Diagnosis

Pulmonary hemorrhage with renal failure may be seen in Wegener's granulomatosis, systemic lupus erythematosus, polyarteritis nodosa, and renal vein thrombosis with pulmonary embolism. These disorders lack the constellation of clinical, pathologic, and immunologic features on which the diagnosis of Goodpasture's syndrome is based.

Treatment & Prognosis

Since the disorder may be rapidly fatal, it is imperative that it be diagnosed and treated promptly. Treatment is directed at removal of circulating anti-GBM antibody, modulation of the inflammatory response, and suppression of new antibody synthesis. This has been effectively orchestrated with plasma exchange to remove anti-GBM antibodies and immunosuppressive drugs (corticosteroids and cytotoxic drugs) to suppress inflammation and new antibody formation. If instituted early in the course of the disease, this type of therapy may halt the progression of the disease and maintain renal function. A number of factors influence the response to treatment. The initial serum creatinine level and the percentage of crescents noted on the original renal biopsy are the best predictors of recovery: the prognosis for recovery is poor when the serum creatinine level is >5 mg/dL and when crescents are present in >50% of glomeruli. Bacterial infections during the recovery period are often associated with relapse. For patients with end-stage renal disease, renal transplantation has been successful after the disappearance of the circulating anti-GBM antibodies. Unfortunately, involvement of the new kidney has occasionally been reported following renal transplantation. Mortality is associated with respiratory failure secondary to pulmonary hemorrhage, complications of renal failure, and infection.

PULMONARY VASCULITIS SYNDROMES

Granulomatous and nongranulomatous vasculitides of unknown etiology affecting the lung are listed in Table 42–6, along with conditions presenting as pulmonary–renal syndromes. Some are discussed fully elsewhere in this chapter or in other chapters.

Wegener's Granulomatosis

This is discussed in Chapter 36. The diagnosis and follow-up of disease activity in Wegener's granulomatosis has been facilitated by the discovery of antineutrophil cytoplasmic antibodies (ANCA), which, however, may be positive in other vasculitic syndromes.

Lymphomatoid Granulomatosis

This was described as a new entity in 1972 and has frequently been confused with Wegener's granulomatosis. Later studies recognized lymphomatoid granulomatosis, involving primarily the lungs, and **polymorphic reticulosis** (or lethal midline granuloma), involving primarily the nose and paranasal sinuses, as histopathologic entities. Recent studies have suggested that these conditions are Epstein-Barr virus-driven lymphoproliferative disorders. Both lymphomatoid granulomatosis and polymorphic reticulosis can involve other tissues, including the skin, central nervous system, and abdominal organs, and both may result in malignant lymphoma. Radiation therapy is successful at treating localized disease.

Clinical manifestations of lymphomatoid granulomatosis include cough, fever, and dyspnea. Most patients are in early middle age, and men predominate. Pulmonary lesions are commonly in the lower lung fields bilaterally in a peripheral location without hilar adenopathy, and they tend to wax and wane. Skin lesions occur in one half of the patients. Glomerulonephritis is absent, but nodular renal lesions occur.

Table 42–6. Granulomatous and nongranulomatous vasculitis syndromes affecting the lung.

Granulomatosis–angiitis syndromes
   Wegener's granulomatosis.
   Lymphomatoid granulomatosis.
   Allergic granulomatosis of Churg and Strauss.
   Sarcoidal vasculitis.
Small-vessel vasculitis
   Leukocytoclastic angiitis.
   Henoch-Schönlein purpura.
   Behçet's disease.
   Collagen-vascular disease.
Pulmonary–renal syndromes
   Goodpasture's syndrome.
   Wegener's granulomatosis.
   Lymphomatoid granulomatosis.
   Allergic granulomatosis of Churg and Strauss.
   Systemic lupus erythematosus.
   Progressive systemic sclerosis (scleroderma).

Nervous system involvement is common and may include central nervous system dysfunction and peripheral neuropathies. Treatment with cyclophosphamide and prednisone has been somewhat successful, but about 50% of patients die of malignant lymphoma.

Small-Vessel Vasculitides

These are discussed in Chapters 33 and 36. As a group, they usually present with cutaneous lesions. The lung is involved uncommonly, with the possible exception of essential mixed cryoglobulinemia, which may present with interstitial pneumonitis and symptoms of asthma, hemoptysis, or pleuritis.

Collagen-Vascular Diseases

These diseases, including their effects on the lung, are discussed in Chapter 33.

PULMONARY MANIFESTATIONS OF IMMUNODEFICIENCY

Immunodeficiency diseases and disorders, including AIDS, are covered elsewhere in this volume (Chapters 20–25 and 53). These diseases increase the risk of specific pulmonary infections, depending largely on the type of defect in the immunocompromised host. Impaired antibody formation or complement deficiency predisposes patients to pneumonia caused by pyogenic organisms, chiefly *Streptococcus pneumoniae* and *Haemophilus influenzae*. Compromise of cellular immunity leads to increased risks for infections with mycobacteria and *Nocardia;* fungi such as *Pneumocystis carinii* (formerly classified as a protozoan), *Candida,* and agents of systemic mycoses; herpes viruses, vaccinia virus, and measles virus; and parasites including *Toxoplasma gondii* and *Strongyloides stercoralis.* Defects in granulocytes commonly result in staphylococcal abscesses that may involve the lung.

LUNG TRANSPLANTATION

Major Immunologic Features

- Class II major histocompatibility complex (MHC) antigens are expressed on bronchiolar epithelium.
- Recipient's helper T lymphocytes are activated when chronic graft rejection occurs.

General Consideration

With the improvement in surgical techniques and a better understanding of the pathogenesis and treatment of rejection and infection, heart–lung transplantation and single-lung transplantation have become life-saving options for patients with end-stage pulmonary hypertension, cystic fibrosis, idiopathic pulmonary fibrosis, and selected cases of chronic obstructive pulmonary disease. The major threats to the success of these procedures have been related to reperfusion injury, airway anastomosis failure, hemorrhage, infection, and rejection. Chronic rejection causing airway obstruction secondary to **obliterative bronchiolitis** is now recognized as a significant complication in up to 50% of patients. Early recognition and treatment of chronic rejection and infection may improve long-term survival.

Immunologic Pathogenesis

Although initial triggers and subsequent immune mechanisms responsible for obliterative bronchiolitis are poorly understood, one hypothesis is that some inhaled stimulus (possibly viral) may induce HLA-DR antigens on bronchiolar epithelium. These class II MHC antigens would then be recognized by the patient's T lymphocytes as foreign, and their activation would subsequently mediate the rejection process. Substances known to induce HLA-DR expression, such as interferon gamma, may play an active role in this process. Pathologically, one sees the characteristic pattern of perivascular lymphocytic infiltrates and mucosal inflammation with lymphocytic bronchiolitis.

Clinical Features

The process of obliterative bronchiolitis secondary to chronic rejection takes a mean of 14 months to develop but can occur as early as 2 months after transplantation. Initial symptoms are bronchitic in nature, with cough and mucopurulent sputum production. Dyspnea follows within months. At this point a chest x-ray is normal in 60% of cases, but high-resolution computed tomography of the chest may reveal peribronchial infiltrates. Serial pulmonary function testing has proved valuable in detecting the onset of this process. Consistent, progressive reduction in vital capacity (VC), total lung capacity (TLC), and forced expiratory volume in 1 second (FEV_1) is the rule. The fall in flow rates is usually not responsive to bronchodilators. Hypoxemia and mild decrease in diffusion are common.

Diagnosis

It was initially hoped that serial bronchoalveolar lavage might predict early rejection by changes in the cellular and phenotypic analyses. Unfortunately, increasing cell counts, increased numbers of activated CD4 cells, and increased CD4/CD8 ratios have not proved to be sufficiently discriminating. The use of serial transbronchial biopsies is currently the best method for confirming early rejection, with sensitivities ranging from 70 to 84% and specificities of 100%. These bronchoscopic procedures have been successful in differentiating opportunistic infection from rejection.

Differential Diagnosis

The usual diagnostic dilemma centers on differentiating opportunistic infection from chronic rejection.

This can be difficult since certain viruses (eg, cytomegalovirus) are known to play a role in acute and chronic rejection. Other causes of obliterative bronchiolitis include toxic injury from the oxides of nitrogen, hypersensitivity pneumonitis, lung injury secondary to collagen vascular diseases (particularly rheumatoid arthritis and Sjögren's syndrome), and small-airway involvement by various infections.

Treatment & Prognosis

During the early postoperative period, patients are treated prophylactically with cyclosporine, tacrolimus (formerly called FK506), azathioprine, and antilymphocyte globulin to decrease the chance of rejection. Corticosteroids may be used briefly, although they are usually withheld to allow for anastomotic healing. Signs of rejection are treated with high-dose corticosteroids, cyclosporine, and azathioprine. Early treatment has significantly reduced the morbidity of airway obstruction and the mortality of respiratory failure.

ADULT RESPIRATORY DISTRESS SYNDROME

General Considerations

The adult respiratory distress syndrome (ARDS) is a form of acute lung injury characterized by noncardiogenic pulmonary edema from increased vascular permeability. It can occur in the setting of a wide variety of clinical conditions, including sepsis, gastric acid aspiration, pancreatitis, trauma, fat emboli syndrome, and central nervous system insult.

Diagnosis

In the proper clinical setting, a diagnosis of ARDS is made when there are diffuse, bilateral infiltrates on chest x-ray (consistent with pulmonary edema), no evidence of increased pulmonary capillary hydrostatic pressure (this usually requires placement of a pulmonary artery catheter), and refractory hypoxemia that cannot be corrected by high concentrations of oxygen. In the last decade, mortality rates have fallen in most studies to 40–50%. Mortality relates to the underlying etiology of ARDS and to the development of multiple organ failure.

Immunologic Pathogenesis

A putative pathogenetic mechanism is the activation of the complement system with recruitment and sequestration of neutrophils in pulmonary interstitial capillaries. A number of cytokines released from macrophages may play a significant role in the recruitment of neutrophils. **Tumor necrosis factor alpha (TNFα)** is probably the most important cytokine to be synthesized in response to endotoxin. The

actual amount of TNFα released is modulated by the metabolites of arachidonic acid (PGE_2). In the capillaries, neutrophils responding to these signals accumulate and release a number of toxic products including oxygen free radicals and proteinases, which cause endothelial cell damage, interstitial and intra-alveolar edema, hemorrhage, and fibrin deposition.

Treatment

A better understanding of the mediators of the inflammatory process has led to the development of a number of new therapeutic approaches for clinical trials. These treatments include receptor antagonists and monoclonal antibodies directed at specific mediators. These can potentially modulate the cascade of events associated with ARDS and reduce the mortality of this syndrome. At present, treatment of patients with adult respiratory distress syndrome is supportive.

ALLERGIC ASTHMA

Asthma has been classified as extrinsic or atopic asthma due to inhalation of common inhalant allergens (house dust mite, mold spores, pollens, animal danders), occupational asthma secondary to sensitization to a variety of allergens including simple chemicals acting as haptens, and idiopathic or intrinsic asthma of unknown cause. Asthma as an allergic disease is discussed in Chapter 27.

HYPERSENSITIVITY PNEUMONITIS

Hypersensitivity pneumonitis (extrinsic allergic alveolitis) is a pulmonary and constitutional illness that is due to an immunologic reaction to a variety of inhaled antigens. Diagnosis has often been confused with a condition called organic dust toxic syndrome (ODTS) that includes grain fever caused by inhalation of endotoxin, mycotoxins, or other agents. Sensitization is not required in ODTS, and the lung may or may not be affected. These diseases are discussed in Chapter 28.

ALLERGIC BRONCHOPULMONARY ASPERGILLOSIS

Allergic bronchopulmonary aspergillosis (ABPA) usually presents as an eosinophilic pneumonia in patients with long-standing atopic asthma, is associated with allergy to *Aspergillus fumigatus* or occasionally other fungi, may complicate cystic fibrosis, and leads to proximal bronchiectasis and irreversible airways obstruction. It is discussed in Chapter 27.

REFERENCES

DRUG-INDUCED RESPIRATORY DISEASES

Israel-Biet D et al: Drug-induced lung disease: 1990 review. *Eur Respir J* 1991;**4:**465.

Kuhlman JE: The role of chest computed tomography in the diagnosis of drug-related reactions. *J Thorac Imaging* 1991;**6:**52.

Rosenow EC III et al: Drug-induced pulmonary disease. *Chest* 1992;**102:**239.

EOSINOPHILIC PNEUMONIAS

Allen JN, Davis WB: Eosinophilic lung diseases. *Am J Respir Crit Care Med* 1994;**150:**1423.

Allen JN et al: Acute eosinophilic pneumonia as a reversible cause of noninfectious respiratory failure. *N Engl J Med* 1989;**321:**569.

Lopez M, Salvaggio JE: Eosinophilic pneumonias. *Immunol Allergy Clin North Am* 1992;**12:**349.

Umeki S: Reevaluation of eosinophilic pneumonia and its diagnostic criteria. *Arch Int Med* 1992;**152:**1913.

Walker C et al: Activated T cells and cytokines in bronchoalveolar lavages from patients with various lung diseases associated with eosinophilia. *Am J Respir Crit Care Med* 1994;**150:**1038.

OCCUPATIONAL & ENVIRONMENTAL LUNG DISEASES

Epler GR: Clinical overview of occupational lung disease. *Radiol Clin North Am* 1992;**30:**1121.

Grammer LC, Patterson R: Occupational immunologic lung disease. *Ann Allergy* 1987;**58:**151.

Kreiss K: The sick building syndrome in office buildings: A breath of fresh air (editorial). *N Engl J Med* 1993;**328:**877.

Reed CR: Hypersensitivity pneumonitis and occupational lung diseases from inhaled endotoxin. *Immunol Allergy Clin North Am* 1992;**12:**819.

SARCOIDOSIS

DeRemee RA: Sarcoidosis. *Mayo Clinic Proc* 1995;**70:**177.

Girgis RE et al: Cytokines in the bronchoalveolar lavage fluid of patients with active pulmonary sarcoidosis. *Am J Resp Crit Care Med* 1995;**152:**71.

Semenzato G et al: Cellular immunity in sarcoidosis and hypersensitivity pneumonitis. Recent advances. *Chest* 1993;**103**(suppl):139S.

Thomas PD, Hunninghake GW: Current concepts of the pathogenesis of sarcoid. *Am Rev Respir Dis* 1987;**135:**747.

IDIOPATHIC PULMONARY FIBROSIS

Cherniack RM et al: Current concepts in idiopathic pulmonary fibrosis: A road map for the future. *Am Rev Respir Dis* 1991;**143:**680.

duBois RM: Idiopathic pulmonary fibrosis. *Annu Rev Med* 1993;**44:**441.

Goldstein RH, Fine A: Potential therapeutic initiatives for fibrogenic lung diseases. *Chest* 1995;**18:**848.

Kelly J: Cytokines of the lung. *Am Rev Respir Dis* 1990;**141:**765.

GOODPASTURE'S SYNDROME

Hellmark T et al: Characterization of anti-GMB antibodies involved in Goodpasture's syndrome. *Kidney Int* 1994;**46:**823.

Johnson JP et al: Therapy of antiglomerular basement membrane antibody disease: Analysis of prognostic significance of clinical, pathologic and treatment factors. *Medicine* 1985;**64:**219.

Kelly PT, Haponik EF: Goodpasture's syndrome: Molecular and clinical advances. *Medicine* 1994;**73:**171.

GRANULOMATOSIS–VASCULITIS SYNDROMES

Davenport A et al: Clinical relevance of testing for antineutrophil cytoplasm antibodies (ANCA) with a standard indirect immunofluorescence ANCA test in patients with upper or lower respiratory tract symptoms. *Thorax* 1994;**49:**213.

deRemee RA et al: Lesions of the respiratory tract associated with the finding of anti-neutrophil cytoplasmic autoantibodies with a perinuclear staining pattern. *Mayo Clin Proc* 1994;**69:**819.

Koss MN: Pulmonary lymphoid disorders. *Semin Diagn Pathol* 1995;**12:**158.

Staples CA: Pulmonary angiitis and granulomatosis. *Radiol Clin North Am* 1991;**29:**973.

Strickler JG et al: Polymorphic reticulosis: A reappraisal. *Hum Pathol* 1994;**25:**659.

LUNG TRANSPLANTATION

Bierman MI et al: Critical care management of lung transplant recipients. *J Intensive Care Med* 191;**6:**135.

Burke CM et al: Lung immunogenicity, rejection, and obliterative bronchiolitis. *Chest* 1987;**92:**547.

Keenan RJ et al: Clinical trial of tacrolimus versus cyclosporine in lung transplantation. *Ann Thorac Surg* 1995;**60:**580.

ACUTE RESPIRATORY DISTRESS SYNDROME

Kollef MH, Schuster DP: The acute respiratory distress syndrome. *N Engl J Med* 1995;**332:**27.

Lewis JF, Jobe AH: Surfactant and the adult respiratory distress syndrome: State of the art. *Am Rev Respir Dis* 1993;**147:**218.

MacNaughton PD, Evans TW: Management of adult respiratory distress syndrome. *Lancet* 1992;**339:**469.

Repine JE: Scientific perspectives on adult respiratory distress syndrome. *Lancet* 1992;**339:**466.

Reproduction & the Immune System

43

Karen Palmore Beckerman, MD

Perhaps, then, the zoologist is right to think of placentation as one of the more easily understood innovations of vertebrate phylogeny. But as it happens, not all the problems of viviparity have been satisfactorily solved. The relationship between mother and foetus is still in some degree teleologically inept, and it will be argued that certain trends in the evolution of viviparity raise special immunological difficulties for the foetus. (PB Medawar, 1952)

The purpose of this chapter is to acquaint the reader with basic principles of the immune response relevant to reproductive processes. Although many issues discussed here relate directly to contemporary cellular immunology, most of the questions are far from new, and, in fact, have remained essentially unanswered since they were first articulated by Medawar and his predecessors in the first half of this century.

The reader is introduced to the field of reproductive biology with a brief overview of the anatomy and histology of the male and female genital tracts. Recent findings regarding genital mucosal immunity are presented, followed by examination of the immune status of ovarian and testicular tissues, and, of course, the remarkable immune privilege enjoyed by tissues of the fetus. Topics receiving significant attention in scientific and lay journals, such as immune causes of infertility and abortion are discussed critically.

Two areas of maternal–fetal medicine are presented in some detail because of their clinical relevance and their importance to contemporary immunologic understanding of cellular interactions during gestation and parturition. The relatively well understood phenomenon of Rh-isoimmunization and anti-Rh immunoglobulin prophylaxis are examined first. Then we examine the perinatal transmission of HIV infection, which, although less completely understood, effectively illuminates neglected areas of investigation that have become indispensable to our understanding of the dynamics of maternal and fetal immune interactions.

REPRODUCTIVE TRACT ANATOMY AND IMMUNITY

ANATOMY

Female

The mucosa of the vagina and outer portion of the uterine cervix (or **ectocervix**) is made up of a highly vascularized submucosa and a superficial, nonkeratinized, stratified squamous epithelium (Fig 43–1). This squamous epithelium abruptly changes to simple stratified columnar epithelium at the **transitional zone,** which marks the beginning of the inner portion of the cervix (or **endocervix**). This is the site of hormonally regulated secretion of specialized mucous that facilitates sperm transport. The endocervix ends in the uterine cavity, the lining of which is referred to as either **endometrium** in the nonpregnant state or **decidua** during pregnancy. Depending on the hormonal stimulation, the endometrium varies from 1 to 6 mm in thickness and is made of several glandular layers. The innermost layer, the **stratum functionale,** grows and thickens prior to and after ovulation. If pregnancy and implantation occur, it hypertrophies further to become the nutrient-rich, intensely glandular decidua; if pregnancy does not occur, this layer is shed at the time of menses.

The site of fertilization is the fallopian tube, a muscular membranous structure lined by a highly vascular mucosa **(endosalpinx),** consisting of ciliated and secretory cells. The endosalpinx is thrown into numerous, branched, slender longitudinal folds and is ideally suited to the maintenance, nutrition, and transport of the conceptus during its 5-day journey to the uterus.

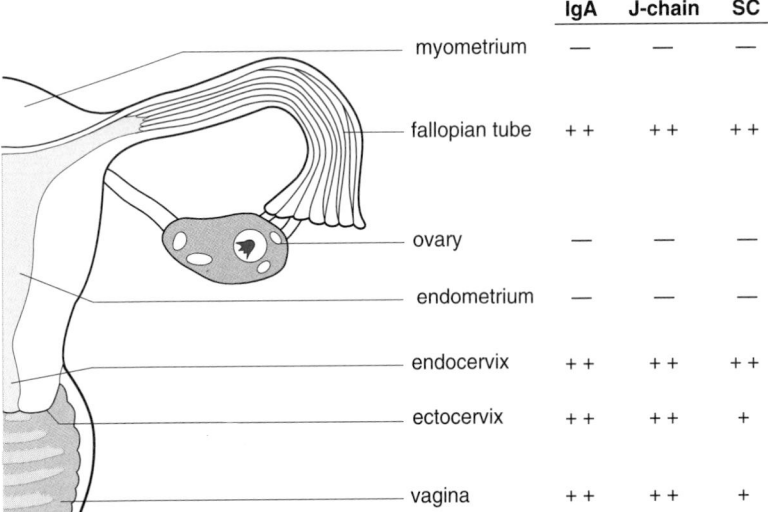

	IgA	J-chain	SC
myometrium	—	—	—
fallopian tube	+ +	+ +	+ +
ovary	—	—	—
endometrium	—	—	—
endocervix	+ +	+ +	+ +
ectocervix	+ +	+ +	+
vagina	+ +	+ +	+

Figure 43–1. The secretory immune system of the female genital tract. Immunofluorescence was used to analyze tissue from the uterus, fallopian tube, ovary, endocervix, ectocervix, and vagina. Note that fallopian tube and endocervix are the only sites strongly positive for the presence of IgA, J-chain, and secretory component (SC). –, negative; +, weakly positive; ++, strongly positive. (Reproduced, with permission, from Kutteh WH et al: *Mol Androl* 1993;**4**:183.)

Male

The character of the penile urethral epithelium varies in different places. The most distal portion of the urethra lies in the glans penis and is termed the **fossa navicularis.** The urethral mucosa in this section is lined by stratified squamous epithelium. The remainder of the penile urethra **(pars cavernosa)** is composed of pseudostratified columnar epithelium. Both sections are surrounded by a highly vascular submucosa. Penile periurethral tissue contains many small, branched, tubular glands lined by columnar mucus-secreting cells **(glands of Littré),** which can become chronically infected after urethritis. Nearer to the bladder, the urethra is lined by transitional epithelium characteristic of the bladder itself.

MUCOSAL IMMUNITY

The mucosa of the female genital tract (see Fig 43–1) is an anatomic and immunologic barrier of critical importance to host defenses against the spread of sexually transmitted diseases, including HIV infection. It is composed of immunologically reactive tissues capable of mounting local responses to foreign antigens in a manner similar to other immunologically active surfaces such as the respiratory and gastrointestinal tracts. Inductive sites for mucosal immunity of the reproductive tract consist of the cervix; vagina; large intestine and rectum; and the obturator, iliac, and inguinal lymph nodes that drain these structures. Immunoglobulin A (IgA)-containing plasma cells have been demonstrated in the lamina propria of the fallopian tube, endometrium, endocervix, and vagina, sup-

porting an immune effector role for these structures. Unique distributions of Langerhans' cells, dendritic cells, CD4 and CD8 T lymphocytes, and plasma cells have been described in surgical specimens of normal fallopian tube, cervix, vagina, and vulva.

The greatest number of intraepithelial and subepithelial lymphocytes is seen in the cervical transitional zone, suggesting that this site is an area of enhanced immune activity similar to other mucosal surfaces exposed to the external environment. As in the ileum, it appears that intraepithelial T cells of the fallopian tube and cervix are predominantly CD8, whereas subepithelial populations are CD4. The functional result of this tissue distribution is not entirely clear. Taken together, however, these findings support an important inductive role for cervical and fallopian tube lymphoid tissues in host mucosal defenses.

Vaginal immunization results in the appearance of specific IgA and IgG in vaginal secretions and IgG in the uterine cavity. Nasopharyngeal and intramuscular immunization induces low-level secretion of IgG (but not IgA) in the vagina and uterus coincident with increasing serum IgG titers. There is general agreement that cervical IgG is serum-derived, whereas cervical IgA is locally produced. Along with the cyclical hormonal effects on mucosal integrity and mucous production, it is apparent that immunoglobulin levels in the cervix vary markedly during the menstrual cycle.

To date, although mucosal immunity has been well studied in the lower gastrointestinal tract, immune responses in the male genital mucosa have been less well characterized. It may be reasonable to assume that as the spread of sexually transmitted diseases is studied in further detail, similar mechanisms of mucosal immune defenses in the male will be described.

DEFENSE AGAINST PATHOGENS VERSUS TOLERANCE OF SPERM "INVASION"

Covering, as it does, more than 400 m² of mucosa, the mucosal immune system is the largest component of a host's immune apparatus and contains the majority of the body's antibody-producing plasma cells. Much as in gut-associated lymphatic tissues, resident populations of macrophages, Langerhans' cells, dendritic cells, and T cells have been characterized in the superficial submucosa of the female genital tract. Antigen that reaches the cervical or vaginal submucosa is thought to be phagocytosed by antigen-presenting cells (presumably the resident macrophages and Langerhans' cells), which migrate to regional lymph nodes where processed antigen is presented. Once activated, T cells and B cells migrate to mucosal effector sites by specific binding to local postcapillary venule adhesion molecules. After arriving at mucosal tissues, B cells undergo clonal expansion as a result of activation by antigen, antigen-presenting cells, T-cells, and cytokines to become IgA plasma cells. These cells contain J chain, and the IgA produced is largely polymeric. In addition, vaginal and cervical epithelium produces secretory component for transport of immunoglobulin into reproductive tract secretions. Despite the regular, repetitive inoculation of millions of foreign spermatozoa into sexually active women, the immune system of the female reproductive tract is typically unresponsive to sperm antigen. Several factors are postulated to account for this. First, the ejaculate contains factors that inhibit immune responses. It is also thought that characteristics unique to female genital mucosal immunity must play an essential role in tolerance to sperm antigen. Different studies have reported a 1–12% incidence of antisperm antibodies in fertile women, whereas sperm-reactive antibodies are formed in 75% of men engaged in oral–genital intercourse, suggesting that in the case of antisperm antibodies at least, the inductive arm of mucosal immunity in the cervix and the vagina is uniquely tolerant to sperm antigen.

THE OVARY AND TESTIS

The Testis

The observations that germ cell antigens can behave more as foreign than as self and that in the male, haploid germ cells do not develop until puberty, long after the fetal or neonatal period when self tolerance is established, led to the development of the theory that sperm autoantigens are sequestered behind a strong blood–testis barrier. Although tight junctional barriers between the supporting Sertoli cells that surround cells involved in spermatogenesis can be demonstrated, the immune privilege that must be enjoyed by male germ cells in the testis is not complete. The normal testis contains numerous class II-negative resident macrophages in the interstitial spaces between the seminiferous tubules. In the mouse, these cells can be induced to upregulate their class II expression, and early germ cells, which lie outside the blood–testis barrier, can be immunogenic to their host, as discussed later in the section on infertility.

The Ovary

Unlike the testis, the ovary is clearly not a site of immune privilege. First, meiosis is not complete until just after sperm penetration of the egg, so that haploid female gamete antigens have little opportunity to be expressed. Still, ovarian antigens can produce autoimmune disease, as discussed later. Within the ovary, resident macrophages are a major component of the interstitial ovarian compartment, there is an influx of leukocytes around the time of ovulation, and numerous macrophages are observed in the corpus luteum after follicular rupture. Macrophage-secretory products have been shown to influence ovarian cells in vitro: tumor necrosis factor alpha (TNFα) inhibits steroid secretion by ovarian granulosa cells, whereas interleukin 1b (IL-1b) is cytotoxic to ovarian cell dispersates. Gonadotropin-dependent IL-1b gene expression has been identified in the human ovary prior to ovulation, along with expression of IL-1 receptor and IL-1 receptor antagonist. These and other observations have led some investigators to describe ovulation as an inflammatory-like reaction, with IL-1b as its centerpiece.

FERTILIZATION, IMPLANTATION, & THE IMMUNE RESPONSE TO FETAL TISSUES

SPERM–EGG FUSION

Fertilization is achieved following the successful completion of a complex sequence of events involving a spermatozoon and an egg. Although much of the cell biology of this process is well beyond the scope of this chapter, certain aspects of sperm–egg interactions deserve consideration. Fusion of gametes must require mutual, species-specific recognition of surface antigen and an initial adhesion step. Contact of gametes signals the **acrosome reaction,** whereby the covering of the head of the sperm is dissolved, activating enzyme systems that make it possible for the sperm to penetrate the cell mass (**cumulus oophorus**) and the thick, acellular mucopolysaccharide layer (**zona pellucida**) that surround the egg.

Complementary adhesion molecules have been characterized on the surface of mouse gametes. An 83,000-MW glycoprotein, murine zona pellucida 3 (mZP3), appears to act as a primary sperm receptor. Adhesion is carbohydrate-mediated via serine–threonine-O-linked oligosaccharides and results in initiation of the acrosome reaction. Another glycoprotein, mZP2, is involved in maintaining sperm binding to the ovum. On the acrosomal membrane of the head of the sperm, a putative 56,000-MW egg-binding protein has been identified as sp-56. It is assumed that homologous molecules regulate the early phases of fertilization in other mammals.

IMPLANTATION

After fertilization is completed and mitotic division is successfully initiated, it takes 6 days for the conceptus, surrounded by the zona pellucida, to traverse the fallopian tube and reach the uterus as an autonomous, cystic, embryonic cell mass known as the preimplantation **blastocyst.** Implantation of the blastocyst is regulated by complex interactions between peptide and steroid hormones that synchronize the preparation of the endometrium with development of the embryo. Progesterone secretion by the corpus luteum of the ovary is a critical component of these interactions and is necessary for decidual maintenance and development. Human chorionic gonadotropin (HCG) is secreted by embryonic tissues by the first day after implantation and is responsible for the conversion of the corpus luteum of the menstrual cycle to the corpus luteum of pregnancy. Thus, the early conceptus is responsible for supporting the ovarian progesterone secretion that is necessary for its own survival. Besides maintaining the endometrium of pregnancy, commonly called the **decidua,** progesterone, first of ovarian origin and later produced by the developing placenta itself, may also play a significant immunosuppressive role at the maternal–fetal interface.

At the time of implantation, the decidua contains numerous leukocytes, including T cells and macrophages. Their cytokine products are thought to be mediators of many of these interactions. For example, estrogen-dependent expression of epidermal growth factor (EGF) and its receptor have been identified in the mouse uterus, where they may regulate uterine angiogenesis and growth. The EGF receptor has been identified on the preimplantation blastocyst and in in vitro embryo cultures; EGF stimulates blastocyst development, suggesting a functional ligand–receptor interaction for EGF during preimplantation events. The colony-stimulating factor family of cytokines (GM-CSF, CSF-1, and IL-3) along with the c-*fms* receptor for CSF-1 have been identified in murine placenta and decidua and in human placental cell lines. Recent data suggest that these cytokines modify blastocyst membrane properties in preparation for im-

plantation. Indeed, the homozygous female CSF-1-deficient osteopetrotic mouse is infertile in matings with homozygous-deficient males but can produce offspring in matings with heterozygotes.

Before implantation, the zona pellucida must be shed. Although it is not clear whether the source of enzymes needed for degradation of the zona pellucida is endometrial or embryonic, it does appear that a burst of uterine expression of the cytokine, leukemia inhibitory factor (LIF) is required for adhesion and implantation of the blastocyst into the endometrium. Female mice lacking a functional LIF gene are fertile, but their blastocysts fail to implant and develop. These concepts are quite viable, however, and can be transferred to pseudopregnant wild-type controls, where they implant and develop normally.

Other cytokines secreted by decidual T cells and macrophages can either facilitate or impede implantation events. In vitro studies show that IL-1b inhibits murine blastocyst attachment but enhances trophoblast outgrowth. Interferon gamma (IFNγ) inhibits trophoblast outgrowth and causes degenerative changes in these cells, suggesting that implantation events may be regulated by the types of cytokines present and the timing of their secretion relative to embryonic development.

TROPHOBLAST INVASION OF MATERNAL TISSUES

Human embryonic development requires rapid access to the maternal circulation. Once attached to the endometrium, a distinct subset of **cytotrophoblast** cells (which now surround the embryonic tissues of the blastocyst and are destined to differentiate into the placenta and the outer layer of the fetal membranes) quickly differentiate into the highly invasive **trophoblast.**

The invasive trophoblast first erodes into endometrial stroma and then invades endometrial arterioles by day 12 of human gestation; it then replaces maternal endothelium and vascular smooth muscle, establishing the maximally dilated, fetal trophoblast-lined, **uteroplacental circulation** (Fig 43–2). Despite the fact that maternal leukocytes are in continuous contact with these fetal tissues now lining maternal vessels of the decidua and placenta, all of these structures continue to transport nutrients and eliminate waste from the fetus for the remainder of the pregnancy without rejection or attack by the immune system of either the fetus or the mother.

THE PLACENTA AS AN IMMUNE ORGAN

The placenta is a unique, short-lived organ. While producing protein and steroid hormones that regulate physiologic activities of pregnancy, it also acts as the

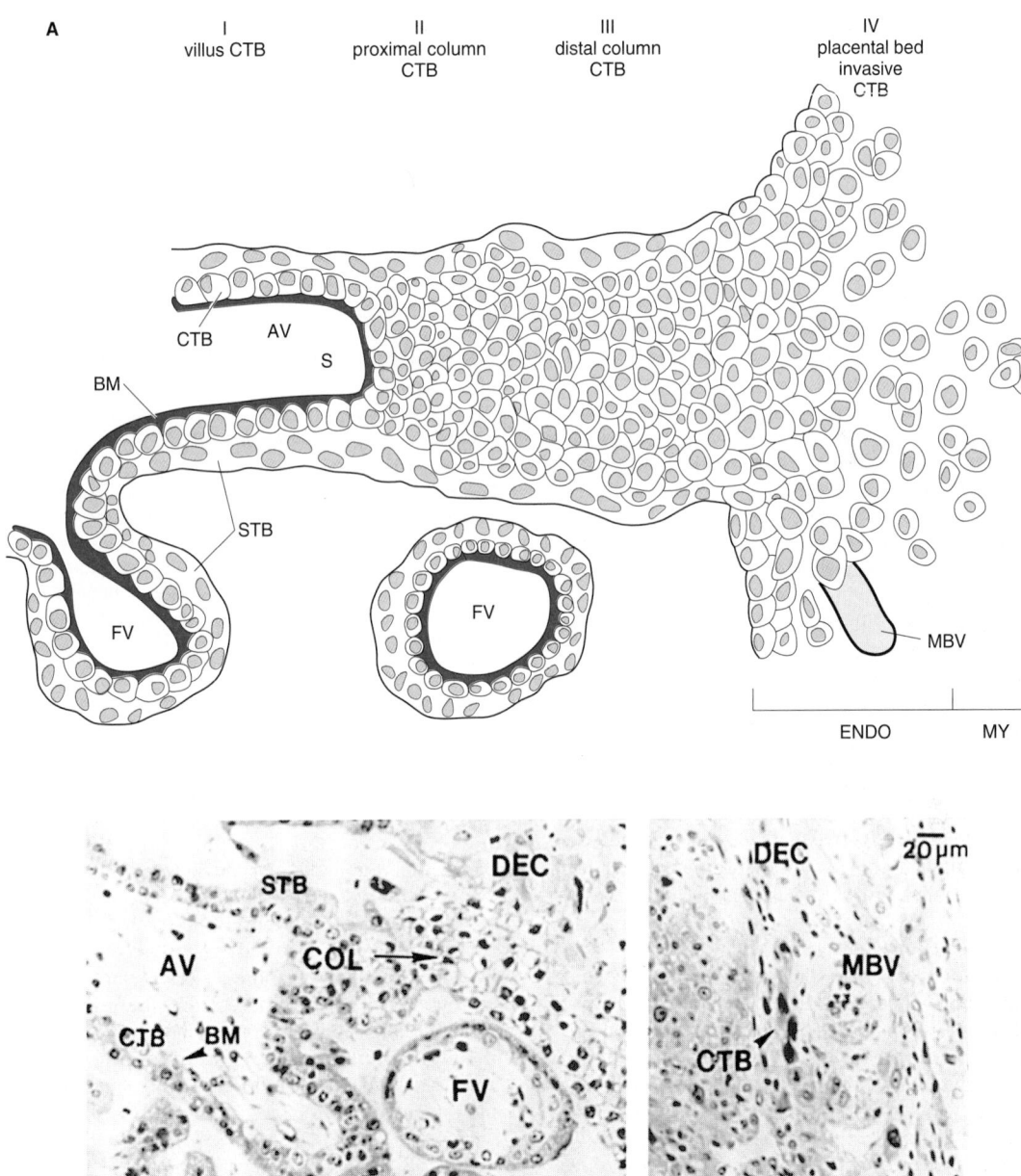

Figure 43–2. Trophoblast invasion at the maternal–fetal interface in the 10-week-old human placenta. **A:** Diagram showing floating villi and an anchoring villus with an associated cell column invading endometrium and myometrium of the uterine wall. The spatial organization of this tissue recapitulates the differentiation of cytotrophoblast along the invasive pathway. Zone I contains floating villi where mononuclear cytotrophoblast stem cells fuse to form the overlying syncytiotrophoblast layer past which maternal blood will percolate throughout gestation as part of the uteroplacental circulation. In an anchoring villus, cytotrophoblast form cell columns that connect the fetal and maternal compartments of the placenta (zones II and III). After shallow penetration of the uterine wall, columns spread laterally and break up into clusters of cells that penetrate endometrium (also called decidua) and myometrium layers of the pregnant uterus in zone IV. These invasive cytotrophoblast go on to invade and line maternal blood vessels, replacing endothelium and vascular smooth muscle in vessels of the inner one third of the uterine wall. **B** and **C:** Sections of a 10-week-old human placental bed biopsy showing all stages of cytotrophoblast differentiation along the invasive pathway. FV, floating villi; AV, anchoring villus; ENDO, endometrium; MY, myometrium; CTB, cytotrophoblast; STB, syncytiotrophoblast; MBV, maternal blood vessel. (Reproduced, with permission, from Damsky CH, Fitzgerald ML, Fisher SJ: *J Clin Invest* 1992;**89**:210.)

fetal lung, kidneys, intestine, and liver. Its function as a complex tissue of immunologic significance has received considerable attention in recent years.

Trophoblast

The multinuclear **syncytiotrophoblast** layer of the placenta (see Fig 42–2) was traditionally thought to act as a sort of "shield" for the fetus by serving as a barrier to maternal immune effector mechanisms. This model alone, however, has not been sufficient to explain maternal tolerance of fetal tissues. Trophoblast secretes cytokines that have been primarily associated with mononuclear phagocytes, such as CSF-1 and its receptor, c-*fms,* IL-3, and GM-CSF. Like macrophages, a trophoblast expresses high levels of the LIF receptor (see earlier discussion), is capable of phagocytosis and syncytialization, and expresses FcR, CD4, and CD14. There has been one preliminary reporting of trophoblast expression of IL-10, and it appears from work done in a number of different experimental systems that the trophoblast is responsive to TNFα, IL-1, transforming growth factor beta (TGFβ), and IL-6. Taken together, these findings have led to speculation that the trophoblast could represent part of a network of macrophage-like tissues distributed throughout the body that share common cytokine pathways and other characteristics. Such a model itself may or may not yield meaningful clinical information in the near future; however, the introduction of concepts such as cytokine signaling and other dynamic interactions between maternal and fetal tissues will be critical to further advances in our understanding of trophoblast development and survival.

The Hofbauer Cell

The Hofbauer cell is a macrophage-like cell found within the fetal portion of the placenta (chorionic villus) in the stromal tissue that surrounds the fetal vessels of the villous core (Fig 43–3). It is present early in gestation and is probably of fetal origin. Early in pregnancy this cell may play a significant role in flow dynamics within the fetal villus and later it is actively phagocytic; however, its function in placental development, physiology, and immunity has not been completely characterized.

Placental HLA Expression

It has become quite clear that the trophoblast is distinct from all other cell types in its ability to express human leukocyte antigen (HLA) molecules. The trophoblast does not express class I or class II HLA either constitutively or in response to IFNγ, despite the presence of abundant receptors for IFNγ in placental tissues and despite demonstrable enhancement of RNA synthesis, production of renin, and transferrin receptor expression by first-trimester trophoblast culture in response to the cytokine. The trophoblast does, however, constitutively express the nonclassic HLA class I molecule HLA-G. The HLA-G gene was

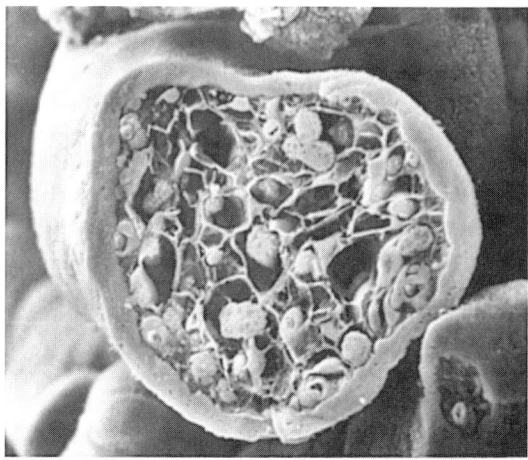

Figure 43–3. Scanning electron micrograph of a cross-fractured 10-week-old floating villus showing the villus core with its fetal vessels and numerous deep compartments formed by cytoplasmic processes of fixed stromal cells. Numerous Hofbauer cells are seen migrating between compartments. (Reproduced, with permission, from Castellucci M, Kaufmann P: *Placenta* 1982;**3**:269.)

originally isolated from a human lymphoblastoid cell line, but it is not expressed on any human cell type except the trophoblast, where it is expressed on the surface of the extravillous cytotrophoblast and secreted in its soluble form. It is nonpolymorphic, associated with β$_2$-microglobulin and can interact with CD8. It is found in highest levels in the first trimester and is markedly decreased in third trimester trophoblast. No function has been identified for HLA-G in human tissues; however, the total absence of polymorphic HLA expression in the trophoblast in the presence of unique expression of nonpolymorphic HLA-G is highly suggestive to many investigators that this molecule plays a significant role in trophoblast invasion and interaction with maternal tissues.

IMMUNITY IN PREGNANCY

BACKGROUND: ALTERED SUSCEPTIBILITY TO INFECTION IN PREGNANCY

With the advent of antimicrobial therapy, many of the dangers posed by infection to maternal health have been obscured. It is difficult to imagine that the single most common indication for therapeutic abortion prior to the late 1950s was tuberculosis. Indeed, infections against which host defenses are primarily cell-mediated, such as diseases caused by viruses, intracellular bacteria, fungi, protozoa, and helminths, have all been reported to be more likely acquired or reactivated and to be of greater virulence during pregnancy.

It is instructive to examine a few of the diseases to which pregnant women are more susceptible than nonpregnant controls. Until the 1960s, clinical poliomyelitis was two to three times more common in pregnancy, and the incidence of residual paralysis was significantly higher in pregnant patients. Hepatitis A occurs more commonly with a more fulminant course in pregnancy. One report from Africa notes a 40% rate of coma with 33% mortality among pregnant women compared with an 8% rate of coma and no mortality in nonpregnant controls. The frequency and severity of hepatitis B is thought to increase greatly during the last trimester. In the 1957 epidemic of influenza A, 50% of women of childbearing age who died in New York City were pregnant, even though they accounted for only 7% of women in that age group.

Pregnant women are much more likely to suffer the serious sequelae of malaria, including cerebral malaria, blackwater fever, acute renal failure, disseminated intravascular coagulation, pulmonary edema, and splenic rupture. In addition, plasmodia have a special affinity for placental tissue: a 46% placental infestation rate has been reported in an affected population that had only 17% positive peripheral blood smears. Interestingly, resistance to malaria is promptly restored following parturition.

In endemic areas, coccidioidomycosis is a leading cause of maternal death. The risk of miliary tuberculosis is threefold higher in pregnancy, and leprosy is reported to progress rapidly in pregnant women. Host defense against the intracellular bacteria *Listeria monocytogenes* is almost entirely cell-mediated. Even though clinically significant infection with this organism usually occurs only in the immunocompromised, up to one third of cases are found in pregnant women, their fetuses, and neonates. Peripartum listeriosis generally starts with a flu-like prodrome and progresses to acute chorioamnionitis, resulting in abortion or premature labor and delivery. Placental histology reveals chorioamnionitis, and fetal autopsy shows gram-positive rods in the fetal liver, lungs, amniotic fluid, and blood. After delivery and evacuation of infected uterine contents, the maternal condition rapidly improves. Important findings in a murine model of placental listeriosis are discussed in the following section.

Proposed Mechanisms of Altered Immunity in Pregnancy

In the face of such impressive historic data on compromised host defenses during gestation, the exact role played by the gravid state in modulation of the immune response has remained elusive. In pregnancy, B-cell immunity is maintained at normal levels, and serum immunoglobulin levels are unchanged. In addition, some manifestations of cell-mediated immunity, such as delayed hypersensitivity, skin reactions, skin

allograft rejection and in vitro responses to mitogen, are unaltered in pregnancy.

Contemporary discussions of immune responses during pregnancy generally embrace a theory of depression of selective aspects of cell-mediated immunity thought to be necessary for maternal accommodation of the so-called "fetal allograft." Unfortunately, many such discussions in the literature are highly speculative.

Local Immunosuppression at the Placenta and Adjacent Tissues

Experiments by Lu and Redline designed to study immunoregulatory mechanisms at the maternal–fetal interface during *L monocytogenes* infection in the pregnant mouse have yielded important information on cell-mediated immunity in pregnancy. Like the human, the adult mouse is able to mount an effective cell-mediated immune response to this intracellular parasite. During pregnancy, the maternal immune response in the liver and spleen was not impaired, even in the presence of overwhelming placental infection. In the placenta itself, large inflammatory infiltrates were identified in the maternal decidua; however, there was no inflammatory response in the fetal spongiotrophoblast and labyrinth layers of the murine placenta, despite the presence of large numbers of bacteria. This led to the conclusion that local events at the fetomaternal interface prevented an effective immune response and that the infected placenta might exert further detrimental effects by providing the listeria a protected environment from which it could seed other maternal and fetal organs. Further work by this group has identified profound local deficits in macrophage function in the placenta, which cannot be accounted for by regional deficits in macrophage-activating cytokines nor by immunosuppressive trophoblast products. These investigators' speculation that mechanisms preventing optimal macrophage function in the murine placenta may have evolved, not to make the fetoplacental unit susceptible to intracellular infections but to protect it from rejection by the maternal immune system, is thought-provoking but as yet unproved.

Secretion of Placental Steroid Hormones

The placenta secretes high levels of estrogens and progesterone, which it synthesizes from maternal and fetal precursors, resulting in extremely high levels in the maternal–placental circulation and causing a marked increase in maternal systemic hormone plasma levels. Free and albumin-bound hydrocortisone, of fetoplacental–placental origin, also increase.

Steroid hormones have been shown in vitro to depress different aspects of cell-mediated immunity in a variety of experimental models, including inhibition of graft rejection and suppression of lymphocyte activation of macrophages. Such experiments generally require high concentrations of hormones, in the 10- to 20-mM range, which is 20–50 times higher than levels found in maternal serum. It is conceivable, however, that such levels may be achieved in the placenta.

Secretion of Placental Proteins

Human chorionic gonadotropin (HCG) is produced by the trophoblast, increases during the first trimester, and decreases through the remainder of pregnancy. Inconsistent experimental data and recent work with purified HCG suggest there is minimal role for HCG alone in suppression of cell-mediated immunity in pregnancy. Alpha-fetoprotein (AFP) is secreted by the fetal liver into fetal serum and amniotic fluid in high levels during the second trimester and then plateaus. Physiologic levels of AFP can depress proliferative T-cell responses.

Intrinsically Decreased Lymphocyte Reactivity in Pregnancy

Although the clinical evidence for depressed cellular immunity during pregnancy is indisputable, there is conflicting opinion regarding changes in T-cell number, distribution, and reactivity during gestation. Some reports suggest a decrease in CD4 cells and others an increase in CD8 cells; cytotoxic activity of natural killer cells is said by others to be defective. Lymphocyte responsiveness to mitogens in vitro is moderately but significantly depressed in some studies but unchanged in others. Thymic involution, observed in other stressful conditions such as malnutrition and infection has been observed in rodents during the latter half of gestation coincident with rising plasma corticosteroid levels. No consistent or significant changes in B-cell immunity has been demonstrated during pregnancy.

Other Theories

Many theories explain the decreased cell-mediated immunity in pregnancy. So-called IgG "blocking antibodies of pregnancy" have been implicated, along with other proteins (eg, the macroglobulin pregnancy-associated α_2-glycoprotein), cell-associated pregnant serum factors, and altered balance between helper and suppressor T cells. To date, all such explanations of the status of cell-mediated immunity during pregnancy are incomplete. Further insight into placental physiology and immunology is needed before new hypotheses can be properly formulated and tested.

INFERTILITY AND SPONTANEOUS ABORTION

With increased numbers of women of childbearing age; the routine availability of pregnancy diagnosis before the first missed menstrual period; and significant numbers of couples electing to delay childbearing until they are older, statistically less fertile, and

somewhat more likely to experience spontaneous pregnancy loss, the public perception that infertility and spontaneous abortion are worsening problems in the United States is not unfounded. However, the rates of infertility and spontaneous abortion in this country are not increasing. Nonetheless, the number of couples seeking medical advice and treatment for infertility is increasing rapidly, to more than a million.

INFERTILITY

Infertility is the inability to establish pregnancy within a certain period of time, usually one year. Primary infertility refers to couples who have never achieved a pregnancy, whereas secondary infertility refers to those who have previously achieved a pregnancy but who are having difficulty doing so now. Documented causes of infertility include pelvic or tubal factors interfering with ovum transport, anovulation, abnormalities of the male reproductive system, and abnormal penetration of the cervical mucous by the sperm. For 10% of couples undergoing evaluation, no cause can be identified.

Immune Causes for Infertility

Antisperm antibodies have been studied since the early 1900s, when it was demonstrated that intraperitoneal injection of sperm into the female guinea pig induced antibody formation. Antisperm antibodies can be found in men and women in blood and lymphatic fluid (primarily IgG) and in local seminal or cervicovaginal secretions (primarily IgA). Development of these antibodies can occur in the male following traumatic or inflammatory disruption of the blood–testis barrier. Vaginal inoculation is far less likely to result in development of antisperm antibodies than is oral–genital intercourse. Interest in this field springs from two different clinical areas: first, identification of a treatable cause of idiopathic infertility, and, second, development of a highly specific contraceptive method by vaccinating individuals "against" pregnancy by inoculation with sperm antigen.

Three types of assays have been used to detect antisperm antibodies: sperm agglutination assays, sperm immobilization assays, and assays that directly detect antibody. The source of sperm antigen determines whether antibodies of possible significance (eg, those directed against a sperm cell surface antigen) or of doubtful significance (those directed against internal antigen) will be detected. Many assays do not measure IgA, the predominant class of antigen in mucosal secretions. Agglutination assays can be falsely positive due the presence of amorphous material in semen or by serum proteins. Immobilization assays may be affected by complement sources (guinea pig sera) that are toxic to sperm. Immunoglobulin-specific techniques, such as enzyme-linked immunoabsorbent and immunofluorescence assays, can be highly quantitative but cannot yield information about the location of an antibody on the sperm surface, but other tests such as immunobead and the mixed antiglobulin reaction with erythrocytes (MAR) can indicate the location of an antibody and can be used to evaluate immunoglobulin isotype, but do not provide quantitative information.

Depending on the assay used, antisperm antibodies are found in 1–12% of fertile women and in 10–20% of women with unexplained infertility. In the male, autoantibodies to sperm can be detected in both the seminal plasma and serum, and one half of men undergoing vasectomy form antisperm antibodies following the procedure. Importantly, data are not available that document significant differences in the presence or titers of antisperm antibodies in fertile and infertile populations.

Autoimmune disease of the testis and ovary is a known cause of infertility in domestic animals and is a likely cause of some forms of human infertility. Granulomatous disease and immune complexes can be found in the testis of infertile men and resemble changes seen in experimental autoimmune orchitis in mice. Ovarian autoantibodies and idiopathic oophoritis have been documented in women with premature ovarian failure. In addition, autoimmune orchitis and oophoritis have been identified as components of human polyendocrine and autoimmunity syndromes. Studies based on experimental autoimmune gonadal disease models have yielded new information on genetic control of organ-specific autoimmune disease and on antigen mimicry at the T-cell receptor.

Experimental autoimmune oophoritis is induced 2 weeks following immunization of rats with bovine ovarian homogenate or immunization with synthetic peptide fragments of ZP3, the sperm receptor protein on the zona pellucida (see the section on sperm–egg fusion). Disease can also be induced 2 days after adoptive transfer of T-cell lines and T-cell clones derived from lymph node cells from immunized, diseased mice to normal untreated recipients. These lines and clones are uniformly CD4 and produce IL-2, TNF, and IFNγ on stimulation. Interestingly, four randomly positioned amino acids in the peptide nanomer ZP3 330–338 are critical for induction of disease and T-cell response, but polyalanine peptide inserted with the critical ZP3 residues is fully capable of eliciting disease.

Experimental autoimmune orchitis is under polygenic control, involving *H*-2- and non-*H*-2-linked genes. Severe disease can be induced only by inoculation with homologous crude testis antigen and by adoptive transfer of T-cell lines and clones derived from lymph nodes of immunized mice. Manipulations of the normal immune system can also cause autoimmune gonadal disease. For example, neonatal murine thymectomy performed between day 1 and day 4 after birth can result in a variety of autoimmune sequelae, including autoimmune disease of the testis, ovary, thyroid, prostate, and stomach, suggesting that the neonatal T-cell repertoire is enriched with self-reactive T cells and

that such novel disease models may be powerful tools for examining and manipulating mechanisms of self tolerance of a wide variety of potential autoantigens.

Immune Therapies for Infertility

Different therapies have been used to treat the infertile couple who show antisperm antibodies identified in either the male or the female. **Condom therapy** has been advocated to reduce exposure to antigen in women with antisperm antibodies. Pregnancy rates following specified periods of condom use vary from 11% to 56%; however, most studies do not include proper control groups. In fact, one study has documented a 44% rate of spontaneous pregnancy in couples who rejected condom contraception as a means of achieving pregnancy. Attempts to **process semen or wash sperm** to reduce the amount of antibody present in the ejaculate has not improved pregnancy rates, and techniques to chemically dissociate antibodies from sperm result in irreversible loss of sperm motility.

Intrauterine insemination (in order to bypass antibody present in the cervical mucous), **corticosteroid therapy, in-vitro fertilization,** and **gamete intrafallopian transfer** have all been reported as successful therapies. Rare but serious and unpredictable complications, such as aseptic necrosis of the femur due to corticosteroids or anaphylactic shock after intrauterine insemination, can occur with these therapies, and none has been demonstrated effective in well-controlled, randomized trials. It would seem that the high spontaneous "cure" rate of this syndrome (that is, pregnancy without intervention), the difficulties involved in meaningful and standardized diagnostic evaluation of affected couples, and the large numbers of couples with unexplained infertility who might be subjected to these therapies would mandate such clinical trials in the near future. Until then, the detection of antisperm antibodies in couples with unexplained infertility can only be considered to be of unknown significance, and couples must be advised that prescribed treatments are of questionable benefit and carry the risk of serious complications.

RECURRENT SPONTANEOUS ABORTION

Background and Definitions

The occurrence of three or more spontaneous consecutive pregnancy losses defines this clinical syndrome. Given that a single clinically documented pregnancy carries a 15–20% chance of loss, some investigators believe that recurrent abortion is a chance phenomenon that occurs in 0.5% of the population, and most clinicians find that no cause can be found for the majority of repetitive losses. Other researchers contend that a cause can be found for losses in over 60% of affected couples. Fetal chromosomal abnormalities account for the largest share of repetitive losses, followed by uterine anatomic abnormalities, endometrial abnormalities, and hormonal abnormalities. Immunologic disorders have been cited as being associated with the large number of couples experiencing recurrent pregnancy loss for whom no specific cause is demonstrable. It is important to note that, for couples with unexplained recurrent pregnancy loss, 60% or more will eventually carry a pregnancy successfully to term with no therapeutic intervention.

HLA Sharing

A large body of literature has appeared in the last decade invoking HLA homozygosity between parents as a cause of pregnancy loss. In theory, HLA sharing has been said to lead to a decreased production of maternal "blocking" antibodies, which may appear in all successful pregnancies. Maternal blocking antibodies have been postulated as a factor needed to suppress the maternal immune response in order to allow survival of the fetal allograft. With limited studies to support such theories, some centers have advocated the immunization of women with paternal lymphocytes. One meta-analysis combining four randomized, controlled trials found that not only did each trial drop from their analysis all the women who received therapy and did not become pregnant, but also the aggregate success rates for immunotherapy were 48% compared with 60% for no treatment. Another recent meta-analysis by the Recurrent Miscarriage Trialists Group of data from 15 different centers around the world suggested an increase in the live birth rate from 60% in placebo-treated controls to 70% in women who received paternal leukocyte immunization, suggesting a modest beneficial effect of such therapy at most. Even those who advocate immunization cite a continuing lack of diagnostic tests to define patients who would most likely benefit from immunotherapy. Still it must be emphasized that because large, properly controlled clinical trials designed to study this treatment have not been performed, data have never existed to justify this "widely accepted" practice. Similarly, in the absence of such data, it has not been possible to discredit or eradicate its use. Serious complications can occur from paternal leukocyte immunization, and graft-versus-host-like reactions have been reported.

The **antiphospholipid antibody syndrome** was first described in the early 1950s in women who were noted to have prolonged bleeding times that were not correctable by addition of normal plasma, history of hypercoagulability, false-positive VDRL, and a history of recurrent pregnancy loss. In the following years, the lupus anticoagulant and the anticardiolipin antibody were characterized as acquired antibodies (IgG, IgA, or IgM), with specific activities against negatively charged phospholipids. They are thought to interfere with synthesis of the potent vasodilatory prostaglandin, prostacyclin, by endothelial cells, which theoretically would predispose to maternal

thrombosis and placental infarction resulting in placental insufficiency and pregnancy loss. For the lupus anticoagulant, diagnosis consists of prolongation of a phospholipid-dependent in vitro coagulation test, such as the activated partial thromboplastin time (aPTT) or the Russell viper venom time. Treatment has included prednisone (40–60 mg/day), low-dose aspirin (80 mg/day), and heparin therapies in varying combinations. Recent data suggest that heparin or prednisone plus aspirin result in greater numbers of viable offspring than no treatment; however, the use of heparin and aspirin alone may have lower morbidity for both mother and fetus.

In normal obstetric populations, one or other of these antibodies are seen in 2% of women tested; in referral populations of women with recurrent pregnancy loss, this figure may approach 15%. The antiphospholipid antibody syndrome, however, must be viewed as quite rare. More importantly, the presence of anticardiolipin antibody is of no significance in women without a history of recurrent (that is, at least three) pregnancy losses, and the presence the even rarer lupus anticoagulant is of unknown significance in women without clinical histories of recurrent thromboses and pregnancy losses. Even in the presence of such histories, patients must be advised that studies showing benefit of therapies have used largely historic controls (often the patients themselves) and are statistically seriously flawed or completely invalid.

Recurrent pregnancy loss and infertility are distressing problems that cause significant grief and suffering. Many couples presenting with these problems are panicked and desperate for a "cure." It is the duty of clinicians and scientists to thoroughly evaluate, educate, and protect these vulnerable individuals from empiric and potentially dangerous therapies whose benefits are largely unproved or have actually been disproved. In the case of therapies that may still be of value, the need for properly performed prospective trials has become imperative.

ISOIMMUNIZATION

HISTORIC BACKGROUND

Pathologic changes associated with **hydrops fetalis,** the syndrome of an abnormal, sometimes massive collection of fluid in fetal tissues, was characterized in the late nineteenth century. In 1932, the critical observation was made by L. K. Diamond that this syndrome was associated with fetal anemia and large numbers of circulating immature red blood cells **(erythroblasts),** and thus the concept of **erythroblastosis fetalis** was introduced. Subsequent characterization of hemolytic disease of the fetus and newborn, the discovery of the rhesus (**Rh;** also referred to as **D** of the CDE blood group system) factor in 1940, and ultimately the development of effective maternal anti-Rh prophylaxis in the early 1960s represent one of the great medical triumphs of the twentieth century. Today, the administration of anti-Rh immunoglobulin prophylaxis may seem routine; however, with the exception of immunization against infectious disease, no other immune therapy has had such a definitive and far-reaching effect on such a common and formerly devastating immune disorder.

PATHOPHYSIOLOGY OF ISOIMMUNE HYDROPS

The precise function of the Rh antigen is unknown. It is a polypeptide embedded in the lipid phase of the red blood cell membrane and may interact with a membrane adenosine triphosphatase (ATPase), functioning as part of a cation or proton pump to control fluid and electrolyte fluxes across the cell membrane. Any individual who lacks a specific red cell antigen is capable of producing antibody to that antigen. To a variable degree, every pregnancy is associated with the passage of fetal blood cells into the maternal circulation; most notably at the time of delivery or after maternal trauma, ectopic pregnancy, abortion, or invasive diagnostic procedures such as amniocentesis and chorionic villus sampling. Of course, isoimmunization can also be the result of transfusion of Rh-positive blood into an Rh-negative individual. Once Rh-positive blood has entered the circulation, a primary immune response may occur, and low levels of anti-Rh antibodies are detected in maternal serum. Significantly, the fetus is at most only mildly affected during a primary isoimmunization. It is the Rh-positive products of subsequent gestations that are at risk for severe compromise from maternally produced antibody.

For incompletely understood reasons, an unimmunized Rh-negative mother has only a 16% chance of becoming immunized against her Rh-positive fetus with any given pregnancy. Explanations that have been proposed include variable "antigenicity," insufficient transplacental passage of antigen, variable maternal response, and protection from isoimmunization by ABO blood type incompatibility (see following section).

Anti-Rh IgG antibodies do not fix complement. Rather, intact Rh-positive cells are apparently sequestered in the maternal spleen and lymph nodes where an anti-Rh immune response is generated or amplified, presumably initiated by processing and presentation of antigen by macrophages and other antigen-presenting cells (Fig 43–4). Once primary sensitization has occurred, subsequent Rh-positive pregnancies elicit a much more potent, secondary maternal immune response, and anti-Rh IgG gains access to the fetal circulation, where it is found bound to fetal red cells and free in serum. Accelerated red blood cell destruction ensues, leading to varying degrees of hemolysis and fetal anemia. Prolonged hemolysis results in erythroid hyperplasia of the bone marrow, extramedullary hematopoiesis in the fetal spleen and liver, and hydrops, which is characterized by varying degrees of hepatomegaly, splenomegaly, and placental edema. With severe hydrops, fatty degeneration, hemosiderin deposition, and engorgement of hepatic canaliculi may also be seen in the liver. Cardiac enlargement, pulmonary hemorrhage, and pleural and pericardial effusions may occur, in addition to massive ascites and subcutaneous edema, which result in severe dystocia. Hydrothorax can compromise neonatal respiratory status after birth.

The exact pathophysiology of progression from hemolysis and mild fetal anemia to the massively hydropic fetus still has not been fully characterized. Different investigators have attributed the cause of hydrops to high-output congestive heart failure secondary to profound anemia, portal and umbilical venous hypertension secondary to disruption of the hepatic parenchyma by extramedullary hematopoiesis, and decreased colloid osmotic pressure secondary to hepatic failure and disruption of capillary endothelial integrity due to anemia and hypoxia. Affected fetuses are subject to a wide range of clinical outcomes. If left untreated, hydropic fetuses may die in utero or in the early neonatal period. Less severely affected infants can appear well at birth and develop hyperbilirubinemia in the neonatal period due to loss of placental clearance of bilirubin from the fetal circulation. If untreated, this can lead to significant central nervous system damage, termed **kernicterus** in pathologic specimens.

ABO INCOMPATIBILITY

ABO hemolytic disease is more common and much milder than Rh disease. A and B antigens are frequently found in nature, and individuals lacking them on their red cells develop anti-A and anti-B antibodies early in life when they are exposed to similar antigens in their intestinal flora. Unlike anti-Rh, anti-A and anti-B bind complement. Whereas transfusion of ABO-incompatible blood produces life-threatening intravascular hemolysis, ABO incompatibility of mother and fetus does not result in an increased rate of stillbirth. ABO isoimmunization is considered a neonatal, not a fetal, problem. Although a firstborn can be affected, at its worst the disease results in moderate neonatal anemia and hyperbilirubinemia, for which management is quite straightforward.

Although 20% of infants have ABO maternal blood group incompatibility, only 5% of these show overt signs of hemolytic disease. Individuals with group A or B blood types produce predominantly IgM anti-B or anti-A, which does not cross the placenta, whereas type O individuals produce predominantly IgG. Also, there are fewer antigen sites on the fetal red cell than on the adult cell, and A and B antigens expressed in

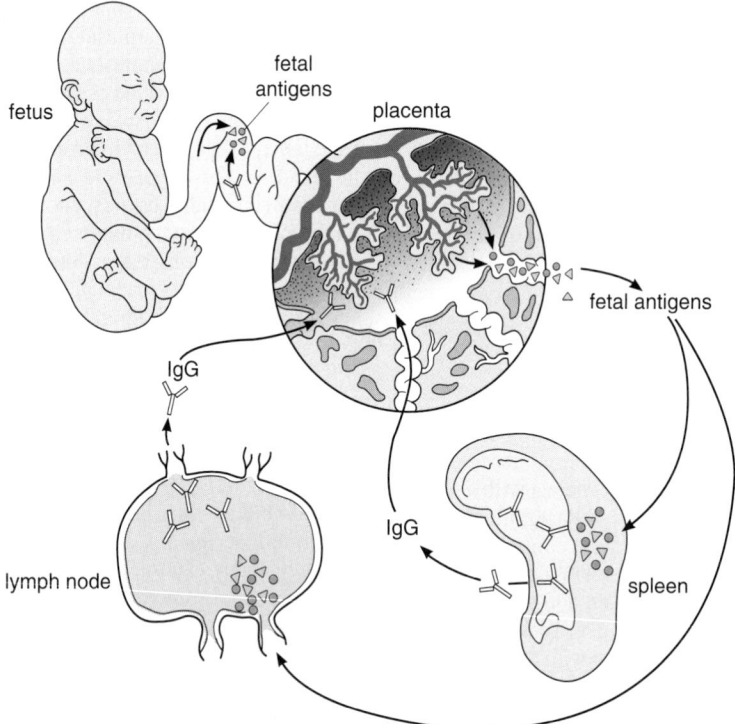

Figure 43–4. Maternal immune activation by fetal antigen. Fetal antigen escapes from or across trophoblast tissues in the placenta, to be sequestered in the maternal spleen or lymph nodes where an immune response is generated. Only maternal IgG can cross the placenta and affect fetal tissues.

other tissues may compete with the fetal erythrocyte for binding of antibody.

Interestingly, ABO incompatibility reduces the risk of Rh isoimmunization from 10–16% to 1.5–2% after delivery of an Rh-positive fetus. This effect is most pronounced in pregnancies in which the mother is type O and the father is type A, B, or AB. Two mechanisms may be responsible for this. At delivery, the number of fetal red blood cells detectable in the maternal circulation is lower in ABO-incompatible pregnancies than in ABO-compatible pregnancies, suggesting that there is increased clearance of ABO-incompatible fetal cells from the maternal circulation before they can be trapped in the maternal spleen and lymph nodes, where an immune response would be initiated. Alternatively, maternal anti-ABO antibody may damage or alter fetal Rh antigen so that it is no longer immunogenic.

ANTI-Rh Ig PROPHYLAXIS

The Use of Rh-Immune Globulin

The incidence of Rh isoimmunization has dramatically decreased in this country since the introduction of passive immunization of Rh-negative women after delivery of Rh-positive infants using anti-Rh immune

globulin (also known by its trade name, RhoGAM) (Fig 43–5). Because initial protocols calling for a single postpartum injection resulted in a low but significant incidence of prophylaxis failures, current recommendations are that anti-Rh immune globulin be administered to all pregnant Rh-negative women at 28 weeks gestation and again postpartum, if the neonate is found to be Rh-positive. In addition, prophylaxis is given at any time of pregnancy loss, ectopic pregnancy, maternal trauma, uterine bleeding, or other evidence of fetomaternal hemorrhage. Because platelets can express the Rh antigen, some researchers recommend prophylaxis for Rh-negative women after platelet transfusion. Following these guidelines, Rh isoimmunization rates should approach zero.

Mechanism of Prophylaxis

Development of Rh isoimmunization prophylaxis in the 1960s was based on the well-recognized phenomenon of antibody-mediated immune suppression (**AMIS**), in which passively administered antibody was known to prevent active immunization by its specific antigen. Even today the mechanism of the AMIS response is not completely understood. Three general theories have been proposed: antigen deviation or diversion; antigen blocking/competitive inhibition; and central inhibition. The first two theories are unsatis-

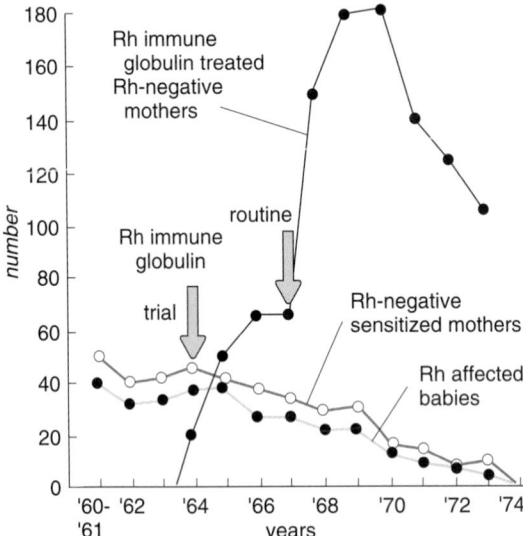

Figure 43–5. Incidence of Rh disease correlated with Rh immune globulin treatment during the years 1960 to 1974. A fairly constant number of sensitized mothers and affected infants was seen at the Columbia-Presbyterian Rh antepartum clinic prior to the first clinical trial with Rh immune globulin in 1964. Thereafter, a steady decline in the incidence of sensitization and hemolytic disease was seen annually. (Reproduced, with permission, from Freda VJ et al: *N Engl J Med* 1975;**292**:1014.)

factory. Although studies of ^{51}Cr-labeled Rh-positive red cells infused into Rh-negative volunteers have shown that Rh-immune globulin increases clearance of Rh-positive cells, the antigen itself is not destroyed. Rather, the intact antibody-coated cells are removed to the spleen or lymph nodes, where an immune response would normally be initiated. Antigen blocking cannot explain AMIS: first, less than 20% of available antigen is bound by Rh immune globulin; second, in murine models of immunization by sheep erythrocytes, F(ab)$'_2$ fragments, which bind avidly to sheep red blood cells, do not suppress the murine immune response, but whole antibody with an intact Fc region does.

Central inhibition may represent a plausible explanation for AMIS. Fetal red cells coated with anti-Rh are filtered out of the maternal circulation by the spleen and lymph nodes, where the increase in local concentration of complexes of anti-Rh antibody bound to Rh antigen is thought to suppress the primary immune response by interrupting T-helper cell-mediated clonal expansion of Rh-specific B cells. Again, the Fc region appears to be required for AMIS; neither F(ab) or F(ab)$'_2$ fragments are effective. This model also is consistent with the observation that neither AMIS nor Rh immune globulin prophylaxis inhibits secondary immune responses.

MANAGEMENT OF THE ISOIMMUNIZED PREGNANCY

Eradication of Rh disease will be achieved by prophylaxis, not by treatment of isoimmunization. Nevertheless, with the dramatically decreased but still significant occurrence of isoimmunization to the Rh antigen and more importantly to the comparatively rare "minor," or "atypical" erythrocyte antigens for which there is no prophylaxis, technologic innovations in the fields of fetal diagnosis and treatment have become exceedingly important.

Screening maternal serum for erythrocyte antibodies is a cornerstone of modern prenatal care. When a low titer of antired cell antibody is first detected in the current pregnancy and remains stable, patients can simply be followed. Even when titers are rising, if the involved antigen is not a proven cause of hemolytic disease of the newborn (such as anti-Lewis), no intervention is necessary. However, if titers of a potentially serious antibody (in addition to anti-Rh this includes the common atypical antibodies: anti-E, anti-Kell, anti-c, anti-c+E, or anti-Fy^a) are detected in a second affected pregnancy or if markedly rising titers are detected in a first pregnancy, more aggressive intervention is warranted. Although diagnostic and treatment protocols are not yet standard, techniques available to most practitioners in major medical centers, such as amniocentesis for DOD^{450} of amniotic fluid (an indirect reflection of severity of disease and fetal anemia), sampling of umbilical cord blood in utero for fetal blood typing and direct fetal hematocrit, and fetal blood transfusion (either intraperitoneally or intravascularly into the fetal umbilical vein), have revolutionized the treatment and prognosis for severely affected isoimmunized fetuses.

NEONATAL ALLOIMMUNE THROMBOCYTOPENIA

Platelet isoimmunization, most commonly against the P1^{A1} antigen is a rare syndrome (less than 0.1% of births) and is analogous to Rh isoimmunization in that the mother forms IgG antibodies to antigen present in paternal and fetal platelets. These antibodies cross the placenta and result in increase platelet sequestration and destruction.

As with Rh isoimmunization, there is a wide range of clinical manifestations. Some infants are mildly affected with only petechiae noted at birth; others present with severe hemorrhage (particularly intracranial), which can lead to neonatal death.

Unlike Rh disease, the firstborn infant can be affected, suggesting that platelet antigen has greater access to the maternal circulation than red cell antigen. Postnatally, therapy is directed at treatment and prevention of hemorrhage. If a couple has previously had a severely affected infant, antenatal diagnostic fetal cord blood sampling may be performed. In utero therapy has been suggested. Although maternal steroid therapy has no place here, maternal infusion of high-dose immunoglobulin G may raise the fetal platelet count, and platelet transfusion into the umbilical vein has been reported. Because this syndrome is rare, the utility of these interventions has not yet been completely evaluated.

HIV INFECTION AND THE REPRODUCTIVE SYSTEM

HETEROSEXUAL TRANSMISSION OF HUMAN IMMUNODEFICIENCY VIRUS

As a disease among women, acquired immunodeficiency syndrome (AIDS) was largely invisible until the late 1980s. Even up to the present day, most research on the disease has focused on adult males whose source of infection was most likely to be homosexual contact or intravenous drug use. Until it became apparent that growing numbers of women were being infected sexually, and that the overwhelming majority of these were of reproductive age, who, when pregnant, were choosing to maintain their pregnancies, the reproductive health aspects of human immunodeficiency virus (HIV) infection and AIDS were not raised as a research priority.

In the United States today, heterosexual transmission of HIV-1 is the most rapidly rising cause of new infection, and women are being infected at a higher frequency than men. Worldwide, heterosexual contact is responsible for 70–80% of HIV infection, despite the inefficiency of this mode of transmission. Whereas one in four individuals exposed to *Neisseria gonorrhoeae* or hepatitis B develop disease, it is estimated that for a single contact, the infectivity of HIV-1 is 0.3%. Still, some individuals become infected after a single or few sexual contacts. Several cofactors have been found to increase the risk of acquiring disease through heterosexual contact. In the United States, male-to-female transmission is more efficient than female to male. It is generally agreed that compromise and alteration of vaginal mucosal immunity appear to have a significant influence on disease transmission. For example, postcoital bleeding, cervical ectopy (that is, migration of glandular endocervical epithelium from the endocervix to the ectocervix), lack of circumcision, genital ulcer disease, and infection with other sexually transmitted diseases have all been shown to be cofactors associated with transmission. In addition, receptive anal intercourse increases the risk of male-to-female dissemination of disease.

Infectivity appears to vary between specific HIV strains, and clinical stage of disease directly influences the amount of viral shedding in secretions.

Susceptibility may be influenced by such unique factors as nutritional status, stage of menstrual cycle, or pregnancy. Both cell-associated and cell-free HIV are present in the cervicovaginal secretions and semen of asymptomatic HIV-infected individuals and AIDS patients. The fate of HIV-infected cells in ejaculate in the vagina is unknown. It is unlikely that infected cells can cross intact vaginal mucosa, and due to low vaginal pH, normal vaginal flora, lysozyme, and proteinases, latently infected cells in the ejaculate are unlikely to survive long enough to produce infectious virions, so that only cells producing infectious HIV particles at the time of inoculation are thought likely to contribute to sexual transmission.

The cellular targets of HIV during genital transmission are unknown. Since only a few CD4 T cells are present in the vaginal submucosa, the most likely targets are macrophages and Langerhans' cells. Cervical biopsies from HIV-infected women show no evidence of epithelial cell infection by HIV. CD4-positive, class-II-bearing Langerhans' cells, dendritic cells, and macrophages present in the vaginal mucosa and submucosa may have a role in the sexual transmission of the virion (Fig 43–6). As antigen-presenting cells, they are well suited to disseminate virus from the mucosa to draining lymph nodes. In vitro, they have been shown to produce virus without exhibiting the cytopathic effects typical of T-cell infection. Thus, it is likely that infection and initial viral replication occurs in these local target cells, followed by further replication in draining lymph nodes before spread to more distant lymphoid tissues. There has been considerable speculation regarding the association of tissue trauma with spread of disease. It is unlikely that virus can gain direct entry into the bloodstream via breaks in the vaginal mucosa. Rather, it is more probable that blood cells (including CD4 T cells) escaping from the vasculature do not reenter the bloodstream but instead travel the same route as Langerhans' cells and macrophages, through the lymphatics to draining lymph nodes. Trauma and infection are likely to be associated with increased numbers of CD4 target cells in genital tissues and thus increase the efficiency of HIV transmission; these conditions, however, are unlikely to alter the route of infection.

Recent studies by A. I. Spira and colleagues of acute simian immunodeficiency virus (SIV) infection have yielded important insights into the sexual transmission of HIV-1. Four female rhesus macaques were inoculated intravaginally with the SIV mac251 strain. In situ polymerase chain reaction (PCR) amplification performed on tissue sections collected during the first 9 days after inoculation showed no evidence of infection of the epithelium itself. By day 2, evidence of infection appeared in cells of the lamina propria close to the basement membrane of stratified squamous epithelium of the vagina and ectocervix and the simple columnar epithelium of the endocervix. These submucosal cells had processes characteristic of antigen-

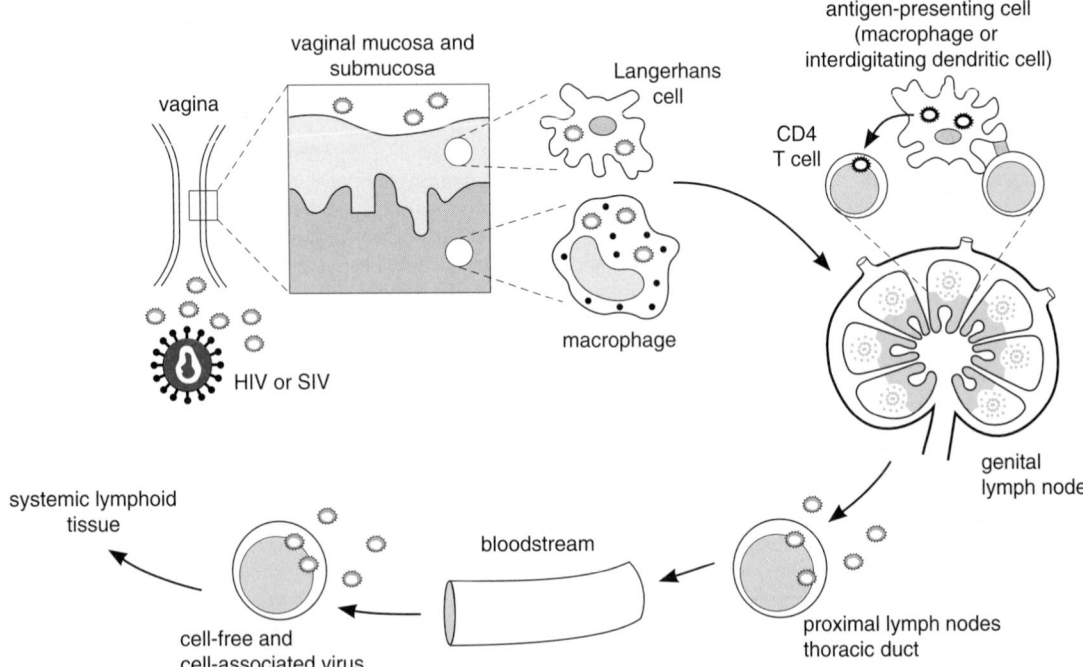

Figure 43–6. Viral dissemination during the genital transmission of HIV. This hypothetical model depicts viral contact with the genital mucosa and infection of target cells, presumably macrophages or Langerhans' cell in the vaginal submucosa. Infected target cells move through lymphatic vessels to draining lymph nodes, enter the CD4 T-cell-rich lymph node paracortex, and present processed antigen, thus initiating an immune response. Viral replication occurs in the lymph node. Cell-free and cell-associated virus then travel via efferent lymphatics to proximal lymph nodes and the thoracic duct into the bloodstream, ultimately resulting in systemic infection. (Reproduced, with permission, from Miller CH et al: *Lab Invest* 1992;**68:**129.)

presenting cells, contained class II antigens, but did not contain CD68, suggesting that they were dendritic cells or dendritic/T-cell syncytia. Provirus was detected in draining internal iliac lymph nodes by day 2, and in peripheral lymph nodes by day 5. Thus, it appears that productively infected submucosal dendritic cells are capable of quick dissemination of the virus to draining lymph nodes followed by systemic dissemination shortly thereafter.

The question remains: if cells of the epithelium are not infected, how does HIV reach the lamina propria? Indeed, this group's observations reflect the inefficiency of HIV-1 transmission, prompting the researchers to suggest that transepithelial transport of HIV-1 is an important rate-limiting factor of HIV-1 transmission efficiency. In addition, they observed that viruses that can demonstrably infect epithelial cells, such as poliovirus, herpesvirus, and rhinovirus, are much more efficiently transmitted than HIV.

Current studies are aimed at demonstrating permeation of epithelium by free virus, Langerhans' cell binding and transport of virus, epithelial disruption by inoculation, and mechanisms not yet observed in the vagina that might be similar to intestinal M-cell transport of virus across epithelial cell barriers.

PERINATAL TRANSMISSION OF HIV

The rate of transmission of HIV from mother to infant varies widely. Diagnosis of HIV infection in the neonate is difficult since serologic studies are biased by the presence of maternally derived antibodies in neonatal serum. Prevalence studies of neonatal infection are based primarily on PCR and virus culture studies and have yielded rates of 11–60% transmission in different parts of the world. For diagnosis in the individual patient, it should be remembered that PCR is quite sensitive but can lack specificity, and virus culture is time-consuming and difficult to perform routinely. Transfer of HIV from mother to infant can occur in utero or after delivery. Even though HIV has been isolated from umbilical cord blood, amniotic fluid, placenta, and other fetal tissues, there is considerable disagreement in the literature about the frequency of HIV infection of fetal tissues. Some investigators find no virus in fetal tissues; others report detection of HIV genomic sequences in 30% of second-trimester abortuses, virtually identical to newborn transmission rates, and conclude that most vertical transmission occurs early in gestation. On the other hand, an observed delay in the ability to isolate

HIV from neonatal serum until after 1 month of life suggests to some that transmission is most likely to occur at parturition, secondary to maternal–fetal transfusion, or fetal exposure to maternal secretions and blood during the delivery process.

Cesarean section has not been shown to alter rates of transmission in the United States, but several European studies suggest a protective effect of abdominal delivery. Although HIV infection via breast milk is considered rare, it has been documented and has been particularly prominent in infants of mothers who are primarily infected postpartum.

The mechanism of in utero transmission of HIV is not understood. Transmission may correlate with absence of maternal antibody to the viral envelope, especially to the third variable region of gp120. Low maternal CD4 counts, maternal viral burden, and p24 antigenemia have all been reported to be associated with vertical transmission. Although HIV has been detected in fetal and placental tissues by in situ hybridization, PCR, and immunohistochemistry, identification of viral particles in highly purified primary trophoblast culture has not yet been reported. In vitro, however, trophoblast cultures and human choriocarcinoma cell lines have been successfully infected by virus or virus-infected cells. The CD4 receptor is identified in some cell populations studied, however, significant literature exists suggesting that infection of the trophoblast can occur independently of the CD4-mediated pathway. Whatever the case, only low-level viral replication can be detected in these in vitro infected cells.

Given transplacental transmission of HIV, the exact route and mechanism of disease induction in the fetus is not clear. After 16–20 weeks gestation, mature T cells can be identified in fetal tissues and CD4, CD8 double-positive T-cell precursors are found even earlier. If early fetal infection occurs, it is unclear why entire T-cell populations with ab receptors are not eliminated. Different investigators speculate that infected T-cell precursors could go on to differentiate while latently infected; alternatively, transmission may occur much later in pregnancy.

PEDIATRIC HIV-1 INFECTIONS

Whatever the mode of transmission, the incubation period for perinatally acquired infection is comparatively short, with early-onset and late-onset patterns of disease presentation being reported. The early-onset group of infected infants develops disease early in life, between 3 and 8 months of age, and have a high mortality rate. For example, for infants in whom HIV is first diagnosed with *Pneumocystis carinii* pneumonia infection, median survival is 1 month; survival is somewhat longer with other initial presentations such as recurrent bacterial infections (50 months) and lobar interstitial pneumonia (72 months). Late-onset disease presents in older children and has a comparatively indolent course, closely resembling a lymphoproliferative disorder. Both late- and early-onset disease are commonly complicated by recurrent bacterial infections, ranging from recurrent otitis media to fulminant bacterial meningitis or pneumonia.

It is now clear that antiretroviral therapy can lower the rate of vertical infection of fetuses and neonates by their HIV-1-infected mothers. The AIDS Clinical Trial Group protocol 076 showed that perinatal transmission was reduced from 25% in placebo-treated controls to 8% when zidovudine was administered to mothers prenatally, intrapartum and to babies in the neonatal period. Further data have appeared to show that viral burden may be highly correlated with vertical transmission rates. Studies of combination drug therapy during pregnancy aimed at decreasing viral burden are only now being initiated. Unfortunately, it seems quite apparent that any such therapies will be out of reach for the vast majority of perinatally infected children, those who live in developing countries where children make up 5–25% of HIV-infected populations.

CONCLUSION

As Medawar noted in 1952, and is still true today, every well-authenticated, clinically significant example of an immunization of the mother by its fetus has implicated antigen derived from either the red blood cell or platelet. Antigens responsible for the rapid and violent reactions provoked by grafting tissues from one individual to another are not part of maternal–fetal interactions. Even with isoimmunization, the challenging question has become not how it occurs, but why it does not occur more often. As with infectious processes, we know that this wrinkle, as it were, in the maternal immune response is located in inductive pathways: once immunized or isoimmunized, pregnancy does not modify a host's response to offending antigen. Precise characterization of the immunobiology of the maternal–fetal relationship properly begins with the detailed examination of the trophoblast and the tissues that it touches; further insight will be gained by attempts to understand the interactions of these tissues in light of contemporary cellular and molecular immunologic models.

REFERENCES

GENERAL

Gill TJ et al (editors): *Immunoregulation and Fetal Survival.* Oxford University Press, 1987.

Grimes DA: Technology follies: The uncritical acceptance of medical innovation. *JAMA* 1993;**269**:3030.

Medawar PB: Some immunological and endocrinological problems raised by the evolution of viviparity in vertebrates. *Symp Soc Exp Biol* 1953;**7**:320.

Strauss JF, Lyttle CR (editors): *Uterine and Embryonic Factors in Early Pregnancy.* Plenum Press, 1991.

REPRODUCTIVE TRACT ANATOMY AND IMMUNITY

Bulmer D: The histochemistry of ovarian macrophages in the rat. *J Anat Lond* 1964;**98**:313.

Edwards JNT, Morris HB: Langerhans' cells and lymphocyte subsets in the female genital tract. *Br J Obstet Gynaecol* 1985;**92**:974.

Kutteh WH, Mestecky J: Secretory immunity in the female reproductive tract. *Am J Reprod Immunol* 1994;**31**:40.

Miller CH et al: Mucosal immunity, HIV transmission, and AIDS. *Lab Invest* 1992;**68**:129.

Ogra PL, Swtantarta SO: Local antibody response to poliovaccine in the human female genital tract. *J Immunol* 1973;**110**:1307.

OVULATION AND SPERMATOGENESIS

Adashi EY: Cytokine-mediated regulation of ovarian function: Encounters of a third kind. *Endocrinology* 1989;**124**:2043.

Adashi EY: Editorial: With a little help from my friends— The evolving story of intraovarian regulation. *Endocrinology* 1995;**136**:4161.

Hurwitz A et al: Interleukin-1 is both morphogenic and cytotoxic to cultured rat ovarian cells: Obligatory role for heterologous, contact-independent cell–cell interaction. *Endocrinology* 1992;**131**:1643.

Kol S, Adashi EY: Intraovarian factors regulating ovarian function. *Curr Opin Obstet Gynecol* 1995;**7**:209.

Yule TD et al: Role of testicular autoantigens and influence of lymphokines in testicular autoimmune disease. *J Reprod Immunol* 1990;**18**:89.

FERTILIZATION, IMPLANTATION, AND THE IMMUNE RESPONSE TO FETAL TISSUES

Castellucci M, Kaufmann P: A three-dimensional study of the normal human placental villous core: II. Stromal architecture. *Placenta* 1982;**3**:269.

Haimovici F et al: The effects of soluble products of activated lymphocytes and macrophages on blastocyst implantation events in vitro. *Biol Reprod* 1991;**44**:69.

Paria BC, Dey SK: Preimplantation embryo development in vitro: Cooperative interactions among embryos and role of growth factors. *Proc Natl Acad Sci USA* 1990;**87**:4756.

Pijnenborg R et al: Trophoblast invasion and the establishment of haemochorial placentation in man and laboratory animals. *Placenta* 1981;**2**:71.

Saling PM: Mammalian sperm interaction with extracellular matrices of the egg. *Oxf Rev Reprod Biol* 1989;**11**:339.

Stewart CL et al: Blastocyst implantation depends on maternal expression of leukemia inhibitory factor. *Nature* 1992;**359**:76.

Wassarman PM: Mouse gamete adhesion molecules. *Biol Reprod* 1992;**46**:186.

IMMUNITY IN PREGNANCY

Castellucci M et al: Mitosis of the Hofbauer cell: Possible implications for a fetal macrophage. *Placenta* 1987;**8**:65.

Hunt JS et al: Evaluation of human chorionic trophoblast cells and placental macrophages as stimulators of maternal lymphocyte proliferation in vitro. *J Reprod Immunology* 1984;**6**:377.

Khayr WF et al: Listeriosis: Review of a protean disease. *Infect Dis Clin Pract* 1992;**1**:291.

Lu CY et al: Pregnancy as a natural model of allograft tolerance. *Transplantation* 1989;**48**:848.

McLean JM et al: Changes in the thymus, spleen and lymph nodes during pregnancy and lactation in the rat. *J Anat* 1974;**118**:223.

Redline RW, Lu CY: Role of local immunosuppression in murine fetoplacental listeriosis. *J Clin Invest* 1987;**79**:1234.

Redline RW, Lu CY: Specific defects in the anti-listerial immune response in discrete regions of the murine uterus and placenta account for susceptibility to infection. *J Immunol* 1988;**140**:3947.

Rocklin RE et al: Immunobiology of the maternal–fetal relationship. *Ann Rev Med* 1979;**30**:375.

Sridama V et al: Decreased levels of helper T cells: A possible cause of immunodeficiency in pregnancy. *N Engl J Med* 1982;**307**:352.

Weinberg ED: Pregnancy-associated depression of cell mediated immunity. *Rev Infect Dis* 1984;**6**:814.

INFERTILITY AND SPONTANEOUS ABORTION

Dudley DJ: Recurrent pregnancy loss and cytokines: Not as simple as it seems. *JAMA* 1995;**273**:1958.

Fraser EJ et al: Immunization as therapy for recurrent spontaneous abortion: A review and meta-analysis. *Obstet Gynecol* 1993;**82**:854.

Haas GG: Immunologic infertility. *Obstet Gynecol Clin North Am* 1987;**14**:1069.

Katz I et al: Cutaneous graft-versus-host-like reaction after paternal lymphocyte immunization for prevention of recurrent abortion. *Fertil Steril* 1992;**57**:927.

Kutteh WH et al: Antisperm antibodies: Current knowledge and new horizons. *Mol Androl* 1993;**4**:183.

Kutteh WH, Carr BR: Recurrent pregnancy loss. In: *Textbook of Reproductive Medicine,* Carr BR, Blackwell Richard E (editors). Appleton & Lange, 1993.

Luo AM et al: Antigen mimicry in autoimmune disease sharing of amino acid residues critical for pathogenic T cell activation. *J Clin Invest* 1993;**92**:2117.

Mishell DR: Infertility. In: *Comprehensive Gynecology.* Herbst AL et al (editors). Mosby Year Book, 1992, pp 1189–1243.

Recurrent Miscarriage Immunotherapy Trialists Group: Worldwide collaborative observational study and meta-analysis on allogeneic leukocyte immunotherapy for recurrent spontaneous abortion. *Am J Reprod Immunol* 1994;**32**:55.

Tung KSK, Lu CY: Immunologic basis of reproductive failure. In: *Pathology of Reproductive Failure.* Kraus FT et al (editors). Williams and Wilkins, 1992, pp 308–333.

Vazquez-Levin M et al: The effect of female antisperm antibodies on in vitro fertilization, early embryonic development, and pregnancy outcome. *Fertil Steril* 1991;**56:**84.

ISOIMMUNIZATION

Branch DW, Scott JR: Isoimmunization in pregnancy. In: *Obstetrics: Normal and Problem Pregnancies.* Gabbe SG et al (editors). Churchill Livingstone, 1991, pp 957–990.

Cunningham FG et al: Hemolysis from isoimmunization. In *Williams Obstetrics* Appleton and Lange, 1989, pp 599–609.

Freda VJ et al: Prevention of Rh hemolytic disease–Ten years' clinical experience with Rh immune globulin. *N Engl J Med* 1975;**292:**1014.

Pollack W: Recent understanding for the mechanism by which passively administered Rh antibody suppresses the immune response to Rh antigen in unimmunized Rh-negative women. *Clin Obstet Gynecol* 1982;**25:**255.

HIV INFECTION, THE REPRODUCTIVE SYSTEM, AND VERTICAL TRANSMISSION

Connor EM et al: Reduction of maternal–infant transmission of human immunodeficiency virus type 1 with zidovudine treatment. *New Engl J Med* 1994;**331:**1173.

Dickover RE et al: Identification of levels of maternal HIV-1 RNA associated with risk of perinatal transmission. Effect of maternal zidovudine treatment on viral load. *JAMA* 1996;**275:**599.

Levy JA: Pathogenesis of human immunodeficiency virus infection. *Microbiol Rev* 1993;**57:**183.

Mestecky J et al: Mucosal immunity in the female genital tract: Relevance to vaccination efforts against the human immunodeficiency virus. *AIDS Res Hum Retroviruses* 1994;**10,**(supp 2):S11.

Miller CH et al: Mucosal immunity, HIV transmission, and AIDS. *Lab Invest* 1992;**68:**129.

Oxtoby MJ: Vertically acquired HIV infection in the United States. In: *Pediatric AIDS: The Challenge of HIV Infection in Infants, Children, and Adolescents,* 2nd ed. Pizzo PA, Wilfert CM (editors), Williams and Wilkins, 1994, pp 3–20.

Spira AI et al: Cellular targets of infection and route of viral dissemination after an intravaginal inoculation of simian immunodeficiency virus into Rhesus macaques. *J Exp Med* 1996;**183:**215.

Mechanisms of Tumor Immunology

44

Philip D. Greenberg, MD

Tumor immunology is the study of (1) the antigenic properties of transformed cells, (2) the host immune responses to these tumor cells, (3) the immunologic consequences to the host of the growth of malignant cells, and (4) the means by which the immune system can be modulated to recognize tumor cells and promote tumor eradication. One potentially important function of the immune system is to provide protection from the outgrowth of malignant cells. This represents a formidable task because tumor cells have many similarities to normal cells, despite exhibiting abnormal propensities to proliferate, to spread throughout the host, and to interfere with normal organ functions. Thus, tumor cells present special problems to the host's immune system beyond those presented by other self-replicating antigens such as bacteria, which can more easily be distinguished as foreign.

Normal cells have a variable capacity to proliferate and to express differentiated functions. These cell activities are tightly coordinated within an organ or tissue, so that the rate of cell loss due to the natural death of mature differentiated cells is equal to the rate of appearance of new cells from the less mature proliferating cell pool. In some pathologic conditions, the stimulus for cell proliferation exceeds the requirement for cell replacement, resulting in organ hypertrophy from polyclonal expansion of cells proliferating in response to growth signals. Once the condition responsible for excess stimulation of cell growth terminates, however, the rate of cell proliferation decreases and the organ hypertrophy resolves. In contrast to this nonmalignant, regulated polyclonal cell growth, an individual cell may undergo a transforming event and acquire the potential to produce daughter cells that proliferate independent of external growth signals. The autonomous growth of such transformed cells of monoclonal origin represents the basis of malignant disease. Many of the properties of tumor cells are summarized in Table 44–1. The protean effects of cancer reflect in large part the unrestrained growth of

Table 44–1. Common properties of tumor cells.

1. Failure to respond to the regulatory signals responsible for normal growth and tissue repair.
2. Autonomous growth without an absolute requirement for exogenous growth signals.
3. Invasive growth through normal tissue boundaries.
4. Metastatic growth in distant organs following entry into blood and lymph channels.
5. Monoclonal origin, although genotypic and phenotypic heterogeneity may develop as tumor mass increases.
6. Differences in appearance and membrane antigenic display from nontransformed cells of the same tissue origin.

tumor cells that locally invade and disrupt normal tissue as well as metastasize and grow in distant organs.

DEVELOPMENT OF TUMORS

The transformation of a normal cell to a malignancy can result from a variety of different causes, the particular nature of which helps determine if the immune system will effectively control the outgrowth of the tumor cells. These transforming events may occur spontaneously by random mutations or gene rearrangements; alternatively, they may be induced by a chemical, physical, or viral carcinogen.

Tumors induced by chemical carcinogens were initially described in the eighteenth century, when chimney sweeps were observed to have an unusually high incidence of carcinoma of the scrotum. Polycyclic aromatic hydrocarbons in soot and tar have since been found to be a major class of carcinogens, and retention of tar in the wrinkles of the scrotum was apparently responsible for these tumors. In fact, painting tar on epithelial cells has become a useful experimental technique for inducing tumors in the laboratory. A second major class of carcinogens, the aromatic amines, was identified following the observation of a high frequency of bladder cancer among factory workers using aniline dyes. The mechanisms by which chemical carcinogens induce neoplastic transformation predominantly reflect the mutagenic activity of these compounds.

Evidence of tumor induction by physical carcinogens accrued rapidly following the discovery of x-rays and radioactivity in the late nineteenth century when many of the early radiologists developed skin cancer. The most dramatic evidence of radiation-induced carcinogenesis has been in survivors of the atomic bomb explosions in Japan, who demonstrated an increased incidence of a wide range of tumors for more than 20 years after the nuclear holocaust. Such ionizing radiation directly injures cellular DNA, resulting in mutations, chromosomal breaks, and abnormal rearrangements. Another physical carcinogen, ultraviolet radiation, induces skin cancer on sun-exposed parts of the body, particularly in people with xeroderma pigmentosum, a disease in which there is a defective repair mechanism for ultraviolet-induced damage to DNA.

Viral oncogenesis is of particular interest in tumor immunology because of the great likelihood that cells transformed by the introduction of viral genes will express new virus-associated antigens that can be recognized by the immune system. Oncogenic viruses can be subdivided into either DNA or RNA types, depending on the genetic information carried by the intact virus. Most cells infected by the potentially oncogenic DNA viruses, which include papovaviruses, herpesviruses, and adenoviruses, express all of the viral genes and support viral replication, which commonly results in cell lysis. Infection of nonpermissive cells, however, can result in integration of viral DNA into the host genome and expression of only some viral genes, so that lytic virus particles are not formed. Transformation results either from direct triggering of host genes by the integrated viral DNA or from aberrant splicing of transcribed viral RNA to produce new proteins that promote transformation. Several human DNA viruses have been found to contain potential oncogenes and have been associated with the development of malignancies. These include links between Epstein-Barr virus (EBV) and Burkitt's lymphoma, Hodgkin's disease and nasopharyngeal carcinoma, and human papillomavirus and cervical anogenital and skin carcinomas.

Oncogenic RNA viruses contain genes for a polymerase called **reverse transcriptase,** which permits the use of the viral RNA as a template for transcription of a DNA copy, which can be integrated into the host genome. Because this is a reversal of the normal DNA-to-RNA transcription of genetic information, these viruses are often referred to as **retroviruses.** RNA tumor viruses, which were first discovered in chicken tumors, appear to be responsible for a large number of naturally occurring cancers in many species. Some of these viruses contain directly transforming oncogenes, whereas others must activate host genetic material. A class of human retroviruses, the human T-cell leukemia viruses (HTLV), are responsible for a subset of T-cell leukemias, particularly cases occurring in a region of southern Japan where the infection is endemic. Many retroviruses, such as feline leukemia virus and HTLV, can spread horizontally from infected to normal hosts, and resistance to tumorigenesis results in part from the generation of an immune response to virus-associated antigens in exposed resistant hosts.

Advances in molecular biology have provided the tools to better understand the events involved in transformation. Analogues to many of the viral oncogenes have been identified in the normal cellular genome, and in vitro studies have demonstrated that activation of these cellular oncogenes can transform normal cells under appropriate conditions. The essential role of many cellular oncogenes in normal growth and development has been demonstrated, but the abnormal maintenance of these genes in an active state can result in transformation. This may occur by mutation, such as ones that interfere with regulation of the transcription or of the activity of the protein; by a translocation that places the oncogene next to an active cellular gene, such as is observed in B-cell tumors with the translocation of the c-*myc* oncogene next to an immunoglobulin V region gene; or by insertion of an active promoter that enhances expression, such as may occur following integration of a slowly transforming retrovirus. Oncogenes code for a wide variety of products including membrane receptors, autocrine growth factors, and regulators of cell cycle progression and gene expression. The expression of at least some of these oncogene products, particularly those representing mutations of the normal protein, can render malignant cells sufficiently disparate from normal cells for detection by immunologic methods and potentially for elimination by immunologically directed attack.

ANTIGENS ON TUMOR CELLS

The field of tumor immunology is based in large part on the supposition that tumors express antigens that permit immunologic separation of malignant from normal cells. Problems in the past demonstrating the immunogenicity of tumor cells in the host of origin led to a great deal of skepticism. More recent efforts, however, have taken advantage of advances in cellular and molecular immunology and convincingly demonstrated that many human tumors express antigens that can induce cellular and humoral responses in the host, as well as elucidated many of the reasons underlying the ineffective and often undetectable response in the primary host. The relevant tumor antigens fall into two major categories. **Unique tumor-specific antigens** are found only on tumor cells and therefore represent ideal targets for an immunologic attack. In contrast, **tumor-associated determinants** are found on tumor cells and also on some normal cells, but qualitative and quantitative differences in antigen expression permit the use of these antigens to distinguish tumor cells from normal cells.

A wide variety of cellular proteins have now been identified to function as tumor antigens. Many distinct molecular mechanisms may result in the production of a tumor antigen. The most straightforward is a transforming event resulting in the production of a new protein, such as would occur following infection with a potentially oncogenic virus such as EBV, HTLV, or human papillomavirus (HPV). Similarly, point mutations or gene rearrangements affecting cellular oncogenes that promote the transformed phenotype, such as reported with *ras* and p53 in breast and colon cancer or bcr-*abl* in chronic myelogenous leukemia, can result in the expression of new epitopes potentially recognizable by the immune system. Unique tumor antigens can also result from uncovering normally nonexposed determinants, as observed with some complex branching glycolipid antigens in which deletion of a branch exposes a new antigenic determinant. Nonunique proteins that may nevertheless serve as tumor antigens can result from the aberrant expression of fetal or differentiation antigens, such as that observed with the expression on human gastric carcinoma cells of ABO blood group antigens disparate from the host ABO blood type or of the melanoma-associated gene (MAGE) antigens in human melanoma cells.

Unique Tumor Antigens

These are antigens that can be detected only on tumor cells and not on other host cells. The best studied unique tumor antigens are the new antigens expressed on tumors induced in inbred mice by oncogenic viruses and chemical carcinogens. Identification of the presence of unique tumor antigens has been difficult with human tumors because of the inability to perform classic tumor transplantation studies but has now become feasible owing to advances in molecular biology. Thus, human retroviruses such as HTLV have been isolated, viral proteins expressed in the tumor identifice, and the unique viral antigens demonstrated to be potentially immunogenic. "Spontaneous" tumors, many of which may have actually been induced by exposure to environmental carcinogens, have no predictable antigenic markers and therefore have been harder to study. Technologic advances have also occurred in lymphocyte isolation and culture, however, and made it possible to expand low-frequency antigen-reactive T cells and antibody-forming cells from tumor-bearing hosts. Thus, tumor-specific T cells and antibodies have been isolated from tumor-draining lymph nodes of patients with melanoma, breast cancer, leukemia, lymphoma, and lung cancer, as well as from lymph nodes following immunization with human colon carcinoma cells in association with an immunoadjuvant. Such tumor-reactive cells and antibodies have been used as immunologic reagents to screen expression

libraries derived from tumor cells to characterize the target antigens.

Elucidation of the processing pathways for presentation of protein antigens in association with major histocompatibility complex (MHC) molecules to T cells has revolutionized our understanding of the potential origin of unique tumor-specific antigens. T cells recognize small peptides derived from intracellular degradation of proteins that are inserted into a peptide-binding cleft in the MHC molecule and are then transported with the MHC molecule to the cell surface (see Chapter 6). Therefore, any abnormal cellular protein, not just proteins detected on the membrane, is a potential immunogen. Thus, the presence in a tumor cell of a truncated or nonfunctional protein product of a mutated allele could result in the immunogenicity of that product. Moreover, the difficulties previously encountered in detecting unique antigens on human tumors with monoclonal antibodies now appear to be predictable; the results do not imply that these tumors do not express unique antigens but, rather, that the use of molecular approaches to probe gene expression rather than surface phenotype are more likely to be productive.

Tumor-Associated Antigens

Although it may not be possible to detect unique tumor antigens on all tumors, many tumors display antigens that distinguish them from normal cells. These tumor-associated antigens may be expressed by some normal cells at particular stages of differentiation, but the quantitative expression or the composite expression in association with other lineage or differentiation markers can be useful for identifying transformed cells. The identification of tumor-associated antigens progressed rapidly with the advent of technology for generating and screening monoclonal antibodies. These monoclonal antibody reagents have permitted the isolation and biochemical characterization of the antigens and have been invaluable diagnostically for distinguishing transformed from nontransformed cells and for definition of the cell lineage of transformed cells.

The best characterized human tumor-associated antigens are the oncofetal antigens. These antigens are expressed during embryogenesis but are absent or very difficult to detect in normal adult tissue. The prototype antigen is **carcinoembryonic antigen (CEA),** a glycoprotein found on fetal gut and human colon cancer cells but not on normal adult colon cells. Since CEA is shed from colon carcinoma cells and found in the serum, it was originally thought that the presence of this antigen in the serum could be used to screen patients for colon cancer. It soon became apparent, however, that patients with inflammatory lesions involving cells of endodermal origin, such as colitis or pancreatitis, as well as patients with other tumors, such as pancreatic and breast cancer, also had elevated serum levels of CEA. Despite these limitations, monitoring the fall and rise of CEA levels in colon cancer patients undergoing therapy has proven useful for predicting tumor progression and responses to treatment. Moreover, studies in mice have suggested that antitumor T-cell immunity can be elicited to tumors expressing CEA, and a human clinical trial in patients with colon cancer is currently evaluating whether a recombinant vaccinia virus vaccine expressing CEA can induce T-cell responses to CEA that will eliminate residual cancer cells. Several other oncofetal antigens have been useful for diagnosing and monitoring human tumors. In particular, **α-fetoprotein,** an alpha globulin normally secreted by fetal liver and yolk sac cells, is found in the serum of patients with liver and germinal cell tumors and can be used as a marker of disease status.

Differentiation and lineage-specific antigens, which are present on normal adult cells, may be aberrantly expressed on some tumor cells. For example, a T-cell antigen, CD5, is commonly expressed on the malignant human B cells found in chronic lymphocytic leukemia, and an erythrocyte blood group antigen is frequently found on human stomach cancer cells. These inappropriately expressed antigens are very useful for identifying transformed cells, and their unexpected presence on tumor cells may ultimately aid in deciphering the regulation and function of such antigens on normal differentiated cells.

Many other tumor-associated antigens, which have unknown function but very limited tissue distribution on normal cells, have now been identified with monoclonal antibodies. Membrane glycoprotein and glycolipid antigens isolated from malignant melanoma cells appear to be relatively specific for these tumors, although some expression on normal cells such as neuronal tissue has been detected. A glycoprotein found on human leukemia cells, called common acute lymphocytic leukemia antigen (CALLA, or CD10), has been detected at low levels on other cells such as granulocytes and kidney cells. Many other similar examples exist, and the use of such antigenic markers for diagnostic and therapeutic purposes has great promise.

The recent successes in isolation and cloning of tumor-reactive T cells from cancer patients, coupled with expression cloning of tumor genes and screening of the transfected targets for recognition by the T cells, has made it possible to identify tumor-associated antigens that unequivocally can induce immune responses. In melanoma, T-cell responses to at least five normal cellular proteins, including MAGE and tyrosinase, as well as a mutated oncogenic protein, have been characterized. Similar strategies have identified immunogenic proteins in breast cancer, ovarian cancer, lung cancer, and pancreatic cancer. A major focus of tumor immunologists is now to devise methods to elicit therapeutic responses to these antigens in patients whose tumor expresses the protein.

IMMUNOLOGIC EFFECTOR MECHANISMS POTENTIALLY OPERATIVE AGAINST TUMOR CELLS

Virtually all of the effector components of the immune system have the potential to contribute to the eradication of tumor cells. It is likely that each of these effector mechanisms plays a role in the control of tumor growth, but a particular mechanism may be more or less important, depending on the tumor and setting. Immunologically specific effector responses are probably most important with highly immunogenic tumors, and nonspecific effector responses are presumably of greater significance with less immunogenic tumors.

T Cells

The T-cell response is unquestionably the most important host response for the control of growth of antigenic tumor cells; it is responsible for both the direct killing of tumor cells and the activation of other components of the immune system. T-cell immunity to tumors reflects the function of the two T-cell subsets: class II-restricted T cells, which largely represent CD4 helper T (T_H) cells that mediate their effect by the secretion of lymphokines to activate other effector cells and induce inflammatory responses, and class I-restricted T cells, which largely represent CD8 cytotoxic T (T_C) cells that can also secrete lymphokines but mediate their effect mostly by direct lysis of tumor cells.

The precise contribution of each T-cell subset and T-cell function to the antitumor response appears quite variable, but tumor-specific T cells from each subset are capable of mediating tumor eradication and have been detected in the peripheral blood of individual patients and in the cells infiltrating human tumors. Most tumor cells, however, express class I but not class II MHC molecules, and the T_H cell subset cannot directly recognize these tumor cells. Therefore, such T_H cell responses depend on antigen-presenting cells such as macrophages to present the relevant tumor antigens in the context of class II molecules for activation. After antigen-specific triggering, these T cells secrete lymphokines that activate T_C cells, macrophages, natural killer (NK) cells, and B cells and can produce other lymphokines, such as lymphotoxin or tumor necrosis factor (TNF), which may be directly lytic to tumor cells (see Chapter 9 and 12). In contrast to T_H cells, the T_C cell subset is capable of directly recognizing and killing tumor targets by disrupting the target membrane and nucleus. Only a minor fraction of class I-restricted T cells are capable of providing helper functions, however, and thus effective T_C cell responses are generally dependent on class II-restricted T_H cell responses to provide the necessary helper factors to activate and promote the proliferation of T_C cells.

B Cells & Antibody-Dependent Killing

A potential role for host antibody responses in human tumor immunity has been suggested by the occasional detection of tumor-reactive antibodies in the serum of patients. Moreover, recent studies in which hybridomas or B-cell lines are formed from B cells derived from lymph nodes draining human tumors have suggested that human tumors may frequently elicit antibody responses to tumor-associated antigens. In addition to secreting antibodies that may contribute to the control of tumor growth, B cells with surface immunoglobulin reactive with tumor antigens may play a role in binding, processing, and presenting tumor antigens for induction of T-cell responses to the tumor.

There are two major mechanisms by which antibodies may mediate tumor cell lysis. Complement-fixing antibodies bind to the tumor cell membrane and promote attachment of complement components that create pores in the membrane, resulting in cell disruption due to loss of osmotic and biochemical integrity. An alternative mechanism is antibody-dependent cell-mediated cytotoxicity (ADCC), in which antibodies, usually of the IgG class, form an intercellular bridge by binding via the variable region to a specific determinant on the target cell and via the Fc region to effector cells expressing Fc receptors. Many potential effector cells can mediate the lytic event, including NK cells, macrophages, and granulocytes. ADCC is a more efficient in vitro lytic mechanism than complement-mediated cytotoxicity, requiring fewer antibody molecules per cell to kill. Immunotherapy studies with monoclonal antibodies of different isotypes (and thus different capacities to fix complement or mediate ADCC) have also suggested that ADCC may be the more important in vivo effector mechanism.

Natural Killer Cells

NK cells can kill a wide range of tumor targets in vitro (see also Chapter 9). The mechanism by which NK cells preferentially recognize and lyse transformed rather than normal targets is not well defined. However, NK cells recognize but receive an off-signal from class I molecules, and thus preferentially lyse target cells with diminished expression of self-class I MHC molecules. Downregulation or loss of class I molecule expression is commonly observed in virus-infected and many transformed cells and may partially explain the therapeutic activity reported with NK effector cells. Cytolysis by NK cells is mediated by the release of a cytotoxic factor(s) and the use of perforins to puncture holes in the target cell membrane. The cytotoxic activity of NK cells can be augmented both in vitro and in vivo with the lymphokines interleukin-2 (IL-2) and interferon, and thus NK activity can be amplified by immune T-cell responses. Recent studies have demonstrated that augmentation of NK activity in visceral organs enhances resistance to the growth of metastases. Therefore, NK cells may represent a first line of host defense against the growth of transformed cells at both the primary and metastatic sites, as well as providing an effector mechanism recruited by T cells (or the pharmacologic administration of cytokines) to supplement specific antitumor responses.

Additional cytotoxic effector cells that bear many similarities to but can be distinguished from classic NK cells have also been identified. Natural cytotoxic (NC) cells kill a somewhat different spectrum of tumor targets than do NK cells, are resistant to glucocorticoids, and respond to IL-3. Lymphokine-activated killer (LAK) cells can be induced by very high pharmacologic doses of IL-2, are phenotypically heterogeneous (including both NK and CD8 T cells), and kill a much broader spectrum of tumor targets than do NK cells, but their role during physiologic antitumor responses remains to be elucidated.

Macrophages

Macrophages are important in tumor immunity as antigen-presenting cells to initiate the immune response and as potential effector cells to mediate tumor lysis. Resting macrophages are not cytolytic to tumor cells in vitro but can become cytolytic if activated with macrophage-activating factors (MAF). MAF are commonly secreted by T cells following antigen-specific stimulation, and therefore the participation of macrophages as effector cells in the absence of administration of cytokines may be dependent on T-cell immunity. This is supported by studies showing that macrophages isolated from immunogenic tumors undergoing regression exhibit tumoricidal activity, whereas macrophages isolated from progressing or nonimmunogenic tumors generally show no cytotoxic activity. T-cell lymphokines with MAF activity include interferon gamma, TNF, IL-4, and granulocyte–macrophage colony-stimulating factor (GM-CSF) (see Chapter 10).

The mechanisms by which macrophages recognize tumor cells and mediate lysis are not defined, but activated macrophages bind to and lyse transformed cells in marked preference to normal cells. Binding by activated macrophages is an energy-dependent process dependent on trypsin-sensitive membrane structures. Several distinct lytic mechanisms may be operative, depending on the MAF responsible for activating the macrophages. These include intercellular transfer of lysosomal products, superoxide production, release of neutral proteinases, and secretion of the monokine TNF.

POTENTIAL MECHANISMS BY WHICH TUMOR CELLS MAY ESCAPE FROM AN IMMUNE RESPONSE

The concept of host immune surveillance, with the immune system providing the function of surveying the body to recognize and destroy frequently developing immunogenic tumor cells, was formally proposed by F.M. Burnet. The failure to demonstrate an increased appearance of immunogenic tumors in immunodeficient hosts incapable of tumor rejection has modified current views of immune surveillance, however. Although antigen-specific responses may provide a surveillance function for the development of certain tumors, such as those induced by oncogenic DNA and RNA tumor viruses, the immune system is much more efficient at recognizing infectious organisms than tumor cells as foreign. Thus, nonspecific effector populations, such as NK cells, rather than tumor antigen-specific immune responses are now believed to be more important in the rejection of newly appearing tumor cells. The failure of the immune system to prevent the emergence of most tumors does not preclude the development of tumor-specific immune responses during the growth of established tumors. Indirect support for the presence of immunity to human tumors includes spontaneous regressions of tumors and regressions of metastatic lesions after removal of large primary tumors. Direct evidence of tumor-specific immunity has been provided by studies using sensitive in vitro methods to detect antibodies or T cells reactive with a tumor from cancer patients. Thus, it seems likely that even though the emergence of many tumors may reflect a failure of immune surveillance and the absence of an immune response during early tumor growth, a potentially detectable but unfortunately ineffective immune response may still be generated during progressive growth of the tumor. Important goals in tumor immunology are to determine why such responses are ineffective and to devise methods to induce effective responses.

Many potential mechanisms permitting escape from immune destruction have been identified. Immunoselection of variant cells has been suggested by analysis of the cells present in a tumor mass, which often reveals heterogeneity with respect to morphology and surface phenotype. Some differences are cell cycle-dependent, but others result from random mutations due to genetic instability in the proliferating cell population. Regardless of the underlying reason, if some of these differences result in a reduction in the expression of a tumor antigen being recognized by the immune system, the cells derived from this clone may have a selective advantage. Moreover, as growth of such a tumor variant proceeds, it becomes the dominant population, which makes it increasingly difficult to identify that a host response to the tumor had been generated.

Antigenic modulation results in similar events to those described earlier, in that an immune response to a tumor antigen selects for the growth of antigen-negative cells. In this setting, however, antigen loss reflects only a phenotypic change in the tumor cell, and if the immune response is ablated, the antigen is reexpressed. Antigenic modulation resulting from antibody responses has been extensively reported, but modulation from T-cell responses has not yet been clearly identified.

As described in Chapter 6, the presentation of antigens by tumor cells for recognition by T cells requires the intracellular processing of proteins, with degradation to small 8–9-amino-acid peptides that are transported to the endoplasmic reticulum and then inserted into a cleft in the class I MHC molecule for subsequent transport to the cell surface. Recent studies have shown that some tumor cells have defective antigen-processing machinery, with the result that class I molecules do not get loaded with peptides and transported to the surface, class I expression is low, and even potentially highly immunogenic tumor antigens cannot be presented to the immune system.

There are many mechanisms by which tumor cells can nonspecifically interfere with the expression of immunity in the host. Some tumor cells can release soluble factors that directly suppress immunologic reactivity. Perhaps the best studied phenomenon is the inhibition of immune responses by macrophages that have modified as a result of residing in hosts bearing progressive tumors. This appears to be mediated largely via the spontaneous secretion of prostaglandins, and in vitro treatment of macrophages with the cyclooxygenase inhibitor indomethacin can overcome the inhibitory effects.

Patients with advanced cancer demonstrate increased susceptibility to opportunistic infections and exhibit global depression of T-cell responses. Analysis of the T-cell receptor-signaling complex from T cells in such patients has demonstrated that this in part reflects the absence of a zeta chain in the T-cell receptor. This defect, as well as the associated abnormal T-cell function, is reversible, providing further support that tumor growth results in release of an immunosuppressive factor. Identification of such factor(s) could not only improve tumor immunity but also possibly provide insights into novel new immunoregulatory compounds. The presence of abnormalities in the T-cell receptor complex with advanced disease has prompted analyses of T cells isolated from tumor sites at earlier stages of disease. Indeed, several studies have shown that T cells from draining lymph nodes or infiltrating tumors often have abnormally phosphorylated or absent zeta chains, which appear functionally nonreactive and would thus make the tumor appear nonimmunogenic.

The presence of tumor-specific suppressor T (T_s) cells may represent another reason for the difficulties in detecting tumor-specific immunity in cancer patients and for the impression that no response has been elicited. For example, even with many of the highly immunogenic animal tumors studied in the laboratory, the presence of T_s cells would prevent the detection of tumor-specific immunity in the host if the presence of immunity was not sought until the tumor had reached a stage comparable to that in which most cancer patients are studied. The major obstacle to understanding the role of T_s cells in tumor immunity has been the difficulty in isolating and characterizing such cells.

Despite this difficulty, the biologic phenomenon of antigen-specific T-cell-mediated suppression has been unequivocally demonstrated in vivo, and future studies will have to elucidate the bases for these observations.

One major reason now emerging to explain the lack of an immune response to tumor cells derives from increased understanding of the functions of antigen-presenting cells (APC). Tumor cells lack many of the essential qualities of professional APC, such as expression of the costimulatory molecules CD80 and CD86 or production of the activating cytokine IL-12. Molecular strategies in which tumor cells are modified to express these functions represent a promising means to elicit antitumor responses.

IMMUNOTHERAPY

Although the host immune system may often be inadequate for controlling tumor growth, the presence of identifiable tumor antigens on most tumor cells, the identification of a detectable but ineffective host response to many tumors, and an improved understanding of the mechanisms by which tumor cells evade immunity suggest that it may be possible to manipulate and amplify the immune system to promote tumor eradication. The recent technologic advances that permit isolation of lymphocyte subpopulations, identification and purification of tumor antigens, growth of selected antigen-specific T cells, amplification of immune responses with cytokines, and targeting of antibody–toxin conjugates to tumors have created a new potential and enthusiasm for the immunotherapy of tumors. Several distinct approaches to immunotherapy are being studied, and it seems likely that at least some of these approaches will soon become important modalities for the treatment of selected tumors.

Immunization with Tumor Cells or Purified Antigens

Immunization of hosts bearing established progressing tumors with tumor cells or tumor antigen has generally been ineffective. This outcome may reflect in part the global immunoincompetence and suppressive state commonly detected in such individuals. Therefore, methods to modify the host–tumor relationship prior to immunization, such as by reduction of the tumor burden, in concert with methods to enhance the immunogenicity of tumor cells and tumor antigens are being explored. One approach has been to directly inject DNA encoding foreign MHC antigens into the tumor, with the hope that the expressed alloantigens will create an immunologic milieu that results in the induction of responses to both the alloantigens and tumor antigens. Studies in mice have been encouraging and have provided the rationale for a current human trial.

An alternative approach has been to isolate tumor cells from a biopsy specimen, introduce cytokine genes or genes encoding accessory molecules expressed by efficient APC, and then use these gene-modified tumor cells to immunize the host. Studies in mice with genes encoding cytokine genes such as IL-2 and GM-CSF or costimulatory accessory molecules such as B7 have provided provocative results—protective T-cell responses to tumor cells previously perceived to be nonimmunogenic have been repeatedly detected. Approaches involving these methods are currently in human trials. Preliminary results of immunization with autologous renal cell tumors expressing GM-CSF have suggested that antitumor responses to established tumors can be achieved.

The identification of tumor antigens shared by many tumors has provided another means of inducing antitumor responses, but studies in animal models have suggested that direct immunization with tumor proteins generally has limited or no apparent efficacy. Consequently, more immunogenic vectors are being evaluated. For example, the gene encoding CEA has been inserted into a recombinant vaccinia virus, and this highly immunogenic vaccine vector is being tested in colon cancer patients. An additional approach being pursued in breast cancer with mucin peptides and in melanoma with immunogenic MAGE peptides is to immunize with the tumor antigen in an adjuvant. A recently developed alternative has been to create a fusion protein in which the gene encoding the tumor protein is fused in frame with an immunostimulatory cytokine such as GM-CSF or IL-2. These approaches offer the potential of eventually developing both protective and therapeutic tumor vaccines.

The recent development of methods to isolate and expand dendritic cells has made it possible to immunize patients with large numbers of this highly efficient professional APC pulsed with tumor antigens. Studies in patients with B-cell lymphoma with dendritic cells pulsed with the tumor idiotype have demonstrated therapeutic antitumor T-cell responses.

Adoptive Cellular Immunotherapy

Animal models have been developed in which hosts bearing advanced tumors can be treated by the transfer of tumor-specific syngeneic T cells. These models, in which syngeneic donor T cells immune to the tumor are used, have served as prototypes of what might be achievable if the host immune response to an autochthonous tumor could be selectively amplified. Complete tumor elimination following adoptive therapy requires an extended period, and the cells transferred must therefore be capable of persisting in the host to be effective. Noncytolytic lymphokine-producing class II-restricted T_H cells, as well as directly lytic class I-restricted T_C cells, mediate antitumor effects in these models. Tumor-specific T cells expanded in vitro by culture with tumor and IL-2 are effective in adoptive therapy, and efficacy can be enhanced by infusing IL-2 after cell transfer, which has been shown to promote in vivo proliferation and survival of the transferred cultured T cells.

These studies are now being applied to the treatment of human cancers by isolating potentially tumor-reactive lymphocytes infiltrating solid tumors, expanding these cells in vitro by stimulation with tumor or IL-2 or both, and then reinfusing the cells into the patients. To enhance the efficacy of such therapy, IL-2 is being administered after transfer. Preliminary results have suggested that these T cells can localize to sites of tumor and can mediate a significant therapeutic effect, particularly with some tumors such as melanoma. Studies with cloned cytolytic T cells specific for human cytomegalovirus have demonstrated that transferred T cells can establish prolonged specific immunity in humans. The methods used to isolate and expand these virus-specific T-cell clones are now being applied to the treatment of tumors, and, with the continued development of methods to identify tumor antigens and to detect and expand the number of tumor-specific T cells from patients, specific adoptive therapy should become an important modality for the treatment of many tumors in the near future.

While the in vitro effects of increasing doses of IL-2 on the generation of tumor-specific T cells were being examined, it was observed that a cytolytic effector cell lacking antigen specificity but displaying a marked preference for transformed cells was induced. These LAK cells, generated only in the presence of exceptionally high, nonphysiologic doses of IL-2, have now been extensively characterized and studied both in vitro and in vivo. LAK cells are phenotypically heterogeneous, but the major effector cell appears to be a non-T cell most similar to an activated NK cell. Administration of cytolytic LAK cells, particularly in association with IL-2, has shown activity in the treatment of some human tumors. Although the efficacy of treatment with LAK cells and IL-2 appears to be limited by a lack of absolute specificity and toxicity to the host, there are many clinical settings, such as isolated pulmonary or liver metastases, in which it may be possible to use these effector cells to achieve a directed and potentially curative antitumor effect. Moreover, approaches are now being explored to improve the specificity of LAK cells, such as by concurrently administering bifunctional antibodies (ie, hybrid or conjugated monoclonal antibodies that have two specificities): one for an antigen that resides on the LAK cell and permits attachment to the effector cell and one for an antigen that resides on the tumor and promotes specific targeting.

Administration of Monoclonal Antibodies

The development of the technology for generating monoclonal antibodies has converted the previously unpromising field of tumor serotherapy into a form of treatment with great potential. Studies with antibodies of different isotypes have demonstrated that ADCC rather than complement-mediated cytotoxicity is the major in vivo effector mechanism following infusion of antibody. Despite occasional reports of exciting clinical results, however, a large number of biologic problems still need to be overcome for this modality to be generally effective. The problem of host immune responses to administered antibodies of murine origin is being resolved by engineering chimeric antibodies with a human backbone as well as transgenic mice that can produce human antibodies. Antibodies and the necessary ADCC effector cells, however, do not appear to penetrate large tumor masses effectively, and tumor escape mechanisms, such as modulation of the target antigen from the tumor cell surface and selection of antigen loss variants, may frequently interfere with monoclonal antibody therapy.

Several approaches are being studied to augment the therapeutic activity of monoclonal antibodies. One approach is to administer antibodies concurrently with cytotoxic chemotherapy, and preliminary studies have suggested this improves response rates. The most promising approaches involve conjugation of cytotoxic drugs, toxins, or radioisotopes to the antibody to deliver a lethal hit directly to the tumor without requiring the participation of host effector cells. Antibody–drug or toxin conjugates may be particularly useful in settings in which the antigen is rapidly endocytosed. In contrast, radioisotopes may be useful with large tumors or in the presence of immunoselection, because radioisotopes kill by emitting ionizing radiation and thus do not need to fully penetrate the tumor to kill all cells and can kill antigen-negative tumor variants in the tumor mass if they are in the proximity of antibody-binding tumor cells. Treatment of patients with B-cell lymphoma with antibody-radioisotope conjugates has yielded some durable complete responses. Most of the tumor-reactive monoclonal antibodies being used in clinical trials recognize tumor-associated rather than tumor-specific antigens and thus are likely to recognize some normal tissues. Consequently, administration of some antibodies or antibody conjugates may prove to be unacceptably toxic to the host. In many instances, however, such as if the antibody recognizes a determinant such as CD19 or CD20 that is expressed both on lymphoma cells and on normal B cells and causes a transient depression of B-cell number, this toxicity may be acceptable if a significant antitumor effect can be achieved. Future studies will need to carefully define the distribution of normal antigens recognized by each antibody to be used in therapy and the potential toxic complications, but recent successes with monoclonal antibody therapy suggest that these reagents will have an increasing role in treatment strategies for a variety of human tumors.

REFERENCES

Anichini A et al: Melanoma cells and normal melanocytes share antigens recognized by HLA-A2-restricted cytotoxic T cell clones from melanoma patients. *J Exp Med* 1993;**177**:989.

Boon T et al: Tumor antigens recognized by T lymphocytes. *Ann Rev Immunol* 1994;**12**:337.

Cheever MA et al: Immunity to oncogenic proteins. *Immunol Rev* 1995;**145**:33.

Dillman RO: Antibodies as cytotoxic therapy. *J Clin Oncol* 1994;**12**:1497.

Fearon ER et al: Interleukin-2 production by tumor cells bypasses T helper function in the generation of an antitumor response. *Cell* 1990;**60**:397.

Finn OJ et al: MUC-1 epithelial tumor mucin-based immunity and cancer vaccines. *Immunol Rev* 1995;**145**:61.

Ghetie MA, Vitetta ES: Recent developments in immunotoxin therapy. *Curr Opin Immunol* 1994;**6**:707.

Greenberg PD: Adoptive T cell therapy of tumors: Mechanisms operative in the recognition and elimination of tumor cells. *Adv Immunol* 1991;**49**:281.

Hsu FJ et al: Vaccination of patients with B-cell lymphoma using autologous antigen-pulsed dendritic cells. *Nature Med* 1996;**2**:52.

Jung S, Schluesener HJ: Human T lymphocytes recognize a peptide of single point-mutated, oncogenic ras proteins. *J Exp Med* 1991;**173**:273.

Klein G: Tumor antigens. *Ann Rev Microbiol* 1966;**20**:223.

Melief CJ, Kast WM: Prospects for T cell immunotherapy of tumours by vaccination with immunodominant and subdominant peptides. *Ciba Found Symp* 1994;**187**:97, discussion 104.

Mizoguchi H et al: Alterations in signal transduction molecules in T lymphocytes from tumor-bearing mice. *Science* 1992;**258**:1795.

Pardoll DM: Paracrine cytokine adjuvants in cancer immunotherapy. *Ann Rev Immunol* 1995;**13**:399.

Peoples GE et al: Breast and ovarian cancer-specific cytotoxic T lymphocytes recognize the same HER2/neu-derived peptide. *Proc Nat Acad Sci USA* 1995;**92**:432.

Restifo NP et al: Identification of human cancers deficient in antigen processing. *J Exp Med* 1993;**177**:265.

Riddell SR, Greenberg PD: Principles for adoptive T cell therapy of human viral diseases. *Ann Rev Immunol* 1995;**13**:545.

Rosenberg SA et al: Treatment of 283 consecutive patients with metastatic melanoma or renal cell cancer using high-dose bolus interleukin-2. *JAMA* 1994;**271**:907.

Rosenberg SA et al: Treatment of patients with metastatic melanoma with autologous tumor-infiltrating lymphocytes and interleukin 2. *J Nat Cancer Inst* 1994;**86**:1159.

Sentman CL et al: Missing self recognition by natural killer cells in MHC class I transgenic mice. A "receptor calibration" model for how effector cells adapt to self. *Semin Immunol* 1995;**7**:109.

Tao MH, Levy R: Idiotype/granulocyte–macrophage colony-stimulating factor fusion protein as a vaccine for B-cell lymphoma. *Nature* 1993;**362**:755.

Townsend SE, Allison JP: Tumor rejection after direct costimulation of CD8+ T cells by B7-transfected melanoma cells. *Science* 1993;**259**:368.

Tsang KY et al: Generation of human cytotoxic T cells specific for human carcinoembryonic antigen epitopes from patients immunized with recombinant vaccinia-CEA vaccine. *J Nat Cancer Inst* 1995;**87**:982.

Urban JL, Schreiber H: Tumor antigens. *Annu Rev Immunol* 1992;**10**:617.

van der Bruggen P et al: A gene encoding an antigen recognized by cytolytic T lymphocytes on a human melanoma. *Science* 1991;**254**:1643.

Walter EA et al: Reconstitution of cellular immunity against cytomegalovirus in recipients of allogeneic bone marrow by transfer of T-cell clones from the donor. *New Engl J Med* 1995;**333**:1038.

Wilder RB et al: Radioimmunotherapy: Recent results and future directions. *J Clin Oncol* 1996;**14**:1383.

45

Cancer in the Immunocompromised Host

John L. Ziegler, MD

In the late 1950s, Sir McFarlane Burnet and Lewis Thomas proposed that the immune system maintains vigil over both alien microorganisms and altered somatic cells. The logic of "immune surveillance," defined more explicitly by Burnet in 1970, finds support in the defense systems of lower organisms, which must resist fusion, invasion, or destructive parasitism to survive. Plants and prokaryotes maintain their integrity through highly conserved cell surface recognition systems. Multicellular eukaryotes evolved a more complex "adoptive" defense system, one impressive feature of which is the ability to discriminate between self and nonself. Other cognate functions, such as immunologic memory, regulatory networks, and a large reperotoire of attack strategies, make the mammalian immune system comparable to the brain in complexity and function. Throughout phylogeny, the role of the immune system in ensuring the autonomy of the host is a basic tenet of evolutionary survival.

IMMUNE SURVEILLANCE

Inferential support for immune surveillance against neoplasia in humans comes from a variety of clinical observations. Patients with congenital immune deficiencies and patients with organ transplants who receive immunosuppressive therapy develop an excess incidence of some forms of cancer. Rare instances of "spontaneous" regression of tumors are ascribed to immune mechanisms. More recently, the discovery of tumor-specific antigens (see Chapter 44) and the observation of tumor-directed immune responses by using autologous lymphocytes and lymphokines provide further evidence for tumor immunity.

Studies of transplantable and spontaneous tumors in animals also lend support to the notion of tumor-directed immunity. For example, surgical removal of a growing tumor in mice renders them resistant to subsequent inocula of the same, but not a different, tumor. Such experiments are more successful when using transplantable tumors rather than spontaneous, autochthonous tumors. Aside from evidence of specific tumor immunity medicated by antibody and T cells, tumor cells can be killed nonspecifically by activated macrophages and natural killer (NK) cells. Finally, examples of "blocking factors" that prevent an immune response are evident in tumor-bearing hosts.

Criteria for Intrinsic Defense

An intrinsic defense against the development of neoplasia might be advantageous to the host. To be successful, it must meet at least four conditions. First, the tumor should express unique antigens that are accessible to the immune system. Second, the host must have a competent immune system and attack the tumor antigen with an appropriate tumor-directed cytotoxic response. Third, there should be no suppressive or blocking influences to obstruct the immune response. Finally, the number of tumor cells should be small enough for the immune attack to locate and eliminate the tumor entirely.

Immunotherapy Research

The 1970s saw an era of empirical immunotherapy, based on the assumptions just listed. The main aims were to augment tumor cell antigenicity and to boost host immunity with various specific or nonspecific vaccines and stimulants. The results of these trials were disappointing, with only rare instances of clinical improvement. By the end of the decade, it was clear that most human tumors were at best only weakly antigenic. It was also obvious that immunotherapy was a "numbers game," with successful killing being dependent on a high lymphocyte-to-target cell ratio. Successful therapeutic manipulation of the immune system demanded a much better appreciation of the intricacies of immunoregulation.

Advances in biotechnology and molecular biology have brought considerable enlightenment to the field of cancer immunology in the 1980s and 1990s. Separate cell populations can be defined by using monoclonal antibodies. The discovery, cloning, and production of purified growth factors permit experiments with high concentrations of purified lymphocytes. Advances in molecular genetics provide techniques to identify tumor clonality. Progress in understanding immunoregulation, mechanisms of immune diversity, and the interactions of the various cellular members of the immune system has opened new doors to pharmacologic and biologic manipulation of the immune response. Finally, the identification of oncogenes and tumor suppressor genes has enabled a better molecular genetic understanding of oncogenesis, including the potential to identify tumor-specific oncogene products.

IMMUNOCOMPROMISE & CANCER

This chapter focuses on the phenomenon of cancer in the immunocompromised human host. **Immunocompromise** is a preferable term to "immunodeficiency" or "immunosuppression." The latter terms imply that the immune system is binary and capable of swaying, like a seesaw, between a normal "replete" state and a suppressed "deficient" state. This notion is clearly oversimplified, given our knowledge of the contextual and integrated nature of immune responses. Immunocompromise should be defined as a state of functional unresponsiveness, due in some circumstances to depletion of specific immune compartments and in others to dysfunction induced by drugs, physical agents, infections, cancer, or autoimmunity.

Oncogenesis

Experimentally, three processes lead to neoplasia: initiation, promotion, and progression (Fig 45–1). **Initiation** involves the alteration of DNA by a chemical, physical, or biologic agent that confers malignant potential onto the cell genotype. "Initiated" cells appear histologically normal but are rendered constitutively susceptible to malignant transformation. **Promotion** is thought to be a process by which the expression of genetic information is altered in the cell. **Progression** is the clonal evolution of established tumors that accounts for heterogeneity and varied phenotypic manifestations, such as invasiveness, drug resistance, and metastatic potential. Thus, cancer is the end stage of a multistep process that evolves over relatively long periods. Its development and behavior in the intact host are driven internally by the renegade genetic program and influenced externally by microenvironmental factors, such as hormonal milieu, vascular supply, and immunity.

Function and Dysfunction of Oncogenes and Tumor Suppressor Genes

Oncogenes are defined as functionally or structurally altered genes that cause neoplastic growth. They are derived from normal genes ("protooncogenes") that govern cell growth, differentiation, tissue renewal, or response to injury. They become altered as a result of mutation, faulty DNA repair, deletion, duplication, or translocation to another part of the genome. Such genetic accidents then lead to enhancement, loss, or critical dysfunction of a gene product. Thus far, over 100 oncogenes have been identified,

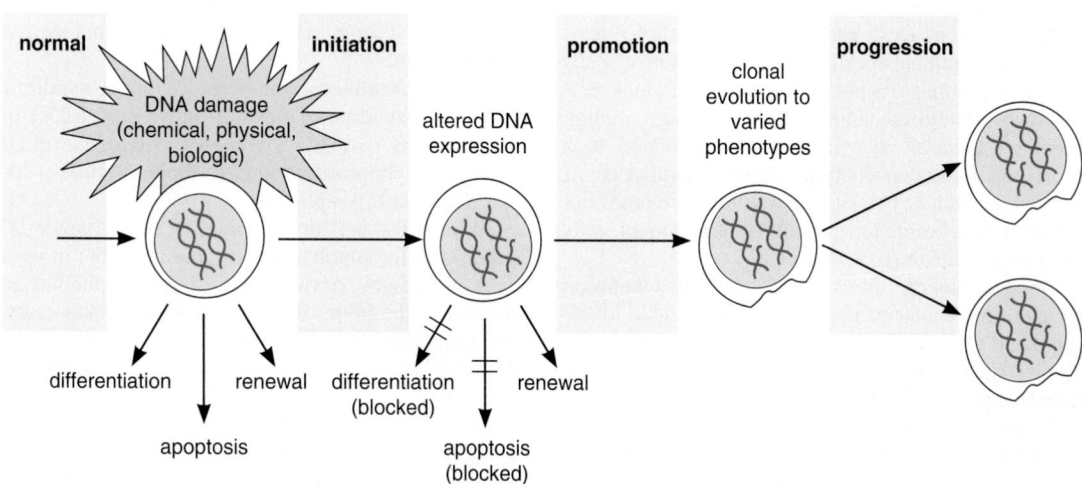

Figure 45–1. Pathogenesis of neoplasia. Normal cells have three choices when dividing: differentiate die, or renew. When certain DNA mutations or chromosomal abnormalities occur, stem cells that are initiated may accumulate in a renewal cycle, due to failure to repair damaged DNA or failure to undergo apoptosis (programmed cell death). These cells are more susceptible to a second genetic accident, and the chance of "promotion" to neoplastic transformation increases over time. As tumor develops, there is genetic drift in the cell renewal compartment, and clones of tumor cells "progress" in different phenotypic directions, producing tumor heterogeneity.

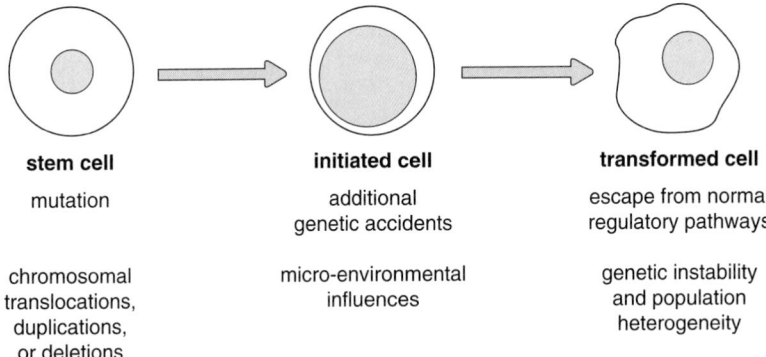

Figure 45–2. Molecular model of malignant transformation. Assuming that cancer is a disease of defective stem cells, there is consensus that the pathway to neoplasia involves multiple "hits" to stem cell DNA, such that the normal signals for self-renewal and differentiation become aberrant or misinterpreted. At the molecular level, these hits presumably alter the expression of regulatory protooncogenes that either stimulate or inhibit cell proliferation.

and appear to code for cellular growth factors or their receptors, cytoplasmic signal transducers, or nuclear regulatory proteins.

One category of oncogenes codes for proteins that regulate DNA repair, cell division, and the programmed death of a cell that has sustained excessive DNA damage, a process called apoptosis. These proteins govern the entry and egress of cells at critical junctures in the cell cycle (eg, cyclins and cyclin-dependent kinases) and afford checkpoints where DNA damage is assessed and repaired. These genes are dubbed "tumor suppressor genes," because their net effect is to halt cell division. The p53 gene is the prototype suppressor and is found to be mutated in over 50% of human malignancies. Normally, p53 activates a decision network that decides the fate of cells with DNA damage: repair or die. p53-Deficient cells are then prone to accumulate DNA damage, raising the likelihood of oncogenesis or progression to a more malignant phenotype. Other regulators of apoptosis (such as bcl-2) are potential oncogenes because their dysfunction permits replication of cells with defective DNA.

Oncogenesis can thus be envisioned as a stepwise series of molecular genetic accidents that lead to unregulated growth of cells with invasive potential (Fig 45–2). These accidents can be aided and abetted by heritable predispositions (eg, defects in DNA repair), endogenous cofactors (eg, chronic inflammation, hormonal stimulation) and by environmental carcinogens (eg, free radicals, radiation, chemicals). Basically, any process that causes cells to proliferate can be potentially oncogenic—the mitogenesis begets mutagenesis hypothesis proposed by Bruce Ames. Our task in this chapter is to understand the development of human cancer in the immunocompromised host.

CONGENITAL IMMUNODEFICIENCY & NEOPLASIA

Table 45–1 indicates the risk of cancer in children with congenital immunodeficiencies. Most of these cancers are seen in four primary disorders: X-linked lymphoproliferative syndrome, Wiskott-Aldrich syndrome, ataxia-telangiectasia, and common variable immunodeficiency disease. Two thirds of the patients were younger than 20 years of age when the tumors were diagnosed. True risk assessment is difficult to measure because the prevalence of the congenital immunodeficiency is unknown. Mild forms of these disorders may be undiagnosed, and many patients with more severe forms may die before cancer develops.

In the X-linked lymphoproliferative syndrome (Duncan's syndrome) Epstein-Barr virus (EBV) infection of B lymphocytes causes progressive oligoclonal lymphoproliferation, leading to Burkitt-like non-Hodgkin's lymphoma.

In the Wiskott-Aldrich syndrome (see Chapter 23), extranodal immunoblastic lymphoma occurs in up to 16% of patients. About half of these lymphomas are located in the brain, which may act as a "sanctuary" for lymphoproliferation. In a minority of patients. Hodgkin's disease and acute myelocytic leukemia are also found.

In ataxia-telangiectasia (see Chapter 23), both Hodgkin's disease (the major subtype being lymphocyte depleted) and non-Hodgkin's lymphoma occur, in a ratio of about 1:5. The latter cases are of histologic types associated with the 14q+ chromosomal abnormality characteristic of lymphocytes in patients with ataxia-telangiectasia. Patients with this disorder manifest a defect in the repair of gamma radiation-induced DNA damage, possibly accounting for an

Table 45–1. Risk of cancer in congenital immunodeficiency syndromes.[1]

Syndrome	Immune Defect	Malignant Tumors	Percent Risk Overall	Median Age of Onset (years)
X-linked immunode-ficiency syndrome	Impaired B-cell responses to EBV antigens.	NHL	35	10
Wiskott-Aldrich syndrome	Complex, multicompartment defects.	NHL, AML HD	15–37	6
Ataxia-telangiectasia	Complex, multicompartment defects; defective DNA repair after gamma irradiation.	ALL, NHL, HD, nerve, ovarian, skin, stomach cancers	12	9
Common variable immunodeficiency	Cellular and humoral defects.	NHL, stomach cancer	8	16

[1] These data are drawn from the University of Minnesota registry on Immunodeficiency and Cancer and from elsewhere in the literature.
Abbreviations: NHL = Non-Hodgkin's lymphoma; AML = acute myeloid leukemia; HD = Hodgkin's disease; ALL = acute lymphoblastic leukemia.

excess of epithelial neoplasms (skin, ovarian, and stomach cancers) among older patients.

A small proportion of patients, predominantly females (2.5–8.5%, depending on survival) with common variable immunodeficiency develop non-Hodgkin's lymphoma. In longer surviving patients, a 50-fold excess incidence of stomach cancer is also found.

Other heritable immunodeficiencies associated with an excess of malignancies are the hyper-IgM syndrome (abdominal lymphoproliferative disease and malignancy) and IgA deficiency (thymona, lymphoma, esophageal, and lung cancer). Patients with adenosine deaminase and nucleotide phosphorylase deficiency (see Chapter 23), both rare disorders, are also associated with lymphoid malignancy. In general, the prevalence of lymphoid tumors in the congenital immunodeficiencies must reflect a complex interplay of immune dysregulation (inadequate control of dividing lymphocytes), antigenic stimulation, and activation of endogenous viruses (eg, EBV).

CANCER IN ORGAN TRANSPLANT RECIPIENTS

Recipients of organ allografts must receive drugs to suppress the immune response to alloantigens in order to avoid graft rejection. Over the past three decades, various forms of immune suppression have been used. The earlier "broad-spectrum" regimens included both corticosteroids and azathioprine. The introduction of cyclosporin in the 1970s has led to more effective T-cell-specific immunosuppression.

Cancer trends in allograft recipients are reminiscent of the experience in patients with primary immunodeficiency syndromes. In general, there is a threefold increase of neoplasms in this population compared with age-matched controls. The average time from transplantation to development of all tumors is 60 months; for lymphomas it is 37 months, and for Kaposi's sarcoma, 23 months.

Skin Cancer

The most common tumors are carcinomas of the skin, which account for 1238 (38%) of 3251 transplant-associated cancers from the Cincinnati registry. This represents a 4- to 21-fold increase over the expected skin cancer incidence. These tumors are also unusual in the overrepresentation of squamous cell carcinomas compared with the more common basal cell type and with melanomas. Skin cancers are diagnosed with higher frequency in younger persons.

In one study, male renal transplant recipients were more likely than controls to have dysplastic lip lesions (O.R. = 90) or carcinoma of one lip (O.R. = 15). In addition to immune suppression, sun exposure was a major risk factor; women wearing lipstick were protected from premalignant lesions. Other risk factors for skin cancer include smoking, infection with human papillomavirus (HPV) and human leukocyte antigen (HLA) phenotype.

Anogenital Cancer

The second most common tumor in transplant recipients is carcinoma of the anogenital tract. Cervical carcinomas account for 16% of cancers (including 80% in situ lesions). Carcinoma of the vulva, perineum, scrotum, penis, and anus occurs in 3% of recipients with cancer. Taken together, anogenital tumors are increased more than 100-fold compared with the incidence in the age-matched general population.

A possible explanation for this excess is the association of anogenital neoplasia in general with HPV, especially with "oncogenic" types 6, 11, 16, 18, 32, 35, and 37. Perhaps immunocompromise permits the activation of latent papillomavirus in anogenital tissues, and the resulting dysplastic epithelial lesions progress to neoplasia.

Two HPV proteins in the oncogenic subtypes E6 and E7 bind specifically tumor suppressor proteins (p53 and RB, respectively) and could promote neoplasia. Because these are virus-associated tumors, there may be some degree of immune surveillance in the immunocompetent host that is directed to virus-specific antigens on the epithelial cell surface. This response would normally identify and eliminate early papillomavirus-associated tumors. In an immunocompromised host, such immunity would be impaired and a higher frequency of tumors might result.

Non-Hodgkin's Lymphoma

Non-Hodgkin's lymphoma constitutes 14% of cancers in transplant recipients. The major histologic types are diffuse large cell and immunoblastic. In addition, a small proportion of lymphomas are unclassified. The majority of tumors classified by modern immunologic techniques are of B-cell origin; lymphomas of T-cell origin account for 12%. As with lymphomas found in patients with primary immunodeficiencies, the majority are extranodal, with one third involving the central nervous system. In individual transplant series, these lymphomas are oligoclonal and are associated with EBV. They may regress on withdrawal of immunosuppressive therapy, treatment with antiviral agents, or infusion of antiB-cell monoclonal antibodies.

Kaposi's Sarcoma

Kaposi's sarcoma is 400–500 times over-represented among transplant recipients compared with the general population. This rare and unusual tumor is of endothelial origin and occurs sporadically in caucasian men of eastern European descent. A polymorphic variety is endemic in certain central African countries. Like non-Hodgkin's lymphomas, this tumor may regress when immunosuppressive therapy is stopped. Although spontaneous Kaposi's sarcoma usually appears on the skin and runs an indolent course, transplant-associated tumors tend to involve internal organs, and the mortality rate is 25%.

In a study of transplant recipients, no unusual epidemiologic features distinguished the subgroup with Kaposi's sarcoma, with the exception that one third of the patients were women. Kaposi's sarcoma predominates among males, and women made up approximately one third of the transplant series. Thus, the usual 9:1 male-to-female ratio became 2:1 in the transplant series.

It is difficult to find control groups for organ transplant series. One study followed 3823 renal transplant recipients and compared them with 1349 patients who received azathioprine, cyclophosphamide, or chlorambucil for nonmalignant conditions. A 60-fold increase of non-Hodgkin's lymphoma and excess skin and mesenchymal cancers were observed in transplanted patients; a similar but less dramatic excess was noted in controls. The author concluded that immunosuppressive drugs alone do not produce the excess of cancers, and that, by inference, transplantation of foreign antigens might also contribute to the risk of malignancy.

The immunostimulation hypothesis of Prehn holds that certain tumors may be promoted by immune stimulation. The experimental model for this theory is the mouse mammary tumor, caused by a retrovirus MMTV. In this system, immunosuppression paradoxically reduces the incidence of breast cancer and prolongs life. To test this hypothesis, a very large series of women who received renal transplants ($n = 25,914$) was examined for cancer incidence. Breast cancer was the only tumor found to be lower than expected in this series, by the same order of magnitude observed in mice. This finding does not have an obvious explanation, and we must keep an open mind about the inevitability of cancer excess among immunosuppressed transplant recipients and about the implications for immunity and oncogenesis.

CANCER IN PATIENTS WITH AUTOIMMUNE DISORDERS

The true prevalence of cancer in patients with autoimmune disorders is not known. Under certain conditions, chronic inflammation per se may predispose to neoplasia, possibly caused by the DNA-damaging effects of free radicals produced at the site. Because autoimmune disorders are treated with immunosuppressive drugs, the additional effect of immunosuppression over a "baseline" of cancer susceptibility cannot be ascertained.

Most series of cancer prevalence in patients with any particular autoimmune disease are small. There is an increased risk of lymphoma in patients with celiac disease, Crohn's disease, and Sjögren's syndrome. Patients with rheumatoid arthritis are not at increased cancer risk unless given long-term treatment with cyclophosphamide or chlorambucil. Patients with Felty's syndrome, however, have a threefold increased risk for cancer and a 19-fold increase risk for lymphoma. One large series that includes patients with many autoimmune disorders treated with immunosuppressive drugs disclosed a 12-fold increase of Hodgkin's disease, a fivefold excess of squamous cell carcinoma of the skin, and a modest excess of other tumor types. Although limited in epidemiologic value, these series concur generally with the clinical experience of immunosuppressed organ transplant recipients.

SECOND TUMORS IN CANCER PATIENTS

Cancer patients, who are already partially immunocompromised by their tumors, may receive immunosuppressive anticancer therapy (ie, chemotherapy or radiotherapy or both) that worsens their already immunocompromised state. Long-term follow-up of cancer survivors treated with cytotoxic drugs discloses a high incidence of second cancers. Most of these are acute leukemias of myeloid or monocytic origin and non-Hodgkin's lymphomas. They occur an average of 4–6 years after treatment of the primary tumor. The most extensive follow-up has been performed in long-term survivors of Hodgkin's disease. Their overall risk of a second cancer is sixfold, with an actuarial risk of approximately 1% per year up to 10 years, after which a plateau is reached. Alkylating agents contribute to the risk of leukemia, whereas radiation therapy is associated with the development of solid tumors.

Interpretation of the epidemiologic data in these groups is confounded by the direct carcinogenic effects of the anticancer treatment, the extent and duration of immunocompromise, and the possibility of a neoplastic predisposition. In contrast to the cancers in patients with autoimmune disorders and transplant recipients, second cancers in surviving cancer patients appear more closely related to the direct carcinogenic effects of therapy.

HUMAN IMMUNODEFICIENCY VIRUS INFECTION & THE DEVELOPMENT OF CANCER

Immunopathogenesis of the Acquired Immunodeficiency Syndrome

More than a decade of intensive research has yet to define clearly the cause of progressive immune deficiency in persons infected with the human immunodeficiency virus (HIV) type 1. The pathogenesis of helper T (CD4) lymphocyte depletion appears to result from a complex and dynamic interaction between the host and the virus.

Early immunity to the virus gradually fails, and a phase of immune activation (during which there is nonspecific stimulation of B lymphocytes and cytotoxic/suppressor [CD8] T lymphocytes) gives way to a progressive lysis of lymphoid follicles and CD4 lymphocytes. This process is mediated in part by an increasing viral burden and by acceleration of lymphocyte apoptosis (programmed cell death) induced by HIV and its protein products. Meanwhile, the virus itself is becoming more pathogenic and, in later stages of disease, takes on a virulent, syncytium-forming phenotype. Viral replication is enhanced in a positive-feedback loop when infected lymphocytes become activated by opportunity infection. The net result is an immune system at first diverted and later destroyed by HIV.

Kaposi's Sarcoma

Kaposi's sarcoma was the first clinical manifestation of the acquired immunodeficiency syndrome (AIDS) to be recognized. Throughout the epidemic, this tumor has predominated in homosexual men, being present in 40% of new cases of AIDS in the early years of the epidemic but falling below 20% by the mid-1980s. Other risk groups in the USA and in Europe have a much lower prevalence of Kaposi's

sarcoma. In Africa, where Kaposi's sarcoma is endemic, HIV-infected patients develop a widespread and aggressive form of the disease, with a much higher incidence in women than was encountered before the AIDS epidemic.

The epidemiology of Kaposi's sarcoma has suggested that it is caused by a sexually transmitted agent. In homosexual men, the tumor is most prevalent among those who practice oral–anal contact, implying a possible infectious route of the agent.

In December 1994, Chang et al described unique DNA sequences detected in Kaposi's sarcoma tissues but not in controls. These sequences are homologous to gamma herpesviruses, with closest relationship to herpes saimiri and EBV. Since this discovery, the sequences have been detected in over 95% of Kaposi's sarcoma tumors from many geographic regions, from both AIDS and HIV-negative subjects. Interestingly, the sequences are also seen in rare AIDS-associated lymphomas confined to body cavities, and in Castleman's disease. Studies in controls show a very low frequency of detection, although sequences are present in other tissues (eg, peripheral blood leukocytes, normal skin) from patients with Kaposi's sarcoma. Other evidence suggests that the agent, now called Kaposi's sarcoma herpesvirus (KSHV), occurs in HIV-infected subjects who later develop Kaposi's sarcoma. Although the virus has not been seen or cultured, the molecular epidemiology, taken together, provides a convincing story that KSHV is a novel herpesvirus, possibly sexually transmitted, and is causally related to Kaposi's sarcoma.

Pathogenesis of AIDS-Associated Kaposi's Sarcoma

Despite its anomalous geographic distribution (Africa, Mediterranean countries) and its polymorphic clinical appearance (plaques, nodules, and florid tumors), the histologic appearance of Kaposi's sarcoma is remarkably consistent. The predominating picture is of a mixed cell type, with abortive endothelial vascular "slits" admixed with mesenchymal-appearing spindle cells and a modest inflammatory infiltrate. Early lesions are dominated by the endothelial component.

Kaposi's sarcoma cells can now be grown in tissue culture with the aid of certain growth factors, particularly fibroblast growth factor and interleukin (IL)-6. Cultured cells also produce a range of autocrine growth factors and induce Kaposi-like lesions when injected into nude mice. Experimental evidence for an indirect role of the HIV *tat* protein include the observation of growth stimulation when *tat* is added to Kaposi tissue cultures and the appearance in male *tat*-transgenic mice of Kaposi-like lesions. Taken together, the evidence suggests that Kaposi's sarcoma begins as a multifocal, paracrine angiogenic proliferation and progresses to neoplastic transformation with invasive and even metastatic potential. In one sense, the tumor represents a nonhealing wound.

A role for other cofactors in the genesis of Kaposi's sarcoma remains speculative. One model posits infection with KSHV (either newly acquired or latent), which becomes reactivated under conditions of immunocompromise, either local (eg, in the skin of the feet and legs) or generalized (eg, induced by corticosteroids of HIV). The route of infection is presumably oral–genital and the cell target lymphocytes and endothelial cells. Activated KSHV induces angiogenesis in multiple sites, which fails to regress owing to autocrine growth or inhibition of apoptosis. In early stages, lesions may wax and wane depending on the immune status of the host. The hormonal milieu may also influence progression, as men are more susceptible than women, and pregnancy exacerbates the disease regression occurs after parturition. The anatomic sites of Kaposi's sarcoma may be a combined result of KSHV distribution and local immunity: lymphadenopathic and widespread visceral and orocutaneous lesions reflect widely disseminated KSHV, whereas localized lesions are manifestations of localized infection. These factors are summarized in an etiologic model shown in Figure 45–3.

Non-Hodgkin's Lymphoma in HIV-Infected Persons

Soon after the initial reports of AIDS-associated opportunistic infections and Kaposi's sarcoma, non-Hodgkin's lymphoma was found in homosexual men with AIDS. As the AIDS epidemic progressed, the incidence of lymphoma rose commensurately, predominating in the homosexual and intravenous drug-abusing risk groups. As the survival of AIDS patients increases with improved therapy, a higher incidence of lymphoma is being reported. The majority of well-characterized lymphomas are of B-cell origin, about evenly divided between intermediate-grade large cell, high-grade immunoblastic, and small non-cleaved cell types. AIDS-associated lymphomas can be conveniently classified as systemic lymphomas and primary central nervous system lymphomas.

Systemic Lymphoma: Clinically, the systemic lymphomas are extranodal in distribution, with a high frequency of central nervous system and bone marrow involvement. In addition, homosexual men have an excess of oral and rectal tumors. All series report a poor response to treatment and a high mortality rate. The major determinants of poor prognosis are a prior AIDS diagnosis, low CD4 lymphocyte counts, presence of extranodal tumor, aggressive cytotoxic chemotherapy regimens, and poor clinical condition.

Primary Central Nervous System Lymphomas: As seen in congenital immunodeficiency and transplant recipients, primary central nervous system (CNS) lymphoma occurs in vast excess among AIDS patients. The presenting features are similar to those in immunocompetent subjects (neurologic deficit, mental status changes, headache, seizures), but other clinical features differ (Table 45–2). AIDS-associated primary CNS lymphomas predominate in

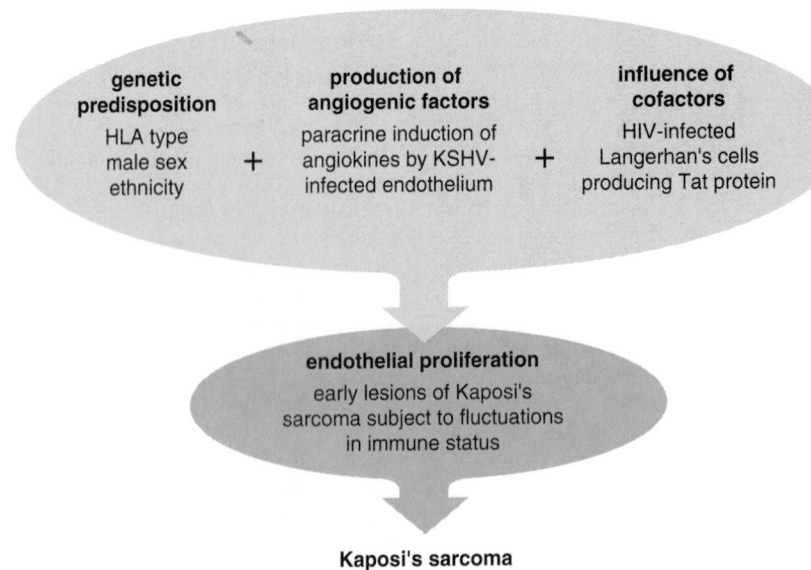

Figure 45–3. Suggested pathogenesis of Kaposi's sarcoma in immunocompromised patients. Kaposi's sarcoma is thought to begin as a vascular reaction to local angiokine production, which can be induced by infection with Kaposi's sarcoma herpesvirus (KSHV) (see text). The paracrine release of angiogenic factors (most probably those in the fibroblast growth factor [FGF] family) causes endothelial cell proliferation and spindle cell formation. Initially, these proliferative lesions may respond to immune control of KSHV. With time, however, the lesions become autonomous and produce their own sustaining growth factors. Yet to be explained in this pathway are the roles of genetic predisposition, gender, and local cofactors (see text).

Table 45–2. Clinical features of primary central nervous system lymphoma in immunocompetent hosts and patients with AIDS.[1]

Features	Immuno-competent	Immuno-compromised
Male/female ratio	1.35	7.38
Mean age	55.2 years	30.8 years
Tumor imaging Solitary lesion Multiple lesions	72% 25%	48% 52%
Histology		
Large cell Immunoblastic Small noncleaved cell	50% 18% 4%	37% 35% 25%
Median survival	18.9 months	2.6 months

[1] Summarized from data on 792 cases reviewed by Fine and Mayer (see References).

Table 45–3. Molecular characteristics of AIDS-associated non-Hodgkin's lymphoma.

Histology	Per Cent[1]			
	Mono-clonal	Poly-clonal	EBV	C-*MYC*
Large cell	50	50	30	15
Immunoblastic	85	15	90	30
Burkitt's (small non-cleaved)	98	2	45	75
Primary central nervous system	100	0	85	0

[1] Data summarized from 95 cases from Herndier et al (see References).

younger men, are more often multifocal and have a poorer prognosis than those seen in immunocompetent patients. Moreover, the histology of the lymphomas favor immunoblastic and small noncleaved subtypes. In AIDS patients, primary CNS lymphomas often mimic cerebral toxoplasmosis, and a stereotactic brain biopsy is usually required for diagnosis.

T-Cell Lymphomas in HIV-Infected Persons

About 5% of the lymphomas associated with AIDS are of T-cell origin. As with the B-cell tumors, these lymphomas are heterogeneous, including T-cell lymphoproliferative syndromes, cutaneous T-cell lymphomas, lymphoblastic lymphoma, and T-cell chronic lymphocytic leukemia. Thus far, only a single patient with a T-cell lymphoproliferative syndrome has been shown to be dually infected with HIV-1 and human T-cell lymphotropic virus (HTLV)-I. Because these two viruses may synergistically coinfect the same host, more T-cell neoplasms may appear as the epidemic progresses, particularly among intravenous drug abusers who are at higher risk for HIV-1 and HTLV-I coinfection.

Molecular Heterogeneity of AIDS-Associated Lymphoma

Table 45–3 shows a summary of molecular features of AIDS lymphomas by histologic type. Large-cell lymphoma is often polyclonal, whereas immunoblastic, Burkitt's (small noncleaved cell) and primary CNS lymphomas are usually monoclonal. These data must be interpreted with caution, as lymphomas tend to evolve from oligoclonality to monoclonality in immunocompromised hosts. Also, polyclonal tumors can exhibit malignant clinical behavior indistinguishable from monoclonal tumors. Association with EBV is highly variable, being highest in the immunoblastic subtype and in primary CNS lymphomas.

Rearrangement of the c-*myc* oncogene is also variable, noted most frequently in Burkitt's lymphomas. The molecular heterogeneity points to a multifactorial and complex pathogenesis.

Pathogenesis of AIDS-Associated Lymphoma

In a manner similar to the situation in immunosuppressed transplant recipients, AIDS-associated lymphoma is presumed to result from renegade growth of B cells, starting with polyclonal and progressing to oligoclonal proliferation. The latter condition may manifest clinically as malignant lymphoma, although most lymphomas are monoclonal by the time of clinical presentation.

Multiple factors conspire to stimulate polyclonal B-cell proliferation in HIV-infected persons: HIV antigens, growth factors from T cells and macrophages, EBV infection, and antigenic stimulation from concomitant infections. Some investigators have described a "premalignant" condition of oligoclonal B-cell hyperplasia and c-*myc* rearrangements followed by a stepwise progression to full-blown malignant lymphoma.

Aside from central nervous system lymphomas, a definitive role for EBV cannot be confirmed at this time, even though experimental c-*myc* transfection into virus-infected B cells produces frank malignant lymphoma. Presumably, EBV is one of several stimuli that induce B-cell proliferation. Other candidates include another retrovirus or DNA virus (either exogenous or B-cell tropic), activation of another protooncogene such as the c-*ras* protooncogene, chronic antigenic stimulation from HIV-infected follicular dendritic cells, or induction of autocrine B-cell growth factors in selected lymphocyte clones.

Hodgkin's Disease & Other Neoplasms in HIV-Infected Persons

Oncologists who care for HIV-infected persons with Hodgkin's disease report a more aggressive natural history, with a predilection for tumor sites in unusual locations such as the rectum and parotid gland.

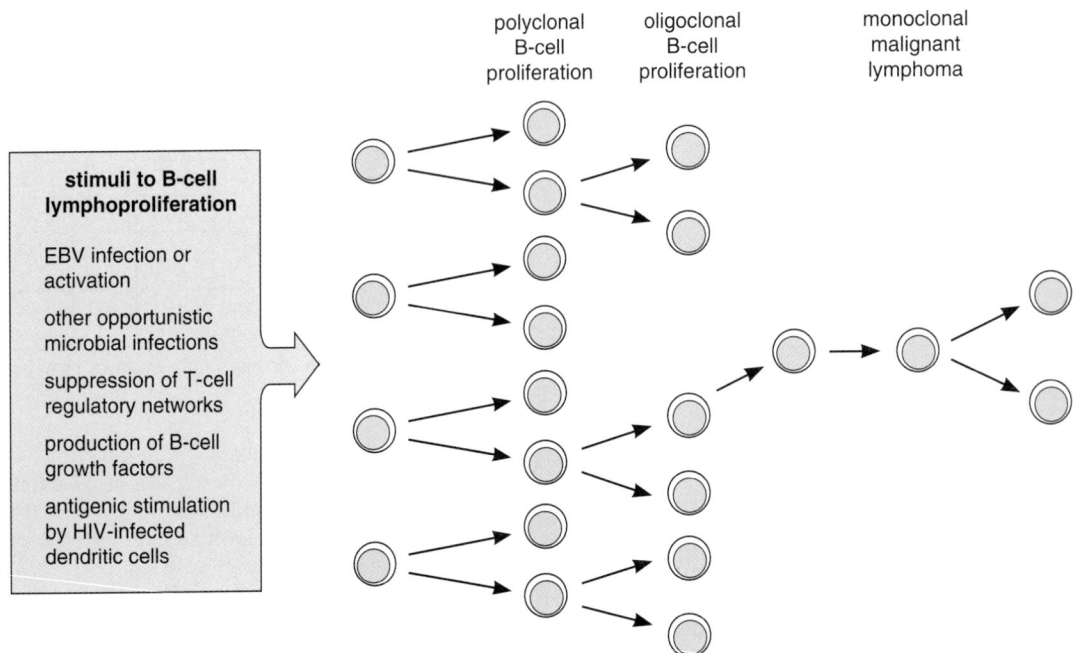

polyclonal
B-cell
proliferation

oligoclonal
B-cell
proliferation

monoclonal
malignant
lymphoma

stimuli to B-cell lymphoproliferation

EBV infection or activation

other opportunistic microbial infections

suppression of T-cell regulatory networks

production of B-cell growth factors

antigenic stimulation by HIV-infected dendritic cells

Figure 45–4. Suggested pathogenesis of B-cell lymphoma in immunocompromised patients. Multiple pathways for B-cell proliferation exist in the immunocompromised patient. These include direct viral activation (EBV) and indirect mitogenic stimuli from infecting microorganisms. In addition, the regulatory networks that normally hold B-cell proliferation in check are impaired, and unrestrained B-cell growth results. In this polyclonal population, the chances of autonomous growth of several clones increases over time, leading to oligoclonal and ultimately monoclonal lymphoma (see text).

A majority of patients have advanced stages of disease, with noncontiguous anatomic spread. Most patients display the mixed cellularity histopathologic subtype, but the tumors are depleted of CD4 lymphocytes. HIV-infected patients with Hodgkin's disease have a very high (~90%) prevalence of EBV in tumor tissue because the highest frequency of Hodgkin's disease occurs in the age group predominantly affected by HIV, an absolute excess prevalence cannot yet be inferred.

An increased prevalence of anal carcinoma occurs in HIV-infected homosexual men, who also have a high prevalence of HPV-associated anal dysplasia. There are as yet no reports of excess cervical carcinoma in HIV-infected women.

Other Cancers in HIV-Infected Persons

Several unusual neoplasms are now associated with HIV infection. Leiomyoma and leiomyosarcoma in young people are reported in excess among AIDS patients and organ transplant recipients. In both situations, there is a strong association with latent EBV infection in the tumor cells. Molecular evidence points to a clonal outgrowth of smooth muscle cells previously infected by EBV, suggesting causality. HIV infection, by means of the transactivating transcription protein *tat,* enhances expression of insulin-like growth factor II in leiomyosarcoma cell lines—an

effect that could implicate a cofactor role for HIV gene products in oncogenesis. Further, HIV infection increases microsatellite instability, reflecting errors in DNA repair which could also potentiate neoplastic transformation.

In Rwanda and Uganda, squamous cell carcinoma of the conjunctiva has increased at least sixfold in the era of AIDS, and 75–82% of cases are HIV-seropositive, versus 19–27% in controls with other ocular conditions (odds ratios 11:13). Squamous cell carcinomas of the skin are associated with ultraviolet light exposure and with immunosuppression. Other studies show that conjunctival carcinomas contain HPV-16, which might become activated in HIV-infected persons. Further work is required to clarify the relationship between HIV and conjunctival cancer in the tropics.

CONCLUSIONS

This survey of neoplasia in immunocompromised patients permits several general inferences about oncogenesis and the immune system. The first is that neoplasia of compartments of the lymphoreticular system (eg, non-Hodgkin's lymphomas from lymphocytes, Kaposi's sarcoma from endothelial cells) predominates in all immunocompromised states. A plausible explanation is dysregulation of the natural proliferative program of these cells, induced stepwise by paracrine or autocrine growth factors, viruses, and genetic accidents.

Second, if a general theory of immune surveillance were correct, we might predict an excess of nonhematopoietic cancers in immunocompromised individuals. These would represent "escape" of nascent tumor cells from the expected immune response. With few exceptions, these cancers are not encountered, and the exceptions can be accounted for by the presence of codeterminants in the persons at risk. For example, epithelial carcinomas in ataxia-telangiectasia may reflect defective DNA repair of radiation-induced damage. Stomach cancer, associated with *Helicobacter pylori*-induced atrophic gastritis, could be a result of defective immune control of *H pylori*. Anogenital carcinomas in immunosuppressed transplant patients may reflect activation of papillomavirus infection.

To date, the experimental and clinical literature supports isolated specific instances of immune surveillance but does not validate a general theory. Thus, certain virus-associated tumors are antigenic to their host and evoke a tumor-directed immune response.

For example, virus-associated tumors, such as the EBV-associated African Burkitt's lymphoma, evoke immune responses to viral antigens expressed on the tumor cell. These tumor-directed responses may be responsible in part for spontaneous remissions and long-term survival of treated patients.

Certain human tumors seem to be antigenic to their host. A tumor-specific antigen has been found in patients with melanoma, and specific T-cell responses to transitional carcinoma of the bladder, malignant glioma, and carcinomas of the skin are reported. Carcinoma of the kidney and malignant melanoma are particularly susceptible to nonspecific killing by activated natural killer (NK) cells. Other tumors express tumor-associated antigens of oncofetal origin, but these do not appear to evoke a protective immune response.

The majority of human cancers, however, are not strongly antigenic, presumably owing to such mechanisms as modification of histocompatibility antigens, cell surface glycosylation, or the production of blocking factors. Whatever the mechanism, the immune system fails to recognize most spontaneous tumors, not because of an immune defect, but because the tumors themselves are relatively nonantigenic.

REFERENCES

Ateenyi-Agaba C: Conjunctival squamous-cell carcinoma associated with HIV infection in Kampala, Uganda. *Lancet* 1995;**345**:695.

Bedi GC et al: Microsatellite instability in primary neoplasms from HIV+ patients. *Nature Med* 1995;**1**:65.

Beral V et al: Kaposi's sarcoma among persons with AIDS: A sexually transmitted infection? *Lancet* 1990;**335**:123.

Burnet FM: Immunologic surveillance in neoplasia. *Transplant Rev* 1971;**7**:3.

Casabona J et al: Epidemiological aspects of HIV infection and cancer. In: *HIV Epidemiology: Models and Methods*, A Nicolosi (editor). Raven Press, 1994.

Chang Y et al: Identification of herpes-like DNA sequences in AIDS-associated Kaposi's sarcoma. *Science* 1994;**266**:865.

Delli Bovi P et al: An oncogene isolated by transfection of Kaposi's sarcoma DNA encodes a growth factor that is a member of the FGF family. *Cell* 1987;**50**:729.

Ensoli B et al: Pathogenesis of AIDS associated Kaposi's sarcoma. *Hematol Oncol Clin North Am* 1991;**5**:281.

Ensoli B et al: Synergy between basic fibroblast growth factor and HIV-1 *tat* protein in induction of Kaposi's sarcoma. *Nature* 1994;**371**:674.

Fine HA and Mayer, RJ: Primary central nervous system lymphoma. *Ann Int Med* 1993;**119**:1093.

Frizzera G et al: Lymphoreticular disorders in primary immunodeficiencies. *Cancer* 1980:**46**:692.

Hanto DW et al: Epstein-Barr virus (EBV) induced polyclonal and monoclonal B-cell lymphoproliferative diseases occurring after renal transplantation. *Ann Surg* 1983;**198**:356.

Herndier BG et al: Pathogenesis of AIDS lymphomas. *AIDS* 1994;**8**:1025.

King GN et al: Increased prevalence of dysplastic and malignant lip lesions in renal transplant recipients. *N Eng J Med* 1995;**332**:1052.

Kinlen LJ: Incidence of cancer in rheumatoid arthritis and other disorders after immunosuppressive treatment. *Ann Intern Med* 1985;**78**(suppl):44.

Kinlen LJ et al: Collaborative United Kingdom–Australasian study of cancer in patients treated with immunosuppressive drugs. *Brit Med J* 1979;**4**:1461.

Knowles DM et al: Lymphoid neoplasia associated with the acquired immunodeficiency syndrome (AIDS). *Ann Intern Med* 1988;**108**:744.

Kripke ML: Immunoregulation of carcinogenesis: Past, present, and future. *J Natl Cancer Inst* 1988;**80**:722.

Lee ES et al: The association of Epstein-Barr virus with smooth muscle tumors occurring after organ transplantation. *N Engl J Med* 1995;**332**:19.

Lombardi I et al: Pathogenesis of Burkitt lymphoma: Expression on an activated c-*myc* oncogene causes the tumorigenic conversion of EBV-infected human B lymphoblasts. *Cell* 1987;**49**:161.

Lymphoma in organ transplant recipients. (Editorial.) *Lancet* 1984;**1**:601.

Macmahon EME et al: Epstein-Barr virus in AIDS-related primary central nervous system lymphoma. *Lancet* 1991;**338**:1991.

McClain KL et al: Association of Epstein-Barr virus with leiomyosarcomas in young people with AIDS. *N Engl J Med* 1995;**332**:12.

Melbye M et al: High incidence of anal cancer among AIDS patients. *Lancet* 1994;**343**:636.

Moore PS et al: Detection of herpesvirus-like DNA sequences in Kaposi's sarcoma in patients with and those without HIV infection. *N Engl J Med* 1995;**332:**1182.

Morris JDH et al: Viral infection and cancer. *Lancet* 1995;**346:**754.

Nair BC et al: Identification of a major growth factor for AIDS-Kaposi's sarcoma cells as oncostatin M. *Science* 1992;**255:**1430.

Penn I: Tumors of immunocompromised patient. *Annu Rev Med* 1988;**39:**63.

Purtilo DT: Opportunistic cancer in patients with immunodeficiency syndromes. *Arch Pathol Lab Med* 1987; **111:**1123.

Rosen F et al: The primary immunodeficiencies. *N Engl J Med* 1995;**333:**431.

Stewart T et al: Incidence of de novo breast cancer in women chronically immunosuppressed after organ transplantation. *Lancet* 1995;**346:**796.

Tucker MA et al: Risk of second cancers after treatment for Hodgkin's disease. *N Engl J Med* 1988;**318:**76.

Vogel J et al: The HIV *tat* gene induces dermal lesions resembling Kaposi's sarcoma in transgenic mice. *Nature* 1988;**335:**606.

Wahman A et al: The epidemiology of classic, African and immunosuppressed Kaposi's sarcoma. *Epidemiol Rev* 1991;**13:**178.

Ziegler JL: Endemic Kaposi's sarcoma in Africa and local volcanic soils. *Lancet* 1993;**342:**1348.

Ziegler JL, Dorfman RK (editors): *Kaposi's Sarcoma, Pathophysiology and Clinical Management.* Marcel Dekker, 1988.

Neoplasms of the Immune System

46

Susan K. Atwater, MD

GENERAL CONSIDERATIONS

Neoplasms of the immune system involve lymphocytes of B, T, and natural killer (NK) lineage; histiocytes; and antigen presenting cells and are similar to other neoplasms in many respects with some important differences. First, neoplastic lymphocytes may circulate in the peripheral blood and lymphatics, like their nonneoplastic counterparts; hence, many lymphoid neoplasms are disseminated at diagnosis. A traditional feature of benign tumors is that they remain localized and neither invade adjacent tissues nor metastasize. In other tissue types, tumors that disseminate throughout the body are characterized by an aggressive growth pattern and poor outcome. Neoplasms of the immune system, however, may not fit this pattern, chiefly the chronic lymphoid leukemias and low-grade lymphomas. These diseases frequently present with widespread systemic dissemination but remain slow-growing, indolent processes for many years.

A second feature of neoplasms of the immune system is that they may retain some functional characteristics of their normal counterparts (see Chapter 1). Neoplastic T cells may secrete cytokines; neoplastic plasma cells usually secrete immunoglobulins. Their functional behavior does not occur in response to a physiologic stimulus, however, as is true for normal cells. Hence, these cellular functions become autonomous and serve no useful purpose, often contributing to the ill health of the patient.

Hematologic neoplasms encompass not only the cell types already mentioned but disorders of myeloid cells and their precursors as well. Myeloid neoplasms are beyond the scope of this chapter, but the interested reader can find information about these disorders in some of the general references.

The purpose of this chapter is to focus on immunologic features of these neoplasms. Some general information is also provided, but for more detailed clinical or pathologic description the reader should consult oncology–hematology texts.

CHARACTERISTICS OF MALIGNANT LYMPHOID CELLS

Clonality

Our current understanding of neoplasia is that it is a clonal process, in which a single cell undergoes malignant transformation via some genetic change and passes this change on to its progeny (see Chapter 44). The progeny are thus monoclonal, having a common cell of origin. Although neoplasia may involve a single transformative event in some instances, it is most commonly thought to be a multistep process, in which the first "hit" leads to a preneoplastic proliferation, and one or more additional genetic changes are required for definitive neoplasia. Even in an overt neoplasm, additional genetic changes may occur and lead to the development of drug resistance, or a more aggressive type of tumor.

Although neoplasms are clonal processes as a general rule, exceptions occur in which polyclonal proliferations may behave aggressively in a manner similar to high-grade neoplasms, such as in lymphoproliferations following solid organ transplantation. Such exceptions are uncommon, however. Conversely, clonal populations of lymphoid cells may be noted when traditional clinical and histologic data show no evidence of a malignant process. Although many such proliferations may be preneoplastic, their clinical significance is often uncertain. Given these limitations, however, the establishment of clonality is an important component of the diagnostic evaluation of many lymphoid neoplasms.

Lineage Association

In general, hematologic neoplasms tend to show features of a particular cell lineage and can be recognized as T cell, B cell, or myeloid in nature. Also, to some degree, neoplasms tend to resemble discrete stages in normal cell development: for example, myeloma cells resemble normal plasma cells, leukemic lymphoblasts resemble normal T and B precursors, and so forth

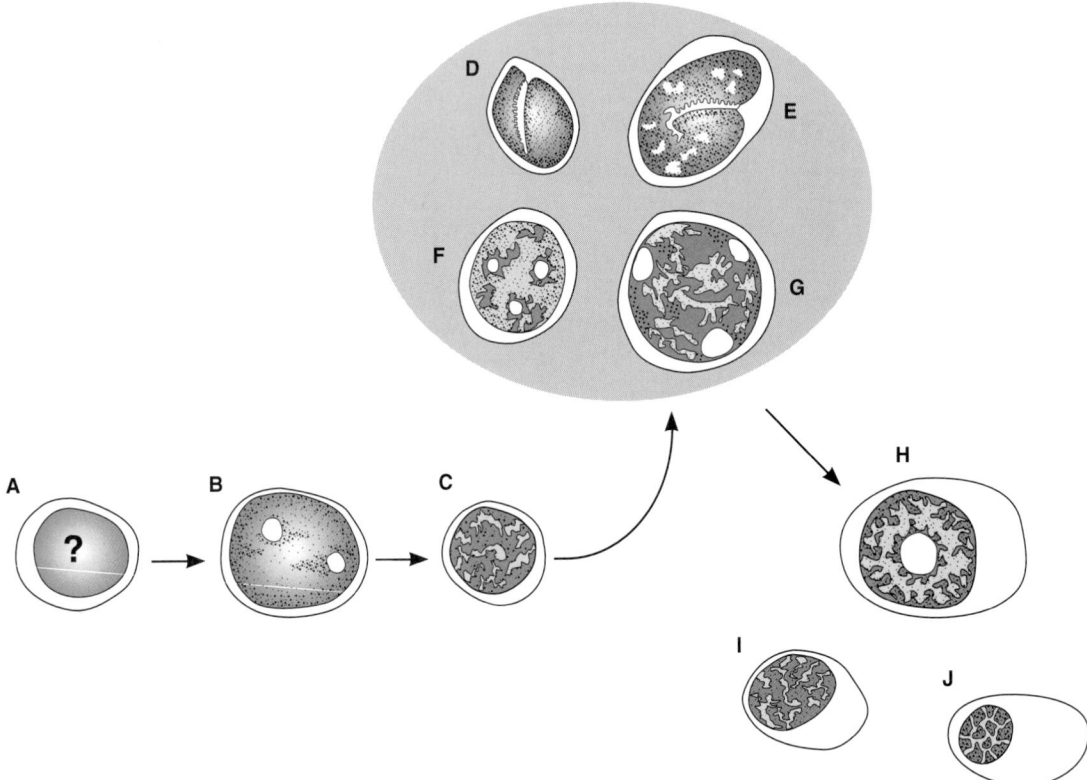

Figure 46–1. B-cell development. Lymphomas and leukemias of B lineage generally resemble cells, at some stage of normal B-cell development, both morphologically and immunophenotypically, to some extent. A simplified scheme of B-cell development is shown here. **A:** Pluripotent hematopoietic stem cells give rise to **B:** B precursors or B lymphoblasts in the bone marrow. Several immunophenotypic stages of B-precursor development are described in Table 46–1. **C:** Mature B cells may respond to an antigen stimulus by proliferating in germinal centers, giving rise to **D:** small cleaved, **E:** large cleaved, **F:** small noncleaved, and **G:** large noncleaved cell types. **H:** Immunoblasts, **I:** plasmacytoid lymphocytes, and **J:** plasma cells are found in terminal B-cell differentiation.

(Fig 46–1 and Tables 46–1 and 46–2). The greater the number of features one compares between normal and neoplastic cell populations, however, the more differences can be found between the two. For example, neoplastic cells often express antigens from more than one cell lineage. In some cases, particularly with acute leukemias, multiple markers from each of two lineages may be present on the cells, producing a hybrid myeloid–lymphoid phenotype. Such mixed phenotypes are called **bilineal** if two or more populations are present within the neoplasm, each of a different lineage, and **biphenotypic** if a single population is present, showing coexpression of myeloid and lymphoid markers on the same cells. In other cases (eg, anaplastic large-cell lymphoma), cells may have lost the surface markers that indicate their lineage of origin, so

Table 46–1. Immunophenotypic stages of early B-cell differentiation.

Stage	Antigen(s)/Immunophenotype
0	CD34, HLA-DR
I	CD34, HLA-DR, TdT, CD19, CD10
II	HLA-DR (brighter), CD19, CD10 (dimmer)
III	HLA-DR, CD19, CD10, CD20, sIgM
IV	HLA-DR, CD19, CD20, CD21, CD22, ± sIgD

Table 46–2. Immunophenotypic stages of early T-cell differentiation.

Multipotential thymic progenitors	CD7, CD13, CD33, CD34, CD45RA
Bipotential T/NK progenitors	CD7, cyCD3, CD13, cD33, CD34, CD38, CD45RA, ± CD2, ± CD5
Committed T-cell progenitors	CD1, CD2, cyCD3, CD5, CD7, CD13, CD28, CD34, CD38, CD45RA
Immature single-positive	CD1, CD2, cyCD3, CD4, CD5, CD7
Immature double-positive	CD1, CD2, cyCD3, CD4, CD5, CD7, CD8
Mature T cell	CD2, sCD3, CD5, CD7 and either (CD4+/CD8−) or (CD4−/CD8+)

that lineage determination then requires molecular diagnostic techniques.

When a cell population that has undergone malignant proliferation shows a combination of antigens that is not known to occur in normal cells, several possibilities are present: either a normal cell counterpart exists but too few of these are present to have been detected during normal development, or no such normal cell counterpart exists. Often, the discovery of the normal cell counterpart is triggered by the recognition of the aberrant phenotype on neoplastic cells, as was the case for CD5+ B cells and chronic lymphatic leukemia (CLL).

Aberrant Features

Just as neoplastic cells can express markers from more than one lineage, they may also express combinations of lineage-associated antigens that are not detectable, or present only on extremely rare cells, during normal cell development. For example, many leukemias of B lymphoblasts coexpress CD34, an antigen present on primitive hematopoietic progenitor cells and the very earliest normal B cells, along with CD22, a B-lineage-associated antigen present on the surface only of mature B cells. This combination is detectable only on an extremely small percentage of normal B-cell precursors in bone marrow. Such differences can be useful in determining whether a proliferation of immature B cells in a bone marrow is due to an increase in normal B precursors or acute leukemia.

Leukemia Versus Lymphoma

The term "leukemia" describes a hematologic neoplasm in which malignant cells are present in the bone marrow and the blood, whereas "lymphoma" describes a localized proliferation of lymphoid cells forming a solid tissue mass. Many hematologic neoplasms show both patterns of involvement, to varying degrees. Clinically, the neoplasm is usually described according to which growth pattern is predominant. For example, acute lymphoblastic leukemia, a disease that usually fills the bone marrow and gives rise to many circulating blasts, commonly also infiltrates lymph nodes. If a biopsy were performed on a sample from such a lymph node, a diagnosis of **lymphoblastic lymphoma** might be rendered if the pathologist had no knowledge of the blood or bone marrow findings. In this case, however, the best diagnosis for the patient is still acute lymphoblastic leukemia. In contrast, a lymphoma growing in a lymph node but only focally involving the marrow, with no peripheral blood involvement, is still called a lymphoma. In clinical practice, distinctions between leukemia and lymphoma may thus be somewhat arbitrary. More important is the characterization of the type of neoplastic cell and the establishment of the correct diagnosis, so that appropriate therapy can be selected.

APPROACH TO DIAGNOSIS

A pathologic diagnosis is often regarded as "the answer," despite the fact that wide variation exists in how neoplasms are diagnosed. Ancillary diagnostic modalities, such as immunophenotyping and cytogenetic and molecular analysis, may be essential to accurately characterize some neoplasms, although morphologic examination may suffice for others. Equally important is the judicious weighing of all available data in a final assessment, especially when some data "fit the picture" better than others.

Morphologic Examination

Morphologic diagnosis has been the mainstay of diagnostic pathology for many decades. Although pathologists are often most familiar with hematoxylin–eosin-stained sections from paraffin-embedded tissue blocks, other preparations are often equally valuable, such as air-dried smears of blood or bone marrow cells stained with Wright's stain. In fact, hematopathologists consider these two techniques to be complementary, because each highlights different morphologic features of cells. For example, air-dried preparations are essential for the accurate diagnosis and classification of most leukemias. In contrast, examination of histologic sections is more important for the diagnosis and classification of non-Hodgkin's lymphomas, because sections provide information about the architecture of the tissues involved and the patterns of infiltration by abnormal cells. For example, the nodular growth pattern of a follicular center lymphoma would be seen histologically but cannot be appreciated if only a smear of cells were stained and examined.

Immunophenotypic Analysis

Cells can be characterized by detecting antigens in the cell membrane, cytoplasm, or nucleus using monoclonal antibodies directed against them. These antibodies are tagged with some compound to render them visible, usually either fluorochromes requiring analysis with either a flow cytometer or fluorescence microscope, or enzymes such as horseradish peroxidase or alkaline phosphatase that give rise to colored reaction products detectable in visible light under the microscope (see Chapters 14 and 15). Various methods of immunophenotypic analysis are available (Table 46–3), each with its advantages and drawbacks. In practice, it is best to have more than one method available and to select whichever method(s) give the most useful information for a given patient.

Monoclonal antibodies have been developed for a wide and ever-increasing variety of cell surface molecules; many of these are useful in clinical diagnosis. Five international workshops on human leukocyte differentiation antigens have been held, in which a standardized **cluster of differentiation,** or **CD,** nomenclature has been developed (see Appendix for CD table). Various antibodies recognizing the same antigen

Table 46–3. Comparison of immunophenotyping methods.

Technique	Advantages	Disadvantages
Immunoperoxidase staining of frozen tissue sections.	Tissue architecture visible. Wide range of antibodies available.	Cytomorphology not as good as with paraffin sections. Technically difficult; not widely available.
Immunoperoxidase staining of paraffin-embedded tissue sections	Tissue architecture visible. Good cytomorphologic detail. Widely available.	Fewer antibodies available than with frozen sections or flow cytometry. Surface immunoglobulin often fails to stain. Two-color staining not widely available.
Immunoperoxidase or immunoalkaline phosphatase staining of cytocentrifuge preparations.	Excellent cytomorphology. Cytoplasmic staining visible. Good results with very few cells in sample.	Tissue architecture not examined. Two-color staining not widely available.
Immunofluorescence by flow cytometry.	Wide range of antibodies available. Large numbers of cells examined. Excellent immunoglobulin staining. Ability to selectively analyze cell subpopulations. Results available quickly. Two- or three-color studies easy to perform.	Tissue architecture not examined. Cytomorphologic detail visible only indirectly on cytocentrifuge preps from sample.

are grouped together within a cluster and referred to by the same CD number. Table 46–4 summarizes several commonly used antigens.

Immunophenotypic analysis using a variety of monoclonal antibodies can give information about how many cell populations are present within a sample, what the cell lineage and differentiation stage is of each population, and whether any of these populations show abnormal features (Tables 46–5 and 46–6). Answering these questions usually requires multiparametric analysis of some sort, in which several different parameters are measured for any given cell. Analysis using two simultaneous fluorochrome-tagged antibodies, each with a different color, is now commonplace in flow cytometry (see Chapter 15), and three- and four-color analysis are becoming more widely available. These allow precise dissection of cell types within a sample, maximizing the information obtained from the cell sample.

Clonality can be assessed in B-cell proliferations if the B cells express surface or cytoplasmic immunoglobulin. A reactive B-cell population contains a mixture of kappa-positive and lambda-positive B cells, and the ratio of kappa+ to lambda+ cells can be calculated. Nonneoplastic B-cell populations typically show $\kappa{:}\lambda$ ratios from 1:1 to 2.5:1, whereas a monoclonal population contains light chains of only one type (Fig 46–2). Mixtures of monoclonal and polyclonal B cells can occur and increase or decrease the light-chain ratio in proportion to the number of monoclonal cells present. Light scatter properties of cells allow flow cytometric data to be examined selectively, looking at light-chain ratios of larger or smaller cells. Figure 46–3 shows a flow cytometric analysis of lymph node cells in which the smaller cells show a mixture of both light-chain types, but the larger cells are virtually all kappa-positive, indicating

the presence of a monoclonal population within a mixed background of polyclonal lymphocytes.

DNA Analysis

DNA of individual cells can be stained with a fluorescent dye and measured by a flow cytometer or image analyzer so that the amount of total DNA per cell can be quantified. With this technique, the percentage of cells in S and G2/M phases of the cell cycle can be measured, and this measurement taken as an indicator of the proliferative activity of a cell population. Also, aneuploid populations in which more than one chromosome is gained or lost appear as separate peaks to the right or left of the diploid peak in a sample. Aneuploidy is measured with the DNA index (ratio of the fluorescence intensity of the aneuploid peak relative to the diploid peak). Aneuploidy is seen in some malignant neoplasms, and its presence in a clinical sample can confirm the presence of a malignancy.

In malignant lymphomas, the percentage of cells in S phase correlates with histologic grade and hence with biologic behavior and clinical outcome. It is used by some but not all laboratories in diagnostic evaluation of lymphomas. Detection of aneuploidy in acute lymphoblastic leukemia (ALL) is useful in that hyperdiploid ALL (51 or more chromosomes by karyotype, or a DNA index of greater than 1.16) has a favorable prognosis compared with other groups. Since the karyotype provides equivalent prognostic data, however, DNA analysis is not uniformly carried out on acute leukemic patients at diagnosis.

Cytogenetic Analysis

Malignant cells are grown in short-term culture, and the chromosomes of cells in metaphase are spread out on a glass slide and stained with Feulgen's DNA stains so that the chromosomes show alternating

Table 46–4. Antigens useful in immunophenotypic analysis of lymphomas and lymphocytic leukemias.

Designation	Description
	B-Cell-Associated Antigens
sIg	Surface immunoglobulin, present on mature B cells and their neoplastic counterparts as well as on L3 ALL. Absent on plasma cells.
cIg	Cytoplasmic immunoglobulin, present in plasma cells, some plasmacytoid lymphocytes and some immunoblasts.
CD10	Also known as CALLA, the common *ALL* antigen, this antigen is present on many normal B-cell precursors and most cases of B-precursor ALL, but is also present on germinal center B cells and many cases of follicular center lymphomas, as well as on some T-ALL and T-LBL. However, it is not significantly present on mature circulating B cells.
CD19	Expressed on B cells and their precursors from very early in development, but absent on plasma cells.
CD20	Similar to CD19, though expression begins later in early B-cell development.
CD22	Present in the cytoplasm in very early B-cell precursors, but not expressed on the surface until late in B-cell precursor development. Also present on mature B cells and their neoplastic counterparts, but absent on plasma cells.
CD23	IgE Fc receptor; increased on EBV-infected B cells. Useful in distinguishing CLL (usually CD23+) from mantle cell lymphoma (usually CD23–).
CD79a	*mb*-1 protein, expressed in association with surface IgM. Highly specific marker for B lineage.
	T- and NK Cell-Associated Antigens
CD1	Present on some normal thymocytes as well as Langerhans' cells; also on many T-lymphoblastic leukemias–lymphomas and Langerhans' cell histiocytosis.
CD2	Sheep RBC "receptor"; present on thymocytes, mature T cells and mature NK cells. Present on most T- and NK-lineage neoplasms and occasional myeloid leukemias.
CD3	Present in the cytoplasm of early thymocytes; expressed on the surface on mature T cells. Present in most T-lineage neoplasms. Cytoplasmic CD3 is detectable in nearly all T-lymphoblastic neoplasms.
CD4	Helper–inducer T-cell subset, monocytes–macrophages and some dendritic cells; present on many T-lineage neoplasms.
CD5	Immature and mature T cells and neoplasms.
CD7	Immature and mature T and NK cells and neoplasms; also on 15–20% of acute myelogenous leukemia.
CD8	Cytotoxic–suppressor T-cell subset; also many NK cells.
CD16	IgG Fc receptor III; present on NK cells and granulocytes.
CD56	NK cells, small T-cell subset, most T/NK angiocentric lymphomas; also some nonhematopoietic tumors.
CD57	Some NK cells; also some nonhematopoietic tumors, especially of neuroendocrine origin.
	Myeloid Lineage-Associated Antigens
CD11c	Monocytes–macrophages and NK cells. Although absent on mature resting B cells, CD11c is strongly expressed on hairy cell leukemia cells, and less strongly on some other low-grade B-cell neoplasms.
CD13	Granulocytes, monocytes–macrophages, and their precursors; also on most acute myeloid leukemias.
CD14	Monocytes–macrophages and their precursors; also on many myelomonocytic or monoblastic leukemias.
CD15	Granulocytes, monocytes—macrophages, Reed-Sternberg cells of Hodgkin's disease.
CD33	Granulocytes, monocytes–macrophages, and their precursors; also on most acute myeloid leukemias.
	Miscellaneous
TdT	Terminal deoxyribonucleotidyl transferase is a nuclear enzyme that is active during rearrangement of immunoglobulin and T-cell receptor genes. It is found in nearly all lymphoblastic leukemias and lymphomas, but is not seen in mature B- or T-lineage neoplasms. It is also present in approximately 25% of acute nonlymphocytic leukemias.
HLA-DR (Ia)	Class II HLA antigen; found on B lymphocytes and their precursors, monocyte–macrophage lineage cells, and activated mature T cells, as well as their neoplastic counterparts.
Fc receptors	Receptors for Fc portion of immunoglobulin molecule. Plasma immunoglobulin binding nonspecifically to Fc receptors may interfere with measurement of light-chain expression patterns on B cells.
CD25	IL-2 receptor; present on activated T cells. Generally expressed on adult T-cell leukemia–lymphoma cells but often absent or weak on Sézary cells.
CD30	Ki-1 antigen, present on some activated B or T cells, and on the majority of anaplastic large-cell lymphomas and Hodgkin's disease.
CD34	Present on multipotent hematopoietic stem cells and committed progenitors, but absent on more mature precursors. Expressed on many cases of ALL, lymphoblastic lymphomas, or AML, but absent in non-Hodgkin's lymphomas of mature B or T cells.
Ki-67	Nuclear antigen expressed during the cell cycle but absent in G_0 cells. Fraction of Ki-67+ cells correlates with histologic grade in non-Hodgkin's lymphoma.

regions of lightly and darkly staining DNA. Chromosomes can then be identified, and any rearrangements of chromosomes can be detected.

Using these methods, karyotypic abnormalities can be detected in almost all malignant neoplasms. These are somatic genetic changes, which are not present in nonneoplastic cells of that individual. In general, all of the cells within a tumor show the same or related chromosome abnormalities. This evidence strongly supports the notion that most neoplasms arise from a single altered cell, in which the somatic genetic changes somehow lead to a selective growth or survival

Table 46–5. Immunophenotypic characteristics of normal cell populations.

Cell Type and Source	Characteristics
Mature B cells (blood or lymph node)	Express CD19, CD20, CD22, HLA-DR, sIg. Polytypic pattern of light-chain expression. TdT-negative. CD5 present on minority of cells. CD10 absent in blood, present in germinal center B cells from lymph node. CD11c is present only on small minority.
Mature T cells	Express CD3, CD2, CD5. 80–90% also express CD7. Mixture of CD4+ and CD8+ cells (CD4:CD8 ratio varies with clinical status of patient) TdT-negative.
Bone marrow B cells	Many coexpress CD19 and CD10; some also express TdT. Fewer are CD20+ or surface CD22+. These cells may be increased in number in some reactive settings.
NK cells	Express CD2, CD7. Lack CD3. Express CD16, CD56, or CD57. Express CD11c.
Thymocytes	Spectrum of differentiation stages; many coexpress CD4 and CD8, and express CD1. CD3+ and CD3– cells present; however, nearly all express CD2, CD5, and CD7.

advantage for the progeny of the original "mutant" cell. However, although neoplasms represent clonal growth from a single cell or origin, they are frequently not homogeneous, since subpopulations evolve from the original clone because of the genetic instability of the neoplastic cells. **Primary** genetic changes are thought to occur early in the neoplastic process and may indeed be the event that causes the original neoplastic transformation. **Secondary** changes may or may not occur later in the disease and in some instances may be associated with disease progression.

Translocations are a common finding in hematologic malignancies and historically have provided clues to the location of oncogenes or tumor suppressor genes within the genome. Translocations involve breaks in two separate chromosomes (eg, chromosomes 14 and 18) and the rejoining of part of one chromosome to part of the other. These translocations are often reciprocal, with rejoining of the other halves as well. These events bring two different genes in close proximity to each other, often resulting in activation of one normally dormant gene by its close proximity to one that is actively being transcribed. The translocations may create fusion genes, coding for hybrid proteins whose amino and carboxy termini originate from the two different genes. It is believed that most of these translocations are primary, in the sense that the fusion genes produced as a result of the translocation are integral to the pathogenesis of that particular leukemia or lymphoma. Table 46–7 shows several common cytogenetic abnormalities in lymphoid neoplasms along with their molecular correlates.

Table 46–6. Commonly encountered immunophenotypic patterns and their significance.

Pattern	Significance
Light-chain restriction	A population of sIg+ or cIg+ B cells expressing only one light-chain type. This finding indicates the presence of a monoclonal population. However, this finding in and of itself is not tantamount to a diagnosis of malignancy (see text).
Polytypic light-chain expression	Both kappa+ and lambda+ B cells are present. Depending on other findings, results might either be most likely reactive, or suspicious for the presence of a small monoclonal population.
T-cell antigen loss	When a majority population of T cells fails to express one or more pan T antigens, this finding is strong evidence for an abnormal and probably neoplastic process. Smaller populations with this finding are harder to interpret.
CD5+ B cells	Normally present in blood in small numbers. However, if a majority of B cells are strongly CD5+, this suggests either CLL, small lymphocytic lymphoma, mantle cell lymphoma or (less likely) another process.
CD11c+ B cells	Strong expression of CD11c on a majority population of B cells suggests the diagnosis of hairy cell leukemia, especially if CD22 is also strongly expressed. Weak CD11c expression on B cells is less specific.
bcl-2+ germinal center B cells	bcl-2 protein (detectable in paraffin sections) is strongly expressed in the neoplastic follicular structures of follicular lymphomas, but is generally absent in reactive germinal centers.
Mixture of normal-appearing T and B cells in a lymph node	Although this picture shows no evidence of an abnormal population, and indeed is a common result when reactive lymph node aspirates are analyzed, it may also be seen when neoplastic cells are a small minority of the total (as in Hodgkin's disease), or when a neoplasm is associated with fibrosis and not well represented in the sample sent for analysis.

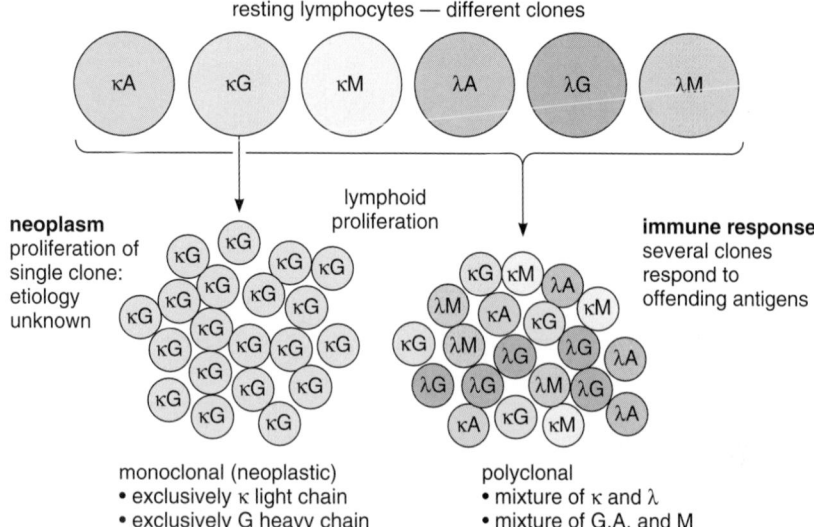

Figure 46–2. Monoclonal versus polyclonal proliferation of B lymphocytes. The monoclonal population contains one type of light and heavy chain in the example given κ and G chains), whereas the polyclonal population consists of lymphocytes containing both κ and λ light chains and several different heavy chains. (Reproduced, with permission, from Chandrasoma P, Taylor CR: *Concise Pathology.* Appleton & Lange, 1991.)

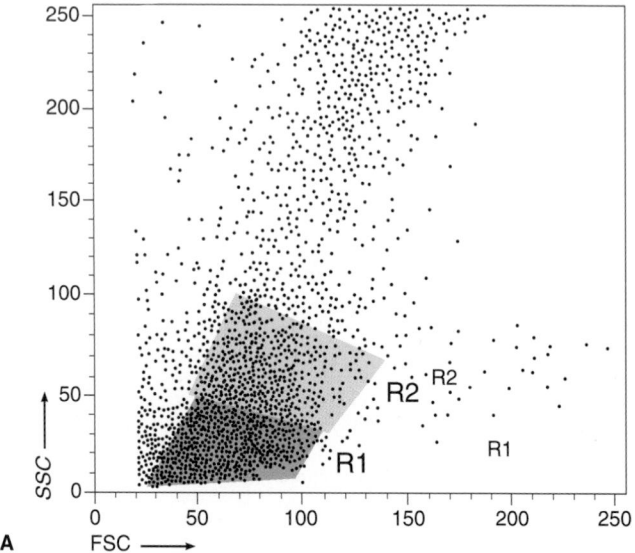

Figure 46–3. Immunophenotypic analysis of a B-cell lymphoma. A 48-year-old man complained of an enlarged, nontender cervical lymph node that has been increasing in size over the past month and was 6 cm in diameter at the time of examination. A fine-needle aspiration biopsy of this mass showed scattered lymphocytes, mostly small and round with a few larger lymphocytes, within a bloody background. Since morphologic review was nondiagnostic, a sample was submitted for an immunophenotypic study. Cells were incubated with various fluorochrome-tagged monoclonal antibodies directed against B- or T-lymphoid cell membrane proteins and then analyzed on a flow cytometer. As each cell passes through the laser beam, scattered light is measured, as is light emitted by fluorochromes. Forward light scatter (FSC) is proportional to cell size, and side scatter (SSC) is proportional to the internal complexity of cells. Light scatter properties thus allow the user to correlate flow phenotypic findings with morphologic data. *A:* shows a plot of forward versus side scatter. Neutrophils, which appear in the upper half of the diagram, have high side scatter due to their granule content. A single broad population is present in the lower half of the diagram, where lymphocytes normally appear. Two analysis regions, or "gates," have been somewhat arbitrarily drawn, dividing this population into smaller, less complex cells (R1) and larger, more complex cells (R2).

(continued on page 658)

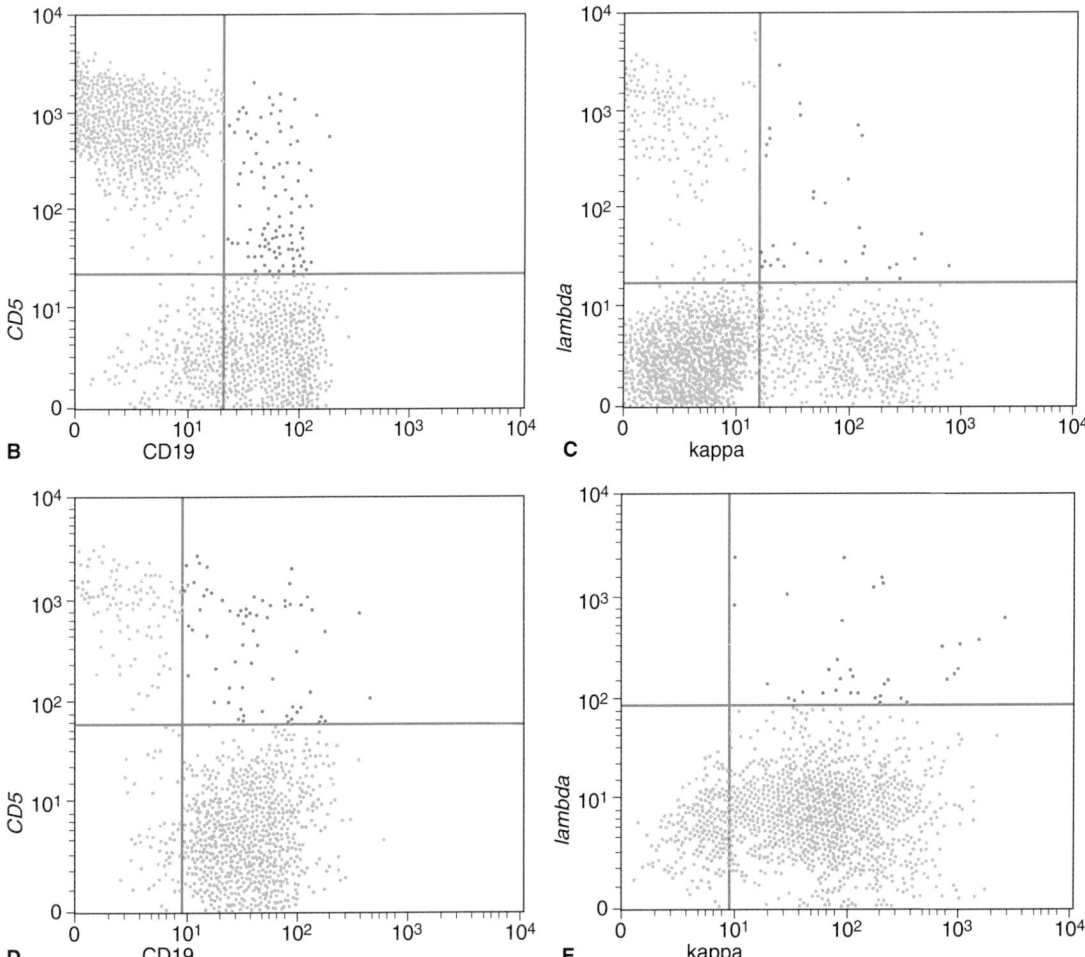

Figure 46–3. *(continued) B & C:* Smaller lymphoid cells within analysis region R1 are predominantly T cells expressing CD5; a lesser number express the B-cell-associated antigen CD19. These contain both kappa- and lambda-positive cells, with a κ:λ ratio of 2:1. ***D & E:*** The region containing larger cells contains mostly B cells, and virtually all of these express surface kappa light chains. The findings indicate the presence of a monoclonal population of large B lymphocytes within a background of smaller B and T lymphocytes. It is likely that nonneoplastic lymphocytes from the peripheral blood were admixed with lymphocytes from the neck mass. Although monoclonal B-cell populations may rarely be present in patients without overt malignancy, the clinical signs in this patient strongly favor a diagnosis of lymphoma. Further evaluation would be necessary to accurately characterize this process.

Burkitt's lymphoma and its leukemic counterpart, L3 ALL, provide examples of such recurring translocation. In nearly all cases of Burkitt's lymphoma or L3 ALL, translocations involving the long arm of chromosome 8 are seen, with the breakpoint occurring at 8q24. In most cases, the other chromosome involved is 14, with the breakpoint occurring at the locus of the immunoglobulin heavy-chain gene, 14q32. Breakpoints involving the kappa and lambda gene loci on chromosomes 2 and 22 are sometimes seen, however. This finding led to the identification of the c-*myc* protooncogene at 8q24. It is thought that when the c-*myc* oncogene is translocated adjacent to an immunoglobulin gene, the active enhancer of the latter gene deregulates the expression of c-*myc* resulting in its constitutive activation. Overexpression of c-*myc*, which encodes a protein active in mitogenesis, is thought to be the primary event in neoplastic transformation of Burkitt's lymphoma.

Cytogenetic information can help confirm the diagnosis of leukemia or lymphoma if a clonal karyotypic abnormality is found, although the absence of abnor-

Table 46–7. Common cytogenetic abnormalities in lymphoid malignancies and their molecular correlates.

Cytogenetic Finding	Molecular Lesion	Diseases
t(14;18)(q32;q21)	Juxtaposition of *bcl*-2 adjacent to IgH gene with consequent *bcl*-2 overexpression.	Follicular lymphomas, some diffuse B-cell lymphomas.
t(8;14)(q24;q32) t(2;8)(p12;q24) t(8;22)(q24;q11)	Juxtaposition of c-*myc* with Ig heavy- or light-chain genes with consequent c-*myc* overexpression.	Burkitt's lymphoma, L3 ALL.
t(11;14)(q13;q32)	Fusion of *bcl*-2 (cyclin D1 gene) with Ig H gene.	Mantle cell lymphoma.
t(9;22)(q34;q11)	*bcr/abl* fusion.	CML, some ALL.
t(1;19)(q23;p13)	*E2A/PBX*1 fusion.	Pre-B ALL (sIg–, cIg+).
12p13 abnl	Abnormalities involving *TEL*.	Many B-precursor ALL.
11q23 abnl	Fusion of *MLL/HRX* gene with various partners.	Infant ALL, AML.
14q11 abnl	α/δ T-cell antigen receptor gene.	T-cell neoplasms.
Trisomy 12	??	CLL.
Hyperdiploidy	??	B-precursor ALL.
3q27 abnl	*bcl*-6.	Large-cell lymphomas.
7q35 abnl	β T-cell antigen receptor gene.	T-cell neoplasms.
t(2;5)(p23;q35)	*NPM/ALK* fusion.	Anaplastic large-cell lymphoma.

malities does not exclude a diagnosis of neoplasia. A normal karyotype may be seen either when the neoplastic cells themselves have no visible karyotypic changes, or when normal cells have preferentially grown out in short-term culture and the neoplastic cells have not been sampled for study.

Certain nonrandom chromosomal abnormalities are so characteristic for a given diagnosis that they help establish this diagnosis (eg, the t(8;14) translocation of Burkitt's lymphoma or the t(14;18) translocation seen in follicular center lymphomas). In addition, many abnormalities provide prognostic information, as seen in B-precursor ALL, in which both the t(9;22) and t(4;11) translocations have been shown to connote a particularly poor prognosis. In fact, in many cases, an ALL patient whose leukemic cells carry either of these translocations is often treated with bone marrow transplantation in first remission, in contrast to patients with good-prognosis ALL who are generally not transplanted at that point.

Molecular Genetic Analysis

Molecular analysis of DNA or RNA offers additional tools for detecting clonal populations and translocations (see Chapter 18). Its ability to detect clonal T-cell populations is especially critical, since immunophenotypic methods for detecting T-cell clonality are not easily available. Detection techniques for B and T cells exploit the fact that during cell development, the immunoglobulin heavy chain undergoes somatic rearrangement within each B cell, giving rise to a slightly different rearranged gene for each cell. A similar process occurs in T cells in which T-cell receptor genes are rearranged.

In the Southern blot assay (see Chapter 18) to detect immunoglobulin gene rearrangements, DNA is first extracted and digested by restriction enzymes, and then run on a gel to separate DNA fragments by size. These are incubated with a DNA probe that binds to the joining region of the immunoglobulin genes, whether these are germline or rearranged. In a population of reactive B cells, the B cells are polyclonal, and each has its own rearranged gene with a unique size. Hence, a smear of different fragment lengths binds the probe and is detected on the autoradiograph. In contrast, a monoclonal proliferation of B cells has identical rearranged immunoglobulin genes, and a single band is seen on the autoradiograph. A similar assay can detect monoclonal patterns of beta T-cell receptor gene rearrangement.

Translocations can be detected by Southern blot analysis as well, if a probe directed against the fusion gene is available. Translocations are also detectable by PCR (see Chapter 18) if primers on either side of the breakpoint are available and if the regions the primers recognize are not too widely separated. PCR detection of translocations is extremely sensitive, and its ability to detect minimal residual leukemia or lymphoma after therapy is the subject of many recent and ongoing research trials. PCR methods of detecting clonal populations via amplification of rearranged genes are also available now.

Integrating the Data

Patients whose clinical presentations are classic textbook examples of a disease are the exception rather than the rule. More commonly, most of the available data seem to fit one possible diagnosis, but some data do not fit the picture. Deciding how much weight to give each piece of information requires considerable experience.

THERAPY

Therapy and prognosis are interrelated. When response to a therapy varies, there is great interest in determining why so that the poor responders can be given alternative treatments. Prognostic indicators are developed that identify good and poor responders. In contrast, if a new treatment is found that cures everybody, the old prognostic indicators no longer predict outcome and lose their value. New therapies for neoplasms of the immune system are constantly being developed and compared with each other, and although no neoplasm is 100% curable at the present time, significant advances have been made in the past few decades.

The therapy for treating neoplasms of the immune system is a combination of managing symptoms and signs (supportive therapy) and attempting to eradicate neoplastic cells through chemotherapy, radiation therapy, or surgical excision. Most patients are treated on prescribed protocols, which vary somewhat from center to center and have differing degrees of success depending on the type of neoplasm, the involved organ(s), and the extent of tumor spread.

Cytotoxic or other antitumor drugs in general affect DNA synthesis and are used in combination and in various delivery sequences to affect the maximum number of cells in S phase. The fact that proliferating cells are more vulnerable to cytotoxic therapy may explain why cure rates may be better with aggressive neoplasms than with low-grade ones. The latter may have an indolent, prolonged course in which remission may be readily induced but is often short-lived.

The selection of appropriate therapy is based on two major factors: cytologic–histologic type and extent of disease. The latter is determined by staging in Hodgkin's disease and the non-Hodgkin's lymphomas. The Ann Arbor Staging Classification for Hodgkin's disease defines four major stages (I–IV) extending from involvement of a single lymph node region (stage I) to disseminated involvement of distant extranodal organs (stage IV). Systemic symptoms such as fever, night sweats, and weight loss provide subcategories for the stages. Staging for non-Hodgkin's lymphomas is similar and uses history; physical examination; surgical and needle biopsies; and x-rays, including tomography, radioisotope scans, CT scans, and lymphangiograms. Because leukemias, by definition, involve bone marrow and peripheral blood, staging is not a factor, but cell type is.

Radiation Therapy

Radiation therapy is more central to the therapy of Hodgkin's disease than of the non-Hodgkin lymphomas. It plays an important role in localized dis-ease, may be the only treatment used for low-grade lymphomas, and may be used in conjunction with chemotherapy in intermediate- and high-grade lymphomas.

Chemotherapy

The alkylating agent chlorambucil has been used alone since 1955 to treat indolent lymphomas and chronic lymphatic leukemia (CLL). It is toxic, however, and may produce irreversible marrow suppression; it is also leukemogenic. Other drugs such as cyclophosphamide are also effective but are toxic. To increase effectiveness and reduce toxicity, combination chemotherapy was developed at the National Cancer Institute. The rationale for multiagent therapy is that drug-resistant cells arise spontaneously, and acquired resistance to a drug results from genetic mutation. Thus, exposure to several drugs may prevent the survival and proliferation of resistant cells. In addition, tumor cell death is related to dose intensity of drugs, so that a maximum dose of a maximum number of drugs over the shortest period should be most effective. This does not, however, avoid toxicity, and careful monitoring is required.

Bone Marrow Transplantation

Because of the ineffectiveness of radiation and chemotherapy in many patients with intermediate- and high-grade lymphomas or acute leukemias, a new therapeutic approach was needed. Both allogeneic and autologous bone marrow transplantation (see Chapter 57) have extended survival in some patients, particularly children.

Eradication of lymphomas or leukemic cells with high-dose chemotherapy and total-body irradiation (purging) is followed by the introduction of marrow-replenishing "stem cells." Techniques for purification of these multipotential cells from autologous marrow or peripheral blood have steadily improved, so that repopulation of the hematopoietic system is increasingly effective.

Other Agents

Purine nucleoside analogues are potent inhibitors of adenosine deaminase and have been found to be effective in several lymphoid malignancies. 2-Deoxycoformycin (pentostatin) and 2-chloro-2'-deoxyadenoside (2-CDA) are particularly effective in treating hairy cell leukemia, with clinical remissions seen in the majority of patients following treatment with either of these two agents. Fludarabine is especially effective in treating chronic lymphocytic leukemia, commonly inducing partial responses as well as some complete remissions even in patients whose disease is refractory to chlorambucil.

Therapy with monoclonal antibodies alone or coupled with radioisotopes or cellular toxins directed at lymphoma or leukemia antigens theoretically has great appeal, and has been the subject of many clinical trials. These trials have had variable results, however, and currently this therapy is still investigational.

NEOPLASMS OF B & T LYMPHOCYTES

CLASSIFICATION OF LYMPHOMAS

"The urge to classify," wrote A. T. Hopwood in 1957, "is a fundamental human instinct; like a predisposition to sin, it accompanies us into the world and stays with us to the end." And while hematopathologists and their clinical colleagues alike share an interest in classifying lymphoid neoplasms, the two groups approach the task from slightly different perspectives. Pathologists, who see visual patterns in the different tumor types, are interested in a classification system that identifies these differing patterns as separate entities, which hopefully will lead to an increased understanding of what these patterns signify. Clinical hematologists and oncologists must decide how to treat the patient and want a simple, easy to use classification that reliably separates patients into prognostic categories.

Many classification systems for the non-Hodgkin's lymphomas have arisen over the past few decades, chief among them the Rappaport, Lukes-Collins, and Kiel classification systems. The International Working Formulation for Clinical Use was developed in 1982 as a way of communicating diagnoses across different systems (Table 46–8). It was not originally intended as a classification system itself but in practice has come to be used as such. It has proven useful in categorizing patients for multicenter clinical trials. More recently, in 1994, the International Lymphoma Study Group has developed the Revised European-American Lymphoma (REAL) classification, in which several provisional diagnostic entities are described (Table 46–9). This system is mainly descriptive rather than proscriptive, in that it describes what

Table 46–9. Revised European-American lymphoma (REAL) classification with corresponding working formulation subtypes.

Subtype	Working Formulation Equivalents
B-Cell Neoplasms	
Precursor B-lymphoblastic lymphoma—leukemia	LBL
B-cell CLL/PLL/SLL	SL, SL/CLL
Lymphoplasmacytoid lymphoma	SL-P
Mantle cell lymphoma	SL, DSC, FSC, DM, DL
Follicle center lymphomas, follicular	
Grade I	FSC
Grade II	FM
Grade III	FL
Follicle center lymphoma, diffuse	DSC, DM, DL
Marginal zone B-cell lymphomas	SL, DSC, DM
Hairy cell leukemia	—
Plasmacytoma–myeloma	—
Diffuse large B-cell lymphoma	DLC, IBL, DM
Burkitt's and Burkitt-like lymphomas	SNC-B, DLC, IBL
T-Cell Neoplasms	
Precursor T-lymphoblastic leukemia–lymphoma	LBL
T-cell CLL/T-cell PLL	SL, DSC, —
LGL leukemias (T and NK types)	SL, DSC, —
Mycosis fungoides/Sézary syndrome	—
Peripheral T-cell lymphomas, unspecified	DSC, DM, DL, IBL
Angioimmunoblastic T-cell lymphoma	DM, DL, IBL
Angiocentric lymphoma	DSC, DM, DL, IBL
Intestinal T-cell lymphoma	DSC, DM, DL, IBL
Adult T-cell leukemia–lymphoma	DSC, DM, DL, IBL
Anaplastic large-cell lymphoma	IBL

Table 46–8. International working formulation of Non-Hodgkin's lymphomas.

1. ML, small lymphocytic (SL)
   1a. Plasmacytoid (SL-P)
   1b. Consistent with CLL (SL/CLL)
2. ML, follicular, predominantly small cleaved cell (FSC)
3. ML, follicular, mixed small cleaved and large cell (FM)
4. ML, follicular, predominantly large cell (FL)
5. ML, diffuse, small cleaved cell (DSC)
6. ML, diffuse, mixed small cleaved and large cell (DM)
7. ML, diffuse, large cell (DL)
8. ML, large cell, immunoblastic (IBL)
9. ML, lymphoblastic (LBL)
10. ML, small noncleaved cell (SNC)
    10a. Burkitt's (SNC-B)
    10b. Non-Burkitt's (SNC-NB)

hematopathologists are currently doing in their diagnostic practice. Although this system is sometimes viewed as more unwieldy than the Working Formulation, it describes several lymphoma types with distinct clinical and morphologic features, for which the question is whether they also will respond to treatment in a distinctive way. Both the Working Formulation and the REAL classification are referred to in this chapter. These two systems complement each other at the present time. Authors of the REAL classification have indicated the most important immunophenotypic, cytogenetic, and molecular features of each entity to be taken into consideration at diagnosis; these are summarized in Table 46–10.

Table 46–10. Immunophenotypic and molecular features important in diagnosis of non-Hodgkin's lymphomas.

Subtype	Features Important in Definition of Entity[1]
B-Cell Neoplasms	
Precursor B-lymphoblastic lymphoma–leukemia	CD19+, TdT+, CD79a+, CD10±.
B-cell CLL/PLL/SLL	B-cell assoc. antigen+, CD5+, CD23+, weak surface IgM.
Lymphoplasmacytoid lymphoma	Cytoplastmic Ig+ (some cells), CD5–, CD10–.
Mantle cell lymphoma	B-cell associated antigen+, CD5+, CD23–, presence of t(11;14) and/or cyclin D1 overexpression.
Follicle center lymphomas	CD5–, CD43–, CD10±, usually surface Ig+, presence of t(14;18).
Marginal zone B-cell lymphomas	Cytoplasmic ig+ (in 40%), CD5–, CD10–.
Hairy cell leukemia	CD5–, CD10–, CD23–, CD11c+ (strong), CD25+ (strong), FMC7+, CD103+.
Plasmacytoma–myeloma	sIg–, cIg+, negative for most B-cell-associated antigens.
Diffuse large B-cell lymphoma	B-cell associated antigen+, CD45±.
Burkitt's and Burkitt-like lymphomas	sIgM+, B-cell-associated Ag+, CD10+, CD5–.
T-Cell Neoplasms	
Precursor T-lymphoblastic leukemia–lymphoma	CD7+, cCD3+, TdT+, Ig–, B-cell-associated Ag–.
T-cell CLL/T-cell PLL	T-cell-associated Ag+.
LGL leukemias (T and NK types)	Both types: CD2+, CD16+, CD57±.
	T-cell type: CD3+, CD56–.
	NK type: CD3–, CD56±.
Mycosis fungoides/Sézary syndrome	CD2/CD3/CD5+, CD4+, CD7– in most cases.
Peripheral T-cell lymphomas (PTL), unspecified	Variable T-cell-associated antigen expression with frequent antigen loss.
Angioimmunoblastic T-cell lymphoma	Same as for PTL.
Angiocentric lymphoma	Same as for PTL.
Intestinal T cell lymphoma	CD3+, CD7+, CD103+.
Adult T-cell leukemia–lymphoma	Usually CD4+, CD7–, CD25+ caused by HTLV-1.
Anaplastic large-cell lymphoma	CD30+, EMA+ t(2;5) translocation.

[1] Characteristic cell morphology is an essential component of defining these entities and is described in the text. Key to immunophenotypic designations; +: over 90% of cases positive; ±: over 50% of cases positive; ∓: less than 50% of cases positive; –: less than 10% of cases positive.

Acute Lymphoblastic Leukemia and Lymphoblastic Lymphoma (ALL and LBL, B- and T-cell Types)

Clinical Features: Acute lymphoblastic leukemia (ALL) and lymphoblastic lymphoma (LBL) affect both children and adults. In childhood, ALL accounts for the majority of acute leukemia cases. As discussed earlier, ALL and LBL describe differing clinical presentations, both of which involve a proliferation of neoplastic lymphoblasts. Patients frequently present with cytopenias and circulating lymphoblasts in the blood. Lymph nodes are frequently enlarged, and in the case of T-ALL/LBL, an anterior mediastinal mass is commonly present. Within this group are several different types of ALL/LBL, each with distinctive immunophenotypic and cytogenetic features, which also differ in their clinical presentation. For example, the majority of infants with B-precursor ALL have a rearrangement of the MLL transcription factor at 11q23; these infants have a poor prognosis on conventional therapy and are often scheduled for bone marrow transplantation in first remission. In contrast, children with B-precursor ALL between 1 and 10 years of age usually have a favorable prognosis, especially in cases where the blasts are hyperdiploid (with 51 or more chromosomes) and CD34+. These children are not generally offered bone marrow transplantation in first remission at this time, since they often enjoy long-term clinical remissions, and the morbidity of the transplant procedure could lead to a worse outcome.

Morphologic Features: Lymphoblasts are of intermediate or large size, often with very high nuclear–cytoplasmic (N:C) ratios (eg, Fig 46–4A). Their chromatin is more finely distributed than the chromatin of mature lymphoid cells but may not be as smooth as is seen in myeloblasts. Nucleoli may or may not be present, and nuclear contours may be irregular in some cases. In a small minority of cases, ALL blasts may have abundant deeply basophilic cytoplasm with frequent cytoplasmic vacuoles and multiple distinct nucleoli. This morphologic pattern is

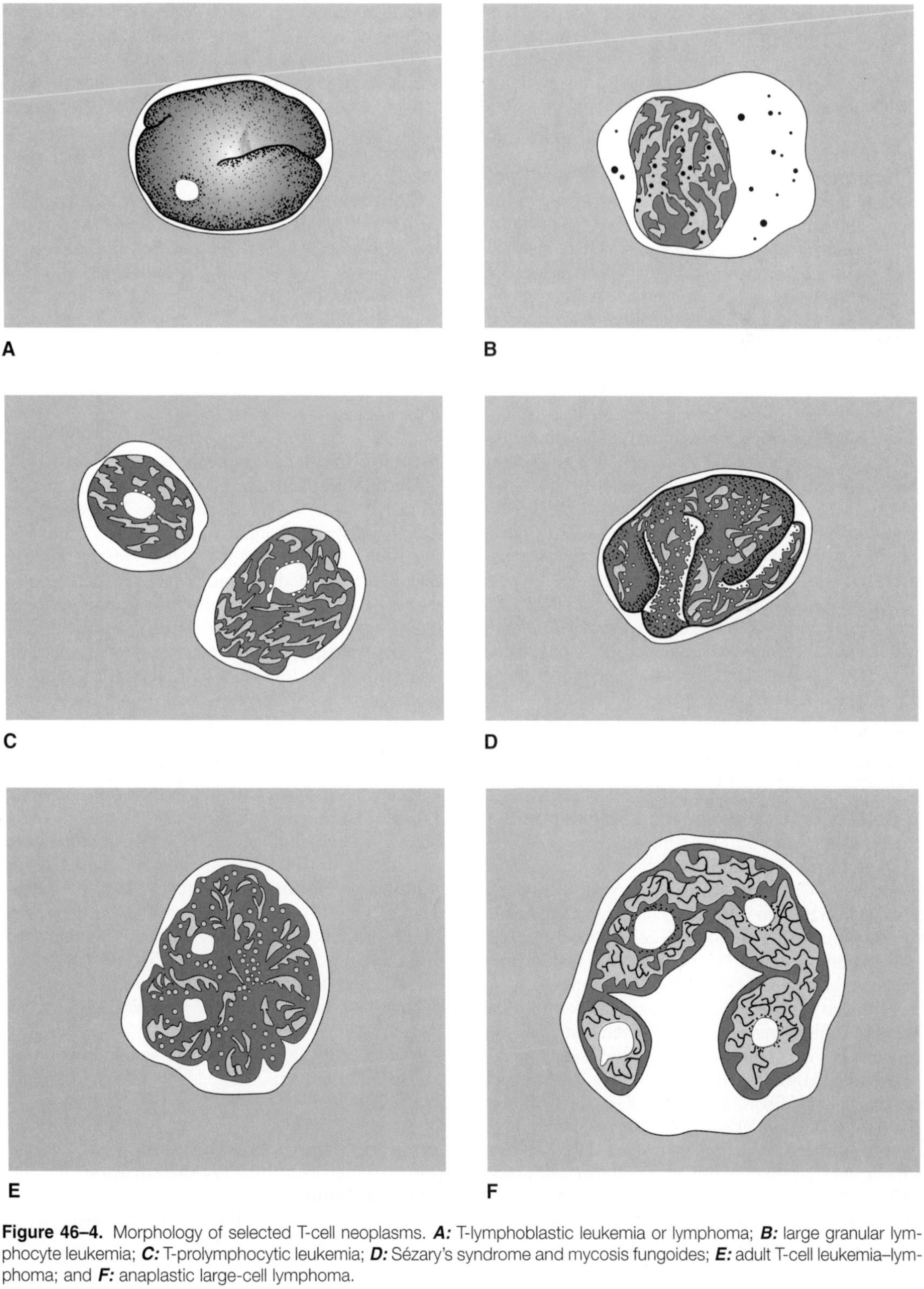

Figure 46–4. Morphology of selected T-cell neoplasms. **A:** T-lymphoblastic leukemia or lymphoma; **B:** large granular lymphocyte leukemia; **C:** T-prolymphocytic leukemia; **D:** Sézary's syndrome and mycosis fungoides; **E:** adult T-cell leukemia–lymphoma; and **F:** anaplastic large-cell lymphoma.

associated with surface membrane immunoglobulin expression and c-*myc* rearrangements and is known either as ALL of FAB L3 type, or as Burkitt's lymphoma, depending on the clinical presentation. In both cases, the cells have an extremely high proliferative rate. Formerly, patients with this subtype responded poorly to conventional therapy, but more aggressive therapy protocols have led to markedly improved survival rates.

Immunophenotypic, Cytogenetic, and Molecular Features: Within the category of "acute lymphoblastic leukemia" are a variety of morphologically similar but biologically distinctive diseases, each with characteristic molecular, phenotypic, and clinical features. L3 ALL with surface immunoglobulin positivity and c-*myc* translocations have been alluded to earlier. Some B-precursor ALL show a t(1;19) translocation involving the E2A and PBX genes; these typically express cytoplasmic *my* heavy chains but lack surface Ig, and have an intermediate prognosis. Philadelphia-positive ALL showing either the t(9;22) translocation or its molecular equivalent (a *bcr/abl* fusion gene) carry a particularly poor prognosis and are frequently treated more aggressively. Translocations involving the *MLL* (or *HRX*) gene at 11q23 may involve several partner genes, are frequently present in infant ALL, and connote a poor prognosis. One subtype of ALL with a relatively favorable outcome is characterized by *hyperdiploidy,* with a modal chromosome number of 51 or greater; this type of disease typically has a precursor-B (SIg-) phenotype often with weak or absent CD45 as well as CD34 positivity, is common in young children but not in infants, and responds well to conventional ALL therapy.

B-Cell Chronic Lymphocytic Leukemia and Small Lymphocytic Lymphoma

Clinical Features: B-cell chronic lymphocytic leukemia (B-CLL) and small lymphocytic lymphoma (SLL) represent two different clinical presentations of this neoplasm of mature CD5+ B cells. Patients are typically elderly or middle-aged adults who may or may not have associated peripheral cytopenias, organomegaly, or lymphadenopathy. Both diseases have an indolent clinical course, in which overall survivals of several years are commonplace. Despite its low rate of progression, however, the cells have low proliferative activity, and the disease is difficult if not impossible to eradicate with chemotherapy. Patients with anemia or thrombocytopenia at presentation have reduced survival rates compared with those with normal peripheral counts. Transformation to prolymphocytic leukemia or large-cell lymphoma supervenes in a number of patients and is associated with a poor prognosis.

Morphologic Features: Lymphocytes are usually small, with coarsely clumped chromatin, lacking nucleoli. Occasional patients may have larger cells that show the same characteristic nuclear features.

Immunophenotypic, Cytogenetic, and Molecular Features: The neoplastic cells have a mature B phenotype, in which surface immunoglobulin is present but typically very weak in staining intensity. CD5 is also characteristically positive, giving rise to speculation that B-CLL/SLL is the neoplastic counterpart of the few normal B cells that also express CD5. Pan B antigens CD20 and CD22 are weakly expressed as well. CD10 is absent, and CD11c is either absent or weakly expressed.

Comments: The diagnosis of B-CLL requires a peripheral lymphocytosis and the demonstration of a monoclonal CD5+ B-cell population in the blood or bone marrow. In addition, some individuals may have monoclonal CD5+ B cells present in their blood without an absolute lymphocytosis or other clinical sequelae. This has been termed "monoclonal lymphocytosis of uncertain significance," and its true incidence is unknown; it is likely on a clinical spectrum with biologic similarity to B-CLL.

Prolymphocytic Leukemia

Clinical Features: Patients with prolymphocytic leukemia (PLL) are adults and typically present with splenomegaly and a high white blood cell count with many circulating prolymphocytes. Other peripheral counts are often decreased. Many patients present with de novo PLL; others have had a history of CLL that is undergoing a transformation to PLL.

Morphologic Features: Prolymphocytes are intermediate to large cells with clumped chromatin, moderate to low N:C ratios, and a prominent single central nucleolus. T-PLL cells tend to have irregular contours more often than B-PLL cells (eg, see Fig 46–4C). A small-cell variant of T-prolymphocytic leukemia has been described in which cells are small, and nucleoli may be less prominent than in classic T-PLL, appearing similar to CLL cells in some cases (see section on T-cell chronic lymphocytic leukemia.

Immunophenotypic, Cytogenetic, and Molecular Features: Eighty percent of the cases of PLL is of B lineage, with bright surface immunoglobulin expression; many are also CD5+. Twenty percent are of T lineage, and most of these are CD4+. All are mature and lack terminal deoxynucleotidyl transferase (TdT).

Comments: Prolymphocytic leukemia is an aggressive disease that responds poorly to currently available therapies.

Lymphoplasmacytoid Lymphoma (Immunocytoma) and Waldenström's Macroglobulinemia

Clinical Features: Patients with lymphoplasmacytoid lymphoma may or may not have the typical clinical picture of Waldenström's macroglobulinemia, in which an excess of soluble monoclonal IgM circulates in the blood, increasing plasma viscosity and causing clinical symptoms. Most patients do have a monoclonal paraprotein of some kind, however. Patients are adults, who typically present with lymphadenopathy or organomegaly (or both), but who usually lack the lytic bone lesions or renal failure that are seen with plasma cell myeloma.

Morphologic Features: The lymphoid infiltrate consists of a mixture of small mature lymphocytes and plasmacytoid lymphocytes, with cytologic features intermediate between lymphocytes and plasma cells. A few typical plasma cells may also be present. Inclusions consisting of immunoglobulin may be present in the nucleus (Dutcher's bodies) or cytoplasm (Russell's bodies).

Immunophenotypic, Cytogenetic, and Molecular Features: Cells are of mature B lineage and typically lack CD5 or CD10 expression. Cells containing cytoplasmic immunoglobulin are typically present and correspond morphologically to cells showing plasmacytoid features.

Comments: Severe hyperviscosity is a medical emergency, often presenting with symptoms such as neurologic symptoms or visual loss due to retinal hemorrhages. Plasmapheresis is effective in reducing the amount of circulating IgM and reducing clinical symptoms.

Mantle Cell Lymphoma

Clinical Features: Mantle cell lymphoma (MCL) affects older adults, with a marked male predominance. The lymphoma is frequently disseminated at diagnosis, with frequent involvement of blood and bone marrow. A subset of patients present with multifocal involvement of the GI tract known as lymphomatous polyposis. This appearance may mimic that of familial polyposis on colonoscopic examination.

Morphologic Features: The neoplastic cells in most cases are small to medium-sized with somewhat irregular nuclear contours and a mature chromatin pattern without nucleoli. The degree of nuclear irregularity is intermediate between the smooth contours of CLL/SL lymphocytes and the small cleaved cells of follicular lymphomas. Large cells are not seen within this infiltrate, in contrast to the case in follicular lymphomas. Also, proliferation centers are not seen, in contrast to the case in CLL/SL. A blastic variant is also described in which neoplastic cells appear similar to lymphoblasts but share the immunophenotype of other MCL. Histologically, many show a mantle zone pattern, in which neoplastic cells form widely expanded mantle zones around histologically benign germinal centers; however, a diffuse pattern is also recognized.

Immunophenotypic, Cytogenetic, and Molecular Features: Neoplastic cells have a mature B phenotype, expressing monotypic surface IgM and B-cell-associated antigens. They express the CD5 antigen; however, in contrast to CLL/SL, CD23 expression is characteristically absent. CD10 is usually although not always absent, and CD43 is usually positive. Many cases of MCL are associated with a t(11;14) translocation involving the immunoglobulin heavy-chain locus and the *bcl*-1 locus on chromosome 11. This latter locus involves the *PRAD*-1 gene, which encodes for cyclin D1, a cell cycle regulatory protein. MCLs lacking the t(11;14) on karyotypic analysis often show molecular evidence of *bcl*-1 gene rearrangement or cyclin D1 overexpression (or both). This translocation is thought to be a primary event in the pathogenesis of this lymphoma.

Comments: This type of lymphoma has been described under other names, including **mantle zone lymphoma, intermediate lymphocytic lymphoma,** and **centrocytic lymphoma.** It is thought that the neoplastic cells are the neoplastic equivalent of the cells in the mantle zone of a normal lymphoid follicle. It was not included in the Working Formulation, and many cases have probably been misdiagnosed as CLL/SL or **diffuse small cleaved** lymphomas. Recognition of the frequency of t(11;14) translocations, and the relative specificity of this molecular lesion for MCL, have led to increased understanding of the biology of this lymphoma subtype. This lymphoma has a median survival of 3 years, considerably less than for low-grade lymphomas. Although 30–50% of patients show complete clinical responses to initial treatment, there is no evidence that any chemotherapy regimen produces durable long-term complete remissions.

Follicular Center Lymphomas

Clinical Features: These lymphomas are most common in adults, presenting only rarely in children. Disseminated disease is frequently present at diagnosis, with multiple enlarged lymph nodes and frequent involvement of bone marrow and peripheral blood.

Morphologic Features: These lymphomas may show a nodular or diffuse pattern or show both patterns simultaneously. The nodules resemble normal germinal centers to an extent but are usually more closely packed, lacking normal mantle zones or polarity. A characteristic feature is a decrease in the number of mitoses or tingible body macrophages compared with normal germinal centers, suggesting a lower proliferative activity than is seen in reactive settings. The infiltrates consist of a mixture of small cleaved cells (with irregular or cleaved nuclei) and larger cells that may have cleaved or noncleaved nuclei. The proportion of large cells is correlated with the aggressiveness of the lymphoma.

Immunophenotypic, Cytogenetic, and Molecular Features: The neoplastic cells are of mature B lineage and have a similar phenotype to reactive germinal center B cells, being frequently CD10-positive. Surface immunoglobulin is typically bright when present although some may lack sIg. Most of these lymphomas have a rearrangement involving the *bcl*-2 oncogene and the immunoglobulin heavy-chain gene. Most but not all of these also result in a t(14;18) translocation visible on karyotype. The *bcl*-2 gene codes for a protein that protects cells against apoptosis. When this gene comes under the influence of the IgH promoter, the gene is constitutively activated and the high *bcl*-2 levels effectively immortalize the cells. Thus, even in neoplasms with very low proliferative activity, the cells accumulate progressively and may be hard to eradicate with conventional chemotherapy.

Marginal Zone B-Cell Lymphomas

Two distinct clinicopathologic entities are recognized within this group: (1) extranodal lymphomas of mucosa-associated lymphoid tissue (MALT) and (2) node-based monocytoid B-cell lymphomas. A third provisional category involves splenic marginal zone lymphomas, many of which may have circulating lymphocytes with cytoplasmic projections (the so-called **splenic lymphomas with villous lymphocytes**).

MALT Lymphomas

Clinical Features: Adults are affected with MALT lymphomas, and there is a slight female predominance. Tumors are most often localized extranodal masses involving sites with glandular epithelium, most commonly the GI tract, salivary glands, thyroid, orbit, or lung. Most patients with salivary gland MALT lymphomas have a history of Sjögren's syndrome. Also, patients with gastric MALT lymphomas have a high incidence of infection with *Helicobacter pylori*.

Morphologic Features: The neoplastic cells, often called centrocyte-like cells, are small, with irregular nuclei somewhat similar to those of small cleaved follicular center cells but with more abundant pale-staining cytoplasm. They are similar to normal cells seen in the splenic marginal zone. MALT lymphomas show distinct histopathologic features similar to those seen in normal mucosa-associated lymphoid tissue (eg, small intestinal Peyer's patches). These include (1) the presence of neoplastic lymphocytes infiltrating epithelial structures, forming **lymphoepithelial lesions,** (2) concentration of plasma cells and plasmacytoid cells adjacent to epithelium, and (3) **follicular colonization,** or the presence of neoplastic centrocyte-like cells within otherwise reactive-appearing germinal centers. Mitoses are few, and most MALT lymphomas are low grade. Some, however, may show predominantly large cells.

Immunophenotypic, Cytogenetic, and Molecular Features: The neoplastic B cells typically express monotypic surface immunoglobulin and B-lineage-associated antigens. Because they lack CD5, CD10, or CD11c, they can be distinguished immunophenotypically from the neoplastic cells of most other lymphoproliferations of small B lymphocytes. Many cells also contain cytoplasmic immunoglobulin, in keeping with the frequent histologic finding of plasmacytoid differentiation. Trisomy 3 has been reported in many cases. Rearrangements of *bcl*-1 and *bcl*-2 are not seen.

Comments: Recently, an association of gastric MALT lymphomas with *Helicobacter pylori* infection has been reported, after which some patients with MALT lymphoma were treated with antibiotics. Surprisingly, many MALT lymphomas regress following eradication of the accompanying *H pylori* infection. The association between MALT lymphomas, *H pylori* gastritis, and Sjögren's syndrome has given rise to speculation that chronic antigenic stimulation plays an important role in pathogenesis of these neoplasms. Indeed, removal of the antigenic stimulus (as with eradication of *H pylori* infection) has led to regression of some of these lymphomas, suggesting that proliferation may often be largely dependent on ongoing antigenic stimulus, thus calling into question our current understanding of the boundary between reactive and neoplastic lymphoid proliferations.

Nodebased Monocytoid B-Cell Lymphomas

Clinical Features: Most of the monocytoid B-cell lymphomas occur in patients with Sjögren's syndrome or extranodal MALT lymphomas; in fact, these may be the lymph nodal equivalent of MALT lymphomas. These also have an indolent clinical course.

Morphologic Features: Centrocyte-like cells, similar to those previously described for MALT lymphomas, are seen in parafollicular, perisinusoidal, or marginal zone pattern of distribution, altering but usually not effacing the nodal architecture.

Immunophenotypic, Cytogenetic, and Molecular Features: These features are similar to those of MALT lymphoma.

Comments: MALT lymphomas and monocytoid B-cell lymphomas are two clinical syndromes apparently involving the same type of neoplastic cell. Differing clinical presentations may be associated with different homing patterns of individual neoplastic clones.

Hairy Cell Leukemia

Clinical Features: Hairy cell leukemia affects adults, with a male predominance. Patients typically experience peripheral cytopenias and splenomegaly.

Morphologic Features: Neoplastic cells are medium-sized to large, with low N:C ratios, abundant pale cytoplasm, and bland round to oval-shaped nuclei without nucleoli. On smear preparations, these cells may or may not show villous, or "hairy," cytoplasmic projections. Electron microscopy shows that these cells have interdigitating cytoplasmic processes, demonstrating that the projections seen on smear preparations are not merely due to technical artifact. In tissue sections, these cells often show a cytoplasmic "halo" of clear cytoplasm with distinct cell borders between adjacent cells.

Immunophenotypic, Cytogenetic, and Molecular Features: The cells have a mature B-lineage phenotype, with expression of B-lineage antigens and abundant surface immunoglobulin. They characteristically coexpress the monocyte/NK-associated antigen CD11c, usually with bright intensity, as well as the IL-2 receptor CD25.

Comments: For much of its history, hairy cell leukemia was referred to by the ungainly name of **leukemic reticuloendotheliosis**, and its cell of origin was not known. Although we now know that this is a B-cell disease, a normal counterpart to the hairy cell has yet to be definitively identified. The disease has an indolent course, and whereas formerly it was considered impossible to eradicate from the marrow, newer treatment with purine analogues 2-chloro-2′-deoxyadenosine (2-CDA) and 2-deoxycoformycin result in clinical remission in 80–90% of patients. A few variant forms of hairy cell leukemia have been described; these also have been shown to respond well to these agents.

Diffuse Large B-Cell Lymphoma

Clinical Features: Large-cell lymphomas constitute 30–40% of non-Hodgkin's lymphomas in adults and may also be seen in children. Patients typically present with a single nodal or extranodal mass that may be rapidly enlarging. Although these tumors are aggressive neoplasms often with high proliferative activity, many are curable with chemotherapy.

Morphologic Features: All large-cell lymphomas have in common the presence of large lymphoid cells constituting the majority of cells present; most have some admixture of smaller lymphocytes. Traditionally, pathologists have recognized centroblastic and immunoblastic variants of large-cell lymphoma. Even when a group of expert pathologists attempts to make distinctions between these entities, however, reproducibility of subclassification is poor. Hence, these entities are grouped together in the REAL classification.

Immunophenotypic, Cytogenetic, and Molecular Features: Large-cell lymphomas may be of B- or T-cell type. Many T-cell lymphomas with distinct clinicopathologic features are described separately, however. All large-cell lymphomas are of mature type, lacking TdT expression. Many B-lineage large-cell lymphomas may show *bcl*-2 rearrangements, as has been described for follicular lymphomas; these patients have a less favorable outcome compared with patients whose cells lack *bcl*-2 rearrangements. In contrast, large-cell lymphomas containing rearrangements of the *bcl*-6 oncogene on chromosome 3q27 have a relatively favorable prognosis.

Burkitt's and Burkitt-Like Lymphomas

Clinical Features: Burkitt's lymphoma occurs in an endemic form in Africa, where it commonly affects the jaw or other facial bones, and a sporadic form in other parts of the world where patients typically present with intra-abdominal tumors. In both cases, children are most commonly involved, and tumors tend to be rapidly expanding masses. Epstein-

Barr virus (EBV) shows a strong association with the endemic form, and the EBV genome can be detected in over 90% of these tumors. A much lower proportion of sporadic cases are associated with EBV. Burkitt's and Burkitt-like lymphomas are also found in patients with acquired immunodeficiency syndrome (AIDS) or other patients with a history of immunosuppression.

Morphologic Features: Burkitt's lymphoma cells are medium-sized with low N:C ratios, deeply basophilic cytoplasm with abundant vacuoles, and nuclei with multiple nucleoli. Diffuse monomorphic sheets of these tumor cells also contain abundant mitoses and tingible-body macrophages; these latter cells appear pale at low power and give rise to the typical "starry-sky" pattern often seen in this and other lymphomas. Burkitt-like lymphomas have similar features but may show larger cells or more pleomorphism, so that the distinction between Burkitt's and large-cell lymphoma is problematic.

Immunophenotypic, Cytogenetic, and Molecular Features: Burkitt's and most Burkitt-like lymphomas are of mature B-cell type, expressing surface immunoglobulin and lacking TdT. CD10 is expressed in most cases as well. Most contain a molecular rearrangement of the c-*myc* oncogene with an immunoglobulin gene, most often the heavy-chain gene. Many of these translocations are visible on cytogenetic examination as translocations involving 8q24 (see Table 47–7). These tumors show some of the highest proliferative activities seen in non-Hodgkin's lymphomas, as one would expect from the histologic appearance.

Comments: Burkitt's lymphoma and the L3 subtype of ALL are differing clinical presentations of the same cell type, with similar phenotypic and molecular features.

Clonal Plasma Cell Disorders

Plasma cell myeloma, or **multiple myeloma,** was recognized as a distinct clinicopathologic entity long before it was known that plasma cells were terminally differentiated B lymphocytes. Because plasma cells secrete immunoglobulin, clonal proliferations of plasma cells usually result in the excessive production of a single immunoglobulin type or often only a single light or heavy chain. These monoclonal paraproteins are detectable by serum electrophoresis or immunofixation as single sharp bands or peaks standing out from the background of reactive immunoglobulins. Often, the presence of monoclonal light chains is detectable in the urine whether or not a serum monoclonal paraprotein is present. These urine paraproteins have been referred to as Bence Jones proteins and may require urine immunofixation for detection (see Chapter 14).

The term **plasma cell dyscrasia** has been used as a generic term indicating any clinical syndrome in which an abnormal plasma cell population is found, whether or not the disease has obvious clinical signs of neoplasia or not. Clonal plasma cell proliferations form a clinical spectrum encompassing indolent and aggressive forms of disease. In many instances, the monoclonal paraprotein is responsible for the majority of clinical symptoms. Clinical evaluation of these syndromes should include routine laboratory tests, a measurement of serum viscosity, radiologic examination for the presence of lytic bone lesions, serum and urine electrophoresis, and renal function tests. Serum should be separated at 37 °C, since some paraproteins are cryoglobulins and precipitate at low temperatures (see Chapter 14).

Plasma Cell Myeloma

Clinical Features: Plasma cell myeloma usually affects only older adults; the disease is virtually unknown in children. Plasma cells form localized lytic bone lesions visible on x-ray, and usually secrete a monoclonal immunoglobulin that can be detected on serum electrophoresis. Immunoglobulin light chains are frequently present in the urine (Bence Jones proteins). Anemia and renal failure are common clinical symptoms.

Morphologic Features: Infiltrates of plasma cells show a monomorphic appearance within any given patient, although wide morphologic variation is seen between patients. Plasma cells range from innocuous, normal-appearing plasma cells, to larger cells with prominent nucleoli, to cells with prominent cytoplasmic inclusions or other changes. In some instances, cells may be difficult to distinguish from plasmacytoid immunoblasts.

Immunophenotypic, Cytogenetic, and Molecular Features: Neoplastic plasma cells are similar to their normal counterparts in that most lack surface immunoglobulin; express abundant cytoplasmic Ig, CD38, and PC-1; and lack most if not all surface B-cell antigens or CD45. In contrast, myeloma cells may express CD56, an adhesion molecule that is absent on normal plasma cells. Many myeloma populations show aneuploidy and a variety of cytogenetic abnormalities, including frequent abnormalities involving the immunoglobulin heavy-chain locus at 14q32.

Comments: Traditional therapy has been largely supportive, although aggressive cytotoxic therapy may prolong survival in selected patients. Autologous bone marrow transplantation is under investigation as a treatment modality. This procedure involves harvesting circulating CD34+ stem cells from the peripheral blood. Most myeloma patients, however, have circulating small lymphocytes that can be shown to be monoclonal, expressing surface immunoglobulin of the same type as the myeloma cells. These cells are present in conventional stem cell harvests but may be absent from samples in which only CD34+ cells have been selected for storage.

Solitary Plasmacytoma

When a single plasmacytoma is found, the patient is assessed for other features of plasma cell myeloma. If no other sites of disease are identified, the patient is said to have a solitary plasmacytoma. These may occur in bone or soft tissue sites. The former has a high prevalence of paraproteinemia and is associated with a poorer prognosis as a result of pregression to plasma cell myeloma. Extramedullary soft tissue plasmacytomas tend to have a more indolent course, usually show nonparaprotein, and only occasionally progress to plasma cell myeloma. Solitary plasmacytomas are usually treated with surgical excision or local radiotherapy.

Monoclonal Gammopathy of Undetermined Significance

A small percentage of otherwise healthy elderly people have small monoclonal paraproteins in either their serum or urine but lack other clinical features of myeloma. Although some of these people eventually develop myeloma, many do not, hence the name **monoclonal gammopathy of undetermined significance (MGUS).** Patients with MGUS are commonly followed by hematologists at regular intervals to detect any evidence of progression to myeloma. Increasing levels of serum or urine paraprotein, or decreasing levels of normal immunoglobulins, often indicate progression to myeloma.

Amyloidosis

Deposits of amyloid may be associated with plasma cell neoplasms and dyscrasias. Amyloid is a complex substance containing fragments of an immunoglobulin light chain, especially the V region. Antibodies directed against this light chain may react with Bence Jones proteins. A nonimmunoglobulin component has a molecular weight of approximately 8000, with 76 amino acids, and is of unknown origin. Another component is a glycoprotein related antigenically to an α_1 globulin present in small amounts in normal human plasma.

Amyloid may arise from (1) the catabolism by macrophages of antigen–antibody complexes; (2) synthesis in situ of whole immunoglobulins or of light chains with reduced solubility; (3) genetic deletions of the light-chain gene, producing an anomalous protein with reduced solubility; of (4) separate synthesis of discrete regions of the light chain. Amyloid deposits may be detected in tissues by light microscopy as eosinophilic material on hematoxylin-eosin-stained sections. These deposits are birefringent with polarized light, and electron microscopy shows nonbranching fibrils, 8.5 nm wide and of various lengths. Special stains selectively stain the material.

A suggested classification of amyloidosis is presented in Table 46–11.

Table 46–11. Classification of amyloidosis.

	Clinical Type	Sites of Deposition
Familial	Amyloid polyneuropathy (Portuguese, dominant inheritance).	Peripheral nerves, viscera.
	Familial Mediterranean fever (recessive).	Liver, spleen, kidneys, adrenals.
Generalized	Primary.	Tongue, heart, gut, skeletal and smooth muscles, nerves, skin, ligaments.
	Associated with plasma cell dyscrasia.	Liver, spleen, kidneys, adrenals.
	Secondary (infection, inflammation).	Any site.
Localized	Lichen amyloidosis.	Skin.
	Endocrine-related (eg, thyroid carcinoma).	Endocrine organ (thyroid).
Senile		Heart, brain.

Heavy-Chain Diseases

Patients with this rare disease complex have paraproteins of one of the three major types of heavy chain (γ, μ, or α) in blood and urine; α-chain disease is the most common. Immunoelectrophoresis demonstrates that heavy chains, but not light chains, are present. There may be partial deletion of the Fc portion of the heavy chain, deletion in the hinge region, or a combination of the two.

α-Chain Disease: Patients commonly present with a severe malabsorption syndrome accompanied by chronic diarrhea, steatorrhea, weight loss, and hypocalcemia. They may have lymphadenopathy. The small intestine is infiltrated with plasma cells, lymphocytes, and histiocytes; these may appear to be benign initially, but as the disease progresses the plasmacytoid cells appear cytologically less mature and extend beyond the lamina propria. α-Chain disease is associated with abdominal lymphomas in patients living in the Mediterranean area, but the disease may occur in other geographic areas as well. Rare cases of involvement of the respiratory tract instead of the gastrointestinal tract have been reported.

γ-Chain Disease: Some patients with this disease may die within weeks of onset, and others may survive for more than 20 years. Commonly, the patients have a lymphoproliferative disorder with hepatosplenomegaly, lymphadenopathy, and uvular and palatal edema. Infection is common and is the usual cause of death. The patients have recurrent fevers, anemia, leukopenia, and atypical circulating lymphocytes.

μ-Chain Disease: IgM heavy-chain disease is seen in patients with long-standing B-CLL with progressive hepatosplenomegaly.

Cryoglobulinemia

A variety of serum and plasma proteins precipitate at low temperature. Some of these are nonimmunoglobulin cryoproteins such as cryofibrinogen, C-reactive-protein-albumin complex, and heparin-precipitable protein. The cryoimmunoglobulins may precipitate at temperatures as high as 35 °C, so that during collection of blood, the specimen must be maintained at 37°C to avoid loss of a cryoprecipitated globulin (see Chapter 14). The rate at which the cryoglobulins precipitate may vary from minutes to days. Therefore, detection of cryoglobulins requires observation of the serum at 4 °C for at least 72 hours.

Small amounts of polyclonal serum cryoglobulin is normally present in healthy individuals. Three types of pathologic cryoglobulins have been identified: type I (25%) includes monoclonal immunoglobulins (IgM and occasionally IgG and rarely IgA or Bence Jones protein); type II (25%) includes mixed cryoglobulins with a monoclonal IgM or occasionally IgG or IgA complexed with autologous normal IgG; and type III (50%) includes mixtures of polyclonal IgM and IgG. Patients with monoclonal type I cryoglobulins usually suffer from the symptoms of their underlying disease (eg, multiple myeloma or Waldenström's macroglobulinemia). Patients with type II or III cryoglobulins may have immune complex disease with purpura, arthritis, and nephritis. These immune complexes often fix complement in vivo and in vitro.

Benign Hypergammaglobulinemic Purpura

This is a rare disease usually seen in young and middle-aged women. It is characterized by a dependent purpuric rash brought on by exercise or alcohol. Some of these patients have autoimmune disorders, particularly systemic lupus erythematosus or Sjögren's syndrome. The patients characteristically have a monoclonal IgG-κ paraprotein that acts as a rheumatoid factor, forming complexes with circulating IgG. Serum levels of IgA and IgM are normal or increased, and there are no findings of multiple myeloma. Treatment is directed at prevention and correction of the underlying autoimmune disorder. Severe symptoms may warrant plasmapheresis.

Large Granular Lymphocyte Leukemias

Clinical Features: Large granular lymphocytic leukemias (LGLL) are mostly indolent chronic leukemias that involve adults and produce an absolute increase in circulating large granular lymphocytes, usually with an absolute overall lymphocytosis as well. Peripheral cytopenias are common, especially neutropenia in T-cell cases. Many patients with T-cell LGLL have a history of rheumatoid arthritis or splenomegaly, and there is probably some overlap with Felty's syndrome in many cases. NK cell proliferations may be indolent or aggressive, and an association with EBV or systemic immunosuppression is often seen in the latter cases.

Morphologic Features: Most frequently, cells are similar to normal large granular lymphocytes, with low N:C ratios, clumped chromatin, and scattered distinct azurophilic granules (eg, see Fig 46–4B). In some cases, irregular nuclei, atypical nuclear features, or abnormal granules may be seen. If cell numbers are low, the peripheral smear may appear similar to the picture seen in acute viral reactions.

Immunophenotypic, Cytogenetic, and Molecular Features: Most cases of LGLL are of T-cell type, expressing CD3 as well as other pan T antigens, CD8, CD16, and usually CD56 or CD57 (or both). These are nearly always clonal and exhibit rearrangements of beta or less commonly gamma T-cell receptor genes. NK-LGLL are less common and lack CD3 expression; most are CD8+, but some are CD4–/CD8–. Clonality of NK-LGLL is difficult to study, since T-cell receptor genes are uninformative. Some show clonal karyotypic abnormalities; these cases usually follow an aggressive clinical course.

T-Cell Chronic Lymphocytic Leukemia

Clinical Features: T-cell lymphocytic leukemia (T-CLL) is an extremely rare chronic leukemia that occurs in older adults, is associated with a high WBC in most cases, and follows a more rapidly progressive course than B-lineage CLL. It also has a poorer prognosis.

Morphologic Features: Cells are small mature lymphocytes as seen in B-CLL. Nucleoli and cytoplasmic granules should be absent.

Immunophenotypic, Cytogenetic, and Molecular Features: Cases currently diagnosed as T-CLL have a mature phenotype and should lack phenotypic features of T-LGL leukemias. Cytogenetic abnormalities involving the beta-T-cell receptor locus at 14q11 are frequently found.

Comments: T-CLL was once thought to be more common, although most previously diagnosed cases of T-CLL would now be classified either as LGLLs or as T-prolymphocytic leukemia. Some authors have argued that the term "T-CLL" be abandoned, since the category is vague, and it is essential to distinguish the indolent LGLLs from the more aggressive cases of T-PLL. Rare cases of T-CLL seem to exist, however.

Mycosis Fungoides and Sézary Syndrome

Clinical Features: These indolent cutaneous lymphoproliferations occur in adults and may present as localized plaques or tumors (mycosis fungoides) or generalized erythroderma (Sézary syndrome). Scaling

and fissuring of the skin on the palms and soles are common. Circulating neoplastic T cells are an expected component of Sézary syndrome and may either be absent or present in low numbers in mycosis fungoides. Mycosis fungoides may become more generalized and Sézary-like over time. Some patients go on to develop a more aggressive large-cell lymphoma.

Morphologic Features: The skin is densely infiltrated with lymphocytes, most with irregular nuclear contours, which occur adjacent to the epidermis and encroach on it (epidermotropism), and may form intraepithelial collections of lymphocytes known as Pautrier's microabscesses. On peripheral smears and touch preparations, lymphocytes have multiple nuclear infoldings producing a characteristic "cerebriform" appearance (eg, see Fig 46–4D). These infoldings are easier to appreciate in thin sections or in transmission electron micrographs. Mitoses are uncommon.

Immunophenotypic, Cytogenetic, and Molecular Features: Cells are of mature T-cell type, expressing pan T antigens but lacking TdT. Most are CD4+, and most also lack expression of the pan T antigen CD7. CD25, the IL-2 receptor, is usually absent, although occasional cases may show weak CD25 expression. However, CD25 expression (especially if bright) should suggest the diagnosis of adult T-cell leukemia–lymphoma. A variety of cytogenetic abnormalities have been described, none of which are characteristic for this disease.

Adult T-Cell Leukemia–Lymphoma

Clinical Features: This disease occurs in adults and is most common in Japan, the Caribbean, and to a lesser extent the southeastern US. The disease is defined as a T-cell neoplasm caused by infection with human T-lymphotropic virus-1 (HTLV-1), a retrovirus; patients typically have circulating antibodies to HTLV-1, and their neoplastic lymphocytes can be shown to contain viral genomes. The acute form of this leukemia–lymphoma syndrome is by far the most common, in which patients usually present with hypercalcemia, a high WBC, organomegaly, lymphadenopathy, and frequent central nervous system involvement. Median survival is less than 1 year. A subacute form is described but is much less frequent.

Morphologic Features: Neoplastic lymphocytes show a variety of cell sizes, mostly medium-sized to large, and are characterized by frequently multilobated nuclei, sometimes showing a radial pattern (eg, see Fig 46–4E). Cells may also appear similar to cerebriform cells seen in cutaneous lymphomas. Chromatin is typically heavier than is seen in lymphoblastic malignancies, but both cell types may show prominent nucleoli.

Immunophenotypic, Cytogenetic, and Molecular Features: Cells have a mature T-cell phenotype, and although nearly all are CD4+, some have been shown to have a suppressor function in vitro. Many lack CD7 or other pan T antigens.

Expression of CD25 is characteristic. T-cell receptor genes are rearranged, and clonal integration of the HTLV-1 genome can be found.

Peripheral T-Cell Lymphomas

Peripheral T-cell lymphomas (PTL) includes a few distinct entities described in the following sections, as well as nondescript peripheral T-cell lymphomas not fitting these descriptions. All are neoplasms of mature T cells, and commonly show pleomorphic histologic features in which atypical cells with irregular contours are present in a range of sizes.

Angioimmunoblastic T-Cell Lymphoma

Clinical Features: Patients are adults who usually present with systemic symptoms, including fever, weight loss, a skin rash, generalized lymphadenopathy, and polyclonal hypergammaglobulinemia. Although these lymphomas may pursue an aggressive clinical course, spontaneous remissions have been described.

Morphologic Features: Histopathologic features are similar to angioimmunoblastic lymphadenopathy and include effacement of the nodal architecture; a hypocellular, or "pink," appearance at low power; absent or regressively transformed ("burnt-out") germinal centers; and a proliferation of small, branching blood vessels. Pleomorphic lymphocytes in a mixture of cell sizes are present in a background of histiocytes, eosinophils, and plasma cells and form sheets or aggregates in at least part of the infiltrate.

Immunophenotypic, Cytogenetic, and Molecular Features: Abnormal lymphocytes are of mature T lineage, showing variable loss of T-cell-associated antigens, and are usually CD4+. T-cell antigen receptor genes show a clonal rearrangement pattern, and EBV genomes can be detected in many of these tumors. Although no specific cytogenetic findings are described, trisomies 3 and 5 are often found.

Comments: The clinicopathologic spectrum between these lymphomas and angioimmunoblastic lymphadenopathy with dysproteinemia (AILD) suggest that cases of AILD without obvious lymphoma are nonetheless preneoplastic in nature. AILD and AILD-lymphomas may represent two aspects of a single biologic disorder of clonal T cells, in which only some cases fulfill traditional histopathologic criteria for a diagnosis of lymphoma.

Angiocentric Lymphoma

Clinical Features: Rare in the US, this disorder is common in Asia among adults, and frequently involves extranodal sites, especially the nose and paranasal sinuses. There is a clinical spectrum from indolent to aggressive behavior, and the proportion of marge cells in the infiltrate may have some bearing on clinical behavior. Patients often develop hemophagocytic syndromes, for which the outcome is poor.

Morphologic Features: These tumors characteristically show an angiocentric and angioinvasive histologic pattern, with atypical lymphocytes invading vessel walls and forming cuffs around them. Not surprisingly, vessel lumina frequently become occluded, and ischemic necrosis is frequently noted in these tumors.

Immunophenotypic, Cytogenetic, and Molecular Features: These neoplasms have a mature T/NK phenotype, frequently lacking CD3 but expressing the NK-related antigen CD56. EBV genomes are frequently detectable in these cells.

Comments: These lymphomas bear some similarity to aggressive NK leukemias and may in fact represent their tissue counterpart.

Intestinal T-cell Lymphoma

Clinical Features: Frequently patients with this lymphoma have had a history of gluten-sensitive enteropathy, and in fact the worldwide incidence pattern follows that of the enteropathy. Patients commonly present with abdominal pain or perforation and are found to have multiple intestinal ulcers. The clinical course is aggressive.

Morphologic Features: The intestinal ulcers consist of a pleomorphic admixture of small, medium, or large atypical cells that may infiltrate the overlying epithelium. Reactive histiocytic infiltrates or villous atrophy in adjacent mucosa may or may not be present.

Immunophenotypic, Cytogenetic, and Molecular Features: Cells have a mature T phenotype; many also express CD103. This latter feature is helpful in establishing the diagnosis.

Comments: Cases formerly described as "malignant histiocytosis of the intestine" are most likely examples of this type of T-cell lymphoma.

Anaplastic Large-Cell Lymphomas

Clinical Features: Anaplastic large-cell lymphomas (ALCL) affect both children and adults. Two clinical presentations are described: a primary cutaneous form localized to the skin without extracutaneous spread at diagnosis, and a systemic form involving lymph nodes and other organ sites as well as the skin in some cases. Some examples of the primary cutaneous form may regress, and this form may be difficult to distinguish from lymphomatoid papulosis in some cases.

Morphologic Features: Neoplastic cells are larger than most large lymphoma cells and show marked nuclear pleomorphism, with frequent wreath-like, horseshoe- or ring-shaped nuclei as well as multinucleated cells (eg, see Fig 46–4F). These cells may show a predominantly sinusoidal distribution pattern in lymph nodes. Neutrophils or macrophages may be present among neoplastic cells in some cases.

Immunophenotypic, Cytogenetic, and Molecular Features: Most cases of ALCL are of mature T lineage, showing clonal rearrangements of T-cell antigen receptor genes, although many lack T-lineage-associated antigens and can be difficult to characterize immunophenotypically. Strong expression of CD30 is a characteristic feature. A t(2;5) translocation has been identified in many cases and is relatively specific for this tumor type. The translocation involves a fusion of the *NPM* and *ALK* genes on chromosomes 5 and 2, respectively.

Comments: Prior to recognition of this lymphoma type, cases were often diagnosed as malignant histiocytosis or lymphocyte depletion Hodgkin's disease. Since lymphoma cells can show a somewhat cohesive appearance and are present in lymph node sinuses, confusion with metastatic carcinoma or melanoma is possible.

HODGKIN'S DISEASE

Hodgkin's disease comprises a group of lymphomas with unique clinical and histopathologic features, accounting for about one third of all lymphomas. Histologically, all forms of Hodgkin's disease are characterized by the presence of Reed-Sternberg cells and their variant forms. Reed-Sternberg cells (Fig 46–5) are very large cells with two or more nuclei or nuclear lobes, each of which contains a single large eosinophilic nucleolus. Their exact lineage is unknown. Variant forms have a single nucleus containing a similar nucleolus. Reed-Sternberg cells and variants are the neoplastic cells of Hodgkin's disease, and are characteristically present in a background of reactive cells (lymphocytes, histiocytes, eosinophils, and plasma cells). In most cases, the reactive cells far outnumber the neoplastic cells. It is believed that the reactive cells represent the host response to the neoplastic cells.

For many years, the disease was considered to be infectious rather than neoplastic because of its clinical course and pathology. The disease is now considered to be neoplastic, since nonrandom chromosome abnormalities have been found in Hodgkin's disease tissue. An association with EBV has been found for some forms of Hodgkin's disease.

Clinical Features: The most common clinical presentation is one or more enlarged, nontender lymph nodes, most commonly in the cervical or supraclavicular node groups. Systemic symptoms, such as fever, chills, night sweats, or weight loss, also known as "B symptoms," are often present and imply a worse prognosis. Patients may also experience pruritus or pain in lymph nodes following ingestion of ethanol for reasons that are unclear. Splenomegaly is present in less than 20% of patients. Progression of disease is predictable, spreading first to adjacent nodal groups before involving more distant sites. This is in contrast to the progression of non-Hodgkin's lymphomas, in which noncontiguous sites may be involved with sparing of intervening node groups. Dissemination into parenchymal organs may occur later in the course of the disease. Clinical stage, or extent of tumor spread, is determined by physical examination, chest x-ray, lymphangiogram, abdominal computed tomography (CT), and liver-spleen scan. Clinical stage is a lightly significant predictor of outcome and is used to determine the therapeutic approach. Histologic pattern is another important prognostic factor.

Morphologic Features: Four broad histologic subtypes are delineated by the Rye classification (Table 46–12): lymphocyte predominance, mixed cellularity, lymphocyte depletion, and nodular sclerosis. A nodular subtype of lymphocyte predominance Hodgkin's disease is recognized and is also known as the nodular L&H (lymphocytic and histiocytic) subtype. This subtype has an unusually indolent course and may represent a fundamentally different type of Hodgkin's disease (see later discussion). The mixed cellularity subtype shows typical Reed-Sternberg (RS) cells and their mononuclear variants within a background of lymphocytes, histiocytes, eosinophils, and plasma cells. The nodular sclerosis subtype shows broad bands of collagen fibrosis dividing the infiltrate into nodules at low power. Typical RS cells are admixed with lacunar RS variants, multilobated large cells with smaller nucleoli that may show retraction artifact in formalin-fixed sections. The lymphocyte-depletion variant shows abundant RS cells and variants with few background cells. Many cases formerly diagnosed as this subtype would now be considered to be anaplastic large-cell lymphoma.

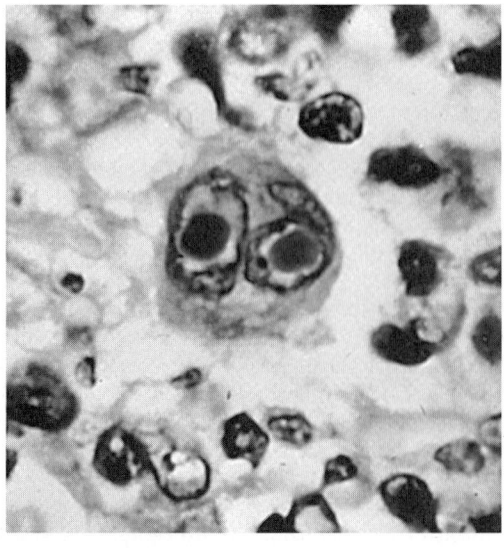

Figure 46–5. Hodgkin's lymphoma. High magnification of a classic Reed-Sternberg cell with two nuclei containing the typical nucleoli. (Reproduced, with permission, from Chandrasoma P, Taylor CR: *Concise Pathology.* Appleton & Lange, 1991.)

Table 46–12. Rye classification of Hodgkin's disease.

Histologic Subtype	Percentage of US Cases	Predominant Features	Prognosis
Lymphocyte predominance	10	Young adult males, stage 1 or 2 at diagnosis; few Reed-Sternberg cells, good lymphocyte host response, connective tissue bands minimal.	Excellent
Nodular sclerosis	60	Young females, stage 1 or 2 at diagnosis; predominant nodules due to wide bands or birefringent collagen, mediastinal mass, "lacunar" variants of Reed-Sternberg cells.	Excellent
Mixed cellularity	20	Majority with stage 3 or 4 at diagnosis; abdominal involvement common, lymphocytes, plasma cells, eosinophils mixed with Reed-Sternberg cells, diffuse involvement of nodes.	Good
Lymphocyte depletion	10	Older males, stage 3 or 4 at diagnosis; systemic symptoms, prolonged fever of unknown origin, abdominal and bone marrow involvement, numerous Reed-Sternberg cells, diffuse fibrosis, and few lymphocytes, indicating poor host response.	Relatively poor

Many cases of lymphocyte predominance Hodgkin's disease have a nodular pattern and are characterized by frequent "L&H cells" or "popcorn cells," an RS-like cell with less conspicuous nucleoli and a multilobated popcorn-like nuclear contour. Typical RS cells are extremely rare. Other cases within this subtype have a diffuse histologic pattern and may or may not have L&H cells.

Immunophenotypic, Cytogenetic, and Molecular Features: Except for the L&H cells of nodular lymphocyte predominance Hodgkin's disease, Reed-Sternberg cells and variants have a characteristic phenotype, expressing CD30 and usually also expressing CD15, but typically lacking CD45. B- and T-associated antigens are also absent, and this feature is especially important in differentiating between lymphocyte depletion Hodgkin's disease and large-cell anaplastic lymphoma. In contrast, L&H cells of nodular lymphocyte predominance Hodgkin's disease are CD45+ and express B-lineage-associated antigens, and although they may or may not express CD30, they lack CD15 expression. These findings have given rise to the idea that nodular lymphocyte predominance Hodgkin's disease is a B-cell neoplasm, distinct from other forms of Hodgkin's disease. The cell of origin for Reed-Sternberg cells has been the subject of debate for some time, and although most investigators consider these cells to be of probable lymphoid origin, the matter is far from settled.

NEOPLASMS OF MONONUCLEAR PHAGOCYTES AND ANTIGEN-PRESENTING CELLS

Cells broadly characterized as **histiocytes** are of two types: mononuclear phagocytes and antigen-presenting cells. The former are derived from blood monocytes and differentiate into phagocytic cells.

The latter comprise the dendritic and interdigitating reticulum cells found in lymphoid tissues, and Langerhans' cells present in the skin. Neoplasms of mononuclear phagocyte type with immature morphologic features are the monoblastic leukemias and the extramedullary myeloid tumors of monoblastic origin. These are discussed more fully in references covering acute nonlymphoid leukemias.

LANGERHANS' CELL HISTIOCYTOSIS

Langerhans' cell histiocytosis (LCH), also known as histiocytosis X, is by far the most common neoplasm of antigen-presenting cells. Until recently, it was unclear whether the etiology was neoplastic or reactive; however, clonality of the neoplastic cells has been demonstrated using an X chromosome inactivation assay. All share a similar histologic appearance characterized by the presence of plump Langerhans' cells with longitudinal nuclear grooves and abundant cytoplasm, admixed with eosinophils, lymphocytes, and rare plasma cells. Three clinical presentations are classically described and are briefly explained here, but the disease can present along a continuous clinical spectrum, frequently in a systemic manner in infants and in a more localized form in older children and adults. **Eosinophilic granuloma** typically presents as a solitary, slow-growing bone lesion in older children and adults, and has a benign clinical course. **Hand-Schüller-Christian** syndrome is a multifocal presentation occurring in children and showing involvement of the pituitary, with resulting diabetes insipidus. **Letterer-Siwe** syndrome describes the systemic multiorgan pattern of involvement seen in infants and carries the worst prognosis. Immunophenotypically, LCH cells are similar to normal Langerhans' cells in that they express the S100 antigen, CD1a, and CD4. Birbeck granules are visible by transmission electron microscopy.

Sarcomas of dendritic and interdigitating reticulum cells have been described and are extremely rare, presenting usually as localized masses in lymph nodes. Many have a spindle cell appearance similar to other soft tissue sarcomas. Immunohistochemical stains are required to demonstrate phenotypic features of reticulum cell origin.

MALIGNANT HISTIOCYTOSIS

Malignant histiocytosis (MH), a rare disease, is now considered to be even rarer than previously thought, since many cases formerly diagnosed as MH would now be diagnosed as anaplastic large-cell lymphomas. In addition, a nonneoplastic proliferation of benign-appearing phagocytic histiocytes (described later in the chapter) has sometimes been confused with MH. The disease occurs in both children and adults and is characterized by widespread disease affecting the reticuloendothelial system, with frequent skin, bone, and GI tract involvement as well. Lymph nodes show a sinusoidal infiltrate of large cells with malignant nuclear features exhibiting phagocytosis. Diagnosis requires not only the characteristic morphologic findings and demonstration of histiocytic antigens (CD68, CD11c, CD14) via immunologic methods but also absence of B- and T-lineage-associated antigens.

HEMATOLOGIC PROLIFERATIONS IN IMMUNOSUPPRESSED PATIENTS

Patients with decreased systemic immune function, whether due to congenital immunodeficiency, HIV infection, or immunosuppressive therapy, have an increased risk of developing malignant lymphomas or lymphoma-like lymphoid proliferations (see Chapter 45). Each of these clinical settings is associated with distinct histopathologic and biologic findings. Patients on systemic immunosuppression following solid organ transplantation frequently develop B-cell proliferations. The risk for developing such a lesion is highest in patients with combined heart–lung transplants and is roughly correlated with the intensity of immunosuppression. Patients receiving cyclosporine or OKT3 therapy are at higher risk than other posttransplant patients. Although many of these lesions are monoclonal, many regress when immunosuppressive drugs are stopped, without the aid of cytotoxic chemotherapy. These are hence called **lymphoproliferative disorders** instead of malignant lymphomas. Epstein-Barr virus is present in the B lymphocytes and is thought to drive the proliferation of B cells unchecked by the usual immune surveillance, which limits B-cell proliferation in healthy people.

These posttransplant lymphoproliferative disorders show a spectrum of histopathologic changes. Most recently, three categories are recognized. **Plasmacytic hyperplasia** is a polyclonal proliferation without cytologic atypia, commonly involves the oropharynx, and generally regresses when immunosuppressive therapy is stopped. **Polymorphic hyperplasia** and **polymorphic lymphoma** show a mixed infiltrate of atypical lymphoid cells, small lymphocytes, and plasma cells; are generally monoclonal; and may or may not regress following cessation of immunosuppression. **Immunoblastic lymphomas** and **myeloma** are not only monoclonal but frequently contain additional genetic changes as well, such as c-*myc* translocations or *ras* oncogene mutations. These generally do not regress when immunosuppression is halted.

It is hypothesized that immunosuppression leads to reactivation of latent EBV infection, or perhaps an unchecked primary EBV infection, with expansion of multiple EBV-infected clones, producing at first a polyclonal proliferation. Clones with a selective growth advantage eventually overgrow the others, producing a monoclonal infiltrate. In some such proliferations, additional genetic changes to tumor suppressor genes or oncogenes may result in a fully malignant clonal neoplasm. This sequence of events is in keeping with the multistep pathogenesis that has been proposed for many other cancers.

HIV-infected individuals have an increased risk of developing lymphomas, and although all subtypes may be seen, three patterns are most common. The largest histologic subgroup is diffuse large-cell lymphomas of B lineage, with or without immunoblastic features. Although all are histologically malignant, both monoclonal and polyclonal varieties have been described. A second group consists of Burkitt's or Burkitt-like lymphomas. This group is associated with the t(8;14) translocation involving the c-*myc* oncogene, or its two variant translocations, as is also true for Burkitt's lymphomas in non-HIV-infected individuals (see Table 46–7). Central nervous system lymphomas comprise the third group and tend to occur later in the course of HIV/AIDS in patients with lower absolute CD4 counts than is true for the other lymphoma subtypes. Virtually all CNS lymphomas are associated with EBV infection, whereas other lymphoma subtypes contain both EBV+ and EBV– cases.

HIV infection in lymph nodes is associated with disruption of germinal center architecture, with follicular lysis, and eventual loss of germinal centers. HIV infection of antigen-presenting cells within germinal centers, with ensuing B-cell dysregulation, has been proposed to play a role in the pathogenesis of node-based HIV-related lymphomas. B cells in polyclonal lymphomas may possibly be proliferating in response to cytokines secreted by another cell population, possibly antigen-presenting cells.

BENIGN CONDITIONS MIMICKING OR ASSOCIATED WITH NEOPLASMS OF THE IMMUNE SYSTEM

A variety of lymphadenopathies may mimic lymphoma either clinically or morphologically. Some are considered truly benign, with little or no increased risk of subsequent lymphoma. This group includes typical follicular hyperplasia, most cases of angiofollicular lymph node hyperplasia (Castleman's disease), the lymphadenopathy seen in systemic lupus erythematosis, dilantin-associated lymphadenopathy, and most viral syndromes. Others may contain small clonal populations of T or B cells and are associated with an increased risk of subsequent lymphoma. These include the lymphoproliferations associated with Sjögren's syndrome and Hashimoto's thyroiditis and angioimmunoblastic lymphadenopathy. All of these may also show concomitant lymphoma at the time of diagnosis.

The hemophagocytic syndromes are a group of histologically benign but clinically aggressive disorders in which histiocytes show phagocytosis of erythrocytes, leukocytes, or platelets. Unlike malignant histiocytosis, the phagocytic cells have benign cytologic features. Patients typically present with fever, peripheral cytopenias related to increased cell destruction, lymphadenopathy or organomegaly, and frequently a component of chronic disseminated intravascular coagulation. The syndrome is associated with infection from a wide variety of agents, most commonly Epstein-Barr virus, and is often present in the setting of an underlying immune deficiency. Familial forms of hemophagocytic syndrome have been described and probably reflect a subtle familial immunodeficiency. T- or NK cell lymphomas and leukemias, most commonly angiocentric lymphomas, are frequently associated with a hemophagocytic syndrome. In these cases, EBV-infected neoplastic T cells are thought to release one or more cytokines, which stimulate reactive histiocytes and cause them to exhibit increased phagocytosis. The pathogenesis of infection-associated hemophagocytic syndromes probably involves release of similar cytokine(s) by reactive T lymphocytes.

REFERENCES

GENERAL
Aisenberg AC: *Malignant Lymphomas: Biology, Natural History and Treatment.* Lea & Febiger, 1991.

Brunning RD, McKenna RW: *Tumors of the Bone Marrow* (Atlas of Tumor Pathology series). Armed Forces Institute of Pathology Press, 1993.

Brunning, RD: Bone marrow. In: *Ackerman's Surgical Pathology,* 8th ed. Rosai J (editor). Mosby, 1996.

Foucar K: *Bone Marrow Pathology.* ASCP Press, 1994.

Jaffe ES: *Surgical Pathology of the Lymph Nodes and Related Organs.* W. B. Saunders, 1995.

Knowles DM: *Neoplastic Hematopathology.* Williams and Wilkins, 1992.

Stamatoyannopoulos G et al: *The Molecular Basis of Blood Diseases,* 2nd ed. W. B. Saunders, 1994.

Warnke RA, et al: *Tumors of the Lymph Nodes and Spleen* (Atlas of Tumor Pathology series). Armed Forces Institute of Pathology Press, 1995.

APPROACH TO DIAGNOSIS
Bain BJ: Routine and specialised techniques in the diagnosis of haematological neoplasms. *J Clin Pathol* 1995;**48:**501.

Batata A, Shen B: Diagnostic value of clonality of surface immunoglobulin light and heavy chains in malignant lymphoproliferative disorders. *Am J Hematol* 1993; **43:**265.

Bentz M, et al: Comparative genomic hybridization in chronic B-cell leukemias shows a high incidence of chromosome gains and losses. *Blood* 1995;**85:**3610.

Borowitz MJ et al: Predictability of the t(1;19)(q23;p13) from surface antigen phenotype: Implications for screening cases of childhood acute lymphoblastic leukemia for molecular analysis: A Pediatric Oncology Group study. *Blood* 1993;**82:**10.

Chappuis PO, Sappino AP: Lymphoid neoplasms— Molecular characterization of non-Hodgkin's lymphomas: Impact on patient management. *Semin Hematol* 1995;**32:**237.

European Group for the Immunological Characterization of Leukemias (EGIL): Proposals for the immunologic classification of acute leukemias. *Leukemia* 1995;**9:**1783.

Gelb AB et al: Detection of immunophenotypic abnormalities in paraffin-embedded B-lineage non-Hodgkin's lymphomas. *Am J Clin Pathol* 1994;**102:**825.

Hurwitz CA et al: Asynchronous antigen expression in B lineage acute lymphoblastic leukemia. *Blood* 1988; **72:**299.

Hurwitz CA, Mirro J: Mixed-lineage leukemia and asynchronous antigen expression. *Hematol/Oncol Clin North Am* 1990;**4:**767.

Knapp W et al: Flow cytometric analysis of cell-surface and intracellular antigens in leukemia diagnosis. *Cytometry* 1994;**18:**187.

Loken MR et al: Flow cytometric analysis of human bone marrow. II. Normal B lymphocyte development. *Blood* 1987;**70:**1316.

National Committee for Clinical Laboratory Standards. *Clinical Applications of Flow Cytometry: Immunophenotyping of Leukemic Cells; Proposed Guideline.* NCCLS Document H43-P, December 1993.

Pinto A et al: New molecules burst at the leukocyte surface: A comprehensive review based on the 5th International Workshop on Leukocyte Differentiation Antigens. *Leukemia* 1994;**8**:347.

Pui C-H et al: Clinical and biologic relevance of immunologic marker studies in childhood acute lymphoblastic leukemia. *Blood* 1993;**82**:889.

Raimondi SC: Current status of cytogenetic research in childhood acute lymphoblastic leukemia. *Blood* 1993; **81**:2237.

Romana SP: High frequency of t(12;21) in childhood B-lineage acute lymphoblastic leukemia. *Blood* 1995; **86**:4263.

Segal GH et al: CD5-expressing B-cell non-Hodgkin's lymphomas with *bcl*-1 gene rearrangement have a relatively homogeneous immunophenotype and are associated with an overall poor progosis. *Blood* 1995;**85**:1570.

Spits H et al: Development of human T and natural killer cells. *Blood* 1995;**85**:2654.

Sullivan MP et al: Clinical and biological heterogeneity of childhood B cell acute lymphoblastic leukemia: Implications for clinical trials. *Leukemia* 1990;**4**:6.

Taniwaki M et al: Interphase and metaphase detection of the breakpoint of 14q32 translocations in B-cell malignancies by double-color fluorescence in situ hybridization. *Blood* 1995;**85**:3223.

MALIGNANT DISORDERS
OF B & T LYMPHOCYTES

Bennett JM et al: Proposals for the classification of chronic (mature) B and T lymphoid leukemias. *J Clin Pathol* 1989;**42**:567.

Dohner H et al: p53 gene deletion predicts for poor survival and nonresponse to therapy with purine analogs in chronic B-cell leukemias. *Blood* 1995;**85**:1580.

Harris NL et al: A revised European-American classification of lymphoid neoplasms: A proposal from the International Lymphoma Study Group. *Blood* 1994; **84**:1361.

National Cancer Institute Sponsored Study of Classifications of Non-Hodgkin's Lymphomas. *Cancer* 1982; **49**:2112.

Zukerberg LR et al: Diffuse low-grade B-cell lymphomas: Four clinically distinct subtypes defined by a combination of morphologic and immunophenotypic features. *Am J Clin Pathol* 1993;**100**:373.

1. Acute Lymphoblastic Leukemia
& Lymphoblastic Lymphoma (B- & T-cell Types)

Cimino G et al: prognostic relevance of ALL-1 gene rearrangement in infant acute leukemias. *Leukemia* 1995;**9**:391.

Copelan EA, McGuire EA: The biology and treatment of acute lymphoblastic leukemia in adults. *Blood* 1995; **85**:1151.

Pui C-H et al: Biology and treatment of infant leukemias. *Leukemia* 1995;**9**:762.

Pui C-H et al: Childhood leukemias. *New Engl J Med* 1995; **332**:1618.

2. B-Cell Chronic Lymphocytic Leukemia
& Small Lymphocytic Lymphoma

Caligaris-Cappio F: B-chronic lymphocytic leukemia: A malignancy of anti-self B cells. *Blood* 1996;**87**:2615.

O'Brien S et al: Advances in the biology and treatment of B-cell chronic lymphocytic leukemia. *Blood* 1995;**85**:307.

Rozman C, Montserrat E: Chronic lymphocytic leukemia. *New Engl J Med* 1995;**333**:1052.

3. Mantle Cell Lymphoma

Banks PM et al: Mantle cell lymphoma. A proposal for unification of morphologic, immunologic, and molecular data. *Am J Surg Pathol* 1992;**16**:637.

Coiffier B et al: Mantle cell lymphoma: A therapeutic dilemma. *Ann Oncol* 1995;**6**:208.

De Boer CJ et al: Cyclin D1 protein analysis in the diagnosis of mantle cell lymphoma. *Blood* 1995;**86**:2715.

Norton AJ et al: Mantle cell lymphoma: Natural history defined in a serially biopsied population over a 20-year period. *Ann Oncol* 1995;**6**:249.

4. Monocytoid B Cell & MALT Lymphomas

Dierlamm J et al: Marginal zone B-cell lymphomas of different sites share similar cytogenetic and morphologic features. *Blood* 1996;**87**:299.

Du M et al: The accumulation of p53 abnormalities is associated with progression of mucosa-associated lymphoid tissue lymphoma. *Blood* 1995;**86**:4587.

Isaacson PG, Spencer J: The biology of low grade MALT lymphoma. *J Clin Pathol* 1995;**48**:395.

Fisher RI et al: A clinical analysis of two indolent lymphoma entities: Mantle cell lymphoma and marginal zone lymphoma (including the mucosa-associated lymphoid tissue and monocytoid B cell subcategories): A Southwest Oncology Group study. *Blood* 1995;**85**:1075.

Bayerdorffer E et al: Regression of primary gastric lymphoma of mucosa-associated lymphoid tissue type after cure of *Helicobacter pylori* infection. MALT Lymphoma Study Group. *Lancet* 1995;**345**:1591.

5. Follicular Center Lymphomas

Symmans WF et al: Transformation of follicular lymphoma. Expression of p53 and *bcl*-2 oncoprotein, apoptosis and cell proliferation. *Acta Cytol* 1995;**39**:673.

6. Hairy Cell Leukemia

Bouroncle BA: Thirty-five years in the progress of hairy cell leukemia. *Leukemia Lymphoma* 1994;**14**:1.

Chang KL et al: Hairy cell leukemia: Current status. *Am J Clin Pathol* 1992;**97**:719.

7. Plasma Cell Dyscrasias

Ruiz AG, San MJ: Cell surface markers in multiple myeloma. *Mayo Clin Proc* 1994;**69**:684.

Chen BJ, Epstein J: Circulating clonal lymphocytes in myeloma constitute a minor subpopulation of B cells. *Blood* 1996;**87**:1972.

8. Lymphoplasmscytoid Lymphoma
& Waldenström's Macroglobulinemia

Dimopoulos MA, Alexanian R: Waldenström's macroglobulinemia. *Blood* 1994;**83**:1452.

9. Diffuse Large-Cell Lymphoma

Hermine O et al: Prognostic significance of *bcl*-2 protein expression in aggressive non-Hodgkin's lymphoma. *Blood* 1996;**87**:265.

Offit K et al: Rearrangement of the *bcl*-6 oncogene as a prognostic marker in diffuse large-cell lymphoma. *New Engl J Med* 1994;**331**:74.

10. Burkitt's & Burkitt-like Lymphomas

van Hasselt EJ, Broadhead R: Burkitt's lymphoma: A case file study of 160 patients treated in Queen Elizabeth Central Hospital from 1988 to 1992. *Paediatr Haematol Oncol* 1995;**12:**283.

11. LGL Leukemias

Loughran TP Jr: Clonal diseases of large granular lymphocytes. *Blood* 1993;**82:**1.

12. T-Prolymphocytic Leukemia & T-Cell CLL

Foon KA, Gale RP: Is there a T cell form of chronic lymphocytic leukemia? *Leukemia* 1992;**6:**867.

Matutes E et al: Clinical and laboratory features of 78 cases of T-prolymphocytic leukemia. *Blood* 1991;**78:**3269.

Matutes E, Catovsky D: Mature T-cell leukemias and leukemia/lymphoma syndromes: Review of our experience in 175 cases. *Leukemia Lymphoma* 1991;**4:**81.

13. Cutaneous T-Cell Lymphoma

Weinberg JM et al: The clonal nature of circulating Sézary cells. *Blood* 1995;**86:**4257.

14. Adult T-Cell Leukemia–Lymphoma

Shimoyama M: Diagnostic criteria and classification of clinical subtypes of adult T-cell leukemia-lymphoma. A report from the Lymphoma Study Group (1984–87). *Br J Haematol* 1991;**79:**428.

15. Peripheral T-Cell Lymphomas

Horning SJ et al: Clinical and phenotypic diversity of T cell lymphomas. *Blood* 1986;**67:**1578.

Cheng A-L et al: Direct comparison of peripheral T cell lymphoma with diffuse B-cell lymphoma of comparable histologic grades: Should peripheral T cell lymphomas be considered separately? *J Clin Oncol* 1989;**7:**725.

16. Anaplastic Large-Cell Lymphoma

Filippa DA et al: CD30 (Ki-1)-positive malignant lymphomas: Clinical, immunophenotypic, histologic and genetic characteristics and differences with Hodgkin's disease. *Blood* 1996;**87:**2905.

Kadin ME: Ki-1/CD30+ (anaplastic) large cell lymphoma: Maturation of a clinicopathologic entity with prospects of effective therapy. *J Clin Oncol* 1994;**12:**884.

Lamant L et al: High incidence of the t(2;5)(p23;q35) translocation on anaplastic large cell lymphoma and its lack of detection in Hodgkin's disease. Comparison of cytogenetic analysis, reverse transcriptase-polymerase chain reaction, and P-80 immunostaining. *Blood* 1996;**87:**284.

17. Other T-Cell Neoplasms

Jaffe ES: Classification of natural killer (NK) and NK-like T cell malignancies. *Blood* 1996;**87:**1207.

HODGKIN'S DISEASE

Pan LX et al: Nodular lymphocyte predominance Hodgkin's disease: A monoclonal or polyclonal B cell disorder? *Blood* 1996;**87:**2428.

Weber-Mattiesen K et al: Numerical chromosome aberrations are present within the CD30+ Hodgkin and Reed-Sternberg cells in 100% of analyzed cases of Hodgkin's disease. *Blood* 1995;**86:**1484.

HISTIOCYTIC MALIGNANCIES

Willman CL et al: Langerhans-cell histiocytosis (Histiocytosis X)—A clonal proliferative disease. *New Engl J Med* 1994;**331:**154.

Cline MJ: Histiocytes and histiocytosis. *Blood* 1994;**84:**2840.

CYTOKINE EXPRESSION BY CLONAL T-CELL PROLIFERATIONS

Cogan E et al: Brief report: Clonal proliferation of type 2 helper T cells in a man with the hypereosinophilic syndrome. *New Engl J Med* 1994;**330:**535.

HEMATOLOGIC PROLIFERATIONS IN IMMUNOSUPPRESSED PATIENTS

Herndier BG et al: Pathogenesis of AIDS lymphomas. *AIDS* 1994;**8:**1025.

Knowles DM et al: Correlative morphologic and molecular genetic analysis demonstrates three distinct categories of posttransplantation lymphoproliferative disorders. *Blood* 1995;**85:**552.

47

Mechanisms of Immunity to Infection

John Mills, MD

The environment in which we live is populated by microorganisms, many of which are capable of causing disease. The immune system probably evolved primarily as a defense against infection by these omnipresent pathogenic microorganisms. Nonimmunologic defenses against infectious disease (Table 47–1) are at least as important as immunologic defenses, however, especially in preventing early stages of infection. Collectively, these immunologic and nonimmunologic defense mechanisms are responsible for keeping our internal milieu free of microorganisms and for maintaining the sterility of distal portions of the "external" portions of the host despite continuous exposure to contamination. The best example of an external domain kept sterile is the respiratory tract, in which the tracheobronchial tree distal to the carina is normally sterile.

As our understanding of the immune system has improved, the boundary between specific and nonspecific immune resistance to infection has blurred. For example, natural killer (NK) cells and macrophages function in nonspecific immune defense mechanisms, but they may be activated by lymphokines produced as a result of the specific interaction between immune lymphocytes and antigens. These cells may also become specific effectors through cooperation with antibody.

Host defenses against infection—whether specific or nonspecific—are also characterized by considerable redundancy. This may explain why profound defects in one sector of host defenses ordinarily result in only a minimal increase in the overall susceptibility to infection.

NONIMMUNOLOGIC DEFENSES AGAINST INFECTION

Host Defenses at Body Surfaces

For an invading pathogen to produce infection, it must first slip through an impressive barrier of surface defenses that operate wherever intact body tissues interface with the environment. These barriers—the skin and mucosal epithelial surfaces—are largely nonspecific and nonimmunologic, but they constitute a vital component of host defense. Normal skin is virtually completely resistant to infection and generally only becomes infected when disrupted by trauma. The mechanisms by which skin resists infection are incompletely understood but probably are related to the dry, acidic environment, antibacterial fatty acids, and the presence of normal flora.

Many pathogens initiate infection by attaching to mucosal epithelial cells. All epithelial cells are covered with a mucous layer, which serves in part to prevent microorganisms from attaching to the cell surface. Coordinated movement of the underlying cilia sweeps organisms entrapped in the mucous layer out of the body. This process may be assisted by coordinated movements of these organs, such as coughing or peristalsis. Intestinal epithelial cells have a short (30-hour) half-life, which also limits the efficiency of infection. If the invading microorganism happens to attach to a desquamating epithelial cell, infection does not occur. Exposure of epithelial cells to many microorganisms triggers a coordinated response in the cell, which may augment host resistance to infection.

Many substances coating body surfaces serve as local disinfectants and antimicrobial substances. The skin has a high content of fatty acids, which are inhibitory to bacteria and fungi. The stomach secretes hydrochloric acid with a pH between 1 and 2, which is sufficient to kill most gastrointestinal pathogens. Factors that reduce gastric acidity, such as treatment with antacids or H_2 blockers, can increase the susceptibility of the host to enteric pathogens. A number of specific bactericidal or fungicidal proteins are formed on body surfaces. For example, the enzyme lysozyme, which is present in tears and many other mucosal secretions, is bactericidal for many gram-positive bacteria. Most of the bacteria susceptible to lysozyme are classified as nonpathogens, but it may be that they are nonpathogenic because of the large amounts of

Table 47–1. Nonimmunologic host defense mechanisms.

Surface defenses
  Mucus
  Coughing/peristalsis
  Epithelial cell turnover
  Local disinfectants (gastric acid, skin lipids)
  Normal microbial flora
Inflammatory reaction
  Cells
    Phagocytic cells
      PMN
      Monocyte-macrophages
    NK cells
  Complement (alternative pathway)
  Collectins
  Fibronectin
  Prostaglandins and leukotrienes
  Cytokines (interferons, IL-1, etc)

Abbreviation: IL-1 = interleukin-1.

The normal flora clearly serve a protective role. For example, elimination of the anaerobic component of the gastrointestinal normal flora by antimicrobial therapy has been shown to increase the susceptibility of patients to infection by enteric pathogens such as *Shigella* and *Salmonella.* However, the extent to which the normal flora participate in host defense and the mechanisms by which they prevent colonization or infection by pathogens are incompletely defined. Some mechanisms that have been identified include stimulation of antibodies and T cells cross-reactive with pathogenic microorganisms, nonspecific stimulation (priming) of the immune system, competition for nutrients, competition for receptor sites on epithelial cells, and secretion of substances toxic to pathogens (eg, secretion of bactericidal short-chain fatty acids by intestinal anaerobes).

Inflammation

Immunoglobulins and phagocytic cells play a major role in host defenses at external surfaces; they are also critical to host defenses within the body.

Cells whose major function is phagocytosis of foreign materials and killing of microorganisms are frequently referred to as "professional phagocytes," to differentiate them from other cells, including epithelial cells, that have some capacity to ingest foreign material (Table 47–3). These cells include neutrophils, basophils, eosinophils, and cells of the monocyte–macrophage series, including blood monocytes and tissue macrophages such as Kupffer's cells and alveolar macrophages. Professional phagocytes also have specialized surface receptors (eg, for the Fc portion of IgG and IgA, complement, and the products of inflammation) that are essential to their function, and they contain proteins in granules that kill eukaryotic and prokaryotic cells. NK cells are lymphoid cells that have surface Fc receptors, but they are nonphagocytic and do not contain microbicidal systems such as lysosomes. They primarily mediate lysis of virus-infected cells (see later discussion and Chapter 53).

Invasion of a host by a pathogen that is able to evade the surface defenses previously described usually results in an inflammatory response. The components of this response include phagocytic cells, soluble factors (eg, complement, arachidonic acid metabolites), and the response of local host tissues and organs (eg, the vascular tree; see Chapters 11 and

lysozyme in secretions. Many other mucosal proteins with specific activity against microorganisms (eg, lactoferrin) have been described. Lactoferrin is an iron-binding protein that maintains the concentration of free iron necessary for bacterial replication below levels at which most bacteria grow.

Most animal and human surfaces that are exposed to the environment are colonized by nonpathogenic (or weakly pathogenic) bacteria and fungi collectively known as the normal flora. Sites populated by the normal flora include the mouth, skin, and gastrointestinal tract (Table 47–2). Anaerobic bacteria are important components of the normal flora at all sites. The density of the normal flora also varies greatly depending on the location; for example, the gastrointestinal tract at the stomach and proximal small bowel is virtually sterile, whereas the contents of the distal colon may contain 10^{11} bacteria/g of contents.

Table 47–2. The normal flora.

Site	Representative Organisms
Oral mucosa	Viridans streptococci Anaerobic streptococci
Vagina	Anaerobic streptococci *Lactobacillus*
Dental plaque	*Fusobacterium* (anaerobes) *Veillonella* (anaerobes) Actinomycetes (anaerobes) Spirochetes (anaerobes)
Colonic mucosa	*Bacteroides* (anaerobes) *Fusobacterium* (anaerobes) *Escherichia coli* (anaerobes) *Clostridium* (anaerobes) *Lactobacillus* Anaerobic streptococci and staphylococci
Skin	*Propionibacterium* (anaerobes) *Staphylococcus epidermidis* *Corynebacterium* *Pityrosporum, Malassezia*

Table 47–3. Phagocytic cells.

Neutrophilic leukocytes
Eosinophilic leukocytes
Basophilic leukocytes
Blood monocytes
Tissue macrophages
Kupffer's cells of the liver
Alveolar macrophages
Astroglial cells

12). In viral infections, NK cells and interferons (see Chapters 9 and 10) are probably important in early nonspecific defense mechanisms. Invasion by microorganisms produces changes in the host that attract phagocytic cells (especially polymorphonuclear neutrophils [PMN]); in addition, some substances produced by pathogens (eg, the *N*-formyl peptides produced by bacteria) are chemotactic (attractive for phagocytic cells) in themselves. The PMNs, which are usually the first cells at the site of infection, attack the invading pathogen and simultaneously produce chemoattractants to call in additional phagocytic cells, both PMNs and monocyte–macrophages. PMN products also produce important changes in host tissues (eg, vasodilatation). Monocyte–macrophages and other cells produce cytokines, such as interleukin-1 (IL-1), tumor necrosis factor (TNF), and interferons. These cause fever and further augment the inflammatory reaction by attracting additional cells, augmenting the activity of these cells, and inducing vasodilatation (see Chapter 10).

Several other types of inflammatory response proteins also play a role in nonspecific host defenses. Collectins are C-type lectins with a collagen-binding domain, having many of the opsonic and microbicidal properties of antibodies but with relatively nonspecific binding determined by carbohydrate recognition. Collectins are found in blood (mannose-binding protein), alveolar-bronchial fluid (SpA and SpD), and at other sites. Fibronectin and laminin, which are proteins secreted by endothelial cells, indirectly augment phagocytosis by polymorphonuclear leukocytes and macrophages. Bacterial lipopolysaccharide-binding protein (LPS-BP) mediates binding of endotoxin to monocyte–macrophages and augments cytokine release from these cells.

Fever

Elevation of body temperature (fever) in response to infection is nearly universal in humans and other animals; this response has been highly conserved during evolution. It is therefore reasonable to conclude that fever is an important host defense mechanism. This contention has been difficult to prove, however. The main problem in proving the role of fever in antimicrobial defense in homoiothermic animals has been in dissociating the effects of the endogenous pyrogens (IL-1, TNF) that produce fever from the complex effects of fever per se. Fever has a salutory effect on the course of infection, whereas hypothermia has deleterious effects. Although these data would argue for not reducing fever in patients with infections (eg, through tepid sponging or antipyretic drugs such as aspirin), high fever itself may be deleterious. In addition, the role of fever as a host defense mechanism is probably adjunctive rather than central, and it becomes insignificant if effective antimicrobial chemotherapy is being administered.

IMMUNOLOGIC DEFENSES AGAINST INFECTION

Immunologic defenses are, by definition, those host defense mechanisms that are specific for the invading pathogen and that are augmented on second and subsequent exposures. The specificity of the host response to invading microorganisms is determined primarily by immunoglobulins and T lymphocytes; however, the response frequently requires recruitment of otherwise nonspecific components, such as complement and phagocytic cells.

Antibody-Mediated Host Defenses

Antibodies serve a variety of important host defense functions, both alone and in conjunction with nonspecific effectors (Table 47–4) (see Chapter 7). Functions of antibodies include neutralization of the biologic activity of microbial toxins (the mechanism by which tetanus and diphtheria toxoid vaccines protect against disease), inhibition of enzyme activity (eg, the neuraminidase of influenza virus), blocking of the adherence of microorganisms to mucosal surfaces, and inhibition of the growth of some prokaryotes such as *Mycoplasma*. Viruses may be neutralized in the presence of antibody alone, but many enveloped viruses are neutralized more efficiently if complement is also present. Although in vitro lysis of virus-infected cells by specific antibody and complement has been documented, the overall role of this phenomenon in host defense is unclear. Opsonization—preparing material for ingestion by phagocytic cells—also may occur with antibody alone, although the combination of antibody and complement usually increases the efficiency of ingestion. Killing of gram-negative bacteria by IgM antibody has an absolute requirement for complement.

T-Lymphocyte-Mediated Host Defenses

Although T lymphocytes play a central and critical role in the generation of the immune response to invading microorganisms (see also Chapter 3), their role is predominantly one of recruiting, facilitating, and augmenting other effectors, especially macrophages, rather than of directly attacking the pathogens themselves. Viruses are the major exception to this generalization, because the T-lymphocyte-mediated attack on virus-infected cells constitutes a major host defense against established viral infection. The specific T-cell response to virus-infected cells is mediated by CD8 cytotoxic T lymphocytes (CTLs); in addition, for some viral infections (eg, by herpes simplex virus) NK cells and macrophages are important in recovery from infection. Secretion of lymphokines, especially interferon gamma, by immune lymphocytes is responsible for augmented NK and CTL activity. Lymphokines (especially interferon gamma) also activate macrophages, which constitute a major host defense against many bacterial, fungal, and parasitic

Table 47–4. Principal antibody-mediated host defenses.

Immunologic Function	Pathogens Affected	Principal Antibody Classes Involved	Nonspecific Cofactors Required
Opsonization	V, B, F	IgG, IgM	Phagocytic cells and complement (in some cases)
Neutralization	V	IgG, IgM, IgA	Complement (in some cases)
Inhibition of binding	B, F(?)	IgA	None
Cytolysis	V,[1] B, P	IgG, IgM	Complement
Toxin neutralization	B	IgG	None
Enzyme inhibition	V, B(?)	IgG	None
ADCC	V, F(?), ?P(?)	IgG, IgA	None
Growth inhibition	*Mycoplasma* B[2]	IgG, IgA IgA	None Lactoferrin

Abbreviations: V = viruses; B = bacteria; F = fungi; P = parasites; ADCC = antibody-dependent cell-mediated cytotoxicity; Ig = immunoglobulin.
[1] Lysis of virus-infected cells.
[2] IgA against bacterial nonbinding proteins synergistically inhibits growth with lactoferrin.

infections. Interferons produced by virus-infected cells that are not a part of the immune system (eg, interferon alpha from fibroblasts) have a direct antiviral effect, but they also augment NK cell and macrophage function.

In vitro testing has shown that T cells may play a direct role in defense against prokaryotic and eukaryotic pathogens by a number of mechanisms. Sensitized T lymphocytes have been shown to lyse certain bacteria, fungi, and parasites both directly and in the presence of antibody (antibody-dependent cell-mediated cytotoxicity [ADCC]). Macrophages infected with some intracellular bacterial pathogens are recognized and lysed by specific T-cell clones (both CD4 and CD8 types). The in vivo significance of these mechanisms, however, has generally not been validated. In some experimental bacterial infections T cells have been shown to have a direct protective effect, perhaps by secreting poorly characterized bactericidal proteins or lymphokines.

Complement

Complement acts by inactivating microorganisms, through lysis, and by facilitating phagocytosis (opsonization); in both roles it is often assisted by antibody (see Table 47–4) (see Chapter 11). In addition, complement breakdown products induce vasodilation and are chemoattractants. The alternative complement pathway alone can be stimulated to kill some gram-negative bacteria and inactivate some viruses in the absence of antibodies. Specific antibody, however, is required for activation of the classic complement pathway, which plays an important role in host defenses to bacterial and other infections (see Table 47–4). Early in infection, prior to synthesis of specific antibodies, the ability of the alternative complement pathway to nonspecifically opsonize or kill certain bacteria may be critical to recovery from infections.

Complement also limits tissue damage from immune complexes by accelerating their clearance.

The importance of complement as an early nonimmune host defence mechanism is most strikingly seen in patients deficient in terminal complement components, who have a markedly increased risk of fulminant neisserial infections (see Chapter 25).

Phagocytic Cells

Phagocytic cells fulfill a number of important functions in host defense (Table 47–5) (see Chapters 1 and 12). They subserve nonspecific roles such as phagocytosis and secretion of monokines and enzymes, but these functions are often augmented by lymphokines secreted as the result of a specific immune response, as described earlier. Many organisms have extracellular products (eg, the polysaccharide capsule on pneumococci) that inhibit phagocytosis. Once ingested by phagocytic cells, the microorganisms are attacked by a variety of microbicidal systems (Table 47–5; Chapter 1). Organisms that can survive and replicate within the professional phagocyte are termed "facultative intracellular pathogens."

In addition, Fc-bearing phagocytic cells and NK cells may have immunologic specificity imposed on them by antibody: the so-called ADCC reaction (see Table 47–4). When coated with specific IgG antibody, virus-infected cells and perhaps fungi and other eukaryotic pathogens become susceptible to killing by these NK cells and macrophages (and perhaps by PMN in some cases). The immunologic specificity of this reaction is wholly imparted by the antibody. The importance of the ADCC mechanism has been demonstrated conclusively in some experimental viral infections (eg, adult and neonatal murine herpes simplex virus infection), but it is thought to play some role in many other infections.

Table 47–5. Functions of phagocytic cells thought to be important in host defenses.

Chemotaxis
Phagocytosis
Nonfacilitated
Facilitated (opsonization)
Killing
Intracellular
Oxygen-dependent
Oxygen-independent
Extracellular
Nonfacilitated
Antibody-facilitated (ADCC)
Secretion
Monokines (IL-1, TNF, etc)
Enzymes (proteinases, etc)
Inflammatory mediators (kinins, prostaglandins, etc)
Growth factors

Abbreviations: ADCC = antibody-dependent cell-mediated cytotoxicity; IL-1 = interleukin-1; TNF = tumor necrosis factor.

THE SPLEEN IN HOST DEFENSES

The spleen is a critical organ for host defense against infection, especially bacterial infections and serves as a phagocytic filter for the bloodstream and also as an important organ for generating T-cell and B-cell immune responses. The importance of the spleen in host defenses is most clearly highlighted in patients lacking a spleen because of surgery or disease (eg, sickling hemoglobinopathies). Such patients show a marked increase in susceptibility to overwhelming infection by encapsulated bacteria, such as pneumococci and *Haemophilus influenzae,* and by erythrocytic parasites, such as *Babesia microti.*

IMMUNOPATHOLOGY OF INFECTION

Disease may result directly from injury induced by a pathogen, for example, the paralysis and death caused by secretion of tetanus toxin by *Clostridium tetani.* In other cases, however, the host response to the pathogen may contribute to the resulting disease and, in a few instances, may be solely responsible for the resulting clinical findings. In addition, the host immune response may facilitate or augment infection in some cases, such as the antibody-mediated enhancement of dengue virus and human immunodeficiency virus (HIV) infection of Fc-bearing cells such as macrophages. Lastly, some pathogens, particularly viruses, may injure the immune system itself, producing transient or even longstanding immunosuppression. Infection with HIV is the most important example of this type of host–parasite interaction (see Chapter 53).

Nonspecific host immune responses to invading pathogens (ie, the inflammatory response or some component of it) may be injurious in many cases. Release of inflammatory mediators causes pain and swelling, and the enzymes secreted by PMN and macrophages may produce permanent tissue damage. In most instances the beneficial effects of the local inflammatory response far outweigh any deleterious ones. For the patient suffering from the discomfort of a large staphylococcal abscess, however, this may be a difficult point to make!

Endotoxin-mediated host injury, which clinically results in the sepsis syndrome, or septic shock, is usually consequent to severe infection by gram-negative bacteria such as meningococci. In this instance, much of the resulting disease is attributable to the host response to the endotoxin, not to direct injury by the endotoxin itself. The most important host response to endotoxin is probably direct stimulation of IL-1 and TNF synthesis by macrophages, which results from binding of endotoxin to specific receptors on the macrophage surface. TNF is quite probably the principal mediator of the lethal action of endotoxin, since pretreatment of animals with antibodies to TNF reduces the mortality from experimental endotoxic shock. Some of the effects of TNF itself may also be indirect, mediated through other products of inflammation, such as arachidonic acid metabolites or kinins.

There are many examples of host injury secondary to the humoral immune response to a pathogen. The most important examples occur in immune-complex disease (see Chapter 29). Poststreptococcal glomerulonephritis results from formation of complexes between streptococcal antigens and host IgG antibody, which are deposited in the kidney, attracting complement and inflammatory cells. Chronic antigen–antibody complex disease may occur in hepatitis B virus infection, with a clinical syndrome of polyarteritis nodosa. Incorporation of complement in immune complexes accelerates their clearance and reduces tissue damage.

Infection by *Mycoplasma pneumoniae* induces antibody to the I blood group antigen on erythrocytes, even though the I antigen is not found on the organisms. In some patients who develop high titers of this antibody, hemolytic anemia may develop.

Clear examples of host injury secondary to the cellular immune response are more difficult to identify. It is likely that some of the clinical features of tuberculosis are attributable to delayed hypersensitivity to the proteins of *M tuberculosis,* but as the organism itself produces injury, this has been difficult to prove. Liver cell damage by hepatitis B virus is probably due wholly or partly to the CTL response to viral antigens (see Chapter 49), but direct proof of this point is also lacking.

One mechanism by which microbes can trigger a deleterious cellular response is through synthesis of **superantigens** (see Chapter 9). These microbial proteins, examples of which include staphylococcal enterotoxins and the rabiesvirus nucleocapsid, directly bind to a large set of major histocompatibility complex (MHC) class II molecules, linking them relatively nonspecifically with the T-cell receptor (TCR) on antigen-presenting cells and inducing release of inflammatory cytokines such as TNFα. Superantigen-triggered cytokine release is thought to be a major contributor to illness in the staphylococcal toxic shock syndrome.

REFERENCES

Burton DR, Woof JM: Human antibody effector function. *Adv Immunol* 1992;**51:**1.

Densen P et al: Granulocyte phagocytes. In: *Principles and Practice of Infectious Diseases,* 4th ed. Mandell GL et al (editors). Wiley, 1995.

Dinarello CA, Wolf SM: The role of interleukin-1 in disease. *N Engl J Med* 1993;**328:**106.

Elsbach P, Weiss J: The bactericidal/permeability-increasing (BPI) protein, a potent element in host-defense against gram-negative bacteria and lipopolysaccharide. *Immunobiology* 1993;**187:**417.

Gabay JE, Almeida RP: Antibiotic peptides and serine protease homologs in human polymorphonuclear leukocytes: Defensins and azurocidin. *Curr Opin Immunol* 1993;**5:**97.

Galanos C, Freudenberg MA: Mechanisms of endotoxic shock and endotoxin hypersensitivity. *Immunobiology* 1993;**187:**246.

Halmskov U et al: Collectins: Collagenous C-type lectins of the innate immune defense system. *Immunol Today* 1994;**15:**67.

Kluger MJ: Fever revisited. *Pediatrics* 1992;**90:**846.

Locksley RM, Wilson CB: Cell-mediated immunity and its role in host defense. In: *Principles and Practice of Infectious Diseases,* 4th ed. Mandell GL et al (editors). Wiley, 1995.

Tramont EC: General or nonspecific host defense mechanisms. In: *Principles and Practice of Infectious Diseases,* 4th ed. Mandell GL et al (editors). Wiley, 1995.

Ulevitch RJ: Recognition of bacterial endotoxins by receptor-dependent mechanisms. *Adv Immunol* 1993;**53:**267.

Urbaschek B (editor): Perspectives on bacterial pathogenesis and host defense: Proceedings of a Symposium. *Rev Infect Dis* 1987;**9:**S431.

Wick MJ et al: Molecular cross talk between epithelial cells and pathogenic microorganisms. *Cell* 1991;**67:**651.

48

Bacterial Diseases

John L. Ryan, MD, PhD

Immunity to bacterial infections is mediated by both cellular and humoral mechanisms. Bacteria express many different surface antigens and secrete a variety of virulence factors (eg, toxins) that may trigger immune responses. Since the topic of bacterial immunity is vast, attention in this chapter focuses on three principal types of immunity to bacteria, with examples for which pathogenesis and host responses are well characterized.

(1) The first is immunity to **toxigenic bacterial infections.** Bacterial exotoxins and endotoxins are important in the pathogenesis of specific diseases. Exotoxins are the sole virulence factor in certain toxigenic bacterial infections, and immunity directed against these toxins can completely prevent disease.

(2) The second is immunity to **encapsulated bacteria.** These organisms evade phagocytosis by coating themselves with innocuous polysaccharide. Encapsulated bacteria may be gram-positive or gram-negative, and vaccines containing purified capsular antigens generate protective immunity.

(3) The third is immunity to **intracellular bacteria.** These bacteria avoid the host immune response because they grow inside cells, particularly phagocytes. The same evasive mechanism is used by many fungal and parasitic pathogens. Cellular immunity mediated by macrophages that are activated by specific lymphocytes and their products is the critical mode of host defense against this group of bacteria.

SERODIAGNOSIS

Serodiagnosis of bacterial diseases is of value only in specific circumstances. IgG antibody is long-lived, and its presence, while indicative of previous infection or immunization, gives little or no information on current bacterial infection. IgM antibody is usually produced within days to a few weeks after exposure to antigen, and thus its presence suggests recent exposure in most cases. As with viral diseases, serial determina-tions of antibody levels with rising titers are of greater diagnostic value, but because of the time intervals required, they are usually of little clinical value.

In general, culture of specific pathogens is required to confirm the diagnosis of a bacterial disease. Serologic tests may aid in diagnosis when diseases are caused by bacteria that are difficult to grow. *Brucella* is one such species. These organisms are difficult to culture from patients' specimens, and there is no useful delayed hypersensitivity skin test. A serum agglutination test for antibodies using *B abortus* antigen is often used to help diagnose brucellosis. Most mycobacteria are also difficult to grow, but antibody titers are not helpful in diagnosis. Thus, in contrast to viral and fungal pathogens, the serologic tests in bacterial infections remain primarily a tool for epidemiologic studies rather than for clinical diagnosis. Nevertheless, most bacteria induce specific antibody responses, which, in most cases, can be easily measured in serum. As discussed later on, these antibody responses are often critical in determining the host response to an infecting agent.

EXOTOXINS & ENDOTOXINS

Exotoxins are noxious proteins that are secreted by many bacteria. These toxins are often heat-labile and thus can be heat-inactivated for use as vaccines to prevent toxigenic bacterial disease. Many bacteria produce more than one protein exotoxin, making vaccine development more difficult. Endotoxins are somatic lipopolysaccharide–protein complexes. These complex antigens are located in the outer membrane of all gram-negative bacteria. Toxicologic activity is associated with the lipid A component of the endotoxin, whereas the serologic determinants are polysaccharides. Antibody directed against specific polysaccharides can be protective both by enhancing phagocytosis directly and by fixing complement for lysis. Unfortunately, from an immune standpoint, there are antigenic differences in the polysaccharide components of endotoxins among strains of bacteria. Thus, in general, infection with one strain does not generate protective immunity to reinfection with a different strain of the same species. IgM and IgG antibodies directed against the lipid. A component of lipopolysaccharide have different capacities to neutralize the infectivity of gram-negative bacteria. It appears that IgM is a more potent neutralizing antibody than IgG. This is particularly true for cross-reacting antibody directed against core polysaccharide or lipid A determinants of gram-negative bacteria. Passive administration of human or murine IgM directed against core determinants of endotoxin has been attempted for treatment of gram-negative sepsis. These attempts have not been efficacious except in selected subgroups of patients.

TOXIGENIC BACTERIAL DISEASES

In this section, two groups of toxigenic diseases are considered. In the first group, an exotoxin is the sole virulence determinant, and vaccines directed at the exotoxin can generate effective immunity. In the second group, toxins are major virulence factors, but other pathogenic factors exist, making specific immune responses less effective in disease prevention (Fig 48–1). Antibody to toxins can neutralize the toxin by several mechanisms, including enhancing clearance by macrophages or blocking binding sites on toxin for its cellular receptors.

Clostridium Species

Clostridia are obligate anaerobic, spore-forming gram-positive rods, which cause a variety of clinical diseases. *Clostridium tetani* is the cause of tetanus. Disease occurs when spores are introduced into wounds from contaminated soil or foreign bodies. After these spores germinate, a potent neurotoxin called tetanospasmin is produced. Tetanospasmin binds to specific glycolipids in nerve cells in the peripheral nervous system and ascends to the spinal cord from nerves in the periphery. The toxin blocks normal postsynaptic inhibition of spinal reflexes, leading to generalized muscular spasms, or "tetany." A vaccine prepared from the inactivated toxin, termed "toxoid," prevents disease by generating antibodies that neutralize the toxin. It is recommended that all children be immunized with tetanus toxoid soon after birth (see Chapter 55). Subsequent boosts of immunity to toxoid are required every 10 years during adult life to maintain a protective level of antibody. There does not appear to be significant antigenic variation in tetanus toxins, since the single vaccine is protective.

Clostridium botulinum is another exotoxin-producing species for which immunity requires neutralizing antibodies to the toxin (antitoxin). *C botulinum* causes botulism, which is primarily a food-borne disease, occurring when spores or toxin are ingested from contaminated food. The botulinum toxin acts by inhibiting the release of acetylcholine neurotransmitter at the neuromuscular junctions. This produces diplopia, dysphagia, and, in severe cases, respiratory arrest. Botulism is treated with antitoxin, which is equine antiserum

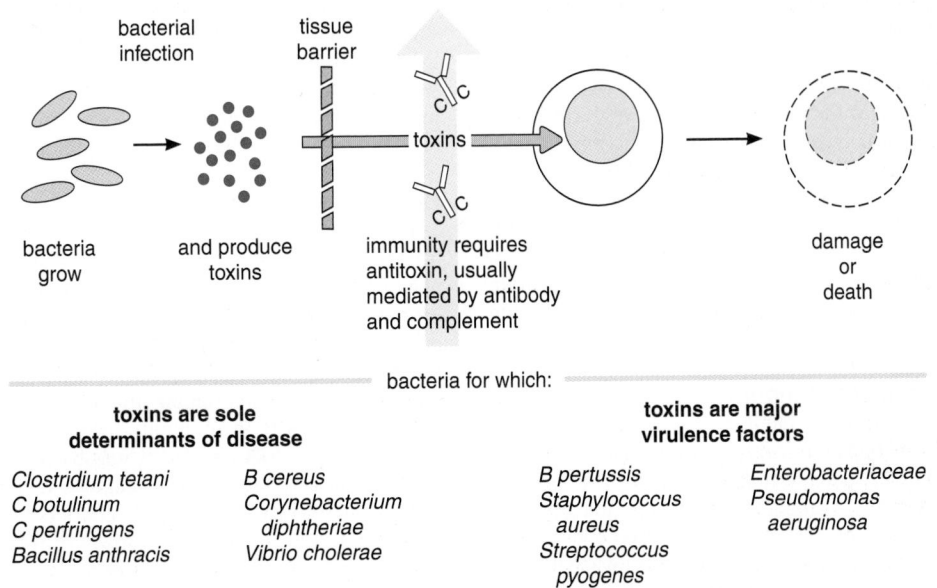

toxins are sole determinants of disease		toxins are major virulence factors	
Clostridium tetani	B cereus	B pertussis	Enterobacteriaceae
C botulinum	Corynebacterium	Staphylococcus	Pseudomonas
C perfringens	diphtheriae	aureus	aeruginosa
Bacillus anthracis	Vibrio cholerae	Streptococcus	
		pyogenes	

Figure 48–1. Toxigenic bacterial infections. In this group of bacterial infections, antibody to protein toxins and complement play a protective role in enhancing survival.

directed against the three most common toxin serotypes: A, B, and E. A pentavalent toxoid (A, B, C, D, E) is distributed by the Centers for Disease Control and Prevention (CDC). This toxoid is prepared from formalin-treated toxins, which are adsorbed to aluminum phosphate to enhance immunogenicity. Natural immunity does not occur, because immunogenic doses of these toxins are lethal.

Several other *Clostridium* strains cause pyogenic infections that are mediated, in part, by cytopathic exotoxins. The most common are soft tissue infections caused by *Clostridium perfringens,* which releases a potent lecithinase called α toxin. This toxin has been associated with massive intravascular hemolysis in uncontrolled infection. It is associated with clostridial myonecrosis or, "gas gangrene." *C perfringens* also secretes several other toxins, including an enterotoxin that is an important cause of food poisoning. Therapy with antitoxins has not been useful in treating diseases caused by *C perfringens,* because the organism secretes such a wide variety of toxins.

Bacillus Species

Bacillus species are facultative anaerobic gram-positive rods that can form spores. They are similar to clostridia, except for their facultative anaerobic metabolism. One of the first pathogenic bacteria to be studied was *Bacillus anthracis,* the only nonmotile species in the genus. The disease anthrax is caused by human contact with animal products contaminated by *B anthracis.* Animals are infected by ingestion of the bacteria or spores in the environment. Pathogenicity depends on toxin production, and the disease can be prevented by vaccination against attenuated bacteria. Pasteur was the first to show that vaccination could prevent anthrax in animals. The anthrax exotoxin is complex, consisting of at least three components: protective antigen, edema factor, and lethal factor. The protective antigen, which is not toxic alone, induces immunity and is the major component of current vaccines. *B anthracis* has also been shown to have a polysaccharide capsule, which may contribute to the virulence of this organism.

Bacillus cereus represents another important toxigenic *Bacillus* species. It is a common cause of food poisoning. Several toxins, including a pyogenic toxin and two enterotoxins, are produced. Little is known about protective immunity to these bacteria.

Corynebacterium diphtheriae

Corynebacteria are facultative anaerobic gram-positive rods that do not form spores. The most important species is *Corynebacterium diphtheriae,* the cause of diphtheria. This organism colonizes the mucous membranes of the posterior pharynx and elaborates a potent exotoxin. The toxin kills cells by covalently linking adenosine diphosphoribose to elongation factor 2, which is required for cellular protein biosynthesis. Immunity to diphtheria depends on the presence of antibody to the toxin. Diphtheria toxoid, a formalin-inactivated toxin preparation, is currently used worldwide to vaccinate infants against diphtheria. Immunity to diphtheria is assessed by using the Schick test. In this test, small amounts of toxin and toxoid are injected intradermally at different sites. If no response is observed at either site after 48 hours, the patient is immune to the toxin (has circulating antitoxin) and is not hypersensitive to the toxoid. If there is necrosis at the toxin site and response at the toxoid site, the patient does not have protective antibody. An immediate reaction at both sites indicates allergy to the proteins. A delayed reaction at one or both sites indicates cellular immunity to the proteins. The Schick test has been very useful in assessing immunity to *C diphtheriae.* It is no longer used very often and has been replaced with antibody titers. Nevertheless, it has provided insight into the importance of maintaining adequate circulating antibody to toxin to ameliorate or prevent clinical infection.

Vibrio cholerae

The vibrios are curved, gram-negative bacilli with polar flagellae. Infection with *Vibrio cholerae,* the agent of cholera, occurs after ingestion of contaminated water. Organisms multiply in the gut and release an enterotoxin, which binds to epithelial cells and triggers massive secretion of fluid and electrolytes. Severe diarrhea may occur within hours after infection, and the fluid loss is often life-threatening, particularly in infants and young children. Cholera is unique among the toxigenic diseases in that antibody to the toxin does not fully prevent disease. Infection with *V cholerae* induces systemic and mucosal antibody. Mucosal IgA, which prevents attachment of the bacteria in the gut, may be the most important form of immunity. Cholera vaccines induce short-term protection and elicit only IgM and IgG responses unless administered orally. Neither IgM nor IgG functions well in the intestinal lumen. Extensive research is under way to develop an oral cholera vaccine that will confer lifelong immunity.

Bordetella pertussis

Pertussis (whooping cough) is caused by mucosal infection with *Bordetella pertussis,* a small, gram-negative coccobacillary organism that replicates in bronchial mucosa. Infection is characterized by paroxysmal coughing, which can result in significant morbidity in young children. *B pertussis* contains several antigens that may elicit immune responses, but the critical factors in immunity to this organism are not fully understood. Killed whole bacteria are currently used as a vaccine, but acellular vaccines containing three to five components are under active development and have been proven efficacious in clinical trials. Pertussis vaccine is given in combination with diphtheria toxoid and tetanus toxoid (DPT) to infants at 2, 4, and 6 months of age, with boosters usually given 1 year later and again before the children begin to attend school. Immunity to pertussis is relatively short-lived, lasting only 3 years after completion of primary immunization or boosting. Antibody that prevents attachment of the bacteria to respiratory epithelium appears to be the first line of defense, with antitoxin providing further protection against a protein exotoxin produced by the bacteria.

The presence of *B pertussis* in the DPT combination vaccine may enhance the antibody response to both protein toxoids (DT). The lipopolysaccharide in the outer membrane of *B pertussis* is a potent immune adjuvant. Thus, it is advantageous as well as convenient to use the combined vaccine, but the acellular form is more tolerable, producing fewer adverse reactions while maintaining efficacy.

Staphylococcus aureus

Staphylococci are facultative anaerobic, nonmotile gram-positive cocci that are most often seen as clusters in gram-stained specimens. *Staphylococcus aureus* is probably the single most prevalent pathogen in skin and soft tissue infections. Its virulence has been studied intensively, but the mechanism remains obscure. The primary line of defense against staphylococci is the polymorphonuclear leukocyte, which phagocytoses and kills the bacteria. *S aureus* produces a vast number of virulence factors, including toxins, which may contribute to its pathogenicity. Production of coagulase, a factor that can bind and activate fibrinogen, defines the species *S aureus*. At least four separate hemolysins are also produced. A nonhemolytic leukocidin is cytotoxic for granulocytes. In addition, *S aureus* secretes several enterotoxins, an exfoliative toxin associated with epidermal necrolysis, and an exotoxin associated with the toxic shock syndrome.

The immune response to *S aureus* infections is inadequate in that previous infection does not protect the host from reinfection. The few strains of *S aureus* that have significant capsules do generate protective antibody, but these strains are not commonly pathogenic. Most staphylococci contain small amounts of capsular polysaccharides that do not generate protective antibody. Conjugation of these polysaccharides to protein carriers, however, may elicit protective antibody. Similarly, antibodies to the toxic shock exotoxin and to the exfoliative exotoxins seem to prevent the specific clinical syndromes caused by these toxins. Pyogenic *S aureus* infections occur, however, despite the presence of multiple antibodies against cellular components in the host. Only the number and functional capacity of granulocytes are critically important in the defense against *S aureus*.

Another *Staphylococcus* strain associated with human disease is *S epidermidis*. This strain produces few toxins and is associated primarily with bacteremias in patients with plastic catheters or other foreign objects in the bloodstream. *S epidermidis,* as the name implies, is one of the most common bacteria of the skin flora. It adheres to catheters or other materials by means of an extracellular polysaccharide slime, which inhibits the ability of granulocytes to function properly. Protective immunity to this organism does not appear to develop, since repeated infections may occur in susceptible hosts.

Streptococcus Species

Streptococci are a diverse group of catalase-negative, facultatively anaerobic gram-positive cocci, which cause a variety of toxigenic and pyogenic infections in humans. *Streptococcus pyogenes* is the most important bacterial cause of pharyngitis. Late sequelae, such as rheumatic fever and glomerulonephritis, may follow infection with certain strains of this species.

Most streptococcal infections do not confer immunity unless the syndrome is mediated by toxins, such as the streptococcal pyogenic exotoxins associated with scarlet fever. The antigenic composition of streptococci is complex, with approximately 18 group-specific carbohydrate antigens lettered A–R. These antigens are useful for classifying streptococci, but they do not elicit protective immunity. Group A streptococci contain another set of type-specific M antigens, known as M proteins (more than 80 types exist). These proteins are antiphagocytic factors and enhance the virulence of group A streptococci. The M proteins do generate protective IgG antibody, but since there are many serotypes of M protein, reinfection with another strain is common.

Streptococci of groups A, B, C, F, and G produce many extracellular products that may elicit protective immunity. Streptolysins O and S are cytopathic proteins that inhibit phagocytosis and killing by leukocytes. A variety of proteinases exist, including streptokinase and other degradative enzymes such as hyaluronidase and deoxyribonuclease, which enhance the pathogenicity of the organism. Antibodies may be produced to all of these factors during infection. The widely used Streptozyme test is a hemagglutination procedure that detects a variety of antibodies against streptococcal enzymes.

Group D streptococci have recently been reclassified as enterococci and are antigenically distinct from other streptococci in that they do not possess a group-specific carbohydrate antigen, but they do have a group-specific glycerol teichoic acid antigen. Because of their innate resistance to most antibiotics, enterococci have emerged as a leading cause of nosocomial infections in the United States.

Most of the streptococci that normally colonize the human oropharynx do not possess group-specific antigens and are classified in the viridans group. Many individual strains may be defined by biochemical tests, but none of these streptococci are prominent toxin producers. They are active in causing periodontal diseases and are the most common causes of infective endocarditis. Little is known about protective immunity to this diverse group of organisms.

Gram-Negative Rods

Gram-negative rods produce a variety of toxins and are responsible for many infectious diseases. The family Enterobacteriaceae comprises five major genera: *Escherichia, Klebsiella, Proteus, Yersinia,* and *Erwinia.* These are all glucose-fermenting, nonspore-forming bacilli. All members of the family Enterobacteriaceae, but particularly *Escherichia* and *Salmonella,* have undergone extensive immunologic analyses. They are serotyped on the basis of O antigens (polysaccharides associated with the lipopolysaccharide component of the outer membrane), K antigens (polysaccharide capsular components), and H antigens (proteins associated with flagella).

Some of these organisms are partially responsible for contributing to the immune pathogenesis of the spondyloarthropathies. The well-known association of the major histocompatibility complex (MHC) class I molecule human leukocyte antigen (HLA)-B27 and ankylosing spondylitis, as well as the association of the disease with preceding enteric infection, has stimulated a search for molecular mimicry, that is, identity between epitopes on a bacterium and one in the human host. The immune response to *Klebsiella pneumoniae* elicits antibody that can bind to HLA-B27 on the surface of synovial lining cells. Similar molecular mimicry has been shown for *Shigella flexneri,* which produces an arthritogenic epitope that is shared by HLA-B27 antigen. Thus, the immune response to certain members of the Enterobacteriaceae may result in autoimmune disease in selected hosts.

Each member of the family Enterobacteriaceae contains an endotoxin. This endotoxin is a lipopolysaccharide–protein complex in the outer membrane and contains the O-specific serologic group. The biologically active components of the endotoxin are the lipid A and certain lipoproteins associated with the lipopolysaccharide.

Enterotoxins are also produced by many members of the Enterobacteriaceae, particularly *Escherichia coli. E coli* has at least two enterotoxins: an immunogenic heat-labile toxin and a nonimmunogenic heat-stable toxin. More typical exotoxins are also related to certain strains of *E coli, Shigella,* and *Yersinia.*

Immunity to the Enterobacteriaceae is achieved early in life after colonization of the gut with *E coli.* Antibodies against K and O antigens are generated and are protective against autologous serotypes. Prior to the development of antibody, the neonate is susceptible to systemic and particularly to central nervous system infection by *E coli.* In adult life, these bacteria cause opportunistic as well as enteric diseases. Attempts to transfer passive immunity with antiserum to *E coli* have proved effective in both animal and some human studies. Antibodies directed against the endotoxin component may be able to help prevent the morbidity and mortality associated with sepsis in certain patient groups, but clinical trials to establish this have not yet been done.

Pseudomonas aeruginosa is the most clinically important nonfermenting gram-negative rod and has been the subject of extensive immunologic analysis. It characteristically produces exotoxin A, a cytolytic factor with a similar mechanism of action to diphtheria toxin. Antibodies directed against exotoxin A as well as the lipopolysaccharide appear to be important in immunity to infection with *P aeruginosa.* Different serotyping schemes have been used to define *P aeruginosa* for epidemiologic purposes. Multivalent vaccines containing several serotypes to protect immunocompromised patients from invasive *Pseudomonas* infection are under investigation. *Pseudomonas* is a virulent opportunistic pathogen that commonly invades immunocompromised patients. The role of antibody to endotoxin in ameliorating human disease has been shown in animals by using homologous and heterologous antisera to protect them against lethal *P aeruginosa* infections.

ENCAPSULATED BACTERIA

Bacteria that express capsular polysaccharide present a unique problem for the immune system. Capsular polysaccharide inhibits phagocytosis by both macrophages and polymorphonuclear leukocytes. Effective phagocytosis requires functional leukocyte receptors for the Fc region of immunoglobulin and C3b or C3bi (Fig 48–2). Opsonization of encapsulated bacteria with antibody and complement is necessary for phagocytes to efficiently ingest and kill these pathogens. The charge and hydrophilicity of unopsonized encapsulated bacteria inhibit phagocytosis by interfering with attachment of leukocytes and bacteria. Immaturity of humoral immunity in the very young and decline of humoral immunity in the elderly probably account for the susceptibility of individuals at these stages of life to invasive disease by encapsulated bacteria.

Bacterial vaccines hold great promise for enhancing immunity against encapsulated bacteria. Since polysaccharides are relatively poor immunogens, particularly in infants, complexes of protein with polysaccharides have proven to be more effective vaccines. Coupling of weak antigens with other types of adjuvants may also improve the efficacy of vaccines.

Streptococcus pneumoniae

Streptococcus pneumoniae strains, commonly called pneumococci, differ from other streptococci in that they contain complex polysaccharide capsules that determine the major virulence determinant in the species. Pneumococci are respiratory pathogens that colonize upper airways and cause bronchitis or pneumonia after aspiration of respiratory secretions. The capsule inhibits alveolar macrophage phagocytosis and allows the pneumococcus to multiply in the lung. Patients with abnormal mucociliary reflexes or de-

A

B

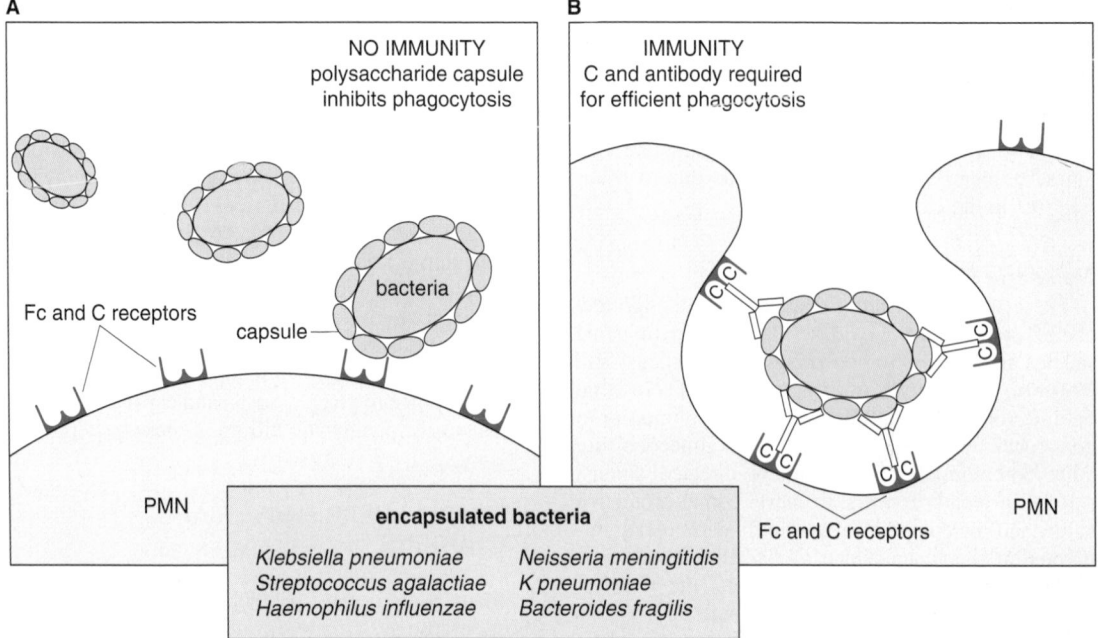

Figure 48–2. Encapsulated bacteria. Polysaccharide capsules allow bacterial multiplication by avoiding receptor-mediated phagocytosis. If specific antibody to the capsule is present, both antibody and complement serve as opsonins to enhance the uptake of bacteria by host phagocytes.

creased alveolar macrophage function are more susceptible to pulmonary infection. Patients with decreased systemic clearance of bacteria are susceptible to disseminated disease.

Type-specific antibody is elicited and is protective, but there are more than 80 serotypes of pneumococci. Thus, reinfection with a different serotype is common in susceptible persons. The polysaccharide capsule is sometimes cross-reactive with the capsular polysaccharides of different genera, including *Haemophilus* and *Klebsiella.* A vaccine containing capsular polysaccharide from the 23 most prevalent or virulent serotypes is available for adult patients at high risk for pneumococcal disease. Conjugated protein–polysaccharide vaccines containing the most common infecting serotypes are under development to prevent disease in infants.

Streptococcus agalactiae (Group B)

The group B streptococci are a leading cause of neonatal meningitis. Most disease occurs because of colonization of the infant by members of the vaginal flora during parturition. Group B organisms contain four major capsular serotypes. Sialic acid, one of the carbohydrate components of group B streptococcal capsular polysaccharide, can block complement activation. This prevents a key nonspecific defense mechanism in infants who are without adequate antibody levels. Type-specific antibodies are protective for group B streptococcal disease. Both passive immunization with IgG antibody to capsular polysaccharides and active immunization with polysaccharides and protein–polysaccharide conjugates to prevent group B streptococcal disease in the neonatal period are under investigation.

Haemophilus influenzae

Of the several species of *Haemophilus* that are known, *Haemophilus influenzae* is the most prevalent pathogen. Several distinct capsular serotypes have been defined, but type b *H influenzae* is responsible for most clinical disease. *H influenzae* is a respiratory pathogen that colonizes the oropharynx and causes bronchitis, pneumonia, or disseminated infection when local or systemic host defense factors are compromised. The type b capsule is a polyribitol phosphate. The susceptibility of a given host to infection is directly related to serum levels of bactericidal antibody. Maternal IgG is lost within a few months after birth, and natural antibody is acquired by 3–4 years of age. The development of natural antibody may be related to colonization and subsequent immunization with nonpathogenic members of the family Enterobacteriaceae that contain cross-reactive capsular polysaccharides. *H influenzae* type b capsular polysaccharide (polyriboseribitol phosphate, PRP) is a weak immunogen, and vaccines have not been effective in children younger than 2 years. Recently, conjugate vaccines with diphtheria toxoid, tetanus toxoid, and outer membrane proteins linked to PRP have proven effective in immunizing children between 6 months and 2 years of age. There are few bacterial diseases in which the protective role of antibody has been so clearly demonstrated as in *H influenzae* type b disease. The widespread use of the new conjugate vaccines has nearly eradicated meningitis due to *H influenzae* in the United States.

Neisseria Species

These are gram-negative cocci containing high levels of cytochrome *c* oxidase. The two pathogenic species are *Neisseria gonorrhoeae* (gonococcus) and *Neisseria meningitidis* (meningococcus). There is no definite role of anticapsular antibody in immunity to gonococci. Repeated infections with gonococci are quite common. Mucosal antibody directed against surface proteins appears to have some protective value, and the complement system is particularly important in the maintenance of bactericidal activity. The meningococcus normally inhabits the pharynx without producing disease. This provides a reservoir for outbreaks and produces some immunity in the host. The critical antigenic components of the meningococcus are capsular polysaccharides, and 13 distinct serotypes can elicit group-specific protective antibody. IgM antibody appears to be more protective than does IgG, perhaps because of its more potent complement-fixing activity. Patients deficient in the terminal complement components C6, C7, C8, or properdin are susceptible to recurrent neisserial infections. A polyvalent vaccine containing polysaccharide from groups A, C, Y, and W-135 is available. Group B capsular polysaccharides are cross-reactive with *E coli* capsular polysaccharides (K1 antigens), and no vaccine is available against this strain. The importance of antibody in protection against meningococcal disease is underscored by the peak incidence of disease, which occurs at about 1 year of age, when maternal antibody has waned and acquired antibody has not yet been produced.

Klebsiella pneumoniae

Klebsiella species are members of the family Enterobacteriaceae that are characterized by polysaccharide capsules with more than 70 serotypes. Although they are predominantly intestinal organisms that cause opportunistic infections, they are also associated with primary pneumonias. This is probably related to the ability of these bacteria to avoid phagocytosis in the absence of antibody. The capsular polysaccharides found in *Klebsiella* are related to those in *Streptococcus* and *Haemophilus*. The role of specific anticapsular antibodies in *Klebsiella* has not been elucidated. Immunity appears to be multifactorial, with disease most commonly occurring in debilitated patients with depressed host defenses.

Bacteroides fragilis

Bacteroides fragilis and closely related species are obligate anaerobic, nonspore-forming, gram-negative rods, which colonize the intestinal tract and are often associated with intra-abdominal abscess formation. Unless the mucous membrane barrier of the gastrointestinal or respiratory tract is damaged, *B fragilis* is a member of the harmless normal flora. In the presence of tissue necrosis or trauma, *B fragilis* may be released into a relatively low-oxygen environment, allowing growth and elaboration of several enzymes that potentiate tissue damage. *B fragilis* also contains a capsular polysaccharide that is a key virulence factor in animal models of infection. The capsule mediates resistance to phagocytosis, and capsular antibody enhances the phagocytic killing of these bacteria.

INTRACELLULAR BACTERIAL PATHOGENS

Many bacteria have developed the ability to avoid host defense systems by invading cells so that serum antibody and complement cannot harm them and granulocytes cannot recognize them (Fig 48–3). These bacteria induce T-lymphocyte-mediated immunity in the same fashion as fungi, parasites, and viruses. Serum antibody and complement are not markers of resistance for these bacteria. The presence of sensitized T lymphocytes and activated macrophages is the key factor in immunity. Microbial antigens are expressed on the surface of macrophages after the antigens are processed, in conjunction with products of the major histocompatibility complex. In this configuration, macrophages interact with T lymphocytes to produce macrophage-activating factors such as interferon gamma. This complex series of events is required for the expression of effective immunity to intracellular pathogens.

Salmonella Species

Salmonella species are members of the family Enterobacteriaceae and cause a significant proportion of enteric disease. Three major species (*Salmonella typhi, Salmonella choleraesuis,* and *Salmonella enteritidis*) exist. Based on serologic reactions, there are more than 1700 types of *S enteritidis*. Most invasive disease, such as typhoid fever, is caused by *S typhi,* and it is of great interest that this is the only species of *Salmonella* with a surface capsular antigen. This capsule, therefore, is a key virulence factor for *S typhi.* Antibody against the capsule is not protective, and many typhoid carriers have circulating antibody. This reflects the ability of salmonellae to reside within cells of the reticuloendothelial system. Salmonellae usually enter the body by ingestion and cause enterocolitis if they are present in sufficient numbers to survive the acidic environment of the stomach. If they invade mucosal tissues, they can cause disseminated disease.

A

macrophage (containing intracellular bacteria);
antibody and C do not have access

B

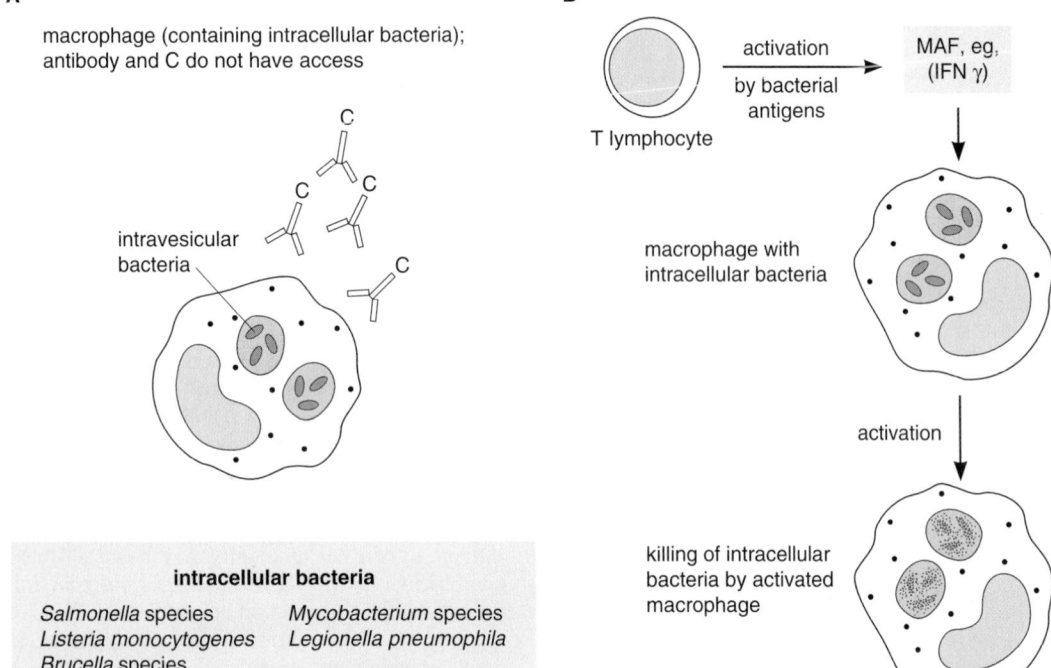

Figure 48–3. Intracellular bacterial pathogens. Antibody and complement have no access to intracellular pathogens. Lymphokines mediate macrophage activation, which allows the killing of these bacteria by both oxidative and nonoxidative mechanisms.

Immunity to *Salmonella* involves activation of macrophages by sensitized T lymphocytes through lymphokine secretion. Circulating antibodies do not penetrate the cell to eradicate intracellular bacteria. Thus circulating antibody represents a marker of infection, but not of immunity.

Other Intracellular Bacterial Pathogens

Bacterial strains other than *Salmonella* that are intracellular pathogens include *Legionella, Listeria,* and *Brucella. Legionella pneumophila* and related strains are obligate intracellular parasites of macrophages. These bacteria exhibit optimal growth only within cells. Antibodies to serogroup-specific antigens are produced and are useful for diagnostic or epidemiologic studies, but they have not proved to be protective. Antigen-specific T-lymphocyte activation with release of interferon gamma and other macrophage-activating factors enhances immunity to *Legionella.*

Listeria monocytogenes is a gram-positive rod similar to *Corynebacterium;* it causes meningeal infections or sepsis in adults and a variety of infections in neonates. Although antibody may play some role in preventing invasion, it is clear that the macrophage is the primary mode of defense against these bacteria. Investigations in animal models have demonstrated that T-lymphocyte function is important in macrophage activation for immunity to *Listeria.*

Brucella species are small coccobacillary gram-negative bacteria that resemble *Haemophilus* in appearance and are spread to humans through contact with animals (zoonosis). Three species are pathogenic for humans and cause systemic disease that may be chronic or subacute. The first is *Brucella abortus* from cattle, the second is *Brucella suis* from pigs, and the third is *Brucella melitensis,* usually from goats and sheep. Diagnosis is often made by serology, but antibody does not confer immunity. Immunity to *Brucella* species is conferred by activated macrophages produced by specifically sensitized T lymphocytes and lymphokines derived from them. The specific antigens that elicit cellular immunity to brucellosis have not been defined.

Mycobacterium Species

The genus *Mycobacterium* comprises a unique group of bacteria characterized by a lipid-rich cell wall that contains *N*-glycolylneuraminic acid. The major pathogenic strain is *Mycobacterium tuberculosis,* although *Mycobacterium avium* complex (MAC) has emerged as a significant pathogen in patients with acquired immunodeficiency syndrome (AIDS). Tuberculosis has been one of the great infectious scourges of humankind throughout history and remains a major world health problem today. One reason is that despite decades of excellent research into the immune mechanisms relating to tuberculosis, an effective vaccine has not been found. Bacillus Calmette-Guérin (BCG), an attenuated *Mycobacterium bovis* strain, has been used for more than 60 years and is able to confer delayed cutaneous hypersensitivity but no clear-cut cellular immunity. Serum antibody plays no role in immunity to mycobacterial diseases. Sensitized T lymphocytes and activated macrophages are the critical factors in immunity. The components of the cell wall of *M tuberculosis* that may confer immunity have been analyzed in detail. Both proteins and polysaccharides have immunogenic potential, and there are data supporting a substantive role for the polysaccharide components as the key epitopes for cellular immunity. A purified protein derivative is used as an intradermal antigen to measure delayed hypersensitivity to *M tuberculosis*. A positive delayed skin test demonstrates previous exposure to the bacteria and is often correlated with immunity. There is not a one-to-one correlation between a positive skin test and immunity, however, and further definition of the protective antigens in the tubercle bacillus is needed before immunity to *M tuberculosis* can be understood.

The need to develop more effective vaccines against *M tuberculosis* has been accentuated by the recent striking increase in the incidence in AIDS patients of tuberculosis due to bacteria with multiple drug resistance.

Immunity to mycobacteria such as MAC and *M leprae* (the agent of Hansen's disease, ie, leprosy) is also mediated by cellular immunity, with serum components playing an insignificant role. The common occurrence of MAC infections in AIDS patients underscores the critical importance of cell-mediated immunity in resistance to mycobacterial infections.

CONCLUSIONS

Immunity to bacterial infections is extremely complex because of the diverse virulence factors used by bacteria to enhance their survival. Primary nonspecific defense against bacterial infections is afforded by granulocytes, which ingest and kill most potential pathogens. Specific immunity is needed for protection against encapsulated or intracellular bacteria. This requires the development either of antibody, which can enhance killing by its opsonic or complement-fixing activity, or of T-cell immunity, which can activate the microbicidal activity of macrophages. In many infections, a complex interaction of immune mechanisms is required to achieve protective immunity. Thus, antibody, complement, granulocytes, lymphocytes, and macrophages are all needed to permit the development of protective immunity to many bacterial pathogens.

REFERENCES

GENERAL

Braude AI (editor): *Infectious Diseases and Medical Microbiology,* 2nd ed. WB Saunders, 1986.

Mandell GL et al (editors): *Principles and Practice of Infectious Diseases,* 4th ed. Churchill Livingstone, 1995.

Sherris JC (editor): *Medical Microbiology: An Introduction to Infectious Diseases.* Elsevier, 1984.

SPECIFIC

Bloom BR et al: Tuberculosis: Commentary on a reemergent killer. *Science* 1992;**257:**1005.

Daniel DM: Antibody and antigen detection for the immunodiagnosis of tuberculosis: Why not? What more is needed? Where do we stand today? *J Infect Dis* 1988;**158:**678.

Densen P et al: Familial properdin deficiency and fatal meningococcemia. *N Engl J Med* 1987;**316:**922.

Dezfulian M et al: Kinetics study of immunologic response to *Clostridium botulinum* toxin. *J Clin Microbiol* 1987;**25:**1336.

Fattom A et al: Laboratory and clinical evaluation of conjugate vaccines composed of *Staphyloccus aureus* type 5 and type 8 capsular polysaccharides bound to *Pseudomonas aeruginosa* recombinant exotoxin A. *Infect Immun* 1993;**61:**1023.

Fierer J: *Pseudomonas* and *Flavobacterium.* In: *Infectious Diseases and Medical Microbiology,* 2nd ed. Braude AI (editor). WB Saunders, 1986, p. 314.

Gazapo E et al: Changes in IgM and IgG antibody concentrations in brucellosis over time: Importance for diagnosis and follow-up. *J Infect Dis* 1989;**159:**219.

Greenman RL et al: A controlled clinical trial of E5 murine monoclonal antibody to endotoxin in the treatment of gram-negative sepsis. *JAMA* 1991;**266:**1097.

Griffiss JM et al: Vaccines against encapsulated bacteria: A global agenda. *Rev Infect Dis* 1987;**9:**176.

Harriman GR et al: The role of C9 in complement-mediated killing of *Neisseria. J Immunol* 1981;**127:**2386.

Johnston RB: Recurrent bacterial infections in children. *N Engl J Med* 1984;**310:**1237.

Kasper DL: The polysaccharide capsule of *Bacteroides fragilis* subspecies *fragilis:* Immunochemical and morphologic definition. *J Infect Dis* 1976;**133:**79.

McCabe WR et al: Immunization with rough mutants of *Salmonella minnesota:* Protective activity of IgM and IgG antibody to the R595 (Re Chemotype) mutant. *J Infect Dis* 1988;**158:**291.

Orskov F, Orskov I: Enterobacteriaceae. In: *Infectious Diseases and Medical Microbiology,* 2nd ed. Braude AI (editor). WB Saunders, 1986, p 292.

Ryan KJ: *Corynebacteria and Other Non-Spore Forming Microoganisms. An Introduction to Infectious Diseases.* Sherris JC (editor). Elsevier, 1984.

Santosham M et al: The efficacy in Navajo infants of a conjugate vaccine consisting of *Haemophilus influenzae* type b polysaccharide and *Neisseria meningiditis* outer-membrane protein complex. *N Engl J Med* 1991;**324:**1767.

Schwimmbeck MD, Oldstone MBA: Molecular mimicry between human leucocyte antigens B27 and *Klebsiella Am J Med* 1988;**85**(suppl 6A):51.

Ziegler EJ et al: Treatment of Gram-negative bacteremia and septic shock with HA-1A human monoclonal antibody against endotoxin. *N Engl J Med* 1991;**324:**429.

49

Viral Infections

John Mills, MD

The interactions between viruses and the host immune system are not only complex and fascinating but also critical in determining the outcome of infection and strategies for its prevention.

With all other pathogens, viruses share the qualities of being complex, replicating immunogens that stimulate both cellular and humoral immune responses, which then influence the outcome of the infection. Virus infections may be broadly classified into those in which the host immune response eliminates the virus from the body (eg, influenza virus and poliovirus) and those in which the virus is able to persist despite the host immune response. Viruses may persist as a latent infection, with or without intermittent replication (eg, herpes simplex virus), or as a chronic infection (eg, HIV or hepatitis C virus). Viral genomes may be maintained either by integration into the host genome (eg, HIV) or independently within the cell (eg, herpes simplex virus).

Because viruses parasitize cellular metabolic processes during their own replication, they have a unique capacity to directly alter cell structure and function. Although it was once thought that the viral genome only specified those proteins required for intracellular replication as determined in vitro, it is now clear that many (if not most) viruses also carry genes that are dispensable for replication in cell culture but which play critical roles for in vivo pathogenesis. These "virulence factors" appear to act chiefly by modulating the host immune response to infection, by a variety of mechanisms (Table 49–1). The role of these viral proteins in pathogenesis is currently a topic of intense investigation.

The clinical features of infection by a specific virus are determined primarily by which cells are infected and by the cellular pathology induced by infection (eg, cytolysis). For many viruses, however, the host immune response to viral antigens induces additional injuries, called **immunopathic effects,** which are qualitatively different from directly **viropathic effects** and which may involve cells or organs that are uninfected by the virus. Much of the disease morbidity associated with some viruses is, in fact, secondary to the host immune response. Other viral infections may have late immunologic sequelae (Table 49–2).

INFLUENZA VIRUS

Major Immunologic Features
- Viral surface proteins show marked antigenic variation, resulting from mutation and recombination.
- In the naive host, cytolytic T lymphocytes (CTL) are responsible for elimination of virus after infection.
- Serum antibodies to viral surface proteins mediate resistance to pneumonia; mucosal (IgA) antibodies protect against rhinotracheitis.

General Considerations
Influenza is a respiratory infection with systemic manifestations; it is caused by influenza viruses. The disease occurs chiefly in epidemics, predominantly during the winter months. Although all age groups are affected, the severity of the illness is greatest at the extremes of age, and the mortality rate is highest in the elderly and in individuals with underlying chronic cardiorespiratory disease. Recurrent epidemics of influenza contribute significantly to the premature death of patients in these risk groups.

Virology
Influenza virus has an envelope and an antisense RNA genome, which is segmented (seven to eight pieces) rather than continuous, as is found in most viruses. The virus has several important structural proteins (Table 49–3), and, in general, each genome segment specifies one protein.

Three types of influenza virus—A, B, and C—are known; the classification is based on the antigenic characteristics of the ribonucleoprotein and matrix proteins, as well as other features. Influenza A virus is

Table 49–1. Examples of strategies used by viruses to evade the host immune response.

Virus	Gene or Protein	Immunopathologic Effect
Many viruses, eg, herpes simplex	Those that are targets of the immune response.	Downregulation of viral protein synthesis as viral infection becomes low-grade and persistent, or latent.
Many RNA viruses, eg, HIV, influenza	Those that are targets of the humoral or cellular immune response.	Immune evasion. High rate of error in RNA-dependent polymerases (including reverse transcriptases) generates mutations that are selected through pressure of the immune system.
HIV	Various, probably multiple.	Destruction of CD4 lymphocytes ultimately causes profound cellular and humoral immunodeficiency.
HIV	Nef.	Downregulates CD4 and IL-2 receptor expression on infected lymphocytes, perhaps by inhibiting Lck kinase, inhibiting proliferative responses.
Herpes simplex (and other herpesviruses)	gC, gE, gI.	Homologues of Fc and complement receptors; block humoral cytolysis (eg, by ADCC).
Epstein-Barr virus	BCRF-1.	An IL-10 homologue that stimulates B-cell replication and transformation and suppresses T-cell responses to EBV.
Epstein-Barr virus	LMP-1.	Induces the protooncogene *bcl*-2 which inhibits apoptosis of B cells, augmenting virus replication.
Vaccinia	Soluble IL-1 receptor.	Diminishes host local inflammatory response, augmenting virus replication.
Adenovirus	19-kd E3 protein.	Decreases MHC class I transport to cell surface, decreasing susceptibility of virus-infected cells to CTL lysis.

Abbreviations: HIV = human immunodeficiency virus; Nef = negative effector factor; BCRF = B cell replacing factor; LMP = latent membrane protein; ADCC = antibody-dependent cell-mediated cytotoxicity; EBV = Epstein-Barr virus; MHC = major histocompatibility complex; CTL = cytolytic T lymphocytes.

unique in part because it infects both humans and many other animals (pigs, horses, birds, and seals) and because it is the principal cause of pandemic influenza. When a cell is infected by two different influenza A viruses, the segmented RNA genomes of the two parental virus types mix during replication, so that virions of the progeny may contain RNA and protein from both parents (so-called "recombinants," even though they are really reassortants). Influenza A virus thereby varies its surface hemagglutinin and neuraminidase molecules by recombining with other strains (including animal strains) as well as by mutation. Like other viruses with an RNA genome, influenza virus has a high rate of mutation, which underlies its rapid antigenic variation. These phenomena result in new epidemic strains (Fig 49–1). Influenza B virus does not have an animal reservoir from which it can select novel hemagglutinin types, and thus the

range of antigenic variation observed is narrower than that for influenza A virus. Influenza C virus appears to have only one serotype and differs from types A and B in some other features as well.

The principal targets for influenza virus infection are the ciliated epithelial cells of the upper and lower respiratory tract. Influenza virus infection kills these cells, which regenerate slowly during convalescence. Virus shedding terminates with recovery from infection, and neither chronic nor latent infection occurs.

Clinical Features

Influenza is spread through both aerosols and fomites. The clinical features of influenza are fever, cough, myalgia, headache, and malaise. Mild

Table 49–2. Viral infections with immunologic sequelae.

Acute Viral Infection	Immunologic Sequelae
Measles virus	Encephalitis (early), subacute sclerosing panencephalitis (SSPE) (late).
Rubella virus	Encephalopathy, arthritis.
Hepatitis B virus	Polyarteritis nodosa, glomerulonephritis.
Respiratory syncytial virus	Asthma (unproved association).
Epstein-Barr virus	Guillain-Barré syndrome.

Table 49–3. Major structural proteins of influenza virus.

Protein	Location	Function
Hemagglutinin	Surface (envelope)	Acts as ligand for cell receptor acetylneuraminic acids.
Neuraminidase	Surface (envelope)	Releases progeny virus from cell.
Matrix protein	Internal	Stabilizes virus coat.
RNA polymerase	Internal	Replicates RNA genome.
Nucleoprotein	Internal	Stabilizes RNA within virion.

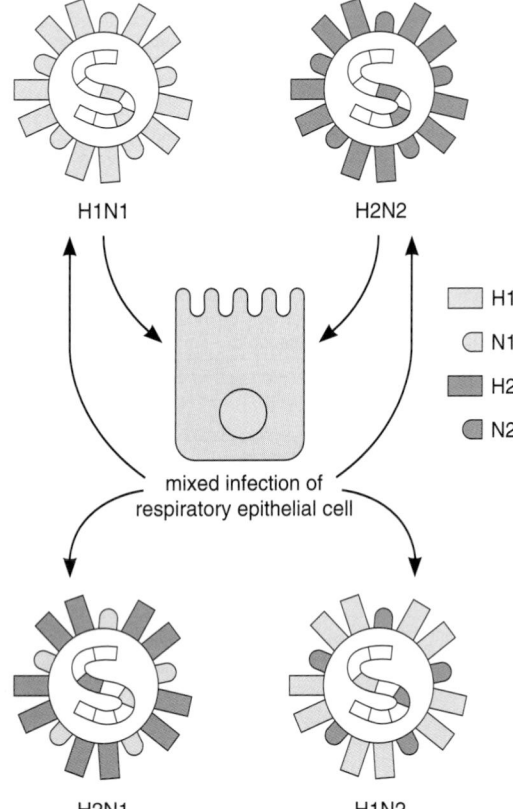

H1N1   H2N2

H1

N1

H2

N2

mixed infection of
respiratory epithelial cell

H2N1   H1N2

Figure 49–1. Schematic reproduction of genetic reassortment in influenza viruses. Shown are the major surface proteins and their corresponding gene segments.

pharyngeal or conjunctival irritation is common, and gastrointestinal symptoms may occur as well, especially in children. There are no characteristic abnormalities on routine laboratory testing. Influenza may be diagnosed by culture of the virus from nasopharyngeal or pulmonary secretions, by direct detection of viral antigens on desquamated respiratory epithelial cells with labeled monoclonal antibodies, or by demonstration of an antibody response to the virus in convalescent-phase sera.

Immunologic Pathogenesis

Although influenza virus stimulates a vigorous host immune response, including specific antibodies and cytotoxic T cells, most of the clinical findings are probably due to the cytopathic effects of this virus and to vigorous stimulation of interferon alpha production. In animal models of influenza, immunosuppression has a variable effect on the course of the infection, but virus replication is invariably prolonged. Patients with a wide variety of immunodeficiency disorders do not clearly show increased symptoms following influenza virus in-

fection, although virus shedding may be prolonged, particularly in the context of cellular immune deficiency.

Cellular immunity, measured by either skin test reactivity or in vitro lymphocyte activation to antigens, is slightly depressed during acute influenza. This transient immunosuppression appears to have no clinical effects and does not alter antiviral immune responses. The mechanism is unknown, although it may be related to production of inhibitors of interleukin-1 (IL-1). In contrast, influenza virus infection suppresses normal pulmonary antibacterial defenses, so that patients recovering from influenza have a greatly increased risk of developing bacterial pneumonia. The mechanism of this effect is unknown, but it may be the disruption of the mucociliary escalator combined with impaired function of pulmonary alveolar macrophages or neutrophils.

Infection with influenza virus stimulates interferon synthesis and also a vigorous CTL response, and both contribute to eradicating the virus. Antibody is also produced, but this appears to have only a marginal role in recovery from infection. Nude mice (which lack cellular immunity) cannot control influenza infection, and administration of antibody results in only transient cessation of virus shedding. In contrast, reconstitution of infected nude mice with cloned influenza-specific CTL eradicates the infection. Natural killer (NK) cells do not appear to play an important role in resistance to influenza.

Immunity to influenza is subtype-specific, long-lasting, and largely antibody-mediated. Antibodies directed against hemagglutinin and neuraminidase surface proteins are critical determinants of host resistance to influenza virus. Some antibodies to the M_2 protein may be protective as well. Antibodies to the hemagglutinin prevent the virus from attaching to cells and neutralize infectivity. Alone, they can prevent infection. Antibodies to neuraminidase inhibit the release of virus from cells and its subsequent spread to other cells within the host or to other people. Although antineuraminidase antibodies do not prevent infection, they ameliorate disease. In mice, serum antibodies to influenza prevent pulmonary infection but not rhinotracheitis; in contrast, mucosal IgA antibody (to the hemagglutinin and neuraminidase) is primarily responsible for resistance to upper respiratory infection. The limited data available from humans suggest that this is true in humans as well.

Influenza is associated with a number of postinfectious disorders including encephalitis (see Chapter 40), myopericarditis (see Chapter 36), Goodpasture's syndrome (see Chapters 38 and 42), and Reye's syndrome. The pathogenesis of these complications is unknown.

Treatment

Amantadine and rimantadine are cyclic amines that arrest influenza A virus replication in vitro and are effective clinically for both prophylaxis and treatment. The utility of these drugs, however, is limited by a relatively high incidence of adverse reactions, their narrow antiviral spectrum (influenza A virus only), and the propensity of this virus to become resistant.

Prevention

As mentioned earlier, serum (IgG) antibody to the major influenza surface proteins, the hemagglutinin and neuraminidase, prevents pulmonary infection, whereas mucosal (IgA) antibody is required to prevent infection of the upper respiratory tract and trachea. The presence of influenza-specific CTL also limits influenza virus infection. Although the protective antibody response is highly serotype-specific, the CTL response tends to be much broader (so-called heterotypic immunity), in part because it is directed toward viral proteins (eg, the nucleoprotein), which are much more highly conserved among strains than are the hemagglutinin and neuraminidase.

Vaccines against influenza virus were developed within a few years after identification of the virus in 1933. Current vaccines are made from virus inactivated with formalin or β-propiolactone, but the viral antigens are separated from egg proteins to avoid sensitization or reaction to egg proteins. Vaccines are standardized by hemagglutinin concentration, the only viral antigen found in significant amounts in the vaccine. Influenza vaccine is given parenterally and thus stimulates serum IgG antibody but not mucosal IgA antibody or CTL. The strains of influenza A and B viruses used for vaccine production (influenza C virus is not included because of its minor public health importance) are changed annually to reflect the antigenic characteristics of current isolates, on the recommendations of the Centers for Disease Control and Prevention.

When given annually, influenza vaccines induce protection against both severe and mild influenza. Protection against infection per se is usually minimal or nonexistent. Protection is due entirely to the stimulation of antibodies directed against the hemagglutinin protein (see Table 49–3). The efficacy of the vaccine is limited by continuing antigenic variation in influenza A and B viruses, especially the extreme antigenic changes that occur in influenza A virus.

Influenza vaccines are relatively free of serious side effects, although painful local reactions are relatively common. At least one type of influenza virus—the swine influenza virus—has been associated with production of Guillain-Barré syndrome (see Chapter 40) when administered as a vaccine. No other influenza virus type has yet been associated with this complication.

Research on improving influenza vaccines centers on development of live attenuated vaccines, insertion of hemagglutinin and neuraminidase genes into other vectors such as vaccinia virus, and attempts to find protective epitopes on molecules that are not subject to antigenic variation.

RESPIRATORY SYNCYTIAL VIRUS

Major Immunologic Features

- There is moderate antigenic variation of viral surface proteins.
- Immunity is imperfect, resulting in repeated infections throughout life.
- Infection of infants causes bronchospasm, perhaps as a result of IgE antibodies to respiratory syncytial virus.

General Considerations

Respiratory syncytial virus (RSV) causes respiratory infections in children and adults. Infections occur in annual epidemics, commonly during the winter or rainy months. The disease causes severe pneumonia and bronchiolitis in infants, whereas upper respiratory infection predominates in adults.

Virology

Respiratory syncytial virus is an enveloped virus with a continuous, negative-stranded RNA genome. On the basis of antigenic and sequence analysis of the virion surface glycoproteins, F and G, two major groups (A and B) have been identified, and there are subgroups of both, although the exact number is still uncertain. Most of the observed antigenic variation is in the G protein. The virus infects respiratory epithelium and causes extensive cytopathology, including characteristic syncytia. Recovery from infection is complete, and neither latent nor chronic infection occurs.

Clinical Features

The virus is spread through airborne droplets and by interpersonal contact through fomites. In infants 2–24 months of age, RSV infection is frequent and is often associated with lower respiratory tract disease. It is the most common cause of bronchiolitis–pneumonia associated with bronchospasm and air trapping (Fig 49–2). The severity of disease is greatest in premature infants and those with underlying chronic cardiorespiratory conditions. Infection is diagnosed by recovery of the virus in tissue culture, by identification of viral antigens on desquamated respiratory epithelial cells with monoclonal antibodies, or by documentation of a serum antibody response. Precise virologic diagnosis is important because chemotherapy is available.

Immunologic Pathogenesis

Infection with RSV stimulates both humoral and cellular immunity. Eradication of established infection is primarily a function of intact CTL, since patients with defective cellular immunity may become persistently infected with the virus. Antibody (against the F and G proteins) appears to partially protect against reinfection and disease, and maternal IgG antibody transferred transplacentally to the fetus confers some protection against disease early in life. Passive

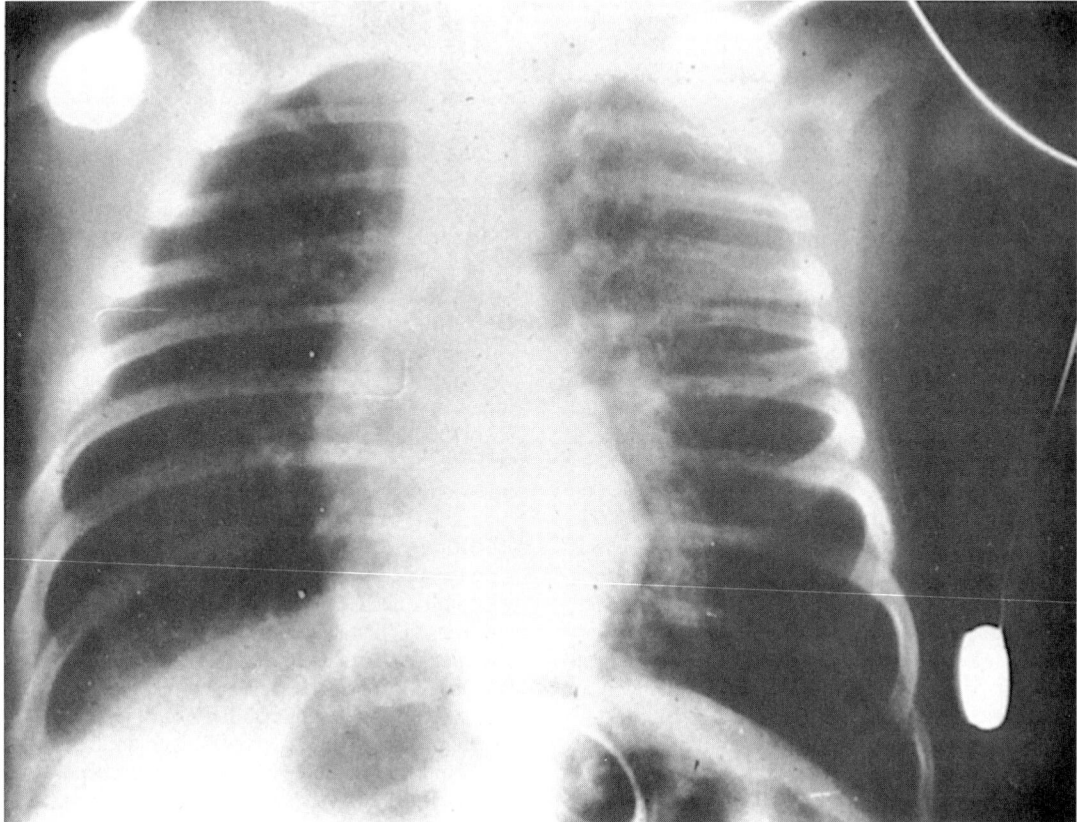

Figure 49–2. Chest x-ray of 1-year-old child with bronchiolitis due to respiratory syncytial virus, showing diffuse hyperinflation and air trapping with a left upper lobe infiltrate.

transfer of antibody to both the F and G proteins, but particularly the former, is protective in experimental respiratory syncytial virus infection and in infants.

The pathogenesis of the wheezing and air trapping associated with respiratory syncytial virus infection in infancy is not fully understood. Allergy to the virus is one possibility, since infection stimulates virus-specific IgE antibody, which can result in mast cell degranulation. The severity of bronchiolitis is directly proportionate to the quantity of mast cell products in respiratory secretions. Some of the histopathologic changes are probably due to the CTL response to RSV. In experimental animals, administration of CD4- and CD8-expressing respiratory syncytial virus T-cell lines worsens pulmonary lesions. An immunopathogenic mechanism for RSV bronchiolitis is also supported by results of a clinical trial conducted in the 1960s showing that infants who had received a parenterally administered, formalin-inactivated, highly immunogenic RSV vaccine paradoxically had worse disease following RSV infection than infants who had received a placebo. In vitro studies have also shown that RSV infection of lymphocytes and macrophages can directly depress the function of these cells, perhaps restricting the protective antiviral immune response.

Treatment

A nucleotide analogue, ribavirin, has been shown to accelerate the recovery of children with RSV infection and is licensed for this indication in the USA. The drug is aerosolized and administered by inhalation. Because of its high cost and marginal efficacy, this drug is generally used only for children who are at risk for severe morbidity or mortality from RSV infection.

In experimental animals, passive administration of antibodies to the F and G proteins (particularly the former) accelerates resolution of disease, and preliminary studies in infants are promising. Passive immunotherapy with various RSV antibodies (high-titer human immune globulin and a humanized mouse anti-F monoclonal) are in progress.

Prevention

Many efforts to produce a vaccine have been made because of the morbidity and mortality rates associated with RSV infection in infants. An immunogenic, formalin-inactivated whole RSV vaccine was field-tested in the 1960s. In this placebo-controlled trial, vaccine recipients had more severe disease after RSV infection than did those receiving the placebo. Studies of RSV infection in animal models have shown that the CTL response to this virus is both critical to recovery from infection and a major determinant of severity of illness. A formalin-inactivated vaccine similar to that used in the clinical trial produced a feeble CTL response in mice and accentuated disease after RSV challenge. This vaccine also produced a vigorous humoral response to the F and G proteins, but the antibodies lack potent virus-neutralizing activity. Thus, although the mechanism(s) is still not wholly clear, the paradoxic response to this inactivated RSV vaccine appears to have been immunologically mediated.

Promising new approaches to the prevention of RSV infection include passive immunoprophylaxis with antibodies to the F (or F and G) virion surface proteins, an F protein subunit vaccine, and live, attenuated RSV vaccines. Clinical studies using these approaches are currently in progress.

MEASLES VIRUS

Major Immunologic Features

- There is a single viral serotype; either infection or immunization results in lifelong immunity.
- Acute infection depresses cellular immunity.
- The rash is due to the cellular immune response to virus in the skin.
- "Unbalanced" immune response to inactivated measles vaccine may produce atypical and severe disease after natural infection.

General Considerations

Measles virus causes an important acute exanthem of childhood and, rarely, a chronic, slowly progressive neurologic disease, subacute sclerosing panencephalitis (SSPE), which may follow decades after an acute infection. The highly infectious virus is spread via respiratory secretions. Acute infection is associated with significant morbidity and mortality, especially in individuals in developing countries. An effective live, attenuated vaccine is available; if used widely, it could prevent nearly all cases.

Virology

Measles virus is a paramyxovirus with an envelope and a negative-stranded RNA genome. There is only one serotype, although minor sequence changes may occur in the surface glycoproteins of the virus. The virus has internal proteins, including a ribonucleoprotein and an RNA-dependent RNA polymerase, a matrix protein, and two envelope proteins, the fusion protein and a hemagglutinin. Acute infection of cells results in their death, commonly accompanied by syncytial giant-cell formation.

Clinical Features

After an incubation period of 9–11 days, during which the virus undergoes subclinical replication at unknown sites, perhaps in the lymphoreticular system, viremia occurs (virus is carried primarily in monocytes) and patients develop fever, cough, coryza, and conjunctivitis. Within 1 or 2 days, an erythematous, maculopapular rash develops, which quickly spreads over the entire body. In malnourished children, the disease is severe, and enteritis is prominent. The main complications are bacterial superinfections, such as otitis media and pneumonia, and a postinfectious encephalomyelitis.

Decades after the primary infection, a very small proportion of individuals develop SSPE, a chronic, progressive neurologic disorder due to persistent infection of the central nervous system. SSPE is caused by clonal variants of measles virus with defects that interfere with virion assembly and budding. As a consequence, extracellular virus is not produced, and infected cells do not produce viral antigens on their surface and thus are not removed by immune surveillance. A low-grade, persistent infection results in gradual neurologic injury by unknown mechanisms. SSPE is particularly common in those who acquired measles before the age of 2 years, and is very rare after measles vaccine.

In children who are vaccinated with inactivated measles virus vaccine, an "atypical" form of measles can occur, with acute infection, characterized by pleomorphic skin eruptions, including a vesicular rash, and pneumonitis. This condition is thought to be due to an unbalanced immune response to the virus (see next section).

The diagnosis of measles can be made clinically in most cases. Lymphopenia is a characteristic laboratory abnormality in acute cases. The diagnosis may be confirmed by recovering the virus from blood or oropharyngeal secretions in tissue culture, by demonstrating viral antigen on leukocytes or respiratory epithelium, or by documenting the development of IgG antibodies to the virus during convalescence. The presence of IgM antibody to measles virus during the illness also confirms the diagnosis.

Immunologic Pathogenesis

Acute measles viral infection is associated with both immune activation and immunosuppression. There is polyclonal B-cell activation, increased expression of T-cell activation markers, generation of measles-specific CD8 CTL, and elevated cytokine concentrations in plasma; concurrently there is a generalized depression of cellular immunity as measured by clinical or laboratory testing (see Chapter 15). Measles-induced immunosuppression may result in reactivation of some latent infections such as tuberculosis. The mechanism of the immunosuppression is unclear but is probably related to a direct effect of the virus on B and T lymphocytes and monocytes. The postviral encephalitis that rarely complicates measles is probably due to the host immune response to viral antigens, perhaps cross-reacting with neural antigens.

Control of measles virus replication is predominantly a function of cellular immunity although antibody does contribute to recovery from infection. Patients with defects in cellular immunity often develop progressive, fatal infections. In contrast, the virus is quickly eradicated in patients with intact cellular immunity, including those with hypogammaglobulinemia. Immunodeficient patients usually fail to develop a rash, suggesting its dependence on T-cell immunity.

Resistance to measles virus infection is primarily due to humoral immunity, specifically antibodies to the viral envelope proteins. Evidence for this is that resistance to measles virus may be conferred by passive administration of human IgG containing antibodies to the virus. Protective antibodies elicited by infection persist for life. Antibodies that develop in response to immunization may not persist as long, particularly if the vaccine was administered before 1–2 years of age.

The first measles vaccines were made from inactivated virus. Natural infection following such vaccination often resulted in severe disease but with very atypical clinical features such as pneumonitis and vesicular skin rash. These early vaccines stimulated antibody to the viral hemagglutinin but not to the fusion protein—in contrast to live virus vaccines or natural infection, in which a vigorous antibody response occurs to both proteins. This "unbalanced" immune response may be responsible for the atypical disease. Because the inactivated vaccine has not been used for decades, cases of atypical measles should now be rare.

Prevention

Resistance to disease following measles virus infection is predominantly a function of serum antibody, which results from natural infection, infection with attenuated vaccine strains of measles virus, or passive immunization. Passive administration of pooled human IgG (immune serum globulin [ISG] or intravenous immunoglobulins [IVIG]) is not a long-term control measure but is useful for postexposure prophylaxis of nonimmune subjects. It prevents measles even if given up to 1 week after exposure.

Current measles vaccines are live, attenuated viruses given parenterally. They are extremely effective and prevent disease in more than 95% of those immunized. Because measles virus is extremely infectious and highly communicable, however, herd immunity requires that more than 98% of the population have protective antibodies. Thus, control of the disease requires high compliance with immunization guidelines. All children should be immunized unless they have a congenital or acquired defect in cellular

immunity contraindicating live virus vaccination (see Chapter 55).

HEPATITIS B VIRUS

Major Immunologic Features

- There is a single viral serotype, with eight major subtypes.
- Liver damage is secondary to antiviral cellular immune response.
- Acute and chronic immune complex disease may occur.
- Infection and immunization usually result in long-lasting, complete resistance to infection.
- Perinatal transmission can be prevented by passive antibody administration followed by active immunization.

General Considerations

Hepatitis B virus (HBV) is a major cause of acute and chronic hepatitis as well as hepatic carcinoma. The virus causes either acute, self-limited infection or a chronic infection that may be lifelong. Chronic carriers may remain infectious for life and are the major reservoir for the virus. It is estimated that there are more than 200 million chronic hepatitis B carriers worldwide.

Virology

HBV is a nonenveloped DNA virus with a unique structure and mode of replication. It is related to several other animal hepatitis viruses, which collectively are known as hepadnaviruses. They contain double-stranded DNA with a nicked or single-stranded region, and they replicate via an RNA intermediate. Virion genomic DNA is synthesized from the RNA intermediate by a virion-encoded RNA-dependent DNA polymerase, structurally closely related to the reverse transcriptases of retroviruses, which are enveloped viruses with an RNA genome. The major proteins of HBV are the surface antigen (HBsAg) and core antigen (HBcAg). Although over eight subtypes of the virus are recognized, this distinction is rarely of clinical importance. Following infection, the virus replicates primarily in hepatocytes, with production of large amounts of excess surface antigen, HBsAg, which then circulates in the blood. Acute infection may resolve, with complete elimination of the virus or may be followed by chronic persistent infection in which viral cDNA persists and replicates either as an episome or integrated into the host genome. Persistent infection is associated with a high risk of hepatic carcinoma.

A defective RNA virus, hepatitis delta virus (HDV), can replicate only in HBV-infected cells, and thus causes infection only in patients with HBV infection. The delta virus genome codes for only one protein, delta antigen, and following replication, genomes of the progeny are packaged in HBsAg.

HDV may be cotransmitted with HBV or may super-infect patients with chronic HBV infection.

Clinical Features

HBV is transmitted almost exclusively by sexual contact; parenteral inoculation of blood or blood products through transfusion, parenteral drug abuse, tattooing, or acupuncture; and from infected mothers to their infants during birth (perinatal transmission). The incubation period varies from 3–4 weeks to nearly 6 months; however, it is generally 1–2 months. The majority of infections are asymptomatic, although laboratory testing reveals "chemical" hepatitis with elevated transaminase levels and the presence of HBV infection (see next section). Some 10–20% of infected patients have symptomatic hepatitis, and about 1% of those develop fatal fulminant hepatitis. A proportion of patients who recover from acute infection then go on to chronic infection, which, in turn, may be asymptomatic or associated with chronic hepatitis. Chronic infection is a major risk factor for the development of hepatoma; the incubation period may be up to 40 years.

Age and ethnicity are major variables in determining the outcome of HBV infection. Infection of the neonate during birth is rarely associated with acute hepatitis, but more than half of those children become lifelong carriers of HBV. In contrast, although hepatitis occurs in 10–20% of HBV infections acquired in adult life, chronic carriage occurs in fewer than 5% of cases. Asians appear to be at higher risk than whites for developing chronic carriage.

HDV is transmitted primarily by intravenous drug use, although some infections have been transmitted by sexual contact, particularly between homosexual men. HDV coinfection with HBV usually results in more severe disease than HBV infection alone; in some instances, the course of the disease is bimodal. HDV superinfection of patients chronically infected with HBV often results in marked worsening of the chronic hepatitis.

HBV infection was initially recognized and now is most frequently diagnosed by detection of the excess HBsAg present in serum during both acute and chronic infection. This antigen can be detected by a variety of standard immunologic tests; all are highly sensitive and specific. More than 95% of patients with

acute and chronic infection have antigen detected by these techniques. Screening of blood donors for HBsAg, as well as exclusion of paid donors, has dramatically reduced the incidence of HBV infection among recipients of blood and blood products.

Another useful test for the diagnosis of acute HBV infection is detection of the IgM antibody to core antigen (IgM anti-HBcAG), which, unlike HBsAg, is present only in patients with acute HBV infection. This test is useful for differentiating acute and chronic HBV infection and infection by other hepatitis viruses (Table 49–4). The antibody response to HBsAg tends to be delayed for several months following infection and hence is seldom used for diagnosis. The presence of either anti-HBsAg or anti-HBcAg indicates past infection, however, Figure 49–3 shows the time course of HBV serologic markers and the resulting host immune response in relation to infection.

Immunologic Pathogenesis

The prodromal symptoms of hepatitis (fever, myalgia, malaise) may be due to induction of interferon-alpha or IL-1 by this virus. Hepatic damage due to HBV infection is attributable primarily to the cellular immune response to the virus, chiefly CD8 CTL. HBV infection of hepatocytes by itself is noninjurious, and the clinical and laboratory findings of hepatitis do not appear unless virus-specific CTLs are generated. Thus, infection in patients with reduced cellular immunity (eg, neonates) tends to be asymptomatic. Resolution of the acute infection and elimination of the virus, however, also depend on the same cellular immune response; hence, immunodeficient patients also have a much higher incidence of chronic persistent infection.

HBV infection is associated with overproduction (occasionally massive) of HBsAg. In some patients with acute HBV infection, simultaneous synthesis of anti-HBsAg results in immune-complex disease, manifested by fever, skin rashes, arthralgia, and arthritis. Glomerulonephritis is rare. These findings wane as HBsAg antibody levels increase and HBsAg levels fall, resulting from control of the infection by the cellular immune response. A small proportion of patients with chronic HBV infection develop other complications of antigen–antibody complex disease, including polyarteritis nodosa, membranous glomerulonephritis, and Gianotti-Crosti syndrome of children.

Table 49–4. Use of HBV markers for the diagnosis of hepatitis.

Markers Present in Serum			
HBsAg	IgM Anti-HBcAg	Anti-HBsAg	Diagnosis
+	+	−	Acute HBV infection.
−	+	−	Acute HBV infection (after HBsAg has disappeared).
+	−	±	Chronic HBV infection.
−	−	+[1]	Past HBV infection or HBV vaccination. Indicates immunity.

[1] IgG-class anti-HBcAg also present if infection has occurred (not present following immunization).

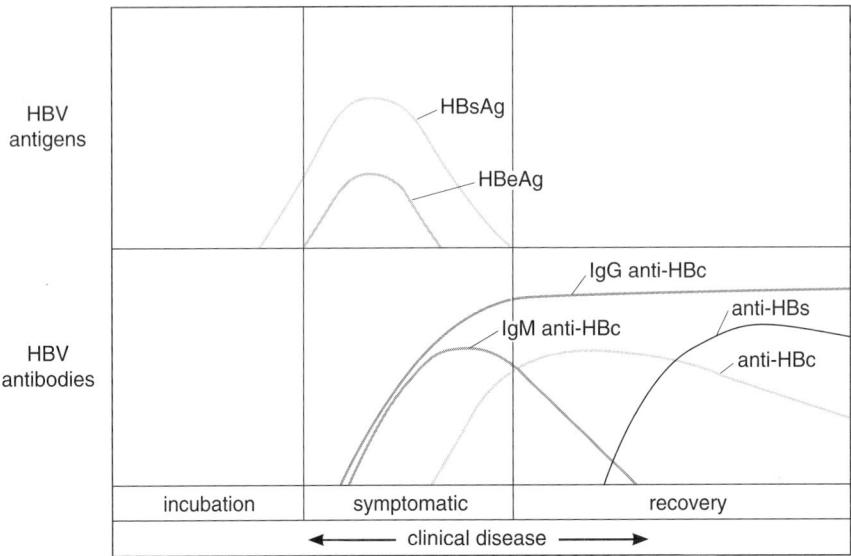

Figure 49–3. Schematic diagram showing temporal pattern of viral markers, illness, and antibody response in acute HBV infection.

Treatment

Chronic HBV infection is associated with considerable morbidity and mortality, and given the large number (>200 million) of chronic carriers known globally, there is an obvious need for chemotherapy. Interferon alpha has been licensed for treatment of chronic HBV infection in many countries, and with one or more courses of treatment about 50% of patients temporarily clear HBsAg and up to 25% appear to be cured. Interferon is not primarily an antiviral agent for HBV but instead acts by increasing the expression of class I human leukocyte antigen (HLA) antigens on the surface of the hepatocytes, which facilitates their recognition by cytotoxic T lymphocytes. Several nucleoside analogues (including ganciclovir, famciclovir, and lamivudine) have shown anti-HBV activity in clinical trials and will probably be useful adjuncts to interferon alpha therapy in the future.

Prevention

Cytotoxic T lymphocytes are critical to recovery from HBV infection and elimination of the virus. In contrast, resistance to HBV infection is mediated effectively by antibody to HBsAg alone. Either passive administration of antibody to HBsAg, or eliciting anti-HBsAg by immunization with inactivated or recombinant HBsAg confers resistance to infection.

Preventive measures for HBV infection employ either pooled human immune serum globulin with high titers of antibody to HBsAg (hepatitis B immune globulin [HBIG]) or HBV vaccine. The latter consists of HBsAg, either purified from the plasma of chronic carriers or prepared by recombinant DNA techniques. Both types of vaccines are extremely safe and induce protective antibodies in more than 95% of individuals immunized.

Control measures may be implemented either in anticipation of infection or after infection has already occurred; the latter is known as "postexposure prophylaxis." Postexposure prophylaxis is highly effective and is indicated when a susceptible individual has been exposed to someone with active infection (ie, a patient with HBsAg in the blood), for example through sexual contact or a needle-stick injury. It is also indicated postpartum to infants born to mothers with HBV infection. Passive immunity is achieved immediately by administration of HBIG. Then active immunity is stimulated by administration of HBV vaccine. The only circumstance in which antigenic variation in HBV has been clinically significant is in postexposure prophylaxis of infants born to HBV-infected mothers, where vaccine-induced escape mutants have occasionally been observed.

Preexposure immunization against HBV infection was formerly recommended only for individuals at high risk of HBV infection, but there is now a reasonable consensus that universal hepatitis B immunization has a favorable cost-benefit ratio and should be instituted in most countries, including the USA. HBIG has no role in preexposure prophylaxis.

HEPATITIS A VIRUS

Hepatitis A virus (HAV) is closely related to other picornaviruses (small, nonenveloped RNA viruses) such as poliovirus. There is only a single serotype.

HAV is transmitted primarily by the fecal–oral route. Following ingestion, the virus travels via the bloodstream to the liver, probably the exclusive site of virus replication. Replication in the liver results in a brief period of viremia (5–10 days) and shedding of virus in the stools for 1–2 weeks. The infection resolves completely in all cases, except for rare instances of fatal infection. In contrast to HBV, chronic or latent infection does not occur. Resolution of infection is dependent on intact cellular immunity, since patients with cellular immunodeficiency may experience prolonged virus shedding and disease, similar to the case with other enteroviruses (see the section on Poliovirus).

The incubation period of HAV infection averages 30 days and ranges from 10 to 50 days. Most infections, especially those in children, are asymptomatic, although evidence of "chemical" hepatitis is usually found on laboratory testing. Liver cell injury is thought to be due primarily to the host cellular immune response, as in HBV infection. The mortality rate during acute infection is about 0.1% overall, but it is lower in children and increases with increasing age.

HAV infection generates a vigorous antibody response, which protects against reinfection and serves as the basis for diagnosis. Detection of the transient anti-HAV IgM response is the single most useful test for acute infection, whereas detection of the long-lasting anti-HAV IgG response is the best marker for past infection and resistance to subsequent infection. Infection may also be documented by demonstrating the development of IgG antibody response by comparing acute- and convalescent-phase serum specimens. This approach is cumbersome, however, and may yield false-negative results, especially if the acute-phase serum specimen was obtained too long after the initial antibody response; thus, it is little used today. Unlike HBV, there is no serologic test for HAV antigen.

Resistance to HAV infection is mediated solely by serum antibody to the virus. This has been demonstrated by studies showing passive transfer of protection by immune globulin that contains antibody to HAV. Protection from HAV infection can be achieved with pooled human ISG given every 3–6 months. The intramuscular preparation is usually used, although intravenous immune globulin is also effective. Protection from illness may also be achieved by administration of ISG within 1 week following exposure to HAV. An inactivated HAV vaccine grown in cell culture is now licensed in many countries; it is entirely safe and provides longlasting protective antibodies. At present it is recommended primarily for residents of developed countries who are traveling to developing countries and who otherwise would have received immune globulin for protection. In the future, it may become part of the recommended panel of vaccines for universal immunization.

RABIES VIRUS

Rabies virus infection is enzootic in many wild animal species, including foxes, skunks, and bats. It can infect many domestic animals (dogs are the most commonly infected), although infection of domestic animals is unusual in developed countries because of the widespread application of control measures. When rabies virus infects humans, generally as the result of an animal bite, the resulting disease is virtually 100% fatal. Hence, preventive measures are of the utmost importance.

Rabies virus is an enveloped RNA virus that is related to several other animal viruses. Although only one serotype is detectable by the usual clinical criteria, studies with monoclonal antibodies have identified strains with differing geographic and host ranges. Following a bite wound, the virus replicates in muscles and nerves, extends centripetally along peripheral nerves over a period of days to months or even years, finally reaching the spinal cord and central nervous system. At this stage the hyperexcitability and hydrophobia characteristic of rabies occur. There are no effective antiviral drugs, and even with maximum supportive care, virtually every affected individual dies.

Because of the tremendous epidemiologic and public health implications of a case of rabies, the clinical diagnosis of rabies must be supported by laboratory data. Viral antigens can be detected by immunofluorescence with specific antisera or monoclonal antibodies in the brains of animals and humans and in corneal epithelial cells of humans. This technique is more sensitive than the histopathologic demonstration of Negri bodies. A diagnosis can also be made by demonstrating a rise in antibody titer following infection, although this is less useful clinically.

Animal data support a role for the host immune response in the pathogenesis of rabies. Although immunosuppression of animals prior to infection shortens the latency period and increases the mortality rate, immunosuppression after infection may delay mortality, even though brain virus titers are increased. In immunosuppressed animals with high brain virus titers, administration of rabies hyperimmune serum markedly worsens disease, further supporting the role of the immune system in production of illness.

Antibody to the virus surface glycoprotein (G protein) is protective. Individuals with serum antibody elicited by immunization are resistant to infection, and protection from disease can be achieved even after infection by administration of hyperimmune animal or human antibodies. These antibodies are effective only if given shortly after infection, and their efficacy is increased by local administration around the site of the bite wound, suggesting that they act by local neutralization of the virus.

The first rabies vaccines were prepared by Pasteur, who used virus that had been adapted to growth in rabbit neural tissue and then inactivated by heating and drying. Currently, many rabies vaccines are available; however, the only one used widely in developed countries is inactivated virus grown in human fibroblasts. This vaccine is highly immunogenic, protective if given either before or immediately after infection, and relatively free of serious side effects. Although animal-derived vaccines from rabbit or monkey brain or embryonated egg are effective in preventing rabies and are still available in many developing countries, the nervous tissue antigens present in these products may cause allergic encephalitis in vaccine recipients. A vaccinia virus recombinant expressing the rabies virus G protein infects animals if given orally (food bait laced with vaccine) and has proven effective in control of rabies in wildlife. G-protein vaccines made by recombinant DNA technology may be available for humans in the near future.

POLIOVIRUS

Poliovirus is the cause of poliomyelitis, an acute encephalomyelitis that results in asymmetric paralysis with muscle atrophy. Although cases of paralysis almost certainly due to poliovirus have been recognized for thousands of years, the 20th century has seen a marked increase in the incidence of the disease and a change from endemic to epidemic spread. Development of poliovirus vaccine in the middle of the 20th century and its widespread application in developed countries have resulted in the virtual elimination of the disease in vaccinated populations.

Poliovirus is a member of the picornavirus family, which consists of small, nonenveloped positive-stranded RNA viruses and includes other enteroviruses (echovirus, coxsackievirus, etc), rhinoviruses, and HAV. Although closely related by structure, mode of replication, and RNA sequence homology, these viruses exhibit tremendous antigenic diversity, and there is little or no serologic relatedness or cross-resistance among them. Poliovirus has three noncross-reactive serotypes: serotypes 1, 2, and 3. Infection generates a vigorous cellular and humoral immune response to the coat proteins of the virus.

Patients infected with poliovirus and the other enteroviruses shed large amounts of virus in the feces, often for periods of weeks or months. Infection is transmitted when a susceptible individual ingests food or water contaminated by infected feces. The virus replicates in the intestinal tract, and viremia occurs; this is followed by seeding of the spinal cord and central nervous system. Although most patients (>99%) recover without sequelae, the remainder suffer some degree of motor nerve dysfunction, which varies from minimal weakness of an extremity to severe paralysis

of all major muscle groups. Partial or complete recovery may occur after the acute illness.

Resolution of infection and elimination of the virus appear to require intact cellular immune mechanisms, since patients with defective cellular immunity continue to shed poliovirus as well as other enteroviruses for months or years after infection. Antibodies, however, play some role in recovery from infection, since patients with isolated hypogammaglobulinemia have persistent enterovirus infections. Resistance to disease is mediated by serum-neutralizing antibody to virion surface antigens. Administration of pooled human ISG containing antibodies to poliovirus prevents the disease, even if given a few days after exposure. In addition, inactivated vaccines that stimulate humoral but not cellular immunity are also highly protective. Intestinal infection can still occur in the presence of serum antibodies; however, viremia with seeding of the central nervous system does not occur. Intestinal mucosal IgA (coproantibody) antibody to poliovirus is stimulated by natural infection and immunization with live attenuated (Sabin-type) vaccine and prevents infection.

The first poliovirus vaccine consisted of tissue culture-grown suspensions of poliovirus types 1–3, which were inactivated with formalin. Although inactivated (Salk) vaccine is highly effective for preventing paralytic poliomyelitis, it has several disadvantages. It requires parenteral injection (hence, there is an increased cost for needles and syringes); booster doses are required to maintain immunity; and it does not displace wild-type poliovirus circulating in the community. Live, attenuated (Sabin) vaccine can be given orally; it does not routinely require booster doses; and when immunization is widespread in a community, the vaccine virus displaces the wild-type virus in the environment, thus reducing the risk of paralytic disease among the unimmunized. Live poliovirus may rarely revert to virulence, however, producing paralytic disease in vaccinees or their contacts.

Both inactivated and live attenuated poliovirus vaccines are manufactured and used today, although either one or the other is usually selected by national vaccination programs. Although the choice between live and inactivated virus vaccine is often the subject of heated debate, either type of vaccine virtually eliminates paralytic poliomyelitis if used extensively. Widespread polio immunization has already eradicated poliomyelitis in the Americas and Australasia; the World Health Organization has set in place a program to eradicate poliovirus infection worldwide by early in the 21st century. Active investigation is also under way to improve both the live attenuated and inactivated vaccines.

REFERENCES

GENERAL

Spriggs MK: One step ahead of the game: Viral immunomodulatory molecules. In: Paul WE et al (editors). *Ann Rev Immunol* 1996;**14**:101.

Tyler KL, Fields BN: Pathogenesis of viral infections. In: *Virology,* 3rd ed. Fields BN et al (editors). Lippincott-Raven Publishers, 1996, p. 173.

Whitton JL, Oldstone MBA: Immune response to viruses. In: *Virology,* 3rd ed. Fields BN et al (editors). Lippincott-Raven Publishers, 1996, p. 345.

INFLUENZA VIRUS

Bender BS, Small PA: Influenza: Pathogenesis and host defense. *Semin Respir Infect* 1992;**7**:38.

Klenk HD, Rott, R: The molecular biology of influenza virus pathogenicity. *Adv Virus Res* 1988;**34**:247.

Murphy BR, Webster RG: Orthomyxoviruses. In: *Virology,* 3rd ed. Fields BN et al (editors). Lippincott-Raven Publishers, 1996, p 1397.

RESPIRATORY SYNCYTIAL VIRUS

Collins PL et al: Respiratory syncytial virus. In: *Virology,* 3rd ed. Fields BN et al (editors). Lippincott-Raven Publishers, 1996, p 1313.

Mills J: Immunotherapy and immunoprophylaxis of respiratory syncytial virus infections. *Curr Opin Infect Dis* 1995;**8**:473.

MEASLES VIRUS

Griffin DE, Bellini WJ: Measles virus. In: *Virology,* 3rd ed. Fields BN et al (editors). Lippincott-Raven Publishers, 1996, p 1267.

HEPATITIS B VIRUS

Chisari FV: Hepatitis B virus biology and pathogenesis. *Mol Genet Med* 1992;**2**:67.

Ferrari C et al: Immune pathogenesis of hepatitis B. *Arch Virol Suppl* 1992;**4**:11.

Hollinger FB: Hepatitis B virus. In: *Virology,* 3rd ed. Fields BN et al (editors). Lippincott-Raven Publishers, 1996, p. 2738.

HEPATITIS A VIRUS

Hollinger FB, Ticehurst JR: Hepatitis A virus. In: *Virology,* 3rd ed. Fields BN et al (editors). Lippincott-Raven Publishers, 1996, p 735.

Lemon SM: Hepatitis A virus: Current concepts of the molecular biology, immunobiology and approaches to vaccine development. *Rev Med Virol* 1992;**2**:73.

RABIES VIRUS

Dietzschold B et al: Rhabdoviruses. In: *Virology,* 3rd ed. Fields BN et al (editors). Lippincott-Raven Publishers, 1996, p 1137.

King AA, Turner GS: Rabies: A review. *J Comp Pathol* 1993;**108**:1.

POLIOVIRUS

Melnick JL: Enteroviruses: Polioviruses, coxsackieviruses, echoviruses, and newer enteroviruses. In: *Virology,* 3rd ed. Fields BN et al (editors). Lippincott-Raven Publishers, 1996, p 655.

50

Fungal Diseases

Thomas F. Patterson, MD, & David J. Drutz, MD

Infectious disease caused by fungi are called **mycoses.** Fungi, like mammalian cells, are eukaryotes; that is, they possess a true nucleus containing several chromosomes, bounded by a nuclear membrane. In contrast, bacteria are prokaryotes, with a single linear chromosome and no true nucleus. The principal sterol of the mammalian cell membrane is cholesterol; that of fungi is ergosterol. Ergosterol is the target of amphotericin B and the antifungal azoles and triazoles. Fungal cell walls have no counterpart in mammalian cells, and they differ from those of bacteria by lacking peptidoglycans, teichoic acids, and lipopolysaccharides (endotoxin). In their place are the external and antigenic **peptidomannans** embedded in matrices of α- and β-**glucans;** structural rigidity is provided by sheets, disks, or fibrils of **chitin** (poly β-1,4-*N*-acetylglucosamine). RNA typing studies and electron microscopic analysis have been used to characterize exceptional organisms that are not clearly classified as fungi. For example, RNA typing studies have established a relationship between true fungi and *Pneumocystis carnii,* an organism initially classified as a protozoan based on growth characteristics. Although, *P carnii* has chitin and β-glucans in its wall and contains a fungal-specific protein elongation factor 3. It differs from fungi in that it lacks ergosterol, responds poorly to most traditional antifungal agents, and appears morphologically distinct from fungi. Although data establish the molecular similarity of *P carnii* to fungi, differences clearly exist so that additional classification is still needed. Other organisms that lack an in vitro culture system such as *Loboa loboi* and *Rhinosporidium seeberi* are presumed to be fungi, but molecular analysis is needed to identify their correct phylogeny.

Although there are thousands of fungi in nature, relatively few are pathogenic for normal humans. Table 50–1 lists common mycoses according to the usual sites of infection. Superficial mycoses usually occur on the body external to common immunologic influences. Cutaneous mycoses produced delayed hyper-

sensitivity responses to the local presence of keratinolytic fungi. Subcutaneous and systemic mycoses represent successful challenges to major immunologic host defense mechanisms. Some systemic mycoses (eg, blastomycosis, coccidioidomycosis, histoplasmosis, and paracoccidiodomycosis) are due to primary pathogens, theoretically capable of infecting anyone present in an endemic area. Others (eg, candidiasis, cryptococcosis, aspergillosis, and mucormycosis [zygomycosis]) are due to opportunistic pathogens, which seldom cause life-threatening tissue invasion in the absence of impaired host defense. Most fungal infection occurs from exogenous acquisition of the organism from environmental sources. Other fungi, such as *Malassezia* and *Candida* spp., may produce infection that results from endogenous colonizing sources. Yeasts such as *Candida albicans, C glabrata, C tropicalis,* and *Candida* spp., however, have been associated with acquisition of infection from environmental sources and may be associated with nosocomial transmission, frequently through hand carriage. Most primary invasive mycoses are acquired by the inhalation of specialized forms (conidia and spores) that are progeny of filamentous soil forms of the fungi. Once inhaled, some fungi reproduce in the body in the original filamentous (mycelial, hyphal) form. Others adopt specialized forms (yeasts, spherules, and endospores) more suitable for host survival and tissue invasion. Opportunistic fungi, however, can cause overwhelming infection in the increasing number of patients with impaired host defenses, including patients with acquired immunodeficiency syndrome (AIDS), organ and bone marrow transplants, and hematologic malignancy. Mycoses that exist in nature as an infectious mould and invade tissues as a yeast (or yeast-like form such as spherules or endospores) are called **dimorphic fungi.** Table 50–1 indicates the forms assumed by common fungi when invading host tissues. A major attribute of all opportunistic filamentous fungi is the tendency to invade blood vessels (**angioinvasion**), with resultant tissue infarction (Table 50–2).

Table 50–1. Common mycoses according to usual sites of disease production.

Site and Disease	Etiologic Agents	Origin	Invasive Form	Pathophysiologic Basis	Principal Clinical Features
Superficial mycoses Pityriasis (tinea) versicolor	*Malassezia furfur*	Hair follicle (yeasts)	Yeasts and/or mycelia	Decreased epithelial turnover allows normal flora to produce disease.	Hypopigmented or hyperpigmented macular skin lesions.
Malassezia	*Malassezia furfur*	Hair follicle (yeasts)	Yeasts	Obstructed hair follicles are damaged by follicular flora.	Acneiform folliculitis.
Tinea nigra	*Exophiala werneckii*	Soil (mycelia)	Mycelia	Hyperhidrosis permits infection from environment.	Brown-black nonscaly macules (especially on palms).
White piedra	*Trichosporon beigelii*	Soil, skin (mycelia)	Mycelia and yeasts	Poor personal hygiene permits infection from environment or by normal flora.	Soft whitish nodules on hair shaft.
Black piedra	*Piedraia hortae*	Soil (mycelia)	Mycelia	Poor personal hygiene permits infection from environment.	Hard gritty black nodules on hair shaft.
Cutaneous mycoses Dermatophytosis	*Epidermophyton, Trichophyton,* and *Microsporum* spp	Soil and animal fur (mycelia)	Mycelia	Etiologic agents are keratinolytis; infection is potentiated by warmth, moisture, and occlusion; cutaneous inflammation is due to delayed-hypersensitivity reaction.	Tinea pedis (scaly, vesicular, ulcerative), tinea cruris (dry, red, scaloped, expanding), tinea corporis (ringworm); tinea barbae (suppuration, beard), tinea capitis (scalp; resembles seborrhea), tinea unguium (nails).
Subcutaneous mycoses Chromoblastomycosis	*Cladosporium, Fonsecaea, Philaophora,* and *Rhinocladiella* spp	Soil (mycelia)	Mycelia and sclerotic bodies	Traumatic implantation.	Papules, warty tumors, plaques, cauliflower-like growths.
Mycetoma	*Acremonium, Exophiala, Leptosphaeria, Madurella, Microsporum, Neotestudina,* and *Pseudallescheria* spp	Soil (mycelia)	Mycelia and grains	Traumatic implantation.	Swelling, draining fistulae, pus, and grains.
Sporotrichosis	*Sporothrix schenckii*	Vegetation (mycelia)	Yeasts	Traumatic implantation.	Subcutaneous nodules along lymphatics.

(continued)

Table 50–1. Common mycoses according to usual sites of disease production *(continued)*.

Site and Disease	Etiologic Agents	Origin	Invasive Form	Pathophysiologic Basis	Principal Clinical Features
Systemic invasive mycoses Primary pathogens Blastomycosis	*Blastomyces dermatitidis*	Soil (mycelia)	Yeasts	Inhalation of conidia.	Pulmonary, spreading to skin, bones, male reproductive tract.
Coccidioidomycosis	*Coccidioides immitis*	Soil (mycelia)	Spherules and endospores	Inhalation of arthroconidia.	Pulmonary, spreading to skin, bones, joints, meninges.
Histoplasmosis	*Histoplasma capsulatum*	Soil (mycelia)	Yeasts	Inhalation of microconidia.	Pulmonary, spreading to reticuloendothelial system, mucous membranes, adrenals.
Paracoccidioidomycosis	*Paracoccidioides brasiliensis*	Soil (mycelia)	Yeasts	Inhalation of conidia.	Pulmonary, spreading to reticuloendothelial system, skin, mucous membranes, adrenals.
Opportunistic pathogens Candidiasis	Principally *Candida albicans, C tropicalis,* and *C glabrata*	Mucosal surfaces (yeasts, pseudomycelia)	Yeasts, pseudomycelia, mycelia	Local extension; bloodstream invasion from colonization sites (mucosal disruption).	Mucosal site, spreading to eyes, skin, kidneys, myocardium, other sites.
Cryptococcosis	*Cryptococcus neoformans*	Soil (yeast, basidiospores [sexual form])	Yeasts	Inhalation of desiccated yeasts or basidiospores.	Pulmonary, spreading to meninges, brain, bone skin.
Aspergillosis	*Aspergillus fumigatus, A flavus, A terreus,* and *A niger,* principally	Soil (mycelia)	Mycelia	Inhalation of conidia.	Invasive pulmonary or sinus disease, leading to hematogenous dissemination.
Mucormycosis (zygomycosis)	*Rhizopus, Rhizomucor, Absidia, Cunninghamelia, Mortierella, Saksenaea* and *Mucor* spp	Soil (mycelia)	Mycelia	Inhalation of spores.	Invasive sinus or pulmonary disease, leading to hematogeneous dissemination.

(continued)

Immunity to the mycoses is principally cellular, involving neutrophils, macrophages, lymphocytes, and probably natural killer (NK) cells. With the possible exception of the dermatophytes and *Rhizopus arrhizus,* the principal etiologic agent of mucormycosis (zygomycosis), fungi are not susceptible to direct killing by antibody and complement. Patients with neutropenia or defective neutrophil function appear

Table 50–1. Common mycoses according to usual sites of disease production *(continued)*.

Site and Disease	Etiologic Agents	Origin	Invasive Form	Pathophysiologic Basis	Principal Clinical Features
Pneumocystosis	*Pneumocystis carinii*	Unknown	Cysts and trophozoites	Inhalation of infective particles or arousal from latency.	Progressive interstitial lung disease with or without cysts, pneumothorax.
Phaeohyphomycosis	Approximately 40 genera of pigmented fungi (eg, *Alternaria, Bipolaris, Cladosporium, Exserohilum, Phialophora, Wangiella*)	Soil (mycelia)	Mycelia	Inhalation or implantation of common environmental fungi (pigmented; dematiaceous).	Invasive sinus or pulmonary disease, leading to hematogenous dissemination.
Hyalohyphomycosis	Diverse nonpigmented fungi (eg, *Fusarium, Paecilomyces, Pseudallescheria, Scopulariopsis*)	Soil (mycelia)	Mycelia	Inhalation or implantation of common environmental fungi (nonpigmented).	Invasive sinus or pulmonary disease, leading to hematogenous dissemination.

predisposed to hematogenously disseminated infection with yeast-like fungi (eg, *Candida* spp, *Trichosporon beigelii*), or with filamentous fungi (eg, *Aspergillus,* agents causing mucormycosis, and *Fusarium* spp). Patients with defective cell-mediated immunity (CMI) (eg, patients with AIDS) are predisposed to mucosal candidiasis or hematogenously disseminated cryptococcosis, histoplasmosis, and coccidioidomycosis (Table 50–3). Allergy to fungi is discussed in Chapters 26–30.

Salient features of the superficial, cutaneous, and subcutaneous mycoses may be found in Tables 50–1 to 50–4. The major systemic invasive mycoses found in the Western hemisphere are described in the following section.

SYSTEMIC INVASIVE MYCOSES: PRIMARY PATHOGENS

BLASTOMYCOSIS

Major Immunologic Features

- Yeasts are large, single, and broad-based and commonly exceed the size of phagocytes.
- Islands of suppuration (microabscesses) amid granulomas are produced.
- Both neutrophils and CMI may play important and concomitant roles in host defense.
- Severe, widely disseminated infection may occur

in patients with defective CMI, including those with AIDS.

General Considerations

Blastomycosis is an inhalation-acquired mycosis that can produce primary pulmonary infection or hematogenously disseminated disease involving predominantly skin, bones, and the male genitourinary tract. *Blastomyces dermatitidis,* the cause of this disease, is a spherical multinucleated yeast with thick walls and single broad-based buds. The mycelial form of *B dermatitidis* is a soil organism found on river banks predominantly in the south-central USA and around the Great Lakes. A closely related fungus occurs in Africa. Infection occurs by inhalation of fungal microconidia in endemic areas (eg, by hunters, trappers, campers, or boaters). Hunters and their dogs have been simultaneously infected. There are sporadic and occasionally common-source outbreaks with the organism isolated from soil collected from damp areas such as a beaver dam and along a river bank. Areas where the disease is endemic are defined by the occurrence of cases and by seroconversions. However, there is no reliable skin test to gauge population exposures and establish the epidemiology of infection. No convincing sex or age prevalence is apparent in common-source outbreaks. Men are more susceptible than women to progressive pulmonary or hematogenous disease. There is no known genetic predisposition. Although overwhelming disseminated infection may occur as a late complication of AIDS, blastomycosis is an infrequent complication in that population.

Table 50–2. Pathologic features of subcutaneous and systemic mycoses.

Mycosis	Predominant Location of Fungi	Suppuration	Granulomas	Caseation	Fibrosis	Calcification	Other
Subcutaneous Chromo-mycosis	Extracellular (sclerotic bodies)	Dominant	Dominant	Rare	Dominant	Rare	PH; transdermal elimination.
Mycetoma	Extracellular (grains)	Dominant	Dominant	Rare	Dominant	Rare	Grain color varies by etiologic agent; grains surrounded by amorphous material reflecting immune complex deposition (Splendore-Hoeppli phenomenon).
Sporotrichosis	Intracellular and extracellular (yeasts)	Dominant	Dominant	Occasional	Occasional	Rare	Asteroid bodies with Splendore-Hoeppli phenomenon.
Systemic Primary pathogens Blastomycosis[1]	Extracellular (yeasts)	Dominant	Dominant	Rare	Occasional	Occasional	PH.
Coccidio-idomy-cosis	Extracellular (spherules)	Dominant (endospores)	Dominant (spherules)	Rare	Occasional	Occasional	PH.
Histoplas-mosis	Intracellular (yeasts)	Rare	Dominant	Occasional	Dominant	Dominant	Proliferative end-arteritis (lungs).
Paracocci-dioidomy-cosis[1]	Extracellular (yeasts)	Dominant	Dominant	Rare	Dominant	Occasional	PH.
Opportunistic pathogens Cryptococcosis[1]	Extracellular (yeasts)	Rare	Dominant	Rare	Rare	Rare	Extensive accumulation of extracellular capsular material may produce local anatomic distortions.

(continued)

Table 50–2. Pathologic features of subcutaneous and systemic mycoses *(continued)*.

Mycosis	Predominant Location of Fungi	Suppuration	Granulomas	Caseation	Fibrosis	Calcification	Other
Candidia-sis[2]	Intracellular (yeasts), extracellular (pseudomy-celia, mycelia)	Dominant	Rare	Rare	Rare	Rare	Granuloma formation common only with chronic mucocutaneous candidiasis.
Aspergill-osis[2]	Extracellular (mycelia)	Dominant	Rare	Rare	Rare	Rare	Angioinvasion and infarction.
Mucormy-cosis (zygom-ycosis)[2]	Extracellular (mycelia)	Dominant	Rare	Rare	Rare	Rare	Angioinvasion and infarction.
Pneumo-cystosis	Extracellular (trophozoites, cysts)	Rare	Rare	None	Occasional	Rare	Foamy intra-alveolar infiltrate and alveolar epithelial damage.

Abbreviations: PH = pseudoepitheliomatous hyperplasia of skin and mucosal lesions; CMI = cell-mediated immunity.

[1] Severely depressed CMI is often associated with poor granuloma formation and increased suppuration with increased numbers of microorganisms (blastomycosis, coccidioidomycosis, paracoccidioidomycosis) or with gelatinous masses of encapsulated fungi (cryptococcosis).

[2] Severe neutropenia is often associated with loss of suppurative tissue response.

Pathology

See Table 50–2.

Clinical Features

A. Signs and Symptoms: Primary exposure may be asymptomatic, or it may produce an influenza-like syndrome. Pneumonia, pleuritis, pulmonary cavitation, and mediastinal adenopathy may occur. Hematogenous dissemination may occur in the presence or absence of apparent pulmonary disease. Favored sites of metastic infection include skin (papules, pustules, or verrucous granulomas that heal centrally and extend peripherally); bone (lytic lesions, especially vertebrae and long bones, with or without draining sinuses); and prostate, testis, and epididymis. Central nervous system infection occurs in about 5% of cases, but this increases to 40% in patients with AIDS. Disseminated, progressive infection with extensive pulmonary involvement occurs in patients with AIDS. Gastrointestinal tract involvement almost never occurs.

B. Laboratory Findings: These include leukocytosis, abnormal chest x-ray, and evidence of specific organ dysfunction at metastatic loci. Diagnosis is established by finding large budding yeasts on smears or histologic sections and by recovering the fungus in culture.

C. Immunologic Diagnosis: See Table 50–4. With the possible exception of antibody directed against the A antigen, immunologic tests lack either sensitivity or specificity. Other antigens, including a 160-kd antigen extracted by B. S. Klein and colleagues, may be more useful for establishing a serodiagnosis of infection, but their utility remains experimental.

D. Differential Diagnosis: This includes diverse granulomatous infectious diseases (eg, other mycoses and tuberculosis), sarcoidosis, and pulmonary cancer.

E. Treatment: Itraconazole is highly effective and has fewer side effect than ketoconazole when used to treat chronic, indolent forms of blastomycosis. For patients with meningitis or acute life-threatening infections, intravenous amphotericin B is preferable.

F. Prevention: No vaccine is available.

G. Complications and Prognosis: Untreated extrapulmonary blastomycosis carries a 20–90% mortality rate, depending on the individual series. The mortality rate with therapy in most patients is less than 10%; however, mortality rates in AIDS patients with disseminated infection are high. Most relapses occur within 1 year of treatment, but they have been documented after as long as 9 years.

Table 50–3. Effect of common immunologic abnormalities on disease course of common mycoses.

Mycosis	Reduction in PMN[1]	Reduction in CMI[2]	Other
Superficial Pityriasis (tinea) versicolor	None	None	Lipid hyperalimentation therapy is associated with *Malassezia furfur* and pulmonary vasculitis, especially in infants.
Pityrosporum folliculitis	None	None	Treatment
Tinea nigra	None	None	
White piedra	Hematogenous dissemination of *Trichosporon beigelii*[4]	None	
Black piedra	None	None	
Cutaneous Dermatophytosis	None	Increased severity and chronicity of *T rubrum* infection	
Subcutaneous Chromomycosis	None	None	
Mycetoma	None	None	
Sporotrichosis	None	Increased in severity and likelihood of dissemination	
Systemic, invasive **Primary pathogens** Blastomycosis	None	Increase in severity and likelihood of dissemination	Frequency of meningitis is increased in patients with AIDS.
Coccidioidomycosis	None	Definite increase in severity and dissemination	Possible increase in severity and dissemination in second and third trimesters of pregnancy.
Histoplasmosis	None	Definite increase in severity and dissemination	
Paracoccidioidomycosis	None	Probable increase in severity or likelihood of dissemination	
Opportunistic pathogens Candidiasis	Hematogenous dissemination	Increased severity of mucosal disease	
Cryptococcosis	None	Definite increase in severity and dissemination	
Aspergillosis	Invasive paranasal sinus and respiratory infection, and hematogenous dissemination	Possible increase in severity	
Mucormycosis (zygomysosis)	Invasive paranasal sinus and respiratory infection, and hematogenous dissemination	Possible increase in severity	Diabetic ketoacidosis predisposes to invasive paranasal sinus infection.
Pneumocystosis	None	Drastic incraese in incidence and severity in AIDS	
Phaeohyphomycosis	Invasive paranasal sinus infection and hematogenous dissemination	None	
Hyalohyphomycoses	Invasive paranasal sinus infection and hematogenous dissemination	None	

Abbreviations: AIDS = acquired immunodeficiency syndrome; CMI = cell-mediated immunity.

[1] <500 PMN/dL.

[2] Principally AIDS. Histoplasmosis, coccidioidomycosis, and cryptococcosis also occur with increased severity and/or extent of dissemination in patients with other causes of depressed CMI (eg, immunosuppression for organ transplantation).

[3] *Malassezia* is a lipophilic fungus. Lipid hyperalimentation therapy allows them access to the bloodstream. Patients with *Malassezia* fungemia do not have tinea versicolor or folliculitis.

[4] Patients with *Trichosporon beigelii* sepsis do not necessarily have white piedra.

Table 50–4. Immunologic diagnosis of subcutaneous and systemic mycoses.

Mycosis	Serologic Tests		Delayed-Hypersensitivity Skin Test[1]	Comments[2]
	Antibody	Antigen		
Subcutaneous Chromoblasto-mycosis	None	None	None	Chromoblastomycosis is diagnosed by its characteristic clinical appearance (warty plaques, nodules, and cauliflower-like excrescences), together with the demonstration of characteristic pigmented sclerotic bodies in histologic sections. Specific etiologic diagnoses must be established by culture.
Mycetoma	None	None	None	Mycetoma is diagnosed by its characteristic clinical picture (sinuses discharging pus and grains). Specific etiologic diagnosis rests upon microscopic examination of grains and cultures of grains and biopsy material.
Sporotrichosis	EIA, TA, LPA (sensitive/specific) CF, ID (less sensitive)	None	Investigational only	Serologic tests are generally valuable only in extracutaneous and disseminated infection. A slide latex agglutination titer of ≥1:8 is presumptive evidence of disseminated or systemic infection.
Systemic Primary pathogens Blastomycosis	ID, CF (blastomycin as antigen); ID, CF EIA (A antigen)	None	Blastomycin (mycelial phase), BASWS (investigational only)	The blastomycin skin test and serologic tests lack sensitivity and specificity; there is major cross-reactivity with histoplasmosis. Tests for antibody to A antigen are more specific (especially ID and EIA).
Coccidioido-mycosis	IgM (TP, IDTP, LPA); IgG (CF, IDCF) (coccidioidin as antigen)	Experimental only	Coccidioidin (mycelial phase), spherulin (spherule phase)	IgM tests are positive early and transiently; IgG tests are positive later and more persistently A CF antibody titer in blood >1:16 suggests hematogenous dissemination, especially if skin tests are negative. A positive CF titer in the cerebrospinal fluid is virtually diagnostic of meningitis.
Histoplasmosis	CF (whole yeast cells as antigen); CF (histoplasmin as antigen); ID (histoplasmin as antigen); LPA (histoplasmin as antigen)	Useful for antigen detection in urine serum CSF (see text); available in Indianapolis commercially	Histoplasmin (mycelial phase), histolyn CYL (yeast phase)	A positive histoplasmin skin test can artificially elevate CF antibody titers and produce a positive ID test ("m" band). Histolyn YCL is less likely to do this. An ID antibody "h" band suggests active infection. An LPA antibody titer ≥1:32 suggests active infection. A CF antibody titer ≥1:32 or a fourfold titer rise suggests active infection.

(continued)

COCCIDIOIDOMYCOSIS

Major Immunologic Features
- Inhaled arthroconidia have an antiphagocytic surface and are highly infectious.
- Spherules exceed the size of phagocytes and have an antiphagocytic surface.
- Endospores are released in packets that exceed the size of phagocytes.
- Mixed granulomas and suppuration occur.
- Primary infections may be signaled by erythema nodosum or erythema multiforme.

Table 50–4. Immunologic diagnosis of subcutaneous and systemic mycoses *(continued).*

Mycosis	Serologic Tests		Delayed-Hypersensitivity Skin Test[1]	Comments[2]
	Antibody	Antigen		
Paracoccidioi-domycosis	ID, CIE (simple, more specific); CF, EIA (sensitive; less specific)	None	Various "paraco-ccidioidins" (mycelial phase), investigational only	Elevated precipitin titers (transient) precede elevated CF titers (more persistent). The number and duration of precipitin bands are directly proportional to disease activity. The CF titer is directly proportional to the severity of illness. The skin test is commonly negative with active disease.
Opportunistic pathogens Cryptococco-sis	IFA, EIA, TA	Capsular polysaccharide (LPA, EIA)	"Cryptococcin" (investigational only)	Cryptococcal skin tests and tests for antibody lack sensitivity and specificity. The LPA for cryptococcal antigen is highly sensitive and specific. Rare (low-titer) cross-reactivity with *Trichosporon beigelii*. A positive cerebrospinal fluid test is diagnostic of cryptococcal meningitis.
Candidiasis	Multiple, diverse serologic tests (precipitins, agglutinins most common); CIE, IHA, IFA, RIA, ID, LPA	Mannan (LPA, EIA, RIA, coagglutination), enolase 48-kd cytoplasmic protein (LIA, EIA, DIA), undefined heat-labile glycoprotein antigen (LPA), D-arabinitol, D-mannose (GLC)	Oidiomycin	Skin tests lack diagnostic value (healthy persons are positive). Antibody tests lack sensitivity and specificity, especially in immuno-suppressed patients. Mannan antigen tests are positive in low titer, generally too late in the course of illness to be useful diagnostically. Heat-labile antigen lacks sensitivity and specificity in immunocompromised patients. Tests for mannose and arabinitol are not of proven diagnostic efficacy.
Aspergillosis	Multiple, diverse serologic tests (precipitins most common)	Galactomannan and related antigens (RIA, EIA)	"Aspergillin"	More than 90% of patients with ABPA have positive *Aspergillus* skin tests and precipitin titer elevation. More than 90% of patients with aspergilloma have precipitin titer elevation. Serologic tests for antibody lack sensitivity and are without value in patients with invasive aspergillosis. Galactomannan antigen is not of proven efficacy in diagnosis. Other antigen tests are experimental.
Mucormycosis (zygomycosis)	EIA, ID	None	None	Serologic tests for zygomycosis have been unsuccessful owing to poor antibody response to the antigens that have been tested. The disease moves with such rapidity that death may occur before characteristic antibody uses can be documented.

Abbreviations: BASWS = an alkali-soluble, water-soluble blastomycosis skin test preparation; BF = bentonite flocculation; CIE = counterimmunoelectrophoresis; CF = complement fixation; DIA = dot immunoassay; EIA = enzyme immunoassay; ID = immunodiffusion; IDCF = immunodiffusion with the CF antigen; = IDTP = immunodiffusion with the TP antigen; IFA = indirect immunofluorescence assay; IHA = indirect hemagglutination; GLC = gas–liquid chromatography; LIA = liposomal immunoassay; LPA = latex particle agglutination; PHA = passive hemagglutination; RIA = radioimmunoassay; TA = tube agglutination; TP = tube precipitin; YCA = whole yeast cell agglutination.

[1] Skin tests are predominantly of epidemiologic importance, defining loci of endemicity. A positive skin test indicates only that infection has occurred in the past. Some skin tests (especially histoplasmin) can influence serologic test results.

[2] In vitro correlates of CMI (eg, lymphocyte blastogenesis and migration inhibition) have been studied extensively, but are insufficiently standardized for routine diagnostic use.

- Negative skin test (coccidioidin, spherulin) and high complement fixation antibody titer suggest hematogenous dissemination.
- Disease is much more severe with defective CMI (including in AIDS).
- Infection confers solid immunity.

General Considerations

Coccidioidomycosis is an inhalation-acquired mycosis that can produce primary pulmonary infection, progressive pulmonary disease, or hematogenously disseminated disease involving predominantly skin, subcutaneous tissues, bones, joints, and meninges. It is caused by *Coccidioides immitis,* a fungus characterized uniquely by large spherules that rupture to release hundreds of endospores, which, in turn, mature to more spherules. The mycelial form of *C immitis* is a soil organism found in semidesert areas of the USA (eg, California, Arizona, and Texas), contiguous areas of Mexico, and scattered areas of Central and South America. Infection occurs by inhalation of arthroconidia in endemic areas (eg, by tourists, travelers, farmers, archeologists, or construction engineers).

Sporadic and, occasionally, common-source outbreaks occur (eg, dust storm in central California). Endemic areas are defined by skin test (coccidioidin, spherulin) reactivity. Susceptibility to hematogenous dissemination is greatest at the extremes of age. It is also positively correlated with male sex, race (blacks and Filipinos are the commonest victims), deficient CMI, and hormonal status (it occurs more often in the second and third trimesters of pregnancy than in the first). The growth of *C immitis* is stimulated by estrogen. There is a suspected HLA-related susceptibility to infection (HLA-A9).

Pathology

See Table 50–2.

Clinical Features

A. Signs and Symptoms: Primary exposure may be asymptomatic (60%) or associated with an influenza-like syndrome. In some patients (especially white women) there may be transient arthralgias, erythema nodosum, or erythema multiforme (also known as valley fever, and desert rheumatism). Similar immunologic phenomena have been observed with histoplasmosis and blastomycosis. Pneumonia, pleuritis, and pulmonary cavitation may occur; cavitary lung disease may be chronic or progressive. Hematogenous dissemination usually occurs in the absence of apparent pulmonary disease. Among the usual manifestations of metastatic infection are skin lesions, including nodules, ulcers, sinus tracts from deeper loci, and verrucous granulomas. Also involved are bones, joints, tendon sheaths, and meninges. Meningitis may be the sole apparent locus of metastasis. The gastrointestinal tract is rarely involved.

In patients with AIDS, disease is more acute and more severe. Manifestations of fungemia, including hematogenous (miliary) pneumonia, adult respiratory distress syndrome (ARDS), cellulitis, and papulopustular skin lesions in a hematogenous pattern, may dominate. Meningitis is commonly present.

B. Laboratory Findings: These include leukocytosis, eosinophilia (including cerebrospinal fluid), abnormal chest x-ray, and evidence of specific organ dysfunction at metastatic loci. Diagnosis is established by demonstrating endosporulating spherules on smears and histologic sections and by recovering the fungus in cultures.

C. Immunologic Diagnoses: See Table 50–4. Immunologic tests are useful in diagnosis and prognosis. Negative delayed-hypersensitivity skin tests and an elevated (or rising) complement fixation (CF) titer suggest hematogenous dissemination. An elevated CF titer in the cerebrospinal fluid is virtually diagnostic of coccidioidal meningitis, which is often culture-negative. An immunodiffusion test for complement fixing (IDCF) IgG antibody to *C immitis* correlates well with traditional CF tests and is commercially available for routine clinical use. Positive antibody tests are detected 2–6 weeks after onset of infection and parallel the extent of infection. Coccidioidin (and presumably spherulin) skin testing in a patient with active erythema nodosum may produce a violent, necrotic skin test reaction.

D. Differential Diagnosis: This includes diverse granulomatous infectious diseases (eg, mycoses, tuberculosis), sarcoidosis, and cancers.

E. Treatment: Amphotericin B is the drug of choice in immunocompromised patients acutely ill with hematogenous dissemination; it must be given intrathecally for meningitis. Ketoconazole, itraconazole, and fluconazole are useful for long-term maintenance therapy of nonmeningeal disease. Fluconazole and itraconazole have both been used successfully in patients with disseminated infection, including that of the central nervous system (CNS), but slow response and eventual relapse after discontinuation of azole therapy is common. Even in nonmeningeal disease, azole therapy must be continued for 6–12 months after resolution of infection. The poor efficacy of amphotericin B in managing meningeal disease has lead to the use of fluconazole, which offers the potential advantage of high cerebrospinal fluid (CSF) levels, or itraconazole in patients with CNS infection. Lifelong azole therapy for meningeal disease is usually required because relapses are very common.

F. Prevention: A spherule vaccine has failed to demonstrate effective protection.

G. Complications and Prognosis: Most patients recover spontaneously from primary infection. Erythema nodosum and erythema multiforme are considered particularly good prognostic signs. Some 2–4% of primary infections go on to progressive cavitary lung disease (poorly responsive to antifungal drugs; adjunctive surgery may be required) or hematogenously disseminated disease. Meningitis is fatal without therapy. AIDS-associated infections require lifelong suppressive therapy to prevent relapse.

HISTOPLASMOSIS

Major Immunologic Features
- It is a reticuloendothelial system disease in which tiny yeasts reside in macrophages.
- Granulomas with or without caseation are present.
- Cavitary lung disease may have a partial immunologic basis (subintimal arterial proliferation; pulmonary infarction).
- The disease is more severe in patients with defective CMI (including those with AIDS).
- Reactivation of latent infection may occur in patients with AIDS.
- Prominent calcification and fibrosis occur during healing.
- Immunity to reinfection occasionally wanes.

General Considerations
Histoplasmosis is an inhalation-acquired mycosis that can produce primary pulmonary infection, progressive pulmonary disease, or hematogenously disseminated disease involving predominantly the reticuloendothelial system, mucosal surfaces, and adrenal glands. It is caused by *Histoplasma capsulatum,* a tiny intracellular yeast. *H capsulatum* is a soil saprobe (mycelial form) that is found worldwide. In the USA it is particularly common in river valleys of the southeastern and central states. It grows particularly well in soil fertilized by bird droppings and bat guano, especially in caves. Infection occurs by inhalation of microconidia in areas where the infection is endemic, for example, by farmers, cave explorers, tourists, or construction workers. Sporadic and, occasionally, common-source outbreaks occur (eg, during construction in Indianapolis). Reactivation of latent infection is common in patients with advanced AIDS, so that patients living in nonendemic regions may develop active histoplasmosis from exposure to *H capsulatum* in an endemic area many years earlier. A positive delayed-hypersensitivity skin test is extremely common in endemic areas. Hematogenous dissemination is especially common at the extremes of age. Progressive pulmonary disease, strongly resembling tuberculosis, is especially common in white men with chronic obstructive pulmonary disease. There is no known genetic predisposition.

Pathology
See Table 50–2.

Clinical Features
A. Signs and Symptoms: Primary exposure may be asymptomatic or associated with a flu-like syndrome. Pneumonia, pleuritis, pulmonary cavitation and mediastinal adenopathy may occur. Except in infants, hematogenous dissemination usually occurs in the absence of apparent pulmonary disease. Favored sites of metastatic infection include the reticuloendothelial system (hepatosplenomegaly; lymphadenopathy; bone marrow involvement with anemia, leukopenia, and thrombocytopenia); mucous membranes (oronasopharyngeal ulcerations); gastrointestinal tract (malabsorption); and adrenals (adrenal insufficiency). An intense fibrotic response during healing may lead to fibrous mediastinitis. Calcification is common at healed loci ("buckshot" granulomas of the lungs; splenic calcifications). A presumed ocular histoplasmosis syndrome is described in persons in endemic regions, which may represent a hyperactive immunologic response to histoplasmin antigen or to delayed-hypersensitivity skin test reactions in general. In patients with AIDS, disease is more acute and may be fulminating, resembling bacterial septicemic shock. Manifestations include hematogenous (miliary) pneumonia, ARDS, disseminated intravascular coagulation (DIC), hematogenously distributed papulopustules, and meningitis.

B. Laboratory Findings: These include leukocytosis or leukopenia, thrombocytopenia, and anemia. There is evidence of specific organ dysfunction at metastatic loci. Diagnosis is established by the presence of intracellular yeasts on smears (eg, buffy coat smears in AIDS patients); histologic specimens (eg, mucosal biopsies); or cultures of sputum, blood, bone marrow, and liver biopsy material.

C. Immunologic Diagnoses: See Table 50–4. Serologic tests may be useful in assessing disease activity and, less frequently, in establishing the diagnosis. A positive histoplasmin skin test may spuriously elevate antibody titers detected serologically. The detection of polysaccharide antigen in urine, blood, or CSF may be especially helpful in diagnosis and in assessing the response to therapy. Histoplasma antigen is measured commercially by Wheat and colleagues in Indianapolis.

D. Differential Diagnosis: This includes diverse granulomatous infectious diseases (eg, mycoses, tuberculosis, leishmaniasis, and toxoplasmosis), sarcoidosis, Whipple's disease and other causes of malabsorption, and lymphohematogenous cancer. *Penicillium marneffei,* a dimorphic fungus with a yeast-like intracellular form, is an emerging pathogen in AIDS patients in Southeast Asia. The disease, penicilliosis, and the fungus, bear a superficial resemblance to histoplasmosis and its causative fungus.

E. Treatment: Amphotericin B is the drug of choice in treating immunocompromised patients acutely ill with hematogenous dissemination. Itraconazole is highly effective for nonmeningeal, non-life-threatening forms of the disease and has a superior side effect profile to that of ketoconazole. Fluconazole is less active than itraconazole, but at higher doses it may be used in patients intolerant of itraconazole. AIDS-associated infections require life-long suppressive therapy to prevent relapse.

F. Prevention: No vaccine is available.

G. Complications and Prognosis: Most primary infections resolve spontaneously. Progressive cavitary pulmonary disease is difficult to treat and may contribute to death from underlying pulmonary insufficiency. Hematogenous dissemination is generally fatal in the absence of therapy. Relapses are common in those with severe underlying immunodeficiency. Adrenal insufficiency may occur years after the original disease is quiescent.

PARACOCCIDIOIDOMYCOSIS

Major Immunologic Features

- Large, multiply budding yeasts may exceed the size of phagocytes.
- Mixed granulomas and suppuration occur.
- It may be more severe with defective CMI.

General Considerations

Paracoccidioidomycosis is an inhalation-acquired mycosis that can produce primary pulmonary infection or hematogenously disseminated disease involving predominantly the skin, mucous membranes, reticuloendothelial system, and adrenals. It is caused by *Paracoccidioides brasiliensis,* a large, spherical, uninucleate yeast with highly characteristic multiple buds attached by narrow necks (wagon-wheel appearance). The mycelial form of *P brasiliensis* is a soil saprobe that has only rarely been recovered from the environment in the area where it is endemic in tropical and subtropical forests of Latin America, particularly Brazil, Venezuela, and Colombia. Paracoccidioidomycosis is the most common systemic mycosis in South America. Infection occurs by inhalation of conidia and is most common among agricultural workers. The disease is sporadic. Skin test surveys suggest that men and women are equally susceptible. Men, however, are 12–48 times as likely to experience hematogenous dissemination as women, perhaps because physiologic concentrations of estrogen can prevent the conversion of conidia to invasive yeasts. In Brazilians, HLA-B40 antigen is more common in patients than in controls; in Colombians, HLA-A9 and -B13 are more common. Paracoccidioidomycosis is uncommon in AIDS patients.

Pathology

See Table 50–2.

Clinical Features

A. Signs and Symptoms: Primary exposure may be asymptomatic, or pneumonia, pleuritis, pulmonary cavitation, and mediastinal adenopathy may occur. Hematogenously disseminated disease occurs in two main forms: juvenile and adult. In the juvenile pattern (3–5% of cases), the primary pulmonary infection disseminates rapidly, with predominant reticuloendothelial system involvement. In the adult form (90% of cases), fungi, presumably aroused from latency, give rise to progressive localized lung disease, skin lesions, mucocutaneous lesions, reticuloendothelial system infection, and adrenal involvement. Oropharyngeal mucosal invasion is characteristic, with ulcerating lesions that involve most of the oral adventitia. Lesions are so painful that eating is difficult; tooth loss is common. Involvement of the gastrointestinal tract may lead to malabsorption; adrenal involvement can produce adrenal insufficiency.

B. Laboratory Findings: These include leukocytosis and evidence of specific organ dysfunction at metastatic loci. Diagnosis is established by demonstrating multiple-budding yeasts on smears or histologic sections and by recovering the fungi in culture.

C. Immunologic Diagnosis: See Table 50–4. Serologic tests are of use in monitoring the course of established disease.

D. Differential Diagnosis: This includes diverse granulomatous infectious diseases (eg, mycoses, tuberculosis, leishmaniasis, yaws, and syphilis), sarcoidosis, and cancer.

E. Treatment: Both ketoconazole and itraconazole are useful for the treatment of paracoccidioidomycosis. Itraconazole has become the drug of choice because of its improved side effect profile and shorter required duration of therapy. Sulfonamides have traditionally been used and offer a less expensive alternative.

F. Prevention: No vaccine is available.

G. Complications and Prognosis: Disseminated paracoccidioidomycosis is generally fatal in the absence of therapy. Disease that was originally acquired asymptomatically may present as disseminated infection years after the infected individual has emigrated from the area where the infection is endemic. Length of therapy is critical because relapses are common. Most patients require 1–2 years of therapy, which may be guided by serial serology.

SYSTEMIC INVASIVE MYCOSES: OPPORTUNISTIC PATHOGENS

CANDIDIASIS

Major Immunologic Features

- The source of the infection is usually the normal host flora.
- Intact mucosal barriers represent the major nonspecific host defense mechanism.
- Phagocytes ingest yeasts but attack pseudomycelia and mycelia by extracellular apposition.

- Neutropenia predisposes to hematogenous dissemination.
- Defective CMI predisposes to invasive mucosal disease.
- Thrush, esophagitis, and vaginitis are major presenting features of AIDS.
- Chronic mucocutaneous candidiasis is a specific syndrome in patients with defective immunoregulation.

General Considerations

Candidiasis is a general term for diseases produced by *Candida* species and encompasses colonization, superficial infection (eg, thrush, vaginitis, cystitis, and intertrigo), deep local invasion (eg, esophagitis), and hematogenous dissemination (eg, to the eyes, skin, kidneys, and brain). The species that most commonly cause candidiasis are *C albicans* (yeasts, pseudomycelia, and mycelia), *C tropicalis* (yeasts and pseudomycelia), and *C (torulopsis) glabrata* (yeasts only). *Candida* species are found in nature, but human infection usually arises from normal flora. *C albicans, C tropicalis,* and *C glabrata* are commonly found on mucous membranes (eg, vagina, and gastrointestinal tract) but rarely on the skin. Vaginal colonization is increased by diabetes mellitus, pregnancy, and the use of oral contraceptive agents. Carriage at all sites is increased by antibiotics. Hematogenous dissemination occurs most commonly in a setting of neutropenia or gastrointestinal mucosal disruption after repeated abdominal surgery. Neonates may be colonized or infected by passage through a colonized birth canal; premature infants in intensive care units are at particularly high risk of life-threatening *Candida* sepsis. Nosocomial transmission of candidal infection may occur with hand carriage, a common exogenous source of the organism. Vaginal colonization occurs after menarche. Disseminated infection occurs in both sexes and at all ages as a function of immunologic impairment. Chronic mucocutaneous candidiasis, characterized by extensive infection of skin, mucous membranes and nails, shows a familial tendency in about 20% of cases. In about 50% of cases there is associated endocrinopathy (eg, hypoparathyroidism, hypoadrenalism, hypothyroidism, or diabetes mellitus). The cause of this association is not known.

Pathology

See Table 50–2.

Clinical Features

A. Signs and Symptoms: Mucosal candidiasis is characterized by thrush, laryngitis, esophagitis, gastritis (especially in patients with drug-induced hypochlorhydria), vaginitis, cystitis, and intestinal candidiasis (the assumed source of hematogenous dissemination in most neutropenic patients). Vulvovaginitis is probably the most common overall manifestation of *Candida* infection. Chronic mycocutaneous candidiasis is manifested by persistent infection of skin, scalp, nails, and mucous membranes and is often accompanied by chronic dermatophyte infections. Associated findings include alopecia, depigmentation, cheilosis, blepharitis, keraconjunctivitis, corneal ulcers, and cutaneous horn formation. Hematogenously disseminated candidiasis can be either acute or chronic. The acute syndrome is characterized by involvement of the eyes (chorioretinitis), muscles (myalgias), skin (macronodular skin lesions), and kidneys (parenchymal destruction, papillary necrosis, and bezoar formation). Hematogenous (miliary) pulmonary infection is common, but *Candida* aspiration pneumonia is rare. Other manifestations include myocardial abscesses, meningitis, cerebral abscesses, and arthritis. Chronic disseminated candidiasis occurs most commonly in patients recovering from neutropenia who remain febrile despite broad-spectrum antibacterial therapy. Imaging studies reveal abscesses in the liver, spleen, lungs, and kidneys. The former designation of this syndrome as "hepatosplenic" candidiasis is not adequately descriptive and should be dropped.

B. Laboratory Findings: These include leukopenia or leukocytosis and evidence of specific organ dysfunction at metastatic loci. Diagnosis is established by direct histologic demonstration of fungal tissue invasion or recovery of fungi in culture from normally sterile areas (or both). Candidemia should be regarded as indicative of invasive infection in all but the most exceptional circumstances. Candiduria indicates cystitis more frequently than it indicates progressive renal infection.

C. Immunologic Diagnosis: See Table 50–4. Serologic tests are not helpful in neutropenic patients.

D. Differential Diagnosis: This includes diverse septicemic syndromes (eg, *Staphylococcus aureus* and *Pseudomonas aeruginosa* infections) and diverse opportunistic infectious diseases of neutropenic patients, including mycoses.

E. Treatment: Topical imidazoles are used for treating thrush and vaginitis, ketoconazole or fluconazole for vaginitis or progressive mucocutaneous infection, amphotericin B for deep local invasive infection or hematogenous dissemination, and amphotericin B plus flucytosine (depending on renal function) for managing disseminated infections that involve the eyes or central nervous system. Fluconazole may be useful as prolonged follow-up therapy for treating acute or chronic disseminated candidiasis. Fluconazole has been demonstrated to have similar efficacy in the treatment of candidemia in nonneutropenic patients, but amphotericin B remains the standard therapy for neutropenic patients and those with complicated infections. Candiduria can usually be cured by removal of a urinary catheter plus a short course of intravesicle amphotericin B or oral or intravenous fluconazole.

F. Prevention: Prophylactic administration of nystatin or ketoconazole to immunocompromised patients has not been clearly shown to prevent *Candida* infections. Prophylactic ketoconazole may actually predispose to infection by *C tropicalis, C glabrata,* or *Aspergillus* spp, which are not susceptible to ketoconazole. Similarly, prophylactic fluconazole may predispose to infections with *C krusei* or *C glabrata.* The use of fluconazole prophylaxis in patients undergoing bone marrow transplantation or induction chemotherapy for hematologic malignancy, however, has decreased the incidence of candidemia in many centers.

G. Complications and Prognosis: Chronic mucocutaneous candidiasis can be ameliorated but not cured by chronic ketoconazole therapy. *Candida* endocarditis is essentially incurable without valve replacement. Empirical amphotericin B therapy in febrile neutropenic patients has led to an improved prognosis for recovery in these patients, whose illness is otherwise extremely difficult to diagnose and who often die untreated. Reversal of neutropenia is the most important single predictor of recovery from infection.

CRYPTOCOCCOSIS

Major Immunologic Features

- Unencapsulated environmental yeasts acquire a capsule in the lungs.
- Encapsulated yeasts evade phagocytosis.
- Free capsular polysaccharide triggers suppressor cells, downregulating host defenses.
- Disease is much more common and severe in patients with defective CMI, particularly patients with AIDS.
- Detection of free capsular polysaccharide is extremely helpful in diagnosis.

General Considerations

Cryptococcosis is an inhalation-acquired mycosis that is initiated by symptomatic or asymptomatic pulmonary infection. In patients with altered CMI, dissemination to the meninges is common. Less common sites of hematogenous dissemination include skin, bones, eyes, and prostate. It is caused by *Cryptococcus neoformans,* an encapsulated yeast with four serotypes (A, B, C, and D) based on antigenic differences in the capsular polysaccharide. Virulence is linked to encapsulation and the capacity to synthesize melanin. Cryptococci are ubiquitous, and the disease occurs worldwide. Serotypes A and D are most commonly found in avian habitats (eg, in pigeon dung); serotypes B and C may be associated with eucalyptus trees. Serotype A causes most disease worldwide; serotype D is common only in Europe. Disease caused by serotypes B and C is found predominantly in subtropical areas (most commonly Australia but also including southern California). Serotypes A and D are the most common causes of cryptococcal infection in immunocompromised patients and are over-

whelmingly the most common serotypes recovered from patients with AIDS. Studies with poorly standardized "cryptococcin" skin tests suggest that asymptomatic infection may be common. Immunosuppression (including AIDS) causes the disease to emerge from apparent latency. Some 6–13% of AIDS patients develop a *C neoformans* infection. Cryptococcosis is more common in males, even excluding the current AIDS population. Infection is rare in children. The disease is sporadic. There is no known genetic predisposition. Most patients with infection have underlying immunosuppression.

Pathology

See Table 50–2.

Clinical Features

A. Signs and Symptoms: Cryptococcal infection commonly presents as isolated meningitis. Disease of the lungs is generally not apparent, even though this is the site of fungal entry. In patients who do present with pulmonary infection, however, meningeal involvement may be inapparent or absent. The most common manifestations of pulmonary cryptococcosis are solitary or multiple infiltrates or nodules. Cryptococcal meningitis is commonly a subtle or subacute process characterized by headache, impaired mentation, optic neuritis or papilledema, cranial nerve palsies, and seizures. Hydrocephalus may lead to progressive mental deterioration. In patients with AIDS, meningeal involvement may also be subtle, despite disproportionately huge numbers of fungi in the cerebrospinal fluid. In addition, manifestations of widespread hematogenous dissemination may also be present (eg, diffuse skin lesions, miliary pulmonary infiltrates, ARDS) and may lead rapidly to death. Other sites of hematogenous dissemination include the skin (particularly prominent in AIDS patients), bones, prostate, kidneys, and liver.

B. Laboratory Findings: Meningitis is usually low grade, with lymphocytosis and low sugar levels in cerebrospinal fluid. The diagnosis is usually established by cryptococcal antigen detection, India ink stains, and positive cultures of the cerebrospinal fluid. Organisms may also be cultured from blood, skin lesions, urine, and prostatic secretions.

C. Immunologic Diagnosis: See Table 50–4. Demonstration of cryptococcal antigen in cerebrospinal fluid or blood is extremely helpful in establishing the diagnosis. In AIDS patients, antigen titers are extremely high.

D. Differential Diagnosis: The differential diagnosis of pulmonary cryptococcosis includes diverse infections and cancers. Cryptococcal meningitis may be confused with diverse chronic hypoglycorrhachic syndromes, including tuberculosis or coccidioidomycosis. Symptoms may be erroneously attributed to a primary psychiatric disorder. In AIDS patients the differential diagnosis includes the gamut of opportunistic infections commonly encountered in this disorder.

E. Treatment: Because of its rapidity of action, amphotericin B, with or without flucytosine, should be used to initiate therapy. Fluconazole may be substituted once the infection has stabilized. AIDS-associated infection requires lifelong suppressive therapy to prevent relapse.

F. Prevention: The widespread use of fluconazole in patients with AIDS appears to have resulted in an overall decreased incidence of cryptococcal infections. Fluconazole prophylaxis significantly reduced the number of cryptococcal infections in a prospective clinical trial, but long-term prophylaxis is expensive and may lead to the emergence of fluconazole-resistant yeasts.

G. Complications and Prognosis: Patients with any alteration in mental status at the time of presentation are more likely to die than those with normal mentation. Elevated intracerebral pressures have been associated with increased morbidity and mortality associated with cryptococcal meningitis. Large-volume spinal taps and even pharmacologic measures (eg, steroids or acetazolamide) may be needed to reduce intracranial pressures. The likelihood of cure is inversely proportional to the severity of underlying immunosuppression. Although the cryptococcal antigen test is very helpful in establishing a diagnosis, the decrease in antigen titer may not be proportionate to the extent of clinical therapeutic response. Thus, disappearance of antigen from cerebrospinal fluid may not be a realistic therapeutic goal.

ASPERGILLOSIS

Major Immunologic Features

- Infection is caused by inhalation of conidia (common environmental contaminants).
- Conidia are ingested and killed by alveolar macrophages.
- Phagocytes attack mycelia by extracellular apposition.
- Neutropenia or neutrophil dysfunction predisposes to respiratory tract invasion, angioinvasion, and hematogenous dissemination.
- Balls of fungi may colonize previously damaged respiratory tissues (aspergilloma).
- Allergy may develop to inhaled conidia or to fungi colonizing the bronchial tree (atopic asthma, extrinsic allergic alveolitis, allergic bronchopulmonary aspergillosis).

General Considerations

Aspergillosis is a poorly descriptive term, which includes disease processes characterized by colonization, allergy, or tissue invasion. In addition, *Aspergillus* spp produce mycotoxins. Aflatoxin *(A flavus)* is linked epidemiologically to hepatocellular carcinoma; gliotoxin *(A fumigatus)* is toxic to macrophages and cytotoxic T cells. The focus of this section is on invasive aspergillosis. Allergic bronchopulmonary aspergillosis (ABPA) is discussed elsewhere (see Chapter 30). *Aspergillus* spp are among the most common environmental saprophytic fungi. Only a few thermotolerant species are pathogenic for humans, most notably *A fumigatus, A flavus, A terreus,* and *A niger. Aspergillus* infections occur worldwide. Outbreaks of invasive aspergillosis have followed exposure to conidia released by hospital construction, contaminated air-conditioning ducts and filters, and fireproofing materials above false ceilings. Invasive infection occurs in both sexes at all ages, as a function of immunologic impairment. There is no known genetic predisposition.

Pathology

See Table 50–2.

Clinical Features

A. Signs and Symptoms: Invasive pulmonary aspergillosis occurs characteristically in immunosuppressed, neutropenic patients. Widespread bronchial ulceration, parenchymal invasion, and angioinvasion lead to patchy necrotizing pneumonia, thrombosis, and infarction. Clinical features suggestive of invasive pulmonary aspergillosis include the development of pleuritic chest pain with hemoptysis in a febrile, neutropenic patient on broad-spectrum antibiotics. Widespread metastatic infection may occur. Infarcted lung tissue may contain necrotic sequestrae that resemble aspergillomas. A similar process may take place in the paranasal sinuses, resulting in a clinical picture identical to that of rhinocerebral mucormycosis (see the following section). An indolent, semi-invasive pulmonary infection occasionally occurs in immunocompetent patients with underlying chronic obstructive pulmonary disease. Ulcerative tracheobronchitis occurs in patients with AIDS and as a complication of lung transplantation. This syndrome is characterized by ulcerative endobronchial lesions that may only be diagnosed by bronchoscopy.

B. Laboratory Findings: These include neutropenia, abnormal chest or sinus x-rays, and evidence of specific organ dysfunction at metastatic loci. Diagnosis depends on histologic demonstration of tissue invasion by an exclusively mycelial fungus. Cultivation of *Aspergillus* spp from respiratory secretions may reflect only transient colonization, but in a high-risk patient (eg, febrile, neutropenic patient with pulmonary infiltrates) cultivation may be an important clue to the diagnosis of infection; blood cultures are rarely positive.

C. Immunologic Diagnosis: See Table 50–4. Serologic tests for antibody are not useful in diagnosis for invasive aspergillosis; antigen and polymerase chain reaction (PCR) tests are promising, but still experimental. Delayed-hypersensitivity skin tests and precipitin titers may be quite helpful in diagnosis of ABPA.

D. Differential Diagnosis: This includes diverse opportunistic pulmonary infections (bacterial and fungal), pulmonary infarction, diverse septicemic syndromes, and rhinocerebral mucormycosis.

E. Treatment: Amphotericin B is the only drug of proven therapeutic value for treating severely immunosuppressed patients. It must be used early and aggressively if the patient is to survive. Itraconazole may be useful for long-term follow-up therapy or in treating patients whose disease is not acutely life-threatening. Liposomal forms of amphotericin B reduce the toxicity of amphotericin therapy and allow higher doses of drug to be given, which may improve the outcome of some patients with this disease.

F. Prevention: Hospital rooms with enclosed filtered ventilation systems provide some degree of protection from environmental fungi.

G. Complications and Prognosis: Invasive aspergillosis is commonly fatal. An aggressive approach to diagnosis and treatment is essential. Surgical debulking of infected, infarcted tissues may be of particular value. Empirical amphotericin B therapy in febrile neutropenic patients who are not responding to broad-spectrum antibacterial agents is commonly used in an attempt to prevent this and other opportunistic mycoses. Reversal of neutropenia is the single most important predictor of recovery from this infection.

MUCORMYCOSIS (ZYGOMYCOSIS)

Major Immunologic Features

- Infection is caused by inhalation of spores.
- Spores are ingested and prevented from germinating by alveolar macrophages.
- Phagocytes attack mycelia by extracellular apposition.
- Acidotic states predispose to invasive paranasal sinus infection.
- Neutropenia predisposes to paranasal sinus, pulmonary, and disseminated infection.

General Considerations

Mucormycosis is a suppurative opportunistic mycosis that produces predominantly paranasal sinus (rhinocerebral) disease in patients with acidosis and rhinocerebral, pulmonary, or disseminated disease in patients with neutropenia. The most common etiologic agent is *Rhizopus arrhizus;* others include *Rhizomucor, Absidia, Cunninghamella, Mortierella, Saksenaea* spp and, rarely, *Mucor.* These are all common environmental contaminants. Colonization and infection are uncommon in healthy persons; mucormycosis is less common than invasive aspergillosis in immunocompromised patients. Infection occurs sporadically; clusters of infection occur sporadically but are rare. Wound infections may occur, and CNS infection may complicate intravenous drug abuse. Invasive infection occurs in both sexes and at all

ages as a function of acidosis or immunosuppression. There is no known genetic predisposition.

Pathology

See Table 50–2.

Clinical Features

A. Signs and Symptoms: These are virtually identical to those of invasive aspergillosis. Rhinocerebral mucormycosis accounts for about 50% of all cases of mucormycosis; more than 75% of cases occur in patients with acidosis, especially diabetic ketoacidosis. Increasing numbers of cases are being seen, however, in association with neutropenia and immunosuppression. Early clinical features include nasal stuffiness, bloody nasal discharge, facial swelling, and facial and orbital pain. Later manifestations include orbital cellulitis, proptosis, endophthalmitis, orbital apex syndrome, cranial nerve palsies, and cerebral extension.

B. Laboratory Findings: These include acidosis (principally diabetic ketoacidosis), neutropenia, abnormal paranasal sinus or chest x-rays, and evidence of specific organ dysfunction at sites of local extension (central nervous system) or metastatic loci. Diagnosis depends on histologic demonstration of tissue invasion by an exclusively mycelial fungus. Cultures are positive in fewer than 20% of patients, and even positive cultures may represent the presence of fungal contaminants.

C. Immunologic Diagnosis: See Table 50–4. There are no useful tests available.

D. Differential Diagnosis: This includes diverse opportunistic paranasal sinus infections (aspergillosis, phaeohyphomycosis, hyalohyphomycosis) and diverse opportunistic pulmonary bacterial and fungal infections.

E. Treatment: Amphotericin B is the only drug of proven value. Aggressive surgical debridement is required for paranasal sinusitis or rhinocerebral mucormycosis. Hyperbaric oxygen has been used for treating devitalized tissues, but its efficacy remains controversial.

F. Prevention: No effective preventive measures are known.

G. Complications and Prognosis: Rhinocerebral mucormycosis advances at an extremely rapid rate; an aggressive approach to diagnosis and treatment is essential. Survival is more likely in the setting of diabetic ketoacidosis than that of neutropenia.

PNEUMOCYSTOSIS

Pneumocystis carnii, the etiologic agent of pneumocystosis, has been considered a protozoan organism based on it morphologic appearance. Molecular evidence shows that it is not a protozoan and that it shares homology with fungi. Distinct differences between true fungi and *P carnii* exist, however (eg, lack of ergosterol in the cyst wall, distinct morphologic characteristics, lack of response to antifungal agents), suggesting that additional classification is needed.

Major Immunologic Features

- Infection is apparent only in patients with impaired CMI or in infants with severe protein-calorie malnutrition (marasmus).
- It is the most common index diagnosis for AIDS.
- Disease is predominantly alveolar and interstitial; extrapulmonary spread is distinctly rare.

General Considerations

Pneumocystis carinii pneumonia (PCP) is an apparently inhalation-acquired disease, but the environmental form of the pathogen has never been identified. PCP occurs predominantly in patients with impaired CMI and is classically the defining opportunistic infection for AIDS. *P carinii* is a unicellular eukaryote with a proposed life cycle consisting of trophozoites and cysts. It can be maintained transiently in cell culture but has never been cultivated independently in cell-free media. Seroepidemiologic studies indicate that more than two thirds of normal children have acquired antibody to *P carinii* by 3–4 years of age. Clinical attributes of the presumed infecting event are unknown, and autopsy studies have failed to provide evidence of residual pulmonary microorganisms in persons who have died of unrelated causes. The occurrence of PCP in immunocompromised adults could represent either new infection or arousal of inapparent disease from latency. When PCP occurs in infants with AIDS or marasmus, it is assumed to represent primary infection. Common-source outbreaks of PCP have occurred, suggesting that infection may be spread by aerosol. Most cases, however, appear to be sporadic. Diverse animal species harbor *P carinii,* as evidenced by spontaneous occurrence of PCP in response to immunosuppression. There is no evidence of spread from animals to humans; there are antigenic differences among human and animal strains. Prevalence is directly related to the occurrence of marasmus or impaired CMI. Neutropenia is not a risk factor. There is no independent age or sex-related susceptibility. Approximately 75% of AIDS patients experience at least one episode of *P carinii* pneumonia if no prophylaxis is given. There is no known genetic predisposition.

Pathology

See Table 50–2.

Clinical Features

A. Signs and Symptoms: These include fever, cough, and shortness of breath, especially in patients with prolonged fatigue and weight loss.

B. Laboratory Findings: These include CD4 T-cell counts of generally less than 200/mL; elevated nonspecific serum lactic dehydrogenase level; and diffuse alveolointerstitial infiltrates on chest x-ray, sometimes with cystic changes or pneumotoceles. Hypoxemia and alveolar-to-arterial O_2 tension differences are common, especially in response to exercise. Gallium lung scanning is sensitive but not specific. Diagnosis is established by visualizing characteristic organisms, in expectorated sputum, induced sputum, bronchoalveolar lavage specimens, or lung biopsy specimens obtained transbronchially or by open thoracotomy.

C. Immunologic Diagnosis: See Table 50–4. There are several experimental techniques for detecting an antibody response to *P carinii* or free *P carinii* antigen. These are not of current clinical value, however. An immunofluorescent antibody test using a monoclonal antibody specific for *P carinii* has enhanced recognition of the organism (over that by Giemsa and fast silver stains) in clinical specimens.

D. Differential Diagnosis: This includes the gamut of diseases caused by the opportunistic pulmonary pathogens in patients with AIDS or profoundly depressed CMI. Among these are tuberculosis, histoplasmosis, cryptococcosis, toxoplasmosis, cytomegalovirus infection, bacterial pneumonia, lymphomas, and Kaposi's sarcoma.

E. Treatment: Trimethoprim-sulfamethoxazole (TMP-SMZ) and intravenous pentamidine isethionate are both effective for the treatment of *P carinii;* however, TMP-SMZ is associated with fewer and less severe side effects, particularly in patients without AIDS. Other drugs shown to be effective include dapsone, TMP-dapsone, trimetrexate, clindamycin-primaquine, and atovagnone. Corticosteroids are useful in the prevention and treatment of *P carinii*-induced ARDS.

F. Prevention: *P carinii* prophylaxis is central to the clinical management of AIDS. A regimen of TMP-SMZ given daily or three days per week is highly effective. Aerosolized pentamidine administered once monthly is also effective. No vaccine is available.

G. Complications and Prognosis: Aggressive use of prophylaxis in AIDS patients is decreasing the frequency of PCP as an index diagnosis. Aerosolized pentamidine may delay or change the presentation of PCP to less easily recognized forms (eg, apical cystic disease and hematogenously disseminated disease, both of which are extremely rare at present). Pneumothorax is a late but important complication of PCP.

REFERENCES

GENERAL
Anaissie E et al: Focus on fungal infections: An update on diagnosis and treatment. *Clin Infect Dis* 1992;**14:**S-1.

Armstrong D: Treatment of opportunistic fungal infections. *Clin Infect Dis* 1993;**16:**1.

Beck-Sagué CM et al: Secular trends in the epidemiology of nosocomial fungal infections in the United States, 1980–1990. *J Infect Dis* 1993;**167:**1247.

Chandler FW, Watts, JC: *Pathologic Diagnosis of Fungal Infections.* ASCP Press, 1987.

Cox GM, Perfect JR: Fungal infections. *Curr Opin Infect Dis* 1993;**6:**422.

Cox RA: *Immunology of the Fungal Diseases.* CRC Press, 1989.

Gradon JD et al: Emergence of unusual opportunistic pathogens in AIDS: A review. *Clin Infect Dis* 1992;**15:**134.

Kwon-Chung KJ: Phylogenetic spectrum of fungi that are pathogenic to humans. *Clin Infect Dis* 1994;**19:**S1-7.

Kwon-Chung KJ, Bennett JE: *Medical Mycology.* Lea & Febiger, 1992.

Kaufman L, Reiss E: Serodiagnosis of fungal diseases. In: *Manual of Clinical Laboratory Immunology,* 4th ed. Rose NR et al (editors). American Society for Microbiology, 1992, p. 506.

SUPERFICIAL MYCOSES
Pityrosporum & Malassezia
Danker WM et al: *Malassezia* fungemia in neonates and adults: Complication of hyperalimentation. *Rev Infect Dis* 1987;**9:**743.

Marcon MJ, Powell DA: Human infections due to *Malassezia* spp. *Clin Microbiol Rev* 1992;**5:**101.

White Piedra; *Trichosporon beigelii*
Anaissie E et al: Azole therapy for trichosporonosis: Clinical evaluation of eight patients, experimental therapy for murine infection, and review. *Clin Infect Dis* 1992;**15:**781.

Walsh TJ: Trichosporonosis. *Infect Dis Clin North Am* 1989;**3:**43.

SUBCUTANEOUS MYCOSES
Dermatophytosis
Feingold DS: What the infectious disease subspecialist should know about dermatophytes. In: *Current Clinical Topics in Infectious Diseases.* Vol 8. Remington JS, Swartz MN (editors). McGraw-Hill, 1987, p. 154.

Chromomycosis
Fader RC, McGinnis MR: Infections caused by dematiaceous fungi: Chromoblastomycosis and phaeohyphomycosis. *Infect Dis Clin North Am* 1988;**2:**925.

Mycetoma
McGinnis MR, Fader R: Mycetoma: A contemporary concept. *Infect Dis Clin North Am* 1988;**2:**939.

Sporotrichosis
Penn CC et al: *Sporothrix schenckii* meningitis in a patient with AIDS. *Clin Infect Dis* 1992;**15:**741.

Winn RE: Sporotrichosis. *Infect Dis Clin North Am* 1988;**2:**899.

SYSTEMIC INVASIVE MYCOSES
Blastomycosis
Al-Doory Y, DiSalvo AF: *Blastomycosis.* Plenum, 1992.

Bradsher RW: Clinical considerations in blastomycosis. *Infect Dis Clin Pract* 1992;**1:**97.

Pappas PG et al: Blastomycosis in patients with the acquired immunodeficiency syndrome. *Ann Intern Med* 1992;**116:**847.

Coccidioidomycosis
Ampel NM et al: Coccidioidomycosis during human immunodeficiency virus infection: Results of a prospective study in a coccidioidal endemic area. *Am J Med* 1993;**94:**235.

Einstein HE, Johnson RH: Coccidioidomycosis: New aspects of epidemiology and therapy. *Clin Infect Dis* 1993;**16:**349.

Histoplasmosis
Dismukes WE et al: Itraconazole therapy for blastomycosis and histoplasmosis. *Am J Med* 1992;**93:**489.

Wheat LJ et al: Disseminated histoplasmosis in AIDS: Clinical findings, diagnosis and treatment, and review of the literature. *Medicine* 1990;**69:**361.

Wheat LJ et al: Effect of successful treatment with amphotericin B on *Histoplasma capsulatum* variety *capsulutum* polysaccharide antigen levels in patients with AIDS and histoplasmosis. *Am J Med* 1992;**92:**153.

Penicillium marneffei
Supparatpinyo K et al: *Penicillium marneffei* infection in patients infected with human immunodeficiency virus. *Clin Infect Dis* 1992;**14:**871.

Paracoccidioidomycosis
Brummer E et al: Paracoccidioidomycosis: An update. *Clin Microbiol Rev* 1993;**6:**89.

Candidiasis
Crislip MA, Edwards JE Jr: Candidiasis. *Infect Dis Clin North Am* 1989;**3:**103.

Rex JH et al: A randomized trial comparing fluconazole with amphotericin B for the treatment of candidemia in patients without neutropenia. *N Engl J Med* 1994;**331:**1325.

Walsh TJ et al: Detection of circulating *Candida* enolase by immunoassay in patients with cancer and invasive candidiasis. *N Engl J Med* 1991;**324:**1026.

Cryptococcosis
Chuck SL, Sande MA: Infections with *Cryptococcus neoformans* in the acquired immunodeficiency syndrome. *N Engl J Med* 1989;**321:**794.

Patterson TF, Andriole VT: Current concepts in cryptococcosis. *Eur J Clin Microbiol* 1989;**8:**457.

Powderly WG: Treatment of cryptococcal meningitis. *Infect Dis Clin Pract* 1992;**1:**164.

Saag MS et al: Comparison of amphotericin B with fluconazole in the treatment of acute AIDS-associated cryptococcal meningitis. *N Engl J Med* 1992;**326:**83.

White M et al: Cryptococcal meningitis: Outcome in patients with AIDS and patients with neoplastic disease. *J Infect Dis* 1992;**165:**960.

Aspergillosis

Denning DW, Stevens DA: Antifungal and surgical treatment of invasive aspergillosis: Review of 2,121 published cases. *Rev Infect Dis* 1990;**12:**1147.

Denning DW et al: NIAID mycoses study group multicenter trial of oral itraconazole therapy for invasive aspergillosis. *Am J Med* 1994;**97:**135.

Minamoto GY et al: Invasive aspergillosis in patients with AIDS. *Clin Infect Dis* 1992;**14:**66.

Patterson TF et al: The utility of antigen detection in the diagnosis of invasive aspergillosis. *J Infect Dis* 1995; **171:**1553.

Tang CM, Cohen J: Invasive aspergillosis: Diangosis, treatment, and prevention. *Infect Dis Clin Pract* 1992;**1:**217.

Mucormycosis (Zygomycosis)

Paparello SF et al: Hospital-acquired wound mucormycosis. *Clin Infect Dis* 1992;**14:**350.

Rinaldi MG: Zygomycosis. *Infect Dis Clin North Am* 1989;**3:**19.

Pneumocystosis

Edman JC et al: Ribosomal RNA sequence shows *Pneumocystis carinii* to be a member of the fungi. *Nature* 1988;**334:**519.

Huges WT: *Pneumocystis carinii* infection: An update. *Medicine* 1992;**71:**175.

Phaeohyphomycosis & Hyalohyphomycosis

McGinnis MR, Hilger AE: Infections caused by black fungi. *Arch Dermatol* 1987;**123:**1300.

Parasitic Diseases

51

James McKerrow, MD, PhD

Parasitic diseases such as malaria, schistosomiasis, and leishmaniasis are among the most prevalent and important health problems in developing countries. Not only is an understanding of the immunology of parasitic disease essential to control these diseases by immunization, but also the study of the host response to parasites continues to lead to important discoveries about the immune response itself. For example, the response to schistosome (blood fluke) eggs by infected mice represents one of the best experimental models for studying the formation and regulation of granulomatous inflammation. Immature schistosomes (schistosomula) and eggs have also provided an in vitro experimental model for elucidating the function of the eosinophil. New models of regulation of cytokine production and the role of cytokines in the immune response have come from studies of leishmaniasis, a protozoan parasite infection.

Immune responses to the complex antigenic structures of parasites have diverse manifestations and do not always lead to complete protective immunity. Unfortunately, as is often the case with infectious diseases, the immune response to parasites can even produce more serious disease than the parasite itself. Examples are the hepatic granulomas of schistosomiasis, antigen–antibody complex glomerulonephritis in quartan malaria, and antibody-mediated anaphylactic shock from a ruptured hydatid cyst or from too-rapid killing of filarial microfilariae by drugs.

Some of the most fascinating and perplexing aspects of parasitic disease are the variety of mechanisms by which the parasite evades the immune response (Fig 51–1). A parasite can "hide" within a host's own cells, as in leishmaniasis, produce successive waves of progeny with different surface antigens, as in African trypanosomiasis, or disguise itself as a host cell by incorporating host antigens, as occurs in schistosomiasis. Nonspecific immunosuppression, due to a variety of stimuli, is characteristic of a number of parasitic infections. The ability of parasites to adapt to the host environment is the essence of suc-

cessful parasitism, and it increases immeasurably the difficulty of developing immunization procedures against parasitic infection.

IMMUNE RESPONSE TO PROTOZOA

Protozoa are important agents of worldwide disease. Falciparum malaria, for example, is still considered one of the most lethal diseases in humans despite massive efforts at eradication and control. These parasites also offer unlimited immunologic challenges, the immune responses induced being as diverse as the protozoa themselves. In developing countries, especially in Africa, malaria and trypanosomiasis take enormous tolls of life and are significant barriers to economic development. Amebiasis, giardiasis, and toxoplasmosis are widespread even in highly developed countries. The use of immunosuppressive drugs to treat cancer and to prevent rejection of transplanted organs has resulted in activation of otherwise subclinical infections with protozoa such as *Toxoplasma* or has induced an overwhelming systemic infection with the nematode *Strongyloides stercoralis*. Finally, the global epidemic of acquired immune deficiency syndrome (AIDS) has led to exacerbation of preexisting parasitic infections as well as complicated multiple infections by protozoa such as *Cryptosporidium, Toxoplasma,* and Microsporidium.

MALARIA

Major Immunologic Features
- Complex partial humoral and cellular immunity occurs with multiple exposure.
- Nonimmune individuals in areas where malaria is endemic have significantly higher mortality rates from cerebral malaria.

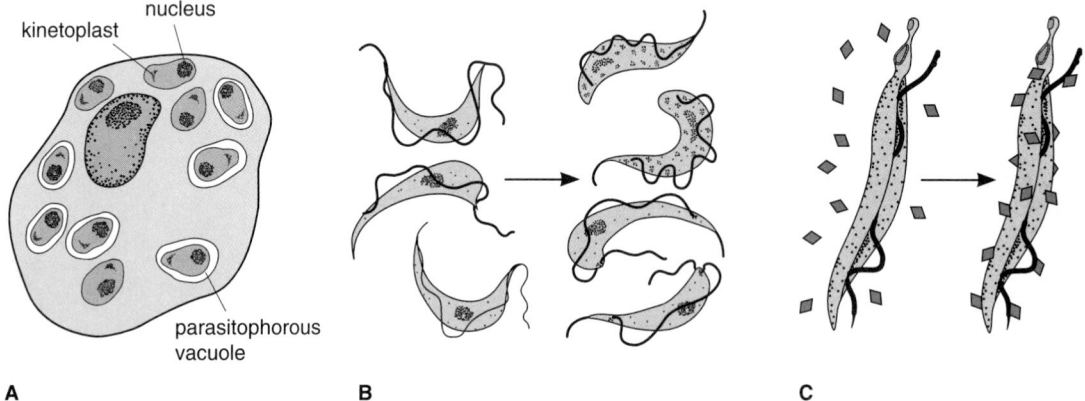

Figure 51–1. Some of the devious ways in which parasites evade the host immune response. **A:** Living within a host cell (*Leishmania* living in macrophage within a parasitophorous vacuole). **B:** Rapidly changing surface antigens (trypanosomes). **C:** "Camoflaging" surface with host antigens.

- Species-specific protective IgG antibody is produced against merozoites after multiple infections.
- Host variability in immune response to specific parasite antigens has hindered vaccine development.
- Parasites elude clearance in the spleen by expressing variant adhesion molecules on infected red blood cell surfaces (Fig 51–2).

General Considerations

Human malaria is caused by species of *Plasmodium*. It is transmitted by female anopheline mosquitoes that ingest the sexual forms of the parasite in blood meals. The infective sporozoites develop in the mosquito and are injected into the definitive (human) host when bitten by the insect. In the human, the parasites first develop as an exoerythrocytic form, the sporozoite, multiplying within hepatic cells without inducing an inflammatory reaction. The progeny, or merozoites, invade host erythrocytes to begin the erythrocytic cycle and initiate the earliest phase of clinical malaria. The gametocyte is the sexual stage taken up by the mosquito.

Destruction of erythrocytes occurs on a 48-hour cycle with *Plasmodium vivax* and *Plasmodium ovale* and every 72 hours with *Plasmodium malariae*. The characteristic chills-fever-sweat malarial syndrome follows this cyclic pattern, being induced by synchronous rupture of infected erythrocytes by the mature asexual forms (schizonts), releasing merozoites that quickly invade new erythrocytes. *Plasmodium falciparum,* although classically thought to occur on a 48-hour cycle, is, in fact, frequently not synchronous. In contrast to the exoerythrocytic stage, the erythrocytic merozoites induce an array of humoral responses in the host, as demonstrated by complement fixation, precipitation, agglutination, and fluorescent antibody reactions.

In *P vivax* and *P ovale* infections, relapse after a period of dormancy may result from periodic release of merozoites from the liver (hypnozoites), owing to the

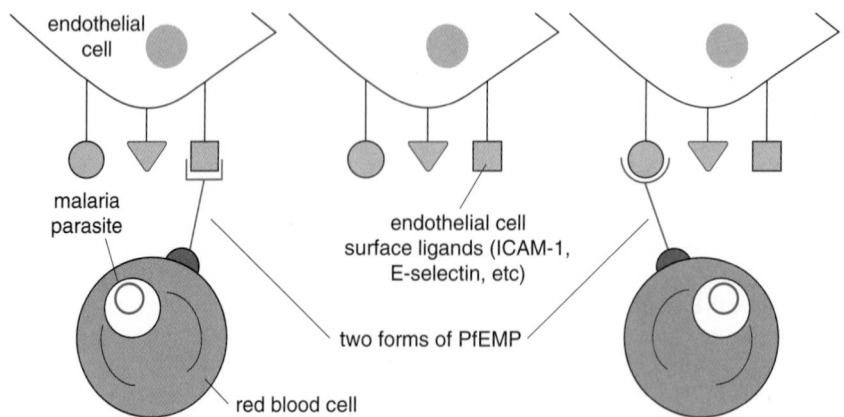

Figure 51–2. Expression of variant endothelial cell adhesion molecules by malaria-infested red blood cells. It shows two types of *P falciparum* erythrocyte membrane protein (PfEMP).

lack of an immune response to the intracellular parasites. When the erythrocytic cellular and humoral protection is deficient (from concurrent infection, age, trauma, or other debilitating factors), the reappearing blood stage forms induce a new round of clinical malaria until the erythrocytic cycle is again controlled by a humoral and T-cell host response. This is a true relapse, as opposed to a recrudescence of erythrocytic infection. Relapses can occur for up to 5 years with some strains of *P vivax* and possibly 2–3 years for *P ovale. P malariae* appears to recur only as a recrudescent erythrocytic infection, sometimes appearing 30 or more years after the primary infection. *P falciparum* may have a short-term recrudescence but does not develop a true relapse from liver-developed merozoites.

Blackwater fever, formerly a common and rapidly fatal form of falciparum malaria among European colonists in Africa, has declined in frequency with reduction in quinine therapy. It is associated with repeated falciparum infection, inadequate quinine therapy, and possibly genetic factors more frequently found in white persons. The resulting rapid, massive hemolysis of both infected and uninfected erythrocytes is thought to result from autoantibodies from previous infections that react with autoantigens (perhaps an erythrocyte–parasite–quinine combination) derived from a new infection with the same falciparum strain. With increased use of quinine to prevent or treat chloroquine-resistant falciparum malaria, blackwater fever may again increase in frequency.

Quartan malaria, caused by *P malariae,* has been associated with a serious complement-dependent immune complex glomerulonephritis and nephrosis in African children, resulting in edema and severe kidney damage unless the disease is arrested early. After resolution of the edema, persistent symptomless proteinuria or slowly deteriorating renal function is common. Stable remissions with corticosteroid therapy occur when proteinuria is restricted to only a few classes of protein and histologic changes are minimal. Patients with poorly controlled generalized proteinuria, however, probably do not benefit from antimalarial or immunosuppressive therapy. Chronic *P malariae* infection probably triggers autoimmunity, perpetuating the immune complex glomerulonephritis, but the antigen involved is not yet identified.

Innate, nonacquired immunity to malaria is well demonstrated. Africans or African Americans lacking Duffy blood group antigen Fy(a–b–) are immune to *P vivax,* as the Duffy surface protein is necessary for successful merozoite penetration of the human erythrocyte by this plasmodial species. Intracellular growth of the malaria parasites is also affected by the molecular structure of hemoglobin. Sickle cell (SS) hemoglobin inhibits growth of *P falciparum.* The sickle cell gene is widespread in areas of Africa, hyperendemic for falciparum malaria. Although the prevalence of infection appears unaffected by the sickling trait, *severe* infections in individuals with hemoglobin A/S (sickle cell trait) are very much reduced compared with those in nonsickling homozygous individuals. Similarly, *P falciparum* growth is retarded in erythrocytes with the fetal hemoglobin (F)—hence the selective advantage of β-thalassemia heterozygotes, in whom postnatal hemoglobin F declines at a lower than normal rate. Other red cell abnormalities such as glucose-6-phosphate dehydrogenase deficiency appear to be protective of the erythrocyte and thereby reduce the severity of plasmodial infection.

Immunity to *P falciparum* malaria is species- and strain-specific. If immune individuals migrate to other, geographically distinct areas of endemicity, they may acquire new disease. Both acquired and innate specific or nonspecific resistance to malaria are influenced by a number of genetic traits that reflect strong selective pressure in areas with specific mosquito–human–*Plasmodium* combinations. A very gradual long-term resistance to hyperendemic falciparum malaria is acquired in African populations. The resistance develops years after the onset of disease among nearly all children over 3 months of age. Initial passive protection is present owing to transplacental maternal IgG. Nonetheless, there are estimates of a million malaria deaths a year in Africa, chiefly among children under 5 years of age. Even after surviving a childhood infection, a large proportion of adults remain susceptible to infection and show periodic parasitemia, while their serum contains antiplasmodial antibodies, some with demonstrated protective action. Susceptibility to a low-level chronic infection provides the population with a protective **premunition** or prevention of subsequent infection. It is believed that in areas of Africa, where malaria is hyperendemic, nearly all residents harbor throughout their lives a continuous series of falciparum infections of low to moderate pathogenicity. Antibodies are produced that inhibit the entry of merozoites into erythrocytes. All immunoglobulin classes are elevated in the serum of malaria patients, but IgG levels appear to correlate best with the degree of malaria protection (or control of acute manifestations).

Despite evidence for human immunity, the malaria parasite has been very successful. The World Health Organization estimates over 200 million people are infected worldwide, resulting in 1–2 million deaths annually. How does the parasite manage to elude clearance by the host? First, like several other protozoan parasites, it hides within host cells. Very shortly after injection into the bloodstream by the mosquito, the sporozoite form enters and replicates inside of the liver cells. During the erythrocytic cycle, most of the parasite's metabolism is carried out within host red blood cells. A second problem the parasite faces, however, is the mechanism for clearing abnormal red blood cells in the host spleen. To circumvent this problem, the parasite expresses a group of surface proteins whose function has been most extensively studied in the *Plasmodium falciparum* species. They are collectively known as PfEMP-1 (*P falciparum*-infected erythrocyte membrane protein 1). Rather than being expressed on the surface of the parasite, these proteins are synthesized by the parasite but transported and expressed on the surface of the infected erythrocytes. Here they mediate interaction between erythrocytes and endothelial cell adhesion molecules, such as ICAM-1, E-selectin, and VCAM-1. This allows parasite-infected red blood cells to stick to endothelial cells and not circulate into the spleen where they would be recognized and destroyed. This parasite mechanism mimics the adhesion of leukocytes during host inflammatory reactions. Leukocyte surface molecules are bound by the same endothelial cell adhesion molecules that the parasite is exploiting. The parasite, in essence, has made an erythrocyte act like a leukocyte.

Although avoiding clearance in the spleen, the expression of a parasite protein on the surface of the erythrocyte presents a second problem for the parasite. The host's immune response can now recognize a foreign protein on the infected cell. In fact, a distinctive structure called the "knob" forms on the surface of the infected erythrocytes in the region where the PfEMP-1 protein is immunolocalized. To circumvent this problem, the parasite can synthesize a repertoire of PfEMP-1 proteins from a gene cluster known as the "var" genes. This theme of antigenic variation is similar to that of the African trypanosome, but the mechanism by which different members of the gene family are expressed by different clones of parasites is presently unknown. Nevertheless, it is clear that different members of the PfEMP-1 family can bind to different endothelial cell adhesion molecules.

In addition to the variables of parasite genetics, it is clear that there is significant variability within human populations in the ability to mount an immune response to the malaria parasite. This has somewhat dampened the optimism for early development of a subunit vaccine against malaria. Preliminary clinical trials of the first vaccine candidate were disappointing, raising fears that subunit vaccines would be poorly immunogenic in many individuals of a target population. Genetic variability in induction of immune response by a vaccine is by no means a new observation. Even in a very effective recombinant vaccine such as that against hepatitis B, one finds a bell-shaped curve of response, with some individuals failing to produce sufficient levels of antibodies in the standard vaccination protocol. The situation in malaria is even more complex, and variation in response is seen in inbred strains of mice as well as in "outbred" human populations. In mice, the variability in immune response is linked to variability in the major histocompatibility complex (MHC). Is it apparent, however, that immune response to malaria in humans is probably also regulated by genes outside the MHC region that have yet to be defined.

The failure to induce protective antibodies in vaccinated individuals led research investigators to focus on the role of cell-mediated immunity, and especially T-cell-derived cytokines, already known to be important in control of other parasitic diseases. One striking observation was that in areas where there is a high proportion of both malaria and human immunodeficiency virus (HIV), no significant effect of HIV infection on the course of malaria or, for that matter, of malaria on the course of HIV infection has been noted. This occurred even when individuals with low T-cell counts and malaria infections were studied. Humoral immunity may indeed be important in control of malaria, or other types of T cells, for example γd T cells, generate cytokines that can control malaria and are not affected in HIV infection.

TOXOPLASMOSIS

Major Immunologic Features
- Specific antibody is present.
- There is a nonspecific increase in serum immunoglobulins.
- Natural acquired immunity is widespread; cell-mediated immunity is probably the major mechanism.
- Disseminated toxoplasmosis is a frequent complication in HIV-infected individuals with low T-cell counts.

General Considerations
Toxoplasma infection in humans is generally asymptomatic; it has been estimated that as much as 40% of the adult population worldwide is infected, as well as all species of mammals that have been tested for the presence of this ubiquitous parasite. Clinical disease, which develops in only a small fraction of those infected, ranges from benign lymphadenopathy to an acute and often fatal infection of the central nervous system. The developing fetus and the aged or otherwise immunologically compromised host are most vulnerable to the pathologic expression of massive infection and resulting encystation in the eye or brain. Damage to the fetus is greatest during the first trimester, when the central nervous system is being organized, and nearly all such instances end in fetal death. Infection of the mother during the second trimester may produce hydrocephaly, blindness, or various lesser degrees of neurologic damage in the fetus. Most cases of fetal infection occur during the third trimester, resulting in chorioretinitis or other ophthalmic damage, reduced learning capacity or other expressions of central nervous system deficit, or asymptomatic latent infection that may become clinically apparent years later. Women exposed *before* pregnancy are thought to be unable to transmit the infection in utero.

In most cases, the diagnosis of toxoplasmosis is made by serology. Positive tests for IgM appears approximately 5 days after infection, and IgG approximately 1–2 weeks after. Because an IgG reaction may persist for months to years, IgM is diagnostically more useful, since a single high titer is indicative of acute infection. For confirmation, two specimens are generally drawn at a 3-week interval and tested simultaneously. A serial rise in titer is a reliable indication of recent infection.

In ocular toxoplasmosis, no rise in titer is observed, but a negative serologic test can be used to rule out chorioretinitis. The IgM serologic test can also be used during pregnancy and on cord blood, but serologic positivity may be suppressed by immunosuppressive therapy or acquired immunodeficiency syndrome (AIDS).

Many potential sources of infection have been suggested, including tissue cysts in raw or partially cooked pork or mutton and oocysts passed in feces of infected cats (the true final hosts). These sources seem insufficient to account for such large numbers of infections, however. The major reservoirs of infection are therefore unknown. *Toxoplasma* infection usually occurs through the gastrointestinal tract, and the protozoa can apparently penetrate and proliferate (as rapidly multiplying tachyzoites) in virtually every cell in the body. They ultimately produce cysts filled with minute slow-growing infective bodies (bradyzoites) that remain viable for long periods. Following successful cellular and humoral immune response, only encysted parasites can survive.

The tachyzoites of *Toxoplasma* and the promastigotes of *Leishmania* (discussed in the next section) are two examples of parasite protozoa that replicate inside human macrophages. *Toxoplasma* invades a cell in a process that is independent of normal phagocytosis. The tachyzoite attaches to the cell membrane and induces changes in membrane topology as well as secretion from the specialized parasite structures called rhoptries. The parasite enters the cell through a moving membrane junction and forms a parasitophilus vacuole in the cytoplasm. This vacuole is a specialized structure that is probably the result of rhoptry secretions and which contains no recognizable host membrane proteins. The "parasite nature" of the vacuole prevents it from becoming acidified or fusing with host cell lysosomes. Before invasion, parasites become coated with extracellular matrix protein such as laminin, which, by interacting with host cell integrins (cell surface receptors), inhibit phagocytosis and the oxidative burst of macrophages that could result in parasite killing.

The ability of macrophages to kill intracellular parasites is greatly increased if the parasites are first exposed to antibody. In that case, the antibody-coated *Toxoplasma* is recognized by the Fc receptors of the macrophage. This triggers normal phagocytosis and the formation of reactive oxygen and nitrogen intermediates that ultimately kill the parasite.

An intact immune system is necessary for protection against *Toxoplasma;* thus, immunosuppression to control transplant rejection or malignancies, or infection with HIV, may result in active toxoplasmosis. This phenomenon may result either from the elimination of sensitized lymphocytes previously limiting an apparent infection or from inability of the immunosuppressed host to mount an adequate protective response to new infection.

LEISHMANIASIS

Leishmania is a genus of obligate intracellular parasites that infect macrophages of the skin and viscera to produce disease in both animals and humans. Sandflies, the principal vectors, introduce the parasites into the host while taking blood meals. In leishmaniasis, a range of host responses interact with a number of parasite leishmanial species and strains to produce a panoply of pathologic and immunologic responses. Leishmaniasis represents two important lessons: (1) how different species or strains of the same parasite can produce drastically different diseases in a given host, and (2) how genetic differences in the host can also lead to vastly different immune responses to infection by the same parasite.

1. CUTANEOUS LEISHMANIASIS

Major Immunologic Features
■ Cell-mediated immunity is a critical factor.
■ There is little or no specific serum antibody.

General Considerations
Old World cutaneous leishmaniasis, or tropical sore, is caused by several species of *Leishmania: L tropica, L major,* and *L aethiopica.* These agents induce an immune response characterized by nonprotective antibody but strong cell-mediated immunity. In cutaneous leishmaniasis, it is chiefly the patient's immune response to the infection that determines the form taken by the clinical disease; however, the strain of parasite may also determine part of the host response. If the human host mounts an adequate but not excessive cell-mediated immune response to the parasite, healing of the ulcerative lesions and specific protection result. If cell-mediated immunity to the parasite is inadequate or suppressed, however, the result may be diffuse cutaneous disease, in which there is little chance of spontaneous cure. In the Old World, this condition is due chiefly to *L aethiopica* in East Africa. A similar form, caused by *L mexicana* subsp *pifanoi,* occurs in Venezuela, again in specifically anergic patients. On the other hand, an excessive cell-mediated immune response produces lupoid or recidiva leishmaniasis, caused by *L tropica,* in which nonulcerated lymphoid nodules form at the edge of the primary lesion; these lesions persist indefinitely, although parasites are not easily demonstrated. Recidiva leishmaniasis may occur from 2 to 10 years

after the initial lesion. Thus, a spectrum of host responses to cutaneous leishmaniasis exists, ranging from multiple disseminated parasite-filled ulcers or nodules (anergic response) to single, spontaneously cured immunizing sores, to recidiva hyperactive host responses with few or no parasites (allergic response).

Cutaneous leishmaniasis of the New World is caused by a number of leishmanial pathogens now divided into two species complexes: *L mexicana* (subdivided into four or more subspecies) and *L braziliensis* (subdivided into four or more subspecies). The parasite subspecies (considered distinct species by many specialists) are distinguished on the basis of growth characteristics in the vector and in culture, isoenzyme electrophoresis patterns, kinetoplast DNA analysis, lectin-binding specifities, excreted factor serotyping, and monoclonal antibody probes. Geographic factors, hosts, and the character of the disease produced in humans are also important.

The most significant clinical distinction in the *L mexicana* complex is the high frequency of ear cartilage lesions (chiclero ulcer) and rare diffuse cutaneous leishmaniasis. In the *L braziliensis* complex, metastatic lesions develop, usually within 5 years of healing of the initial ulcer, which itself may be large, persistent, and disfiguring. Nasal cartilage and other nasopharyngeal tissues are attacked and destroyed by the subsequent massive ulceration (espundia), which may erode away much of the face and cause death by septic bronchopneumonia, asphyxiation, or starvation. This manifestation of American leishmaniasis is frequently nonresponsive to treatment. Parasites are abundant in the early stages of espundia but subsequently are rare, whereas persistent infiltration of giant cells, plasma cells, and lymphocytes is characteristic. Delayed and perhaps immediate hypersensitivity and circulating antibody levels are higher in espundia than in cases of the primary lesion alone. The mucocutaneous form is thought to be an allergic or abnormal immunologic manifestation of infection with the type subspecies *L braziliensis.*

A skin test (Montenegro test) is rapidly positive with cutaneous leishmaniasis, particularly the New World forms. Assays for lymphocyte proliferation or production of cytokines such as interferon gamma are also positive. Dermal response to kala-azar is slower, becoming positive only after cure of the visceral infection. Serodiagnosis of cutaneous leishmaniasis is still unsatisfactory because of low serum antibody levels and, in Latin America, because of cross-reactions with Chagas' disease antibodies. An important advance in field analysis of species (*L mexicana* versus *L braziliensis* complexes) has been the application of nonradioactive species-specific DNA probes. Using the polymerase chain reaction (PCR), the *Leishmania* species infecting a patient can be determined from a small amount of parasite material in a cutaneous lesion.

The varying clinical courses that infection with *Leishmania* species can produce constitute a paradigm for the immune response to intracellular parasites. *Leishmania* parasites enter cells by a different pathway from that used by *Toxoplasma* organisms discussed previously. *Leishmania* promastigotes enter passively through phagocytosis into macrophages. One of the unusual features of this infection is the predilection of the organisms for infection of the macrophage, a cell that is itself key to the host immune response. *Leishmania* have adapted to replication in an unusual environment, the phagolysosomal vacuoles. Nevertheless, in cases of spontaneous cure of cutaneous leishmaniasis, parasite killing does occur. Studies of a mouse model of infection helped to shed light on this interplay between host and intracellular parasite. First, a single dominant genetic locus, called *Bcg,* appears to govern whether mice are resistant to infection by *Leishmania* as well as *Mycobacterium.* This locus includes a gene that codes for a membrane channel protein that may be key in the transport of precursors of nitric oxide or oxygen radicals used by the macrophage for parasite killing. It is noteworthy that lessons from studying the immune response to intracellular parasites can cross-fertilize research on host response to mycobacteria and other fungal or bacterial infections in which macrophages play a key role. T-cell products are also key to a successful host response to *Leishmania.* Interferon gamma is critical to parasite killing. In *L major* infections of mice, two CD4 T-cell subtypes have been identified (Fig 51–3). In genetically resistant mice, the T_H1 subtype predominates. This is a T-cell population that produces interferon gamma in its cytokine repertoire. In contrast, genetically susceptible mice have a predominant T_H2 T-cell subtype response with no production of interferon gamma but IL-5, IL-4, and IL-10 instead. Although the existence of distinct T-cell subtypes in human infections is more controversial, the mouse studies point out how a particular cytokine profile is key to activating infected macrophages to successfully kill the intracellular parasites. This work has had practical application administration of recombinant interferon gamma enhances patient response to chemotherapy in cases of visceral leishmaniasis.

2. VISCERAL LEISHMANIASIS

Major Immunologic Features

- Delayed hypersensitivity occurs only after spontaneous recovery or chemotherapy.
- Increased nonspecific immunoglobulin levels.
- Causes polyclonal B-cell hypergammaglobulinemia.
- Parasites in cells throughout the body produce systemic disease, characterized by leukopenia and splenomegaly and release of TNFα.

General Considerations

The immune response to visceral leishmaniasis (kala-azar)—caused by various subspecies of *L dono-*

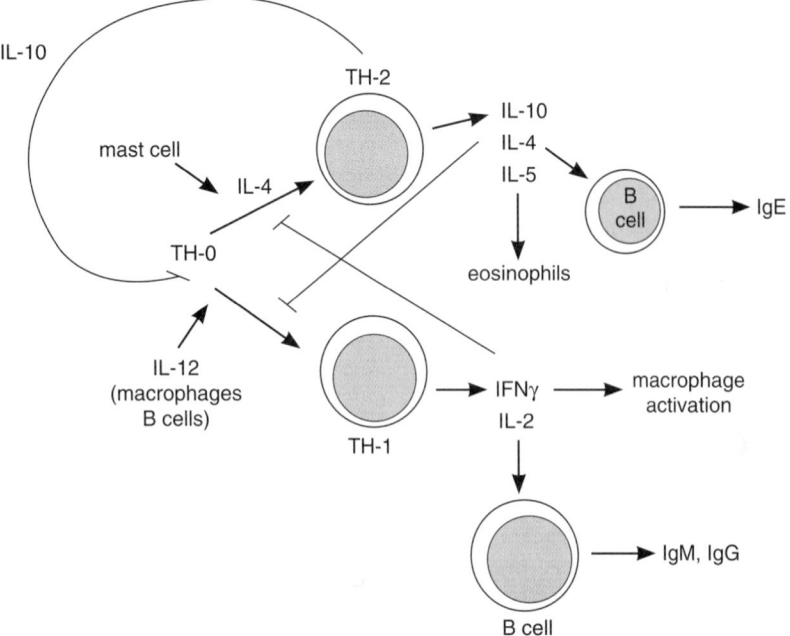

Figure 51–3. Cytokine production by T_H1 and T_H2 subtypes of CD4 T cells.

vani (considered separate species by some authors)— is significantly different from that of cutaneous leishmaniasis, although the parasites are distinguishable only by enzyme analysis with zymodemes or other forms of molecular characterization. Massive polyclonal hypergammaglobulinemia with little or no evidence of cell-mediated immunity is the rule in visceral leishmaniasis. There is no quantitative relationship between the elevated serum immunoglobulin levels and antiparasite antibodies, which are, moreover, not species-specific. The immunoglobulin level diminishes rapidly when treatment begins. Delayed cutaneous hypersensitivity to parasite antigens becomes demonstrable only after spontaneous recovery or treatment, which suggests that cell-mediated mechanisms play a role in the resolution of the infectious process. Under certain circumstances, postkala-azar dermal "leishmanoid" occurs. Nodules containing many parasites form papules as a result of incomplete or defective cell-mediated immunity or a persistent allergic reaction to parasite antigens. Many cases of severe disseminated infection in HIV-infected individuals have now been reported in Mediterranean countries. This underscores the importance of cell-mediated immunity in controlling disease.

AFRICAN TRYPANOSOMIASIS

Major Immunologic Features

■ There is a succession of parasite populations in the bloodstream, each with a different antigenic coating.

General Considerations

Trypanosoma brucei subsp *gambiense,* also called *T gambiense,* is the agent of chronic Gambian, or West African, sleeping sickness. *Trypanosoma brucei* subsp *rhodesiense,* also called *T rhodesiense,* is the agent of acute Rhodesian, or East African, sleeping sickness. Both cause human disease, and the Rhodesian form is the one most responsible for denying vast areas of Africa to human occupation, chiefly in the flybelt regions where the tsetse fly vectors are found. Tsetse-borne trypanosomes (*T brucei* subsp *brucei* as well as several other species) infect domestic animals with similar or even greater virulence. The effect of this dual threat—one to humans and the other to domestic animals, especially cattle—has had an enormous influence on human history in Africa. The great herd of wild herbivores, once abundant everywhere, have survived in this region because of their natural tolerance to heavy infections. The trypanosomes multiply extracellularly in successive waves in the human and animal bloodstream but produce very little disease in spite of their numbers. Only when the parasites enter the central nervous system does the ravaging disease sleeping sickness develop. It is this pathologic phase of an otherwise harmless chronic or recurrent infection to which humans and domestic animals succumb and which most native antelope and other herbivores resist.

Greatly increased levels of immunoglobulins, especially of the IgM class, are regularly present in infected humans and animals. The increased immunoglobulin levels, which do not correlate positively with protection, may result from B-cell stimulants produced by the trypanosomes themselves or by the increased IgG production by helper T cells, which act nonspecifically to increase immunoglobulin levels. A large proportion of the immunoglobulin in infected hosts is nonspecific in nature.

Although trypanosomes are continually exposed to the host immune system in the bloodstream, they evade the host defenses. The first hint of how this is accomplished was noted in 1910, when the periodicity of fever in patients with trypanosomiasis was correlated with a sharp rise and fall in the number of trypanosomes found in the blood. More recently, it was discovered that when individual organisms are cloned in culture, each clone displays a unique antigenic surface protein. When organisms first enter the host (Fig 51–4), the host immune system generates antibodies against the predominate surface antigen (called a variable surface glycoprotein [VSG]). Antibodies can kill over 90% of the original infecting trypanosome population. The reason why not all of the trypanosomes are killed is that some have switched on a different VSG antigen not recognized by the initial immune response. This switch occurs spontaneously and can be detected in immune-deficient mice. It is therefore not dependent on the host immune response. The switch is very rapid, so that by 5 days into an infection, parasites with more than one antigen type can be detected. By 6 days, as few as 15% of the trypanosomes may still have the initial surface VSG. This switching from one VSG to another explains the waves of parasitemia and periodicity of the fever characteristic of trypanosomiasis. The potential VSG repertoire is not known, although parasites derived from a single parent trypanosome have been found with more than 100 distinct VSGs.

What is the mechanism by which the trypanosome switches its surface coat? Some steps in the process are clear. One copy of the VSG gene is located on a specific chromosome (Fig 51–5). If that VSG is to be expressed, a copy of the gene is made and translocated to another chromosome close to the telomere. In this new location, and only in the new location, it is transcribed into a precursor messenger RNA, which is processed by transsplicing of a 35-nucleotide sequence that was itself transcribed from yet another genomic site. There are as many as 1000 VSG genes to choose from, and the repertoire can be expanded in chronic infection by point mutations or partial gene replacements. Some of the VSGs are derived from genes that are already near the telomere and do not translocate before expression. Although some steps in the mechanism of "gene jumping" and subsequent expression have been elucidated, the entire mechanism by which one VSG is switched to another is still unclear. Understanding of this switching mechanism might provide a means of interrupting the ability of trypanosomes to change their antigenic disguises.

Specific antibodies to trypanosomes can either lyse the parasites or clump them. Clumping allows for more efficient removal of the parasites by the reticuloendothelial system. It is controversial whether humans or domestic animals living in areas where the infection is endemic develop resistance to infection, although epidemiologic observations suggest that resistance does arise. The fact that there are healthy human carriers of *T rhodesiense*—which usually pro-

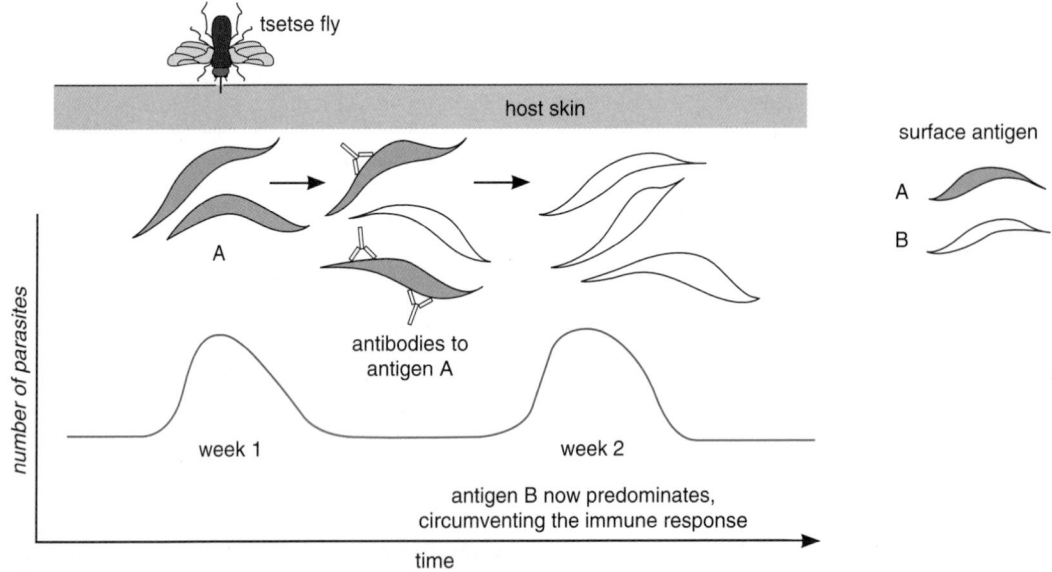

Figure 51–4. Antigenic variation and parasitemia in trypanosomiasis.

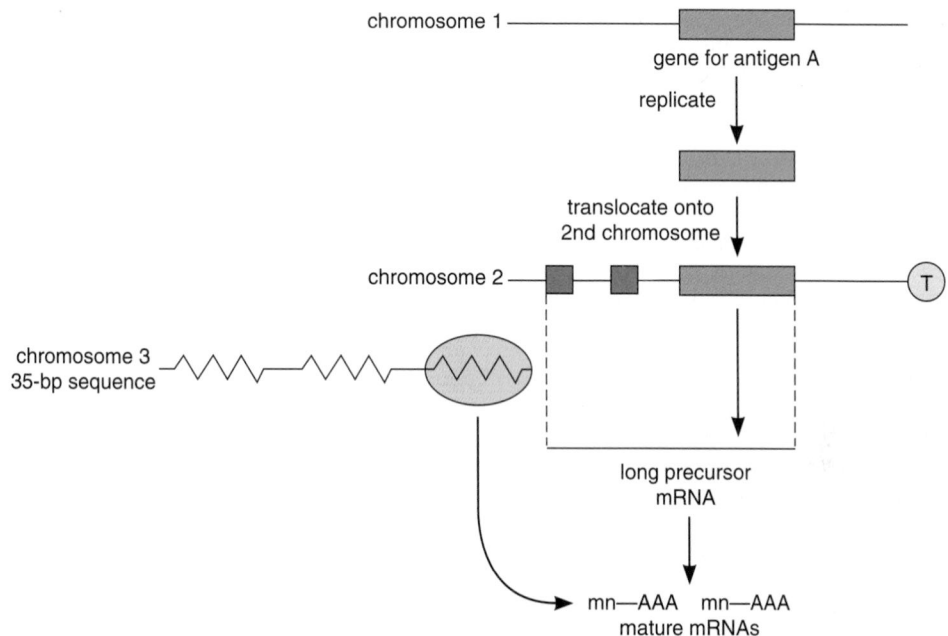

Figure 51–5. Molecular mechanism of antigenic diversity in trypanosomiasis.

duces a fatal infection—implies that some protective mechanism must exist.

The multiplicity of antigenic variants observed during field studies in bovines makes vaccination an unlikely solution to trypanosomiasis unless common antigens can be found.

THE IMMUNE RESPONSE TO HELMINTHS

Multicellular parasites, by reason of their size, more complex tissue and organ structure, and varied and active metabolism, include very complex host responses. Further complicating the picture is the fact that several forms of the parasite may be present in the host, each eliciting a unique immune response.

The primary antigens of helminths may often be metabolic by-products, enzymes, or other secretory products. For example, the eggs of *Schistosoma mansoni* have been shown to secrete unique antigens that induce granuloma formation; the various stages of developing nematodes have stage-specific antigens, often molting fluids, to which the host responds in various ways; and the granules in the stichocytes, special cells located in the "neck" of *Trichuris trichiura* elicit specific antibody.

Trematodes, cestodes, and nematodes probably all share common antigens. The two most frequent responses to helminths—eosinophilia and reaginic antibody (IgE)—are both T-cell-dependent. Moreover, certain helminths have been shown to potentiate the immune response to other antigens, perhaps by common metabolic by-products acting as nonspecific adjuvants.

TREMATODES

Trematodes are important pathogens of humans and domestic animals. Fascioliasis debilitates and kills domestic animals in large numbers and renders the livers unfit for human consumption. Schistosomiasis is a major disease of humans. The lung flukes of the genus *Paragonimus* cause central nervous system complications in humans if they encyst in the brain. In the lungs, considerable mechanical damage results. *Clonorchis sinensis,* the fish-borne Chinese liver fluke, produces infection that may last the lifetime of the host.

1. SCHISTOSOMIASIS

Major Immunologic Features

- Response to invading worms is both humoral (IgE, IgM, IgG) and cellular (eosinophils, lymphocytes, macrophages).
- A serum sickness-like acute disease (Katayama fever) may develop.
- Chronic disease occurs owing to granulomatous reaction to eggs with subsequent fibrosis.
- Developing larvae and adult worms evade immune response by camouflaging their surface with host antigens.

Schistosomiasis in humans is caused by *Schistosoma mansoni, S japonicum, S haematobium,* and *S mekongi.* The advent of new high dams in many areas of the world, especially Africa, has increased the prevalence of schistosomiasis, because the additional irrigation made possible by the dams has vastly enlarged the habitat of the freshwater snails that serve as intermediate hosts to the worms. The life cycle of this parasite depends on skin penetration of the definitive host by infective larvae produced in large numbers in the snail. Because attempts to reduce snail populations have largely failed, infection has become rampant in these areas. *S mansoni,* now widespread in Africa and the Middle East, has also spread extensively in South America. *S haematobium* is found in all watered areas of Africa and the Arabian peninsula. *S japonicum* is found in the Yangtze River watershed in China, where it has been subjected to a vast control effort but is still common in Szechwan province and may be returning to the main river valley. It is also common in the central Philippines. A purely animal-infecting (zoophilic) form is found in Taiwan. *S mekongi,* a newly described species similar to *S japonicum,* causes human disease in Thailand, Laos, and Cambodia, with a scattering of cases in Malaysia, recently described as *S malaysiensis.* There is also a focus of *S japonicum* in Sulawesi (Celebes) that may prove to be a distinct species.

In brief, the life cycle of the schistosomes that infect humans is as follows. Infected humans and animals excrete eggs that hatch in water, releasing miracidia; these actively penetrate snails, in which several generations of multiplying larvae (sporocysts) develop. These in turn produce great numbers of fork-tailed cercariae, the stage infective for humans, which leave the host snail at a rate of 300–3000 per day. The cercariae penetrate the skin of the definitive host, leaving the tail outside, and enter the bloodstream as minute motile immature schistosomula, which migrate in 3–8 days to the lungs and eventually to the liver. Further development and adult worm pairing take place about 5 weeks after skin penetration. The paired mature schistosomes then migrate against the venous flow into the mesenteric or vesical venules, where eggs are deposited. Some investigators have suggested that the granuloma produced by the host around the egg "chaperones" it through the wall of the intestine. Egg movement is also probably aided by peristalsis of the intestine or contractions of the bladder.

Unfortunately, not all the eggs reach the lumen of the intestine or bladder. Some become trapped in the submucosa, and others do not leave the bloodstream but instead are carried with the venous flow to the liver portals or by collateral circulation to other organs of the body. Because of their size, eggs reaching the liver become trapped in the portal venules and do not enter the sinusoids. When eggs are trapped in the liver, the wall of the intestine, or the bladder, they elicit a granulomatous inflammation that is the hallmark of the chronic stage of schistosomiasis. An early infiltrate of neutrophils and lymphocytes may be seen around eggs, but distinctive granulomas containing a core of macrophages and eosinophils, surrounded by a cuff of lymphocytes, appear shortly. The early stages of inflammation may be seen by 6 weeks, but granulomas reach their maximal cellularity within 9–12 weeks. Later, an increasing number of fibroblasts or lipocytes (Ito cells) can be seen in association with the granulomas, and the cellular lesion becomes slowly replaced by collagen. In the liver, older lesions become periportal scars. Since numerous eggs are deposited, a circumferential periportal fibrosis called Symmer's clay pipestem fibrosis develops, particularly well demarcated in *S mansoni* infection. This fibrosis blocks normal blood flow from the portal venous system to the sinusoids, resulting in portal hypertension and its complications.

The factors that initiate granuloma formation are soluble proteins secreted through pores in the eggshell by the embryonic micracidium. These soluble egg products, some of which have been purified, are used in one serodiagnostic test for schistosomiasis. As might be expected from the complex group of cells that form the granuloma, the mechanisms of granuloma formation, modulation, and subsequent fibrosis are complex. Pleiotropic cytokines are involved, as well as factors from the egg itself that may be both chemotactic and mitogenic for fibroblasts. The importance of cellular immunity in granuloma formation has been underscored by the observation that both the granulomatous reaction to schistosome eggs and subsequent periportal fibrosis are absent or significantly diminished in thymic-deficient ("nude") mice and in mice with severe combined immunodeficiency (SCID). SCID mice have no functional T and B cells, and in the absence of a granulomatous response, schistosome eggs produce a frequently fatal acute hepatotoxic effect. The predominant, but not exclusive, cytokine response to schistosome eggs is T_H2 (see Fig 51–3). The importance of this cytokine phenotype to the pathogenesis of hepatic fibrosis in schistosomiasis is supported by the observation that vaccination with egg antigens accompanied by IL-12 decreased fibrosis in infected mice. IL-12 shifts the cytokine phenotype from T_H2 to T_H1. An unexpected observation from studies of infection in SCID mice was than an intact cellular immune response was necessary for egg production by schistosome females and passage of eggs through the intestinal wall. Injection of supernatant from cultures of T-cell clones led to reconstitution of the host granulomatous response as well as egg production and transmission. This suggested that specific T-cell-derived cytokines were required as key elements in the host–parasite interplay. These observations confirm that the host–parasite relationship is an extremely intricate, complicated, and highly evolved phenomenon in which elements of the host immune response are sometimes subverted by the parasite for its own replication and transmission.

Although the immune response to schistosome eggs is the central immunopathologic mechanism in chronic schistosomiasis, it is not the only immune response of importance in schistosome infection. In some previously infected individuals, invading cercariae may elicit a dermatitis with features of both immediate and delayed hypersensitivity. This is similar to the "swimmers' itch" produced by nonhuman schistosomes that enter the skin of previously sensitized individuals. Some schistosomes species may produce any acute form of schistosomiasis (Katayama fever) characterized by fever, eosinophilia, lymphadenopathy, diarrhea, splenomegaly, and urticaria. This appears to be an anaphylactic (IgE) or serum sickness (IgG) reaction. In fact, cases of glomerulonephritis secondary to schistosome antigen–antibody complexes have been reported.

An important unresolved question is whether protective immunity to schistosomiasis develops in humans after infection. Studies in Kenya and Gambia have shown that schistosome-infected individuals in an area of endemicity who had been treated with antischistosome drugs showed an age-dependent resistance to reinfection. Children were much more easily reinfected than were adults, suggesting that true human immunity can be acquired with age. Identification of "resistant" groups of children may help to identify important parasite antigens. Augmentation of the response to these antigens would be one rational approach to vaccine development.

The question of immunity to reinfection has been studied intensively in two animal models. In the first of these, called the **concomitant immunity model,** mice are infected with 20–30 normal *S mansoni* cercariae 6 weeks prior to challenge. In the second, called the **attenuated vaccine model,** mice are immunized with 400–500 cercariae attenuated by 2–5 Gy of gamma radiation 2 weeks before challenge. The mechanisms by which the host eliminates the challenge infection may be different in each of these two models. Studies with the concomitant immunity model in mice or in rats, a naturally nonpermissive host, emphasized the importance of specific antiparasite immunoglobulin and eosinophils. In fact, these models help to elucidate many of the cellular functions of eosinophils. Eosinophilia is a common denominator in helminth parasite infections, and histologic examination of parasites and host tissue invariably confirms the presence of numerous eosinophils around dead or dying organisms. On the other hand, studies with attenuated vaccine model pointed to macrophages as the principal effector cells in elimination of the challenge infection. Whether one or both of these mechanisms is key in the human immune response to schistosome infection remains an active area of research and debate.

By comparing normal with various immune-deficient mouse strains, the cellular and antibody requirements of vaccine immunity have been investigated.

Vaccinated mice with T-lymphocyte deficiencies, as well as mice immunosuppressed from birth, have a sharply diminished resistance to challenge infection. On the other hand, mice deficient in complement, mast cells, natural killer (NK) lymphocytes, and IgE show no difference in resistance compared with normal controls. In a theme common to many parasitic infections, CD4 T cells secreting interferon gamma and macrophages appear key to killing of larvae in vaccinated mice.

CESTODES

There are two types of immune response to cestodes. One is directed against the intestinal lumen-dwelling adult tapeworms such as *Diphyllobothrium latum* and *Taenia saginata,* which have restricted, nonhumoral immunogenic contact. The response is chiefly cell-mediated, is induced primarily by the scolex, affects growth and strobilation of challenge worms, and varies considerably with the host species. The other is directed against migratory tissue-encysting larval tapeworms such as *Hymenolepis nana* (in its intravillous larval phase), *Echinococcus granulosus* (hydatid cysts), and *Taenia solium* (cysticercosis), which have intimate and continuous tissue contact and induce a strong parenteral host response detectable as serum antibody and strongly protective against reinfection. Serodiagnostic tests are available only for the larval tissue cestode parasites, and humoral responses that protect the challenged host have only recently been described for this form of cestode parasitism. Enzyme-linked immunosorbent assay (ELISA) for serodiagnosis of cysticercosis—with some cross-reactivity—has been developed.

1. ECHINOCOCCOSIS

Major Immunologic Features
- IgE elevated.
- Anaphylaxis may occur after rupture of hydatid and release of cyst fluids.
- Casoni skin test of questionable use.
- Diagnostic antibody present.

General Considerations
The most serious human cestode infection is that caused by *Echinococcus.* These tiny tapeworms do not produce pathologic lesions in the definitive host, the dog, but severe complications occur when their eggs are ingested by humans and other animals. The larval form of the tapeworm hatches from the egg in the intestine of the intermediate host (humans) and then claws its way through the intestinal mucosa and is transported through the lymphatic and blood vessels to sites in which it grows to enormous proportions, although it is enclosed by a heavy cyst wall laid

down by both the host and the parasite. In humans, *Echinococcus* normally forms fluid-filled cysts in the liver, but these can also occur in the lungs, brain, kidneys, and other parts of the body. Hydatid cysts are highly immunogenic and result in production of higher titers of IgE and other immunoglobulins. If a cyst is ruptured, anaphylactic response to the cyst fluid can cause death. Little or no immune protection is elicited by this highly immunogenic cestode, because the hydatid cysts remain alive for years and, in animals, can be shown to increase in number as the host ages. Humans are usually a dead-end host, for the cysts must be eaten by a canid to become sexually mature. There is some evidence that complement-mediated lysis of protoscoleces (the numerous future scoleces in hydatid fluid or "hydatid sand") might be protective in the infected human or other intermediate host.

The Casoni skin test indicates past or present echinococcosis. It consists of intradermal injection of hydatid cyst fluid, resulting in both immediate and delayed hypersensitivity. The specificity of this test is in doubt because of cross-reactions with other helminths. Heating the cyst fluid slightly increases the specificity of the test. Serodiagnosis can be made by hemagglutination, complement fixation, and flocculation tests, ELISA, and radioimmunoassay, using serum from the patient and specially fractionated antigenic components made from cyst fluid. These tests are not species-specific.

NEMATODES

Nematodes are the commonest, varied, and widely distributed helminths infecting humans. As with other parasites, immunogenicity is a reflection of the degree and duration of parasite contact with the host's tissues. Even with the intestinal lumen dwellers such as *Ascaris,* there is a migratory larval phase in which such contact is made—in most cases, in the pulmonary capillaries and alveolar spaces. The hookworms of humans (*Ancylostoma duodenale* and *Necator americanus*) also migrate, except that the infective larvae enter via the skin or buccal mucosa rather than as hatchlings in the small bowel. *Strongyloides stercoralis,* the small intestinal roundworm of humans, undergoes a similar hookworm-like migration (as well as a stage of internal autoinfection or reinvasion via the mucosa of the large intestine or perianal skin).

The immature stages are particularly immunogenic, probably because of their high production of antigens from secretory glands and of enzymes or other products from these metabolically active stages. Commercially prepared vaccines are available only for nematodes, and all are living larval worms, irradiated to arrest their development but not their immunogenicity. These are the cattle and sheep lungworms *Dictyocaulus viviparus* and *Dictyocaulus filaria* and the dog hookworm *Ancylostoma caninum.*

Another important group of human parasites are the filariae (chiefly *Wuchereria bancrofti, Brugia malayi, Loa loa, Onchocerca volvulus,* and the related guinea worm, *Dracunculus medinensis*). Diagnosis of these infections is often difficult, in part because of the presence of common antigens that preclude highly specific immunologic tests. Hypersensitivity reactions may occur after drug treatment (such as with diethylcarbamizine for *Onchocerca*), when large numbers of dead or dying microfilariae produce severe skin reactions and edema or dangerous reactions in the eye and (with *Loa*) when dead adult worms induce severe central nervous system reactions.

1. TRICHINOSIS

Major Immunologic Features

- Skin tests for immediate and delayed hypersensitivity positive.
- Diagnostic antibody present.

General Considerations

Trichinosis is acquired by ingestion of the infective larvae of *Trichinella spiralis* in uncooked or partially cooked meat. Pork is the primary source of infection in humans. The larvae are released from their cysts in the meat during digestion and rapidly develop into adults in the mucosa of the host's small intestine. After copulation in the lumen, the males die and the females return to the intestinal mucosa, where for about 5–6 weeks they produce 1000–1500 larvae per female, which migrate through the lymphatic system to the bloodstream. These larvae travel in the blood to all parts of the body and develop in voluntary muscles, especially in the diaphragm, tongue, masticatory and intercostal muscles, larynx, and the eye. Within the sarcolemma of striated muscle fibers, the larvae coil up into cysts whose outer walls are rapidly laid down by host histiocytes. Larvae may remain viable and infective for as long as 24 years, even though the cysts calcify. The encysted larvae apparently do not elicit immune protection. The migrating larvae and adult forms of the parasite excrete antigens that appear to be responsible for induction of the strong protection from subsequent challenge infections. An important expression of host resistance is active expulsion of developing or adult worms from the gut of a parasitized host—the so-called self-cure phenomenon. This occurs when a new infection initiates a host response, resulting in elimination of the old one—the opposite of concomitant immunity.

The expulsion of *T spiralis* in humans appears to follow the mechanism proposed by B Ogilvie and coworkers for the rodent hookworm, *Nippostrongylus brasiliensis.* A two-step mechanism is proposed: antibody-induced metabolic damage that blocks feeding by the worms followed by worm expulsion induced by activated lymphocytes. Both antibodies and cells are probably required for full expression of intestinal resistance, and the effect is synergistic rather than additive. As in the case of leishmaniasis, discussed earlier, T_H1 subtype CD4 lymphocytes may be key in cellular immunity via their production of interferon gamma.

Trichinella infection sometimes presents characteristic clinical symptoms, such as edema of the eyelids and face, but often presents less specific clinical signs such as eosinophilia, which can also be suggestive of several other parasitic infections. Specific immunodiagnostic tests may thus be of great importance. The bentonite flocculation test for human trichinosis is of value because of its high degree of specificity. A skin test (Bachman's intradermal test) produces both immediate and delayed responses.

In humans, infection with *Trichinella* initially elicits IgM antibody followed by an IgG response. IgA antibody has been reported, which is not surprising, because the female worms are in the intestinal mucosa, although the locally produced protective gut antibodies probably are IgG rather than IgA or IgM. This antibody reaction against the feeding worms is complement-independent and, as noted, precedes the rapid expulsion of the antibody-damaged worms by T lymphocytes.

Although *Trichinella* is extremely immunogenic in its hosts, it can also exert an immunosuppressive action. Certain viral infections are more severe during infection with this parasite, and skin grafts show delayed rejection. On the other hand, cellular immunity to bacillus Calmette-Guérin (BCG) seems to be potentiated when *T spiralis* is present, and *T spiralis*-infected mice are less susceptible to *Listeria* infections.

2. ASCARIASIS

Major Immunologic Features
- Specific antibody detectable.
- Elevated IgE.

General Considerations

Ascaris, the giant roundworm in humans, is a lumen-dwelling parasite as an adult and causes little inconvenience to the host except in the heaviest infections, though even single adult worms may produce mechanical damage by entering the bile or pancreatic ducts. Ingestion of eggs is followed by their hatching and penetration of the mucosa by the larvae, which eventually reach the lung via the bloodstream. In a previously infected host, hypersensitivity reactions in the lung resulting from high levels of IgE can cause serious pneumonitis. Acute hypersensitivity to *Ascaris* antigens often develops in laboratory workers and makes it virtually impossible for them to continue working with the nematode.

Cases of sudden death in Nigeria have been ascribed to *Ascaris*-induced anaphylactic shock syndrome, heretofore rarely diagnosed or recognized. Death probably resulted from the release of a mast cell degranulator by the worms, since degranulated mast cells were found throughout the body tissues in these children, or from a reagin–*Ascaris* allergen interaction at the mast cell surface. Allergy to ascariasis may underlie many of the symptoms of *Ascaris* infection, including abdominal pain.

3. FILARID NEMATODES

Major Immunologic Features
- Induction of host immune response to adults or microfilariae leads to disease.

General Considerations

Filarid nematodes are introduced into the human host by insect vectors. Those of the genus *Brugia* or *Wuchereria* are spread by a mosquito vector, whereas *Onchocerca volvulus* is transmitted by a blackfly. Although the stages of each life cycle are similar, the type of disease produced varies considerably. A common theme is that morbidity is due primarily to the host immune response to the parasite rather than any toxic product of the parasite itself.

O volvulus is the causative agent of onchocerciasis, or African river blindness. This is the major cause of blindness in endemic areas of West Africa and Central America. Infectious larvae that are deposited by a blackfly bite migrate in the subcutaneous tissue and develop into adults in approximately 1 year. The adults elicit an unusual fibrogenic host response, resulting in a subcutaneous collagenous nodule in which the worm lives. The female produces large numbers of microfilariae, which migrate out of the nodule and are distributed widely in subcutaneous tissue. This dispersal of microfilariae increases the likelihood that they will be picked up again by the insect vector to continue the life cycle. Humans react to migrating microfilariae by production of both circulating antibody and cellular immunity. An intense delayed hypersensitivity-like reaction to dead or dying microfilariae can lead to a disseminated skin reaction or a more serious eye disease. Microfilariae can enter all chambers of the eye and elicit a keratitis or retinitis, which, over a period of years, can lead to total blindness.

Parasites of the genera *Brugia* and *Wuchereria,* in contrast, produce lymphatic filariasis. In this case, the damaging response is due to adult worms residing in lymphatics, most commonly in the groin. Over a period of time, the lymphatic lumen may be compromised by scarring, leading to blockage of lymph drainage from the lower extremities and production of a disfiguring condition called "elephantiasis" that characterizes severe chronic disease.

REFERENCES

GENERAL

Reiner SL, Locksley RM: The worm and the protozoa: Stereotyped responses for distinct antigens? *Parasitol Today* 1993;**9**:258.

SERODIAGNOSTIC TESTS

Centers for Disease Control: *Reference and Disease Surveillance.* Center for Infectious Diseases, CDC, 1985.

LEISHMANIASIS

Reiner SL et al: T_H1 and T_H2 cell antigen receptors in experimental leishmaniasis. *Science* 1993;**259**:1457.

Scott P, Sher A: A spectrum in the susceptibility of leishmanial strains to intracellular killing by murine macrophages. *J Immunol* 1986;**136**:1461.

MALARIA

Borst P et al: Antigenic variation in malaria. *Cell* 1995;**82**:1.

Butcher GA: HIV and malaria: A lesson in immunology? *Parasitol Today* 1992;**8**:307.

Greenwood B et al: Why do some African children develop severe malaria? *Parasitol Today* 1991;**7**:277.

Riley EM et al: The immune recognition of malaria antigens. *Parasitol Today* 1991;**7**:5.

Sinigaglia F, Pink JRL: A way round the "real difficulties" of malaria sporozoite vaccine development? *Parasitol Today* 1990;**6**:277.

SCHISTOSOMIASIS

Cheever AW: Schistosomiasis: Infection versus disease and hypersensitivity versus immunity. *Am J Pathol* 1993;**142**:699.

Hagan P, Wilkins HA: Concomitant immunity in schistosomiasis. *Parasitol Today* 1993;**9**:3.

Scott P: IL-12: Initiation cytokine for cell-mediated immunity. *Science* 1993;**260**:496.

Stadecker MJ, Colley DG: The immunobiology of the schistosome egg granuloma. *Parasitol Today* 1992;**8**:218.

Wynn T et al: An IL-12-based vaccination method for preventing fibrosis induced by schistosome infection. *Nature* 1995;**376**:594.

TRYPANOSOMIASIS

Borst P, Rudenko G: Antigenic variation in African trypanosomes. *Science* 1994;**264**:1872.

Donelson JE, Turner MJ: How the trypanosome changes its coat. *Sci Am* 1985;**252**:44.

Spirochetal Diseases

52

Charles S. Pavia, PhD, & David J. Drutz, MD

Spirochetes are a highly specialized group of motile gram-negative bacteria, with a slender and tightly helically coiled structure. They range from 0.1 to 0.5 μm in width and from 10 to 50 μm in length. One of the unique features of spirochetes is their motility by rapidly drifting rotation, often associated with a flexing or undulating movement along the helical path. These bacteria belong to the order Spirochaetales, which includes two families: Spirochaetaceae and Leptospiraceae. Important members of these groups include *Treponema, Borrelia,* and *Leptospira.*

Spirochetal infections leading to such diseases as syphilis and the other treponematoses, Lyme disease, relapsing fever borreliosis, and leptospirosis are important worldwide health problems. A better understanding of the immunobiology of the disease-causing spirochetes has become crucial in efforts to develop effective vaccines, because there has been no significant modification in sexual activity, personal hygiene practices, or vector control—factors essential to the transmission of these infectious agents. Further knowledge of immune responses to spirochetes is essential for their eventual control by immunization, and studies of the host–spirochete relationship have led to important new insights into the immune system itself. Serologic techniques have now become indispensable diagnostic tools for detection of many of the spirochetal diseases, especially syphilis and Lyme disease (Fig 52–1) and potential vaccines for Lyme disease are currently in the testing phase for clinical efficacy. Unfortunately, the immune response to spirochetal infections, as in other infections, may paradoxically cause immunologically induced disease in the host, such as aortitis, immune-complex glomerulonephritis, the gummatous lesions of syphilis, and the neuropathies and arthritis of Lyme disease.

SYPHILIS

Major Immunologic Features

- Both nonspecific, anticardiolipin, and specific antitreponemal antibodies are detectable following primary infection.
- Cell-mediated immunity becomes activated during or after the late secondary stage.
- Immunosuppression occurs during various phases of the disease.
- A complex state of partial immunity develops late following an untreated primary infection.

General Considerations

Treponema pallidum is the spirochetal bacterium responsible for the sexually transmitted disease syphilis, which can have severe pathologic consequences if untreated and for which there is no vaccine. The organism is noncultivable, highly motile, and infectious, and it replicates extracellularly in vivo.

With the institution of antibiotic therapy in the mid-1940s, the incidence of syphilis fell sharply from a high of 72 cases per 100,000 in 1943 to about 4 per 100,000 in 1956. From 1987 to 1991, however, the Centers for Disease Control and Prevention reported significant increases in primary and secondary syphilis cases, which were attributed, in part, to changing life-styles, sexual practices, and other factors, such as an unusually high prevalence and resistance to antibiotics in patients with acquired immunodeficiency syndrome (AIDS). The recent estimated annual rate per 100,000 has decreased gradually nationwide from a decade high of 20.1 cases in 1990 to 8.1 cases in 1994. Despite these periodic fluctuations in incidence over the past 10 years, syphilis still continues to rank annually as the third or fourth most frequently reported communicable disease in the USA.

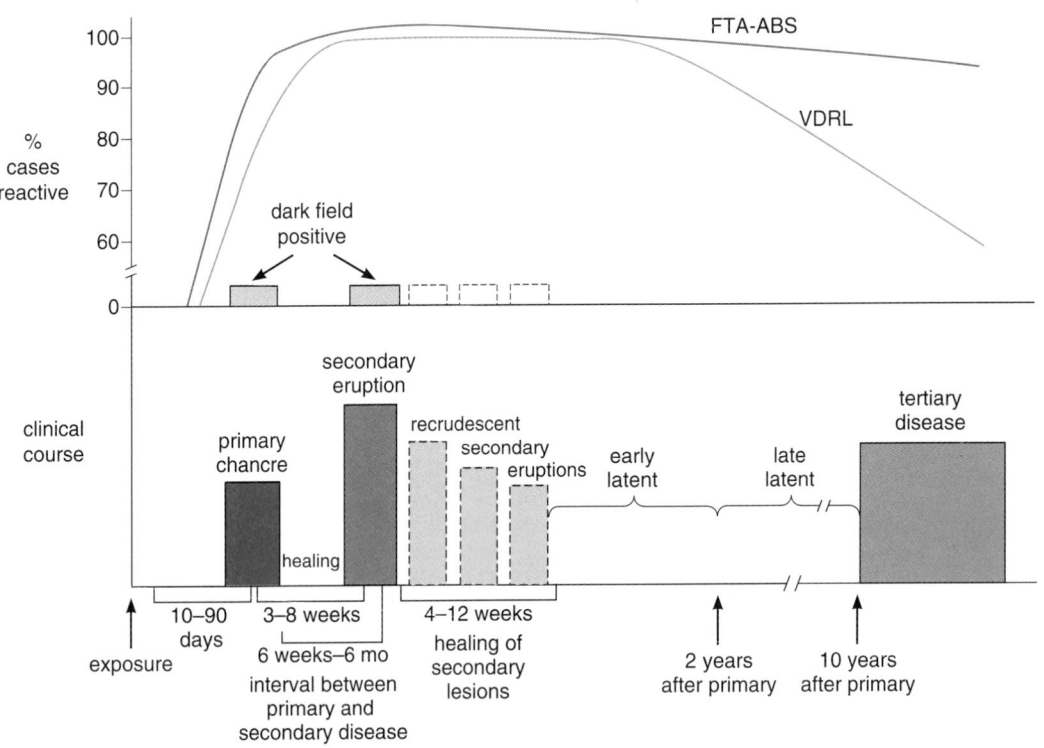

Figure 52–1. The course of untreated syphilis. (Reproduced, with permission, from Joklik WK et al (editors). *Zinsser Microbiology,* 20th ed. Appleton-Century-Crofts, 1992.)

The course of syphilis in humans is marked by several interesting phenomena. Without treatment the disease usually progresses through several well-defined stages. This is unlike most other infectious diseases, which are ultimately eliminated by the host's immune system or, in severe cases, result in death. The relatively slow generation time of treponemes, which is estimated at 30–33 hours, contributes to this unique course. During the first two stages (primary and secondary syphilis) there is almost unimpeded rapid growth of *T pallidum,* leading to an early infectious spirochetemic phase of disease. The third stage (tertiary syphilis) occurs much later, following a prolonged latency period. Alterations in this stage are due primarily to tissue-damaging immune responses elicited by small numbers of previously deposited or disseminated spirochetes.

Syphilis activates both humoral and cell-mediated immunity, but this protection is only partial. The relative importance of each type of immune response is not fully known. Protective immunity against reexposure is incomplete, especially during early stages, when it develops relatively slowly. Evidence for the participation of humoral immunity in syphilis is as follows:

1. A variety of nonspecific "reaginic," or Wassermann, cardiolipin and specific antibodies are routinely present in the sera of patients with syphilis.
2. *T pallidum*-immobilizing antibodies (TPIA) are regularly present in the sera of syphilitic patients.
3. The frequency with which TPIA are found increases as syphilis progresses to latent and tertiary infection.
4. Partial immunity can be conferred in experimentally infected laboratory animals by passive transfer of serum from syphilis-immune donors. This protection is apparent when treponemes are injected intradermally into these animal hosts. Chancres may be either prevented or delayed, and dissemination of treponemes from the primary focus of infection may be reduced by passive immunization.

Interestingly, humans who have been experimentally infected with *T pallidum* also develop increased local resistance to rechallenge at a cutaneous site. This local resistance is referred to as **chancre immunity.** Chancre immunity persists if primary infection remains untreated and syphilis progresses to a latent stage. Although chancre immunity is indicative of heightened local resistance, it does not prevent the systemic spread of *T pallidum* from the site of initial challenge. Chancre immunity may be attributable to antibody, because both the immunity and reaginic antibodies wane after treatment of primary syphilis. The time required depends on the titer of antibody and the severity of the illness. For several reasons, it is not likely that the antibodies are completely protective:

1. Treponemes from the initial infection persist systemically during latent syphilis, even though there is resistance to a second challenge. This suggests that the organism has found sanctuary in some sort of privileged residence, where it resists or is unaffected by host defenses.
2. Some antibodies are nonspecific and are found in other diseases, such as systemic lupus erythematosus. They might even be directed against host rather than treponemal antigens.
3. By preventing the attachment of treponemes to cells in tissue culture, antibodies might, in fact, aid the organism in escaping host defense mechanisms.
4. Circulating immune complexes are formed during infection with *T pallidum.* They are demonstrable in sera of both rabbits and patients with syphilis. They may be composed of cardiolipin–anticardiolipin as well as of treponemal antigen/antitreponemal antibody. Experimentally, they may act to depress the synthesis of IgG against independent antigens, such as sheep erythrocytes. It is conceivable that circulating immune complexes prevent the host from synthesizing treponemicidal antibody during primary syphilis or from synthesizing antitreponemal antibody that might act in concert with cell-mediated immunity against *T pallidum.*
5. The patterns of antibody production change during the course of untreated syphilis. Patients with secondary syphilis have antitreponemal antibody as well as anticardiolipin antibody. These antibodies are of both IgG and IgM classes. As the disease enters latency, antitreponemal IgM antibody production ceases and patients are left with antitreponemal IgG and anticardiolipin IgM and IgG. The clinical significance of this sequence of events is uncertain.

Observations in both infected humans and laboratory animals have implicated cell-mediated immunity as a critical element in host response to *T pallidum.* Evidence for the participation of cell-mediated immunity in syphilis is as follows:

1. Passive transfer of syphilis immune serum is only partially protective and does not follow classic models of humoral immunity.
2. Syphilis progresses through the primary and secondary stages despite the presence of antibodies that immobilize the infecting organism.
3. Delayed hypersensitivity to treponemal antigens is absent in primary and early secondary syphilis but develops late in secondary infection and is regularly present in latent and tertiary syphilis.
4. Granulomatous lesions characterize tertiary syphilis.
5. Immunization with killed microorganisms is usually unsuccessful, whereas immunization with live attenuated organisms has produced immunity.
6. In vitro lymphocyte reactivity to treponemal and nontreponemal antigens and T lymphocyte counts are suppressed during primary and secondary syphilis.
7. Infecting rabbits with *T pallidum* stimulates acquired cellular resistance to *Listeria;* this reaction is mediated by T lymphocytes.
8. Both T and B cells are effective in conferring antisyphilis immunity when transferred from nonimmune recipients to normal challenged recipients.

It is puzzling why so much time is required for patients to develop humoral and cellular immunity to syphilis. Although immune mechanisms are currently unclear, one theory holds that the mucoid envelope of *T pallidum* renders it highly resistant to phagocytosis; only after the treponemes have remained in the host for some time is the mucoid coat broken down sufficiently for phagocytosis to occur. (Treponemal mucopolysaccharides also suppress lymphocyte blastogenic response to concanavalin A.) As a result, treponemal proliferation outstrips the rate of antigenic processing for stimulation of humoral and cellular immune mechanisms; a condition of "antigen overload" then occurs, with production of secondary immunosuppression. An alternative explanation is that sensitization with treponemal antigen leads primarily to generation of antibodies that then block antigenic sites, thereby inhibiting an appropriate cell-mediated immune response.

Clinical Features

The severe late manifestations or complications of syphilis occur in the blood vessels and perivascular tissues. Sexual contact is the common mode of transmission, however, with inoculation on the mucous membranes of genital organs.

The first clinically apparent manifestation of syphilis (primary syphilis) is an indurated, circumscribed, relatively avascular and painless ulcer (chancre) at the site of treponemal inoculation. Spirochetemia with secondary metastatic distribution of microorganisms occurs within a few days after onset of local infection, but clinically apparent secondary lesions may not be observed for 2–4 weeks. The chancre lasts 10–14 days before healing spontaneously.

The presence of metastatic infection (secondary syphilis) is manifested by highly infectious mucocutaneous lesions of extraordinarily diverse description as well as headache, low-grade fever, diffuse lymphadenopathy, and a variety of more sporadic phenomena. The lesions of secondary syphilis ordinarily go on to apparent spontaneous resolution in the absence of treatment. Until solid immunity develops, however—a matter of about 4 years—25% of untreated syphilitic patients may be susceptible to repeated episodes of spirochetemia and metastatic infection.

Following the resolution of secondary syphilis, the disease enters a period of latency, with only abnormal serologic tests to indicate the presence of infection. During this time, persistent or progressive focal infection is presumably taking place, but the precise site remains unknown in the absence of specific symptoms and signs. One site of potential latency, the central nervous system, can be evaluated by examining the cerebrospinal fluid, in which pleocytosis, elevated protein levels, and a positive serologic test for syphilis are indicative of asymptomatic neurosyphilis.

Only about 15% of patients with untreated latent syphilis go on to develop symptomatic tertiary syphilis. Serious or fatal tertiary syphilis in adults is virtually limited to disease of the aorta (aortitis with aneurysm formation and secondary aortic valve insufficiency), the central nervous system (tabes dorsalis, general paresis), the eyes (interstitial keratitis), or the ears (nerve deafness). Less frequently, the disease becomes apparent as localized single or multiple granulomas known as "gummas." These lesions are typically found in skin, bones, liver, testes, or larynx. The histopathologic features of the gumma resemble those of earlier syphilitic lesions, except that the vasculitis is associated with increased tissue necrosis and often frank caseation. *T pallidum* can infect the fetus of an infected mother via placental transmission especially during the latter half of pregnancy. This can lead to fetal death or, when there is a live birth, the appearance in the baby of numerous symptoms and disease manifestations indicative of symptomatic infection.

Immunologic Diagnosis

In its primary and secondary stages, syphilis is best diagnosed by dark-field microscopic examination of material from suspected lesions. Diagnostic serologic changes do not begin to occur until 14–21 days following acquisition of infection. Serologic tests provide important confirmatory evidence for secondary syphilis but are the only means of diagnosing latent infection (Fig 52–1; Table 52–1). Many forms of tertiary syphilis can be suspected on clinical grounds, but serologic tests are important in confirming the diagnosis. Spirochetes are notoriously difficult to demonstrate in the late stages of syphilis.

Two main categories of serologic tests for syphilis (STS) are available: tests for reaginic antibody and tests for treponemal antibody.

A. Tests for Reaginic Antibody: This is an unfortunate and confusing designation; there is no relationship between this antibody and IgE reaginic antibody. Patients with syphilis develop an antibody response to a tissue-derived substance (from beef heart) that is thought to be a component of mitochondrial membranes and is called cardiolipin. Antibody to cardiolopin antigen is known as Wassermann's, or reaginic, antibody. Numerous variations (and names) are associated with tests for this antigen. The simplest and most practical of these are the Venereal Disease Research Laboratory of the US Public Health Service (VDRL) test, which involves a slide microflocculation technique and can provide qualitative and quantitative data, and the rapid plasma reagin (RPR) circle card test. Positive tests are considered to be diagnostic of syphilis when there is a high or increasing titer or when the medical history is compatible with primary or secondary syphilis. The tests may also be of prognostic aid in monitoring the response to therapy, because the antibody titer reverts to negative within 1 year of treatment for seropositive primary syphilis or within 2 years of that for secondary syphilis. Because cardiolipin antigen is found in the mitochondrial membranes of many mammalian tissues as well as in diverse microorganisms, it is not surprising that antibody to this antigen should appear during other diseases. A positive VDRL test may be encountered, for example, in patients with infectious mononucleosis, leprosy, hepatitis, and systemic lupus erythematosus.

Table 52–1. Serologic tests for syphilis.

Antigen	Antigen Source	Tests	Percent Reactivity During		
			Primary Stage	Secondary Stage	Tertiary Stage
Nontreponemal	Extracts of tissue (cardiolipin-lecithin-cholesterol	Complement fixation (Wassermann, Kolmer) Flocculation (VDRL, Hinton, Kann)	78	90	77
Treponemal	*T pallidum* Reiter strain *T pallidum*	RPCF TPI FTA-ABS MHA-TP	61 56 85 85	85 94 99 98	72 92 96 95

Source: Reproduced, with permission, from Joklik WK et al (editors). *Zinsser Microbiology,* 20th ed. Appleton-Century-Crofts, 1992.
Abbreviations: FTA-ABS = Fluorescent treponemal antibody-absorption; MHA-TP = microhemagglutination assay for *T pallidum;* RPCF = Reiter protein complement fixation: TPI = *T pallidum* immobilization; VDRL = Venereal Disease Research Laboratory.

Although the VDRL test lacks specificity for syphilis, its great sensitivity makes it extremely useful.

B. Tests for Treponemal Antibody: The first test used for detecting specific antitreponemal antibody was the *T pallidum* immobilization (TPI) test. Although highly reliable, it proved to be too cumbersome for routine use. A major test development was the fluorescent *T pallidum* antibody (FTA) test. If virulent *T pallidum* from an infected rabbit testicle is placed on a slide and overlaid with serum from a patient with antibody to treponemes, an antigen–antibody reaction occurs. The bound antibody can then be detected by means of a fluoresceinated antihuman immunoglobulin antibody. The specificity of the test for *T pallidum* is enhanced by first absorbing the serum with nonpathogenic treponemal strains. This modification is referred to as the FTA-ABS test. (If specific anti-IgM antibody to human gamma globulin is used, the acuteness of the infection or the occurrence of congenital syphilis can be assessed. This test, however, is sometimes falsely positive or negative in babies born of mothers with syphilis.)

The FTA-ABS test is reactive in approximately 80% of patients with primary syphilis (versus 50% for the VDRL test). Both tests are positive in virtually 100% of patients with secondary syphilis. Whereas the VDRL test shows a tendency to decline in titer after successful treatment, the FTA-ABS test may remain positive for years. It is especially useful in confirming or ruling out a diagnosis of syphilis in patients with suspected biologic false-positive reactions to the VDRL test. Even the FTA-ABS test, however, may be susceptible to false-positive reactions, especially in the presence of lupus erythematosus.

The microhemagglutination-*T pallidum* (MHA-TP) test, a simple passive hemagglutination test, is a satisfactory substitute for the FTA-ABS test. Its principal advantages are economy of both technician time and money. Its results correlate closely with those of the FTA-ABS test, except during primary and early secondary syphilis, when both the VDRL and FTA-ABS are more likely to show reactivity. The VDRL test is the only one that can be used with reliability in the evaluation of cerebrospinal fluid.

The interpretation of serologic data from patients with syphilis may be extremely complex in some cases. For example, a prozone phenomenon may be encountered in secondary syphilis; serofastness may characterize late syphilis; and the VDRL test may be negative in up to one third of patients with late latent syphilis.

Differential Diagnosis

Syphilis produces sufficiently diverse clinical manifestations that a textbook of general internal medicine should be consulted for a discussion of the differential diagnosis.

Prevention

If used properly, condoms can be an effective barrier against the sexual transmission of syphilis. Early treatment with antibiotics is the only way known to prevent the later ravages of syphilis.

Treatment

Penicillin is the drug of choice for treating syphilis in all its stages. Because the lesions of tertiary syphilis may be irreversible, it is crucial to identify and treat the disease before tertiary lesions begin. AIDS patients with syphilis must be treated more intensively with penicillin. This reinforces the notion that curing syphilis depends on interactions between an intact immune system and the treponemicidal effects of antibiotics.

Complications & Prognosis

The most frequent complication of treatment is the **Jarisch-Herxheimer reaction,** which occurs in up to half of patients with early syphilis and is manifested by fever, headache, myalgias, and exacerbation of cutaneous lesions. The intensity of a Jarisch-Herxheimer reaction reflects the intensity of local inflammation prior to treatment and is thought to result from the release of antigenic material from dying microorganisms. The reaction is of short duration (2–4 hours) and is generally not harmful, although shock and death have been attributed to this reaction in tertiary forms of the disease. (The Jarisch-Herxheimer reaction has also been described in the treatment of louse-borne borreliosis, brucellosis, and typhoid fever.)

Other immunologic complications of syphilis include paroxysmal cold hemoglobinuria and nephrotic syndrome.

It is estimated that one in 13 patients who receive no treatment for syphilis develop cardiovascular disease, one in 25 become crippled or incapacitated, one in 44 develop irreversible damage to the central nervous system, and one in 200 become blind.

NONVENEREAL TREPONEMATOSES

The causes of yaws (*T pallidum* subsp *pertenue*), pinta (*T carateum*), and bejel (*T pallidum* subsp *endemicum*) are human pathogens responsible for this group of contagious diseases, which are endemic among rural populations in tropical and subtropical countries. Unlike syphilis, these diseases are transmitted not by sexual activity but primarily by direct contact, mostly among children living under poor hygienic conditions. These three treponemal species are morphologically and antigenically similar to *T pallidum* yet give rise to slightly different disease manifestations. Pinta causes skin lesions only; yaws causes skin and bone lesions; and bejel (so-called endemic syphilis) affects the mucous membranes, skin, and bones. They do resemble venereal syphilis by virtue of the self-limiting primary and secondary lesions, a latency period with clinically dormant disease, and late lesions that are frequently highly destructive. The serologic responses for all three diseases are indistinguishable from one another and from that of venereal syphilis, and there is the same degree of slow development of protective immunity associated with prolonged, untreated infection.

LYME DISEASE

Major Immunologic Features

- Multisystem spirochetal disease involves inflammation of skin, joints, and nervous system.
- Specific antibody is diagnostic following infection.
- Cell-mediated immunity is activated during or shortly after the early stage of disease.

General Considerations

In the mid-1970s a geographic clustering of an unusual rheumatoid arthritis-like condition involving mostly children and young adults occurred in northeastern Connecticut. This condition proved to be a newly discovered disease, named Lyme disease after the town of its origin. The arthritis is characterized by intermittent attacks of asymmetric pain and swelling primarily in the large joints (especially the knees) over a period of a few years. Epidemiologic and clinical research showed that the onset of symptoms was preceded by an insect bite and unique skin rash probably identical to that of an illness following a tick bite, first described in Europe at the turn of the century. The beneficial effects of penicillin or tetracycline in early cases suggested a microbial origin for what was initially called Lyme arthritis.

Lyme disease is now the most common tick-transmitted illness in the USA, and it has been reported in at least 43 states. Since recently being classified as a reportable disease, cases of Lyme disease have increased steadily over the past few years, reaching a peak incidence of 5.0 cases per 100,000 in 1994. It occurs primarily, however, in three geographic regions: the coastal areas of the Northeast from Maine to Maryland, the Midwest in Wisconsin and Minnesota, and the far West in parts of California and Oregon. These geographic areas parallel the location of the primary tick vector of Lyme disease in the USA—*Ixodes scapularis* (formerly *dammini*) in the East and Midwest and *Ixodes pacificus* in the far West. Lyme disease has been reported in many other countries, especially in western Europe, corresponding to the distribution of *Ixodes ricinus* ticks. The greatest concentration of cases is in the northeastern USA, particularly in New York state, where the disease is endemic on Long Island and just north of New York City in neighboring Westchester County.

In the early 1980s spirochetal organisms were isolated and cultured from the midguts of *Ixodes* ticks taken from Shelter Island, NY (an endemic focus), and shortly thereafter they were cultured from the skin rash site, blood, and cerebrospinal fluid of patients with Lyme disease. This newly discovered spirochete, called *Borrelia burgdorferi,* is microaerophilic, resembles other spirochetes morphologically, and is slightly larger than the treponemes. Unlike the pathogenic treponemes, *B burgdorferi* can be readily cultivated in vitro in a highly fortified growth media.

As with syphilis, protection against *B burgdorferi* may develop slowly and it is unclear whether resistance to reinfection occurs. Experimental animal studies have shown that immune sera can transfer protection to normal recipients challenged with *B burgdorferi.* Monoclonal antibodies to borrelial outer surface proteins are also protective and have thus become the major target antigens for a vaccine.

Clinical Features

Lyme disease is an illness having protean manifestations with symptoms that include (1) an erythematous expanding red annular rash with central clearing; (2) fever, headache, stiff neck, nausea, and vomiting; (3) neurologic complications such as facial nerve (Bell's) palsy and meningitis; (4) carditis and heart block; and (5) arthritis in about 50% of untreated patients. These symptoms occur most frequently from May to November, when ticks are active and numerous and people are engaged in many outdoor activities. The most characteristic feature of early Lyme disease is a skin rash, often referred to as erythema migrans (EM), which appears shortly (3–32 days) after a bite from an infected tick. The lesion typically expands almost uniformly from the center of the bite and is usually flat or slightly indurated with central clearing and reddening at the periphery. It is noteworthy, however, that many Lyme disease victims do not recall being bitten by a tick or do not notice the development of classic EM. On the other hand, at various intervals after the initial rash, some patients develop similar but smaller multiple secondary annular skin lesions that last for several weeks to months. Biopsy of these skin lesions reveals a lymphocytic and plasma-cytic infiltrate. Various flu-like symptoms, such as malaise, fever, headache, stiff neck, and arthralgias, are often associated with EM. The late manifestations of Lyme disease may include migratory and polyarticular arthritis, neurologic and cardiac involvement with cranial nerve palsies and radiculopathy, myocarditis, and arrhythmias. Lyme arthritis typically involves a knee or other large joint. It may enter a chronic phase, leading to destruction of bone and joints if left untreated. Interestingly, Lyme arthritis is less common in Europe than in the USA but neurologic complications are more prevalent in Europe. Unique strain variations expressing antigenic subtypes between European and North American isolates of *B burgdorferi* probably explain these dissimilarities.

In most cases, humoral and cell-mediated immune responses are activated during borrelial infection. Antibody, mostly of the IgM class, can be detected shortly after the appearance of EM; thereafter, there is a gradual increase in overall titer and a switch to pre-dominant IgG antibody response for the duration of an untreated infection. Most notably, very high levels of antibody have been found in serum and joint fluid taken from patients with moderate to severe arthritis. Although the presence of such high antibody titers against *B burgdorferi* may reduce the spirochete load somewhat, they appear not to ameliorate the disease process completely and, indeed, may actually con-tribute to some of the pathologic changes. These sero-logic responses form the basis of laboratory tests to aid in the diagnosis of Lyme borreliosis. On the basis of lymphocyte transformation assays, peripheral blood T cells from Lyme disease patients respond to borrelial antigens primarily after early infection and following successful treatment. Also, addition of anti-gens to synovial cells in vitro from infected patients triggers the production of interleukin-1, which could account for many of the harmful inflammatory reac-tions associated with this disease. Human mononu-clear and polymorphonuclear phagocytes can both in-gest and presumably destroy *Borrelia.* Thus, borrelial antigen-stimulated T cells or their products may acti-vate macrophages, limiting dissemination and result-ing in enhanced phagocytic activity and the eventual clearance of spirochetes from the primary lesion.

Immunologic Diagnosis

Successful isolation and culture of *B burgdorferi* from skin lesions, blood, and joint and cerebrospinal fluid in suspected cases of Lyme disease has been done but is rarely used for diagnostic purposes. Con-sequently, procedures based on the polymerase chain reactions (PCR) have been developed (as they have been for other difficult-to-culture microorganisms) for sensitive detection of *B burgdorferi* in certain patient specimens. Antibody responses important in diagnosis typically begin to occur 3–5 weeks after the onset of EM, but they can be obliterated by early antibiotic therapy. Serologic tests provide important confirma-tory evidence for all stages of Lyme disease and may be the only way of diagnosing atypical cases. There is some evidence that a small percentage of untreated pa-tients with Lyme disease produce few or no detectable antibodies throughout the course of infection. The most commonly used serologic tests are the enzyme-linked immunosorbent assay (ELISA) and indirect flu-orescent antibody assay (IFA). Because of its sensitiv-ity, adaptability to automation, and ease of quan-titation, the ELISA is probably the preferred method. Standard indirect IFA and newer quantitative solid-phase IFAs are available. Although not standardized, commercial Western immunoblot test kits are now being offered for further confirmation of a serologic response to specific borrelial antigens. Most of these tests are designed to detect total serum antibody to *Borrelia* without differentiating between IgG or IgM antibodies. Some have been developed for specifically

detecting IgM where this class of antibody usually shows preferentially elevated levels early in primary infection or relapse and in sera of newborn infants fol-lowing transplacentally acquired infections. For all these assays, false-positive reactions are relatively rare but can occur if a patient has syphilis, infectious mononucleosis, systemic lupus erythematosus, or rheumatoid arthritis. Serum from Lyme disease pa-tients is sometimes reactive in specific treponemal an-tibody tests but is consistently negative for the nontre-ponemal (VDRL) tests. In the absence of the hallmark skin rash or with an unclear clinical presentation, lab-oratory serologic testing assumes a vital role in estab-lishing or confirming the diagnosis.

Differential Diagnosis

Like syphilis, Lyme disease produces such a di-verse number of clinical symptoms that a textbook of general internal medicine should be consulted for a detailed account of differential diagnosis. Patients with Lyme disease are usually distinguished by their characteristic skin lesions and diagnostic serologic changes. Distinctions must be made from syphilis, rheumatoid arthritis, and chronic fatigue syndrome, which produce similar symptoms.

Prevention

Avoiding *Borrelia*-infected ticks or tick-infested areas guarantees protection against Lyme disease. For those living in areas where the infection is endemic, a few simple precautions help minimize possible expo-sure. These include wearing clothing that fully pro-tects the body and using repellents that contain deet (diethyltoluamide). If a tick does attach to the skin, careful removal with tweezers shortly after it attaches followed by application of alcohol or another suitable disinfectant makes borrelial transmission unlikely.

Considerable attention is being paid to the develop-ment of a vaccine for Lyme disease. A canine vaccine consisting of whole inactivated organisms (bacterin) has existed for a few years, whereas those being de-veloped for humans consist of recombinant outer sur-face proteins of *B burgdorferi*. One such vaccine is now undergoing phase I and phase II clinical trials, and other prototypes for both humans and dogs are in the early developmental or testing stages.

Treatment & Prognosis

Early disease is adequately treated with a 2–3 week course of penicillin or tetracycline. Later complica-tions such as arthritis and the neuropathies may re-quire more intense and prolonged antibiotic therapy. There are, however, some concerns regarding the uni-versal efficacy of treatment. Despite the use of very aggressive and repeated antibiotic therapy, there are reports of some patients with persisting Lyme dis-ease-like symptoms, indicating that irreversible dam-age may have occurred in a manner analogous to late-stage syphilis. It is unclear whether this phenomenon is due at least in part to persistence of pathogenic *Borrelia*, possibly because of antibiotic resistance.

RELAPSING-FEVER BORRELIOSIS

Relapsing fever is an acute febrile disease of worldwide distribution and is caused by arthropod-borne spirochetes belonging to the genus *Borrelia*. Two major forms of this illness are louse-borne relapsing fever (for which humans are the reservoir and the body louse, *Pediculus humanus*, is the vector) and tick-borne relapsing fever (for which rodents and other small animals are the major reservoirs and ticks of the genus *Ornithodorus* are the vectors). *B recurrentis* causes louse-borne relapsing fever and is transmitted from human to human following the ingestion of infected human blood by the louse and release of newly acquired organisms onto the skin or mucous membranes of a new host. The disease is endemic in parts of central and east Africa and South America. The causative organisms of tick-borne relapsing fever are numerous and include *B hermsii*, *B turicatae*, and *B parkeri* in North America; *B hispanica* in Spain; *B duttonii* in east Africa; and *B persica* in Asia. Ticks become infectious by biting and sucking blood from a spirochetemic animal. The infection is transmitted to humans or animals when saliva is released by a feeding tick through bites or penetration of intact skin.

After an individual has been exposed to an infected louse or tick, *Borrelia* organisms penetrate the skin and enter the bloodstream and lymphatic system. After a 1–3 week incubation period, spirochetes replicate in the blood, and an acute onset occurs of shaking chills, fever, headache, and fatigue. Concentrations of *Borrelia* can reach as high as 10^8 spirochetes/mL of blood, and these are clearly visible after staining blood smears with Giemsa or Wright's stain. During febrile disease, *Borrelia* organisms are present in the patient's blood but disappear prior to afebrile episodes and subsequently return to the bloodstream during the next febrile period. Jaundice can develop in some severely ill patients as a result of intrahepatic obstruction of bile flow and hepatocellular inflammation; if left untreated, patients can die from damage to the liver, spleen, or brain. The majority of untreated patients, however, recover spontaneously. They produce borrelial antibodies that have agglutinating, complement-fixing, borreliacidal, and immobilizing capabilities and that render patients immune to reinfection with the same *Borrelia* serotype. Serologic tests designed to measure these antibodies are of limited diagnostic value because of antigenic variation among strains and the coexistence of mixed populations of *Borrelia* within a given host during the course of a single infection. Diagnosis in the majority of cases requires demonstration of spirochetemia in febrile patients.

LEPTOSPIROSIS

Leptospirosis is an acute, febrile disease caused by various serotypes of *Leptospira*. Often referred to as Weil's disease, infection with *Leptospira interrogans* causes diseases that are extremely varied in their clinical presentations and that are also found in a variety of wild and domestic animals. Transmission to humans occurs primarily after contact with contaminated urine from leptospiruric animals. In the USA, dogs are the major reservoir for exposure of humans to this disease. After entering the body through the mucosal surface or breaks in the skin, leptospiral bacteria cause an acute illness characterized by fever, chills, myalgias, severe headaches, conjunctival suffuseness, and gastrointestinal problems. Most human infections are mild and anicteric, although in a small proportion of victims, severe icteric disease can occur and be fatal, primarily owing to renal failure and damage to small blood vessels. After infection of the kidneys, leptospiras are excreted in the urine. Liver dysfunction with hepatocellular damage and jaundice is common. Antibiotic treatment is curative if begun during early disease, but its value thereafter is questionable.

Diagnosis of leptospirosis depends on either seroconversion or the demonstration of spirochetes in clinical specimens. The macroscopic slide agglutination test, which uses formalized antigen, offers safe and rapid antibody screening. Measurement of antibody for a specific serotype, however, is performed with the very sensitive microscopic agglutination test involving live organisms. This method provides the most specific reaction with the highest titer and fewer cross-reactions. Agglutinating IgM-class-specific antibodies are produced during early infection and persist in high titers for many months. Protective and agglutinating antibodies often persist in sera of convalescent patients and may be associated with resistance to future infections.

REFERENCES

GENERAL

Barbour AG: Laboratory aspects of Lyme borreliosis. *Clin Microbiol Rev* 1988;**1**:399.

Benach JL, Bosler EM (editors): Lyme disease and related disorders. *Ann NY Acad Sci* 1988;**539**:1.

Schell RF, Musher DM (editors): *Pathogenesis and Immunology of Treponemal Infections.* Marcel Dekker, 1983.

Sigal LH (editor): National Clinical Conference on Lyme Disease. *Am J Med* 1995;**98**(4A):S1.

SYPHILIS

Baseman JB et al: Virulence determinants among the spirochetes. In: *Microbiology—1979.* Schlessinger D (editor). American Society for Microbiology, 1979, p 203.

Baughn RE et al: Detection of circulating immune complexes in the sera of rabbits with experimental syphilis: Possible role in immunoregulation. *Infect Immun* 1980;**29**:575.

Bryceson AD: Clinical pathology of the Jarisch-Herxheimer reaction. *J Infect Dis* 1976;**133**:696.

Hanff PA et al: Humoral immune response in human syphilis to polypeptides of *Treponema pallidum. J Immunol* 1982;**129**:1287.

Lukehart SA et al: Invasion of the central nervous system by *Treponema pallidum:* Implications for diagnosis and treatment. *Ann Intern Med* 1988;**109**:855.

Pavia CS, Niederbuhl CJ: Acquired resistance and expression of a protective humoral immune response in guinea pigs infected with *Treponema pallidum* Nichols. *Infect Immun* 1985;**50**:66.

Pavia CS, Niederbuhl CJ: Adoptive transfer of antisyphilis immunity with lymphocytes from *Treponema pallidum*-infected guinea pigs. *J Immunol* 1985;**135**:2829.

Pavia CS et al: Cell-mediated immunity during syphilis: A review. *Br J Vener Dis* 1978;**54**:144.

Schell RF et al: Endemic syphilis: Passive transfer of resistance with serum and cells in hamsters. *J Infect Dis* 1979;**140**:378.

LYME DISEASE

Barbour AG, Heiland RA, Howe TR: Heterogeneity of major proteins of Lyme disease borreliae: A molecular analysis of North American and European isolates. *J Infect Dis* 1985;**152**:478.

Benach JL et al: Interactions of phagocytes with the Lyme disease spirochete: Role of the Fc receptor. *J Infect Dis* 1984;**150**:497.

Dressler F et al: Western blotting in the serodiagnosis of Lyme disease. *J Infect Dis* 1993;**167**:392.

Ma J et al: Impact of the saponin adjuvant QS-21 and aluminum hydroxide on the immunogenicity of recombinant OspA and OspB of *Borrelia burgdorferi. Vaccines* 1994;**12**:925.

Magnarelli LA: Quality of Lyme disease tests. *JAMA* 1989;**262**:3464.

Magnarelli LA: Cross-reactivity in serological tests for Lyme disease and other spirochetal infections. *J Infect Dis* 1987;**156**:183.

Sadziene A et al: In vitro inhibition of *Borrelia burgdorferi* growth by antibodies. *J Infect Dis* 1993;**167**:165.

Schwartz I et al: Diagnosis of early Lyme disease by polymerase chain reaction amplication and culture of skin biopsies from erythema migrans lesions. *J Clin Microbiol* 1992;**30**:3082.

Steere AC: Lyme disease. *N Engl J Med* 1989;**321**:586.

Steere AC et al: The spirochetal etiology of Lyme disease. *N Engl J Med* 1983;**308**:733.

LEPTOSPIROSIS

Adler B, Faine S: The antibodies involved in the human immune response to leptospiral infection. *J Med Microbiol* 1978;**11**:387.

Alexander AD: Serological diagnosis of leptospirosis. In: *Manual of Clinical Laboratory Immunology,* 3rd ed. Rose NR et al (editors). American Society for Microbiology, 1986, p 435.

RELAPSING FEVER BORRELIOSIS

Meier JT et al: Antigenic variation is associated with DNA rearrangements in a relapsing fever *Borrelia. Cell* 1985;**41**:403.

Southern PM, Sanford JP: Relapsing fever: A clinical and microbiological review. *Medicine* 1969;**48**:129.

53

Virus Infections of the Immune System

Suzanne Crowe, MBBS, FRACP, & John Mills, MD

Although measles virus infection has been recognized for decades as a cause of immunosuppression, Epstein-Barr virus (EBV) was the first pathogen shown to cause immune dysfunction as a result of directly infecting cells of the immune system. Since then, other viruses, especially herpesviruses and retroviruses, have been identified that can infect cells of the immune system and produce immune suppression, immune stimulation, or both. The discovery of the human immunodeficiency virus (HIV), which primarily infects immune cells, has provided additional impetus for understanding the mechanisms by which virus infection results in immune dysfunction.

HUMAN IMMUNODEFICIENCY VIRUS

Major Immunologic Features

- CD4 cells of the immune system, including T lymphocytes, monocyte–macrophages, follicular dendritic cells, and Langerhans' cells, are infected.
- Infection causes progressive global defects of humoral and cell-mediated immunity.
- CD4 (helper/inducer) T lymphocytes are depleted.
- There is polyclonal activation of B lymphocytes with increased immunoglobulin production.
- Disease progresses despite vigorous humoral and cell-mediated responses to the virus.

General Considerations

The acquired immune deficiency syndrome (AIDS) was first recognized in 1981. The identification of HIV as the causative agent of AIDS in 1983–1984 was rapidly followed by characterization of this virus and the target cells that it infects and by elucidation of the multiple consequences of infection. Epidemiologic studies have identified the major populations at risk of acquiring infection and the routes by which the virus can be transmitted. The clinical illnesses associated with HIV infection have been classified, and therapeutic strategies to treat or suppress them have

been designed. By 1985, diagnostic kits had been developed for the detection of antibody to HIV, potentially therapeutic compounds were being screened for in vitro activity against this virus, and clinical trials for safety and efficacy of these potential drugs had begun. In 1987, only 6 years after the initial recognition of the AIDS epidemic and 3 years after identification of the etiologic agent, zidovudine (2'-azido-3'-deoxythymidine [AZT]), the first antiretroviral agent, was licensed by the US Food and Drug Administration for treatment of HIV infection.

Infection with HIV results in an acquired defect in immune function, especially involving cell-mediated immunity. Infected individuals may be asymptomatic or have progressive disease associated with recurrent opportunistic infections, certain cancers, severe weight loss, and central nervous system degeneration.

The recognition of the viral etiology of AIDS has stimulated immunologists to investigate the pathogenesis of the disease. Rational development of effective antiretroviral compounds can be aided by knowledge of the mechanisms by which HIV can damage the immune system. Although research on HIV has probably provided us with more pathogenetic information than we have on any other virus, the genesis of the characteristic and profound immune dysfunction caused by HIV still remains incompletely understood.

Etiology

A. Virology: HIV is a member of the retrovirus family, a group of enveloped viruses possessing the enzyme reverse transcriptase. This enzyme allows the virus to synthesize a DNA copy of its RNA genome. HIV was previously termed *human T-lymphotrophic virus type III* (HTLV-III), *lymph-adenopathy-associated virus* (LAV), and *AIDS-related virus* (ARV). Molecular characterization of these retroviruses demonstrated their relatedness, however and they are regarded as variants of the same virus. HIV has been subclassified within the lentivirus family, a group of nontransforming retroviruses with a long latency pe-

Table 53–1. Classification of retroviruses.

Oncoviruses	Lentiviruses	Spumiviruses
Avian retroviruses	Visna/maedi virus	Human foamy virus
Bovine leukemia virus	Caprine arthritis encephalitis virus	Simian foamy virus
Murine retroviruses	Equine infectious anemia virus	
Feline leukemia virus	HIV-1 and HIV-2	
HTLV-I and HTLV-II	Simian immunodeficiency virus	

Abbreviations: HTLV = human T-cell leukemia virus; HIV = human immunodeficiency virus.

riod from infection to the onset of clinical features similar morphologic features, and nucleotide sequence homology. Other members of the lentivirus family include visna and caprine arthritis–encephalitis viruses, which cause chronic, progressive neurodegenerative disease in sheep and goats, respectively. The clinical picture of lentivirus infection in sheep and goats is fairly similar to that resulting from HIV infection in humans and is characterized by a slow and progressive disorder of the immune system and the brain. HIV is also closely related to simian immunodeficiency virus (SIV), which causes an AIDS-like illness in macaque monkeys. There are two subtypes of HIV: HIV-1 is most prevalent in central Africa, USA, Europe, and Australia, and HIV-2 is found in west Africa, parts of Europe, and less commonly elsewhere. At the molecular level, HIV-2 more closely resembles SIV, supporting data that suggest that HIV originated from primate lentiviruses. When compared with HIV-1, HIV-2 has a longer clinical latency period from the time of infection to the development of symptoms and has a lower rate of vertical transmission (Table 53–1; Fig 53–1).

B. Genomic Organization: HIV consists of an inner core, containing an RNA genome, surrounded by a lipid envelope. The HIV genome (Fig 53–2) contains the standard retroviral structural genes, *env, gag,* and *pol,* encoding the viral envelope proteins, viral core protein, and viral enzymes (reverse transcriptase, integrase, and proteinase), respectively. HIV and SIV possess at least six other genes, a feature that makes them unique among retroviruses. Many of these gene products are made as precursor proteins, which must be cleaved by viral proteinases or cellular enzymes later in the replicative cycle. Within the DNA provirus, the viral genes are flanked by long terminal repeats (LTR) at both the 5′ and the 3′ ends. The LTR contains enhancer and promoter elements, which are necessary for transcription. HIV is initially transcribed into a full-length messenger ribonucleic acid (mRNA), which is translated into the structural Gag and Pol proteins. Production of singly and multiply spliced mRNA is necessary for the synthesis of the envelope proteins and accessory proteins, respectively.

The first of the additional gene products to be recognized was the transactivating protein Tat, a positive-feedback regulator of HIV replication, which can accelerate viral protein production by several thousandfold. Tat-binding protein, a cellular protein, attaches to Tat and thereby can modify its function. Current data suggest that Tat can act via TAR (transactivating response) structures within the LTR at both the DNA and RNA levels. The *rev* gene encodes proteins that regulate viral mRNA expression. The Rev protein permits unspliced mRNA to leave the nucleus

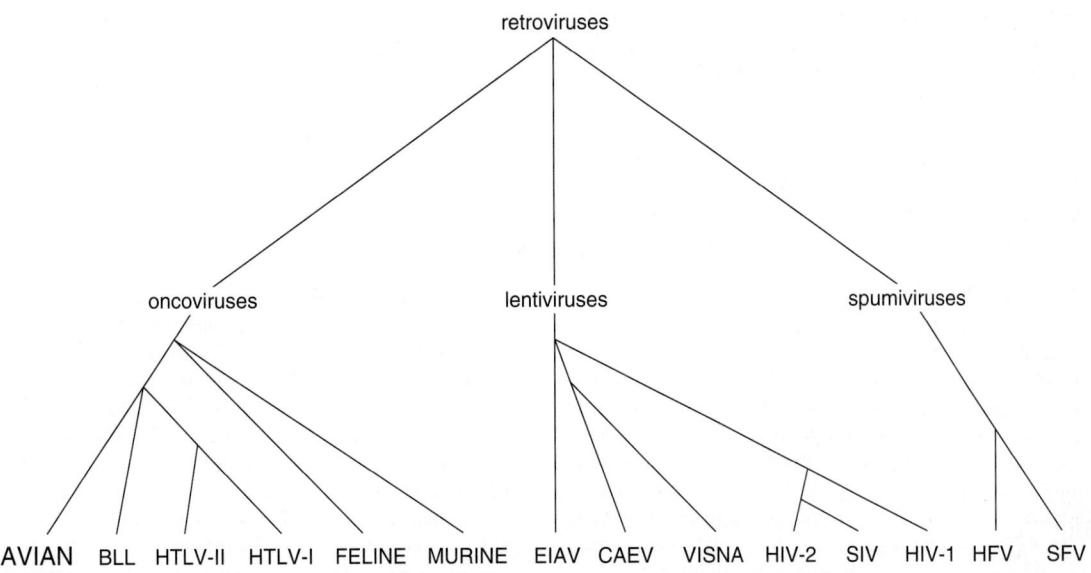

Figure 53–1. Schematic evolutionary relationships among retroviruses.

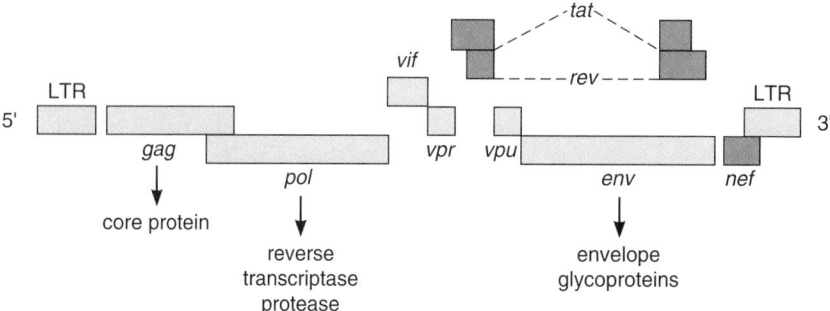

Figure 53–2. Genomic organization of HIV. The 9.6-kb genome of HIV consists of both structural and regulatory sequences (see text for details). HIV has a far more complex genome than that of many other retroviruses.

and thus inhibits transcription of the regulatory genes while enhancing expression of the viral structural genes. Rev protein binds to the Rev-responsive element (RRE), an RNA structure found in all mRNA species that are unspliced. The product of the virion infectivity gene, *vif*, increases viral infectivity and may be responsible for the efficient cell-to-cell transmission observed with HIV. The complete function of the *nef* gene is still being evaluated. It is now clear that Nef modulates cell function and HIV replication. This protein enhances HIV replication, possibly by increasing the activity of nuclear factor kappa B (NFκB) and down-modulating CD4 and IL-2 receptors on the surface of T cells. It also interacts with important cell-signaling proteins, including Lck, Hck, Fyn, and p53. The role of Nef in HIV pathogenesis is clear from experiments both in macaques, in which *nef*-deleted strains of SIV were less pathogenic than wild-type virus, and from data regarding a cohort of HIV-infected long-term nonprogressors who were all infected with a strain of HIV-1 that has deletions in the *nef* region. Two further genes have been described: the *vpr* (viral protein R) gene, and the *vpu* (viral protein U) gene *vpr* is considered to play a role in the regulation of viral and cellular gene expression and may be important in viral assembly and infection of macrophages. It may also induce apoptosis. *vpu* influences release of HIV from the cell surface and contributes to CD4 degradation within the endoplasmic reticulum (see Fig 53–2).

C. Pathogenesis of Infection: HIV infection affects predominantly the immune system and the brain. The dominant immunologic feature of HIV infection is progressive depletion of the CD4 (helper/inducer) subset of T lymphocytes, thereby reversing the normal CD4:CD8 ratio and inexorably causing immunodeficiency. The depletion of CD4 lymphocytes is predominantly due to the tropism of HIV for these and other CD4-bearing cells because the CD4 cell surface molecule functions as a receptor for the virus. The CD4 lymphocyte is necessary for the proper functioning of the immune system. It interacts with antigen-presenting cells, B cells, cytotoxic T cells,

and natural killer (NK) cells (see Chapter 9). Thus, it is easy to see that infection and depletion of this cell population could induce profound immunodeficiency. Early in situ hybridization studies suggested that only very few (about 1 in 10,000) CD4 lymphocytes contain replicating HIV. More recently, studies of peripheral blood lymphocytes have demonstrated that up to 1 in 10 of these cells are infected with HIV, particularly in persons with advanced disease. Although the data are limited, the number of infected cells in tissues appears to be larger than that in peripheral blood.

The finding that the CD4 molecule is present on cells other than helper/inducer T lymphocytes was accompanied by evidence that HIV could infect other cell populations that expressed this molecule on their surface. Other cells susceptible to HIV infection include monocyte–macrophages, microglial cells, Langerhans' cells, follicular dendritic cells, and immortalized B cells. Other molecules, including Fc receptors, complement receptors, adhesion molecules such as leukocyte functional antigen 1 (LFA-1), and galactosyl ceramide receptor, may act as accessory receptors for HIV on some cell types, such as macrophages, fibroblasts, brain astrocytes and oligodendrocytes, and certain gastrointestinal tract cells. Dendritic cells in the blood can transmit HIV infection to T lymphocytes. It is controversial as to whether or not these dendritic cells are susceptible to HIV infection. Although HIV infection of macrophages and T lymphocytes has been clearly demonstrated in vivo, there is less conclusive evidence that blood dendritic cells, Langerhans' cells, CD34 stem cells, or B lymphocytes are infected in vivo (Table 53–2). Monocyte–macrophages are thought to provide a major reservoir for HIV in vivo and may contribute to the pathogenesis of the immune deficiency by functioning abnormally. For example, HIV-infected monocyte–macrophages secrete an inhibitor of interleukin 1 (IL-1), a cytokine of major importance in T-cell proliferative responses, and HIV-infected macrophages poorly phagocytose organisms such as *Candida albicans* (see Chapter 10). Although the pathogenesis of immune dysfunction associated with HIV infection is incompletely understood, it is likely that the process

Table 53–2. Cells infected by HIV.

CD4 T lymphocytes
Monocyte–macrophages
Follicular dendritic cells
Langerhans' cells
Microglial cells
Immortalized B cells
Retinal cells
Colonic mucosal cells
Endothelial cells in brain

occurs through collective dysfunction of both antigen-presenting cells, such as macrophages, and T lymphocytes, especially the CD4 subset.

The loss of CD4 lymphocytes, which is characteristic of HIV infection, may occur as a result of a number of possible mechanisms. These include the death of uninfected CD4 T cells as a result of cell fusion with HIV-infected cells, the development of pores in the cell membrane of the infected lymphocyte as HIV buds from the cell surface, the accumulation of unintegrated viral DNA within the cell cytoplasm, and the killing of both uninfected CD4 T cells (innocent bystanders) which have found free HIV envelope glycoprotein gp120 and HIV-infected cells expressing gp120 by gp120-specific clones of cytotoxic lymphocytes. Recently, apoptosis, or programmed cell death, has been implicated in the depletion of CD4 T lymphocytes. HIV enters the cell through a specific interaction between the V1 region of the CD4 molecule on the cell surface and a specific region within the HIV envelope glycoprotein. Whether HIV is able to infect macrophages or lymphocytes (cell tropism) is determined largely by the amino acid sequence of the HIV envelope. The binding of the gp120 to CD4 results in exposure of the transmembrane protein, gp41, facilitating virus-cell fusion and viral entry. A chemokine receptor, CCR5, facilitates entry into lymphoid cells that coexpress CD4. Other receptors for other chemokines may also play roles in the early phases of HIV-cellular interaction and life cycle. HIV replication within monocyte–macrophages occurs at a leisurely pace compared with that within lymphocytes, with little cytopathology, supporting their role as a viral reservoir in vivo. Resting T lymphocytes can also be infected with HIV, but the virus replication cycle is blocked at the reverse transcription step. If the cell is activated within a few days, infectious virus is produced; otherwise, the infection is aborted. Thus resting or nonactivated lymphocytes provide an additional reservoir of HIV in infected persons. The factors that trigger latently infected cells to produce virus are not completely known. A number of intracellular and viral factors can influence the production of HIV. These include cellular transcription factors such as the DNA-binding protein NFκB, as well as cytokines, including tumor necrosis factor alpha (TNFα) and the colony-stimulating factors GM-CSF and M-CSF, which have been found to augment HIV replication. A number of

viruses (herpes simplex virus, cytomegalovirus, adenovirus, human T-lymphotropic virus type I, Epstein-Barr virus, and hepatitis B virus) stimulate HIV replication in vitro, but these findings have not been substantiated clinically. In addition, HIV regulatory genes themselves can influence viral production.

Recent data show that from the time of infection there is production of huge numbers of virions per day, with rapid turnover of both HIV virions (half-life approximately 8 hours) as well as infected T cells (half-life less than 2 days). Although the level of HIV RNA in plasma may be low during the time of clinical latency, limited data suggest that there is considerable production of virus in tissues, particularly in the lymph nodes.

Early in infection, when the individual is asymptomatic, macrophagetropic strains of HIV are isolated predominantly from peripheral blood. At this stage, the virus generally does not produce the characteristic cytopathology of multinucleated giant cells or syncytia in cell culture and is described as nonsyncytium-inducing (NSI). A change in viral phenotype from NIS to syncytium-inducing (SI) occurs at approximately the same time as decline in CD4 numbers and the onset of HIV-related clinical disease. The tropism of the viral strains also broadens to include T lymphocytes and other cell populations as disease progresses. Another major feature of HIV infection in involvement of the central nervous system. The clinical findigns range from minor memory defects to personality changes to progressive, fatal dementia. The mechanism of brain damage is obscure. As there is no evidence to support direct neuronal infection with HIV, it is more likely that soluble factors such as quinolinic acid or TNFα secreted by infected cells that transport the virus to the brain may alter the function of neurons and contribute to the dementia. In infected brain tissue, HIV has been detected in multinucleated giant cells composed predominantly of monocyte–macrophages, and in microglia, suggesting a major pathogenetic role for these cells. An alternative hypothesis is that HIV may competitively inhibit neuroleukin from binding to neurons. This neurotrophic factor shares homology with a conserved region of the HIV envelope glycoprotein, gp 120.

Epidemiology

HIV infection and AIDS are recognized as a major global health problem. Cases of AIDS have now been reported in all countries. In the USA, Europe, and Australia, transmission of HIV has been documented to occur via sexual contact, administration of infected blood or blood products, artificial insemination with infected semen, exposure to blood-containing needles or syringes, and transmission from an infected mother to her fetus or to the infant during or after birth. Homosexual activity accounts for the majority of sexually transmitted cases in these countries, although transmission among injecting drug users or their sexual

Table 53–3. Individuals at risk of HIV infection.

High risk
Homosexual and bisexual men
Injecting drug users who share needles or syringes
Sexual partners of people in high-risk groups
Children born to infected mothers
Low risk
Health care workers, including nurses, doctors, dentists,
and laboratory staff

partners is of increasing importance in many parts of the world. Male-to-female transmission is more commonly reported than female-to-male transmission. HIV has been detected in up to 30% of seminal and vaginal fluid specimens from HIV-infected persons. Transmission from mother to offspring occurs by transplacental passage of the virus at the time of delivery, in utero or, through breast feeding, with estimates for the prevalence of transmission of HIV from an infected mother to her child varying from 15 to 30%. The diagnosis of HIV in a neonate can be difficult (see the section on neonatal diagnosis). Following the introduction of programs to exclude blood donors who are members of high-risk groups and the serologic testing of donated blood, the risk of acquiring HIV from infected blood or blood products has been virtually eliminated. Thus, the groups presently at highest risk are homosexual and bisexual men, injecting drug users who share needles or syringes, sexual partners of people in high-risk groups, and children born to infected mothers (Table 53–3). Health care workers are at risk of HIV infection, but this risk is considered to be very low (approximately 1:250 HIV-positive needle stick exposures results in infection). Epidemiologic data do not support transmission of HIV by casual contact, insects, or sharing of utensils (tableware, toothbrushes, etc). There are no data to suggest aerosolized transmission of the virus. HIV can be detected in less than 10% of saliva samples from HIV-infected persons, at extremely low titer (less than one infectious particle per milliliter). Similarly, urine, feces, sweat, tears and amniotic fluid are considered unlikely to transmit HIV because of their extremely low viral titers.

In central and western Africa, cases of AIDS are equally distributed among men and women, and heterosexual transmission (especially from infected female prostitutes to their clients) is through to account for the majority of cases. In Africa, risk factors associated with HIV infection in heterosexuals include large numbers of sexual partners, prostitution, sex with prostitutes, a history of sexually transmitted disease such as a gonorrhea or syphilis, and genital ulceration of any cause. Although both bowel mucosa and cervical epithelium can be infected with HIV, the chance of infection is markedly increased if abrasions or ulceration are present. Other risk factors include multiple use of needles or syringes in health clinics and ritualistic practices in which unsterilized instruments are used; these include scarification, tattooing, and ear-piercing.

Exposure to HIV does not always result in infection. One exposure may be sufficient to cause infection, however, depending on inoculum size, route of entry, and perhaps, host factors. The dose to infect 50% of exposed individuals (ID_{50}) is not known for humans, but it is presumed to be low (less than 10–100 virions). Both cell-free and cell-associated viruses are infectious. About 50% of HIV-infected individuals will contract AIDS over 10- to 12-year period from the time of infection. The latency period (from time of infection to onset of disease) may vary according to viral inoculum, virulence of the infecting strain, route of entry, and age of the patient.

Clinical Features

A. Acute HIV mononucleosis: Following infection with HIV, an individual may remain asymptomatic or develop an acute illness that resembles infectious mononucleosis. This syndrome usually occurs within 2–6 weeks after infection, with reported periods ranging from 5 days to 3 months. The predominant symptoms are fever, headache, sore throat, malaise, and rash. Clinical findings include pharyngitis (which may be exudative and may be accompanied by mucosal ulceration); generalized lymphadenopathy; a macular or urticarial rash on the face, trunk, and limbs; and hepatosplenomegaly (Table 53–4). During the acute illness, antibodies to HIV are generally undetectable. Although the illness is often severely incapacitating, requiring bedrest or even hospitalization, some individuals experience only mild symptoms and do not seek medical attention.

Acute infection with HIV has also been associated with neurologic disease, including meningitis, encephalitis, cranial nerve palsies, myopathy, and peripheral neuropathy. These findings are usually accompanied by features of the acute HIV mononucleosis syndrome.

B. Symptomatic HIV Infection: There has recently been a change in nomenclature for HIV-associated disease. Conditions previously referred to as *AIDS-related complex* (*ARC*), are now mostly considered under the more general heading of symptomatic HIV infection without an AIDS-defining illness. The development of HIV-related symptoms is regarded as evidence of progressive immune dysfunction. Constitutional symptoms and signs include persistent fever, night sweats, weight loss (but insufficient weight loss to fulfil the Centers for Disease Control

Table 53–4. Clinical features of acute HIV infection.

Fever and sweats
Myalgia and arthralgia
Malaise and lethargy
Lymphadenopathy and splenomegaly
Pharyngitis
Anorexia, nausea, and vomiting
Headaches and photophobia
Macular rash

and Prevention [CDC] criteria for AIDS) unexplained chronic diarrhea, eczema, psoriasis, seborrheic dermatitis, herpes zoster, oral candidiasis, and oral hairy leukoplakia. The latter two conditions are regarded as poor prognostic indicators and herald progression to AIDS. HIV-related thrombocytopenia (defined as a platelet count of <50,000/μL without other known causes) is found in less than 10% of individuals and usually does not result in a bleeding diathesis.

C. AIDS: The criteria for diagnosis of AIDS have been defined by the CDC and comprise certain opportunistic infections and cancers, HIV-related encephalopathy, HIV-induced wasting syndrome, and a broader range of AIDS-indicative diseases in individuals who have laboratory evidence of HIV infection. The CDC has now altered the definition to include adults and adolescents with diagnosed HIV infection who have a CD4 lymphocyte count of less than 200 cells/μL of blood or a CD4 T-lymphocyte level of less than 14% regardless of clinical symptoms. In addition, pulmonary tuberculosis, recurrent bacterial pneumonia, and invasive cervical cancer have been added to the list of AIDS-defining conditions.

The most common opportunistic infections encountered are *Pneumocystis carinii* pneumonitis; disseminated cryptococcosis; toxoplasmosis; mycobacterial disease (both *Mycobacterium avium* complex infection and tuberculosis); chronic, ulcerative, recurrent herpes simplex virus infection; disseminated cytomegalovirus infection; and histoplasmosis (Table 53–5). Patients with AIDS also have a higher incidence of *Salmonella* bacteremia, staphylococcal infections, and pneumococcal pneumonia. Children with AIDS may develop opportunistic infections such as *P carinii* pneumonia, but they have a higher incidence of lymphocytic interstitial pneumonitis and recurrent bacterial infections than adults do.

The most common cancer diagnosed in AIDS patients is Kaposi's sarcoma, a neoplasm or neoplasm-like disease involving endothelia and mesenchymal stroma. Once common, this tumor is now less frequently seen as a presenting illness. The reason for this is obscure. Preliminary data suggest that a new herpes virus (HHV-8) is the etiologic agent of kaposis sarcoma. Late in the course of immune dysfunction, high-grade B-cell lymphomas are encountered; these are generally resistant to therapy.

Table 53–5. Common opportunistic infections encountered in AIDS patients.

Pneumocystis carinii pneumonia
Toxoplasmosis
Mycobacterium avium complex disease
Disseminated *Mycobacterium tuberculosis* infection
Persistent, ulcerative herpes simplex virus infection
Disseminated cytomegalovirus infection
Cryptococcal meningitis

Laboratory Diagnosis
A. Serology:
1. Seroconversion–During the early phase of the primary illness, antibodies to HIV are not detected in the serum; they generally appear 2–8 weeks after the onset of illness. IgM antibodies, detected by immunofluorescence, generally precede IgG antibody detection by Western immunoblot. During seroconversion, antibodies directed against the various viral proteins do not develop simultaneously. Those directed against HIV p24 (core) and gp41 (transmembrane) proteins can be detected before those directed at the *pol* gene products on Western blot. There may be a "window" period during which time the screening enzyme-linked immunosorbent assay (ELISA) is negative but antibodies can be demonstrated by Western blot. HIV antigenemia (predominantly HIV p24, measured by enzyme immunoassay) usually precedes seroconversion. Following the appearance of antibodies (specifically anti-HIV p24), HIV p24 antigen levels decline. They may later reappear, coincident with a loss of anti-HIV p24 antibody (Fig 53–3). Whereas about 70% of AIDS patients have detectable HIV antigen in their sera, the HIV antigen test is positive in fewer than 20% of asymptomatic individuals. The complexing of p24 antigen with specific antibody is largely responsible for the fluctuation of antigen titer during the course of disease. Newer methods to detect p24 antigen by ELISA involve an acid dissociation technique to remove the antigen from antibody. African patients rarely have detectable HIV antigenemia, perhaps owing to higher antibody levels. Persistence of HIV antigen following the acute infection in an asymptomatic carrier is probably associated with a more rapid progression to symptomatic disease.

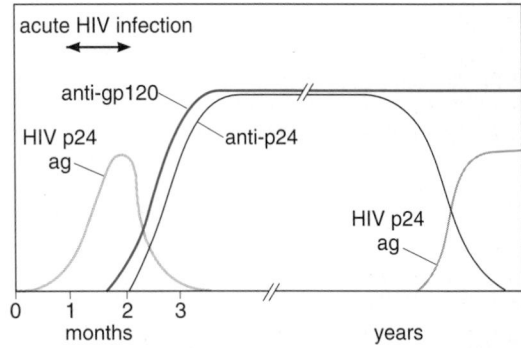

Figure 53–3. Common pattern of serologic response following HIV infection. p24 antigen (p24 ag) may be first detected during the acute HIV mononucleosis phase of infection. The initial antibody to appear in the serum is usually that directed against the HIV envelope glycoprotein gp120 (anti-gp120), and its level remains elevated throughout the course of the disease. Antibody directed against the core protein (anti-p24) appears in the serum coincident with the decline in p24 antigen levels.

By using sensitive methods of detection (eg, polymerase chain reaction [PCR]), HIV can be identified in the peripheral blood mononuclear cells and plasma of virtually all infected persons, regardless of the stage of disease. Quantitative RT (reverse transcriptase)-PCR and branched-chain DNA assays are used to quantify HIV RNA. High levels at the time of seroconversion (>100,000 RNA copies/mL of plasma) predict rapid disease progression. Lower levels of HIV RNA are usually present in blood following HIV seroconversion, remaining low during the asymptomatic phase of infection. As disease progresses and immune function declines, there is an increase in viral load.

2. Screening for HIV–ELISA is the basic screening test currently used to detect antibodies to HIV. Purified native or recombinant virion proteins are immobilized on plastic beads or multiwell trays. Test serum containing antibodies to HIV bind to these viral proteins. An enzyme-linked antihuman antibody added to the reaction binds to the complex and is detected colorimetrically. The ELISA is both highly sensitive (>99%) and highly specific (>99% in high-risk populations). The genomic diversity between HIV-1 and HIV-2 is greatest within the envelope region. As there is significant homology between the *gag* and *pol* gene products of the subtypes of HIV, HIV-2 can usually be detected by HIV-1 ELISAs. The sensitivity of HIV-1 ELISA for HIV-2 is unacceptably low, however, and blood banks should now routinely screen for both HIV-1 and HIV-2 proteins to ensure detection.

3. Confirmatory Tests–A repeatedly reactive ELISA should be confirmed by either a Western blot or, less commonly, a radioimmune precipitation assay, immunofluorescence assay, or ELISA with recombinant antigens. Because of its high sensitivity, a negative ELISA does not usually warrant confirmatory testing. The Western blot detects specific antibodies directed against the various HIV proteins. Purified viral proteins are run on a polyacrylamide gel, transferred to a nitrocellulose membrane, and then reacted with the test serum. Antibodies to HIV present in the serum bind to the specific viral protein (Fig 53–4).

B. Neonatal Diagnosis: Neonates with HIV infection pose a difficult serodiagnostic problem because maternal IgG antibody crosses the placenta. Thus, the infant passively acquires anti-HIV antibody, which may persist for up to 15 months. The predictive value of specific IgM antibodies in the diagnosis of neonatal and perinatal infection awaits clarification. Culture of the virus from peripheral blood or tissue or demonstration of HIV antigen is therefore necessary to be confident of the diagnosis of HIV infection in asymptomatic infants born to HIV-infected mothers. The PCR, which amplifies HIV genome present in cells or serum, provides a useful adjunct to diagnosis.

Immunologic Findings

A. CD4 Lymphocyte Depletion: The immunologic hallmark of AIDS is a defect in cell-medi-

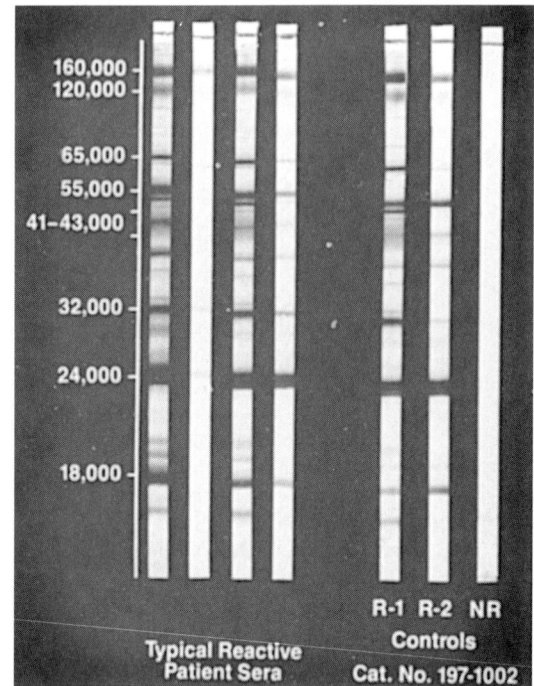

Figure 53–4. Western blot analysis. Reactive sera typically contain demonstrable antibodies to envelope proteins gp160, gp120, and gp41, as well as to core proteins p55 and p24 and to reverse transcriptase p32. Detection of antibody to p24 alone is insufficient to meet the diagnostic criteria for a positive Western blot and may be due to a nonspecific reaction. Alternatively, a reactive band at 24,000 may represent an early serologic response during seroconversion. (Photograph courtesy of Bio-Rad Laboratories, Richmond, CA)

ated immunity, characteristically associated with a decrease in the number and function of the CD4 T lymphocytes. CD4 T lymphocytes are functionally separated into the T_H1 subset, which produces interferon gamma and IL-2, and the T_H2 subset, which produces IL-4, IL-6, and IL-10. In advanced HIV infection, the TH_1 subset is markedly decreased in number.

There is a spectrum of CD4 cell numbers in all clinical stages of HIV infection: occasional asymptomatic individuals have very low counts, whereas rarely the values are normal in individuals with AIDS. Individuals who present with Kaposi's sarcoma frequently have higher CD4 cell counts than those who initially present with AIDS-defining opportunistic infections. This suggests that patients who present with opportunistic infections have more severe immunologic dysfunction than those with Kaposi's sarcoma. CD4 cell levels are of prognostic value: The risk of progression to AIDS in a given time interval increases as the CD4 count declines. The CD4 number can also provide a guide to the risk of development of individual opportunistic infections and malignancies (Fig 53–5). Not unexpectedly, certain infections with

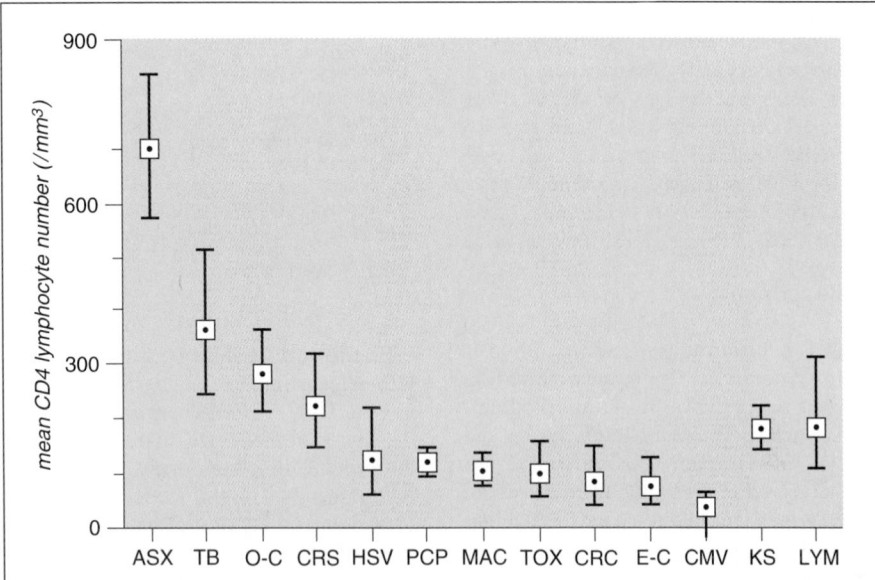

Figure 53–5. The mean CD4 lymphocyte numbers and approximately 95% confidence intervals for individuals with asymptomatic HIV infection, oral candidiasis, or AIDS-defining opportunistic infections or malignancies. Assessments were performed between 2 months preceding or 1 month following diagnosis of the illness, with 55% being determined at the time of diagnosis. A total of 307 events in 222 patients were examined. *Abbreviations:* ASX = asymptomatic infection; TB = disseminated tuberculosis; O-C = oral candidiasis; CRS = cryptosporidium; HSV = recurrent mucocutaneous herpes simplex virus; PCP = *P carinii* pneumonia; MAC = disseminated *M avium* complex; TOX = *T gondii* encephalitis; CRC = cryptococcal meningitis; EC = esophageal candidiasis; CMV = cytomegalovirus retinitis; KS = Kaposi's sarcoma; LYM = lymphoma. (Reproduced, with permission, from Crowe SM et al: Predictive value of CD4 lymphocyte numbers for the development of opportunistic infections and malignancies in HIV-infected persons. *J Acquired Immune Defic Syndr* 1991;**4**:770.)

organisms of high virulence (eg, *Mycobacterium tuberculosis*) are manifest when the CD4 count is well preserved, whereas others with organisms of lower virulence (eg *M avium* complex) tend to occur only when the CD4 number is much lower. In general the CD4 lymphocyte number is less than 200 cells/µL of blood at the time of AIDS diagnosis, and with the routine use of prophylaxis for common opportunistic infections and antiretroviral drugs, the CD4 number is in fact commonly lower than 100/µL at the onset of the first AIDS-defining illness.

The CD4:CD8 ratio invariably becomes inverted primarily as a consequence of CD4 lymphocyte depletion. A variety of other conditions, however, including infection with EBV, hepatitis B virus, and cytomegalovirus (CMV), can cause inversion of the CD4:CD8 ratio, primarily owing to an increase in the CD8 subset. Thus, this ratio is of no diagnostic value.

B. Abnormal Delayed-Type Hypersensitivity Responses: Delayed-type hypersensitivity responses are usually normal in the early phase of HIV infection and decreased or absent in patients with advanced disease.

C. T-Cell Proliferative Responses: The normal in vitro proliferative responses of CD4 T lymphocytes to soluble antigens (such as tetanus toxoid) and mitogens (such as concanavalin A, phytohemagglutinin, or pokeweed mitogen) are impaired in HIV-infected individuals, especially AIDS patients. This abnormality may be due to a selective loss of a subset of CD4 lymphocytes, to defective antigen presentation by monocyte–macrophages, or to direct viral suppression of CD4 lymphocyte function. Current evidence favors a functional defect of this cell population rather than an abnormality of antigen-presenting cells. Responses to mitogens tend to vary and are less severely impaired than responses to antigen. Antigen responses but not mitogen responses strictly require the interaction of the CD4 molecule on the surface of the lymphocyte with the class II major histocompatibility complex (MHC) molecule. The HIV envelope glycoprotein (gp120) binds to the CD4 molecule, and its presence could interfere with the interaction with the class II MHC molecule, thus explaining why mitogen responses are less impaired than antigen responses.

D. Cytotoxic Lymphocyte Responses: Cells infected with HIV provide a target for lysis by the various types of cytotoxic cells, including MHC-restricted cytotoxic lymphocytes, MHC-nonrestricted NK cells, and lymphokine-activated cells. Cytotoxic T lymphocyte (CD8 or CD4) responses and NK cell activity are present but quantitatively defective in cells from HIV-infected individuals with late stages of infection. Although the number of NK cells is relatively normal when compared with that in uninfected controls and binding of these cells to their target is unimpaired, their cytotoxic capacity is moderately diminished. Recent in vitro studies suggest that reduced NK activity may be restored by IL-12. Cytotoxic CD8 cells kills infected cells of the same class I MHC type that express HIV proteins (envelope, core, and some regulatory proteins). In addition to this cytotoxic role, CD8 lymphocytes can suppress HIV replication in CD4 lymphocytes.

E. B-Cell Responses:

1. Polyclonal B-cell activation resulting in hypergammaglobulinemia is commonly found in HIV-infected individuals, resulting predominantly in increases in serum IgG1, IgG3, and IgM levels. This spontaneous secretion of immunoglobulin by B cells is not always present, and in HIV-infected infants panhypogammaglobulinemia may occur.

2. Autoantibodies directed against erythrocytes, platelets, lymphocytes, neutrophils, nuclear proteins, myelin and spermatozoa have been found in patients infected with HIV. In some instances these have been associated with disease (eg, HIV-associated thrombocytopenia and peripheral neuropathy).

3. Antibody capable of neutralizing HIV in vitro is present in low titer in the sera of infected individuals. There is no evidence that this antibody has a protective role, however. Neutralizing antibody is directed against envelope and core proteins.

4. The enhancement of in vitro HIV infection by antibodies has been reported, although the in vivo significance of this phenomenon is uncertain. Antibody-enhanced viral uptake is mediated by Fc and complement receptors.

5. B-cell proliferative responses to T-cell-independent specific B-cell mitogens (such as formalinized *Staphylococcus aureus* Cowan 1 strain) are impaired.

6. Despite depression of helper T-cell function and abnormalities of humoral immunity, HIV-infected individuals at early stages of infection can often mount appropriate antibody responses to commonly used vaccines. A decrease in response to hepatitis B vaccine, pneumococcal vaccine, and influenza vaccine, however, is generally found as HIV disease progresses.

Controversy exists as to whether vaccination (pneumococcal, influenza, etc) increases the viral load in HIV-infected individuals whose immune function allows them to develop a specific response to the vaccine. Some recent studies (but not all) have found that vaccination of HIV-infected individuals, especially those with preserved CD4 counts, can increase HIV RNA in plasma for weeks to months following vaccination.

Table 53–6. Potential role of macrophages in the pathogenesis of AIDS.

Act as target for HIV
Provide reservoir for HIV
Contribute to immune deficiency through abnormal function
Defective phagocytosis
Defective chemotaxis
Defective antigen presentation
Abnormal cytokine production
Contribute to T-cell depletion through a cell fusion process[1]

[1] Shown in vitro only.

F. Monocyte–Macrophage Responses: The HIV-infected monocyte–macrophage is a major reservoir for HIV in vivo. There are conflicting data about the degree of monocyte–macrophage dysfunction and the specific functions that are altered as a result of HIV infection. Current evidence suggests that phagocytosis and killing of organisms, antigen presentation, and chemotaxis are moderately impaired. Infected macrophages produce an inhibitor of IL-1 termed contra-IL-1, which may contribute to the impairment of T-cell proliferative responses observed in HIV-infected individuals (Table 53–6).

G. Other Immunologic Responses: Other abnormal immunologic parameters include decreased lymphokine production (in particular, IL-2 and interferon gamma), decreased expression of IL-2 receptors, and an increase in the level of circulating immune complexes. Elevated serum levels of β_2-microglobulin and neopterin are of some prognostic importance in predicting progression to AIDS.

H. Hematologic Findings: Subjects with acute HIV mononucleosis generally have leukopenia with an atypical lymphocytosis. Transient thrombocytopenia occurs in some patients. With disease progression, the total leukocyte count falls, with an associated lymphopenia, reflecting depletion of CD4 lymphocytes. The hemoglobin and hematocrit decrease as a result of anemia due to chronic disease, the presence of an opportunistic infection, or related to therapy. Mild thrombocytopenia is common.

Differential Diagnosis

Acute HIV mononucleosis must be distinguished from infectious mononucleosis caused by EBV, CMV infection, and less commonly, rubella, secondary syphilis, hepatitis B, human herpesvirus type 6 infection, and toxoplasmosis (Table 53–7). Once there is evidence of immunodeficiency, it should be ascertained that this is an acquired rather than a congenital defect and that there is no other underlying explanation for the clinical and immunologic manifestations, such as hematologic cancer or tissue transplantation. However, any individual with laboratory-confirmed HIV infection and a definitively diagnosed disease that meets the CDC criteria for AIDS is considered to have AIDS, regardless of the presence of other potential causes of immune deficiency.

Table 53–7. Differential diagnosis of acute HIV infection.

EBV infectious mononucleosis
CMV infection
Rubella
Secondary syphilis
Hepatitis B
Toxoplasmosis
Human herpesvirus type 6

Abbreviations: HIV = human immunodeficiency virus; EBV = Epstein-Barr virus; CMV = cytomegalovirus.

Treatment

A. Life Cycle of HIV: The initial phase of the replicative cycle of HIV involves binding of specific epitopes of cell surface CD4 molecules to defined regions of virion gp120. Following this, HIV enters the cell and is uncoated. Viral RNA is then used as a template by reverse transcriptase to make a minus-strand DNA copy, thus forming an RNA–DNA hybrid. Soon thereafter, the RNA strand is degraded by the ribonuclease H activity of reverse transcriptase. A positive DNA strand is synthesized, and the linear double-stranded DNA molecule changes conformation to become circular. Some of this DNA migrates to the nucleus and subsequently becomes integrated into the cellular DNA to form the HIV provirus, through the action of the viral integrase. Further replication of HIV depends on changes within the cell that are only partly understood. Cellular transcription factors that bind to HIV LTR are dependent on the activation of the lymphocyte; differentiation of monocytes into macrophages is associated with increased replication of HIV; cytokines can influence HIV replication through the above mentioned mechanisms as well as by their independent activities. The replication cycle continues with the translation of viral genomic RNA and viral proteins from unspliced, singly spliced, and multiply spliced mRNA species. These proteins undergo posttranslational protein cleavage and glycosylation. Within the cytoplasm the final stage of assembly of viral proteins occurs and is followed by the budding of the mature virion through the cell membrane, with simultaneous acquisition of envelope (Fig 53–6).

B. Antiretroviral Therapy: The complicated machinery used by HIV in its replicative cycle has provided many specific target sites for potential intervention (Table 53–8). Because reverse transcriptase is not normally present in human cells, selective inhibitors of this enzyme have been a major focus of drug development. Zidovudine (AZT) is a thymidine analogue that requires phosphorylation by host nucleoside kinases to the triphosphate derivative within the infected cell for it to be active. Once phosphorylated, the drug inhibits the virus-encoded reverse transcriptase enzyme, since it has about 100 times the affinity for this enzyme as it does for the host DNA polymerase. Zidovudine further prevents HIV replication by becoming incorporated into the transcribed DNA strand and thus preventing further HIV DNA synthe-

sis. In clinical trials, individuals with symptomatic HIV infection treated with zidovudine have had lower mortality rates and less frequent opportunistic infections than those receiving placebo. In asymptomatic HIV-infected persons with a preserved CD4 count, studies to assess the use of zidovudine therapy have provided conflicting data. Many clinicians advocate initiation of antiviral therapy (usually with zidovudine) when the CD4 lymphocyte number falls below 500/mL. Commencement of antiretroviral therapy based on the plasma HIV RNA level rather than CD4 count, however, is likely to be a more useful guide in the future. During zidovudine therapy, CD4 lymphocytes initially increase in number but usually return to baseline levels within 6 months of the start of therapy. Zidovudine resistance develops over a similar period, but the precise clinical significance for this observation remains uncertain. Resistance is due to the development of mutations within the reverse transcriptase gene (codons 67, 70, 215, and 219; mutations in other amino acid positions have also been reported). Recent data from trials in the United States and in Europe and Australia show that zidovudine monotherapy is inferior to combination therapy using zidovudine with didanosine or zalcitabine.

Dideoxyinosine (ddI, didanosine) and dideoxycytidine (ddC, zalcitabine) are related nucleoside analogues with the same mechanism of action as zidovudine; they are licensed for the treatment of HIV-infected persons who are intolerant to or failing zidovudine therapy. Whereas the toxicity of zidovudine is predominantly hematologic (anemia and neutropenia), didanosine and zalcitabine may cause a peripheral neuropathy and pancreatitis. In vitro resistance to didanosine and zalcitabine has been reported but at a lower incidence than that to zidovudine. Lamivudine 2′-deoxy-3′-thiacytadine (3TC) is another related nucleoside analogue, which has only modest efficacy in the treatment of HIV infection when used as monotherapy. It has relatively few side effects. Resistance develops rapidly (within 12 weeks) of commencing lamivudine monotherapy, with the appearance of a mutation within codon 184. This drug has demonstrated considerable efficacy, however, when used in combination with zidovudine, and in many countries has been licensed for the treatment of HIV infection only in combination with other antiretroviral drugs. Stavudine 2′3′-didehydro-3′-deoxythymidine (d4T) another nucleoside analogue, is a potent inhibitor of HIV reverse transcriptase in vitro and is now licensed for use for the treatment of HIV infection in a number of countries. Peripheral neuropathy is the dose-limiting toxicity of this drug. Other reverse transcriptase inhibitors, such as the pyrophosphate analogue foscarnet, do not require cellular phosphorylation for activity and act directly on the enzyme. Second-site reverse transcriptase inhibitors (delavirdine, nevirapine, loviride) are currently being evaluated in clinical trials. The rapid emergence of

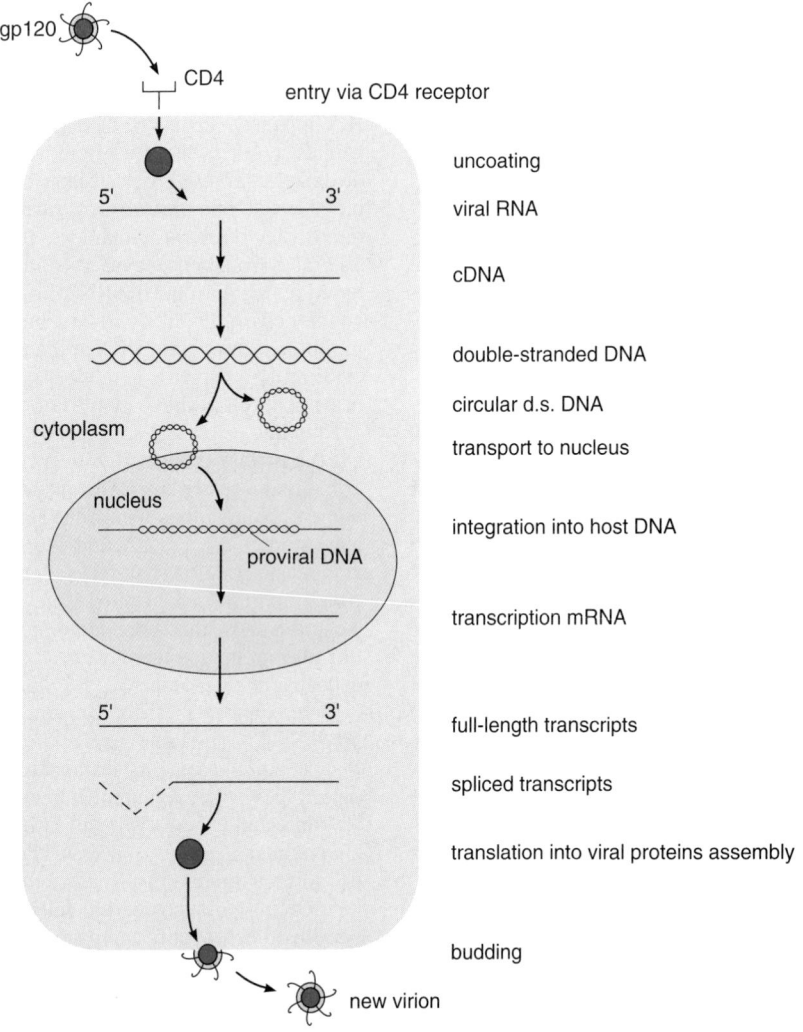

gp120

CD4   entry via CD4 receptor

uncoating

5'   3'   viral RNA

cDNA

double-stranded DNA

circular d.s. DNA

cytoplasm   transport to nucleus

nucleus   integration into host DNA

proviral DNA

transcription mRNA

5'   3'   full-length transcripts

spliced transcripts

translation into viral proteins assembly

budding

new virion

Figure 53–6. Replicative cycle of HIV. Lifelong infection is a consequence of the viral replicative cycle.

resistance in early clinical trials has led to the development of protocols in which these drugs are used in combination with other antiretroviral therapies.

The proteinase inhibitors (including saquinavir, ritonavir, indinavir, and nelfinavir) are perhaps the most potent antiretroviral drugs to date. These compounds are structurally diverse and act to inhibit HIV replication by preventing the proteolytic cleavage of Gag and Gag-Pol precursor proteins into functional protein subunits. The HIV proteinase catalyses this cleavage, and this enzyme is inhibited by the proteinase inhibitors. In clinical trials, therapy with ritonavir and indinavir in particular has been associated with a profound and sustained decrease in HIV RNA in plasma as well as a sustained immunologic response.

Agents acting at other sites in the replicative cycle (including integrase inhibitors are in development.

C. Immunorestorative Therapy: Attempts to restore the defective immune system have to date gen-

Table 53–8. Targets for antiretroviral therapy.

Target	Therapy
HIV binding and cell entry	Soluble recombinant CD4, dextran sulfate, castanospermine, heparin
Reverse transcription	Zidovudine, Didanosine, zalcitabine, lamivudine, stavudine, second-site RT inhibitors (eg, nevirapine)
Regulatory proteins	Tat inhibitors, gene therapy
HIV translation and protein assembly	Ribavirin, proteinase inhibitors (eg, saquinavir, ritonavir, indinavir)
Budding from cell	Interferons

erally been ineffective. The alleged immune stimulator inosine pranobex (Isoprinosine) has been associated with only transitory immunologic benefit; bone marrow and peripheral blood lymphocyte transplantation is not regarded as useful, because the transplanted cells also become infected with HIV. The augmentation of general immune or cytotoxic responses by IL-2 and IL-12 is currently being investigated. Recombinant interleukin-2 has been found in clinical trials to cause a large increase in CD4 lymphocyte numbers, when administered with an antiretroviral agent. Inhibitors of cytokines (such as pentoxifylline, a TNFa inhibitor) may provide additional immune and antiviral benefit. It is possible that combination therapy with an immunomodulatory agent together with one or more antiretroviral agents will be more effective than either alone. In certain patients with Kaposi's sarcoma, administration of high-dose interferon gamma has been beneficial. Interferon inducers such as the mismatched doubled-stranded RNA compound Ampligen are effective in vitro in inhibiting HIV replication. Early clinical trials with this drug suggested temporary clinical improvement with restoration of immune responses, but these studies have not been confirmed. GM-CSF has been used in clinical trials for treating cytopenias occurring in AIDS patients, whether they are due to drugs, opportunistic infections, or HIV itself. This compound, however, may in fact increase viral replication within monocyte–macrophages unless used in combination with an antiretroviral agent. Patients with refractory neutropenia are now more likely to be treated with G-CSF, which has no stimulatory effect on HIV replication.

Passive immunotherapy to enhance HIV-specific humoral immunity is being evaluated in a number of clinical trials. Approaches include the use of humanized monoclonal antibodies directed against either the CD4-gp120-binding site of the viral envelope or the immunodominant V3 loop of HIV gp120. Another approach to boost or augment the immune response to HIV involves using a therapeutic vaccine administered to persons already infected with HIV. Jonas Salk, the polio vaccine pioneer, developed a vaccine made from inactivated HIV (without the envelope); studies to date suggest that it is safe and that it can boost delayed hypersensitivity responses to vaccine antigens. A number of other candidate vaccines are in clinical trial. The immunogens include envelope proteins made in insect and mammalian cell systems, as well as a novel approaches such as HIV core protein produced in such a way that the HIV p24 is presented to the immune system as a virus-like particle. It is anticipated that these vaccines will stimulate both cell-mediated and humoral immune responses, resulting in greater clinical benefit than that provided by immunogens that induce only neutralizing antibodies to HIV.

Prevention

A. Vaccines: The development of an effective

Table 53–9. Obstacles to development of HIV vaccine.

Genomic diversity of HIV strains
Progression of infection despite vigorous immune response
 Transmission of HIV in vivo by cell fusion as well as by
  cell-free virus
Lack of a good animal model
Potential enhancement of HIV replication by neutralizing
 antibody

vaccine has been hampered by the genomic diversity of HIV (Table 53–9). Strains of HIV vary in their nucleic acid sequence by up to 20% as a result of high-frequency point mutations that occur during the replication of the virus. This variation is most evident in the envelope region of HIV. Of interest, certain regions are conserved between different isolates (for example, the region of gp120 that interacts with CD4), and other regions of the envelope are highly variable. Unfortunately, the major antigenic epitopes (and therefore, predictably, the major protective epitopes) are in the regions associated with the highest degree of strain-to-strain variation. This includes the immunodominant third variable loop (V3) within gp120. The V3 loop contains the GPGRA amino acid sequence, which is regarded as the principal neutralizing domain. This genomic diversity is one of the many major obstacles hampering vaccine development, because an effective vaccine should provide protection against all strains of HIV. Another impediment to vaccine development is the fact that HIV is spread from cell to cell via a fusion process as well as by cell-free virus.

Prophylactic vaccines (for HIV-negative persons) containing attenuated virus or inactivated whole virus would meet with ethical concerns because of difficulty in guaranteeing their safety. The discovery, however, in Australia of the attenuated *nef*-deleted strain of HIV-1 in all of the members of a cohort of long-term nonprogressors of HIV infection, together with the findings of lack of progression of disease in macaques infected with the *nef*-deleted strain of SIV, has raised the prospects of a successful prophylactic vaccine using a *nef*-deleted strain of HIV. Recombinant HIV envelope glycoproteins expressed in a cell culture system (eg, mammalian cells, bacteria, or yeasts) and HIV genes inserted into an attenuated vector (eg, vaccinia virus or avipox virus) are currently undergoing trials in chimpanzees. Neutralizing antibodies have been produced to these viral proteins in vaccinated animals. The use of certain HIV genes (eg, *gag-pol*) and genes for certain cytokines (eg, interferon gamma) within a vector in order to direct the immune response toward production of cytotoxic T cells rather than neutralizing antibodies is under investigation. Some of these vaccines have resulted in various degrees of success in providing protection against subsequent challenge with strains of HIV. Because chimpanzees are not an ideal animal model for human HIV infection and because of the shortage of supply of these animals, trial vaccination of humans is now under way. Other strategies in vaccine development include production of anti-idiotype vaccines and construction of synthetic peptides. The recognition of the importance of mucosal immunity, the possible advantages of live vectors such as vaccinia virus or canarypox virus, and the ability of various adjuvants to provide differing immunologic responses are influencing the design of future vaccines.

B. Education: The major thrust of strategies to prevent HIV infection lies in education of individuals about practicing safer sex, in which the transmission of bodily fluids (specifically semen, vaginal secretions, and blood) is prevented, and not sharing needles or syringes.

CYTOMEGALOVIRUS

Major Immunologic Features

- CD8 lymphocyte numbers increase, and there is transient suppression of CD4 lymphocyte numbers and cell-mediated immunity.
- CMV infection of cells decreases MHC class I antigen expression and induces Fc receptors.

General Considerations

Cytomegalovirus (CMV) is a member of the herpesvirus family, a group that includes the human pathogens EBV, herpes simplex virus types 1 and 2, varicella-zoster virus, and human herpesviruses types 6–8, as well as many animal pathogens. Similar to other herpesviruses, CMV is associated with persistent, latent, and recurrent infection, the last being due to reactivation of latent virus. CMV remains latent in monocytes, granulocyte–monocyte progenitor cells, and perhaps in other cell types.

The prevalence of infection within a community varies with socioeconomic status, being as low as 40% in upper strata and approaching 100% in lower groups.

Clinical Features

Infection with CMV can result in a variety of clinical syndromes, depending partially on the immune state of the infected individual (Table 53–10). In healthy subjects, infection is usually subclinical, occasionally causing an infectious mononucleosis-like syndrome resembling that due to EBV or primary HIV infections (however, pharyngitis is unusual).

Table 53–10. Clinical manifestations of CMV infection.

Prenatal infection
Cytomegalic inclusion disease
Immunocompetent host
Subclinical infection
CMV mononucleosis
Immunocompromised host
Disseminated CMV: retinitis, esophagitis, colitis, pneumonitis, other sites

There is a tendency to develop allergic skin rashes to antibiotics, similar to that observed during acute EBV infection. If infection is acquired in utero, following primary maternal infection, the infant may be born with cytomegalic inclusion disease (CID), which has features of hepatosplenomegaly, microcephaly, chorioretinitis, thrombocytopenia, and jaundice. Although only about 5–10% of infants with prenatal infection are born with CID, another 2–5% develop abnormalities such as deafness, spasticity, intellectual retardation, and dental defects within the first 2 years of life. Asymptomatic perinatal infection may be acquired as a result of exposure to CMV in the birth canal or through breast-feeding.

Patients with defective cellular immunity, such as those with AIDS or those being treated with immunosuppressive drugs, are prone to disseminated CMV infection. In this instance, the infection involves predominantly the retinas, gastrointestinal tract (especially the colon, esophagus, and liver), and lungs. Such individuals often have progressive disease, despite high levels of serum-neutralizing antibody. Reactivation of CMV infection also appears to trigger graft-versus-host disease in many cases. Organ transplant recipients develop generalized and occasionally fatal CMV disease more commonly following primary than reactivated infection. In vitro studies have shown clearly that coinfection by CMV and HIV augments HIV replication. Thus, it was speculated that CMV might be a cofactor augmenting the pathogenicity of HIV and shortening the incubation period (between infection and development of AIDS). Although to date there is no clinical evidence that such is the case, this biologically plausible hypothesis remains under study.

Immunologic Findings

A. CMV Serology: IgM antibodies are produced following initial infection and generally persist for 3–4 months. IgG antibodies appear at the same time, peak about 2 or 3 months after infection, and persist for many years and often for life. Although the antibody response is directed against many virion proteins, neutralizing antibodies are primarily directed against the envelope glycoproteins, especially gB and gH. Although neutralizing antibodies play no role in control of established CMV infection, there is good evidence from immunoprophylaxis studies that they may prevent infection.

B. CMV Cellular Immunity: Primary infection is followed by activation of both MHC-restricted cytotoxic CD8 T lymphocytes, whose function is to specifically destroy CMV-infected cells, and MHC-nonrestricted NK cells. The cytotoxic T-lymphocyte (CTL) response to CMV is targeted against a variety of virion antigens. Both the NK and CTL responses appear to play a role in controlling established CMV infection; the role of CTL has recently been reinforced by studies showing protection from CMV infection by passive infusion of CMV-specific CTL in bone marrow transplant recipients. Not surprisingly, there is good evidence that susceptibility to CMV infection is at least partly genetically determined.

CMV infection, however, also results in a general impairment of cellular immunity, characterized by impaired blastogenic responses to nonspecific mitogens and specific CMV antigens, diminished cytotoxic ability, and elevation of the CD8 lymphocyte subset with a moderate but transient decrease in the number of CD4 lymphocytes. Infection with CMV causes down-regulation of MHC class I antigens and selective interference with class I MHC presentation of the major IE (immediate-early) antigen, thus hampering the recognition of infected cells by IE-specific CTL. Thus, there is a delicately balanced relationship between the CMV-mediated immune dysfunction and the ability of the host to control the virologic response. This balance is in part temporal: initially, viral replication and cell-mediated immunopathology occur unhindered, with the immune function being restored during convalescence. Furthermore, the underlying immune status of the infected individual is of major prognostic importance.

In the immunocompetent individual, specific defects in the cell-mediated immune response are restored within a few months following infection. Seropositive individuals, however, may intermittently excrete CMV for many years or perhaps for life, owing to low-grade chronic infection or reactivation of latent infection.

Primary CMV infection in immunocompromised individuals results in a severely blunted immune response to the virus. Contrariwise, reactivation of latent CMV infection usually results from immunosuppression, especially that due to major organ transplantation (eg, heart, lung, bone marrow) and HIV infection. Reactivation of infection in the context of immunosuppression does not result in any predictable changes in CMV serology.

The immaturity of the immune response in infants with congenital or perinatal infection results in chronic excretion of CMV in nasopharyngeal secretions and urine. The immune response in these children is eventually restored coincident with cessation of viral excretion.

Treatment and Prevention

There are now three antiviral agents available for treating CMV infection: ganciclovir, foscarnet, and cidofovir; they are used only for treating severe CMV infections in immunocompromised patients. These drugs are effective for treatment of established CMV infection, as well as for "chemosuppression"—prevention of reactivation of latent infection by long-term therapy. CMV pneumonitis in bone marrow transplant recipients responds poorly to antivirals alone and is usually treated with an antiviral plus CMV intravenous immunoglobulin. CMV pneumonitis probably results from a combination of direct viral cytopathology and a host autoimmune response, and the intravenous immunoglobulin is thought to act as an immunomodulator, not as an antiviral. Use of adjunctive CMV immunoglobulin as treatment for other types of CMV infections has not been beneficial. Reactivation of latent CMV infection and the resulting disease can be largely prevented by a chemosuppression strategy in which patients at risk of reactivation are given antivirals (such as ganciclovir) before and during the period of severe immunosuppression.

Passive immunoprophylaxis with either CMV hyperimmune globulin or CMV-specific CTL has been shown to prevent CMV infection or disease. A live attenuated CMV vaccine (the Towne strain) is apathogenic, but has not clearly shown protective efficacy, and attempts are currently underway to construct subunit CMV vaccines, using the gB and gH envelope glycoproteins.

EPSTEIN-BARR VIRUS

Major Immunologic Features

- B lymphocytes are target cells.
- There is atypical T-cell lymphocytosis.
- Heterophil antibodies are produced.
- There is in vitro transformation of B lymphocytes.

General Considerations

EBV is a member of the herpesvirus family and, as such, can establish persistent and latent infection. EBV also can transform B lymphocytes and has clinically relevant oncogenic potential. Primary infection, which may be subclinical, results in a lifelong carrier state.

Pathogenesis

The virus initially replicates within the pharyngeal epithelium, with subsequent infection of B lymphocytes in subjacent lymphoid tissue. Circulating lymphocytes are responsible for generalized infection. Following the acute infection, EBV remains latent within the B-lymphocyte population; these cells most probably provide a lifelong reservoir of the virus. Intermittent seeding of the pharyngeal epithelia, with low-level replication within these cells, allows potential transmission of infection to susceptible members of the community.

The incubation period varies from 3 to 7 weeks; most commonly adolescents and young adults develop symptomatic infection.

Shedding of EBV from salivary tissue declines following acute infection but probably persists for life. Recently, EBV has been found in both semen and cervical epithelium, suggesting the possibility of sexual transmission. Transmission of EBV by blood transfusion and bone marrow transplantation has been rarely described.

Clinical Features

In 1964, Epstein, Achong, and Barr described the presence of viral particles in fibroblasts cultured from tissue from a patient with Burkitt's lymphoma. Since then, this virus has been causally associated with acute infectious mononucleosis, nasopharyngeal carcinoma, lymphomas in immunocompromised individuals, X-linked lymphoproliferative syndrome (Duncan's syndrome), and two HIV-related conditions (oral hairy leukoplakia and lymphocytic interstitial pneumonitis) (Table 53–11). EBV has been proposed as the cause of the chronic fatigue syndrome, but no evidence supports this association.

Infectious mononucleosis is the most common illness caused by EBV. This disease occurs most frequently in young adults. Typical features include fever; sore throat, often with exudate; generalized lymphadenopathy; and splenomegaly. Chemical hepatitis is present in most patients, and a few develop frank jaundice. About 10% of patients develop a macular rash; therapy with amoxicillin or ampicillin frequently produces an eruption. Rare complications of infectious mononucleosis include hemolytic anemia, aplastic anemia, encephalitis, Guillain-Barré syndrome, myocarditis, nephritis, and hepatic failure.

In immunodeficient patients, primary EBV infection can cause a variety of conditions, including uncomplicated mononucleosis, a benign polyclonal B-cell hyperplasia, and both polyclonal and monoclonal B-cell lymphomas.

EBV is definitely the causative agent of a number of cancers: Burkitt's lymphoma, nasopharyngeal cancer, immunosuppression-induced lymphomas, and Duncan's syndrome. The mechanisms by which EBV causes these tumors are multiple and complex, and beyond the scope of this chapter; however, oncogenesis is uniformly associated with long-standing infection (see Chapter 45).

Laboratory Diagnosis of Infectious Mononucleosis

Usually a mild leukopenia precedes the development of a leukocytosis (and absolute lymphocytosis) during the second to third week of illness. From 50 to 70% of the lymphocytes are atypical. IgM heterophil antibodies, which agglutinate sheep erythrocytes, are present. These antibodies must be distinguished from Forssman's antibodies present in patients with serum sickness, which also agglutinate sheep erythrocytes.

Table 53–11. Diseases associated with EBV.

Infectious mononucleosis
Burkitt's lymphoma
Nasopharyngeal carcinoma
Lymphomas in immunocompromised host
X-linked lymphoproliferative syndrome
Oral hairy leukoplakia[1]
Lymphocytic interstitial pneumonitis[1]

[1] In HIV-infected individuals.

Differentiation of the various heterophil antibodies is based on absorption techniques, with guinea pig kidney and bovine erythrocytes. EBV-associated heterophil antibodies are found in the sera of more than 90% of individuals with infectious mononucleosis. They persist for 3–6 months.

The pattern of antibody response to EBV initially reflects the synthesis of viral antigens involved in cell lysis, notably the early antigens (EA), viral capsid antigens (VCA), and EBV-induced membrane antigens (MA). VCA and MA are classified as late antigens, since their expression is suppressed in the presence of inhibitors of DNA synthesis. The appearance of antibody directed against the EBV nuclear antigen (EBNA) usually occurs weeks to months after infection. EBNA is present in all cells containing the viral genome, whether latently or productively infected (Fig 53–7).

Immunologic Features of EBV Infection

Following EBV infection, most patients mount a vigorous humoral and cellular immune response. The humoral immune response is directed against a variety of viral proteins (see Fig 53–7); antibodies to viral MA and gp350 proteins are neutralizing but probably do

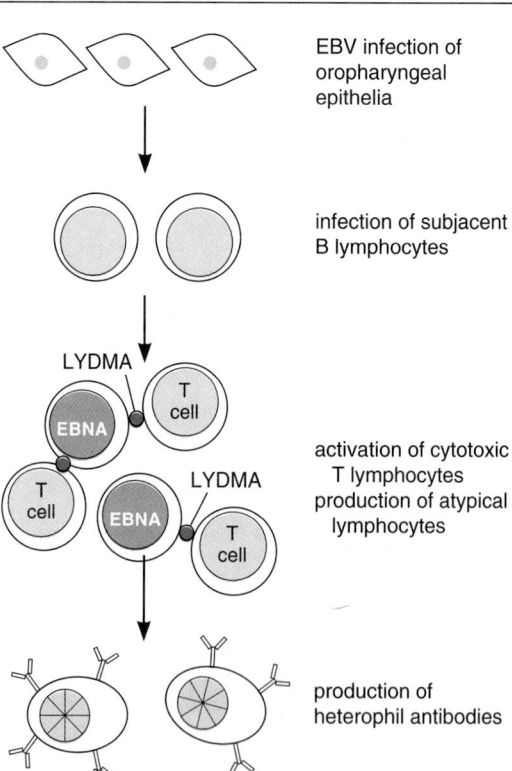

EBV infection of oropharyngeal epithelia

infection of subjacent B lymphocytes

activation of cytotoxic T lymphocytes production of atypical lymphocytes

production of heterophil antibodies

Figure 53–7. Pathogenesis of infectious mononucleosis. Following infection of oropharyngeal epithelia, EBV infection spreads to the subjacent B lymphocytes. Activation of cytotoxic T lymphocytes by EBV antigens results in the appearance of atypical lymphocytes in the peripheral blood.

not play a role in controlling established infection. In addition, perhaps because EBV encodes an IL-10 homologue that stimulates B-cell replication, EBV infection is associated with polyclonal hyperglobulinemia. The cellular immune response to EBV is extremely vigorous; in fact, the atypical lymphocytes that are so characteristic of this disease are primarily activated CD8, EBV-specific cytotoxic T lymphocytes (CTL) and natural killer (NK) cells. Control of acute EBV infection is probably due primarily to the CTL response. Individuals with severe cellular immunodeficiency, such as renal transplant recipients, may develop fulminant EBV infection or B-cell malignancies following primary infection. In addition, there is a rare, X-linked inherited immune defect that predisposes to severe, often fatal EBV infection (Duncan's syndrome; X-linked lymphoproliferative disease).

EBV infects B lymphocytes through binding to the CD21 molecule on the cell surface. CD21 is expressed on a variety of cells besides mature B lymphocyes, including follicular dendritic cells, and pharyngeal and cervical epithelia. CD21 is a receptor for the C3d component of complement as well as for EBV. Following infection, large numbers of atypical lymphocytes appear within the circulation that are not, in fact, virus-infected B cells but result from polyclonal activation of cytotoxic/suppressor (CD8) cells (Fig 53–8). These activated T cells, which are not MHC-restricted or EBV-specific, are responsible for preventing the unchecked expansion of EBV-transformed B lymphocytes. In addition, EBV-specific, MHC-restricted cytotoxic T cells are produced. Of interest, these cells appear to specifically recognize virus-infected B lymphocytes expressing **lymphocyte-determined membrane antigen (LYDMA),** without requiring MHC restriction. The true specificity of cytotoxic T-cell responses in infectious mononucleosis remains to be completely elucidated. The mechanism for viral persistence may involve inhibition of the normal replicative cycle of EBV within B cells prior to the expression of LYDMA, the target antigen for cytotoxic T cells.

Differential Diagnosis of Infectious Mononucleosis

Streptococcal pharyngitis and, less commonly, diphtheria may resemble infectious mononucleosis. In individuals who present with jaundice, hepatitis A, B, C, E, and delta should be considered. The hematologic changes in infectious mononucleosis, together with serology, generally clarify the issue. In persons at risk of HIV infection a negative heterophil antibody test should alert the clinician to the possibility of acute HIV infection. Other causes of mononucleosis-like illness are discussed under the HIV section in this chapter.

Treatment and Prevention

Therapy for infectious mononucleosis is symptomatic. Although EBV is sensitive to acyclovir in vitro,

the drug is of little or no clinical benefit. Oral hairy leukoplakia (an HIV-associated EBV infection), however, responds clinically and virologically to acyclovir. Because EBV-associated tumors carry EBV antigens, scientists are attempting to use EBV-specific CTL to treat these tumors. A subunit vaccine to stimulate EBV CTL in patients with EBV-related lymphomas is undergoing clinical study at present.

Because EBV infection is associated with tumors of public health significance in many parts of the world (eg, Burkitt's lymphoma in Africa; nasopharyngeal cancer in China), efforts are underway to develop vaccines to prevent EBV infection altogether, or to limit EBV replication following infection (and hopefully thereby to decrease the risk of oncogenesis). A subunit vaccine containing EBV gp350 (the major virion membrane protein that stimulates neutralizing antibody) and peptide-based vaccines to stimulate EBV-specific CTL are both under development.

HUMAN T-CELL LEUKEMIA VIRUS TYPES I AND II (HTLV-I AND HTLV-II)

The field of human retrovirology is relatively young. In 1980, the first human retrovirus was isolated in the USA from the T lymphocytes of two black men with aggressive T-cell cancers. This virus, now called HTLV-I, has since been causatively linked with adult T-cell leukemia (ATL) and an incurable progressive neuromyelopathy called tropical spastic paraparesis or HTLV-1-associated myelopathy (HAM). HTLV-II has been associated with unusual T-cell malignancies in humans.

HTLV-I is a type C retrovirus of the oncornavirus family (see Table 53–1). Like other oncornaviruses, HTLV-I may transform (immortalize) cells following infection, although unlike acutely transforming oncornaviruses, it lacks a specific oncogene. HTLV-I preferentially infects T cells, although other cell types can be infected in vitro. Infected T cells are transformed by an unknown mechanism, and it is the proliferation of these transformed cells (which contain the HTLV-I provirus, an integrated DNA copy of the retroviral RNA genome) that results in ATL and perhaps other tumors. The transformed T lymphocytes are usually CD4 (rarely, CD8), express many activation markers, and produce numerous cytokines.

ATL is caused by oligoclonal proliferation of transformed T lymphocytes and is clearly associated with clinically significant immunosuppression. In contrast, HAM is most likely an autoimmune disease, and HTLV-I infection has also been associated with autoimmune arthritis and uveitis. Nothing is known about the immunologic mechanisms involved, however.

Endemic HTLV-I infection exists in parts of the Caribbean region, Japan, and Africa. Worldwide, up to 20 million persons are estimated to be infected with

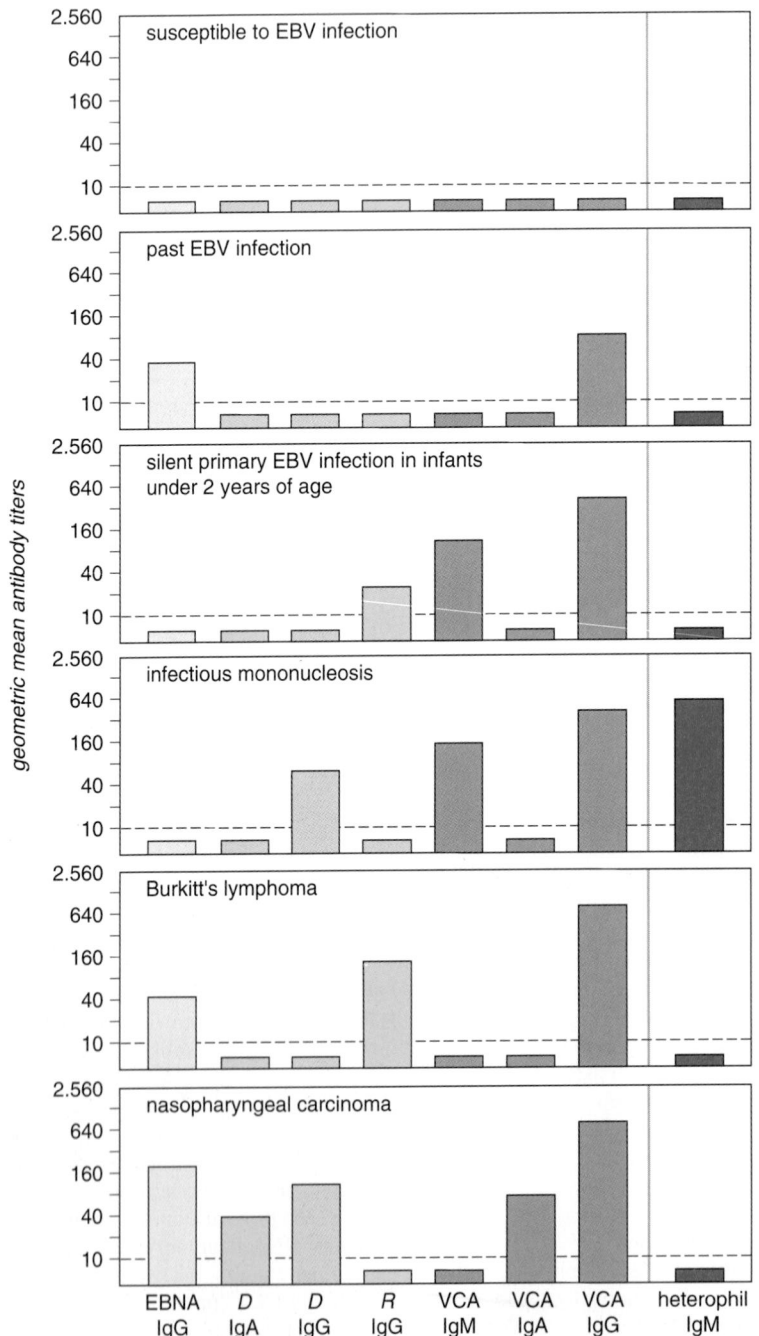

geometric mean antibody titers

Figure 53–8. Serologic response to EBV infection. Typical antibody patterns are observed in different clinical conditions caused by EBV. *Abbreviations:* D = diffuse; R = restricted; EBNA = Epstein-Barr nuclear antigen; VCA = viral capsid antigen; Ig = immunoglobulin.

HTLV-I. The modes of transmission of HTLV-I are virtually identical to those for HIV: via infected blood, through sexual contact, and from mother to child. There is no direct evidence for transplacental transmission of HTLV-I; however, transmission to the infant commonly occurs via the mother's milk, analogous to transmission of bovine leukemia virus.

There is a high rate of infection with HTLV-II in certain populations, including injecting drug users. Screening of blood bank donations in the US for

HTLV-I/II began in 1988. Seroprevalence ranged from 0 to 0.1%. Since HTLV-I is difficult to distinguish serologically from HTLV-II, assays that detect both together have been developed. HTLV-I/II infection is usually detected by enzyme immunoassay, with positives being confirmed by immunoblotting. Differentiation between HTLV-I and HTLV-II infection can be made by immunoblot but is more reliably determined by PCR amplification of provirus.

Human herpesvirus (HHV) 6 is a herpesvirus with a genome closely related to that of human cytomegalovirus, which infects predominantly T lymphocytes. Two variants are recognized, HHV-6A and HHV-6B, which are genetically closely related but clinically and epidemiologically distinct. HHV-6A is not known to cause disease, whereas HHV-6B is the major cause of exathem subitum and other illnesses, primarily in children. HHV-6 infects predominantly the CD4 subset of T lymphocytes, although it does not use CD4 itself as the receptor (unlike HIV). HHV-6 infection of T cells causes cytomegaly and syncytium formation, induces CD4 expression, and may downregulate CD3/T-cell receptor (TCR) expression.

Infection of macrophages suppresses a variety of functions of these cells.

Primary infection with HHV-6 usually occurs in childhood. HHV-6A infection appears to be asymptomatic, whereas HHV-6B causes exanthem subitum (roseola infantum; sixth disease) and undifferentiated febrile illnesses. Primary infection with HHV-6B accounts for 15–40% of children presenting to hospital casualty departments with febrile illnesses. Primary infection of adults with HHV-6 is rare, but infectious mononucleosis-like syndromes have been reported. A variety of other syndromes due to primary HHV-6B infection have been reported involving the respiratory tract, central nervous system, liver, and reticuloendothelial system. Reactivation of latent HHV-6 infection in immunosuppressed patients (especially those receiving bone marrow transplants) has been associated with febrile episodes, pneumonitis, and graft rejection, although the etiologic relationship remains unproven. Interestingly, despite infection of CD4-bearing lymphocytes like HIV, there is no evidence that HHV-6 causes immunosuppression.

REFERENCES

HUMAN IMMUNODEFICIENCY VIRUS

Crowe SM et al: Predictive value of CD4 lymphocyte numbers for the development of opportunistic infections and malignancies in HIV-infected persons. *Acquired Immune Defic Syndr* 1991;**4:**770.

Davis BR, Zauli G: Effect of human immunodeficiency virus infection on haematopoesis. *Baillieres Clin Haematol* 1995;**8:**113.

Ho DD et al: Rapid turnover of plasma virions and CD4 lymphocytes in HIV-1 infection. *Nature* 1995;**373:**123.

Levy JA: *HIV and the Pathogenesis of AIDS.* ASM Press, 1994.

Tinkle BT et al: The pathogenic role of human immunodeficiency virus accessory genes in transgenic mice. *Curr Top Microbiol Immunol* 1995;**193:**133.

CYTOMEGALOVIRUS

Britt, WJ, Alford CA: Cytomegalovirus. In: Fields BN et al (editors). *Virology,* 3rd ed. Lippincott-Raven, 1996, pp. 2493–2523.

Campbell AE, Slater JS: Down-regulation of major histocompatibility complex class I synthesis by murine cytomegalovirus early gene expression. *J Virol* 1994; **68:**1805.

Kondo K et al: Human cytomegalovirus laten infection of granulocyte–macrophage progenitors in SCID-Hu mice and in culture. *Proc Natl Acad Sci USA* 1994;**91:**11879.

Mocarski ES: Cytomegaloviruses and their replication. In: Fields BN et al (editors). *Virology,* 3rd ed. Lippincott-Raven, 1996, pp. 2447–2492.

Scalzo AA et al: CMV-1, a genetic locus that controls murine cytomegalovirus replication in the spleen. *J Exp Med* 1990;**171:**1469.

Sing GK, Ruscetti FW: The role of human cytomegalovirus in haematological diseases. *Bailleres Clin Haematol* 1995;**8:**149.

EPSTEIN-BARR VIRUS

Hanto DW: Classification of Epstein-Barr virus-associated post-transplant lymphoproliferative diseases: Implications for understanding their pathogenesis and developing rational treatment strategies. *Annu Rev Med* 1995;**46:**381.

Moss DJ et al: Potential antigenic targets on Epstein-Barr virus-associated tumors and the host response. *CIBA Foundation Symposium,* 1994;**187:**4.

Rickinson AB, Kieff E: Epstein-Barr virus. In: Fields BN et al (editors). *Virology,* 3rd ed. Lippincott-Raven, 1996, pp. 2397–2446.

Tosato G et al: Epstein-Barr virus as an agent of haematological disease. *Baillieres Clin Haematol* 1995;**8:**165.

HUMAN T LYMPHOTROPIC VIRUS TYPE I

Cann AJ, Chen ISY: Human T-cell leukemia viruses type I and II. In: Fields BN et al (editors). *Virology,* 3rd ed. Lippincott-Raven, 1996. pp. 1849–1880.

Hollsberg P, Hafler DA: Pathogenesis of diseases induced by human lymphotropic virus type I infection. *N Engl J Med* 1993;**328:**1173.

HUMAN HERPESVIRUS TYPE 6

Caserta MT, Hall CB: Human herpesvirus-6. *Annu Rev Med* 1993;**44:**377.

Pellett PE, Black JB: Human herpesvirus 6. In: Fields BN et al (editors). *Virology,* 3rd ed. Lippincott-Raven, 1996, pp. 2587–2608.

54

Immunologic Therapy

Abba I. Terr, MD

Immunologic therapy in its broadest sense encompasses the treatment and prevention of a large number and variety of immunologic and nonimmunologic diseases. Historically, therapeutic immunology began in 1796, well before the dawn of scientific and clinical immunology, when Edward Jenner showed that an ancient viral scourge, smallpox, could be successfully prevented by immunization. Jenner was an English physician who accomplished this feat alone, using only his astute clinical observations. As a result smallpox was completely eradicated as a human disease after the last case was reported in 1977. Ironically, only 3 years later a new and lethal viral disease, acquired immune deficiency syndrome (AIDS), appeared and rapidly became a major worldwide public health problem. The causative virus, human immunodeficiency virus (HIV), infects the CD4 T cell, which is the central focus of the immune response itself. As the subject of widespread research by thousands of immunologists and other scientists, AIDS has generated an enormous expansion of our knowledge of human immunology; however, it has thus far eluded all attempts at successful treatment or prevention by immunization.

The chapters to follow in Section IV discuss major categories of therapy for immunologic diseases and the treatment of these and other diseases by manipulation, alteration, and exploitation of the immune response. Some of these treatment modalities, such as immunization against infections and toxins, allergy desensitization, and certain drugs, arose from empirical clinical observations. Others, such as the use of genetically engineered interleukins, are products of fundamental laboratory investigations. These chapters address pharmacologic properties and mechanisms of well-established and promising new therapies. Clinical indications or details of drug administration are included in the previous sections where specific diseases are discussed.

This chapter is an overview of immunologic therapy. To best understand the mechanisms and clinical indications for the many forms of treatment, the immune system can be divided functionally into two categories: the **immune response** and the **inflammatory response.** Therapy directed at the immune response can be either **antigen-specific** or **antigen-nonspecific.** Some diseases require that the immune response be stimulated, whereas others require suppression. The therapeutic armamentarium to accomplish these diverse goals now includes chemically defined drugs obtained from natural sources, such as fungal products, synthetic chemicals, specific antibodies, and many of the actual cellular and chemical components of the immune system itself. Cloning technology provides large quantities of virtually any new cytokine, adhesion molecule, cell membrane molecule, or receptor in remarkably short time after their discovery.

Increasingly, antibodies are being used as drugs because of their ability to target a particular structure within the body with great specificity. Monoclonal antibodies have largely supplanted the traditional use of serum gamma globulin from animals immunized with the relevant antigen. Although this greatly increases specificity and eliminates the problem of allergic reactions to irrelevant serum proteins, the heterologous monoclonal antibody is itself antigenic and may in time become ineffective by neutralization or by an allergic reaction to it. Even this problem has recently been solved by "humanizing" mouse monoclonal antibodies through substitution of those segments of the immunoglobulin molecule that have a unique murine configuration with the corresponding portions from human immunoglobulin segments. In some cases in which target cell death is the therapeutic goal, the monoclonal antibody has been coupled to a potent toxin such as ricin, diphtheria toxin, or *Pseudomonas* exotoxin A.

MODULATION OF THE IMMUNE RESPONSE

ANTIGEN-SPECIFIC THERAPY

Immune Stimulation

A. Active Immunization: Prophylaxis against the future occurrence of an infectious or toxic disease is possible by means of active immunization. In this case, the natural host immune response to a primary microbial infection is stimulated by immunization with an antigenically active killed or attenuated microorganism, an antigenically cross-reactive but nonpathogenic living organism, an antigenically active product or constituent of the organism, or a modified form of a microbial toxin that is antigenic but nontoxic. The resulting immune response can be transient or lifelong, depending on a number of factors related to the immunizing antigen (often referred to as a vaccine), the host, and the mode of administration of the antigen. The response can generate effector T cells, antibodies, or both. Furthermore, the antibodies produced can include any one or more of the immunoglobulin classes and subclasses (isotypes). The type of immune response determines efficacy in prophylaxis. Chapter 55 details immunization procedures and effectiveness for all of the currently available vaccines.

Immunization to ameliorate **allergic disease** has been clinically successful for many years, but the precise mechanism of the effect is still unknown. The various immunologic changes that ensue from injecting allergen into patients with IgE-mediated diseases are addressed in detail in Chapter 56. These changes include (eventually) both suppression of IgE antibodies and production of IgG antibodies. This shifting of the profile of isotypes of the allergen-specific antibody is presumed to occur because the route of allergen exposure has changed from mucosal absorption to subcutaneous injection. Other explanations may apply, but this one suggests that antigen processing is important in successful allergy desensitization. There is substantial evidence that production of IgE antibodies is associated with a predominance of T helper cells that secrete a T_H2 profile of cytokines, and that the T_H1 cytokines, particularly interferon gamma, inhibit IgE production. Several studies have now shown that allergen desensitization can alter the cytokine profile from T_H2 to T_H1. It is even conceivable that administration of appropriate cytokines with or without antigen could be used to tailor a desired immune response pathway for treatment of allergic and other diseases.

Adjuvants are chemicals added to the immunizing antigen to enhance the host immune response by increasing the availability of the antigen to the antigen-presenting cell (APC), prolonging the persistence of antigen in tissues, or stimulating the APC directly. Examples of adjuvants, discussed in more detail in Chapter 55, are alum (used to insolubilize the antigen), water-in-oil emulsions, muramyl dipeptide, and liposomes.

B. Passive Immunization: The transfer of the active product of the immune response (antibody or effector T cell) from an immune individual to a nonimmune recipient is called passive immunization. The protection afforded in this way is immediate but transient, since no ongoing immune response or memory is involved. The immune donor of the passive antibody can be human or animal. The latter is preferable for producing antibodies to particularly dangerous immunogens, but the resultant antibody is foreign and therefore itself antigenic to the human recipient. The therapeutic benefit of passive immunization is thus limited by immune elimination, neutralization, or possible allergic reaction by the recipient's own immune response to the administered antibody.

Passive human antibody protection is standard therapy for patients with any of the antibody deficiency diseases with or without concomitant cellular immunodeficiency. These conditions are described in Chapters 21 and 23. The treatment usually is given in the form of the gamma globulin fraction of normal human plasma pooled from many donors, yielding a product with a broad range of antibodies. These are almost exclusively IgG antibodies, because ethanol fractionation used in its preparation excludes other immunoglobulin classes. For specific protection of anyone (ie, normal or immunocompromised) with an anticipated exposure to certain infections or toxins, high-titer preparations of the specific antibody are available from hyperimmunized individuals or animals.

Antigen-specific passive cellular immunization by transfer of effector lymphocytes has been demonstrated repeatedly in animal experiments, but to date it has had no role in human treatment. Cellular immunodeficiency diseases are treated instead by adoptive immunity (discussed in the following section).

C. Adoptive Immunity: Transplantation of immunocompetent cells from normal donors is the method used to achieve immune function in children with congenital cellular immunodeficiency. Since the recipient lacks the ability to mount an immune response, rejection of the transplanted cells does not occur, but a graft-versus-host (GVH) reaction is still possible, so histocompatible donors are preferred. The usual source is the bone marrow from which the cells are transfused intraperitoneally or intravenously. Long-term immunologic restoration in children with severe combined immunodeficiency has been achieved in a number of cases. When histocompatible bone marrow is not available, fetal liver or thymus has been used, but to date results have been less satisfactory than with bone marrow.

Rare cases of immunodeficiency arise from congenital deficiency of an enzyme in the purine metabolic pathway, for example, adenosine deaminase or nucleoside phosphorylase. In some cases of adenosine deaminase deficiency, immune competence has been restored by the administration of the enzyme and recently by somatic gene therapy, in which the gene encoding the enzyme is inserted into the genome of bone marrow stem cells by using a viral vector.

Treatment of specific immunodeficiency diseases is covered in Chapters 20–24.

Immune Suppression

A. Active Suppression: A variety of strategies, both tested and theoretical, are designed to actively suppress antigen-specific immune responses. A unique form of highly effective antigen-specific therapy is available for prevention of erythroblastosis fetalis. In this case anti-Rh antibodies are administered to Rh-negative mothers during or promptly after their delivery of an Rh-positive offspring. Although the mechanism is not thoroughly understood, the administered antibody suppresses the ability of the mother to make her own Rh antibody to fetal Rh-positive red cells that enter her circulation during the pregnancy.

In theory, both allergic diseases and disorders caused by autoantibodies to known self-antigens could be cured if a state of specific acquired immunologic tolerance (**anergy**) to the relevant allergen or autoantigen could be permanently induced. As discussed in Chapter 56, the currently used procedure of allergen injection therapy for IgE-mediated atopy or anaphylaxis does create a state of partial immunological tolerance in some patients, so a fully successful application of this therapeutic principle may be possible in the future. Specific therapy for allergy requires a form of allergen administration that avoids systemic reactions, and therapeutic trials involving genetically engineered peptide epitopes have been reported showing some success. In patients with autoimmune diseases the challenge is to identify the autoantigen, which in most of these diseases is unknown. Recently, prevention and reversal of experimental allergic encephalomyelitis in mice, the animal model of human multiple sclerosis, were reported as a result of injections of peptide fragments of myelin basic protein. In theory, therefore, the therapeutically administered peptide epitope can bind to the T-cell receptor (TCR) with the same immunologic specificity as does the complete autoantigen but without activating the T cell.

A possible approach to antigen-specific immune suppression is the elimination of the T cells or B cells bearing the specific TCR or B-cell surface immunoglobulin, respectively, by using an appropriate monoclonal antibody. This is possible only when the antigenic epitope is known, so that the corresponding TCR or immunoglobulin idiotypic specificity can be recognized. This approach has had limited success in certain animal models of autoimmune disease and in treatment of a human B-cell lymphoma.

Another theoretical means of achieving antigen-specific immune suppression would be to prevent the MHC molecule expressed on the surface of the T cell from undergoing its requisite association with the antigen in question. This could be accomplished with anti-MHC monoclonal antibodies. Since there are a number of possible MHC molecules, although the number is much more limited than that of possible antigenic sites, and since presentation of a specific antigen or even a single antigenic epitope may occur in association with more than one MHC molecule, this approach may lack sufficient specificity to avoid eliminating desirable immune responses as well.

Another form of treatment that appears to operate through a "partially specific" mechanism is intravenous normal pooled immunoglobulin (IVIG). Ironically, administration of large amounts of IVIG not only corrects antibody deficiency by passively supplying antibodies from pooled normal plasma but also seems to suppress antibody production when given to patients with certain autoimmune diseases, notably acute idiopathic thrombocytopenic purpura and Kawasaki disease. Although the mechanism of this effect is unknown, current speculation centers on immunomodulation by blocking of Fc receptors for IgG.

B. Passive Suppression: Plasmapheresis consists of repeated removal of blood with replacement of the cells and exchange of patient's plasma for normal plasma, thereby removing circulating antibodies along with other plasma proteins. The procedure does not suppress specific antibody production, but it does selectively remove, albeit transiently, antibodies of the IgM isotype and circulating immune complexes. This makes it a reasonable short-term therapy for certain diseases caused by pathogenic IgM antibodies or antigen–antibody complexes.

ANTIGEN-NONSPECIFIC THERAPY

Immune Stimulation

Techniques for generalized stimulation or upregulation of the immune response are currently being pursued in clinical trials. This general approach to treatment is also called **immune system modulation,** or **biologic response modification.** It is of particular interest in cancer therapy as a means of enhancing the patient's own immunity to the cancer cells. Unfortunately, there are only a few available means to achieve this result, and they are of limited efficacy and often highly toxic, so application of immune stimulation to other conditions with impaired immunity must await development of newer drugs. The current state of knowledge and application is described in Chapter 59.

Adjuvants (see earlier discussion) have been used alone without exogenous antigen in an effort to enhance an endogenous immune response to putative (ie, unknown) tumor cell antigens. To date this experimental form of treatment has been unsuccessful, but future efforts with other adjuvants or modes of administration may prove fruitful.

Certain **cytokines** cloned by genetic engineering technology are potential nonspecific immune stimulators (or inhibitors), because they act as secondary signals in the presence of the antigenic epitope to activate lymphocytes, as discussed in Chapter 10. In fact, clinical trials of various cytokines have been under way in recent years, especially in experimental cancer therapy.

Monoclonal antibodies to various antigenic sites on molecules and cells involved in the immune response can potentially be used in treatment to exploit the ability of the antibody to (1) sterically block a ligand molecule or its receptor to prevent a particular activation or binding step, (2) eliminate the target molecule or lyse the target cell, or (3) stimulate a receptor by acting as a surrogate for the ligand.

The **T-cell receptor/CD3 complex** itself is, of course, the principal site where the immune response is driven, so therapy that sends activation signals to this complex could be nonspecifically immunostimulating, and in fact experiments with an anti-CD3 antibody in mice have yielded antitumor effects. It has been shown in vitro that antigen-mediated activation of T cells is stimulated by monoclonal antibodies to certain **T-cell membrane molecules** such as CD5 and CD28. It remains to be shown whether these antibodies act similarly when administered in vivo and may therefore be of use in treating disease. Monoclonal antibodies to **interleukin receptors** on lymphocytes have the potential for stimulating the receptor by mimicking the action of the interleukin, thereby stimulating the target cell and enhancing the immune response.

Another approach to achieving nonspecific immune stimulation involves the therapeutic use of lymphocytes. In one strategy, natural killer (**NK**) cells are activated by in vitro incubation with interleukin-2 (**IL-2**) to enhance their tumoricidal function. These cells, called lymphokine-activated killer (**LAK**) cells have been used for cancer therapy, although their use has been complicated by IL-2 systemic toxicity. Administration of lymphocytes isolated directly from the patient's own tumor and then incubated with IL-2, called tumor-infiltrating lymphocytes (**TIL**), is another strategy that provides greater tumor cell antigen specificity. These are discussed further in Chapter 59.

Immune Suppression

A variety of immunomodulating techniques are also being used to suppress undesirable immune responses. As the role of the various **cytokines** in immunoregulation becomes clearly delineated, strategies for using cloned cytokines, their receptors, or antibodies to cytokines or their receptors are being developed and tried in animal models of various immunologic diseases to downregulate aberrant or pathologically exuberant immune responses. This approach is particularly appealing as therapy for autoimmune diseases or to suppress graft rejection.

As already discussed, administration of antibodies to lymphocyte membrane molecules can either stimulate or suppress immunity. Originally, the antibodies were produced in animals by injecting purified human cell preparations, but currently monoclonal antibodies to various T-lymphocyte cell surface molecules are being used or undergoing clinical trials. Antibodies to **CD4** are immunosuppressive in animals, and results of limited human trials suggest that they hold promise in treatment of autoimmune disease. There is some evidence that this form of therapy may induce acquired immunologic tolerance as well. Monoclonal antibodies to lymphocytes have also been tried with some success in preventing graft rejection and to a lesser extent in treating GVH reactions.

One way to focus the immunosuppressant effect of antilymphocyte antibodies is to target only cells engaged in an active immune response. For example, activated T cells upregulate their expression of the IL-2 receptor (**IL-2R**) on the cell surface, so anti-IL-2R antibodies have been considered for immunosuppression in graft rejections. Further discussion can be found in Chapter 58.

Certain drugs and ionizing radiation have the ability to destroy cells during cell division. For years the use of **cytotoxic drugs** has been the primary approach to nonspecific immunosuppression, because expansion of nonspecific lymphocyte population by cell division is an essential element in the active immune response. Since all dividing cells are similarly affected, toxicity of this form of treatment reflects the loss of dividing cells in other tissues, as well as the suppression of desirable (eg, antimicrobial) along with the undesirable (eg, autoantibody) immune responses. The types of cytotoxic drugs used for nonspecific immunosuppression and their individual modes of action are discussed in Chapter 58. They are used therapeutically with various degrees of success in many diseases characterized by autoimmune phenomena. During the course of treatment of these diseases, the effect of the cytotoxic drugs on autoantibody production is variable and does not necessarily correlate with clinical improvement in disease activity.

A major breakthrough in nonspecific immunosuppression was the discovery of **cyclosporine,** a drug that selectively blocks T cell activation by downregulating IL-2 synthesis, thereby inhibiting immune responses and immunoregulation. Recently, tacrolimus (formerly called FK506), rapamycin, mycophenolate mofetil, and other immunosuppressant drugs have appeared that have promising therapeutic profiles. Extensive clinical trials will be necessary to determine which drug or drug combination is most effective for each disease.

Corticosteroids are commonly thought of as immunosuppressant, because they are effective therapy for so many human diseases with pathologically overactive immune responses to known or unknown antigens. They apparently do so by interfering with activation of the genes expressing many of the cytokines and adhesion molecules involved in the normal immune response, as described in Chapter 58. Their benefit to these patients, however, may be largely anti-inflammatory, although some of their properties result in modest inhibition of the immune response too. The profound loss of lymphocytes from the peripheral blood circulation that occurs rapidly with pharmacologic doses of glucocorticoids primarily represents a shift of these cells into tissues. Inhibition of IL-1 production from monocytes, however, down-regulates T-lymphocyte synthesis and secretion of IL-2 and T-cell mitosis. Clinically, patients on prolonged steroid therapy may have reduced levels of total serum IgG, although there is little evidence for impaired antibody production when this occurs.

Immune Reconstitution

The success of bone marrow transplantation from donors other than identical twins as a means of restoring a functioning immune system was made a clinical reality with the development of strategies to completely ablate the recipient's own immunity in order to avoid a GVH reaction. Treatment of aplastic anemia and certain leukemias is now routinely accomplished with prospects of a complete cure in many cases. Immunoablation and destruction of the neoplasm are both accomplished by the use of cyclosporine followed by irradiation. Restoration of immune competence by bone marrow transplantation for children with severe combined immunodeficiency can proceed without prior immunoablation. Details are found in Chapters 23 and 57.

MODULATION OF THE INFLAMMATORY RESPONSE

The inflammatory phase of the immune response is one of the effector mechanisms by which the immune response protects the host from infection. The same immune-mediated inflammation, on the other hand, is responsible for the deleterious effects of the allergic diseases, some autoimmune diseases, graft rejection, and the GVH response. Therefore, drugs that reduce or inhibit the inflammatory response are necessary in the treatment of many immunologic diseases. In general, anti-inflammatory therapy is independent of the cause of the inflammation, and therefore these drugs are also useful for tissue inflammation induced by physical injury or toxic insults. Some anti-inflammatory drugs,

such as the corticosteroids, however, have limited immunosuppressive activity as well.

The various types of inflammatory responses are addressed in Chapter 12 as effector consequences of the immune response in vivo. Different immune response pathways lead to different specific pathologic and clinical forms of inflammation. For example, IgE antibody-mediated inflammation is characterized by vasodilation, stimulation of visceral organ smooth muscle contraction, and an eosinophilic infiltrate, whereas effector T-cell inflammation generates tissue infiltration by lymphocytes and monocytes with granuloma formation. Some drugs inhibit only one of these inflammatory pathways, whereas others have a more global anti-inflammatory effect. Most of the inflammation-inhibiting treatments used today have acquired their clinical status empirically, and their precise modes of action are incompletely understood.

The anti-inflammatory mechanisms of steroid (glucocorticoid) and nonsteroid (aspirin and nonsteroidal anti-inflammatory drugs [NSAID]) chemicals share in common the ability to inhibit metabolites of arachidonic acid from inflammatory cell membranes, particularly the prostaglandins. As described in Chapter 60, they do so in quite different ways, however. The NSAIDs inhibit amino acid transport across the cell membrane, whereas the glucocorticoids prevent synthesis of arachidonic acid metabolites by stimulating the cell to synthesize and release lipomodulin, which in turn inhibits phospholipase A_2. Both classes of drugs have other therapeutic actions, side effects, and toxicities, but if the specific property that inhibited cellular inflammation can be pinpointed, there is the possibility in the future of designing a molecule with limited activity, for example, at the level of the arachidonic acid oxygenation products.

Drugs with a more restricted anti-inflammatory effect are available for treatment of IgE-mediated allergic disorders. Cromolyn (disodium cromoglycate) and nedocromil act on the mast cell to prevent mediator release, although the mechanism is unknown. The numerous antihistaminic drugs specifically inhibit histamine H_1 receptors on target cells. Unfortunately, histamine is only one of a number of mast cell-derived mediators in allergy (see Chapters 10 and 11). Zafirlukast, a leukotriene receptor antagonist, has recently been released for treatment of mild or moderate asthma. Other drugs used in allergy, such as sympathomimetic and anticholinergic drugs and theophylline, are indirectly anti-inflammatory because they favorably modulate the function of target tissues involved in the allergic inflammatory process.

REFERENCES

Allison AC, Byars NE: Adjuvant formulations and their mode of action. *Semin Immunol* 1990;**2:**369.

Chatenoud L, Bach J-F: Monoclonal antibodies to CD3 as immunosuppressants. *Semin Immunol* 1990;**2:**437.

Cournoyer D, Caskey CT: Gene therapy of the immune system. *Ann Rev Immunol* 1993;**11:**297.

Gefter M (editor): T cell epitope-based immunotherapy. *Semin Immunol* 1991;**3:**193 (entire issue).

Greenberger PA (editor): Immunotherapy of IgE-mediated disorders. *Immunol Allergy Clin North Am* 1992;**12:**1 (entire issue).

Kahan BD, Ghobrial R: Immunosuppressive agents. *Surg Clin North Am* 1994;**74:**1029.

Oettgen HF: Human cancer immunology II. *Immunol Allergy Clin North Am* 1991;**11:**1 (entire issue).

Schleimer RP: An overview of glucocorticoid anti-inflammatory action. *Eur J Clin Pharmacol* 1993;**45:**(suppl 1):53.

Schreiber SL, Crabtree GR: The mechanism of action of cyclosporin A and FK506. *Immunol Today* 1992;**13:**136.

Waldmann H: Manipulation of T-cell responses with monoclonal antibodies. *Ann Rev Immunol* 1989;**7:**407.

Waldmann T: Immune receptors: Targets for therapy of leukemia/lymphoma, autoimmune diseases, and for prevention of allograft rejection. *Ann Rev Immunol* 1992;**10:**675.

Wofsky D, Carteron NL: CD4 antibody therapy in systemic lupus erythematosus. *Semin Immunol* 1990;**2:**419.

55

Immunization

Moses Grossman, MD

The goal of immunization in any one individual is the prevention of disease. The goal of immunization of population groups is the eradication of disease. Immunization has accounted for some spectacular advances in health around the world. Childhood immunizations have been accepted as part of routine health care; in the USA, the federal government has financed the purchase of vaccines for the public sector and all states have passed legislation requiring proof of immunization as a condition for school entry. As a result, poliomyelitis, diphtheria, and tetanus have all but disappeared in developed nations; measles, rubella, and pertussis have become rare. Smallpox has been eradicated, and the World Health Organization has made poliomyelitis the next target for eradication.

HISTORICAL OVERVIEW

It has been recognized for centuries that individuals who recover from certain diseases are protected from reinfection. The moderately successful but hazardous introduction of small quantities of fluid from the pustules of smallpox into the skin of uninfected persons (variolation) was an effort to imitate this natural phenomenon. Edward Jenner's introduction of vaccination with cowpox virus (1796) to protect against smallpox was the first documented use of a live, attenuated viral vaccine and the beginning of modern immunization. Robert Koch demonstrated the specific bacterial cause of anthrax in 1876, and the causes of several common illnesses were rapidly identified thereafter. Attempts to develop immunizing agents followed (Table 55–1).

TYPES OF IMMUNIZATION

Immunization may be **active,** in which administration of an antigen (usually a modified infectious agent or toxin) results in active production of immunity, or **passive,** in which administration of antibody-containing serum or sensitized cells provides passive protection for the recipient.

ACTIVE IMMUNIZATION

Active immunization results in the production of antibodies directed against the infecting agent or its toxic products; it may also initiate cellular responses mediated by lymphocytes and macrophages. The most important protective antibodies include those that inactivate soluble toxic protein products of bacteria (antitoxins), facilitate phagocytosis and intracellular digestion of bacteria (opsonins), interact with the components of serum complement to damage the bacterial membrane and hence cause bacteriolysis (lysins), or prevent the proliferation of infectious virus (neutralizing antibodies). Newly appreciated are the antibodies that interact with components of the bacterial surface to prevent adhesion to mucosal surfaces (antiadhesins). Some antibodies may not be protective and, by "blocking" the reaction of protective antibodies with the pathogen, may actually depress the body's defenses.

Antigens react with antibodies in the bloodstream and extracellular fluid and at mucosal surfaces. Antibodies cannot readily reach intracellular sites of infection, where viral replication occurs. They are ef-

Table 55–1. Historical milestones in immunization.

Variolation	1721
Vaccination	1796
Rabies vaccine	1885
Diphtheria toxoid	1925
Tetanus toxoid	1925
Pertussis vaccine	1925
Viral culture in chick embryo	1931
Yellow fever vaccine	1937
Influenza vaccine	1943
Viral tissue culture	1949
Poliovaccine, inactivated (Salk)	1954
Poliovaccine, live, attenuated (Sabin)	1956
Measles vaccine	1960
Tetanus immune globulin (human)	1962
Rubella vaccine	1966
Mumps vaccine	1967
Hepatitis B vaccine	1975
Smallpox eradicated	1980
First recombinant vaccine (hepatitis B)	1986
Conjugate polysaccharide vaccine for *H influenzae* B	1988
Poliomyelitis eliminated from Western Hemisphere	1994
Varicella-zoster vaccine	1995

fective against many viral diseases in two ways, however: (1) by interacting with the virus before initial intracellular penetration occurs and (2) by preventing locally replicating virus from disseminating from the site of entry to an important target organ, as in the spread of poliovirus from the gastrointestinal tract to the central nervous system or of rabies virus from a puncture wound to peripheral neural tissue. Lymphocytes acting alone and antibody interacting with lymphoid or monocytic effector K cells may also recognize surface changes in virus-infected cells and destroy these infected "foreign" cells.

Types of Vaccines

The agent used for active immunization is loosely termed "antigen" or "vaccine." It may consist of live, attenuated viruses (measles virus) or bacteria (bacillus Calmette-Guérin [BCG]) or killed microorganisms (*Vibrio cholerae*). It may also be an inactivated bacterial product (tetanus toxoid) or a specific single component of bacteria (polysaccharide of *Neisseria meningitidis*). Such a polysaccharide component may be conjugated to a protein in order to produce immunogenicity at an earlier age (conjugated *Haemophilus influenzae*). It may be a recombinant DNA segment (hepatitis B virus), in which case it would be expressed in another living cell (yeasts, *Escherichia coli*). In each case, it usually contains—in addition to the desired antigen—other ingredients including other antigens, suspending fluids that may be complex and may contain protein ingredients of their own (tissue culture, egg yolk), preservatives, and adjuvants for enhanced immunogenicity (aluminum, protein conjugate). Undesirable reactions may occur not only to the antigen itself but also to these added components.

Active immunization with living organisms is generally superior to immunization with killed vaccines in inducing a long-lived immune response. A single

dose of a live, attenuated virus vaccine often suffices for reliable immunization. Multiple immunizations are recommended for poliovirus in case intercurrent enteroviral infection or interference among three simultaneously administered virus types in the trivalent vaccine prevents completely successful primary immunization. The persistence of immunity to many viral infections may be explained by repeated natural reexposure to new cases in the community, the unusually large antigenic stimulus provided by infection with a living agent, or other mechanisms such as the persistence of latent virus.

All immunizing materials—live organisms in particular—must be properly stored to retain effectiveness. Serious failures of smallpox and measles immunization have resulted from inadequate refrigeration prior to use. Agents presently licensed for active immunization are listed in Table 55–2.

Factors in Immunization

Primary active immunization produces a protective antibody level more slowly than the incubation period of most infections and must therefore be performed prior to exposure to the etiologic agent. By contrast, "booster" reimmunization in a previously immune individual provides a rapid secondary (anamnestic) increase in immunity.

Previous infection can also substantially alter the response to an inactivated vaccine. For example, volunteers who have recovered from cholera or who live in a cholera-endemic area respond to parenteral immunization with an increase in anticholera secretory IgA, which is not seen in immunized control subjects.

The route of immunization may be an important determinant of successful vaccination, particularly if nonreplicating immunogens are used. Thus, immunization intranasally or by aerosol, which stimulates mucosal immunity, often appears to be more successful than parenteral injection against viral or bacterial respiratory challenges.

The route of administration recommended by the manufacturer and approved by the FDA should be used. Vaccines containing adjuvants such as aluminum hydroxide should always be given deep into the muscle and not subcutaneously. The ideal intramuscular injection site is the anterolateral portion of the upper thigh.

The timing of primary immunization, the interval between doses, and the timing of booster injections are based on both theoretic considerations and vaccine trials. The resulting recommendations should be followed closely. Many factors are involved. For instance, the age at which measles immunization is administered in the USA was changed from 12 to 15 months because the persistent maternal antibody, although present in small amounts only, was shown to interfere with active antibody formation by the child. Ironically, now that most mothers have induced immunity rather than naturally acquired measles antibody,

Table 55–2. Materials available for active immunization.

Disease	Product (Source)	Type of Agent	Route of Administration	Primary Immunization[1]	Duration of Effect	Comments
Cholera	Cholera vaccine	Killed bacteria	SC, IM, ID	Two doses 1 week or more apart.	6 months[2]	50% protective; International Certificate may be required for travel.
Diphtheria	DTP, DTaP, DT (adsorbed for child under age 7) also available in combination with conjugated *H influenzae* vaccine; Td (adsorbed) for all others.	Toxoid	IM	Three doses four weeks or more apart, with an additional dose 1 year later for a child under age 7. (Can be given at same time as polio vaccine if doses at least 8 weeks apart.) A fifth dose before entering school is recommended if the fourth dose was given before the fourth birthday.	10 years[3]	Regular booster injections are recommended every 10 years. After the seventh birthday use the adult-type tetanus-diphtheria toxoid (Td). This product has a lower antigenic content and is less likely to produce reactions in older individuals.
Haemophilus influenzae infections	Polysaccharide capsule conjugated with protein	Polysaccharide protein conjugate.	IM	Two or three doses and a booster depending on type of vaccine used.	1 1/2–3 1/2 years	As of 1996, three vaccines are available, conjugated to different proteins. Immunization to be started at 2 months of age. The vaccine can be given at the same time as DPT. A combined product is expected to be available in the future.
Hepatitis A	Hepatitis A vaccine	Inactivated Hepatitis A virus	IM	For children >2 years of age and adults. Different formulations and dosages for adults and children. Simultaneous administration of IgG (but at a different site) does not impair immunogenicity. Protection starts 4 weeks after first dose; second dose necessary for long-term protection.	Four years, and perhaps much longer.	Recommended for travelers to endemic countries (most countries in Asia and Africa and others). Protection starts only 4 weeks after immunization. IgG should be added (at a separate site) for those departing earlier.
Hepatitis B	Hepatitis B vaccine (human carriers). (Recombinant DNA, produced in yeast cells. Human carrier-derived vaccine is no longer being manufactured in the USA but is	Recombinant antigen or formalin-treated purified antigen.	IM	Two doses 1 month apart, followed by a booster given 6 months later. *Do not feeeze vaccine*; this causes aggregation and loss of potency. The simultaneous administration of hepatitis B immune globulin (HBIG) in a separate syringe at	Variable, about 5 years	A stable, adjuvant-supplemented vaccine from highly purified formalin-activated HBsAg harvested from human carriers or recombinant antigen expressed in yeast cells. Recommended for all newborns as a routine immunization. Also for all individuals at high risk of exposure to HBV infection, including health care personnel such as surgeons, anesthesiologists, autopsy staff, phlebotomists, oper-

774

Disease	Type	Form	Route	Dosage	Duration of immunity	Indications and recommendations
	still available commercially.)			a separate site does not appear to impair the effectiveness of the vaccine.		ating room and dialysis nurses, medical technologists, dentists, and other staff exposed to patients with a high rate of HBV carriage; for patients undergoing chronic hemodialysis or repeatedly receiving plasma or clotting factor concentrates for clotting disorders; for sexual and household contacts of HBV carriers (families accepting children from countries with high endemic rates of HBV infection should have the child screened and should be vaccinated if the child is HBsAg-positive); for male homosexuals, intravenous drug abusers, and prison populations with problems of homosexuality and drug use; and other high-risk individuals.
Influenza	Influenza virus vaccine. Monovalent or bivalent (chick embryo). Composition of the vaccine is varied depending on epidemiologic circumstances.	Killed whole or split virus types A and B	IM	One dose. (Two doses 4 weeks or more apart are recommended in individuals who have not previously received the current antigenic components or been otherwise exposed to the current strain of virus. Two doses of the split virus products should be used in persons 12 years of age or under because of fewer side effects.)	1 year	Give immunization by November. Recommended annually for individuals with chronic cardiovascular or pulmonary disease, for residents of nursing homes and other chronic care facilities, for medical personnel who may spread infection to high-risk patients, and for healthy individuals over 65 years of age, as well as for patients with chronic metabolic disorders, renal dysfunction, anemia, immunosuppression, or asthma. Patients receiving chemotherapy for malignant disease are likely to respond better if immunized between courses of treatment.
Japanese encephalitis	Japanese encephalitis vaccine	Inactivated virus derived from mouse brain	SC	Three doses of 1 mL each administered SC on days 0, 7, and 30. Children between 1 and 3 years receive 0.5 mL/dose.		Recommended for travelers to endemic regions in Asia. The risk is principally in rural areas for people whose stay is prolonged (more than 30 days).
Measles[4]	Measles virus vaccine, live (chick embryo)	Live attenuated virus	SC	Two doses, one at 15 months, the other at 6–12 years of age.	Permanent	Usually given as MMR (with mumps and rubella). Two doses are required as proof of immunity for school or college entry and for health care workers. May prevent natural disease if given less than 48 hours after exposure.

(continued)

Table 55–2. Materials available for active immunization. *(continued)*

Disease	Product (Source)	Type of Agent	Route of Administration	Primary Immunization[1]	Duration of Effect	Comments
Meningococcus	Meningococcal polysaccharide vaccine (combination vaccine against groups A, C, Y, and W135).	Polysaccharide	SC	One dose. Since primary antibody response requires at least 5 days, antibiotic prophylaxis with rifampin (600 mg or 10 mg/kg every 12 h for four doses) should be given to household contacts.	?Permanent in older children and adults; transient in children <2 years.	Recommended in epidemic situations, for use by the military to prevent outbreaks in recruits, for patients with anatomic or functional asplenia, for individuals with a congenital deficiency of terminal components of the complement cascade, and possibly as an adjunct to antibiotic prophylaxis in preventing secondary cases in family contacts. Not reliably effective in infants, who require booster injections if antibody is to last for a year (especially antibody to group C). Revaccination may be indicated for individuals at high risk of infection, particularly if first immunized before age 4. A protein-conjugated vaccine that would be immunogenic for infants is being developed.
Mumps[4]	Mumps virus vaccine, live (chick embryo)	Live virus	SC	Two doses	Permanent	Usually given as MMR (with measles and rubella).
Pertussis	DTP, DTaP	Killed bacteria. Also an "acellular" vaccine containing two or more antigens but not the whole cell.	IM	As for DTP	Up to 5 years[3]	The whole-cell vaccine has an efficacy of approximately 80%. It also has some undesirable adverse effects—fever, pain, and tenderness of the injection site; prolonged crying; etc. An acellular vaccine, containing two to four antigenic components, has similar efficacy but fewer adverse effects. It is currently licensed only for children older than 15 months; licensure for infants is expected soon based on favorable field trials. Not generally recommended after the seventh birthday. Contraindications to beginning or continuing pertussis immunization include a history of seizures or the development of seizures before the four-dose primary series is completed. Immunization of these children should be deferred until it can be determined whether an evolving neurologic illness is present. For infants who have received fewer than three doses of DTP, the decision to pursue immunization should be made before 1 year of age; children with seizures have a

(continuation of previous comments column)

higher risk of adverse outcome from pertussis itself and are at increased risk of exposure as they grow older and contact other children. If the neurologic condition is stable and seizures are well controlled, the benefits of immunization outweigh the hazards, although the parents should be warned of an eight-fold increased risk of postimmunization convulsions if febrile convulsions have occurred previously. Definitive contraindications to further administration of DTP include hypersensitivity to the vaccine, an evolving neurologic disorder, or history of a severe reaction.

Disease	Vaccine	Type	Route	Dosage/Schedule	Duration	Comments
Plague	Plague vaccine	Killed bacteria	IM	Three doses 4 weeks or more apart	6 months[3]	Recommended only for occupational exposure and not for residents of endemic area in the southwest USA.
Pneumococcus	Pneumococcal polysaccharide vaccine, polyvalent	Polysaccharide	SC, IM	0.5 mL, if possible before splenectomy or before instituting chemotherapy	Uncertain—probably at least 5 years in adults, but erratic in children under age 5	Recommended for patients with cardiorespiratory disease or other chronic illness, for patients with sickle cell disease, for patients with functional, congenital, or postsurgical asplenia, and for patients with nephrotic syndrome or with cerebrospinal fluid leakage. Also suggested for immunosuppressed or alcoholic patients and for patients aged 65 or older. Only the 23 most common serotypes are incorporated in the vaccine. Children up to age 2, splenectomized children, and some chronically ill patients respond unreliably. *Caution:* Because of a marked increase in adverse reactions following revaccination, booster doses should generally *not* be given, even to recipients of the earlier less comprehensive and less immunogenic vaccine. However, a booster is warranted after 3–5 years for high-risk children and is recommended after 3–4 months off chemotherapy for children first immunized while receiving it. Can be given at the same time as influenza or DTP vaccines. A protein-conjugated vaccine that would be immunogenic for infants is being developed.

(continued)

Table 55–2. Materials available for active immunization. (continued)

Disease	Product (Source)	Type of Agent	Route of Administration	Primary Immunization[1]	Duration of Effect	Comments
Poliomyelitis	Poliovirus vaccine, live, oral, trivalent (monkey kidney, human diploid)	Live virus types I, II, III	Oral	Two doses 6–8 weeks or more apart, followed by a third dose 8–12 months later. (Can be given at the same time as primary DTP immunization.) A fourth dose before entering school is recommended if the third dose was given before age 4.	Permanent	Recommended for adults only if at increased risk by travel to endemic or highly endemic areas or occupational contact. Individuals who have completed a primary series may take a single booster dose if the risk of exposure is high.
	Poliomyelitis vaccine, inactivated	Killed virus types I, II, III	IM	Three doses 4–8 weeks apart, followed by a fourth dose 6–12 months later. A fifth dose before entering school is recommended if the fourth dose was given before age 4. A single booster dose should be given every 5 years until age 18, after which the need is uncertain.	5 years[3]	Killed virus vaccines are preferred for immunologically deficient patients and their household contacts. Adults who have not previously received oral polio vaccine and who are at risk because of travel or, minimally, from immunization of their children should receive the inactivated vaccine. A new "enhanced" inactivated vaccine contains more antigenic material and is more immunogenic.
Rabies	Rabies vaccine (human diploid)	Killed virus	IM or ID (preexposure only)	**Preexposure:** Two doses 1 week apart, followed by a third dose 2–3 weeks later. **Postexposure:** Always give rabies immune globulin as well. If not previously immunized, give a total of five doses, on days 0, 3, 7, 14, and 28 (WHO recommends a sixth dose 90 days after the first dose). If the vaccinee is immunocompromised (or if only DEV is available), a serum specimen should be collected on day 28 or 2–3 weeks after the last dose and tested for rabies	2 years[3] if titer <1:16	Preexposure immunization only for occupational or avocational risk or residence in hyperendemic area. For animal bite, consider antitetanus and other antibacterial measures as well. *Caution:* Several reports document unexpectedly poor response to intradermal immunization. If the intradermal route is used, rabies antibody must be measured 2–3 weeks after the third dose of vaccine. If the antibody titer is <1:16, an additional dose should be given and the antibody level retested 2–3 weeks later. If the antibody response of an individual who has received intradermal vaccine within the past 12 months is unknown, the level should be checked; if more than 12 months have elapsed, a booster should be given and the titer

778

tested 2–3 weeks later. If a rabies exposure takes place following preexposure immunization by the intradermal route and there is no documentation of an adequate antibody level, a full course of HRIG and IM rabies vaccine should be given. Serologic testing does not appear to be necessary if preexposure prophylaxis was given by the IM route.

antibody.[5] If the antibody level is insufficient, a booster should be given and the titer remeasured 2–3 weeks later. *If previously immunized* with diploid vaccine, do not give serum therapy. Give two booster doses, one immediately and one 3 days later. ***Note:*** Unexplained immediate-type (anaphylactic) hypersensitivity reactions have occurred during primary rabies immunization with vaccine from different manufacturers. Immunization of such individuals should be discontinued unless there is actual exposure to rabies virus or inapparent or unavoidable rabies contact is truly likely to occur. In the later situations, the serologic response to rabies should be checked and booster doses omitted if protective titers have already been attained; vaccination should be continued only under careful supervision. Rabies vaccine, adsorbed (RVA Michigan Department of Public Health), a newly licensed vaccine, can be used for both preexposure and postexposure prophylaxis. There is limited experience with and limited availability of this vaccine, but it

(continued)

Table 55–2. Materials available for active immunization. *(continued)*

Disease	Product (Source)	Type of Agent	Route of Administration	Primary Immunization[1]	Duration of Effect	Comments
Rabies *(cont.)*				appears to have a far decreased incidence of hypersensitivity reactions.		
Rubella[4]	Rubella virus vaccine, live (human diploid)	Live attenuated virus	SC	Two doses	Permanent	Give after 15 months of age. Second dose at 6–11 years of age. Usually given as MMR (with measles and mumps) for children. Because a history of rubella is unreliable and because the vaccine is innocuous in immune recipients, unimmunized women of childbearing age should be vaccinated without serologic testing. Vaccination should be avoided during pregnancy on theoretic grounds unless there is a risk of exposure due to an outbreak; however, there is no evidence of vaccine-induced fetal damage in over 200 recipients. Vaccination is contraindicated for those receiving systemic corticosteroids for more than 2 weeks; for leukemic or immunosuppressed patients for at least 3 months after chemotherapy has been discontinued; for recipients of immune globulin treatment other than anti-Rh therapy within the following 2 weeks or prior 3 months; and for individuals with allergy to neomycin but not to eggs or penicillin. If a female is immunized postpartum and has received blood products or Rh immune globulin, serologic testing should be done 6–8 weeks later to confirm successful immunization. Viremia can occur if antibody has fallen to low levels; the frequency and thus the clinical importance of this phenomenon are unknown.
Smallpox	Smallpox vaccine (calf lymph, chick embryo). (Available from CDC[7])	Live vaccinia virus	ID	1 dose	3 years	Smallpox has been eradicated, and smallpox vaccine is no longer available.
Tetanus	DTP, DT (adsorbed) for children under age 7; Td, T (adsorbed) for all others	Toxoid	IM	Three doses 4 weeks or more apart.	10 years[3,5]	Recipients aged 7 or above should be given a third dose 6–12 months after second. (See Table 56–4 regarding use of hyperimmune globulin.)

780

Disease	Vaccine	Type	Route	Dosage	Duration	Comments
Tuberculosis	BCG vaccine	Live attenuated *Mycobacterium bovis*	ID, SC	One dose	?Permanent[6]	Recommended in USA only for PPD-negative contacts of ineffectively treated or persistently untreated cases and for other unusually high-risk groups.
Typhoid	Typhoid vaccine	Killed bacteria	SC	Two doses 4 weeks or more apart, or three doses 1 week apart (less desirable)	3 years[3]	70% protective. Recommended only for exposure from travel, epidemic, or household carrier and not, for example, because of floods.
		Live attenuated bacteria	Oral	Four doses on alternate days	5 years	Oral vaccine has similar effectiveness.
Varicella	Varicella vaccine	Live attenuated virus	SC	One 0.5-mL dose for children. Teens older than 13 years and adults require two 0.5-mL doses given 4–8 weeks apart.	10 years or possibly longer	Recommended as universal immunization for all children to be administered between 12 and 18 months of age, and for adults at risk to exposure who have no demonstrable antibodies. Contraindicated for immunocompromised individuals. May be administered simultaneously with MMR vaccine but in a separate syringe and in a separate site.
Yellow fever	Yellow fever vaccine (chick embryo)	Live virus	SC	One dose	10 years[2]	Certificate may be required for travel. Recommended for residence or travel to endemic areas of Africa and South America. Avoid administration to an immunologically incompetent host or an individual on long-term (>2 weeks) corticosteroid therapy.

Abbreviations: DTP = diphtheria, tetanus, pertussis; DT = diphtheria, tetanus; SC = subcutaneous; IM = intramuscular; ID = intradermal; WHO = World Health Organization; DEV = duck embryo vaccine; HRIG = human rabies immunoglobulin; BCG = bacillus Calmette-Guérin; PPD = purified protein derivative.

[1] Dosages for the specific product, including variations for age, are best obtained from the manufacturer's package insert. Immunizations should be given by the route suggested for the product.

[2] Revaccination interval required by international regulations.

[3] A single dose is a sufficient booster at any time after the effective duration of primary immunization has passed.

[4] Combination vaccines available.

[5] For contaminated or severe wounds, give booster if more than 5 years have elapsed since full immunization or last booster. A single booster any time after primary immunization is effective.

[6] Test for PPD conversion 2 months later, and reimmunize if there is no conversion.

[7] Drug Immunologic and Vaccine Service, Center for Infectious Diseases, Telephone: (404) 329-3311 (main switchboard, day) or (404) 329-3644 (nights and weekends).

their lower antibody titer may require that childhood immunization be changed back to 12 months of age.

Because of the clonal nature of immunity, it is possible—and, in fact, routine practice—to give many different antigens simultaneously. Some antigens are premixed (measles, mumps, rubella [MMR] and diphtheria, tetanus, pertussis [DPT]), whereas others may be given on the same day at different sites (MMR and varicella-zoster [VZV]). Live virus vaccines that are not given on the same day, however, should be given at least 1 month apart.

Splenectomy may markedly impair the primary antibody response to thymus-independent antigens such as bacterial polysaccharides, although many splenectomized patients respond normally to polysaccharide antigens because of priming by natural exposure prior to splenectomy.

Technique of Immunization

When administering vaccines intended for subcutaneous or intramuscular deposition, it is essential to pull back on the syringe before depressing the plunger to make certain that the product will not be injected intravenously, resulting in lessened immunizing effect and increased untoward reactions. It is particularly important to use a sufficiently long needle (usually >1 in.) for intramuscular delivery of adjuvant-containing (eg, alum [aluminum phosphate]-adsorbed) vaccines; subcutaneous inoculation of adjuvants may result in tissue necrosis.

Recent studies of injection techniques suggest that the anterolateral thigh or deltoid site is preferable to the buttocks. Even with the usual precautions, use of the latter site occasionally leads to sciatic nerve damage, and in adults most injections meant for intramuscular delivery are instead delivered into fat.

The intradermal route of immunization is under intensive study as a means of obtaining an earlier or greater immune response with the same amount of antigen or of inducing a satisfactory immune response with a smaller quantity of expensive immunogens, such as the hepatitis B and rabies vaccines.

Adverse Reactions & the Risk-Benefit Ratio

All vaccines approved and licensed in the USA have been shown to be safe and effective. Each of them has also been shown to cause adverse reactions, however. Sometimes these are minimal in occurrence rate and severity, as in tetanus toxoid. Historically, some immunizing agents produced adverse reactions that were so severe they would be unacceptable today; variolation and the original rabies vaccine made from spinal cord material are two examples. Smallpox vaccination with vaccinia virus carried a very acceptable risk at a time when smallpox posed an imminent and serious threat. As the risk of smallpox declined to the point at which the disease was eradicated, however, the risk-benefit ratio of the vaccine has increased and is now infinite. At present, the most controversial vaccine in routine use is the whole-cell pertussis vaccine. It is only about 70% effective for protection, causes very frequent minor reaction, and occasionally produces serious neurologic reactions. It is still used, however, because the risk-benefit ratio is acceptably low. Japan, the United Kingdom, and Sweden have experienced a significant rise in the fatality rate from pertussis since the use of the vaccine was discontinued. This whole-cell vaccine is currently being supplanted by an acellular pertussis vaccine. This latter vaccine is at least as effective but produces fewer side effects.

Unique Hazards of Live Vaccines

Because of their potential for infection of the fetus, live vaccines should *not* be given to a pregnant woman unless there is a high immediate risk (eg, a poliomyelitis epidemic). A pregnant woman traveling in an area where yellow fever is endemic *should* be immunized because the risk of infection exceeds the small theoretic hazard to fetus and mother. If yellow fever vaccination is being performed solely to comply with a legal requirement for international travel, however, the woman should seek a waiver with a letter from her physician. Live vaccines, furthermore, can cause serious or even fatal illness in an immunologically incompetent host. They generally should not be given to patients receiving corticosteroids, alkylating drugs, radiation, or other immunosuppressive drugs or to individuals with known or suspected congenital or acquired defects in cell-mediated immunity (eg, severe combined immunodeficiency disease, leukemias, lymphomas, Hodgkin's disease, and HIV infection). Patients with pure hypogammaglobulinemia but no defect in cell-mediated immunity usually tolerate viral infections and vaccines well but have a 10,000-fold excess of paralytic complications over the usual one case per million recipients, in part because of the frequent reversion of attenuated poliovirus strains to virulence in the intestinal tract. Since live poliovirus is shed by recipients, it should not be given to household contacts of these patients either.

Even in immunocompetent hosts, live vaccines may result in mild or, rarely, severe disease.

The early measles vaccines caused high fever and rash in a significant proportion of recipients. The mild, recurrent arthralgia or arthritis that can follow rubella immunization may represent the consequences of a secondary rather than a primary infection in an individual who has low levels of antibodies not detected by all assays and who has in vitro evidence of cell-mediated immunity.

Because passage through the human intestinal tract occasionally results in reversion of oral attenuated poliovirus vaccine (particularly type III) to neurovirulence, paralytic illness has occurred in recipients or, rarely, their nonimmune contacts, especially adults. The success of live polio vaccines in preventing widespread natural infection has resulted in the paradox that the vaccine itself now accounts for a large fraction of the few cases of paralytic poliomyelitis seen each year in the USA. Killed (Salk) vaccine also appears to be effective in abolishing polio. The major advantages of live (Sabin) vaccine, which sustain its use despite the small risk of paralysis (5 cases per million doses in nonimmune recipients), are its ease of administration and more durable immune response. It is likely that a schedule combining the sequential administration of both vaccines will be introduced within the next few years.

Live vaccines may contain undetected and undesirable contaminants. Epidemic hepatitis resulted in the past from vaccinia and yellow fever vaccines containing human serum. More recently, millions of people received SV40, a simian papavavirus contained in live or inactivated poliovirus vaccine prepared in monkey kidney tissue culture. Although a virus closely related to SV40 has been isolated from the brains of patients with progressive multifocal leukoencephalopathy, a lethal degenerative disease, there is no known history of polio immunization in these cases. An increased incidence of cancer in children of mothers who received inactivated polio vaccine during pregnancy was suggested in two studies but not in a 20-year follow-up of a large number of childhood recipients. SV40 can now be detected and excluded from human viral vaccines, but other undetected viruses might be transmitted by vaccines grown in nonhuman cell lines. Yellow fever vaccine has been reported to be probably contaminated with avian leukosis virus. Bacteriophages and probably bacterial endotoxins have also been shown to contaminate live virus vaccines, although without known hazard thus far.

Live viral vaccines probably do not interfere with tuberculin skin testing, although they depress some measurements of lymphocyte function.

Unlike live vaccines, inactivated vaccines may safely be given to immunocompromised hosts. They may not, however, dependably elicit an adequately protective immune response.

The risk-benefit ratio of live measles vaccine is sufficiently low to recommend its use in patients with human immunodeficiency virus (HIV) infection—even immunocompromised patients.

Other Adverse Effects

Allergic reactions may occur on exposure to egg protein (in measles, mumps, influenza, and yellow fever vaccines) or antibiotics or preservatives (eg, neomycin or mercurials) in viral vaccines. Patients with known IgE-mediated sensitivity to a vaccine component (eg, egg albumin in yellow fever vaccine grown in eggs) should not receive the vaccine unless successfully desensitized (in cases when immunization is essential). Occasionally, the product of a different manufacturer does not contain the offending allergen. Improvements in antigenicity and better purification procedures in vaccine production decrease the amount and number of foreign substances injected and result in fewer side effects.

Reporting Adverse Effects & Legal Liability

Lawsuits arising from adverse reaction to vaccines have led to steep increases in the cost of vaccines in recent years. Because of the high costs of litigation and liability insurance, the threat to development and production of new vaccines prompted the passage of the National Childhood Vaccine Injury Act of 1986. This Act provides for compensation of those injured by adverse reactions and at the same time mandates that certain adverse effects be reported and that physicians use vaccine information pamphlets prepared by the Centers for Disease Control and Prevention (CDC) which provide information on benefits and risks of vaccines. These pamphlets are mandatory when government-purchased vaccine is used and can be obtained by calling (800) PIK-VIPS. Physicians and clinics purchasing their own vaccines may prepare their own information pamphlets.

The reportable events are listed in Table 55–3. Reports are to be made to the Vaccine Adverse Event Reporting System, 1–800–822–7267. Preventable adverse effects can be minimized by reading vaccine labels, storing vaccines carefully, using the correct method of administration at the proper site, and being aware of contraindications, particularly by identifying immunocompromised hosts.

PASSIVE IMMUNIZATION

Immunization may be accomplished passively by administering either preformed immunoreactive serum or cells.

Antibody, either as whole serum or as fractionated, concentrated immune (gamma) globulin that is predominantly IgG, may be obtained from human or animal donors who have recovered from an infectious disease or have been immunized. These antibodies may provide immediate protection to an antibody-deficient individual. Passive immunization is thus useful for individuals who cannot form antibodies or for the nonimmunocompromised host who might develop disease before active immunization could stimulate antibody production, which usually requires at least 7–10 days.

Additionally, passive immunization is useful when no active immunization is available, when passive immunization is used in conjunction with vaccine administration (eg, in rabies vaccination), in the management of specific effects of certain toxins and venoms, and, finally, as an immunosuppressant.

Antibody may be obtained from humans or animals, but animal sera give rise to an immune response that leads to rapid clearance of the protective molecules from the circulation of the recipient and the risk of allergic reactions, particularly serum sickness or anaphylaxis (see later section). Thus, to obtain a similar protective effect, much more animal antiserum must be injected compared with human antiserum (eg,

Table 55–3. Vaccine injury table.

Illness, Diability, Injury, or Condition Covered	Time Period for First Symptom or Manifestation of Onset or of Significant Aggravation After Vaccine Administration
I. DTP; P; DT; Td; or tetanus toxoid; or in any combination with polio; or any other vaccine containing whole-cell pertussis bacteria, extracted or partial-cell pertussis bacteria, or specific pertussis antigen(s):	
A. Anaphylaxis or anaphylactic shock	4 hours
B. Encephalopathy (or encephalitis)	72 hours
C. Any sequela (including death) of an illness, disability, injury, or condition referred to above which illness, disability, injury, or condition arose within the time period prescribed.	Not applicable
II. (a). Measles, mumps, rubella, or any vaccine containing any of the foregoing as a component:	
A. Anaphylaxis or anaphylactic shock	4 hours
B. Encephalopathy (or encephalitis)	5–15 days (not less than 5 days and not more than 15 days) for measles, mumps, rubella, or any vaccine containing any of the foregoing as a component.
C. Residual seizure disorder in accordance with subsection (b)(3)	5–15 days (not less than 5 days and not more than 15 days) for measles, mumps, rubella, or any vaccine containing any of the foregoing as a component.
D. Any sequela (including death) of an illness, disability, injury, or condition referred to above which illness, disability, injury, or condition arose within the time period prescribed.	Not applicable
II. (b). In the case of measles, mumps, rubella (MMR), measles, rubella (MR) or rubella vaccines only:	
A. Chronic arthritis	42 days
B. Any sequela (including death) of an illness, disability, injury, or condition referred to above which illness, disability, injury, or condition arose within the time period prescribed.	Not applicable
III. Polio vaccine (other than inactivated polio vaccine):	
A. Paralytic polio	
In a nonimmunodeficient recipient	30 days
In an immunodeficient recipient	6 months
In a vaccine associated community case	Not applicable
B. Any acute complication or sequela (including death) of an illness, disability, injury, or condition referred to above which illness, disability, injury, or condition arose within the time period prescribed.	Not applicable
IV. Inactivated polio vaccine:	
A. Anaphylaxis or anaphylactic shock	4 hours
B. Any acute complication or sequela (including death) of an illness, disability, injury, or condition referred to above which illness, disability, injury, or condition arose within the time period prescribed.	Not applicable

Abbreviations: DTP = diphtheria, tetanus, pertussis; P = pertussis; DT = diphtheria, tetanus; Td = combined tetanus and diphtheria toxoid (adult type).

3000 units of equine tetanus antitoxin versus 300 units of human tetanus immune globulin).

Human Immune Globulin

This preparation is derived from alcohol fractionation of pooled plasma. The antibody content of immune globulin is almost all of the IgG isotype and reflects the infection and immunization experience of the donor pool. Three types of preparations are available: standard immune gamma globulin for intramuscular use (IMIG), standard immune globulin adapted for intravenous use (IVIG), and special immune globulins with a known high content of antibody against a particular antigen; the last may be available for intravenous or intramuscular use.

Immune globulin should be given only when its efficacy has been established. Although its side effects are minimal, the administration is painful, and rare anaphylactoid reactions have been described. It is not useful for the immunologically normal child or adult with frequent viral infections. There is no evidence that HIV infections can be transmitted by the administration of immune globulin. *Caution:* The intramuscular form should *never* be given intravenously; very serious systemic reactions may result from the presence of high-molecular-weight aggregated immunoglobulins.

IVIG is derived from the same pool of adult donors and also consists almost solely of IgG antibodies. The immune globulin has been adapted to intravenous use by eliminating high-molecular-weight complexes that may activate complement in the recipient. The advantages of the intravenous route are the ability to administer large doses of immune globulin, the more rapid onset of action, and the avoidance of intramuscular injections, which are painful and may be contraindicated because of a tendency to bleed. IVIG is particularly valuable as replacement therapy for antibody deficiency disorders and for the management of idiopathic thrombocytopenic purpura. The cost, however, is approximately five times that of IMIG. Approximately 2.5% of patients receiving IVIG experience side effects of fever or vasoactive phenomena (usually vasodilatation), but these reactions can usually be prevented by slow administration of the material.

Special Preparations of Human Immune Globulin

Many preparations with a high titer of a specific antibody are available. These are prepared either by hyperimmunizing adult donors or by selecting lots of plasma tested for a high specific antibody content. Most of these are available in the intramuscular form; a few are currently being made available for intravenous use (Table 55–4).

Animal Sera & Antitoxins

These preparations are used only when human globulin is not available, because they carry a much higher risk of anaphylactic reactions. They are usually prepared from hyperimmunized horses or rabbits.

No antiserum of animal origin should be given without carefully inquiring about prior exposure or allergic response to any product of the specific animal source. Whenever a foreign antiserum is administered, a syringe containing aqueous epinephrine, 1:1000, should be available. If allergy is suspected by history or shown by skin testing and no alternative to serum therapy is possible, desensitization may be attempted as outlined in Chapter 56.

The various materials available for passive immunization, of both human and animal origin, are detailed in Table 55–4.

Passive Immunization in Noninfectious Diseases

A. Prevention of Rh Isoimmunization: Rh-negative women are at hazard of developing anti-Rh antibodies when Rh-positive erythrocytes enter their circulation. This occurs regularly during pregnancy with an Rh-positive fetus, whether the pregnancy ends in a term or preterm delivery or in abortion. It may also occur with other events listed here. The development of anti-Rh antibodies threatens all subsequent Rh-positive fetuses with erythroblastosis. This can be prevented by administration of Rh immune globulin to the mother.

Rh-negative females who have not already developed anti-Rh antibodies should receive 300 µg of Rh immune globulin within 72 hours after obstetric delivery, abortion, accidental transfusion with Rh-positive blood, chorionic villus biopsy, and, probably, amniocentesis, especially if the needle passes through the placenta. This passive immunization suppresses the mother's normal immune response to any Rh-positive fetal cells that may enter her circulation, thus avoiding erythroblastosis fetalis in future Rh-positive fetuses; it may protect in a nonspecific manner as well, analogous to the "blocking" effect of high-dose IgG in ameliorating autoimmune diseases such as idiopathic thrombocytopenic purpura. Even if more than 72 hours has elapsed after the exposures listed above, Rh immune globulin should be administered, since it is effective in at least some cases. Three of six subjects were protected from the immunogenic effect of 1 mL of intravenous Rh-positive erythrocytes by 100 µg of anti-Rh globulin given 13 days later. Some investigators have also suggested the administration of anti-Rh globulin to Rh-negative newborn female offspring of Rh-positive mothers to prevent possible sensitization from maternal–fetal transfusion.

A significant number of Rh isoimmunizations occur during pregnancy rather than at the time of delivery. This can be almost completely prevented by administration of anti-Rh globulin at 28 weeks of gestation. The American College of Obstetricians and Gynecologists recommends routine administration of 300 µg of Rh immune globulin at 28 weeks of gestation and again at delivery as soon as it is determined that the infant is Rh-positive. Prior to 28 weeks of gestation, any condition associated with fetomaternal hemorrhage (abortion, amniocentesis, ruptured ectopic pregnancy) should be treated with Rh immune globulin (a 50-µg "minidose" is used before 12 weeks and a standard 300-µg dose is used thereafter). A larger dose is necessary when a significant fetomaternal hemorrhage (more than 25 µg/mL of incompatible cells) has taken place.

B. Serum Therapy of Poisonous Bites: The toxicity of the bite of the black widow spider, the coral snake, and crotalid snakes (rattlesnakes and other pit vipers) may be lessened by the administration of commercially available antivenins. These are of equine origin, so the risk of serum sickness is high and the possibility of anaphylaxis must always be considered.

Antisera for scorpion stings and rarer poisonous bites, especially of species foreign to North America, may also be available.

Information on the use and availability of antivenins is often available from Poison Control Centers, particularly those in cities having large zoos, such as New York and San Diego. A Snakebite Trauma Center has been established at Jacobi Hospital in New York ([212] 430–8183). In addition, an antivenin index listing the availability of all such products is maintained by the Poison Control Center in Tucson, Arizona ([602] 626–6016 or 626–6000).

C. Kawasaki Syndrome: This severe disease, a form of generalized vasculitis, produces coronary

Table 55–4. Materials available for passive immunization. (All are of human origin unless otherwise stated.)

Disease	Product	Dosage	Comments
Black widow spider bite	Antivenin widow spider, equine	One vial IM or IV	A second dose may be given if symptoms do not subside in 3 hours.
Botulism	ABE polyvalent antitoxin, equine	One vial IV and one vial IM; repeat after 2–4 hours if symptoms worsen, and after 12–24 hours.	Available from CDC.[1] A 20% incidence of serum reactions. Only type E antitoxin has been shown to affect outcome of illness. Prophylaxis is not routinely recommended but may be given to asymptomatic exposed persons.
Cytomegalovirus	CMV immune globulin		CMV immune globulin may be used intravenously for prophylaxis or for treatment (with an antiviral agent) of CMV infections in the immunocompromised host.
Diphtheria	Diphtheria antitoxin, equine	20,000–120,000 units IM depending on severity and duration of illness.	Active immunization and perhaps erythromycin prophylaxis, rather than antitoxin prophylaxis, should be given to nonimmune contacts of active cases. Contacts should be observed for signs of illness so that antitoxin may be administered if needed.
Hepatitis A	Immune globulin	0.02 mL/μg IM as soon as possible after exposure up to 2 weeks. A protective effect lasts about 2 months.	Modifies but does not prevent infection. Recommended for sexual and household contacts of infected persons including diapered children and their staff contacts in a child care center if one case occurs among them or if cases are recognized in the households with more than two children. (If cases occur in more than three homes, consider prophylaxis for all households with diapered children attending the center.) In centers without diapered children, prophylaxis is recommended only for classroom contacts of an index case. Prophylaxis is also suggested for coworkers of an infected food handler (but not generally for patrons) and for persons exposed to a common source *if* cases have not yet begun to occur. Prophylaxis is not recommended for personal contacts at offices, schools, hospitals, or institutions for custodial care *except* in an outbreak centered in these areas.
		For continuous risk of exposure, a dose of 0.05 mL/kg is recommended every 5 months.	Personnel of mental institutions, facilities for retarded children, and prisons appear to be at chronic risk of acquiring hepatitis A, as are those who work with nonhuman primates. Also recommended for travelers who will remain in endemic areas for more than 2 months.
Hepatitis B	Hepatitis B immune globulin (HBIG)	0.06 mL/kg IM up to a maximum of 5 mL as soon as possible after exposure, preferably within 24 hours, but up to 14 days for sexual exposure. HBV vaccination begun within 7 days of exposure is recommen-	Administer to nonimmune individuals as postexposure prophylaxis following sexual contact with HBsAg-positive individuals (one dose of HBIG appears to be as effective as two doses for sexual

(continued)

Table 55–4. Materials available for passive immunization. (All are of human origin unless otherwise stated.) *(continued)*

Disease	Product	Dosage	Comments
Hepatitis B *(cont.)*		ded in preference to a second HBIG injection 25–30 days after the first.	exposure). For percutaneous or mucosal exposure to known HBsAg-positive or high-risk material, prophylactic strategy depends on testing the source and upon the vaccination history of the exposed person (see Table 55–2). Of no value for persons already demonstrating anti-HBsAg antibody. Administration of various live virus vaccines should be delayed for at least 2 months after this concentrated immune globulin has been given. Pregnant women should be screened before delivery or as soon as possible thereafter, and newborn infants of all carriers should be given HBIG, 0.5 mL, within 12 hours of birth. Immunization with HBV vaccine should be started within the first week of life (see Table 55–2). High-risk mothers include women of Asian, Pacific island, or Alaskan Eskimo descent, whether immigrant or US-born; women boen in Haiti or sub-Saharan Africa; and women with a history of acute or chronic liver disease work or treatment in a hemodialysis unit, work or residence in an institution for the mentally retarded, repeated blood transfusion, frequent occupational exposure to blood in a medicodental setting, rejection as a blood donor, household exposure to an HBV carrier or a hemodialysis patient, multiple episode of sexually transmitted disease, or percutaneous use of illicit drugs. HBIG has no effect upon non-A, non-B hepatitis.
Hypogamma-globulinemia	Immune globulin	0.6 mL/kg every 3–4 weeks.	Give double dose at onset of therapy. Immune globulin is of no value in the prevention of frequent respiratory infections in the absence of demonstrable hypogammaglobulinemia.
	Immune globulin IV	100–150 mg/kg IV about once a month, depending on maintenance of serum IgG levels.	Ordinary immune globulin cannot safely be given intravenously because of complement-activating aggregates. It is difficult to administer sufficient IM globulin to maintain normal IgG levels in immunodeficient children or to passively protect acutely infected individuals who lack a specific antibody. This material contains a very small amount of IgA and can cause an allergic reaction in a sensitive IgA-deficient recipient. The IgE in some preparations may cause some reactions; although one product causes symptoms, particularly if confirmed by skin testing, another preparation may not.

(continued)

Table 55–4. Materials available for passive immunization. (All are of human origin unless otherwise stated.) *(continued)*

Disease	Product	Dosage	Comments
Measles	Immune globulin	0.25 mL/kg IM as soon as possible after exposure. This dose may be ineffective in immunoincompetent patients, who should receive 20–30 mL.	Live measles vaccine usually prevents natural infection if given within 48 hours following exposure. If immune globulin is administered, delay immunization with live virus for 3 months. Do not vaccinate infants under age 15 months.
Rabies	Rabies immune globulin[2]	20 IU/kg, 50% of which is infiltrated locally at the wound site if anatomically feasible, and the remainder given IM. (See also rabies vaccine in Table 55–2.) If the equine produce is used, the dose is 40 IU/kg.	Give as soon as possible after exposure. Recommended for all bite or scratch exposures to carnivores, especially bat, skunk, fox, coyote, or raccoon, despite animal's apparent health, if the brain cannot be immediately examined and found rabies-free. Give also even for abrasion exposure to known or suspected rabid animals as well as for bite (skin penetration by teeth) of escaped dogs and cats whose health cannot be determined. Not recommended for individuals with demonstrated antibody response from preexposure prophylaxis.
Rh isoimmunization (erythroblastosis fetalis)	Rh_o (D) immune globulin	One dose IM within 12 hours of abortion, amniocentesis or chorionic villus biopsy, obstetric delivery of an Rh-positive infant, or transfusion of Rh-positive blood in an Rh_o (D)-negative female.	For nonimmune females only. May be effective at much greater postexposure interval. Give even if more than 72 hours have elapsed. One vial contains 300 μg of antibody and can reliably inhibit the immune response to a fetomaternal bleed of 7.5–8 mL as estimated by the Betke-Kleihauer smear technique. Some groups also recommend administration of 100 μg of antibody at 28 and 34 weeks of pregnancy to prevent prepartum isoimmunization. Transient seropositivity for anti-HAV and anti-HBV antibodies may follow the administration of large doses.
Snakebite	Antivenin coral snake, equine. Antivenin rattlesnake, copperhead, and moccasin, equine.	At least 3–5 vials IV.	Dose should be sufficient to reverse symptoms of envenomation. Consider antitetanus measures as well.
Tetanus	Tetanus immune globulin[3]	Prophylaxis: 250–500 units IM. Therapy: 3000–5000 units IM.	Give in separate syringe at separate site from simultaneously administered toxoid. Recommended only for major contaminated wounds in individuals who have had fewer than two doses of toxoid at any time in the past (fewer than three doses if wound is more than 24 hours old). (See tetanus toxoid in Table 55–2.) There is some evidence that 250 units given intrathecally to mildly affected patients prevents progression to severe disease and death, but intrathecal therapy is not effective in severe cases with generalized repeated spasms.

(continued)

Table 55–4. Materials available for passive immunization. (All are of human origin unless otherwise stated.) *(continued)*

Disease	Product	Dosage	Comments
Vaccinia	Vaccinia immune globulin (Available from CDC[1])	Prophylaxis: 0.3 mL/kg IM. Therapy: 0.6 mL/kg IM. VIG may be repeated as necessary for treatment and at intervals of 1 week for prophylaxis.	Give at a different site if used to prevent dissemination in a patient with skin disease who must undergo vaccination. May be useful in treatment of vaccinia of the eye, eczema vaccinatum, generalized vaccinia, and vaccinia necrosum and in the prevention of such complications in exposed patients with skin disorders such as eczema or impetigo. Also recommended to prevent fetal vaccinia when a pregnant woman must be vaccinated. VIG should rarely be needed, since smallpox vaccination is now limited to military personnel and at-risk laboratory workers.
Varicella	Varicella-zoster immune globulin (VZIG).[4]	One vial/10 kg or fraction thereof, up to a maximum of five vials, given IM within 96 hours of exposure.	It should be administered to nonimmune leukemic, lymphomatous, or immunosuppressed children, children receiving prednisone at ≥2 mg/kg/d for any reason, or other immunoincompetent children <15 years of age who have had household, hospital (same room containing ≤ four beds or adjacent beds in large ward), or playmate (>1 hour play indoors) contact with a known case of varicella-zoster. Should also be given to exposed bone marrow transplant patients regardless of immune history of donor, to exposed infants born before 28 weeks of gestation, and to neonates whose mothers have developed varicella <5 days before or 48 hours after delivery or who are exposed postnatally and whose mothers have uncertain or negative histories of varicella. VZIG should be considered for adults—especially pregnant women and immunocompromised patients—having close contact with a case of varicella-zoster as defined above for children and whose history suggests susceptibility. A negative history for varicella is extremely unreliable (only about 8% of adults who believe they are nonimmune become infected after household exposure) and should if possible be checked by a serologic test such as the fluorescent antibody test against membrane antigen, because of the high cost of VZIG (an adult dose costs approximately $400). Protective antibody levels can be attained using immune globulin IV in a dose of 6 mL/kg if VZIG is unavailable.

(footnotes for this table continue on next page)

Table 55–4. Materials available for passive immunization. (All are of human origin unless otherwise stated.) *(continued)*

Abbreviations: ABE = antibotulinum toxin, equine; CMV = cytomegalovirus; HBV = hepatitis B virus; IM = intramuscular; VIG = vaccinia immunoglobulin.
[1] Available from the Centers for Disease Control and Prevention. Telephone: (404) 329–3311 (main switchboard, day) or (404) 329–3644 (night).
[2] Antirabies serum, equine, may be available but is much less desirable.
[3] Bovine and equine antitoxins may be available but are not recommended. They are used at 10 times the dose of tetanus immune globulin.
[4] Contact the regional blood center of the American Red Cross.
Note: Passive immunotherapy or immunoprophylaxis should always be administered as soon as possible after exposure to the offending agent. Immune antisera and globulin are always given intramuscularly unless otherwise noted. Always question carefully and test for hypersensitivity before administering animal sera.

artery aneurysms that may result in myocardial infarction in a significant number of cases. There is a large and convincing body of evidence that IVIG given during the acute phase of the disease substantially improves the outcome. The dose and duration that have been successful in initial clinical trials are 400 mg/kg daily for 5 days given as early as possible during the acute phase. A single 2-g/kg dose of IVIG administered over 10 hours is equally efficacious.

D. Thrombocytopenic Purpura: In this disease, IVIG is given because it presumably prolongs platelet survival by blocking Fc receptors for IgG on macrophages that ingest antibody-coated platelets.

Hazards of Passive Immunization

Illness may arise from a single injection of foreign serum but more commonly occurs in patients who have previously been injected with proteins from the same or a related species. Reactions range in severity from serum sickness arising days to weeks following treatment to acute anaphylaxis with urticaria, dyspnea, cardiovascular collapse, and even death (see Chapter 28). Typical manifestations of serum sickness include adenopathy, urticaria, arthritis, and fever (see Chapter 29). Demyelinating encephalopathy has been reported.

Rarely, the administration of human immune globulin is attended by similar allergic reactions, particularly in patients with selective IgA deficiency (see Chapter 21). Viral hepatitis may be transmitted by whole human plasma or serum but not by the purified gamma globulin fraction.

The administration of intact lymphocytes to promote cell-mediated immunity is hazardous if the recipient is immunologically depressed. The engrafted donor cells may "reject" the recipient by the graft-versus-host reaction, producing rash, pancytopenia, fever, diarrhea, hepatosplenomegaly, and death (see Chapter 57).

COMBINED PASSIVE–ACTIVE IMMUNIZATION

Passive and active immunization are often undertaken simultaneously to provide both immediate, transient protection and slowly developing, durable protection against rabies or tetanus. The immune response to the active agent may or may not be impaired by the passively administered antibodies if the injections are given at separate sites. Tetanus toxoid plus tetanus immune globulin may give a response superior to that generated by the toxoid alone, but after antiserum has been given for rabies, the course of immunization is usually extended to ensure an adequate response.

Parenterally administered live virus vaccines, such as measles or rubella virus, should not be given until at least 6 (and preferably 12) weeks after the administration of immune globulin.

CLINICAL INDICATIONS FOR IMMUNIZATION

Immunizing procedures are among the most effective and economical measures available for preservation and protection of health. The decision to immunize a specific person against a specific pathogen is a complex judgment based on an assessment of the risk of infection, the consequences of natural unmodified illness, the availability of a safe and effective immunogen, and the duration of its effect.

HERD IMMUNITY

The organism that causes tetanus is ubiquitous, and the vaccine directed against it has few side effects and is highly effective, but only the immunized individual is protected. Thus, immunization must be universal. By contrast, a nonimmune individual who resides in a community that has been well immunized against poliovirus and who does not travel has little opportunity to encounter wild (virulent) virus. Here the immunity of the "herd" protects the unimmunized person since the intestinal tracts of recipients of oral polio vaccine fail to become colonized by or transmit wild virus. If, however, a substantial portion of the community is not immune, introduced wild virus can circulate and cause disease among the nonimmune group. Thus, focal outbreaks of poliomyelitis have occurred in religious communities objecting to immunization.

ANTIGENIC SHIFT
& ANTIGENIC VARIATION

Each immunologically distinct viral subtype requires a specific antigenic stimulus for effective protection. Immunization against adenovirus infection has not benefitted civilian populations subject to many differing types of adenovirus, in contrast to the demonstrated value of vaccine directed against a few epidemic adenovirus types in military recruits. Similarly, immunity to type A influenza virus is transient because of major mutations in surface chemistry of the virus every few years (antigenic shifts). These changes render previously developed vaccines obsolete and may not permit sufficient production, distribution, and use of new antigen in time to prevent epidemic spread of the altered strain. Antigenic variation may also be an important impediment to immunization against HIV infection.

SOME SPECIFIC DISEASES

Pertussis

Several acellular vaccines used in Japan for the past 12 years are saline suspensions of two or more antigens: formalin-treated lymphocyte proliferative factor (pertussis toxin) and filamentous hemagglutinin. The degree of protection afforded by acellular vaccine appears to be about the same as or better than that for the whole-cell product, and minor reactions (fever, pain) are less frequent. Acellular pertussis vaccine (in combination with diphtheria and tetanus toxoids [DT]) has been licensed for children older than 15 months. Licensing for younger children awaits the evaluation of already completed studies.

Poliomyelitis

Two forms of polio vaccine are available. The live, attenuated oral (Sabin) vaccine, used in the USA and many parts of the world, is cheap, effective, and easily administered. Infection causing paralysis occurs in only one per 7 million immunodeficient recipients or members of their households. The killed virus vaccine (Salk) is also effective, particularly in the new "enhanced" form. It requires injection and gives a shorter duration of immunity but is free of the danger of producing paralysis in the recipient or household members. Immunodeficient individuals should receive the killed vaccine. Adults who have never been immunized are protected by herd immunity in developed countries and should therefore be immunized with the killed (Salk) vaccine prior to travel to areas endemic for polio.

Hepatitis B

Vaccine for hepatitis B has been available for some 10 years and is used for special populations—health care workers, infants of surface antigen-positive mothers. A 1992 recommendation for universal immunization against hepatitis B in infancy has been widely adopted.

Cholera

Cholera immunization offers only temporary and incomplete protection. It is of little use to travelers and should be given only when the risk of exposure is high or in fulfillment of local regulations.

Varicella

An attenuated strain of varicella-zoster virus has been in use in Japan for some 12 years. In 1995, this vaccine was licensed in the US and recommended for routine immunization of all children between the ages of 12 and 15 months. It can be administered simultaneously with MMR vaccine but not in the same syringe.

AGE AT IMMUNIZATION

The natural history of a disease determines the age at which immunization is best undertaken. Pertussis, polio, and diphtheria often infect infants; immunization against these diseases is therefore begun shortly after birth. Serious consequences of pertussis are uncommon beyond early childhood, and pertussis vaccination is not usually recommended after 6 years of age. Since the major hazard of rubella is the congenital rubella syndrome, and since nearly half of congenital rubella cases occur with the first pregnancy, it is very important to immunize as many females as possible prior to puberty. In this way the theoretic hazard of vaccinating a pregnant female and endangering the fetus is avoided, although inadvertently immunized fetuses have thus far not been reported to be damaged by their exposure to the attenuated virus.

The efficacy of immunization may also be age-related. Failure may occur because of the presence of interfering antibodies or an undeveloped responsiveness of the immune system. Infants cannot be reliably protected with live measles, mumps, or rubella vaccines until maternally derived antibody has disappeared. Because a proportion of children immunized as late as 1 year of age fail to develop antibody after measles vaccination, the age recommended for measles vaccine administration had been changed to 15 months. Because measles is becoming a rare disease in the US, however, most mothers have shorter lasting vaccine-derived antibodies rather than disease-induced antibodies. Thus it makes sense to go back to the 12-months immunization schedule, particularly if the infant is likely to be exposed, usually through travel. Furthermore, delay in immunization is attended by a decrease in the number of children actually immunized, which approximates the improved rate of seroconversion. Infants frequently develop severe infections with *Haemophilus influenzae* type b, pneumococci, or meningococci, but injecting them

Table 55–5. Recommended ages for administration of currently licensed childhood vaccines[1]—July 1995.

Age → Vaccine ↓	Birth	2 mos	4 mos	6 mos	12[4] mos	15 mos	18 mos	4–6 yrs	11–12 yrs	14–16 yrs
Hepatitis B[5,6]	Hep B-1									
		Hep B-2		Hep B-3					Hep B[6]	
Diphtheria, Tetanus, Pertussis[7]		DTP	DTP	DTP	DTP[4,7] (DTaP at 15+ m)			DTP or DTaP	Td	
Haemophilus influenzae type b[8]		Hib	Hib	Hib[8]	Hib[1,5]					
Polio		OPV	OPV	OPV				OPV		
Measles, mumps, rubella[9]					MMR[4,9]			MMR or MMR		
Varicella-zoster[10] virus vaccine					VZV[10]				VZV[10]	

[1] Vaccines are listed under routinely recommended ages. Solid bars indicate range of acceptable ages for vaccination. Shaded bars indicate new recommendations or vaccines licensed since publication of the *Recommended Childhood Immunization Schedule* in January 1995. This schedule indicates new recommendations for vaccines licensed since publication of the Recommended Childhood Immunization Schedule in January 1995. The Recommended Childhood Immunization Schedule is reviewed and published annually by the Advisory Committee on Immunization Practices, the American Academy of Pediatrics, and the American Academy of Family Physicians. After review and revision, this schedule will be published in the MMWR in January 1996 as the "Recommended Childhood Immunization Schedule, United States—January 1996."

[2] Hepatitis B vaccine is recommended at 11–12 years of age for children not previously vaccinated.

[3] Varicella-zoster virus vaccine is recommended at 11–12 years of age for children not previously vaccinated, and who lack a reliable history of chickenpox.

[4] Vaccines recommended in the second year of life (12–15 months of age) may be given at either one or two visits.

[5] **Infants born to HBsAg-negative mothes** should receive 2.5 μg of Merck Sharp & Dohme (MSD) vaccine (Recombivax HB) or 10 μg of SmithKline Beecham (SKB) vaccine (Engerix-B). The second dose should be given between 1 and 4 months of age, if at least 1 month has elapsed since receipt of the first dose. The third dose is recommended between 6 and 18 months of age.
     Infants born to HBsAg-positive mothers should receive immunoprophylaxis for hepatitis B with 0.5 mL hepatitis B immune globulin (HBIG) within 12 hours of birth, and either 5 μg of MSD vaccine (Recombivax HB) or 10 μg of SKB vaccine (Engerix-B) at a separate site. In these infants, the second dose is recommended at 1 month of age and the third dose at 6 months of age. All pregnant women should be screened for HBsAg during an early prenatal visit.

[6] Hepatitis B vaccine is recommended for adolescents who have not previously received three doses of vaccine. The three-dose series should be initiated or completed at the 11–12 year-old visit for persons not previously fully vaccinated. The second dose should be administered at least 1 month after the first dose, and the third dose should be administered at least 4 months after the first dose.

[7] The fourth dose of DTP may be administered as early as 12 months of age, provided ≥6 months have elapsed since DTP3. Combined DTP-Hib products may be used when these two vaccines are to be administered simultaneously. DTaP (diphtheria and tetanus toxoids and acellular pertussis vaccine) is licensed for use for the fourth and/or fifth dose of DTP vaccine in children ≥15 months of age and may be preferred for these doses in children in this age group. Td (tetanus and diphtheria toxoids, adsorbed, for adult use) is recommended at 11–12 years of age if ≥5 years have elapsed since the last dose of DTP, DTP-Hib, or DT.

[8] Three *Haemophilus influenzae* type b conjugate vaccines are available for use in infants: HbOC [HibTITER] (Lederle Praxis); PRP-T [ActHIB; OmniHIB] (Pasteur Mérieux, distributed by SmithKline Beecham; Connaught); and PRP-OMP [PedvaxHIB] (Merck Sharp & Dohme). Children who have received PRP-OMP at 2 and 4 months of age do not require a dose at 6 months of age. After the primary infant Hib conjugate vaccine series is completed, any licensed Hib conjugate vaccine may be used as a booster dose at age 12–15 months.

[9] The second dose of MMR vaccine should be administered *either* at 4–6 years of age *or* at 11–12 years of age, consistent with state school immunization requirements.

[10] Varicella-zoster virus vaccine (VZV) is routinely recommended at 12–18 months of age. Children who have not been vaccinated previously and who lack a reliable history of chickenpox should be vaccinated by 13 years of age. VZV can be administered to susceptible children any time during childhood. Children <13 years of age should receive a single 0.5-mL dose; persons ≥13 years of age should receive two 0.5-mL doses 4–8 weeks apart.

with purified capsular polysaccharide has failed to reliably yield a good antibody response, despite the excellent activity of the same antigen in older children and adults. This issue has now been addressed by the development of several conjugated *H influenzae* vaccines (polysaccharide conjugated to protein). A similar effort is under way for *Neisseria meningitidis* and *Streptococcus pneumoniae* polysaccharide vaccines.

Recommendations for Childhood Immunization

Despite the extraordinary effect of immunization in the developed world, WHO estimates that of every 1000 children born today, 5 are crippled by poliomyelitis, 10 die of neonatal tetanus, 20 die of pertussis, and 30 die of measles and its complications. A rational program of immunization against infectious diseases begins in childhood, when many of the most damaging and preventable infections normally appear. Table 55–5 summarizes the current guidelines for immunization in childhood recommended by the Advisory Committee on Immunization Practices (A.C.I.P.) and the American Academy of Pediatrics. The need for childhood immunization has increased because unimmunized individuals in a partially immune population are less exposed to such childhood diseases as measles and mumps and therefore develop them later than they otherwise would. When these illnesses do occur in adolescence or adulthood, they are often diagnostically bewildering to the physician unprepared for such illnesses in this age group.

The physician should provide the patient with a clear and up-to-date record of all immunizations, which is useful in future medical encounters and in fulfilling school registration and other institutional requirements. Physicians can improve immunization rates by developing recall systems to identify children who are due for immunizations and by using the occasion of a visit for intercurrent illness to investigate and augment a patient's immune status. It is *not* necessary to restart an interrupted series of vaccinations or to add extra doses. If the vaccine history is unknown and there are no obvious contraindications, the child or adult should be fully immunized appropriately for his or her age. Reimmunization poses no significant risk.

For developing nations in which much preventable serious infection occurs in the first few years of life, WHO recommends an accelerated immunization program: at birth, oral poliovirus and BCG; at ages 6, 10, and 14 weeks, oral poliovirus and DTP; at age 9 months, measles (to be repeated in the second year of life if given before age 9 months).

Immunization of Adults & the Elderly

Childhood immunization programs have significantly decreased the incidence of preventable infections in developed countries. Optimal immunization of adult populations has not yet been achieved, however. Much disease preventable by immunization continues to exist. Table 55–6 lists the most important immunizations for the adult and elderly population.

SIMULTANEOUS IMMUNIZATION WITH MULTIPLE ANTIGENS

The simultaneous inoculation of the nonliving antigens of diphtheria, tetanus, and pertussis (DTP) elicits a response equal to that seen with their separate injection. Similarly, the single injection of a mixture of live, attenuated measles, rubella, and mumps viruses elicits good responses to each component of the mixture. Between 2 and 14 days following the administration of one live virus vaccine, however, there is a period of suboptimal response to a subsequently injected live virus vaccine. Live vaccines that are not given simultaneously should be given at least 4 weeks apart if time permits. The administration of cholera and yellow fever vaccines within 1–3 weeks of each other decreases the antibody response to both agents. Therefore, these immunizations also should be given at the same time or at least 4 weeks apart.

The recent addition of conjugated *H influenzae* vaccine and recombinant hepatitis B vaccine to childhood immunizations has created a serious problem with multiple needle sticks necessary at each well-baby visit. This has stimulated the production of combined vaccines, such as DTP and conjugated *Haemophilus* vaccine. Several combinations are commercially available, and more are under way.

IMMUNIZATION FOR FOREIGN TRAVEL

Planning for foreign travel should include a review of the current immunization status of the traveler and consideration of special immunization requirements in the area to be visited. Infectious diseases such as measles that have become quite rare in the US are rampant in developing countries. Thus, travelers (children, in particular) should be up to date on their routine immunizations and boosters.

National health authorities may require an International Certificate of Vaccination against cholera or yellow fever from travelers, usually depending on the presence of these diseases in countries on their itinerary. Cholera vaccination may be given by any

Table 55–6. Vaccines and toxoids[1] recommended for adults, by age groups, in the USA.

Age group (years)	Vaccine/toxoid					
	Td[2]	Measles	Mumps	Rubella	Influenza	Pneumococcal Polysaccharide
18–24	X	X	X	X		
25–64	X	X[3]	X[3]	X		
≥65	X				X	X

[1] Refer also to sections in text on specific vaccines or toxoids for indications, contraindications, precautions, dosages, side effects, adverse reactions, and special considerations.

[2] Td, tetanus and diphtheria toxoids, adsorbed (for adult use), which is a combined preparation containing <2 flocculation units of diphtheria toxoid.

[3] Indicated for persons born after 1956.

licensed physician; because it is not very effective, it is not generally recommended except when required. The certificate must be completed in all details and then validated with an officially approved stamp. Yellow fever vaccination may be administered and the certificate validated only at an officially designated center, which may be located by contacting the state or local health department. In addition to these legal requirements, all adults are advised to be adequately immunized against measles, tetanus, and diphtheria and to undergo additional immunizations (against poliomyelitis, typhoid, hepatitis A, and meningococcal meningitis) if they are visiting areas where the frequency of illness in the population or the level of sanitation increases the risk of infection. Travelers should be immunized against plague if contact with wild rodents or rabbits in an endemic rural area is anticipated and to hepatitis B if sexual contacts are anticipated in Southeast Asia or sub-Saharan Africa. Japanese B encephalitis is prevalent in a number of Asian countries (China, India, Thailand, Japan, Nepal, and others). It is mosquito-borne, so travelers to these destinations who anticipate exposure to mosquitos should consider immunization. An inactivated vaccine has recently been licensed in the US.

Travelers to malaria-endemic areas should be specifically advised to use mosquito repellents, malaria chemoprophylaxis, and acute therapy of presumptive infections.

No special immunizations are generally recommended for persons traveling from the USA to Western Europe, Canada, Australia, or Japan. Detailed suggestions of the United States Public Health Service (CDC) are given country by country in its *Health Information for International Travel Supplement* (see References).

VACCINES FOR SPECIAL POPULATIONS

The greatest application of vaccines is in routine immunization of children and adults in large population groups. Some vaccines, however, are used only for population groups at greater hazard of disease by virtue of geography, occupation, or special exposure. The armed forces use an oral adenovirus vaccine containing types 4 and 7, as well as a polyvalent meningococcal vaccine, for all recruits.

Veterinarians and animal handlers usually receive preexposure rabies vaccination, whereas postexposure rabies immunization is appropriate for the general public. Hepatitis B vaccine is recommended for those with increased occupational, household, or lifestyle risks.

VACCINES CURRENTLY IN DEVELOPMENT

Many vaccines are currently in various stages of development. New ones produced by recombinant DNA technology can be anticipated. The first of these to be licensed and marketed is hepatitis B recombinant vaccine; many others are in various stages of design and production. Synthetic analogues of antigen and possibly anti-idiotype antibodies may be developed in the future.

An effective vaccine against hepatitis A has been developed, but its application remains to be determined. Vaccines against cytomegalovirus, herpes simplex virus, gonococci, Lyme disease, *Plasmodium, Pseudomonas aeruginosa,* respiratory syncytial virus, rotavirus, *Shigella,* and many other pathogens are undergoing active development in the laboratory and in clinical trials. An effort is under way to conjugate the polysaccharide capsule of pneumococci to protein in a manner analogous to what has been accomplished with *H influenzae.*

Special immunoglobulin pools high in specific antibodies are being developed. The use of monoclonal antibodies in clinical practice is discussed in Chapter 59.

HIV INFECTION

Active efforts are under way to develop a recombinant DNA vaccine using HIV viral components. Candidate vaccines have been targeted both for prevention of HIV infection in uninfected individuals and for boosting the immune response of those already infected. Many obstacles stand in the way of the effort, among them the frequent antigenic shift of this virus (see Chapter 49). The current recommendation for HIV-infected individuals is that they receive all the normal childhood immunizations (see Table 55–4), with the exception that polio immunization be restricted to the inactivated form (Salk). This is principally to protect other members of the household who may be seriously immunocompromised. Live measles vaccine is recommended, despite the theoretic hazard, because of the severe form of measles infection that occurs in HIV-infected children. Vaccines against influenza and *S pneumoniae* should also be administered to the appropriate individuals in this group.

REFERENCES

Ad Hoc Working Group Standards for Pediatric Immunization Practices. *JAMA* 1993;**269:**1817.

American Academy of Pediatrics. *Report of Committee on Infectious Diseases.* 1994 AAP Elk Grove Village, IL 60009-0927.

Barnett ED, Chen R: Children and international travel: Immunizations. *Pediatr Infect Dis J* 1995;**14:**982.

Brewer MA et al: Who should receive hepatitis A vaccine? *Pediatr Infect Dis J* 1995;**14:**258.

Cherry JB: Acellular pertussis vaccines: A solution to the pertussis problem. *J Infect Dis* 1993;**168:**21.

CDC: Recommendations for use of *Haemophilus* b conjugate vaccines and a combined diphtheria, tetanus, pertussis, and *Haemophilus* b vaccine. *MMWR* 1994; **42:**(RR013).

CDC: Recommendations of the international task force for disease eradication. *MMWR* 1993;**42:**RR16.

CDC: *Health Information for International Travel 1994.* HHS Publication. (Revised annually.)

Edwards KM, Decker MD: Combination vaccines: Hopes and challenges. *Pediatr Infect Dis J* 1994;**13:**345.

Gilsdorf JR: Vaccines: Moving into the molecular era. *J Pediatr* 1994;**125:**339.

Katz SL: Prospects for childhood immunizations in the next decade. *Ped Annals* 1993;**22:**733.

Lieu TA et al: Cost effectiveness of a routine varicella vaccination program for U.S. children. *JAMA* 1994;**271:**375.

Loewenson PR et al: Physician attitudes and practices regarding universal infant vaccination against hepatitis B infection in Minnesota: Implications for public health policy. *Pediatr Infect Dis J* 1994;**13:**373.

Nichol KN et al: The effectiveness of vaccination against influenza in healthy working adults. *N Engl J Med* 1995;**333:**889.

Rabinovich R, Robbins A: Pertussis vaccines: A progress report. *JAMA* 1994;**271:**68.

Schmitt HJ et al: Efficacy of acellular pertussis vaccine in early childhood after household exposure. *JAMA* 1996;**275:**37.

Stiehm ER: New developments: Recent progress in the use of intravenous immunoglobulin. *Curr Prob Pediatr* 1992;**22:**335.

Szilagyi PG et al: Missed opportunities for childhood vaccinations in office practices and the effect on vaccine status. *Pediatrics* 1993;**91:**1.

Werzberger A et al: Controlled trial of formalin inactivated hepatitis A vaccine in healthy children. *N Engl J Med* 1992;**327:**453.

West DJ, Margolis HS: Prevention of hepatitis B virus infection. *Pediatr Infect Dis J* 1992;**11:**866.

56

Allergy Desensitization

Abba I. Terr, MD

Allergy **desensitization** is a form of treatment in which allergens are injected into the patient for the purpose of reducing or eliminating the allergic response. It is also called allergen immunotherapy, hyposensitization, or allergy injection therapy. The term "desensitization" is used here to avoid confusion with the use of the term "immunotherapy" elsewhere in this book to describe other forms of therapeutic manipulation of the immune system. It is most often used in IgE antibody-mediated diseases, but it has been used in other forms of allergy as well. Ideally, the treatment goal is the complete abolition of the allergic sensitivity, but in practice the result is usually a significant diminution in symptoms. It is an adjunct to allergen avoidance and symptomatic drug therapy, not the primary mode of treatment or a substitute for avoidance of allergens. Nevertheless, it is usually effective in situations in which allergen avoidance is not possible.

Noon published the first report of desensitization for hay fever in England in 1911. Since then it has been extensively used in allergy practice to treat hay fever and allergic asthma. A sufficient number of controlled clinical trials have been completed to clearly establish its effectiveness in allergic rhinitis and Hymenoptera venom anaphylaxis. So far there have been too few definitive studies of its use in asthma to draw firm conclusions. Short-term desensitization has been accomplished in some cases of penicillin and insulin allergy. Successful oral desensitization has been reported for some drug-induced cutaneous eruptions, but these findings are not based on controlled trials. Desensitization is often attempted in *Rhus* contact dermatitis (poison ivy or poison oak), but as yet it has not been shown to be effective in this disease.

The mechanism of allergy desensitization is still uncertain, but it is immunologically specific to the injected allergens. A variety of specific immunologic responses are induced during desensitization treatment. Promising improvements in the procedure are currently under study.

Ironically, allergy desensitization is widely used by allergists in the USA, but it is now almost never prescribed by allergists in the UK where it originated.

METHODS

The general procedure for desensitization in allergic rhinitis today is similar to the method used originally by Noon. Sterile allergen extracts are administered subcutaneously in increasing doses once or twice a week until a dose is reached that produces a transient small local area of inflammation at the injection site. This dose is then given on a maintenance schedule once every 2–4 weeks. Originally the course of treatment was preseasonal for patients with a single-season pollen allergy for 3–6 months before the expected onset of the season. Because most patients with allergic rhinitis have allergies to different pollens at different times of the year as well as year-round dust or mold allergy, perennial (year-round) injection therapy is the most common schedule used by allergists today. The injections include a mixture of all relevant inhalant allergens, and after the maximum tolerated dose of the mixture is reached, the maintenance injections are continued for several years.

The injections are given subcutaneously. Oral, sublingual, inhaled, and local nasal routes of desensitization have been tried, but none has been clearly shown to be effective in preventing diseases caused by IgE antibodies.

Extracts used in allergy desensitization are the same as those used for testing (see Chapter 26). In most cases they are crude or partially purified aqueous extracts of the common inhalant allergens. Some are now standardized for content of the major allergen to ensure uniformity among different batches of extracts. Purified isolated major allergens, such as ragweed Amb a I, formerly called antigen E, have been used in clinical studies and may be effective in treatment of certain patients with restricted sensitivity to that allergen. Many allergic patients, however, have multiple sensitivities and therefore require the multiple allergens present in crude allergen extracts.

Injection Technique

Details of the proper technique for administering therapeutic allergen injections to patients with atopic or anaphylactic disease are important for the success and safety of the treatment. Because of the risk of systemic reactions, facilities must be available to treat such reactions. Potentially fatal reactions usually begin within 30 minutes after the injection. Treatment should be withheld on a day when the patient is experiencing acute asthma or a fever. Small local swelling with itching at the injection site is acceptable. Excessive local swelling or any systemic reaction requires a reduction in the subsequent dose. The dose should also be reduced if there has been a lapse in treatment.

Duration of Treatment

There are insufficient data to set guidelines for the overall length of desensitization in atopy. The variability in the natural course of disease, the vagaries of environmental exposure for the many different indoor (dust, molds, animals) and outdoor (pollens, molds) allergens, and the effect of nonallergic factors (weather, pollution, infections, stress) make definitive controlled long-term studies technically difficult. The immunologic changes induced by desensitization (see later section), either singly or in combination, do not correlate sufficiently with symptomatic relief to justify in vitro immunologic monitoring to assess the optimal duration of therapy. Clinically, there is a progressive reduction of symptoms of pollen allergy for the first 3 or 4 years of injection therapy, after which the therapeutic effect levels off. There are no data yet on recurrence of symptoms after the injections are stopped. Some allergists recommend that treatment be discontinued after 2 or 3 successive symptomless years.

Desensitization for Hymenoptera venom anaphylaxis has been shown to be highly effective in reducing the risk of reactions from spontaneous stings throughout the period of active treatment at the maintenance dosage. Recent studies strongly suggest that the treatment may be discontinued after 5 years of maintenance injections.

Clinical Results

The results of the first controlled clinical trial of desensitization for allergic rhinitis were published in 1949. Since then, results from dozens of placebo-controlled double-blind studies have shown clearly that desensitization is effective in seasonal and perennial allergic rhinitis when sufficient allergen is given to induce an immunologic response. The effect is immunologically specific. Figure 56–1 shows the results of one such study on patients with seasonal ragweed hay fever. On average, symptoms are considerably reduced, especially at the peak of the pollen season.

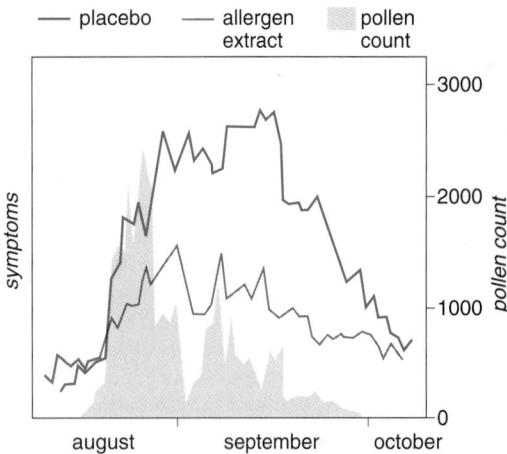

Figure 56–1. Desensitization therapy in patients with allergic rhinitis. Results of a placebo-controlled double-blind trial of ragweed allergen injections on the allergic symptoms of patients with ragweed hay fever during the ragweed pollinating season. (Modified and reproduced, with permission, from Norman PS et al: Trials of alum-precipitated pollen extracts in the treatment of hay fever. *J Allergy Clin Immunol* 1972;**50**:31.)

Similar efficacy has been shown for other pollens and for molds, house dust, dust mites, and cat allergen.

Controlled trials on patients with allergic asthma are more difficult to perform because the disease is exacerbated by so many nonallergic factors, such as respiratory infections, atmospheric irritants, and emotions. Nevertheless, one study showed that desensitization treatment of asthma caused by allergy to cats reduced the bronchoprovocation response to cat allergen inhalation. Two recent studies, however, failed to provide evidence of efficacy in childhood and adult asthma caused by pollen allergy.

Hymenoptera insect venom anaphylaxis responds exceedingly well to desensitization: 95% of treated patients are protected from reactions to deliberate or unintentional stings, whereas about 50% of untreated or placebo-treated controls continue to experience systemic reactions to insect stings. Venom desensitization also appears to be effective in patients who respond to insect stings with urticaria or with consistently large local swellings at the sting site, but these conditions are not considered serious enough to warrant the treatment.

Desensitization has not been evaluated as a treatment for atopic dermatitis because exacerbations of the skin lesions usually do not correlate with inhalant allergen exposure. There is no evidence that desensitization of patients suffering from both allergic rhinitis and atopic dermatitis improves their skin disease. Food allergen injection therapy has not yet been definitively evaluated for efficacy against any of the clinical manifestations of food allergy, including anaphylaxis.

IMMUNOLOGIC EFFECTS

Several different immunologic effects are induced in allergic patients by desensitization therapy.

Hyposensitization

The term "desensitization" implies that the treatment eliminates the preexisting allergen-specific IgE antibody, converts the wheal-and-erythema skin test to negative, prevents the target organ response to the allergen by provocative-dose testing, and cures the disease. In practice, true desensitization is rare, being achieved in only about 5% of patients on an adequate course of therapy. Most treated atopic patients are hyposensitized. That is, immunologic and clinical measures of the specific IgE-mediated allergy are significantly lessened but not eliminated, even after many years of the injection treatment. The level of circulating IgE antibody falls below pretreatment levels only after many months of treatment (Fig 56–2). It is important to note that IgE antibody production is enhanced transiently during the first few months of low-dose allergen injections, and some patients experience a corresponding temporary worsening of symptoms during that time.

Immunization

An allergen-specific IgG antibody is induced by treatment (see Fig 56–2). The antibody is often called "blocking antibody," because it inhibits the effect of IgE antibody in the passive-transfer (Prausnitz-Küstner) skin test and in the passive transfer in vitro histamine release assay. Blocking antibodies of the IgA isotype may also be detected in the serum of treated patients, but blocking activity in secretions does not occur to a significant extent. Some studies suggest that the quantity of blocking antibody of the IgG4 subclass may correlate better with clinical improvement than that of other IgG subclasses. The presence of blocking antibody in serum is sustained as long as the maintenance injections are continued; the level then drops off gradually after treatment is stopped.

Regulation of IgE Antibody Production

There is limited evidence from a few studies that desensitization therapy alters regulatory factors in the production of allergen-specific IgE antibody. Some in vitro experiments indicate that treatment generates specific T cells with suppressor activity on IgE antibody production. Other studies are consistent with a shift in peripheral blood lymphocyte response to allergen from a T_H2 to a T_H1 cytokine profile. One study detected the induction of anti-idiotypic auto-antibodies.

Combination Effects

It is likely that the beneficial effect of desensitization treatment in allergic diseases may derive from an optimal combination of some or all of the immunologic changes already described—and perhaps oth-

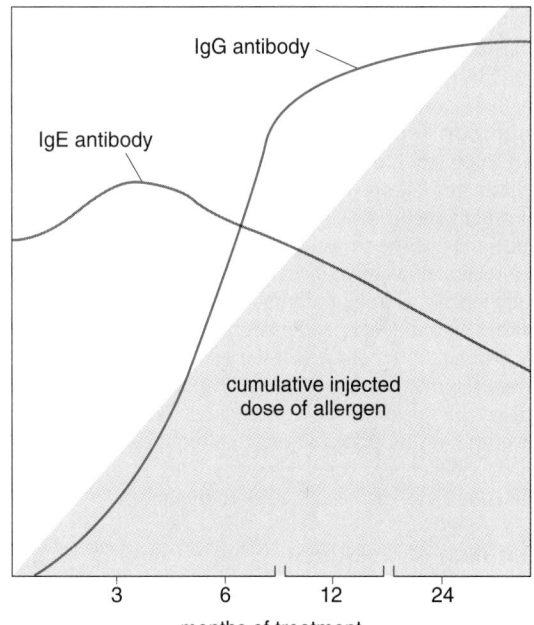

Figure 56–2. IImmunologic changes during prolonged desensitization therapy for IgE-mediated diseases. The level of circulating IgE antibody is initially increased and later decreases below pretreatment levels. IgG antibody appears rapidly after the start of treatment, and its level is sustained while treatment continues.

ers—since no single effect, such as the quantity of blocking antibody, correlates well with clinical improvement. Regardless of the precise mechanism, desensitization is specific for the allergens injected, is dose-related, and requires repeated and prolonged parenteral administration.

ADVERSE EFFECTS

The adverse effects of desensitization are limited to immediate reactions. The immediate hazard is a systemic anaphylactic reaction. The risk is greatest both during the early weeks or months of treatment while the dose is being increased before a significant level of blocking antibody has been achieved and again when the dose is at or near the maintenance level. Systemic reactions are unpredictable and may occur after years of uneventful injections. They are more likely to happen during the patient's pollen allergy season than during the off-season. Fever and physical exercise increase blood flow, causing more rapid absorption of the injected allergen, thereby enhancing the risk of reaction.

The prevalence of systemic reactions is unknown. Between one and five deaths occur per year in the USA from allergy injection treatment or skin testing, some because of dosage errors. About half of these occur in patients with active asthma.

Other immediate adverse effects are the same as for any subcutaneous injection, such as vasovagal reactions, infections, or injury from injecting the needle into the wrong tissue.

There appear to be no late or long-term ill effects from immunotherapy. With the use of aqueous allergen extracts, there is no evidence that repeated injections induce de novo allergic sensitization to components to which the patient was not previously sensitive. There are no proven instances in which allergen desensitization produces systemic immune-complex disease or other late sequelae.

INDICATIONS

Atopy

Desensitization has been used for almost 80 years to treat allergic rhinitis, and today it is widely accepted as beneficial. It is indicated for patients who are allergic to unavoidable inhalant allergens such as pollens and fungi and whose symptomatic periods of illness are severe, prolonged, and not well controlled by antihistamines or other symptomatic medications. House dust and dust mite desensitization is used in conjunction with a program of dust and mite elimination, since the latter may not be completely effective. Allergists are currently divided in their opinion about injections of animal dander extracts for treatment of allergy to pets in the home or for occupational animal allergy. Opponents point out the paucity of controlled studies, presumed excessive risk of systemic reactions, and concern about unknown long-term effects of immunization with animal protein. Although there are insufficient controlled clinical trials for firm recommendations, the indications for desensitization of allergic asthma parallel those for allergic rhinitis. Desensitization is not indicated for treatment of atopic dermatitis or allergic gastroenteropathy. Patients with atopic dermatitis may receive injections for concomitant allergic rhinitis or asthma if indicated, but starting doses should be low and the buildup in dosage should be slow, because injected allergens may cause a flare of the dermatitis. Desensitization is not indicated for food allergy.

Anaphylaxis

Desensitization is indicated for any patient with a history of systemic anaphylaxis from a Hymenoptera insect sting who has a positive skin test to one or more Hymenoptera venoms. Many authorities exclude from treatment those patients whose reaction to the sting is limited to urticaria, regardless of the skin test results, because such patients generally do not have an excessive risk of systemic anaphylaxis on future stings. There is no indication for desensitization treatment of localized swelling from an insect sting, since these re-

sponses also do not predict future anaphylaxis. The injected allergens for treatment of anaphylaxis should include all of the venoms that give a positive skin test, since identification of the stinging insect under field conditions of a spontaneous sting is usually unreliable.

Desensitization for anaphylaxis in response to drugs has been successful for selected cases of penicillin and insulin allergy. In those instances, injection of increasing doses at intervals of approximately 30 minutes achieves a clinical state of desensitization permitting therapeutic use of the drug on a regular basis. If the drug is withdrawn, the patient may again become allergic.

Urticaria

Desensitization has never been shown to be effective therapy for urticaria, and it is not indicated for this condition.

Immune-Complex Allergies

Desensitization is not necessary for treatment of cutaneous Arthus' reactions or for serum sickness. These are self-limited reactions, which subside when the allergen has been eliminated.

Allergic Contact Dermatitis

Oral and subcutaneous desensitization with extracts of *Rhus* oil has been used for many years, but there is no evidence for its effectiveness in prevention of *Rhus* allergic dermatitis (from poison ivy and poison oak), and therefore it is not indicated for these conditions.

Hypersensitivity Pneumonitis

Desensitization is not indicated for this disease.

MONITORING DESENSITIZATION

Desensitization of respiratory atopic disease is a treatment that continues for years. Indications for starting this long-term process are usually clear, but selection of allergens, dosages and frequency of injections, and duration of therapy must be individualized. The beneficial and adverse responses are difficult to predict in advance. It is therefore important to establish a long-term goal and a program for monitoring treatment at the outset.

Changes in serum levels of specific IgE antibody and induced IgG blocking antibody correlate poorly with clinical improvement, so these are not useful monitors of progress in individual cases. Some allergists repeat skin testing at regular intervals, but clinical improvement can occur without change in skin test reactivity. The principal reason for retesting is to diagnose new sensitivities when symptoms worsen or appear with a new seasonal pattern.

Assessing desensitization for effectiveness requires monitoring of symptoms and physical signs of illness, as well as performing objective tests such as pulmonary functions when applicable. It is reasonable to discontinue the injections after 2 or 3 successive disease-free years.

DESENSITIZATION WITH MODIFIED ALLERGENS

There has been a continuing effort to improve the effectiveness of specific injection therapy and to reduce the risk of reactions and the number of injections through the use of adjuvants and by chemical alteration, modification, and polymerization of the allergen.

Adjuvants

Incomplete Freund's adjuvant—an emulsion of aqueous antigen in mineral oil—enhances the immune response by providing an insoluble lipid depot in the subcutaneous tissue from which droplets of allergen are gradually released, thereby simulating repeated injections of allergen over time. In the early 1960s this method of "one-shot" desensitization given preseasonally underwent extensive clinical trials. It was abandoned because of concern about potential carcinogenicity and the development of long-lasting nodules, cysts, and sterile abscesses.

Adsorption of allergens onto alum produces an insoluble antigen that is more efficiently phagocytosed by macrophages. Alum-adsorbed allergens have had limited acceptance in practice for many years. The presumed advantages over aqueous allergens—fewer injections and improved efficacy—have not been achieved.

Allergoids

Formalin treatment of toxic antigens such as tetanus toxin yields a toxoid, a molecule without toxicity that retains antigenicity. Attempts to modify allergens with formalin, propylene glycol, urea, and other chemicals to eliminate or reduce allergenicity and risk of systemic reactions while preserving immunogenicity to the native allergen have been unsuccessful.

Polymerized Allergens

Polymerizing protein allergens with glutaraldehyde covalently links allergen monomers to yield a molecule with low allergenicity in proportion to the degree of polymerization while retaining immunogenicity. Although not licensed for clinical practice, several different polymerized inhalant allergens have been confirmed by therapeutic trials to be clinically effective.

Peptide Epitopes

A radically new approach to desensitization currently in clinical trials is an attempt to induce a state of anergy to an allergen in T lymphocytes by exposing the cell to peptides containing T-cell epitopes prepared in vitro from recombinant allergen protein molecules. In theory, presentation of the peptide epitope to the T cell in the absence of in vivo processing of the intact protein molecule by the APC bypasses costimulatory APC/T-cell signals necessary for the immune response and renders the T cell specifically anergic to the protein allergen, thereby preventing T-cell help necessary for IgE antibody production by the B cell.

Preliminary results of subcutaneous injections of peptides containing the major allergenic T-cell epitopes from the cat allergen Fel d I in a small group of cat-allergic asthmatic patients show partial clinical tolerance to the expected allergic asthmatic response on exposure to cats under controlled experimental conditions. Unexplained mild side effects occurred. Further research is necessary to assess this form of therapy for general use.

REFERENCES

American Academy of Allergy and Immunology Executive Committee: Personnel and equipment to treat systemic reactions caused by immunotherapy with allergenic extracts. (Position statement.) *J Allergy Clin Immunol* 1986;**77:**271.

British Thoracic Society: Guidelines on the management of asthma. *Thorax* 1993;**48:**(suppl)S1.

Canadian Society of Allergy and Clinical Immunology: Guidelines for the use of allergen immunotherapy. *Can Med Assoc J* 1995;**152:**1413.

Castracane JM, Rocklin RE: Detection of human auto-anti-idiotypic antibodies (Ab2). *Int Arch Allergy Appl Immunol* 1988;**86:**295.

Creticos PS et al: Ragweed immunotherapy in adult asthma. *N Engl J Med* 1996;**334:**501.

Grammer LC et al: Modified forms of allergen immunotherapy. *J Allergy Clin Immunol* 1985;**76:**397.

Lichtenstein LM et al: Clinical and in vitro studies on the role of immunotherapy in ragweed hay fever. *Am J Med* 1968;**44:**514.

Lowell FC, Franklin W: A double-blind study of the effectiveness and specificity of injection therapy in ragweed and hay fever. *N Engl J Med* 1965;**273:**675.

National Heart, Lung, and Blood Institute: National Asthma Education Program Expert Panel Report: Guidelines for the diagnosis and management of asthma. *J Allergy Clin Immunol* 1992;**88:**425.

Noon L: Prophylactic inoculation against hay fever. *Lancet* 1911;**1:**1572.

Norman PS: Immunotherapy for nasal allergy. *J Allergy Clin Immunol* 1988;**81:**992.

Norman PS: An overview of immunotherapy: Implications for the future. *J Allergy Clin Immunol* 1980;**65:**87.

Ohman JL: Allergen immunotherapy in asthma: Review of efficacy and current practice. *Med Clin North Am* 1992;**76:**977.

Rocklin RE: Clinical and immunologic aspects of allergen-specific immunotherapy in patients with seasonal allergic rhinitis and/or allergic asthma. *J Allergy Clin Immunol* 1983;**73:**323.

Sherman WB, Connell JT: Changes in skin-sensitizing antibody titer (SSAT) following two to four years of injection (aqueous) therapy. *J Allergy Clin Immunol* 1966;**37:**123.

57

Clinical Transplantation

Marvin R. Garovoy, MD, Peter Stock, MD, Fraser Keith, MD, & Charles Linker, MD

Transplantation of organs today is a significant factor in medical practice. What was once an experimental and life-saving emergency procedure is now a life-enhancing and technologically advanced form of therapy.

The first successful renal transplant was performed in 1954. Subsequently, advances in histocompatibility testing and immunosuppressive drug therapy made renal transplantation a clinical reality in the 1960s. Improved skills and handling of immunosuppressive drugs (prednisone and azathioprine) resulted in a decline in infectious complications and marked reduction in mortality rates. The 1970s witnessed the beneficial effects of blood transfusions and antilymphocyte globulin (ALG) as graft-enhancing treatments. The 1980s may be characterized as the era of cyclosporine and the advent of monoclonal antibody therapy—immunosuppressive agents that have greatly improved the success rate of kidney transplants and have also made possible heart, liver, lung, and pancreas engraftment with better results than before. The 1990s have witnessed the introduction of two additional immunosuppressive agents (tacrolimus and mycophenolate mofetil)—agents that have further strengthened our ability to control graft rejection. Transplant outcome has become so promising that it is now being offered early in the care of many patients with chronic and debilitating diseases.

KIDNEY TRANSPLANTATION

Patients with end-stage renal disease can be considered for renal transplantation. Absolute contraindications are conditions that would interfere with the safe administration of anesthesia or immunosuppressive therapy. These include debilitating cardiopulmonary disease, cancer, and untreated peptic ulcer disease or infection. Preoperative immunologic evaluation includes ABO blood grouping, histocompatibility testing (determination of the patient's and potential

donor's human leukocyte antigens [HLA antigens] and the degree of haplotype matching) (see Chapter 16), state of presensitization to HLA antigens, and viral serology (hepatitis B and C viruses, human immunodeficiency virus [HIV], cytomegalovirus [CMV], and Epstein-Barr virus). Medical evaluation to rule out contraindications to transplantation frequently includes voiding, cystourethrography, dental and pulmonary evaluations, and assessment of cardiac status.

ABO TESTING

ABO testing is performed on all recipients and potential donors. The ABO system is present not only on erythrocytes but also on the vascular endothelium of the graft. The danger of transplanting across the ABO barrier is the production of very rapid graft rejection owing to preformed isohemagglutinins that injure the vascular endothelium and elicit a coagulation reaction in situ. The same rules that apply to blood transfusion compatibility also apply to renal transplantation: For a type O recipient the donor should be type O; for a type A recipient the donor may be type A or O; for a type B recipient the donor may be type B or O; and for a type AB recipient the donor may be type A, B, or O. It is possible to overcome the ABO barrier by plasmapheresis to lower the natural titer of anti-A or anti-B antibodies and by administration of cyclophosphamide to prevent new antibody formation, but long-term graft survival has been disappointing.

Living Related Donor Transplantation

All recipients and their potential donors should have complete testing for HLA-A, -B, -C, -DR, and -DQ antigens (see Chapter 17). On the basis of family typings, it is usually possible to determine the genotype or haplotype (chromosome) assignment for each identified antigen. The value of haplotype matching (zero, one, or two) was established clinically; a sibling matched for two haplotypes and a parent or sibling matched for one haplotype achieve 90% graft survival at 1 year. Because of improved immunosuppression, zero-haplotype-matched family members can now also achieve 90% graft survival at 1 year. Recently, living unrelated (spouse, friend) transplants have become an established and acceptable source of donors. Typically, the donor is highly motivated and altruistic. Provided there is ABO compatibility, a good outcome can be expected. Within this group of donors, further improvement of graft survival is also seen between those recipient–donor pairs who by chance share one or more HLA antigens.

Presensitization

Prior exposure to transplantation antigens can lead to sensitization manifested by the development of cytotoxic antibodies against HLA antigens. Patients who have antibodies to HLA antigens may have a poorer graft outcome. Moreover, patients who are sensitized and receive second and subsequent transplants are more likely to reject these grafts than are those who receive a primary graft. This likelihood is especially increased in patients who rapidly rejected their first graft (in <3 months). Whether repeated rejection is caused by specific sensitization to transplantation antigens or reflects a high immune reactivity of the recipient is under investigation.

Crossmatching

The crossmatch test is used to determine the presence of any preformed antibodies (presensitization) to donor HLA antigens. A crossmatch typically is performed by using the patient's most recent serum and donor lymphocytes (either peripheral blood mononuclear cells or isolated T or B lymphocytes) (see Chapter 17). Positive crossmatches are a contraindication to transplantation, since they are associated with very early and uncontrollable rejection episodes, leading to irreversible graft loss.

Cadaveric Transplantation

When the recipient has no family members as potential donors, the opportunity exists to receive a kidney from a recently deceased individual (cadaveric transplantation). Recipients referred for this type of treatment undergo comparable immunologic evaluation of ABO grouping, HLA typing, and antibody screening and are then placed on a waiting list. The most likely causes of formation of anti-HLA antibodies include pregnancy and previously rejected grafts. To monitor the extent of anti-HLA antibodies produced, serum from each recipient is collected monthly and tested in a manner known as screening. The patient's serum is crossmatched against a panel of lymphocytes obtained from many individuals. The number of individuals whose cells are killed is often expressed as a percentage of the panel (eg, 10% panel-reactive antibody). By this procedure, it is possible to determine the extent of presensitization, that is, the likelihood that the recipient will have a positive crossmatch, assuming that the transplant organ is taken from the same genetic pool of donors as the lymphocyte panel. In addition, knowing which HLA antigens on the lymphocyte panel cells have been lysed makes it possible to analyze the specificities of the antibodies in the serum that are responsible for the positive reactions.

Donor Selection

When a potential cadaveric donor's organs are harvested, a section of spleen, some lymph nodes, and some peripheral blood are collected. The donor ABO blood group and HLA antigens are determined from these samples. The waiting list of recipients can then be crossmatched against the donor tissues, using the patient's current serum and the recipient's highest reacting serum within the past 2 years to exclude the possibility of a positive crossmatch. Recipients who are ABO-compatible and crossmatch-negative become available for further consideration. Often, there may be a second round of crossmatch testing among this smaller pool of recipients, in which additional past sera are chosen to be certain of no hidden presensitization. From among the ABO-compatible, crossmatch-negative recipients, the best matched recipients may then be selected. In programs in which a large enough choice of recipients is not available to find a perfectly matched recipient, additional criteria, such as length of time on the waiting list, urgency of medical condition, and whether this is a first or second transplant, are considered in recipient selection.

Donor Evaluation & Procedures

Candidacy for living donation is determined by evaluating the potential donors for heart disease, renal dysfunction, diabetes, infection, and malignancy. A preoperative angiogram guides selection of the right or left kidney for living donation. Factors that influence the choice of kidney are operating safety for the donor, vascular and internal anatomy, and occasionally differential creatinine clearance by renal scan. The living donor nephrectomy procedure includes a flank incision through which the kidney and vascular pedicle are removed. The ureter and all periureteral soft tissue are removed in order to preserve the ureteral blood supply and to prevent distal ureteral avascular necrosis.

Studies conducted to evaluate a potential living donor include a complete medical evaluation. There is no long-term change in survival or life-style of individuals who have undergone uninephrectomy for donation. Because improved immunosuppression and preoperative conditioning have increased success rates of living donor transplantation, it is now possible to consider living donors who share two, one, or no haplotypes with the recipient. With the increasing demand for kidneys, many centers are now performing transplants from living unrelated donors. Recent results indicate that a 90% 1-year survival rate can be achieved. Evaluation of donor motivation and psychologic factors is necessary.

Cadaveric donors can be considered when they are determined to be neurologically dead from a variety of causes, including spontaneous intracerebral hemorrhage and head trauma. Cadaveric donors must be free from metastasizing tumors, kidney dysfunction, or active infection (particularly with hepatitis viruses or HIV). There are evolving criteria for selecting organs for transplantation from donors who are positive for hepatitis C antibody. Hemodynamic stabilization with volume expansion and the conservative use of vasopressors and desmopressin acetate maintain optimal organ function. Organ recovery from cadaveric donors includes removal of both kidneys with renal arteries and veins frequently left en bloc with the donor aorta and vena cava. Both ureters are removed, including all periureteral soft tissue, in order to include the ureteral blood supply and to prevent distal ureteral avascular necrosis. Samples of spleen and lymph nodes are also removed for donor tissue typing and crossmatching against potential recipients.

Once removed, the kidney is flushed with preservation fluid to remove all donor blood. Cadaveric kidneys can be stored by either of two methods. Cold storage involves storing in ice to maintain subphysiologic temperatures. Alternatively, the aorta or renal arteries are cannulated, and a cold mixed-electrolyte solution is instilled by continuous cold pulsatile perfusion. Cadaver renal transplantation within the first 48 hours after donor nephrectomy is preferred.

Blood Transfusion

In the past, recipient preconditioning with blood transfusion has led to improved graft survival. Explanations for the transfusion effect include the elimination of immunologic responders who will demonstrate cytotoxic antibodies contraindicating transplantation, development of specific and nonspecific immunoregulatory T cells, and generation of blocking or anti-idiotypic antibodies. With improved immunosuppressive protocols, the benefits of pretransplant transfusions have been more difficult to demonstrate. Furthermore, many centers now believe that the infectious risks associated with blood transfusions outweigh the potential benefits.

Transplant Surgery

The operative procedure for the recipient includes an incision over the iliac fossa through which the graft is placed in the retroperitoneal position against the psoas muscle (Fig 57–1). A renal artery anastomosis to either the internal or external iliac artery and renal vein anastomosis to the external iliac vein are standard. Ureteroneocystotomy involving anastomosis of the ureter to bladder mucosa through an anterior cystotomy incision is a usual approach. The ureter is often passed through a short submucosal tunnel

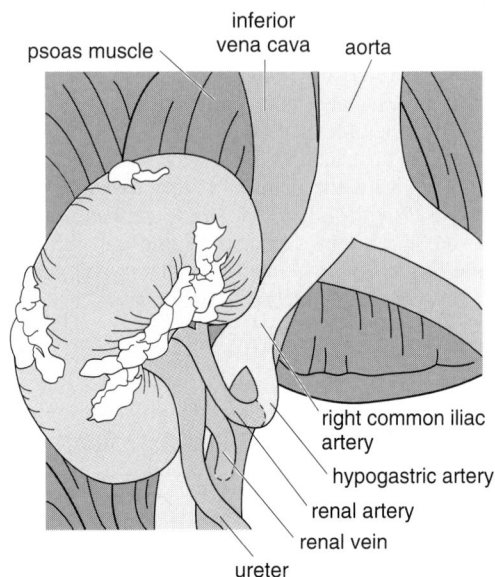

Figure 57–1. Technique of renal transplantation. (Reproduced, with permission, from Way LW (editor): *Current Surgical Diagnosis & Treatment,* 9th ed. Appleton & Lange, 1991.)

in the bladder wall to prevent vesicoureteral reflux.

Postoperatively, hemodynamic stability is achieved with central venous pressure monitoring and careful fluid and diuretic management. Careful monitoring of urine output, electrolytes, blood urea nitrogen, and serum creatinine to evaluate renal function is mandatory. All cadaveric kidneys have some degree of acute tubular necrosis, ranging from very mild to very severe. Dialysis is required in approximately 20% of cadaveric renal transplant recipients during the early period of severe acute tubular necrosis (usually 5–10 days). Acute tubular necrosis is rare in patients receiving related-donor transplants since donor nephrectomy and recipient transplant are performed sequentially, minimizing cold-storage time.

Postoperative Immunosuppression

Postoperative immunosuppression is the most variable aspect of recipient care. Standard immunosuppression to prevent rejection includes corticosteroids, and additional immunosuppression is chosen depending on the type of allograft and tissue match (see Chapters 58 and 60). The use of cyclosporine (5–15 mg/kg/d) has clearly improved long-term allograft success in recipients of cadaveric and some related-donor transplants. Cyclosporine is definitely nephrotoxic, and monitoring of drug dosages and serum drug levels (100–400 µg/mL) is required.

Azathioprine, an antimetabolite that interferes with new DNA formation in proliferating cells, is frequently used (1–2 mg/kg/d) in combination with prednisone and cyclosporine. Azathioprine is potentially

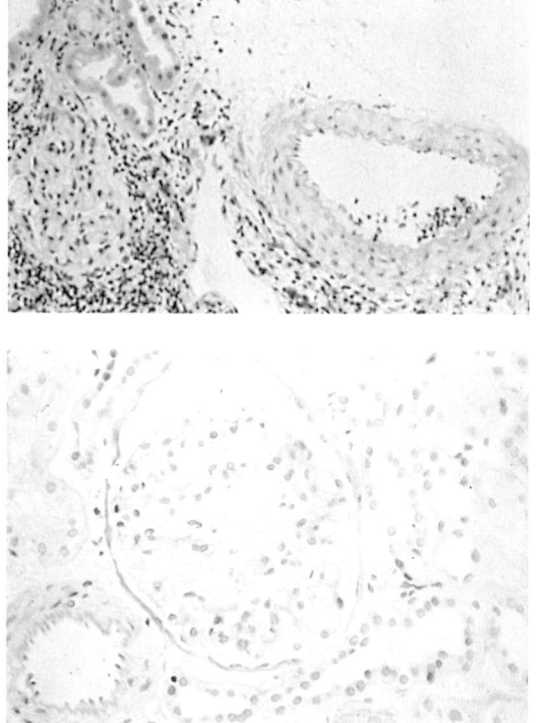

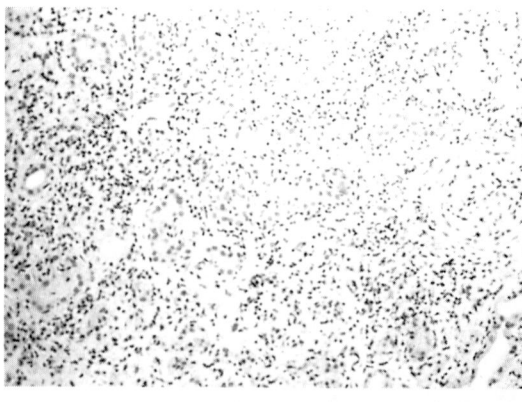

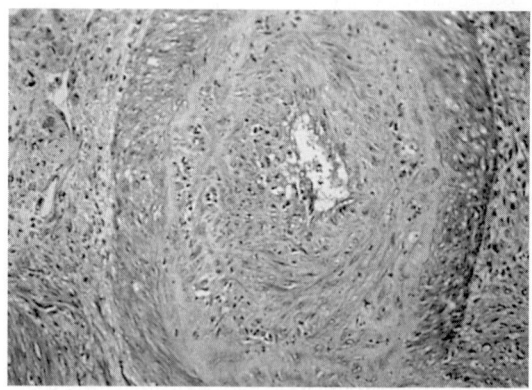

Figure 57–2. ***Top:*** Early acute rejection showing focal mononuclear cellular infiltrate in the interstitium and in the wall of a blood vessel. ***Bottom:*** Appearance of normal renal biopsy specimen with glomeruli, arterioles, and tubules.

Figure 57–3. ***Top:*** Acute rejection—severe. Diffuse mononuclear cellular infiltrate throughout the interstitium. ***Bottom:*** Chronic rejection. Fibroobliterative changes in an arteriole and reduction of vascular lumen.

hepatotoxic, whereas cyclophosphamide is a nonhepatotoxic alternative. Antilymphocyte globulin (ALG; 10–20 mg/kg) and antithymocyte globulin (ATG; 10–20 mg/kg) from serum of animals immunized with human lymphocytes or thymocytes, respectively, are potent immunosuppressive reagents. These heterologous animal proteins can be made in horses, sheep, goats, or rabbits. Monoclonal antilymphocyte antibodies (OKT 3, OKT 4) against specific T-cell subsets are also in clinical use. Lymphoplasmapheresis occasionally is used to remove recipient lymphocytes and immunoglobulin while immunosuppressive drugs are concurrently administered. Local graft irradiation has been used but has not provided reliable immunosuppression. A number of newer immunosuppressive agents with different mechanisms of action have been approved (tacrolimus, formerly called FK 506), and others are in clinical trials (mycophenolate mofetil, 15-deoxyspergualin).

Rejection

Classic signs and symptoms of acute rejection include swelling and tenderness over the allograft and decrease in renal function. Systemic manifestations such as temperature elevation, malaise, poor appetite,

and generalized myalgia can be seen. Decrease in renal function is diagnosed by a decrease in urine volume, increasing blood urea nitrogen and creatinine levels, poorly controlled hypertension, fluid retention, and radiographically by ultrasonography (blurring of corticomedullary junctions, increased resistive index, prominent pyramids) and by radionuclide renal scans showing decreased uptake and excretion of the tracer. In the presence of a decline in renal function, however, the differential diagnosis includes prerenal azotemia and obstruction, acute tubular necrosis, pyelonephritis, and other drug-induced toxicity. In addition, recurrence of the primary renal disease and de novo glomerulonephritis can be late causes of decreased renal function. Renal biopsy is frequently performed to histologically diagnose the cause of graft dysfunction (Figs 57–2, 57–3).

PATHOLOGY OF GRAFT REJECTION

Mechanisms of Rejection

A. Acute: Evidence suggests that at least two pathways of antigen presentation may be operative.

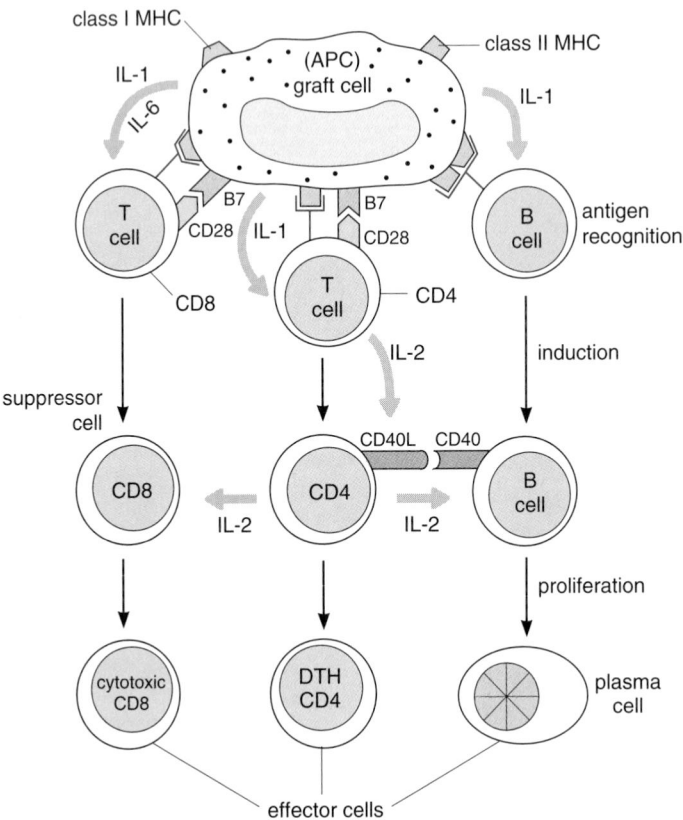

Figure 57–4. Generation of allograft rejection response (primary).

The "direct path" of antigen presentation suggests that blood-borne antigen-presenting cells ("passenger cells") in grafts provide the primary stimulus. These are dendritic cells and monocytes expressing allogeneic class I and II HLA molecules. The "indirect path" of antigen presentation suggests that host (recipient) antigen-presenting cells (APC) can present shed allogeneic class I and II HLA antigens from donor parenchymal cells. Both donor and host antigen-presenting cells provide second signals, interleukin-1 (IL-1), and IL-6, which aid in triggering lymphocyte activation (Fig 57–4). IL-1 not only is involved in the activation of helper/inducer CD4 T cells but probably also is important for the activation of unprimed cytotoxic CD8 T cells and B lymphocytes. The activation of helper/inducer T cells by alloantigen is necessary but not sufficient to the development of cell immune responses against the graft. Also required is a costimulating signal by the interaction of other molecules on the antigen-presenting cell and T lymphocyte. The best studied is the B7 family of molecules on the APC (B7.1/7.2, now called CD80/86), which must bind to the CD28 molecule on T lymphocytes. Together, interaction of the T-cell receptor/MHC (signal 1) with the costimulus (signal 2) is

stabilized by cell adhesion molecules (ICAM-1/LFA-1) supports full T-lymphocyte activation (Fig 57–5).

Once activated, these cells release IL-2, which is an essential cofactor in the activation of both CD8 T cells and B cells. As a consequence of exposure to antigen plus costimulating signals, clonal proliferation and maturation of alloantigen-reactive cells takes place. This leads to the development of effector T cells, which migrate from lymphoid tissue via the blood to all tissues, including the graft, where they mediate damage to antigen-containing sites, and antibody, which is released into the blood or produced locally within the graft, where it has access to these antigens (Fig 57–6).

The precise mechanism by which T cells destroy the graft is still under study. Effector T cells that can destroy graft tissue develop from both CD8 and CD4 subclasses (see Fig 57–6). The results are similar except that CD8 T cells recognize HLA-A and HLA-B antigen-bearing cells, whereas CD4 T cells recognize HLA-DR antigen-bearing cells. Both CD4 and CD8 subclasses of effector cells probably can directly destroy graft cells by classic cytotoxic T-cell mechanisms. Another important consequence of T cell-activation, however, is their release of other lymphokines, especially interferon gamma (IFNγ), which can pro-

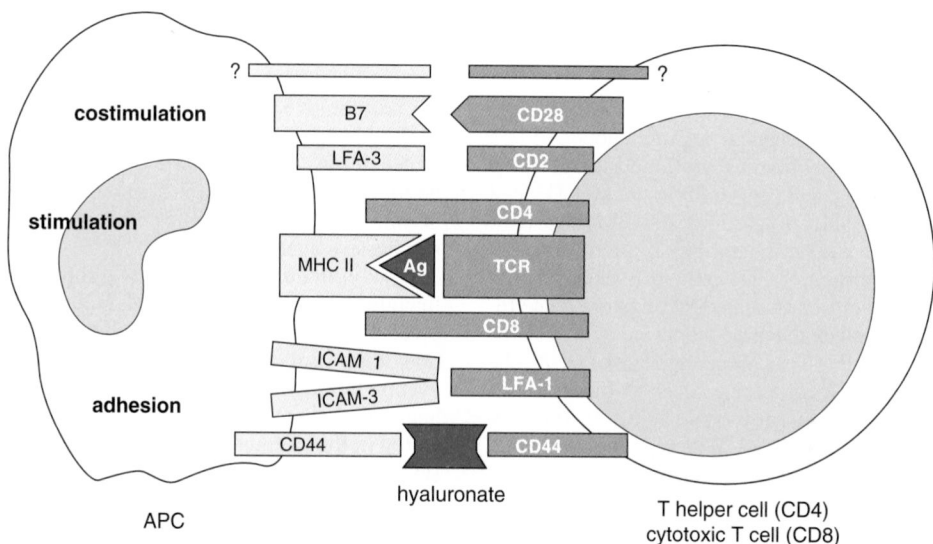

Figure 57–5. Schematic representation of costimulatory and adhesion molecules on the surface of antigen-presenting cells and T lymphocytes.

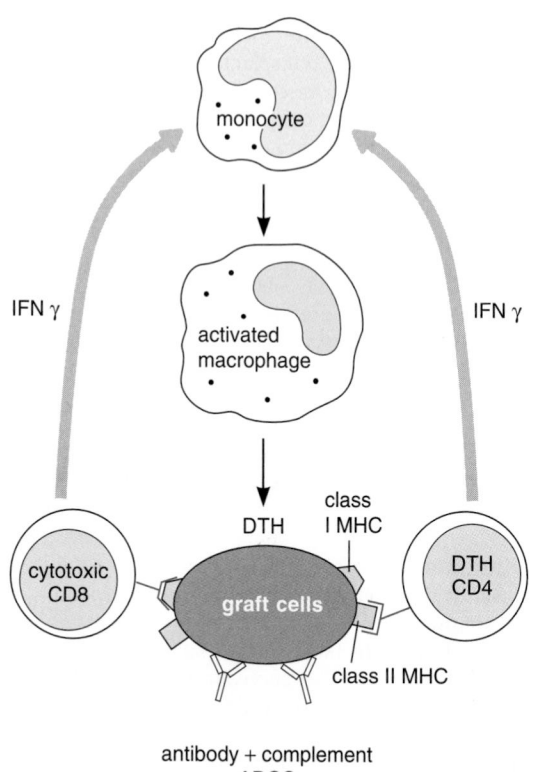

Figure 57–6. Effector mechanisms of allograft rejection.

monocytes to mediate a destructive delayed hypersensitivity response against the graft.

Hence, T cells can directly cause target cell injury or activate macrophages, resulting in nonspecific destruction. Lymphokines in addition to IL-2 and IFNγ are released from activated T cells; they include IL-4 and IL-5, which play a role in directing B-cell production of antibody. Antibody-mediated damage may then take place directly through complement activation or by recruitment of antibody-dependent cell-mediated cytotoxic (ADCC) effector cells (see Fig 57–6). Most of the cells that arrive in the graft early after transplantation are lymphocytes, which migrate out of the capillary and venous beds, but after 4–7 days a remarkably heterogeneous collection of cell types appears. Those of the lymphocytic series predominate over the monocyte–macrophage and include also a few polymorphonuclear neutrophils. Although a variety of cell types are present, there is some evidence that early rejection of solid-tissue allografts is associated with T lymphocytes having direct cytotoxic activity against donor target cells. A significant number of B lymphocytes, null cells, and monocytes also appear in the early infiltrate, and although cytotoxic T-cell activity is easily demonstrated at first, later stages of rejection may involve a non-T killer cell. In all phases, the presence of antibodies and ADCC effector cells makes this mechanism an additional possibility. Macrophages appear to play an effector and suppressor role, whereas some B lymphocytes become activated and begin immunoglobulin synthesis in situ. When the host has been primed to donor antigens before transplantation, an accelerated process, often marked by antibody-mediated vasculitis, may result.

duce two important effects. First, IFNγ induces increased expression of HLA-A, -B, and -DR on graft tissue, which potentially makes the graft more vulnerable to effector mechanisms. Second, it activates

Recent applications of anti-T-cell monoclonal antibodies as diagnostic reagents in staining biopsies and in vivo as therapy add considerable support to the key role of T lymphocytes in most cases of rejection. When immunofluorescence or immunoperoxidase techniques are used with renal graft biopsies, 50–90% of the infiltrating cells generally express CD3 and CD2, with variable proportions of CD4 and CD8 cells. Although the peripheral blood often shows an increased proportion of CD4 cells in association with acute rejection episodes, many investigators relate rejection in the kidney to a preponderance of CD8 cells. More precisely, there is a preponderance of CD8 cells in the blood and perivascular areas in the grafts of patients experiencing irreversible rejection (ratio of CD4 to CD8 cells <1.0). When peripheral blood CD4:CD8 ratios are higher, perivascular ratios are also higher, and rejection usually is reversible with therapy. High-dose corticosteroids, given either intravenously (methylprednisolone, 1 g/d for 3 days) or orally (prednisone, 5–10 mg/kg/d for 5 days) are often used to treat acute rejection. Corticosteroids function through several pathways. They reduce the capacity of antigen-presenting cells to express class II antigens and to release IL-1. They also inhibit the alloactivation of T cells and consequently the release of IL-2. Their effect on migration and function of effector cells, as well as their capacity to release IFNγ, may explain their efficacy in reversing acute rejection. In this regard, they are known to produce lymphocytopenia, especially of CD4 T cells, by delaying transit of lymphocytes through marrow and lymphoid tissues.

If there is no response or only a partial response to corticosteroids, ALG may be given (10–20 mg/kg/d for 5–14 days). ALG lyses lymphocytes, especially T cells, making it an excellent agent for treatment of acute rejection. ALG, however, may cause anaphylaxis, serum sickness, and fever. Biologic effects also vary, since there is no effective measure for standardization.

More commonly, monoclonal antibodies (muromonab-CD3, also known as OKT 3) are used to treat rejection refractory to steroids. This is a mouse IgG2 monoclonal antibody to the human T-cell surface molecule CD3. Not only is it effective for the treatment of initial bouts of rejection, but rejection episodes that are resistant to high-dose steroids usually respond to 5 mg/d intravenously for 10 days. OKT 3 initially causes an acute T-lymphocyte depletion as the antibody-coated T lymphocytes are opsonized and eliminated by the reticuloendothelial system. After 48 hours of therapy, there is a slow return of T lymphocytes to the circulation; however, the T-cell receptor/CD3 complex is modulated (cleared) from the cell surface. Without a sufficient number of CD3 molecules present, T-cell activation is impaired. One side effect of therapy may be the production of antimouse antibodies in a small percentage of patients, which can limit the effectiveness of a subsequent course of therapy. Prolonged or high-dose OKT 3 therapy has been associated with an increased incidence of lymphoproliferative disease. In the future, monoclonal antibodies against lymphokine receptors and adhesion molecules as well as soluble cytokine receptors may be found useful. Figure 57–7 shows the site of action of some new and some currently approved immunosuppressive agents.

B. Hyperacute: Preformed anti-ABO isohemagglutinins or anticlass I HLA antibodies, when present in sufficient quantity, bind to the vascular endothelium and trigger a cascade of immunologic events. Initially, fixation of complement components and complement activation ensues, followed by activation of the clotting pathway. This series of events, if severe enough, can result in microthrombi within glomerular capillary loops and arterioles, leading to severe ischemia and necrosis of the graft. At present, there are no effective means of treating this lesion once it begins. Emphasis is therefore placed on prevention by careful assessment of ABO blood type and donor-specific sensitization to HLA antigens by crossmatch testing prior to transplantation.

C. Chronic: Chronic rejection, which can occur months to years after transplantation, is characterized by a narrowing of the vascular arterial lumen owing to growth of endothelial cells that line the vascular bed (see Fig 57–4). The actual control mechanisms for this response are unknown but may include immunologic injury signals, monocyte release of IL-1, and platelet and endothelial cell release of platelet-derived growth factor. Initially, the proliferating endothelial cell lesion is reversible, but once it progresses to fibrotic changes within the blood vessel wall itself, it is unresponsive to current modes of immunosuppression, leading to graft ischemia, extensive interstitial fibrosis, and ultimate loss of renal function. Since there is no specific therapy for this form of rejection, emphasis is on prevention by seeking the greatest possible degree of histocompatibility between recipients and donors.

Outcome

Survival of patients after renal transplantation is not significantly different from that of patients undergoing dialysis. In most series, patient survival at 2 years is 90–95%. Graft survival, defined as allograft function adequate to maintain life without dialytic treatment, is 85% at 2 years in cadaveric renal allograft recipients treated with corticosteroids and either cyclosporine or ALG/OKT 3. Related-donor transplants have greater than 90% success at 2 years.

Surviving renal allografts have normal function, with mean creatinine levels of less than 2 mg/dL in most series. A functioning allograft therefore affords the recipient an optimal chance for normalization of health and is associated with minimal morbidity and mortality rates.

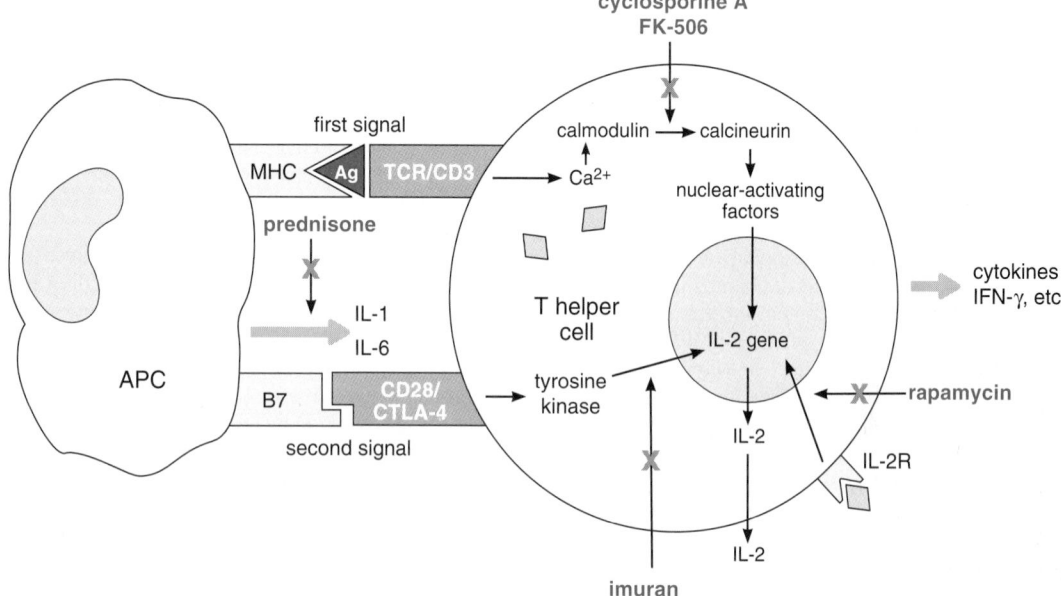

Figure 57–7. Schematic representation of the molecular sites of action of some currently available immunosuppressive agents.

LIVER TRANSPLANTATION

Extensive experimental work in the field of liver transplantation has been performed since the early 1950s. Early investigators, using a variety of animal models, demonstrated that liver transplantation was feasible. The use of large-animal models indicated potential problem areas such as control of the splanchnic circulation during cross-clamping (the predecessor of the venovenous bypass) and rejection in grafts progressing to liver failure in animals untreated with immunosuppressive agents. The first human liver transplant was performed in 1963. Although this and the next several transplants were unsuccessful, liver transplantation later became a successful procedure because of improved surgical techniques, intraoperative management, and methods of immunosuppression. In 1995 more than thirty-five hundred liver transplants were performed in the USA, and over 100 liver transplant centers exist throughout the world at this time.

Although liver grafts were initially thought to be immunologically privileged from results of experimental liver transplantation in animals, rejection is commonly encountered in human liver transplantation. In certain strains of pigs and rats, liver grafts between the same donor and recipient combination have prolonged survival even though allogeneic kidney allografts are rejected within a short time. In addition, animals tolerate subsequent skin grafts from the same donor for prolonged periods but promptly reject third-party skin grafts. These effects are specific to only limited strains. There is evidence that long-term in-

duction of tolerance to the transplanted liver occurs naturally. According to a hypothesis proposed by Dr. Thomas Starzl, lymphoid cells from the donor organ migrate to the periphery and set up a state of chimerism. This chimeric state is associated with the development of host tolerance to the transplanted tissue. Although immunosuppression has been successfully withdrawn in some chimeric recipients, other chimeric patients have rejected the organ following withdrawal of the immunosuppressant treatment. The functional significance of the chimeric state remains unclear, although it appears that it is in some way associated with graft acceptance. There is, however, evidence that liver transplant rejection occurs by substantially different mechanisms from kidney transplant rejection. As a consequence of these different mechanisms and the difference of expression of major histocompatibility complex (MHC) antigens on the surface of liver cells and bile duct cells, the rejection response of the liver is distinctly different from that of other whole organs.

Indications

Liver transplantation is indicated when an individual's disease process is likely to progress to death within 2 years or when the compromise in life-style is so severe as to merit the risk of transplant. Although some diseases are known to be fatal in the long term, it is only recently that longitudinal studies in primary biliary cirrhosis and sclerosing cholangitis have elucidated specific factors that can predict short-term survival. Liver transplantation is usually not indicated until the life expectancy of the individual is less than

2 years. Hepatic dysfunction may be manifested by alterations in either synthetic or regulatory ability.

Signs and symptoms of progressive liver deficiency include malaise, weight loss, encephalopathy, ascites, coagulopathy, hypoalbuminemia, hyperbilirubinemia, and renal insufficiency. Complications of cholestatic disease include intractable pruritus, metabolic bone disease, recurrent biliary sepsis, and xanthomatous neuropathy. In addition, progressive complications of portal hypertension (gastroesophageal bleeding, ascites) in the context of liver deficiency require intervention. With the development of transjugular intrahepatic portasystemic shunts (TIPS), variceal bleeding and refractory ascites can often be managed effectively until a donor organ becomes available. The use of the TIPS is effective in the pretransplant setting in controlling variceal bleeding and refractory ascites. It can, however, exacerbate the encephalopathy and is used most effectively as a bridge to transplantation. At present, many potential liver transplant recipients (particularly children) die before a suitable organ becomes available.

The most common indication for liver transplant in the adult population to date has been non-A, non-B hepatitis virus postnecrotic cirrhosis or chronic active hepatitis. Other diagnoses for which liver transplantation has been performed include primary biliary cirrhosis, sclerosing cholangitis, hepatitis B cirrhosis, hepatitis C cirrhosis, alcoholic cirrhosis, fulminant hepatic failure, hemochromatosis, Wilson's disease, Budd-Chiari syndrome, hepatitis C, and inborn errors of metabolism. Some patients with hepatocellular tumors or cholangiocarcinomas have received transplants, and a few patients have survived long term (3–5 years).

In patients with localized hepatocellular tumors, several centers are proceeding with chemoembolization followed by transplantation. Preliminary data suggest that selected patients can achieve successful transplants using this approach. Patients with antigen-positive chronic active hepatitis B frequently have recurrent hepatitis B antigenemia following transplantation. In the past, large numbers of these patients have developed recurrent hepatitis and cirrhosis, although the rapidity of progression of chronic active hepatitis leading to cirrhosis and liver failure has been questioned. The use of hepatitis B hyperimmune globulin (HBIG) has dramatically improved the results of transplantation for hepatitis B. It remains unclear how long the recipients need to be treated with monthly injections of this agent. For patients who are antigen-positive at the time of transplantation, newer protocols involving the use of the antiviral agent lamivudine are currently being investigated. Patients transplanted for hepatitis C also are at risk for disease recurrence, although progression to end-stage liver failure is less common. To date no therapy has been effective in preventing the recurrence of hepatitis C, although trials with interferon therapy have been attempted. Although liver transplantation in patients with alcohol-related liver failure was initially quite controversial, this indication has become more widely accepted because of the increasing evidence that these patients have results comparable to those of patients with other causes of liver failure. Most transplant centers require that these patients remain abstinent from alcohol for 6–12 months and that they can comply with posttransplant treatment regimens.

The most common diagnosis for which liver transplantation is performed in infants and children is extrahepatic biliary atresia. This disease occurs in between 1:8,000 and 1:12,000 live births in the USA. Children commonly undergo the Kasai procedure, which has long-term effectiveness in one third to one half of all patients. For patients with failed hepaticojejunostomy, liver transplantation is the only viable solution. Other indications for liver transplants in children are inborn errors of metabolism such as α_1-antitrypsin deficiency, tyrosinemia, and Wilson's disease. As outcomes have improved, liver replacement has been used to treat liver-based inborn errors of metabolism that result in extrahepatic organ system failure. For example, one patient with homozygous familial hypercholesterolemia has received a heart–liver transplant, and several patients with α_1-antitrypsin deficiency and renal involvement have received combination liver–kidney transplants. For infants and smaller children, living related donors have been used with increasing frequency. The success of these living related liver transplants approximates that of cadaveric transplantation. Although no immunologic advantage has been noted to date, increased availability of organs has led to more optimal timing of the transplant. This in turn has contributed to a decrease in pretransplantation mortality.

Contraindications to liver transplantation vary from center to center. General guidelines are the exclusion of potential recipients whose disease conditions are associated with poor prognosis (HIV seropositivity, hepatitis B surface or E antigen seropositivity, extrahepatic malignancy, or evidence of metastatic disease). Further contraindications include behavioral and social issues that may predict a poor outcome because of noncompliance. Examples are active substance abuse and the recipient's inability to meet with the rigors of postoperative management (compliance and medication protocol) or postoperative follow-up. Finally, medical contraindications to liver transplantation include advanced cardiopulmonary disease, anatomic considerations that preclude surgical reconstruction, and active infection, especially with fungal pathogens.

Procedure

Orthotopic liver transplantation is the most commonly used method to date. This involves the removal of the host liver and replacement with the transplanted liver in the orthotopic position. Heterotopic transplan-

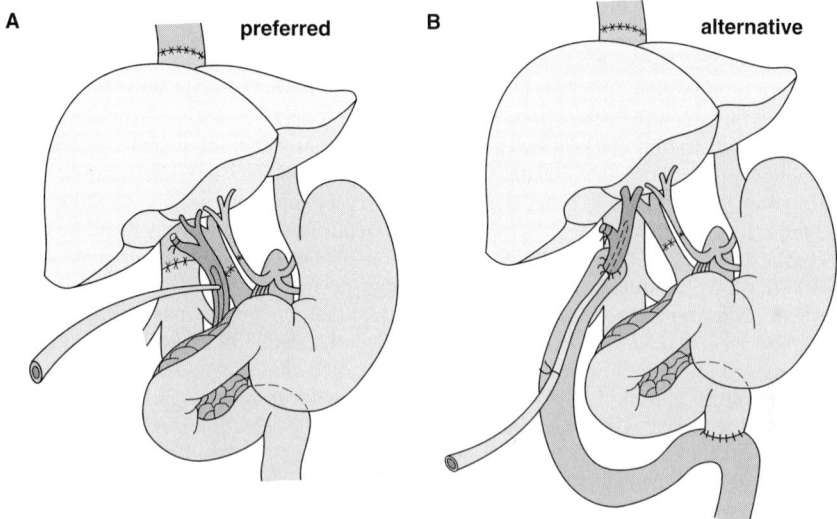

A: preferred   **B:** alternative

Figure 57–8. Liver transplantation. **A:** The preferred method and **B:** the alternative technique are shown. The donor suprahepatic vena cava, infrahepatic vena cava, portal vein, and hepatic artery are anastomosed end to end to the corresponding recipient vessels. When the recipient common duct is intact and the size matches the donor common duct, a choledochocholedochostomy **(A)** is performed. When the recipient duct is not intact (eg, biliary atresia or sclerosing cholangitis), a choledochojejunostomy **(B)** is used.

tation, in which the native liver is left in place and the transplanted liver is placed at an ectopic site, is less frequently performed, because the clinical results have been less successful. After removal from the donor, the donor liver is flushed with heparinized University of Wisconsin (UW) solution and then preserved in preservation solution and stored in the cold. The recently developed UW solution enables the liver to be preserved for more than 24 hours in some cases. This has greatly expanded the ability to transport organs long distances and to use back-up recipients if the first recipient proves unacceptable for transplantation. To minimize the risk of intrahepatic biliary strictures associated with prolonged hepatic preservation time, however, an attempt is made to transplant within 12 hours after harvest. The recipient hepatectomy is technically the most difficult phase of the transplant operation because of frequent portal hypertension, previous surgery, and coagulopathy. Often there is excessive bleeding due to numerous adhesions at the operative site. The liver is mobilized although not removed until the donor organ is brought into the operative field and examined. The anhepatic phase is the time of greatest physiologic stress, because at this point the liver is removed and clamping of the portal vein and vena cava results in decreased venous return to the heart. This may in part be overcome by the use of venovenous bypass, which serves to bypass the splanchnic circulation and the infrahepatic vena caval circulation. Many centers, however, do not use venovenous bypass during the anhepatic phase. The anhepatic phase lasts from the time when the host liver

is removed until the vascular clamps are released, reperfusing the new liver. The revascularization phase requires attention to hemostasis. Revascularization involves supply to the liver via either the portal vein or the hepatic artery, or both, depending on the individual's anatomy and stability on venovenous bypass. The specific type of arterial revascularization depends on the blood supply to the donor organ. Complex revascularization may be required if multiple arteries are supplying the donor liver. The bile duct is reconstructed by using a choledocholedochostomy, preferably when the recipient common duct is of good quality, or a choledochojejunostomy if the recipient duct is poor quality (eg, in biliary atresia) or of marked unequal size compared with the donor's common bile duct (Fig 57–8). Improvements in surgical technique, new technologic advances such as the venovenous bypass, the availability of UW solution, and the ability to control coagulation have decreased operative mortality rates and expanded the preservation time.

Outcome

Early graft failure, also known as primary nonfunction, may be a devastating complication if the patient does not receive a second transplant. Primary nonfunction encompasses a spectrum ranging from no graft function (and certain death without retransplantation) to a liver whose function is mildly impaired at the outset but regains function within the first few days or weeks after transplantation. Factors related to primary nonfunction include the nature of the donor injury, the donor retrieval operation, the preservation solution, the length of preservation, host immunologic factors, the transplant operation, and host cardiovascular factors. One established factor that has been associated with primary nonfunction is the presence of moderate to extensive fat deposits in the donor liver. In cases in which fatty infiltration of the liver is suspected, a biopsy specimen should be taken. The pathologic confirmation of moderate to extensive fat should preclude the use of such livers.

Infectious complications after transplantation are frequent. Survival after infection relates to the type of offending organisms. Bacterial infections from pulmonary, bladder, and vascular sites usually respond to antibiotics, but fungal or viral infections may be associated with higher mortality and morbidity rates. As mentioned previously, the use of HBIG has dramatically improved the results following transplantation for hepatitis B virus. Although recurring hepatitis C is common following transplantation, the disease infrequently progresses to end-stage failure.

Rejection is common after liver transplantation and may be seen in 75% of patients when defined by histologic means alone (see later discussion). Rejection can be readily diagnosed (see later discussion) by frequent percutaneous biopsies and is easily and successfully treated when diagnosed early. Although rejection is common during the early posttransplant period (see later discussion), the rejection is generally easily reversed. Unlike rejection following renal transplantation, early rejection following liver transplants does not usually detrimentally affect the long-term function of the liver. Late failure is due to chronic failure or recurrence of the original disease. A particularly virulent type of rejection that is associated with damage to or disappearance of bile ducts may be connected with early graft loss. The survival rate at 1 year following liver transplantation ranges between 70 and 90% and is about 60% at 5 years.

Crossmatching & Immunosuppression

Decisions regarding the suitability of the donor organ for liver transplantation are currently based on ABO blood matching and organ size. HLA antigen typing is not used to match donors and recipients, although an inverse relationship between matching and survival has been reported. Many liver transplants are performed in children, so the donor liver must be of an appropriate size to fit into the child's abdominal cavity. Recently the use of livers that are made surgically smaller has drastically changed the approach to transplant in small recipients. The use of partial grafts from live donors is an extension of the work with pared-down organs from cadavers. Crossmatches are not routinely performed preoperatively but usually postoperatively. There are only a few reports of hyperacute rejection when the liver recipient has preformed antibodies against the donor. The apparent resistance of the liver to hyperacute rejection is interesting, but its cause is unknown. It has been suggested that perhaps

the liver is not sensitive to preformed antibodies or that the liver mass itself results in dilution of the antibody titer to a level that is not harmful. There have been reports of combination liver and kidney transplants in recipient–donor combinations with a positive crossmatch that becomes negative on completion of the liver transplant. There has been no demonstration of increased antibody fixation to the graft. Loss of cytotoxic antibodies, however, could be due to the formation of soluble immune complexes. Alternatively, it may be that the blood loss associated with the liver transplant operation may dilute the antibody titers. Recently, data from retrospective crossmatches have suggested that positive crossmatches have correlated with poorer long-term graft function.

Although rejection is readily diagnosed by percutaneous biopsy, other causes of hepatic malfunction must be considered. Biliary obstruction, vascular thrombosis, viral hepatitis, drug toxicity, and recurrence of the underlying disease must all be excluded. Signs and symptoms of rejection include fever, abdominal pain, ascites, hepatomegaly, and decreased appetite, all of which are nonspecific. Laboratory abnormalities do not predict for rejection but include elevation of serum bilirubin, alkaline phosphatase, and transaminases. During the first 2 weeks following liver transplant, there is poor correlation between elevation in liver functions, and protocol biopsies are performed to rule out rejection. After this initial period, the decision to perform a biopsy is predicated on abnormal liver function tests.

The histopathologic features that suggest rejection include a mixed cellular portal infiltrate with bile duct epithelial damage and central vein or portal vein endothelial damage. Treatment of rejection includes the use of methylprednisolone, antilymphoblast globulin, or monoclonal antibody OKT 3. More recently, tacrolimus has been used in place of cyclosporine A to treat refractory rejection. The use of these drugs depends on an assessment of the severity of the rejection.

Cyclosporine has had a major effect on the results after liver transplantation. Prior to the cyclosporine era, the 1-year patient survival was in the range of 30–40%. This changed markedly after 1979 with the introduction of cyclosporine. Current protocols at most transplantation centers call for cyclosporine and prednisone with or without azathioprine as prophylaxis against rejection. Tacrolimus, another IL-2 inhibitor, has been used as an alternative to cyclosporine, and in some institutions has been the primary agent. As mentioned earlier, patients have been switched from cyclosporine to tacrolimus for recurrent rejection problems. The antimetabolite Cellcept has been very effective in preventing rejection of cadaveric renal transplants and is currently being evaluated as potential replacement for azathioprine.

Bile salts are necessary for the gastrointestinal absorption of cyclosporine, and if bile output is poor, inadequate absorption may necessitate intravenous administration of the drug. Although hepatotoxicity has been reported with cyclosporine, it is rare, and elevated postoperative liver function tests usually have another cause. The use of cyclosporine and tacrolimus may be limited by their nephrotoxicity, which is compounded in patients with recent hepatorenal syndrome. The bone marrow suppression seen with azathioprine may be more pronounced in patients with hypersplenic cirrhosis. New immunosuppressive agents in clinical trials include tacrolimus, mycophenolate mofetil, 15-deoxyspergualin, and humanized monoclonal antibodies directed against the IL-2 receptor. Advances in the field of immunosuppression are eagerly awaited to avoid the complications of the currently used immunosuppressive agents.

PANCREAS TRANSPLANTATION

Unlike liver transplantation, which often is lifesaving, pancreas transplantation can be considered only life-enhancing at present. The rationale for the use of pancreas transplantation is as prevention of the secondary sequelae of diabetes—nephropathy, neuropathy, and retinopathy—by providing biologically responsive insulin-producing tissue. Pancreas transplantation can be performed with the whole organ, a segmental graft, or dispersed islets of Langerhans. Most uremic diabetic patients improve considerably with a kidney transplant, but other long-term complications of diabetes, such as retinopathy, angiopathy, and neuropathy, do not improve. The autoimmune pathogenesis of type I insulin-dependent diabetes mellitus is evidenced by mononuclear cell infiltrate, which is seen surrounding the islets of Langerhans, and by the presence of circulatory autoantibodies directed against islet cytoplasm and cell surface antigen, which can be found in the sera of some type I diabetics (see Chapter 34). The presence of antibodies to glutamic acid decarboxylase (GAD) has been identified in the sera of some diabetic patients. Recent studies have suggested that GAD may be the principal autoantigen in the pathogenesis of diabetes. There is also a strong association of insulin-dependent diabetes mellitus with other organ-specific autoimmune endocrinopathies, and there is an association with certain HLA types of HLA-DR3 and -DR4 and -DQµ3.2 alleles. Distinguishing recurrent autoimmune disease from rejection in transplanted pancreatic tissue may prove difficult, due to the presence of lymphocytic infiltrate in both situations. Pancreatic tissue appears to be very immunogenic when transplanted into type I diabetic patients, and the contribution of recurrent autoimmune disease following pancreatic transplantation remains to be determined.

Indications

Ideally, pancreas transplantation should be performed before the patient has developed any of the secondary complications of diabetes. Not all diabetic patients suffer from secondary complications, however, and in fact only about 40% of individuals with type I diabetes develop uremia. It has been difficult to balance the risk of long-term immunosuppression against the risks of developing systemic complications of diabetes. Therefore, pancreas transplantation to date has been performed on patients who were uremic and required a simultaneous renal transplant. A few centers, however, now perform pancreas transplants in patients who have neither uremia nor kidney transplantation but have other progressive secondary complications that outweigh the risk of long-term immunosuppression. Solitary pancreas transplantation, either in the nonuremic diabetic patient or following successful renal transplantation, was previously limited by poor results. The poorer graft survival following solitary pancreas transplantation was presumed to be due to an inability to detect rejection without a simultaneously transplanted kidney. With improvements in immunosuppressive regimens as well as better monitoring techniques for rejection, however, results of solitary pancreas transplants have approximated simultaneous pancreas–renal transplants in selected centers. With improvements in the results following solitary pancreas transplants, it can be anticipated that this procedure will be performed with increasing frequency in the patient with poorly controlled diabetes.

Procedure

For the whole-organ or segmental pancreas graft, the pancreas is removed from the donor and preserved in cold storage so that it can be transported from a distant retrieval site to the facility where transplantation is to take place. Preservation time in UW solution has exceeded 20 hours. Pancreas transplantation can either be done simultaneously with implantation of the kidney or sequentially in a postkidney-transplant patient with stable renal function. Simultaneous implantation of the kidney allows the use of kidney function and kidney biopsy as a marker for rejection. Various surgical techniques are used for implantation of the pancreas graft. The grafts are implanted either as a whole organ with a small button of donor duodenum or as a distal segment of the pancreas (Fig 57–9).

Most frequently, the whole organ is transplanted heterotopically to the iliac fossa. The exocrine drainage is via the donor duodenum, which is anastomosed to the recipient bladder. This permits monitoring of the urine amylase, which is important in gauging rejection of the pancreas (see later discussion).

Outcome

The major complications following pancreas transplantation are infection, vascular thrombosis, preservation injury, rejection, and pancreatitis. Overall graft function and patient survival rates have improved steadily since the first clinical pancreas transplant was

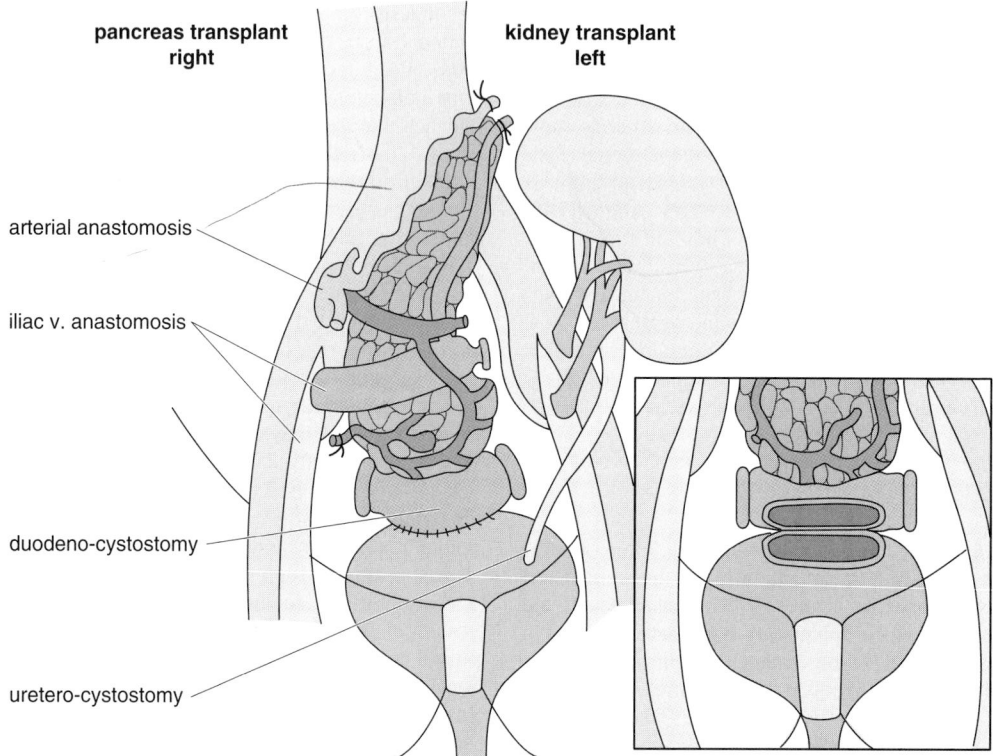

pancreas transplant
right

kidney transplant
left

arterial anastomosis

iliac v. anastomosis

duodeno-cystostomy

uretero-cystostomy

Figure 57–9. Whole pancreatico-duodenal transplantation kidney transplant, as performed in patients with diabetic nephropathy, is also shown.

performed in 1966. The present overall pancreas graft survival at 1 year in patients who have received a simultaneous kidney transplant is over 80%. As mentioned earlier, the survival of solitary pancreas transplants has improved with stricter matching criteria, better techniques for monitoring rejection, and improvements in immunosuppressive regimens. Selected centers have reported graft survival statistics approximating the graft survival observed in simultaneous pancreas–renal transplants.

Crossmatching & Immunosuppression

Pancreas transplant donors and recipients are typed and matched for ABO and HLA antigens, and a transplant is not performed in the face of a positive crossmatch. The exact role of tissue typing has not been clearly defined, largely owing to small numbers of patients. In patients who have received simultaneous pancreas–kidney transplant, both organs are not uniformly rejected, but rejection of their kidney graft can frequently be used to predict ongoing rejection of the pancreas. Nonetheless, in some instances the pancreas has failed (presumably owing to rejection) while the kidney graft continues to function. The benefits of

HLA-DR matching in isolated cadaveric pancreas transplantation have clearly been demonstrated.

Rejection of the vascularized pancreatic allograft is recognized by a loss of control over blood glucose levels. This, however, is unfortunately a relatively insensitive and late finding. Disappearance of insulin from the circulation usually parallels the plasma glucose levels and consequently cannot be used as an early indicator of rejection. Corticosteroids used for immunosuppression also tend to cause diabetogenic effects. Serum amylase levels have not been useful previously in diagnosis of rejection. In transplants drained into the urinary system, however, low levels of urinary amylase are suggestive of graft failure. This finding usually precedes changes in blood glucose levels, therefore allowing time for institution of antirejection therapy.

The current practice at some centers is to perform a biopsy of the graft when there is a question of rejection, even when diagnosis is not ensured. The presence of vasculitis is the only certain histologic evidence for rejection because parenchymal fibrosis and inflammatory-cell infiltrate may be secondary to foreign body reaction, particularly in grafts with polymer-injected ducts or grafts associated with recurrent disease. Successful immunosuppression for pancreas transplantation appears to be more difficult than for kidney or liver transplantation. Rejection is usually treated with intravenous bolus corticosteroids, an increase in the oral prednisone dose, or a course of OKT 3. Currently, many centers are reporting the prevalence of a single rejection episode following simultaneous pancreas–renal transplant at approximately 80%. Although most of these episodes are reversible with the administration of OKT 3, it is clear that these patients initially require more immunosuppression than recipients of only kidney transplants. The addition of tacrolimus (FK 506) and mycophenolate mofetil to the immunosuppression protocols may facilitate management following either solitary pancreas transplantation or simultaneous pancreas–renal transplantation.

Islet Cell Transplantation

A successful placement of isolated islets between nonidentical donor–recipient pairs has been a goal for some time. Initially it was hoped that unmodified islet transplants might display the prolonged survival of other endocrine tissue; however, survival of isolated islet allografts is shorter than survival of allografts of skin, kidney, or heart regardless of placement site. Syngeneic grafts implanted in the liver, under the kidney capsule, produce insulin and are able to reverse hyperglycemia, virally induced diabetes, diabetes induced by beta cell toxins, and spontaneous diabetes in BB rats and NOD mice. Since autografts cannot be used in most clinical situations, the major experimental thrust has been to perfect allograft islet transplantation.

Islet cells are obtained from either adult or fetal pancreas. The fetal pancreas contains less connective tissue, so that the relative yield of viable islets is greater but still not sufficient to render a recipient normoglycemic. The basic method for retrieving islets is via mechanical separation followed by enzymatic digestion, usually with collagenase. Density gradient centrifugation is required to remove as much nonislet tissue as possible. Even purified islets contain dendritic cells and other cells capable of stimulating an immune response. A number of investigators have tried different means of reducing immunogenicity of islet tissue, such as treatment with anticlass II monoclonal antibody or irradiation. Culturing of pure islets in an oxygen-rich atmosphere has been successful in decreasing tissue immunogenicity. An alternative method that has been successful in rats and mice involves encapsulation of individual islets within a semipermeable biologic membrane across which immunocompetent cells cannot pass. More recently, islet tissue derived from genetically manipulated mice deficient for MHC class I antigens has been transplanted across major histocompatibility barriers. This tissue has markedly prolonged survival, demonstrating the potential efficacy of genetic engineering in the field of islet transplantation. All of these experiments have been performed in animal models, with prolonged reversal of the diabetic state when modified islet allografts were used. Although islet transplantation has been slow to develop as a therapy for type I diabetes, success of allotransplanted islets from a single cadaveric donor has been reported. With further improvements in immunosuppressive regimens, methods of tolerance induction, and gene therapy, islet transplantation will reach its full potential.

HEART TRANSPLANTATION

James Hardy attempted the world's first human heart transplant at the University of Mississippi in 1964. Although the operation was described as a technical success the recipient died from inadequate cardiac output a few hours later, likely resulting from the substantial size discrepancy between the donor, a chimpanzee, and the adult human male recipient. Both the second attempt, by Christiaan Barnard at Cape Town, South Africa in 1967, and the third by Adrian Kantrowitz at Columbia University in New York a few days later, were also unsuccessful. Nevertheless these two transplants and the burgeoning clinical experience with cardiac surgery captured the interest of the world's cardiovascular community. In 1968, more than 100 heart transplants were performed. Unfortunately, the 1-year survival rate in this initial group was only 20%, reflecting the primitive state of knowledge about recipient and donor selection as well as immunosuppressive management at the time. These gaps were slowly filled by the few groups that remained clinically active throughout the 1970s. Undoubtedly the most significant factor leading to the resurrection of clinical cardiac transplantation in the 1980s was the development of cyclosporine-based immunosuppressive protocols. Compared with conventional protocols using antilymphocyte sera, azathioprine, and prednisone, cyclosporine markedly reduced the risk of death from acute rejection and infection during the first few months following transplantation. This resulted in an almost exponential worldwide growth in both the number of patients undergoing transplantation and the number of transplant centers, until 1988 when further increases were limited by the available supply of donor hearts.

In 1983, the International Society for Heart and Lung Transplantation (ISHLT) began to maintain a registry of patients undergoing all forms of thoracic organ transplantation. The 1995 report listed 30,297 patients who had undergone cardiac transplantation since the registry began. Annually, about 3500 patients throughout the world undergo transplants in more than 250 centers, most of which are in the USA.

Recipient Selection

Cardiac transplantation is performed in selected patients who are judged to have an imminently life-threatening cardiac disease that is not amenable to conventional medical or surgical treatment. In adults, the main indications are coronary artery disease and idiopathic dilated cardiomyopathy, whereas among children, congenital heart disease and cardiomyopathy are the main indications. All age groups have been transplanted successfully, and operative techniques have been developed to deal with even the most complex congenital cardiac venous and arterial malformations. The current operative mortality rate is less than 10% for most patients. Elevated pulmonary vascular resistance, congenital heart disease, and repeat heart transplantation are some of the most important early risk factors for mortality.

The only absolute contraindications are irreversible pulmonary vascular disease, uncontrollable infection or cancer, and the presence of a separate life-threatening disease. Relative contraindications include age over 65 years, advanced generalized organ dysfunction (CNS, hepatic or renal) as a consequence of poor cardiac function, or a recent pulmonary infarct or a separate disease process that would significantly affect or be affected by immunosuppression (cholelithiasis, peptic ulcer disease, diverticulosis, peripheral vascular disease, etc). Patients with a history of medical noncompliance or those who are at increased risk of noncompliance because of drug or alcohol addiction or psychiatric conditions are not good candidates for any form of organ transplantation.

Donor Selection

Cardiac donors are heart-beating brain-dead cadavers with good cardiac function and without significant history or risk factors for cardiac disease. Donors and recipients are matched for ABO blood group compatibility and body size. Prospective donor–recipient crossmatching is performed only if pretransplant recipient screening reveals an elevated panel-reactive antibody (>15%) or a highly specific HLA antibody specificity. The extreme shortage of cardiac donors in recent years has led to considerable relaxation in the criteria for donor suitability. Currently, donor age >50 years is no longer a contraindication provided cardiac function is satisfactory and any coronary disease is either mild or else amenable to conventional coronary artery bypass or angioplasty. Ventricular hypertrophy, requirement for moderate inotropic support, and short periods of severe hypotension or cardiac arrest are also no longer absolute exclusions provided echocardiographic and visual assessment of cardiac function are satisfactory.

Organ Procurement

Hearts are usually procured during a multiorgan retrieval from the same donor at sites remote from the recipient. The coronary circulation is flushed with a cold electrolyte solution and then the heart is stored in the same solution at 4 °C until it is implanted in the recipient. With current techniques the maximal safe duration of ex vivo preservation is about 6 hours, but most groups try to achieve preservation times of less than 4 hours. Using high-speed civilian jet travel this means that the donor hearts are procured within a radius of 2000 miles from the transplant center.

Operative Procedure

Two operative techniques are used for cardiac transplantation. Both require temporary cardiopulmonary bypass support. In the heterotopic, or piggyback, technique, the recipient's heart remains in its usual location and the donor heart is connected in a parallel configuration, which results in the donor heart being positioned in the right pleural space. In the orthotopic technique the recipient's ventricles are completely excised, and the donor heart is positioned in its normal mediastinal location. The heterotopic technique is technically more difficult, offers few advantages over the orthotopic technique, and is infrequently performed at present. Cardiac function is often impaired in the first few days following transplantation. In most cases this responds to pharmacologic treatment, and in the absence of allograft rejection resting hemodynamics in the late post transplant period are remarkably normal.

Immunosuppression & Allograft Monitoring

The usual maintenance immunosuppressive regimen following heart transplantation consists of a combination of cyclosporine, azathioprine, and corticosteroids. The dosages of the individual drugs are adjusted to produce the desired level of immunosuppression (targeted blood levels, blood white cell count, acute rejection episodes) while producing the minimum toxicity (infections, renal function, hepatic function, bone marrow suppression, malignancy) or side effects. Since chronic corticosteroid use has been implicated in many of the late metabolic, skeletal, and ocular complications, many groups attempt to wean patients from corticosteroids and have successfully done so without increasing alloreactivity or compromising graft function. Tacrolimus, formerly FK 506, and mycophenolate mofetil have both been approved for use in cardiac transplantation in the United States after earlier clinical trials demonstrated their efficacy and safety in this population. Antilymphocyte sera or monoclonal anti-T-cell antibodies are usually reserved for treatment of steroid-resistant rejection or as induction therapy.

The clinical signs of allograft dysfunction (fatigue, dyspnea, fever, hypotension, arrhythmias, added heart sounds, increased jugular venous pressure, pulmonary rales) usually appear late in the course of acute cardiac rejection. Even the EKG findings of acute rejection are nonspecific and in spite of considerable research there does not appear to be a consistently reproducible test of peripheral blood leukocyte function or activation that reliably detects acute rejection in its early stages. Thus monitoring alloreactivity following cardiac transplantation is problematic and depends almost exclusively on the results of histologic examination of small pieces of myocardium removed during transvenous endocardial biopsy. These biopsies are performed at intervals throughout the rest of the recipient's life at intervals that parallel the expected risk of rejection; weekly intervals during the first month or two after transplant and 3–6 month intervals in patients beyond the first year. The biopsies are graded histologically and most groups begin to treat acute rejection once there is evidence of myocyte damage or persistent inflammation.

Chronic rejection in cardiac transplantation is manifested as coronary vasculopathy. It usually presents as heart failure or arrhythmias rather than angina because of the persistent denervation of the allograft. Pathologically there is diffuse concentric intimal hyperplasia affecting both epicardial and intramyocardial vessels. The consequences of acute myocardial infarction and ischemic myocardial dysfunction are the same as those seen with atherosclerotic coronary artery disease. Detection is usually by periodic coronary angiography or, more recently, intracoronary ultrasound.

Complications

Primary graft failure, rejection, infection, and neoplasia are the major obstacles to successful heart transplantation. During the first posttransplant year primary graft failure, acute rejection, and infection account for more than 90% of the deaths. Hyperacute rejection has been documented only rarely and then usually on the basis of postmortem examination. Acute cellular rejection, on the other hand, occurs frequently, and treatment of acute rejection is required in more than 70% of patients during the first year after transplant. Fortunately most episodes resolve with high-dose pulse steroid therapy without any permanent loss of allograft function. As the incidence of acute rejection diminishes to a low but stable level beyond the first year, chronic rejection emerges as the major cause of late mortality. The incidence of angiographically detectable coronary artery disease in the allograft may be as high as 40% at 4 years after transplant. To date no specific treatment has been shown to either prevent or halt the progression of coronary artery disease in the allograft. Interestingly, the disease is seen almost exclusively in recipients who develop HLA antibodies in the posttransplant period, suggesting that humoral rejection mechanisms may be playing an important role and providing some impetus for clinicians to try more effective drugs against that part of the immune response.

Infection continues to be an important early and late cause of morbidity and mortality. The range of opportunistic infections, the sites of infection and the risk factors are quite similar to those seen with other solid organ transplants. The allograft itself seems to be fairly resistant to infection. Although CMV and toxoplasma are occasionally identified on endocardial biopsies, serious bacterial and fungal infections seldom involve the heart except as a terminal event.

Malignancy is also an important cause of morbidity and mortality among this group of transplant recipients. Once again the range of tumors and sites of involvement tend to parallel that observed in other solid organ transplants. The incidence of malignancy seems to correlate more with the overall degree of immunosuppression rather than the specific drugs. Given the generally more intense immunosuppression in heart transplant recipients than in most other recipients it is perhaps not surprising that more tumors are seen in this population.

Results

Currently, the average patient and graft survivals in the ISHLT registry are 78.3, 66.8, and 52.5% at 1, 5, and 10 years, respectively. At 2 years after transplantation 85% of recipients are in New York Heart Association functional class I and 13% are in class II; up to 60% have been able to return to work or school full time.

COMBINED HEART–LUNG & LUNG TRANSPLANTATION

Before 1980, more than 35 attempts at pulmonary transplantation, including 3 combined heart–lung transplants, were performed in humans. The median survival for the entire group was less than 2 weeks. One patient survived for 10 months but the function of the graft in this case was poor. The excellent early results with cyclosporine-based immunosuppression protocols in both animal and human cardiac transplantation in the early 1980s encouraged investigators at Stanford University to reattempt combined heart–lung transplantation first in primates and shortly thereafter in humans. In these early experiments healing of the supracranial tracheal anastomosis was almost always successful, which had not been the case in the previous experience with isolated lung transplantation in which bronchial anastomotic complications (eg, dehiscence or stenosis) were the major cause of death among patients who survived beyond the first week. Thus combined heart–lung transplantation was initially thought to be the safest operative procedure for all patients with end-stage cardiopulmonary or pulmonary disease, and isolated lung transplantation was relegated to the laboratory. Then in a series of well-designed canine experiments, investigators at the University of Toronto defined the adverse effects of high-dose perioperative corticosteroid therapy, the neutral effect of cyclosporine therapy, and the beneficial effect of omental wrapping on bronchial anastomotic healing. They also performed the first successful human single-lung transplant in 1983 in a patient with pulmonary fibrosis and rekindled worldwide interest in single-lung transplantation. In the past decade single-lung transplantation has emerged as the preferred procedure for most types of end-stage pulmonary disease. Patients with pulmonary sepsis (cystic fibrosis, bronchiectasis) require bilateral lung replacement and now undergo either combined heart–lung or simultaneous bilateral single-lung transplantation.

The ISHLT also maintains a registry for patients undergoing combined heart–lung and lung transplantation. In 1995, there were 1708 patients in the registry who had undergone combined heart–lung transplantation (99 centers), 2465 patients who had undergone single-lung transplantation, and 1344 patients who had undergone bilateral lung replacement (111 centers). As in cardiac transplantation the major limiting factor affecting further transplantation remains the limited donor organ availability.

Recipient Selection

The indication for combined heart–lung or lung transplantation is still the presence of an end-stage disease for which there is no alternative treatment that can restore satisfactory survival or function. Major clinical categories include (1) pulmonary vascular disease, either primary pulmonary hypertension or Eisenmenger's syndrome secondary to congenital heart disease; (2) restrictive lung disease, including idiopathic pulmonary fibrosis; (3) obstructive lung disease such as emphysema secondary to α_1-antitrypsin deficiency; and finally (4) diseases such as bronchiectasis and cystic fibrosis that produce a mixed restrictive and obstructive picture. All age groups have undergone transplantation successfully and the indications for single-lung transplantation have been extended to include patients with Eisenmenger's syndrome and correctable intracardiac shunts (atrial septal defect, ventricular septal defect, patent ductus arteriosus).

Absolute contraindications for single or bilateral lung transplantation include concomitant cardiac failure, particularly severe right ventricular dysfunction; uncontrollable infection or cancer; and the presence of a separate life-threatening disease. Preoperative low-dose steroids, prior intrathoracic surgery, and tracheostomy are relative contraindications. A few ventilator-dependent patients have undergone transplantation successfully, but the presence of severe cachexia or multiorgan failure has invariably proven fatal.

Donor Selection

Lung donors are heart-beating, brain-dead cadavers with good pulmonary function, no evidence of pulmonary sepsis, and a negative history or risk factors for pulmonary disease. Obviously, combined heart–lung donors must also satisfy the requirements for cardiac donation. Donors and recipients are matched in terms of approximate size, including thoracic dimensions and ABO compatibility. If pretransplant screening of the recipient for HLA antibodies was positive, a preoperative crossmatch is also performed. For purposes of single-lung transplantation, unilateral lung disease in the donor is not necessarily a contraindication, provided function of the contralateral lung is satisfactory.

Organ Procurement

Combined heart–lung or lung procurement almost always occurs as part of a multiple-organ retrieval from the same donor at a site remote from the recipient. The heart and both lungs can be retrieved as a single block of tissue or separated and used in as many as three recipients. Although several techniques have proven effective for lung preservation, the simplest and most commonly used is the cold flush technique. A potent pulmonary vasodilator, prostacyclin or prostaglandin E_1, is administered prior to flushing the pulmonary circulation with a cold electrolyte or blood–electrolyte solution, and the lungs are inflated and stored in the same solution at 4 °C until they are ready to be implanted in the recipient. Lungs procured in this way can be safely maintained for up to 10 hours, which markedly extends the safe procurement radius over that available for cardiac transplantation, providing additional time for sequential bilateral lung transplantation and HLA typing or crossmatching if they are required.

Operative Procedure

In the combined heart–lung transplant procedure the recipient's lungs, left atrium, and both ventricles are excised and replaced with donor tissue. The airway is then reattached at the lower end of the trachea. This operation requires a major surgical dissection with temporary cardiopulmonary bypass support and can be complicated by bleeding or injury to the phrenic or recurrent laryngeal nerves. Single or bilateral single-lung transplants are technically simpler and do not always require temporary cardiopulmonary bypass support. The pulmonary artery and a cuff of left atrial tissue surrounding the pulmonary veins are used for the vascular anastomoses, and the airway is reattached at the level of the main stem bronchus. In neither technique is the bronchial circulation directly reestablished. The success of single and bilateral lung transplantation in patients with primary pulmonary hypertension has also led to use of pulmonary transplantation combined with simultaneous cardiac repair in patients with congenital heart disease and Eisenmenger's physiology.

Immunosuppression & Allograft Monitoring

Following lung transplantation, the usual maintenance immunosuppression consists of cyclosporine, azathioprine, and corticosteroids. The dosages of the individual drugs are adjusted to optimize immunosuppression and minimize toxicity and side effects. Some groups withhold routine corticosteroid therapy for 2–3 weeks following transplantation to allow for tracheal–bronchial healing; others believe that with modification of the bronchial anastomotic technique, routine postoperative corticosteroid therapy is not detrimental. Both tacrolimus and mycophenolate mofetil have been used successfully in pulmonary transplantation. In addition, the direct access to the allograft epithelium afforded by the airway, has presented an opportunity to try aerosolized delivery of corticosteroids and cyclosporine.

Clinical signs of acute pulmonary rejection (dyspnea, tachypnea, fever, rales, hypoxemia, reduced FEV_1, pulmonary infiltrates) mimic those of pulmonary infection. Differentiation of the two is crucial, although both may coexist within the allograft. Bronchoscopy is extremely useful in this role, and most groups use periodic bronchoscopy as part of their routine posttransplant surveillance. A histologic grading system for both acute and chronic pulmonary rejection has been adopted by most transplant pathologists, and clinicians use this system to determine when to augment immunosuppression. Chronic rejection in lung allografts manifests as bronchiolitis obliterans. This presents as either an asymptomatic decline in expiratory airflow rates on pulmonary function tests or in more advanced cases as unremitting dyspnea. Pathologically there is obstruction and eventually obliteration of small airways by chronic inflammation and fibrosis.

Pulmonary function tests, including exercise oximetry, have also been shown to be an extremely sensitive and reliable way to noninvasively monitor allograft function. Since both pulmonary infection and rejection result in declines in airflow rates and gas transfer, many groups incorporate a program of daily home spirometry with or without oximetry into their surveillance regimen. Technical developments now enable this data to be transmitted over the telephone to the transplant center. This may permit detection of early rejection and infection episodes when treatment may result in recovery or at least prevent any further loss of allograft function.

The role of radiologic techniques (chest x-rays, various types of CT scans, ventilation–perfusion scans) in allograft surveillance is still being defined. There can be no doubt, however, about their usefulness in the diagnosis of mediastinal lymphadenopathy, pleural-based processes, pulmonary nodules, or indeterminate pulmonary infiltrates.

Complications

Technical problems with bleeding and graft dysfunction are important early sources of morbidity and mortality for lung or combined heart and lung recipient. Together with acute rejection and infection, these problems account for more than 90% of the deaths that occur during the first posttransplant year. Recent improvements in operative technique and pulmonary preservation have reduced the operative, or 30-day, mortality over that seen in the 1980s; however, much

remains to be achieved. Acute pulmonary rejection occurs frequently, and asynchronous rejection of the heart and lungs in recipients of combined heart–lung transplantation has been observed. At least 30% of the operative survivors ultimately develop symptoms and signs of chronic pulmonary rejection manifest as obliterative bronchiolitis, and in most it follows a progressively downhill and ultimately fatal course. One of the most important risk factors for the development of obliterative bronchiolitis to have emerged is the frequency and severity of acute pulmonary rejection occurring within the first 6–12 months after transplant. Some combined heart and lung recipients have also developed coronary artery disease in their allograft.

Although infection continues to be an important early and late cause of morbidity and mortality, for all solid organ recipients the lung recipient is particularly predisposed to pulmonary infections. The allograft's normal defense mechanisms are chronically suppressed both as a result of the immunosuppressive drugs and from the airway denervation and abnormal mucociliary clearance resulting from the surgery. In this population primary CMV pneumonitis is a life-threatening illness, leading some groups to recommend donor–recipient CMV matching. Almost all groups now use some form of CMV prophylaxis for recipients at risk during the first few months after transplant. CMV infection may also be a risk factor for the later development of chronic rejection.

Cancer is also a significant long-term risk for the lung recipient, and tumors have arisen within the allograft and elsewhere. Once again the overall degree of immunosuppression is probably more important than any specific immunosuppressive drug. Like heart transplant recipients, these patients are subjected to a generally more intensive immunosuppression than are other solid organ recipients, so it is not surprising that the incidence of tumors is higher.

Results

Currently, the average patient and graft survival in the ISHLT registry are 59% and 42% for combined heart–lung transplantation at 1 and 5 years, respectively; 69% and 62.5% for single-lung transplantation at 1 and 2 years, respectively; and 62% and 51% for bilateral lung transplantation at 1 and 2 years, respectively.

BONE MARROW TRANSPLANTATION

Modern clinical bone marrow transplantation began in 1968, when a small number of patients with severe combined immunodeficiency disease (SCID), Wiskott-Aldrich syndrome, or advanced leukemia received infusions of marrow from HLA-identical siblings. Previous observations in animals had shown that matching the donor and recipient at the MHC loci reduced the incidence of graft-versus-host (GVH)

Table 57–1. Diseases treatable by bone marrow transplantation.

Allogeneic/Syngeneic	Autologous
Aplastic anemia	Leukemia
Leukemia	AML
AML	ALL
ALL	Multiple myeloma
CML	Non-Hodgkin's lymphoma
Myelodysplasia	Hodgkin's disease
Multiple myeloma	Solid tumors
Non-Hodgkin's lymphoma	Breast
Hodgkin's disease	Ovarian
Immunodeficiencies	Testicular
Common variable	Neuroblastoma
SCID	
Wiskott-Aldrich syndrome	
Agranulocytosis	
Osteopetrosis/genetic	
diseases	

Abbreviations: AML = acute myelogenous leukemia; ALL = acute lymphoblastic leukemia; CML = chronic myelogenous leukemia; SCID = severe combined immunodeficiency disease.

disease and improved survival rates. Many patients have now survived for more than two decades after bone marrow transplantation for a variety of malignant and nonmalignant hematologic diseases. Laboratory and clinical advances in such areas as histocompatibility typing, prevention of GVH disease, improved supportive care, and reduction of the risk of relapse have made bone marrow transplantation a realistic and successful form of treatment for several previously uniformly fatal diseases (Tables 57–1 and 57–2).

Until recently, most donors for bone marrow transplantation have been either identical twins (syngeneic) or genotypically HLA-identical individuals (allogeneic). Only 30% of patients, however, can be expected to have an HLA-identical donor, and efforts to use marrow from partially matched family members or phenotypically matched unrelated donors are now increasingly successful. The National Marrow Donor Program (NMDP) now has HLA-typing infor-

Table 57–2. Genetic diseases treatable by bone marrow transplantation.

SCID
Wiskott-Aldrich syndrome
Fanconi's anemia
Kostmann's syndrome
Chronic granulomatous disease
Osteopetrosis
Ataxia-telangiectasia
Diamond-Blackfan syndrome
Mucocutaneous candidiasis
Chédiak-Higashi syndrome
Cartilage–hair hypoplasia
Mucopolysaccharidosis
Gaucher's disease
Thalassemia major
Sickle cell anemia

Abbreviation: SCID = severe combined immunodeficiency disease.

mation on more than 1 million volunteer donors, and 50% of patients with chronic leukemia can now find a suitable donor through this registry. For diseases not involving the marrow, autologous transplantation allows the use of high-dose chemoradiotherapy and avoids the risk of GVH disease. Provocative studies with monoclonal antibodies to leukemic and other malignant cells or with in vitro chemotherapy treatment have given credence to the idea that such marrow "purging" techniques could greatly extend the benefit of autologous transplantation to patients assumed to have indiscernible neoplastic cells remaining in the marrow.

Indications & Results

A. SCID: Bone marrow transplantation is the treatment of choice for children with congenital SCID and its variants. For HLA-matched transplants, no immunosuppressive conditioning is necessary. Partially matched recipients require conditioning, usually with cyclophosphamide and busulfan. The removal of T cells from donor marrow by lectin agglutination or monoclonal antibody and complement lysis enables parents of haploidentical children with these disorders to serve as donors.

B. Aplastic Anemia: Severe aplastic anemia has a mortality rate of 90% when treated with supportive care alone. Allogeneic bone marrow transplantation increases survival to 60% overall and to 80% in patients younger than 30 years. Furthermore, if patients are able to avoid pretransplantation transfusions—and hence presensitization—the overall actuarial survival at 10 years increases to 80–90%. Unlike the case for leukemia, rejection of the donor marrow in patients with aplastic anemia has been a major cause of failure (15–30% versus 1% for leukemia); this is probably due to the underlying autoimmune nature of the aplasia in some patients, to presensitization by transfusions, and to the lack of radiotherapy in the stand and conditioning regimen. New immunosuppressive regimens appear to be beneficial in reducing graft rejection without causing excessive toxicity. These approaches include the addition of either ATG or total lymphoid irradiation to high-dose cyclophosphamide.

For patients without marrow donors or for those over age 60 years, the treatment of choice is immunosuppressive therapy with ATG (possibly combined with cyclosporine). This therapy produces responses and 5-year survival in 60% of patients. Long-term survivors may develop myelodysplasia, however, reflecting underlying bone marrow injury.

C. Acute Myelogenous Leukemia (AML): AML is now a curable malignancy, both in children and adults. With improvements in supportive care, adults up to age 60 should now be approached with curative intent. Once an initial complete remission has been achieved with intensive chemotherapy, several potentially curative options are available. Nonablative intensive chemotherapy offers a 30–40% chance of long-term survival.

For patients with histocompatible siblings, allogeneic bone marrow transplantation in first remission offers a 60% long-term cure rate, which comes, however, at the expense of a 20–25% treatment-related mortality rate in the first 6 months. The improved disease control (15–20% relapse rate compared with 55–65% for chemotherapy) is due both to the high-dose ablative chemoradiotherapy and to an alloimmune function of the marrow graft, "graft-versus-leukemia" (GVL) effect.

For patients without suitable donors or in older patients, autologous bone marrow transplantation offers the advantage of improved disease control from ablative therapy. In the absence of GVL, however, the relapse rate would be expected to be higher than in allogeneic bone marrow transplantation. Autologous bone marrow transplantation is a far less morbid procedure, with treatment-related mortality less than 5%. Preliminary results of autologous bone marrow transplantation show relapse rates of 20–40% and long-term survival in 40–70% of cases. The choice of allogeneic versus autologous transplant depends on risk factors associated with the patient's leukemia.

D. Chronic Myelogenous Leukemia (CML):

For patients with chronic myelogenous leukemia (CML) there had been no hope for cure and no improvement in survival over the past 50 years. Data now clearly show that allogeneic bone marrow transplantation provides a 60–80% relapse-free survival in patients with CML in chronic phase. More favorable results are produced when the transplant is performed within 1 year of diagnosis and when patients are younger than 30 years. For these young favorable patients, disease-free survival is 80%. Results in patients with more advanced CML are inferior. For patients without suitable sibling donors, a search for a matched correlated donor should be performed through the NMDP.

E. Acute Lymphoblastic Leukemia (ALL):

ALL is now a curable malignancy in both children and adults. Conventional nonablative chemotherapy is curative in 60–90% of children and 30–60% of adults, depending on a number of factors. Allogeneic bone marrow transplantation is usually reserved for patients in second remission or in those with high-risk cytogenetics that predict a poor outcome with conventional therapy. Allogeneic bone marrow transplantation offers a 30–50% cure rate in second remission. Autologous bone marrow transplantation is not as successful as in AML but remains on option for patients without donors and should be recommended to patients destined to do poorly with conventional chemotherapy.

Procedure

Unlike other organ transplants, bone marrow aspirated from the iliac crests of a donor is entirely regenerated in 8 weeks. Since the amount harvested is less than 20% of the total, the donor is not harmed immunologically or hematologically. Multiple aspirations of 5 mL each, yielding a total of 10 mL/kg of the recipient's body weight (600–1200 mL), are obtained in a single procedure under general or epidural anesthesia. The marrow is drawn through heparinized needles and placed into heparinized, buffered culture medium. This mixture is then gently filtered through fine stainless steel mesh screens to produce a single-cell suspension. Nucleated-cell counts are checked to ensure the adequacy of the withdrawn marrow. If the donor and recipient are ABO-compatible, 2×10^8 to 6×10^8 nucleated marrow cells/kg of the recipient's weight are infused intravenously together with erythrocytes (erythrocyte volume of 20–30%). If the donor and recipient are not ABO-compatible, the erythrocytes must be removed from the donor's marrow in vitro.

For autologous transplantation, the use of peripheral blood stem cells has virtually replaced the harvest of pelvic bone marrow. Progenitor cells are mobilized and collected (by apheresis) following stimulation with hematopoietic growth factors (granulocyte colony-stimulating factor [G-CSF], granulocyte–macrophage colony-stimulating factor [GM-CSF] either alone or in combination with chemotherapy. The antigen CD34 is expressed on both hematopoietic stem cells and more committed progenitor cells, and measurement of CD34-expressing cells is used to determine collection of adequate numbers of progenitors. The collection of $>5 \times 10^6$/kg CD34-positive cells ensures reliable prompt engraftment. The use of peripheral blood stem cells, as opposed to pelvic bone marrow, has sped engraftment and reduced morbidity and mortality significantly. In the allogenic setting, the use of peripheral stem cells is being explored, with the reservation that peripheral cells contain ten times more of T cells, which may increase the risk of GVH disease.

Except in patients with SCID, destruction of the recipient's immune system is necessary to prevent rejection and to allow transplantation of an entirely new hematopoietic system, including new immunocompetent cells. This is usually accomplished by giving cyclophosphamide, 50–60 mg/kg for 4 or 2 days (the higher dose for patients not receiving total-body irradiation). The dose of total-body irradiation is 1000–1400 cGy, which is usually administered in fractions over 3–5 days rather than in a single dose, to reduce toxicity to the lungs and eyes. This combination of chemotherapy and radiotherapy provides a potent immunoablative and antineoplastic function for most cancer patients.

Following preparative chemoradiotherapy and infusion of the marrow, patients are extremely vulnerable to infections. The early and aggressive use of broad-spectrum antibiotics and amphotericin B is critical. The role of trimethoprim-sulfamethoxazole in preventing *Pneumocystis carinii* pneumonia is clearly established. Ganciclovir is effective in reducing the risk of

CMV infections and pneumonitis. Platelet transfusions, on the other hand, are given to keep the platelet count above 15,000/μL to prevent serious spontaneous hemorrhage. All blood products must be irradiated to prevent GVH disease caused by viable lymphocytes in transfused cellular components or plasma.

Engraftment is heralded by a rising leukocyte count and the appearance of circulating mature neutrophils 2–4 weeks after transplantation. In general, all hematopoietic and immune cells of the recipient are replaced by donor cells, although there are rare examples of mixed "chimerism," most often in children who receive transplants for immunodeficiency diseases. As peripheral counts improve, antibiotics can be discontinued and transfusions become unnecessary. Patients can be discharged when they can be observed closely as outpatients for at least the first 100 days after transplantation.

Posttransplantation Complications

The major obstacles to successful bone marrow transplantation are GVH disease, infections, interstitial pneumonia, venoocclusive liver disease, and relapse of the underlying disease. GVH disease and infections are responsible for 10–30% of morbidity and mortality in the first 100 days following transplantation.

Graft-versus-Host Disease

The presence of immunocompetent donor cells in an immunocompromised host is a prerequisite for graft-versus-host (GVH) disease. In patients who are HLA-identical with their donors, the occurrence of GVH disease is attributed to "minor," presently undetectable differences in histocompatibility.

The clinical syndrome of acute GVH disease in humans consists of skin rash, severe diarrhea, and jaundice. Pathophysiologically, immunocompetent CD8 T cells can be found in biopsy specimens of the skin, intestine, and liver. These tissues appear to be especially at risk because they are rich in surface DR antigens. The skin rash of acute GVH disease usually begins at the time of engraftment, 10–28 days after transplantation. It is a fine, diffuse, erythematous, macular rash often beginning on the palms, soles, or head and spreading to involve the entire trunk and sometimes the extremities. In severe GVH disease, the rash can become desquamative—the clinical equivalent of an extensive second-degree burn. Watery diarrhea is associated with malabsorption, cramps, and gastrointestinal bleeding when severe. Hyperbilirubinemia is due to GVH disease-induced inflammation of small bile ducts and is usually accompanied by an elevated serum alkaline phosphatase level. Elevations of alanine aminotransferase and aspartate aminotransferase are mild to moderate. A staging and grading system for GVH disease developed at the University of Washington has become standard (Table 57–3).

Successful prevention of acute GVH disease began with the use of methotrexate after transplantation.

Table 57–3. Clinical staging of graft-versus-host disease by organ system.

Stage	Skin	Liver	Gastrointestinal Tract
+	Maculopap- ular rash <25% body surface	Serum bilirubin 2–3 mg/dL	>500 mL diarrhea/d
+ +	Maculopap- ular rash 25–50% body surface	Serum bilirubin 3–6 mg/dL	>1000 mL diarrhea/d
+ + +	Generalized erythro- derma	Serum bilirubin 6–15 mg/dL	>1500 mL diarrhea/d
+ + + +	Generalized erythro- derma with bullous formation and des- quamation	Serum bilirubin >15 mg/dL	Severe abdomi- nal pain with or without ileus

Initial studies found that approximately 50% of patients treated with methotrexate alone developed acute GVH disease within 10–70 days after grafting and that up to half of these died. More modern immunosuppressive therapy with both methotrexate and cyclosporine has reduced the risk of acute GVH disease to 20–40%, with only 5–10% of cases being severe (grade III–IV). Cyclosporine is continued for the first 6 months after transplantation. Infusions of ATG, prednisone, and monoclonal antibodies have been used with limited success to treat established acute GVH disease. T-cell depletion of donor marrow is highly successful in reducing GVH disease. Unfortunately, studies of patients receiving T-cell-depleted marrow have shown an increased risk of rejection, higher relapse rate of leukemia, and increased risk of fungal infections. These findings support the concept that donor T cells have an active GVL effect. Efforts to fine-tune T-cell depletion (by elective or incomplete depletion) are under way.

Chronic GVH disease affects 25–45% of patients surviving longer than 180 days. It occurs more frequently in older patients and in those with preceding acute GVH disease. Clinically, it most closely resembles the spectrum of rheumatic or autoimmune disorders, and its main clinical effect is to produce severe immunodeficiency, leading to recurrent and life-threatening infections, much like those seen in the congenital and acquired immunodeficiency syndromes. Treatment with prednisone, alone or in combination with immunosuppressives, can effectively reverse many of the manifestations of chronic GVH disease in 50–75% of affected patients. If the patient survives for 3–5 years, the manifestations of chronic GVH disease usually resolve.

Chronic GVH disease is associated with a beneficial effect of reducing relapse of malignant disease, presumably through an alloimmune process referred to as graft-versus-leukemia (GVL) effect. Infusions of donor lymphocytes as a form of immunotherapy have been used with success in the treatment of relapse of chronic myeloid leukemia after allogenic transplantation.

Venoocclusive Disease of the Liver

High doses of chemoradiotherapy, such as that used to condition patients prior to marrow transplantation, can cause a fibrous obliteration of small hepatic venules, known as venoocclusive disease of the liver. About 20% of patients undergoing bone marrow transplantation develop venoocclusive disease, manifested clinically as hepatomegaly, ascites, hepatocellular necrosis, and encephalopathy within 8–20 days after transplantation. The disease resolves in 60% of patients but is fatal in 5–20%. There is no effective treatment.

The most important risk factor is the presence of hepatitis before transplantation, which, by serology and natural history, is usually non-A, non-B viral hepatitis associated with transfusions. Patients with transaminasemia before bone marrow transplantation are three to four times more likely to develop venoocclusive disease than are those with normal serum liver enzymes. Venoocclusive disease must be distinguished from GVH disease of the liver and from viral and fungal infections.

Infections

Infectious complications following bone marrow transplantation are from the profound lack of granulocytes and lymphocytes following ablation by the pretransplant conditioning regimen. Since full recovery of these two major elements of the immune system occurs separately following transplantation, it is not surprising that the risk of infection can be separated into three distinct phases (Table 57–4).

The first, and most dangerous, phase is the 2–4-week period prior to engraftment, when no circulating leukocytes are present. During this time, patients are at risk for both bacterial and fungal infections, which can advance extremely rapidly and cause death. Clinical experience and trials over the past 15 years have led to the aggressive, empirical use of broad-spectrum antibiotics (both antibacterial and antifungal). The recent increase in infections due to resistant species of staphylococci, especially *Staphylococcus epidermidis* responsive only to vancomycin, is most probably due to the use of tunneled, central intravenous catheters in these patients. As a result, vancomycin is empirically added to the antibiotic regimen.

Two to 4 weeks after transplantation, the marrow begins to export granulocytes successfully to the blood; when the absolute neutrophil count reaches 500/µL and is rising, the greatest threat of bacterial infection is past. The second phase of potential infectious complications is due to the paucity and immatu-

Table 57–4. Sequence of infections after bone marrow transplant.

Phase	Infection
I Up to engraftment	Gram-positive cocci/central lines Gram-negative bacteria *Candida* *Aspergillus*

II
After initial engraftment
	Fungal
	  Aspergillus
	  Candida esophagitis
	Viral
	  CMV
	  Adenovirus
	  EBV
	  Respiratory syncytial virus, enterovirus, parainfluenza, papovaviruses

III Late	Sinopulmonary (sicca syndrome, IgA deficiency) *Streptococcus pneumoniae/Haemophilus influenzae* Varicella-zoster virus

Abbreviations: CMV = cytomegalovirus; EBV = Epstein-Barr virus.

rity of the lymphocytes, and the greatest risk is due to fungal and viral agents during the second and third posttransplant months. An especially prominent and potent pathogen is *Aspergillus fumigatus,* which can cause vascular invasion in the lungs and brain. Although these infections can be treated with amphotericin B, they are difficult to eradicate and may be fatal. The most prominent viral pathogen is CMV. Ganciclovir prophylaxis has had a major effect on this problem. CMV pneumonitis, formerly uniformly fatal, can now be effectively treated with ganciclovir plus intravenous immunoglobulin.

The third phase of infectious complications occurs after the third month and lasts until the maturation of the lymphocytic arm of the immune system. This parallels the neonatal period and takes 6–18 months. During this time, there is an abnormal ratio of CD4 to CD8 T cells, T cells respond poorly to antigens, and immunoglobulin production is abnormal. This leads to a risk of infection by encapsulated bacteria such as pneumococci because of a lack of opsonic immunoglobulins. The higher risk of viral infection diminishes as T-cell function gradually improves. Patients must remain relatively isolated until the immune system has fully recovered. Patients with chronic GVH disease may never recover full function of the immune system. The majority of surviving patients, however, do recover full immunity and lead lives free from infection, requiring no antibiotics or other supplements. Unlike patients with solid organ transplants, they do not need to take immunosuppressive medications to ensure engraftment, since the immune and hematopoietic systems are replaced. Once tolerance is achieved (by about 6 months after transplantation), all medications can gradually be discontinued, and patients are able to live completely normal lives.

BONE TRANSPLANTATION

Bone is more commonly transplanted than any other tissue. In general, bone-grafting operations are performed to promote healing of nonunited fractures, to restore structural integrity of the skeleton, and to facilitate cosmetic repair. Human skull defects larger than 2–3 cm are closed by neurosurgeons to protect the brain and restore bone integrity. Plastic surgeons, oral surgeons, and periodontists use fresh autografts and freeze-dried allografts in oral and maxillofacial surgery. Various bone grafts are used to promote stability of the spine and to correct spinal deformity. Autografts and allografts are used to repair the appendicular skeleton (arms and legs). When autograft sources are insufficient, allogeneic bone may be used but only in combination with an autograft, which provides a greater degree of early repair. Bone is procured for implantation by aseptic removal or by removal and subsequent sterilization by ethylene oxide or gamma irradiation. Except for a fresh autograft, all other bone tissues are used after freezing because of the reduction in immunogenicity achieved by this storage technique.

Posttransplantation Course

After grafting, one of three courses can be followed: (1) the bone graft may become viable, acquiring the mechanical, cosmetic, and biologic characteristics of adjacent bone; (2) it may partially or completely resorb without satisfactory new bone formation, leaving disfigurement or instability; or (3) it may become sequestrated, encapsulated, and treated by the host as a foreign body. The most likely graft to achieve optimal function in humans is the fresh autograft; however, allogeneic implants are becoming more widely used.

A bone graft transferred to a recipient undergoes several adaptive phases before ultimate incorporation into the skeletal system. Osteogenesis from surviving cells of the graft itself is characteristic only of fresh autografts. By contrast, cells from an allograft usually elicit antibody production and cell-mediated immunity and start to decay. These alloimplants slowly revascularize by invasion of capillary sprouts from the host bed during the process of resorption of the old matrix. Finally, in both autografts and allografts, osteoinduction occurs by the process of recruitment of mesenchyme-type cells into cartilage and bone under the influence of a diffusible bone morphogenetic protein derived from the bone matrix. Bone morphogenetic protein is a recently discovered glycoprotein of MW 17,500. The target cell for its activity is an undifferentiated, perivascular mesenchymal cell whose

protein synthesis is reprogrammed in favor of new bone formation.

Temporally, healing of bone grafts follows a well-known pattern. For the initial 2 weeks, an inflammatory response occurs, associated with infiltration of the graft by vascular buds and the presence of fibrous granulation tissue, osteoclast activity, and osteocyte autolysis. There occurs a "creeping substitution" of graft bone, manifested as differentiation of mesenchymal cells into osteoblasts that deposit osteoid over devitalized trabeculae. Dead trabeculae are later remodeled internally. Thus, through appositional new bone formation, the graft is strengthened. In contrast to cancellous bone, cortical bone grafts undergo a somewhat longer period of resorption and slower appositional phases of new bone formation. This results in only half strength being acquired during the first 6 months and full strength 1–2 years after grafting.

Immunologic Rejection

Since bone is a composite of cells, collagen, ground substance, and inorganic minerals, all but the minerals are potentially immunogenic. Cell surface transplantation antigens associated with the MHC are the most potent immunogens within osteochondral allografts and are found on cells of osteogenic, chondrogenic, fibrous, neuronal, fatty, hematopoietic, and mesenchymal origin. Cell-rich marrow contributes significantly to immunogenicity.

Fresh allogeneic bone can sensitize the host and cause the production of circulating antibodies. Nevertheless, cellular immunity is thought to be more important than humoral antibodies in causing rejection of allogeneic bone transplants. Cartilage seems to resist destruction by antibody and cellular resorptive mechanisms, but if an immune response by the recipient develops, this protection is only relative, and a low-grade, slow, immunologically mediated inflammatory response ensues, characterized by an increase in synovial fluid, leukocyte counts, antibody response, and pannus reactions.

Rejection of allogeneic bone (cortical or cancellous) elicits a response that delays healing at the site of osteosynthesis and blocks revascularization, resorption, and appositional new bone formation. Clear-cut rejection or failure of the graft occurs in only about 10% of bone grafts.

Immunosuppression

Temporary systemic immunosuppression has been used, since MHC antigens are present in bone for only 2–3 months after transplantation. Drugs that have successfully allowed bone union include azathioprine, corticosteroids, cyclosporine, and cyclophosphamide. Because of side effects and the low rate of graft failure, these agents are no longer routinely used in human musculoskeletal transplantation. A promising new technique to diminish the antigenicity of grafts is the use of a temporary biodegradable cement that coats the donor bone and hides the bone cell antigens until these cells have died and their MHC antigens have deteriorated.

Clinical Recovery

Early ambulation and mild exercise stimulate blood flow and osteogenesis within the graft. External splinting helps to stabilize the graft. Education of the patients in proper posture, weight-bearing, turning, and exercise has been helpful in allowing sufficient time for healing.

FUTURE OF TRANSPLANTATION

The current shortage of hearts, livers, and lungs is a major impediment to offering transplantation to the growing number of eligible recipients. Stimulated by this urgent need, research into the use of xenogeneic organs (from species other than humans) is proceeding. In addition to the usual rejection problems, a more severe form of hyperacute rejection must be overcome before this approach can become a clinical reality.

Closer to implementation, however, are transplants of specific types of cells that can be used to replace missing genes or enzymes. One can imagine transplanting hepatic parenchymal cells for their synthesis of clotting factors, proteins, and even hematopoietic stem cells.

REFERENCES

KIDNEY TRANSPLANTATION

Cho YW, Terasaki PI: In: *Long Term Survival in Clinical Transplants.* Terasaki P (editor). UCLA Tissue Typing Laboratory, 1988, p 277.

Halloran PF et al: The molecular immunology of acute rejection: An overview. *Transplant Immunol* 1993;**1**:3.

Mizel SB: The interleukins. *FASEB J* 1989;**3**:2379.

Roake J: Dendritic cells and the initiation of the immune response to organ transplants. *Transplant Rev* 1994;**8**:37.

Solez K et al: International standardization of criteria for the histologic diagnosis of renal allograft rejection: The Banff working classification of kidney transplant pathology. *Kidney Int* 1993;**44**:411.

Strom TB, Kelley VE: Toward more selective therapies to block undesired immune responses. *Kidney Int* 1989;**35**:1026.

Terasaki PI et al: High survival rates of kidney transplants from spousal and living unrelated donors. *N Engl J Med* 1995;**333**:333.

Warvariv V, Garovoy MR: Transplantation immunology. In: *Textbook of Internal Medicine.* Kelley WN (editor). Lippincott, 1989, p 752.

LIVER TRANSPLANTATION

Lake JR (editor): Advances in liver transplantation. *Gastroenterol Clin North Am* 1993;**22**:213.

Shaw BW et al: Transplantation of the liver. In: *Surgical Treatment of Digestive Disease.* Moody FG, Carey LC (editors). Yearbook, 1986.

Starzl TE et al: Liver transplantation. *N Engl J Med* 1989;**329**:1014, 1092.

Venook AP et al: Liver transplantation for hepatocellular carcinoma: Results with preoperative chemoembolization. *Liver Transplant Surg* 1995;**1**:242.

Villanil FG, Vierling JM: Recurrence of viral hepatitis after liver transplantation: Insights into management. *Liver Transplant Surg* 1995;**1**:89.

PANCREAS & ISLET CELL TRANSPLANTATION

Osorio RW et al: Major histocompatibility complex class I deficiency prolongs islet allograft survival. *Diabetes* 1993;**42**:1520.

Starzl TE et al: Pancreaticoduodenal transplantation in humans. *Surg Gynecol Obstet* 1984;**159**:265.

Sutherland DER et al: Pancreas and islet transplantation: An update. *Transplant Rev* 1994;**8**:185.

HEART & LUNG TRANSPLANTATION

Bourge RC et al: Pretransplantation risk factors for death after heart transplantation: A multi-institutional study. *J Heart Lung Transplant* 1993;**12**:549.

Hardy JD et al: Lung homotransplantation in man. *JAMA* 1963;**186**:1065.

Hosenpud JD et al: The registry of the International Society for Heart and Lung Transplantation: Twelfth official report—1995. *J Heart Lung Transplant* 1995;**14**:805.

ISHLT: A working formulation for the standardization in the diagnosis of heart and lung rejection. *J Heart Transplant* 1990;**9**:587.

Kaye MP: The Registry of the International Society for Heart and Lung Transplantation. *J Heart Lung Transplant* 1992;**4**:599.

O'Connell JB et al: Cardiac transplantation: Recipient selection, donor procurement, and medical follow-up. *Circulation* 1992;**86**:1061.

Reitz BA et al: Heart and lung transplantation. Autotransplantation and allotransplantation in primates with extended survival. *J Thorac Cardiovasc Surg* 1980;**80**:360.

Reitz BA et al: Orthotopic heart and combined heart and lung transplantation with cyclosporin-A immune suppression. *Transplant Proc* 1981;**1**:393.

Reitz BA et al: Heart-lung transplantation. Successful therapy for patients with pulmonary vascular disease. *N Engl J Med* 1982;**306**:557.

Reitz BA et al: Clinical heart-lung transplantation. *Transplant Proc* 1983;**1**:1256.

The Toronto Lung Transplant Group: Unilateral lung transplantation for pulmonary fibrosis. *N Engl J Med* 1986;**314**:1140.

Trulock EP: Management of lung transplant rejection. *Chest* 1993;**103**:1566.

Veith FJ, Koerner SK: Lung transplantation 1977. *World J Surg* 1977;**1**:177.

BONE MARROW TRANSPLANTATION

Clift RA et al: Marrow transplantation for chronic myeloid leukemia. A randomized study comparing cyclophosphamide and total body irradiation with busulfan and cyclophosphamide. *Blood* 1994;**84:**2036.

Goldman JM et al: Choice of pretransplant treatment and timing of transplants for chronic myelogenous leukemia in chronic phase. *Blood* 1993;**82:**2235.

Gribben JG et al: Immunologic purging of marrow assessed by PCR before autologous bone marrow transplantation for B-cell lymphoma. *N Engl J Med* 1991;**325:**1525.

Kolb H et al: Graft versus host leukemia effect of donor lymphocyte transfusions in marrow grafted patients. *Blood* 1995;**86:**2041.

Linker CA et al: Autologous bone marrow transplantation for acute myeloid leukemia using busulfan plus etoposide as a preparative regimen. *Blood* 1993;**81:**311.

McGlave P et al: Unrelated donor marrow transplantation therapy for chronic myelogenous leukemia: Initial experience of the National Donor Marrow Program. *Blood* 1993;**81:**543.

Mekum FM et al: Pretransplantation burden of leukemia progenitor cells as a predictor of relapse after bone marrow transplantation for acute lymphoblastic leukemia. *N Engl J Med* 1993;**329:**1296.

Snyder DS et al: Fractionated total body irradiation and high dose etoposide as a preparatory regimen for bone marrow transplantation for 99 patients with acute leukemia in first complete remission. *Blood* 1993;**82:**2920.

Storb R et al: Cyclophosphamide combined with antithymocyte globulin in preparation for allogenic marrow transplants in patients with aplastic anemia. *Blood* 1994;**84:**941.

Zihoun RA et al: Autologous or allogenic bone marrow transplantation compared with extensive chemotherapy in acute myelogenous leukemia. *N Engl J Med* 1995;**332:**217.

BONE TRANSPLANTATION

Prolo DJ, Rodrigo JJ: Contemporary bone graft physiology and surgery. *Clin Orthop* 1985;**200:**322.

Immunosuppressive Therapy

58

Alan Winkelstein, MD

The growth of clinical immunology has uncovered increasing numbers of diseases that are due to aberrant immune responses. This has resulted in a search for drugs capable of inhibiting these unwanted responses. Particularly, the technical ability to successfully transplant many organs created a strong impetus for the development of safe and effective immunosuppressive regimens. In addition, more than 40 diseases thought to result from aberrant immune responses are potentially treatable by agents capable of inhibiting immune responses. Over the past two decades, considerable progress has been made in identifying a group of compounds capable of achieving *nonspecific* inhibition of immune response. The eventual goal in this area is to develop *specific* immunosuppression or tolerance directed only at the immune response to selected antigens. This currently remains an elusive goal.

CORTICOSTEROIDS

The glucocorticoid steroid hormones are widely and effectively used to suppress manifestations of numerous inflammatory and immune reactions. The pharmacology and anti-inflammatory effects of corticosteroids are discussed in Chapter 60. Although a clear-cut distinction between the immunosuppressive and anti-inflammatory actions of these drugs is not always possible, this section emphasizes glucocorticoid effects on the cells involved in the immune response.

Clinical research studies have often been confused by a failure to recognize that lymphocytes from different animal species vary in their susceptibility to steroid-induced lysis. In mice, rats, and rabbits, these hormones cause extensive lymphoid destruction. By contrast, normal lymphocytes from guinea pigs, monkeys, and humans are highly resistant to steroid-induced lysis. Not all human lymphocytes, however, are resistant to steroid-induced lympholysis; these drugs effectively kill acute lymphoblastic leukemia cells and are moder-

ately cytolytic for neoplastic B cells in chronic lymphocytic leukemia and non-Hodgkin's lymphomas.

The anti-inflammatory and immunosuppressive activities of corticosteroids can be grouped conveniently into three general categories: the effect of these drugs on leukocyte circulation, their ability to alter specific cellular functions, and other miscellaneous anti-inflammatory activities.

Effects on Cellular Traffic

One of the most important effects of corticosteroids is to alter transiently the number of circulating leukocytes. This is illustrated in Figure 58–1, which depicts the quantitative changes in each cell type following a single intravenous injection of a glucocorticoid. There is a prompt increase in the number of neutrophils and a concomitant decrease in the total number of lymphocytes, monocytes, eosinophils, and basophils. Maximum changes are observed 4–6 hours after injection, and all counts have returned to baseline values within 24 hours.

The neutrophilia resulting from steroid administration appears to be due to at least two distinct activities: release of mature neutrophils from marrow reserves and reduced neutrophil egress from intravascular spaces into inflammatory exudates. As a result, the half-life of circulating neutrophils is increased.

In contrast to the neutrophilia, steroids cause a striking reduction in the number of circulating lymphocytes. This effect results from the sequestration of recirculating lymphoid cells into lymphoid tissues, including the bone marrow. The total numbers of circulating T cells are markedly decreased, B-cell numbers are only modestly reduced, and numbers of null cells are unchanged. Among the T-cell subsets, numbers of CD4 cells are reduced to a greater extent than are numbers of CD8 cells.

One of the important steroid-induced changes is a pronounced monocytopenia. Monocyte counts frequently decline to less than 50 cells/μL, and the reduced availability of these cells has been postulated to

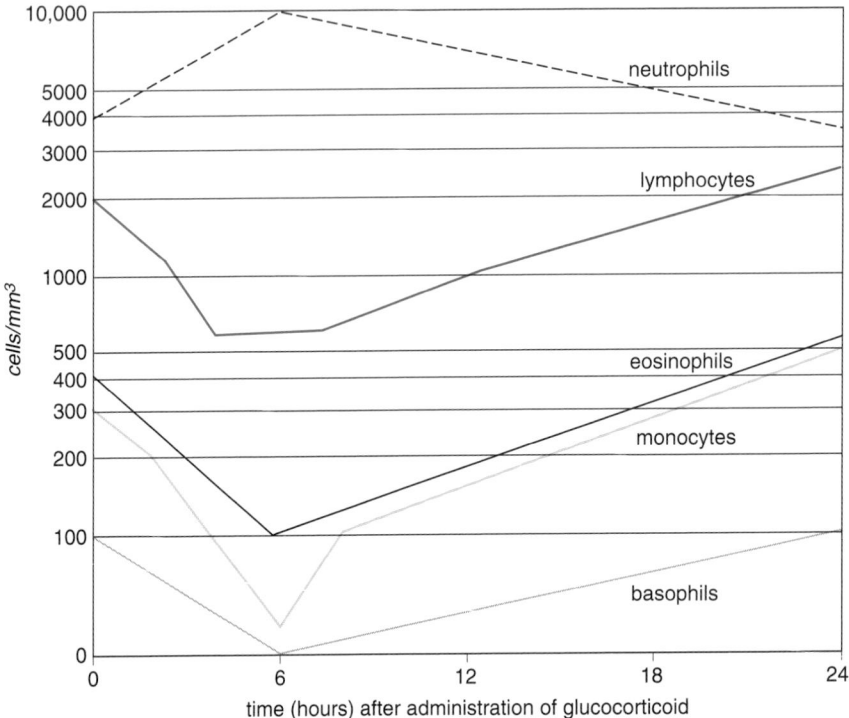

Figure 58–1. Glucocorticoids, whether given as a single dose or repetitively on alternate days, cause a decrease in lymphocyte, monocyte, basophil, and eosinophil counts and a rise in neutrophils within 4–6 hours, with a return to baseline within 24 hours. (Reproduced, with permission, from Claman HN: Glucocorticosteroids. I. Anti-inflammatory mechanisms. *Hosp Pract* 1983;**18**:123.)

be of prime importance in mediating steroid-induced anti-inflammatory activities. Eosinophil and basophil numbers are also reduced in the circulation because of redistribution; the significance of these changes is not known.

Functional Change

In addition to affecting the distribution of leukocytes, corticosteroids alter important functional activities of both lymphocytes and monocytes. Neutrophilic activities such as chemotaxis and lysosomal enzymes are not significantly impaired, but the release of nonlysosomal proteolytic enzymes such as collagenase and plasminogen activator is decreased by steroids.

T-lymphocyte activities are considerably altered by corticosteroids. In vitro lymphoproliferative responses are inhibited, in part from an impairment in the synthesis and secretion of interleukin-2 (IL-2), which is essential for the clonal expansion of activated lymphocytes (Fig 58–2). The decreased availability of IL-2 is most probably an indirect result of suppressed IL-1 production by monocytes. IL-2 receptor expression is not impaired. Steroids do not alter the release of two other lymphokines, interferon gamma and migration inhibitory factor (MIF).

Corticosteroids can block the progression of phyto-

hemagglutinin (PHA)-stimulated lymphocytes through the mitotic cycle (see later section). They inhibit the entry of cells into the G_1 phase and arrest the progression of activated lymphocytes from the G_1 to the S phase.

Corticosteroids have less effect on B lymphocytes. Patients receiving moderate doses of prednisone are able to respond normally to test antigens. On the other hand, high-dose corticosteroid therapy modestly reduces the serum concentrations of IgG and IgA but not IgM. These changes may be observed as early as 2–3 weeks after initiation of the course of steroids and are reversible. In one study using cultured spleen cells from patients with idiopathic thrombocytopenic purpura, steroids inhibited the ability of B lymphocytes to synthesize IgG in vitro. Steroid therapy does not alter the activities of either natural killer (NK) cells or effectors of antibody-dependent cell-mediated cytotoxicity (ADCC).

Paralleling their profound effects on the number of circulating monocytes, corticosteroids induce striking impairment in the functions of monocyte–macrophages in vitro. They suppress the bactericidal activities of these phagocytic cells, thereby lowering resistance to infection. Steroids also interfere with the antigen-presenting function of these cells. Other effects include impaired directed migration in response to chemotactic factors, decreased response to MIF, blocking of the dif-

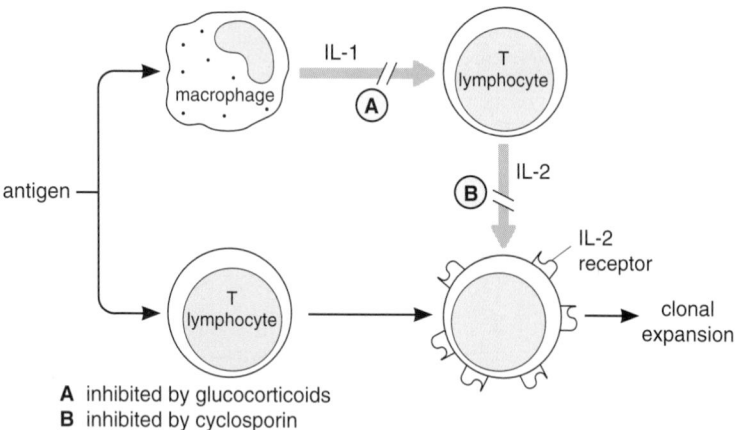

A inhibited by glucocorticoids
B inhibited by cyclosporin

Figure 58–2. Antigen stimulation in vivo induces monocytes to release the cytokine IL-1. This soluble mediator has numerous effects, including inducing helper T cells to synthesize IL-2. Antigen stimulation also induces responsive T cells to express receptors for IL-2. When IL-2 combines with IL-2 receptor (IL-2R)-bearing lymphocytes, these cells undergo clonal expansion. Corticosteroids act primarily to inhibit IL-1 synthesis and release. Cyclosporine suppresses the release of IL-2 and inhibits IL-2R expression. The letters A and B indicate inhibition by glucocorticoids and cyclosporine, respectively.

ferentiation of monocytes to macrophages, and suppression of the capacity of monocytes to express Fc and complement receptors, which may contribute to impaired phagocytic activities.

Steroids suppress the ability of reticuloendothelial cells to phagocytose antibody-coated cells, probably by decreasing the binding of immune complexes to Fc and C3b surface membrane receptors. This impaired binding may account for their beneficial effects in diseases such as idiopathic thrombocytopenic purpura and autoimmune hemolytic anemia.

Delayed-hypersensitivity skin tests to recall antigens are inhibited by prolonged treatment with corticosteroids. In general, these hormones must be administered for 10–14 days before skin test reactivity is impaired.

Recent studies have provided insights into the mechanisms by which corticosteroids suppress immune responses. One of its major activities appears to be mediated by impairing the functions of a transcriptional nuclear factor kappa B (NF-κB), which is a regulator of the genes for many cytokines and cell adhesion molecules. One recently described mechanism that may contribute to the immunosuppressive properties of corticosteroids is their direct binding to NF-κB, thereby preventing it from entering the nucleus.

There is a second, and probably more important, mechanism, however. In the cytoplasm of unstimulated cells, NF-κB is bound to a second protein, IκBα. Signaling of the cell results in phosphorylation of IκBα and the release of NF-κB. This is then translocated to the nucleus where it activates genes producing a variety of cytokines. Glucocorticoids appear to increase the transcription of the gene controlling IκBα, resulting in an increase in its cytoplasmic concentration, a situation that promotes its binding of

NF-κB. As a result, less is available to enter the nucleus and to initiate cytokine gene transcription. Additional mechanisms by which corticosteroids inhibit immunity, such as preventing another transcription factor AP-1 from binding to its target genes, may also be operative (Fig 58–3).

Clinical Use

Pharmacologic quantities of corticosteroids can effectively inhibit a spectrum of clinical manifestations associated with immune-mediated diseases. In numerous circumstances, these effects can be life-saving. The beneficial effects result from a combination of two separate activities, immunosuppressive and nonspecific anti-inflammatory properties. The relative contributions of each cannot be accurately quantified; either can produce the desired therapeutic goal—suppression of the underlying clinical disease. In general, statements to the effect that corticosteroids have "broad immunosuppressive activities" usually refer to this inhibition of disease-associated features, not to the effect of the drug on specific immune responses.

In clinical trials, corticosteroids, as a single therapeutic agent, do not appear to be potent immune inhibitors. By contrast, in combination with other immunosuppressants they have considerable activity as an adjunctive agent. Thus drug combinations containing steroids are extremely useful both in suppressing transplant rejection reactions and in inhibiting manifestations of autoimmune diseases.

Steroid therapy appears to exert differential effects on acute and chronic manifestations of immune-associated diseases. These agents are primarily active in suppressing acute inflammatory reactions and in inhibiting the short-term consequences of aberrant immune responses. In many disorders, however, they do

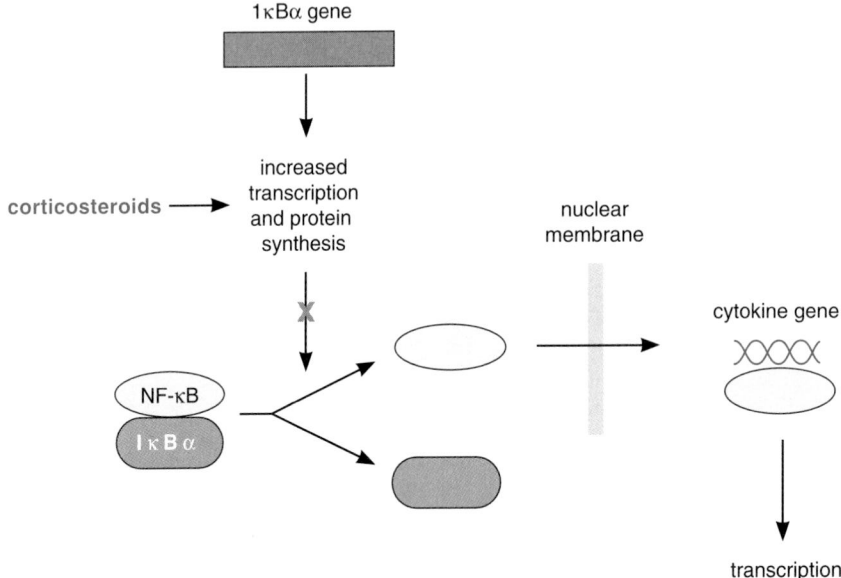

Figure 58–3. Proposed mechanism by which corticosteroids act as an immunosuppressant. It is believed that steroids induce increased transcription of the gene for IκBα. This leads to excessive protein synthesis. As a result, the dissociation of the transcription factor NF-κB from IκBα is suppressed and less NF-κB is able to translocate into the nucleus to initiate transcription of cytokine genes.

not alter the ultimate course of the underlying disease or reduce the concentrations of pathogenic autoantibodies. For example, these hormones are potent inhibitors of acute articular inflammatory reactions in patients with rheumatoid arthritis. By contrast, they do not decrease the incidence of chronic complications such as deforming arthritis. Likewise, steroids can suppress the carditis associated with acute rheumatic fever but do not change the frequency of chronic valvular disease. They inhibit the accelerated cell destruction resulting from autoantibody formation in autoimmune hemolytic anemia or idiopathic thrombocytopenic purpura. These effects often occur without reductions in the concentrations of pathogenic autoantibodies, however, and when the steroid dose is reduced, the cellular destructive processes often recur.

Clinical protocols for corticosteroid administration in immunologic diseases vary with the disease; they are discussed in the relevant chapters. There are three general patterns to steroid therapy protocols, depending on the circumstances. The first is often used if these drugs are to be administered for extended periods. It entails the use of the smallest amount needed to partially suppress disease manifestations. An example of this is the treatment of rheumatoid arthritis with 7.5–10 mg of prednisone daily. The second approach uses larger doses in an attempt to rapidly and completely suppress manifestations of an immunologically mediated disease. Prednisone at 1–2 mg/kg is given daily, in one or divided doses. This type of therapy is often used in disorders such as autoim-

mune hemolytic anemia, idiopathic thrombocytopenic purpura, and various types of immune-induced glomerulonephritis. The third pattern is the pulse administration of very large doses of an intravenous corticosteroid preparation (eg, methylprednisolone at 10–30 mg/kg). These ultralarge doses are generally reserved for unusually severe or potentially life-threatening illnesses. They have also been used successfully in reversing acute allograft rejection reactions. Most studies suggest that the immunologic effects of these massive-dose steroid protocols do not differ significantly from those resulting from more conventional doses. Although the therapeutic superiority of these regimens has not been proven in controlled trials, numerous reports imply effectiveness.

Prolonged therapy with corticosteroids is not innocuous; these drugs have numerous and potentially serious side effects (see Chapter 60). It is important to be aware of these side effects so that high-dose prolonged therapy does not cause greater morbidity than does the underlying disease.

CYTOTOXIC DRUGS

Cytotoxic drugs are a group of chemicals with the pharmacologic property of killing cells capable of self-replication. Immunologically competent lymphocytes make up such a susceptible cell population. These drugs were originally introduced into clinical medicine by R. Schwartz and W. Dameshek in 1959 for anticancer therapy; however, the studies revealed that many also possessed immunosuppressive activities. Thus, their use was extended to treatment of diseases caused by aberrant immune responses and to inhibition of transplant rejection reactions. There are four cytotoxic drugs currently in general clinical use for immunosuppression: cyclophosphamide, azathioprine, methotrexate, and chlorambucil.

Although the antigen-specific cells responsible for the unwanted immune response are potentially susceptible to cytotoxic immunosuppression, it must be recognized that the immunosuppressive activities of these drugs are not limited to a single lymphocyte subset. To various degrees, they can affect all immunologically competent cells, so that therapy leads to a generalized suppression of the immune defense system. As a result, treated patients are more susceptible to both opportunistic infections and certain neoplastic diseases.

Cytotoxic drugs are also not selectively toxic for lymphocytes. They can kill nonlymphoid proliferating cells, including hematopoietic precursors, gastrointestinal mucosal cells, and germ cells in the gonads. Thus, predictable side effects of all these drugs include pancytopenia, gastrointestinal toxicities, and reduced fertility.

The lymphocytotoxic activities of different cytotoxic drugs can be related to their toxicities for cells in specific phases of the mitotic cycle (Fig 58–4). There are four phases in mitosis: G_1 (the pre-DNA synthetic phase), S (the DNA synthetic phase), G_2 (the premitotic phase), and M (the actual mitosis). Cells in a prolonged intermitotic period are considered to be in a G_0 phase. One group of drugs, which includes azathioprine and methotrexate, are termed "phase-specific." These drugs are cytolytic to cells as they enter a selective phase of the mitotic cycle. For example, both azathioprine and methotrexate are cytolytic for cells only when they are in the S (DNA synthetic) phase.

Cyclophosphamide and chlorambucil are classified as "cycle-specific." They are toxic for cells at all stages of the mitotic cycle, including intermitotic (G_0) lymphocytes. They show differential cytolytic activities, however; they are more toxic for actively cycling than for resting (G_0) cells. The third group, the "cycle-nonspecific" compounds, are equally cytotoxic for proliferating and intermitotic cells.

Based on animal experiments, certain principles have been formulated concerning the immunosuppressive activities of cytotoxic drugs. By extension, these principles form the basis for the use of the drugs in clinical situations. They are summarized as follows:

(**1**) A primary immune response is more readily inhibited than is a secondary or anamnestic reaction. Drugs that are effective in suppressing an immune response in an unsensitized animal usually show only minimal inhibitory activity in a sensitized animal. The same effect is observed in patients. For example, the primary immune response elicited by a renal transplant is readily impaired by a combination of azathioprine and corticosteroids. If the recipient has been presensitized to donor histocompatibility antigens, however, this immunosuppressive regimen is relatively ineffective in inhibiting rejection reactions.

(**2**) The stages of an immune response differ markedly in their susceptibility to immunosuppressants. The cellular events associated with an antigenic challenge can be subdivided into two phases, designated the induction phase and the established or effector phase (Fig 58–5). The former is the interval between exposure to antigen (sensitization) and the production of sensitized T cells or mature plasma cells; it is characterized by the rapid proliferative expansion of antigen-sensitive precursors. Thereafter, the reaction is considered to have entered an established phase. Most cytotoxic drugs are effective if the period of drug administration coincides with the induction phase; once the reaction has entered the established phase, they are considerably less active. Furthermore, memory lymphocytes are unresponsive to immunosuppressive drugs. This implies that aberrant immune responses can recur when the individual is reexposed to the inciting antigen.

(**3**) The effectiveness of an immunosuppressive drug in a primary response is highly dependent on the timing of its administration relative to the initial antigenic challenge. On the basis of their effective interval, immunosuppressive agents are divided into three groups:

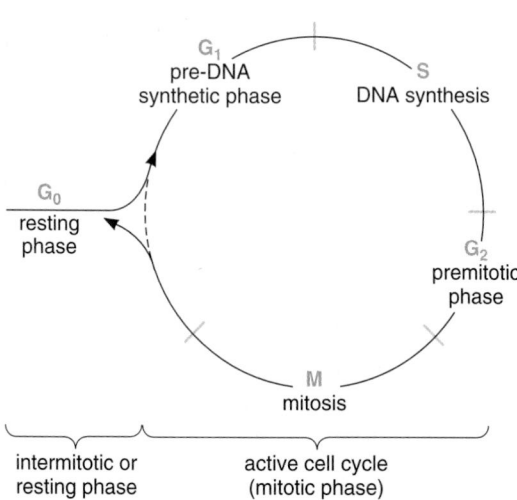

G_1
pre-DNA
synthetic phase

S
DNA synthesis

G_0
resting
phase

G_2
premitotic
phase

M
mitosis

intermitotic or
resting phase

active cell cycle
(mitotic phase)

Figure 58–4. Mitotic cycles. Drugs that are selectively toxic for cells in a discrete phase of their cycle are designated phase-specific agents: most exert their toxicity for cells in the S phase. Examples include azathioprine and methotrexate. Cycle-specific agents, such as cyclophosphamide and chlorambucil, are toxic for both intermitotic and proliferating cells but show greater toxicity for those in active cycle. Cycle-nonspecific agents show equal toxicity for all cells regardless of the mitotic activity. Radiation is considered a cycle-nonspecific therapeutic modality.

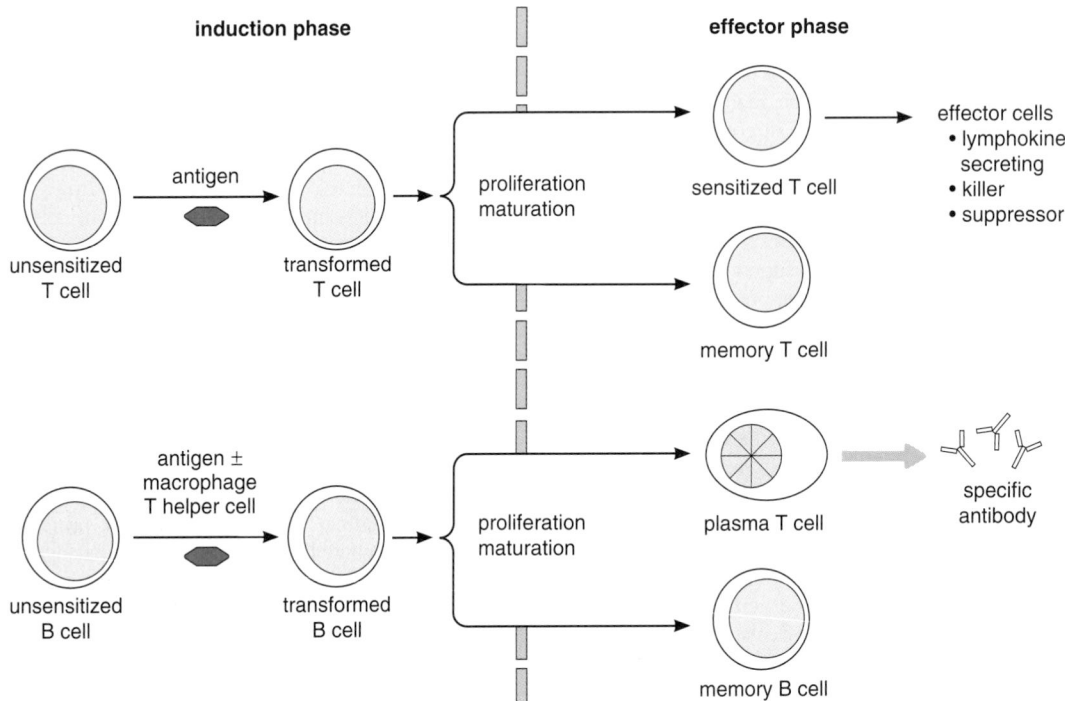

induction phase   **effector phase**

unsensitized T cell → antigen → transformed T cell → proliferation maturation → sensitized T cell → effector cells
• lymphokine secreting
• killer
• suppressor

memory T cell

unsensitized B cell → antigen ± macrophage T helper cell → transformed B cell → proliferation maturation → plasma T cell → specific antibody

memory B cell

Figure 58–5. Development of an immune response. The period from antigenic challenge through the proliferative expansion of transformed lymphocytes is considered the induction phase. The period following cellular expansion is defined as the established (effector) phase.

Group I: This group includes modes of therapy that exert their maximum immunosuppressive activity when administered just before the antigen and are considerably less effective if used after the immunologic challenge. Included in this group are corticosteroids, irradiation, and the cycle-nonspecific cytotoxin, nitrogen mustard.

Group II: This group includes drugs that show immunosuppressive properties only if administered in the period immediately following the antigenic challenge. They do not impair responses if used prior to the antigen. This group includes the phase-specific drugs such as azathioprine and methotrexate.

Group III: This group includes drugs that show inhibitory activity if administered either before or after antigenic stimulation, although these compounds show greater suppressive activities if used after the immune challenge. Pharmacologically, they are cycle-specific drugs; cyclophosphamide is the principal immunosuppressant in this group. The differential effects on immunity are illustrated in Figure 58–6, which shows the response to sheep erythrocytes in mice treated with an immunosuppressant either 24 hours before or 24 hours after antigenic challenge.

(4) Immunosuppressive drugs can exert differential toxicities for T and B lymphocytes. Cyclophosphamide causes a proportionately greater reduction in the number of B cells than of T cells; this correlates with its

greater suppressive effects on antibody responses than on cell-mediated reactions. In clinical usage, cyclophosphamide is considered more effective in suppressing diseases of aberrant humoral immunity, such as idiopathic thrombocytopenic purpura, than in inhibiting transplant rejection reactions. By contrast, azathioprine appears more potent as an inhibitor of T-cell-mediated responses.

(5) In certain circumstances, a paradoxic effect may be elicited by immunosuppressive treatment, namely, augmentation of a specific response. This effect was originally noted with irradiation, which, when administered several days before an antigenic challenge, led to a greater than normal antibody response. Similar effects were then observed with 6-mercaptopurine when used before antigen challenge. With selected treatment protocols, cyclophosphamide can simultaneously suppress humoral responses and augment delayed hypersensitivity reactions to the same antigen. The heightened cellular reactions have been attributed, in part, to its toxicity for suppressor T lymphocytes.

(6) The ability to inhibit manifestations of an immune response may result from pharmacologic activities other than immunosuppression. The expression of many immune responses involves the participation of both immunologically competent cells and nonspecific effector cells, such as neutrophils and monocytes. The numbers or functions of these effector cells can be al-

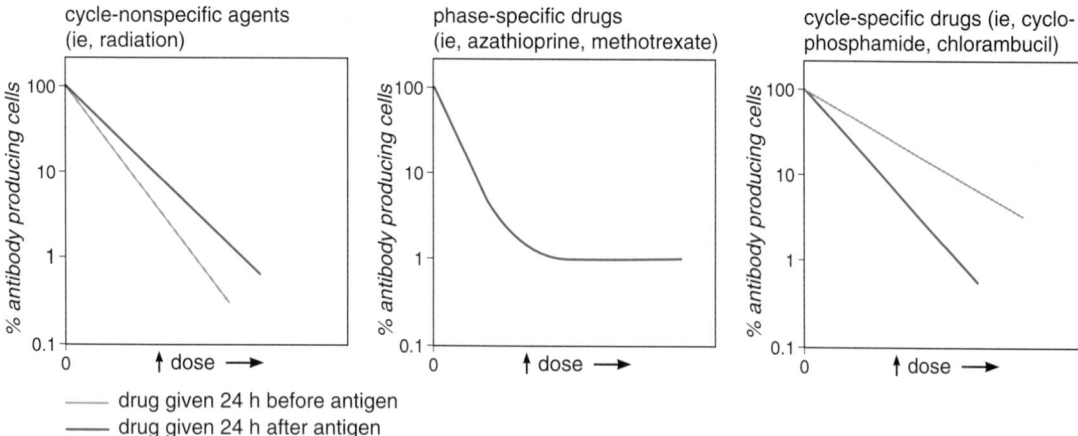

Figure 58–6. Schematic representation of the effects of different classes of immunosuppressants on the numbers of antibody-producing cells. (Reproduced, with permission, from Winkelstein A: Immune suppression resulting from various cytotoxic agents. In: *Clinics in Immunology and Allergy,* Vol 4: *Immune Suppression and Modulation.* Mitchell MS, Fahey JL [editors]. WB Saunders, 1984, p 296.)

tered by immunosuppressive drugs, an effect that can modify or obliterate the expression of a particular response. Therefore, apparent immunosuppression can result from the anti-inflammatory properties of a specific agent. As an example, corticosteroids are potent suppressors of IgE-mediated allergic asthma and T-cell-mediated allergic contact dermatitis. They inhibit inflammation in these diseases without affecting the underlying immune responses.

Clinical Use

These drugs are used to treat many autoimmune disorders. Table 58–1 is a partial list of diseases in which cytotoxic drugs have been reported to be effective.

Despite their usage in these diseases for more than a decade, it is still difficult to ascertain their true effectiveness because there have been only a few controlled clinical trials. Controlled trials are necessary because many autoimmune diseases show unpredictable courses, with both spontaneous remissions and exacerbations. Nevertheless, cytotoxins have

Table 58–1. Some immunologic disorders in which cytotoxic drugs are effective or probably effective.

Rheumatoid arthritis
Systemic lupus erythematosus
Systemic vasculitis
Wegener's granulomatosis
Polymyositis
Membranous glomerulonephritis
Chronic active hepatitis
Primary biliary cirrhosis
Inflammatory bowel disease
Autoimmune hemolytic anemia
Immune thrombocytopenia
Circulating anticoagulants
Multiple sclerosis
Myasthenia gravis

been widely accepted as potentially useful therapy for severe immune-related disorders.

Cytotoxic drugs have been used extensively in the treatment of rheumatic diseases. Table 58–2 compares the activities of each of the commonly used cytotoxic immunosuppressants in these diseases.

Table 58–2. Clinical efficacy of cytotoxic drugs in rheumatic disorders.

Disease	Efficacy of:			
	Azathioprine	Chlorambucil	Cyclophosphamide	Methotrexate
Rheumatoid arthritis	+	+	+	+
Rheumatoid vasculitis	0	+	+	0
Systemic lupus erythematosus	+	+	+	0
Polyarteritis nodosa	+	0	+	0
Polymyositis	+	0	0	+
Psoriatic arthritis	0	0	0	+
Wegener's granulomatosis	+	+	+	0
Reiter's syndrome	0	0	0	+

Source: Adapted from Nashel DJ: Mechanisms of action and clinical applications of cytotoxic drugs in rheumatic disorders. *Med Clin North Am* 1985;**69:**817.
Symbols: ++ = substantial evidence of effectiveness; + = benefit suggested by some studies; 0 = not studied or benefit negligible.

Individual Cytotoxic Drugs

A. Azathioprine: This compound is a phase-specific drug. It is a nitroimidazole derivative of the purine antagonist 6-mercaptopurine and is rapidly converted in vivo to the parent compound (6-mercaptopurine). Although there are conflicting data, most investigators believe that the addition of the imidazole side chain probably enhances its immunosuppressive potency and increases the therapeutic-to-toxic ratio.

Biochemically, both azathioprine and 6-mercaptopurine act by competitive enzyme inhibition to block synthesis of inosinic acid, the precursor of the purine compounds adenylic acid and guanylic acid. Therefore, the major effect is to impair DNA synthesis; this results in a decreased rate of cell replication and explains the phase-specific action of the drug. A second and less important activity is impairment of RNA synthesis.

Azathioprine appears to preferentially inhibit T-cell responses compared with those resulting from activation of B lymphocytes. Nevertheless, both cell-mediated and humoral responses can be suppressed. In addition, azathioprine appears to effectively reduce the numbers of circulating NK cells and lymphocytes bearing Fc receptors for IgG. The latter are responsible for ADCC reactions.

Before the development of cyclosporine (see later section), combinations of azathioprine and corticosteroids were standard therapy for inhibition of transplant rejection reactions. These two agents still maintain an important role in this area. Azathioprine is now frequently used in transplant patients who have developed toxic effects of cyclosporine or in maintaining immunosuppression after discontinuing cyclosporine. In addition, azathioprine is used to treat a spectrum of autoimmune disorders (Table 58–3). There is exten-sive experience with patients who have severe rheumatoid arthritis, for whom this drug is classified as a "disease-remitting" agent. Beneficial effects have also been reported in patients with other connective tissue diseases, autoimmune blood dyscrasias, and immunologically mediated neurologic diseases. This phase-specific drug may also permit the use of reduced amounts of corticosteroids in the treatment of primary biliary cirrhosis, chronic active hepatitis, and inflammatory bowel disease. Azathioprine is administered orally, and the maximum beneficial effects generally require continuous therapy for several weeks.

The primary lymphocytotoxic effects of azathioprine are directed against actively replicating cells. Short therapeutic courses do not reduce the numbers of T or B cells in the peripheral blood, but they do decrease the number of large lymphocytes. These cells are believed to be activated lymphocytes that have entered an active proliferative cycle following exposure to appropriate antigens. Immunoglobulin levels and titers of specific antibodies are only minimally reduced by long-term treatment with azathioprine. The numbers of circulating neutrophils and monocytes are reduced in a dose-dependent fashion because of the drug's cytotoxicity for hematopoietic precursors.

B. Cyclophosphamide: Both experimentally and clinically, this cycle-specific drug is a potent lymphocytotoxic immunosuppressant with a comparatively high therapeutic-to-toxic ratio (Table 58–4). Following pulse administration, there is a dose-dependent reduction in the numbers of both B and T lymphocytes. Cyclophosphamide has diverse effects on immune re-

Table 58–3. Properties and uses of azathioprine.

Trade name	Imuran
Administration	Orally, 1.25–2.5 mg/kg/d
Mechanism of action	S phase toxin (phase-specific agent). Inhibits de novo purine synthesis.
Major indications	Transplant rejection reactions. Chronic graft-versus-host reaction. Rheumatoid arthritis. ? Systemic lupus erythematosus. ? Vasculitis. ? Other connective tissue diseases. Inflammatory bowel disease. Chronic active hepatitis/primary biliary cirrhosis. ? Myasthenia gravis. ? Multiple sclerosis.
Toxicities	Bone marrow depression. Gastrointestinal irritation. Hepatotoxicity (rare). Infections. Cancers.

Table 58–4. Properties and uses of cyclophosphamide.

Trade Name	Cytoxan
Administration	Orally 1–3 mg/kg/d. Intravenously 10–20 mg/kg/every 1–3 months.
Mechanism of action	Cycle-specific agent. Binds and cross-links DNA strands. Affects B cells more than T cells; suppressor T cells more than helper T cells.
Major indications	Rheumatoid arthritis and vasculitis. Systemic lupus erythematosus. Wegener's granulomatosis. Systemic vasculitis. Autoimmune blood dyscrasias. Immune-mediated glomerulonephritis.
Toxicities	Bone marrow depression. Gastrointestinal reactions. Sterility (may be permanent). Alopecia. Hemorrhagic cystitis. Opportunistic infections. Neoplasms (lymphoma, bladder carcinoma, acute myelogenous leukemia). Goodpasture's syndrome.

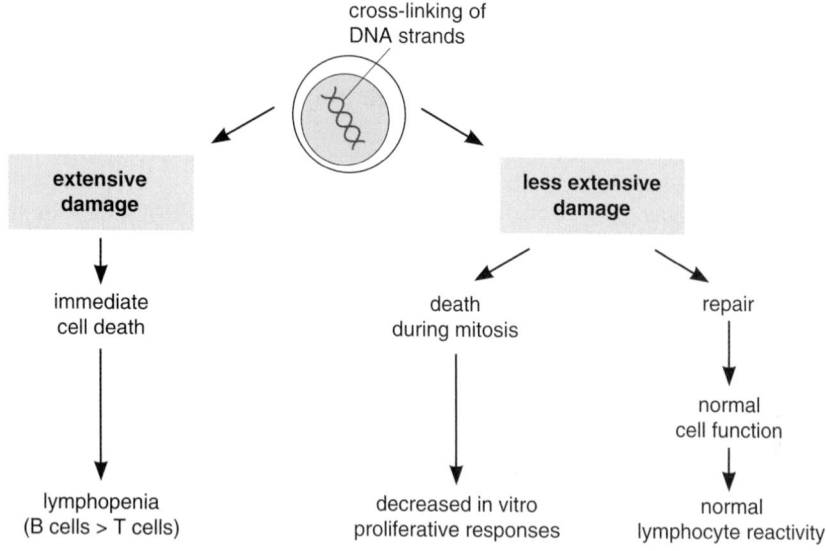

Figure 58–7. The effect of cyclophosphamide on lymphocytes appears to be primarily due to cross-linking DNA strands. This can result in lympholysis and decreased in vitro proliferative response. In cells that are not extensively damaged, repair can occur, and the lymphocyte regains its full proliferative capacity. Because of the slow recovery of B cells, the effect is more pronounced than that on T cells.

sponses in experimental animals. Depending on such factors as the type of antigen, the dose of the drug, and the timing of the drug relative to antigenic challenge, the targeted immune response may be either inhibited or augmented. Cyclophosphamide is an alkylating agent that appears to cause more pronounced suppression of humoral antibody responses than of responses attributed to cellular reactions. This is illustrated by models in which there is pronounced inhibition of both IgG and IgM antibody responses without significant changes in T-cell responses.

The effects of this drug on cell-mediated immune responses are extremely variable. It can prolong the survival of allogeneic skin grafts if administered after grafting. If used before grafting, however, it can be a potent immune enhancer. In part, this augmentation has been attributed to a greater toxicity for suppressor T cells than helper T lymphocytes.

Cyclophosphamide can be administered either orally or intravenously. Recent clinical trials suggest that pulse intravenous therapy, particularly when used with corticosteroids, may be more effective in treating immune-mediated diseases than is daily low-dose oral therapy. The parent drug is inactive until it undergoes hepatic transformation to 4-hydroxycyclophosphamide. This compound is further metabolized to form phosphoramide mustard, acrolein, and other alkylators. These can be found in the circulation for only a few hours after administration. Metabolism is not appreciably altered by either hepatic or renal insufficiency.

The cytotoxic effects of cyclophosphamide are primarily due to its ability to bind and cross-link DNA chains. It may also react with and alter the function of other intracellular macromolecules, however. The DNA-alkylating activity may result in the immediate death of the target cell, or the cell may incur a lethal injury that is expressed during a subsequent mitotic division. In the latter circumstance, the injured cell may function normally in the intermitotic (G_0) phase of its cycle. Conversely, if DNA repair can be effected, the cell will survive and function normally (Fig 58–7). DNA alkylation is a prime mechanism serving to impair the in vitro proliferative responses of residual lymphocytes.

In animal studies, cyclophosphamide causes a depletion of both T and B lymphocytes; its selectivity for B cells appears to result from their delayed recovery. Clinical studies suggest that the effects on different subsets depend on the dose of the drug; comparatively low doses primarily deplete B cells and CD8 lymphocytes, whereas higher doses results in similar reductions in the total numbers of CD4 and CD8 lymphocytes. Patients with rheumatoid arthritis treated with long-term oral cyclophosphamide have reduced serum immunoglobulin levels. Therapy is also associated with a decrease in the titers of many autoantibodies.

Cyclophosphamide has been used successfully in the treatment of disorders believed to result from aberrant immunity. Beneficial effects have been documented in Wegener's granulomatosis, other forms of vasculitis, severe rheumatoid arthritis, the nephritis associated with systemic lupus erythematosus (SLE), autoimmune blood dyscrasias such as idiopathic thrombocytopenic purpura, autoimmune hemolytic anemia, pure erythrocyte aplasia, Goodpasture's syndrome, and immune forms of glomerulonephritis.

Despite a comparatively high therapeutic-to-toxic ratio, cyclophosphamide therapy is associated with serious and potentially lethal adverse reactions. In general, the dose-limiting toxicity is suppression of hematopoiesis. Some studies suggest that this drug has less effect on the bone marrow than do other alkylating agents, and it may have a lower incidence of inducing thrombocytopenia. Other side effects include infertility and gastrointestinal symptoms such as abdominal pain, nausea, and vomiting. Teratogenesis is also a well-recognized complication.

In addition, this alkylating agent induces certain toxic manifestations not observed with other immunosuppressants; these include both hemorrhagic cystitis and alopecia. Cystitis has been reported in 9–17% of rheumatic patients chronically treated with this drug. The delayed toxicities include an increased risk of opportunistic infections and a higher than expected occurrence of cancers, specifically non-Hodgkin's lymphoma, bladder cancer, acute nonlymphoblastic leukemia, and skin cancers. The prevalence of malignancies appears to increase with both the total dose administered and the number of years of treatment. The overall risk for malignancies is difficult to estimate, but two long-term studies (7 and 11 years of follow-up) report that the incidence of neoplastic diseases was 24–25% in the group receiving this alkylating drug compared with 7–13% in the control group. Bladder cancer develops in approximately 10% of patients treated for prolonged intervals with oral cyclophosphamide.

C. Methotrexate: This drug is a specific inhibitor of dihydrofolate reductase, an enzyme required for the conversion of folic acid to its active form, tetrahydrofolate (Fig 58–8). The latter compound serves as a donor of one-carbon fragments for the in vivo synthesis of thymidine. Thus, methotrexate is a potent inhibitor of DNA synthesis and is classified as a phase-specific agent.

Methotrexate was one of the earliest anticancer drugs. Shortly after its introduction into clinical medicine, it was found to be effective in the treatment of psoriasis. The initial trials had to be terminated, however, because of a high risk of hepatic fibrosis. Subsequently, investigators found that lower doses were equally effective in controlling psoriatic manifestations and could be administered for extended periods without inducing hepatic injury. Patients with psoriasis with coexisting arthritis reported concomitant improvement in their joint disease. This led to an evaluation of methotrexate in patients with rheumatoid arthritis, and these studies showed that approximately two thirds of the patients with severe rheumatoid arthritis achieved either partial or complete remissions. Other studies found that methotrexate effectively suppressed manifestations of polymyositis and Reiter's syndrome. It is also of considerable use in preventing graft-versus-host (GVH) reactions in patients undergoing allogeneic marrow transplants (Table 58–5). There are conflicting results from studies of its use in treating steroid-dependent bronchial asthma.

Although animal studies indicate that methotrexate is a potent inhibitor of both humoral and cellular responses with a high therapeutic-to-toxic ratio, the mechanisms by which it exerts its beneficial effects in rheumatic diseases are not well understood. It is unlikely that the small doses used to treat immunologically mediated diseases would significantly inhibit immune responses.

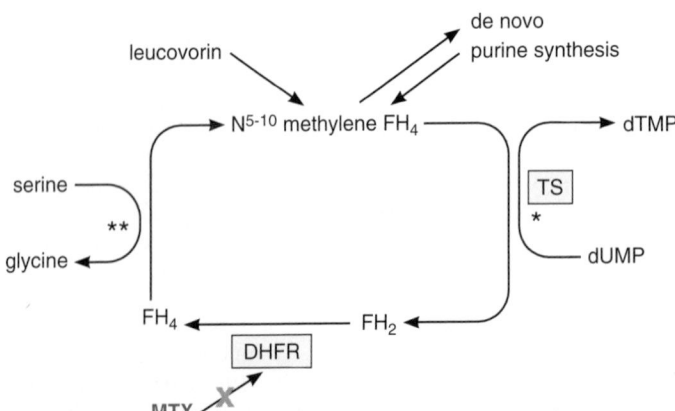

Figure 58–8. The folic acid cycle. Methotrexate (MTX) binds to and inhibits the enzyme dihydrofolate reductase (DHFR), thereby preventing the regeneration of tetrahydrofolate (FH$_4$) from dihydrofolate (FH$_2$). Leucovorin factor can directly antagonize the effects of methotrexate by providing a source of reduced folate. *Abbreviations:* dUMP = 2-deoxyuridylate; dTMP = thymidylate; TS = thymidine synthase. *One-carbon transfer from N^{5,10} methylene FH$_4$ to dUMP; **one-carbon transfer for serine to FH$_4$. (Reproduced, with permission, from Winkelstein A: Immune suppression resulting from various cytotoxic agents. In: *Clinics in Immunology and Allergy,* Vol 4: *Immune Suppression and Modulation.* Mitchell MS, Fahey JL [editors]. WB Saunders, 1984, p. 296.)

Table 58–5. Properties and uses of methotrexate.

Administration	Orally 2.5–5.0 mg every 12 hours × 3 weekly.
Mechanisms of action	S phase toxin (phase-specific). Competitively inhibits dihydrofolate reductase, thereby restricting synthesis of tetrahydrofolate. This is required for one-carbon transfer reactions involved in thymidine synthesis.
Major indications	Rheumatoid arthritis. Psoriasis and psoriatic arthritis. Polymyositis/dermatomyositis. Reiter's syndrome. Prophylaxis for graft-versus-host reaction in bone marrow transplants.
Toxicities	Gastrointestinal (stomatitis, diarrhea, mucositis). Bone marrow (megaloblastic anemia). Hepatic fibrosis. Pneumonitis. Decreased fertility.

A typical treatment regimen for rheumatic diseases consists of administering 2.5 mg of this drug every 12 hours for three doses; this course is repeated weekly. The major toxicity of methotrexate is hepatic fibrosis, which appears to be dose-related. Liver disease is rarely a problem until the total dose exceeds 1.5 g. Of particular note, hepatic fibrosis can occur with maintenance of normal liver function tests.

Other toxic manifestations include hypersensitivity pneumonitis, mucositis, and megaloblastic anemia. With the exception of pneumonitis, these complications are rarely major problems at the doses used to treat rheumatic diseases.

D. Chlorambucil: Chlorambucil is an alkylating drug that has cytotoxic properties similar to those of cyclophosphamide. Most comparative studies suggest that it is less toxic than cyclophosphamide but not as potent an immunosuppressant.

Chlorambucil has been used extensively in Europe to treat immunologically mediated disease, and most reports suggest that it effectively controls these disorders. These include rheumatoid arthritis, SLE, and Wegener's granulomatosis. It is the drug of choice for the treatment of idiopathic cold-agglutinin hemolytic anemia and essential cryoglobulinemia.

Chlorambucil has advantages over cyclophosphamide. It does not cause alopecia or hemorrhagic cystitis and is less irritating to the gastrointestinal tract. Like cyclophosphamide, it causes marrow suppression and interferes with gonadal function. It is also a fetal toxin. It increases the risk of both opportunistic infections and certain cancers.

Combinations of Cytotoxic Drugs

Recent clinical studies have attempted to enhance suppression of the manifestations of immunologically related diseases while minimizing toxicities by using combinations of two or more cytotoxic drugs. Multidrug therapies, which are derived in part from cancer chemotherapeutic protocols, are based on the concept that lower doses of two or more drugs will have an additive or even a synergistic effect on effector lymphocytes. At the same time, the reduced quantities of each agent will result in a decreased incidence of side effects, particularly those that are dose-related. Combinations tested in small series include azathioprine/methotrexate and cyclophosphamide/azathioprine; the initial trials are encouraging, but larger controlled series are required before the ultimate therapeutic role of these combinations is determined.

CYCLOSPORINE

The development of the immunosuppressant cyclosporine has revolutionized the discipline of organ transplantation. This drug is an extremely potent but relatively selective inhibitor of T-cell responses, particularly those responsible for transplant rejection reactions.

Unlike the cytotoxic immunosuppressants, cyclosporine acts not by killing immune effectors but by selectively inhibiting activation and proliferative expansion. The major mechanism responsible for these activities is an interference with the synthesis of IL-2. Specifically, cyclosporine downregulates the transcription of the mRNA of the gene for IL-2. Because of this activity the drug's primary cellular target is the helper T cell. By contrast, it has minimal toxicities for preformed suppressor/cytotoxic T cells, B lymphocytes, granulocytes, or macrophages.

In addition to its potency as an inhibitor of organ transplant rejection reactions, cyclosporine has become a mainstay in the prevention of graft-versus-host (GVH) disease in recipients of MHC-matched allogeneic bone marrow transplants. Although it is active in preventing GVH disease, it is much less effective in suppressing manifestations of ongoing GVH disease. Recently, cyclosporine has been tested for its ability to suppress manifestations of several immune-mediated diseases. Controlled trials indicate that it can be a disease-remitting agent in severe active rheumatoid arthritis. Some reports suggest that it may be useful in other autoimmune diseases, including SLE and inflammatory bowel disease. Nevertheless, the beneficial responses in autoimmune disorders are sufficiently unpredictable that therapy with cyclosporine should be reserved for clinical trials.

Pharmacologically, cyclosporine is a unique cyclic polypeptide consisting of 11 amino acids (Fig 58–9); it is derived from fermentation of a common soil fungus *Tolypocladium inflatum Gams*. The drug is a highly lipid-soluble and, in a suitable vehicle, can be administered orally or parenterally. Absorption from the gastrointestinal tract, however, is highly erratic,

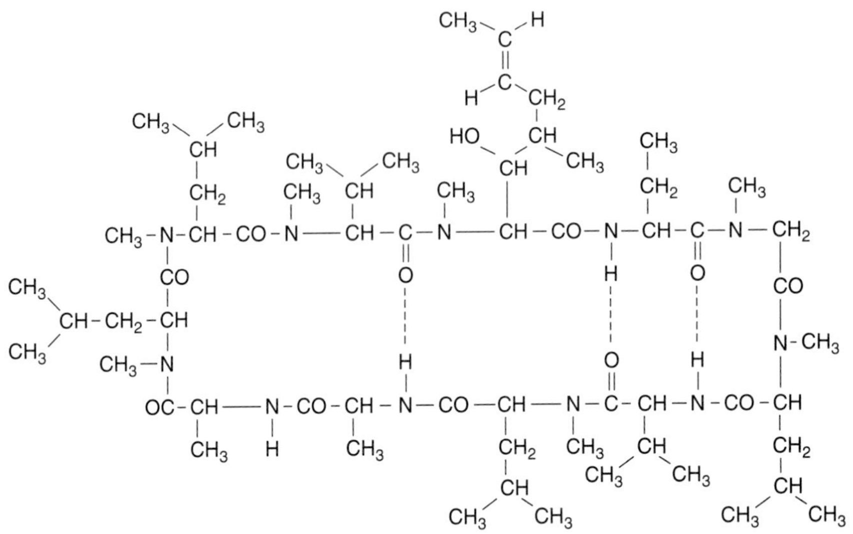

Figure 58–9. Chemical structure of cyclosporine. (Reproduced, with permission, from Cohen DJ et al: Cyclosporine: A new immunosuppressive agent for organ transplantation. *Ann Intern Med* 1984;**101**:667.)

varying from 5–95% (average ≈ 30%) absorption. This results in one of the major difficulties with respect to its clinical use; the blood levels are sufficiently unpredictable that drug concentrations must be carefully monitored. Cyclosporine is widely distributed throughout the body, including fat stores. Over 90% of the drug in the circulation is protein-bound. It crosses the placenta and is present in breast milk. The primary metabolic pathway is through the hepatic cytochrome P-450 enzyme system and is excreted in bile. Blood levels can be appreciably affected by abnormal liver function, by drugs that induce or inhibit hepatic metabolism, or by low bile flow.

The mechanisms by which cyclosporine acts to inhibit T-cell responses has provided valuable information about its pharmacologic properties and the events associated with the activation of normal lymphocytes (Fig 58–10). The principal effect of this drug is to interfere with calcium-dependent signal transduction from the cell membrane to the nucleus. Cyclosporine can be considered to be a prodrug; it enters the cell's cytoplasm and becomes activated only after binding to one of a family of intracellular receptors called **immunophilins.** The specific target of cyclosporine is the immunophilin **cyclophilin.** Cyclophilin has *cis–trans* isomerase activity, which is responsible for protein folding, but this activity appears to be distinct from its immunosuppressive properties. This is due to a drug–protein complex interaction that can bind to an essential intracellular signal transducer, **calcineurin.** Calcineurin is a calcium- and calmodulin-dependent protein phosphatase that is responsible for Ca^{2+}-dependent transmission of signal information from the cell membrane to the nucleus. In the nucleus, the signal induces cell activation. One of the essential processes in activation is the transcription of the genes controlling

the synthesis of IL-2. In vitro studies have shown that cyclosporine does not inhibit Ca^{2+}-independent signaling mechanisms (ie, binding through the CD28 coreceptor) nor does it appear to interfere with the transcription of the genes for the IL-2 receptor.

The intracellular signaling mechanisms for IL-2 gene transcription involve a complex series of events. Interaction of the T-cell receptor with an appropriate ligand results in an increase in intracellular calcium. These ions bind to calmodulin, which, in turn, binds to calcineurin and subsequent activates this phosphatase. The actual signal for IL-2 gene transcription is mediated by another protein, **nuclear factor of activated T cells (NF-AT).** This protein consists of two subunits: one located primarily in the cell's cytoplasm (NF-ATc) and the other, in the nucleus (NF-ATn). Activated calcineurin dephosphorylates NF-ATc, allowing it to be translocated into the nucleus where it combines with NF-ATn. The complete NT-AF molecule then can activate the genes for IL-2, resulting in transcription into mRNA.

The cyclosporine–cyclophilin complex prevents calcineurin from dephosphorylating NF-ATc. As a consequence, a markedly impaired signal is generated, resulting in a profound reduction in the transcription of the IL-2 genes. In the absence of adequate amounts of this growth factor, antigen-stimulated T helper cells are arrested at a G_0/G_1 phase of their proliferative cycle. The targeted lymphocyte population cannot complete their proliferative expansion nor provide the help needed for generating cytotoxic T lymphocytes. Likewise these arrested lymphocytes are unable to activate B cells responsible for T-cell-dependent humoral responses (see Chapter 8). By contrast, this immunosuppressant is ineffective in inhibiting the lytic activities of preformed T cells.

normal signal transduction for IL-2 transcription

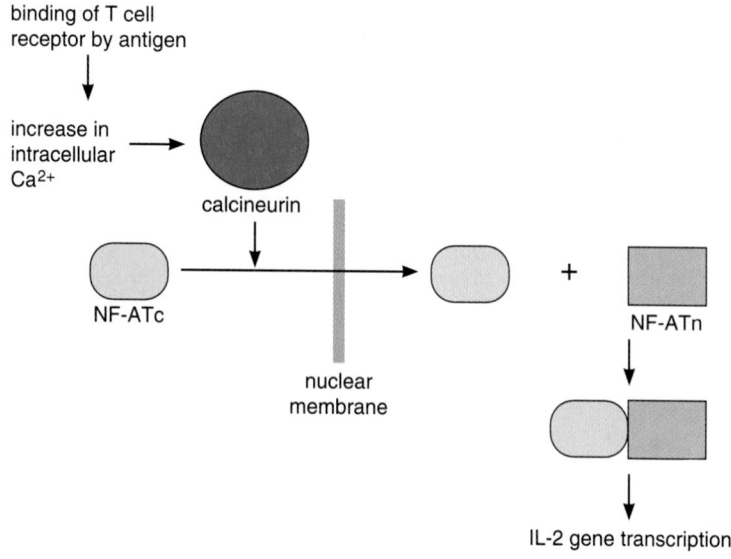

action of cyclosporin A

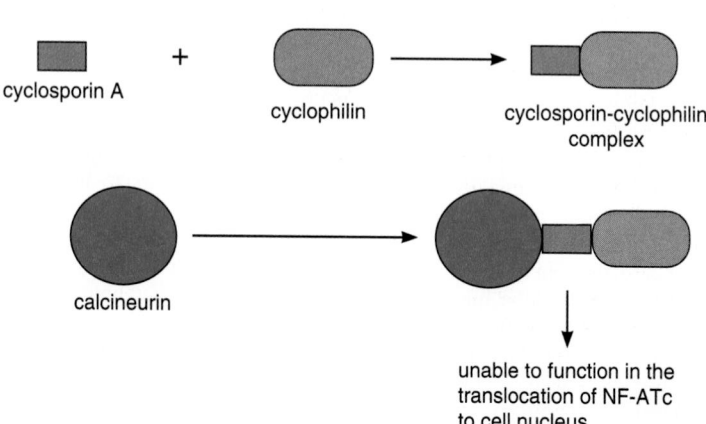

Figure 58–10. Mechanisms involved in normal signal transduction and the action of cyclosporine. Binding of the T-cell receptor by a ligand initiates an increase in intracellular calcium. This interacts with and activates calcineurin, which in turn dephosphorylates the cytoplasmic component of nuclear factor of activated T cells (NF-ATc). NF-ATc is then translocated to the nucleus where it combines with NT-AFn to form a complete molecule that is able to initiate the transcription of the IL-2 gene. Cyclosporine acts as an immunosuppressant by binding to an immunophilin, cyclophilin. This complex in turn binds to calcineurin and prevents it from dephosphorylating NT-AFc.

The immunosuppressive activities of cyclosporine can be augmented by the simultaneous administration of moderate doses of corticosteroids. The two drugs act synergistically. Cyclosporine directly inhibits IL-2 production, whereas steroids indirectly suppress the synthesis of IL-2 by blocking monocyte–macrophage release of IL-1 (see Fig 58–2).

Cyclosporine has a low therapeutic-to-toxic ratio. Unlike cytotoxic drugs, it is not toxic to bone marrow stem cells and therefore does not cause cytopenias. Nephrotoxicity is the most common toxicity; it occurs in two clinical settings. Acute renal failure may occur immediately after transplantation; this appears to be primarily due to decreased blood flow as a result of arteriolar vasoconstriction. This type of failure generally responds to dose reduction. Chronic nephrotoxicity occurs 2–3 months after transplant. The principal pathologic findings are tubulointerstitial fibrosis,

Table 58–6. Properties and uses of cyclosporine.

Administration	Orally, intravenously. Variable dosage, 5–20 mg/kg/d.
Mechanisms of action	Effects primarily limited to helper T cells; not cytotoxic. Inhibits production of IL-2. ? Reduces expression of IL-2 receptors.
Major indications	Inhibition of transplant rejection reactions.
Toxicities	Nephrotoxicity. Hypertension. Hepatotoxicity. ? Epstein-Barr virus-induced lymphomas. Hirsutism, gingival hyperplasia. Neurotoxicity. Hemolytic–uremic syndrome.

tubular atrophy, and glomerulosclerosis. The majority of affected patients experience stable, mild renal failure. In a minority of patients, however, renal failure tends to progress, ultimately resulting in end-stage renal disease.

Another common toxicity of cyclosporine is hypertension due to an increase in renovascular resistance. This drug frequently results in central nervous system dysfunction; manifestations can include tremors, headaches, paresthesias, confusion, and seizures. Reversible hepatotoxicity leading to elevations of the serum bilirubin and transaminase levels is another common side effect. Cyclosporine therapy can increase serum cholesterol, and it is a potential diabetogenic agent. The latter phenomenon results from an inhibition in insulin release from pancreatic islet cells and possibly the occurrence of peripheral insulin resistance. Due to its effects on renal tubular functions, treated patients may develop magnesium wasting and severe hypomagnesemia. Other symptoms of toxicity include nausea, vomiting, diarrhea, abdominal discomfort, gingival hyperplasia, hirsutism, coarsening of facial features, gynecomastia, and visual disturbances. In marrow transplant patients, it can cause a fatal capillary leak syndrome or a hemolytic–uremic syndrome.

Like other immunosuppressants, cyclosporine appears to result in an increased susceptibility to opportunistic infections and certain malignancies. The most frequently encountered neoplasms in organ transplant recipients are skin cancers and non-Hodgkin's lymphoma. The prevalence of lymphoma in transplant recipients has been estimated to be 25–30 times that of an age- and sex-matched control population. The risk from cyclosporine, however, does not significantly differ from that due to other immunosuppressive regimes except that these neoplasms have a shorter latent period. Kaposi's sarcoma constitute a disproportionally high percentage of the skin cancers in treated patients.

TACROLIMUS

Tacrolimus (formerly known as FK 506), a macrolide antibiotic, is also an extremely potent immunosuppressant that shares many characteristics with cyclosporine. It is primarily effective as an inhibitor of T helper cells. Like cyclosporine, tacrolimus suppresses the production of IL-2 by inhibiting gene transcription. In vitro, tacrolimus is 10–100 times more potent than cyclosporine. There is considerable debate, however, as to whether, in vivo, it is either more effective as an immunosuppressant or less toxic than cyclosporine.

Although biochemically unrelated to cyclosporine, tacrolimus acts pharmacologically by a similar mechanism. This drug binds to another immunophilin, the **FK-binding protein (FKBP),** which in turn binds to and interferes with the function of calcineurin. Like the cyclosporine-binding protein, cyclophilin, the tacrolimus-binding protein inhibits protein folding, but this does not appear to be critical to its immunosuppressive activities. Rather, the tacrolimus-binding protein complex binds to calcineurin, thereby preventing the latter from dephosphorylating NT-AFc. Tacrolimus is not lympholytic nor is it toxic for bone marrow progenitors. Furthermore, it does not inhibit target cell killing by preformed cytotoxic lymphocytes.

The toxicity profile of tacrolimus is also similar to that for cyclosporine. Both drugs are nephrotoxic and neurotoxic. Tacrolimus is moderately diabetogenic; it inhibits the release of insulin from islet cells and possibly increases peripheral insulin resistance. Hypertension appears to be less of a problem with tacrolimus than with cyclosporine, and it rarely causes such side effects as gingival hyperplasia, hirsutism, or coarsening of facial features. It also does not cause certain metabolic disturbances such as hyperuricemia and hypercholesterolemia. Long-term complications include both an increased incidence of opportunistic infections and neoplasms such as non-Hodgkin's lymphoma and skin cancers.

RAPAMYCIN

Rapamycin is similar in structure to tacrolimus, but unlike either tacrolimus or cyclosporine, rapamycin appears to effect Ca^{2+} independent-mediated signaling events. Rapamycin binds to FK-BP, the same immunophilin that binds tacrolimus. The complex does not inhibit the action of calcineurin, however. It appears that the rapamycin–FK-BP complex interacts with other intracellular proteins to inhibit a different set of signaling pathways, including those resulting from the interactions of IL-2 with its receptor. Rapamycin also inhibits events mediated via CD-28, protein kinase C, and other lymphokines. Although not extensively tested in clinical situations, immunosuppressive therapy using rapamycin and either cyclosporine or tacrolimus offers potential promise because the combination of agents can sequentially block successive phases of signal transduction.

NEWER IMMUNOSUPPRESSIVE DRUGS

During the last few years, several new immunosuppressive drugs have been developed; many have passed through preclinical tests and are now undergoing clinical trial. One of the most promising is **mycophenolate mofetil,** a prodrug of the antiproliferative agent mycophenolic acid. This agent specifically and reversibly inhibits inosine monophosphate dehydrogenase, thereby blocking the synthesis of guanine. The purine inhibitory effects are more pronounced on proliferating lymphocytes than on myeloid cells because lymphocytes rely primarily on the de novo production of guanine nucleotides rather than synthesis through salvage pathways. In preliminary studies, mycophenolate has been reported to be superior to azathioprine for the prevention of early kidney allograft rejection; this appears to be due, in part, to its higher therapeutic index. Mycophenolate is currently employed as a second-line drug in transplant recipients who become intolerant of cyclosporine or tacrolimus.

Brequinar is another new agent. It serves to inhibit de novo pyrimidine biosynthesis, and preclinical trials suggest it is an extremely potent immunosuppressant.

Likewise the adenosine nucleoside analogues, including fludarabine and 2-chloro-2'-deoxyadenoside (2CDA), compounds that are resistant to an essential lymphocyte enzyme, adenosine deaminase, have been shown to cause a profound depletion of CD4 cells and may be of value as immunosuppressants. These two drugs have proven highly effective in the treatment of low-grade lymphoid malignancies. One of the most notable side effects in the treatment of these neoplasms has been a profound and prolonged depression of cell-mediated immunity.

PLASMAPHERESIS

Diseases due to circulating autoantibodies or toxic antigen–antibody complexes could theoretically benefit from selective removal of the autoantibodies or immune complexes from the plasma. Plasma exchange (plasmapheresis) became clinically feasible with the development of automated cell separators capable of fractionating blood rapidly into its component parts. The procedure has been used experimentally to treat patients with a variety of immunologically related diseases, but there have been insufficient controlled therapeutic trials to ascertain its true effectiveness.

The technique used for plasma exchange is comparatively simple. Blood is removed, the plasma is separated by either centrifugation or membrane filtra-

tion and discarded, and the erythrocytes are reinfused into the patient. Fluid volume is maintained by administering either an albumin solution or fresh-frozen plasma. In most treatment protocols, approximately 50% of the patient's plasma is removed with each exchange procedure.

The ability of plasma exchange to remove a specific group of antibodies is dependent on their immunoglobin class. IgG molecules are distributed in both the intravascular and extracellular spaces, with approximately 40% contained in the vascular system. Thus, a single 50% plasma exchange can, at best, remove only 20% of a specific IgG antibody. By contrast, 85–90% of IgM antibodies are intravascular, so that a single exchange procedure can remove almost half the total quantity of pathogenic IgM antibodies. This accounts for the apparent success of plasma exchange in IgM antibody-related disorders such as idiopathic cold-agglutinin hemolytic anemia, essential cryoglobulinemia, and the hyperviscosity syndrome associated with Waldenström's macroglobulinemia.

Plasma exchange has been most successful for two of the IgG antibody autoimmune diseases: myasthenia gravis and Goodpasture's syndrome. It is noteworthy that both of these diseases are characterized by the presence of highly specific tissue autoantibodies. Plasma exchange has been used, with questionable effectiveness, in intractable rheumatoid arthritis, rheumatoid vasculitis, other forms of vasculitis, lupus nephritis, posttransfusion purpura, bleeding from factor VIII antibodies, and immunologically mediated neurologic diseases such as Guillain-Barré syndrome and multiple sclerosis.

INTRAVENOUS GAMMA GLOBULIN

Replacement therapy with intravenous gamma globulin (IVIG) has become standard treatment for severe humoral immune deficiencies (see Chapters 21 and 23). IVIG has also been found to influence the course of several autoimmune diseases, particularly immune thrombocytopenia, by functioning paradoxically as an immunosuppressant or an immunomodulator. It has been highly effective in treating children with the acute forms of idiopathic thrombocytopenic purpura. Although prolonged remissions in adults are rare, IVIG can often increase platelet counts transiently, which can be potentially life-saving in cases of bleeding diatheses resulting from severe thrombocytopenia. Although the mechanism of action in idiopathic thrombocytopenic purpura is not fully known, IVIG appears to act primarily by blocking FcγR on reticuloendothelial cells, thereby inhibiting the phagocytosis of antibody-coated platelets. In some cases, IVIG may also displace platelet-specific antibodies from the cell surface.

Based on the experience with idiopathic thrombocytopenic purpura, several other immunologically mediated diseases have been treated with IVIG. These include autoimmune hemolytic anemia, autoimmune neutropenia, antibody-mediated pure erythrocyte aplasia, other platelet-destructive diseases, autoantibodies against the blood-clotting factor VIII, myasthenia gravis, and Kawasaki disease. With the exceptions of Kawasaki disease and idiopathic thrombocytopenic purpura, the accumulated experience with these conditions to date is too small to determine the true effectiveness of this method.

Several other mechanisms have been postulated to explain the immune-modulating activities. IVIG has been reported to nonspecifically augment suppressor T-cell activities. It may also inhibit the activities of NK cells and reduce the synthesis of specific immunoglobulins. In addition, it may contain anti-idiotypic antibodies that will serve to inactivate autoantibodies.

ANTILYMPHOCYTE ANTIBODIES

The administration of heterologous antisera against lymphocyte membrane antigens is another mode of achieving nonspecific immunosuppression. Two types of antibody preparations have been used: polyclonal antibodies, which react with multiple membrane determinants, and monoclonal antibodies, which are directed at only a single antigen.

Polyclonal Antibodies

Polyclonal antibodies are generally prepared by immunizing animals with human lymphocytes. If cells from the thymus are used, the preparation is termed **antithymocyte serum (ATS);** this is often further fractionated to obtain the globulin portion, termed **antithymocyte globulin (ATG).** Other antibodies are prepared from thoracic duct lymphocytes, splenic cells, or peripheral blood lymphocytes obtained by leukophoresis. These are referred to as either **antilymphocyte serum (ALS)** or **antilymphocyte globulin (ALG).**

Polyclonal antibodies are effective immunosuppressants in both animal and clinical studies. The primary effect is to inhibit cell-mediated immune responses; this is consistent with their specificities for T lymphocytes. The mechanisms responsible for their immunosuppressive activities are not fully understood, however. They do produce lymphopenia in vivo; this is one postulated mode of action. Clinically, they are used primarily to treat organ graft rejection reactions. More recently, they have been used to treat patients with severe GVH reactions and to promote remissions in some cases of aplastic anemia.

Several major problems are associated with the use of polyclonal antibodies. (1) The preparations are not standardized, and there is no objective measure of in vivo immunosuppressive activity of a particular preparation. Thus, the amount needed to achieve a specific clinical effect cannot be predetermined.

(2) These reagents are not selective for T cells. They cross-react with other types of cells, including platelets, which may lead to a destructive thrombocytopenia. (3) Heterologous antibodies are recognized as foreign proteins by the patient's immune system, thereby eliciting a humoral immune response, which may cause serum sickness (see Chapter 29).

MONOCLONAL ANTIBODIES

Monoclonal antibodies are assuming increasing clinical importance in the treatment of organ graft rejection reactions. Because of their potency, trials have been initiated to assess their activities as a means of prophylactically inhibiting organ rejection and as therapeutic agents for immunologically related diseases. These antibodies are believed to be immunosuppressant by virtue of their ability to bind to and inactive cell surface receptors on T lymphocytes or antibody-presenting cells (APC).

Immunosuppressive monoclonal antibodies can be divided into two general classes: those directed at specific subsets of immune cells and those reactive with antigens selectively present on the lymphocyte subset affecting the targeted immune response. The former includes a series of pan-T-cell antibodies; the one most widely used clinically is OKT3 (muromonab-CD3), a murine antibody with specificity for the ε polypeptide chain of the CD3 antigen. As previously described, the CD3 polypeptide chain is important in signal transduction, which occurs following antigen binding to the T-cell receptor. Figure 58–11 depicts some of the potential targets of monoclonal antibodies.

The OKT3 antibody is an extremely potent immunosuppressant with activity equal to or superior to that of ATG. It is considered the agent of choice for severe rejection episodes in recipients of all types of allografts and, in recent studies, has proven effective as prophylaxis for the prevention of rejection reactions. The mechanisms by which it induces immunosuppression are not completely understood. Shortly after administration, there is a pronounced reduction in blood T lymphocytes. Typically, the lymphopenia persists for several days; it may result from sequestration of targeted cells rather than cell lysis. Once T cells reappear, they show impaired immunologic function.

Despite its success, potential problems are associated with the administration OKT3. One of the most important is its immunogenicity; it induces human antimouse antibodies (HAMA). These antibodies, in high titers, can abrogate its immunosuppressive activities. In an attempt to circumvent HAMA formation, humanized antibodies in which the variable regions of the murine antibody (which contain the antigen reactive site) are coupled with human immunoglobulin-constant regions have been developed. In general, these humanized antibodies reduce but do not abrogate HAMA.

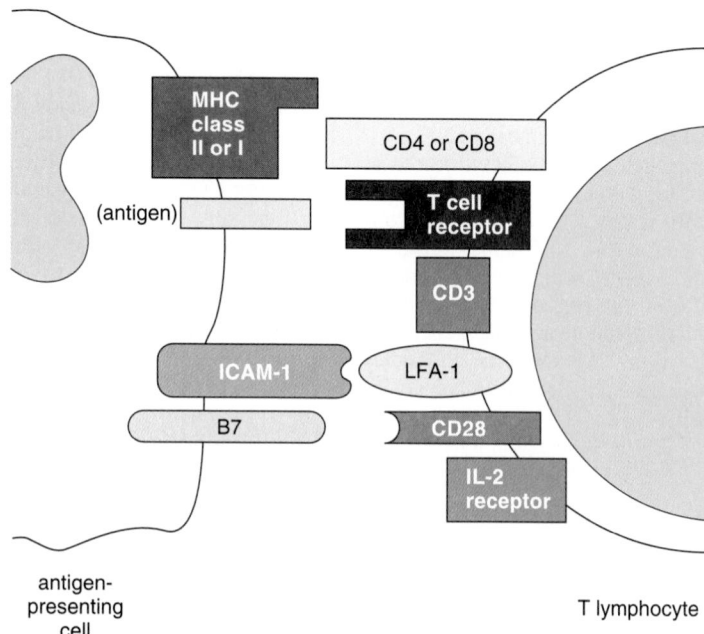

Figure 58–11. Potential targets of monoclonal antibodies. These include the CD3 T-cell receptor complex, antigen-nonspecific coreceptors, and receptors expressed on T-cell activation such as the IL-2 receptor. The antibodies may have specificity for either the receptor on the T cell or its ligand on the antigen-presenting cell.

Another problem with OKT3 is that it may activate cells inducing a profound systemic reaction. This reaction, which occurs during the first and perhaps the second exposure to the drug, appears to result from the massive release of cytokines. It occurs within 1–3 hours after administration. Manifestations may include fever, hypotension, headaches, gastrointestinal symptoms, pulmonary edema, transient acute tubular necrosis, hypercoagulability, aseptic meningitis, and seizures. Clinical manifestations follow the systemic release of cytokines such as TNF-α, IL-2, GM-CSF, and INFγ. Corticosteroids, administered prophylactically, effectively reduce both cytokine release and its clinical manifestations without diminishing its immunosuppressive activities. These reactions generally do not occur after the second or third administration of OKT3.

Other problems with therapy with OKT3 include the long-term consequences of the profound immunosuppression. Treatment predisposes treated patients to opportunistic infections, particularly by CMV and Epstein-Barr virus. Furthermore, prolonged use of OKT3 has been associated with a dramatic increase in the incidence of lymphoproliferative disorders. In addition, rejection reactions commonly occur once therapy is discontinued, indicating that the drug does not induce a state of permanent immune tolerance.

Several other pan-T-cell antibodies have been tested; to date, none have proven more effective than OKT3. Antibodies directed at the α/β chains of the T-cell receptor, however, appear to have activities

equivalent to OKT3 in suppressing rejection reactions and may be less toxic.

An alternative approach to immunosuppression can be achieved with antibodies directed at antigen-nonspecific accessory molecules present on T lymphocytes, APC, or immune targets. As shown in Figure 58–11, T-cell stimulation requires both antigen-specific recognition by the T-cell receptor and the interactions of several adhesion molecules on the lymphocyte with appropriate ligands on antigen-presenting cells. One potentially important coreceptor target is the CD4 complex on T helper/inducer cells. Binding of this complex to MHC class II molecules on APC is a necessary prerequisite for generating an immune response. Early clinical trials suggest that antibodies to the CD4 antigen have considerable immune-inhibitory activities.

Monoclonal antibodies against several other cell membrane constituents also appear to have immunosuppressive properties. An important T-cell interaction is that of the adhesion molecule, leukocyte functional antigen-1 (LFA-1) on the lymphocyte with its ligand, intercellular adhesion molecule-1 (ICAM-1 [CD54]) on antigen-presenting cells. Monoclonal antibodies directed at ICAM-1 have been successfully used in initial clinical trials to inhibit transplant rejection reactions.

Another receptor ligand target for immunosuppression is the interaction between CD28 on T lymphocytes and the B7 antigen present on B lymphocytes and macrophages. Engagement of the T-cell receptor by antigen in the absence of CD28 binding appears to result in T-cell anergy. A fusion protein consisting of a human antibody fragment with high affinity for B7 and a human Fc portion of IgG has significant immunosuppressive activities in preclinical studies.

An alternative approach to antibodies directed at lymphocyte subsets for achieving immunosuppression is to specifically target cells affecting the unwanted immune response. One such target is the interaction between the T-cell growth factor IL-2 and its receptor. Growth factor binding to its receptor is required for T-cell proliferation and the generation of cytotoxic lymphocytes. Monoclonal antibodies against components of the IL-2 receptor are poten-

tially able to selectively inhibit the responses of activated T cells such as those affecting rejection reactions. The IL-2 receptor is a complex consisting of alpha, beta, and gamma chains. To date, only antibodies directed at the p55 alpha chain have been developed and clinically tested. Unfortunately the initial results have not shown consistent immune inhibitory activities, possibly because these antibodies are not specifically targeted to the high-affinity components of the receptor. Hybrid monoclonal antibodies, in which the monoclonal antibody to the alpha chain of the IL-2 receptor is linked to either radionuclides or bacterial or plant toxins, have been proposed as a method that can deliver a toxic injury to specifically targeted cells.

REFERENCES

GENERAL

Bach J-F: Immunosuppressive therapy of autoimmune diseases. *Immunol Today* 1993;**14**:322.

Barry JM: Immunosuppressive drugs in renal transplantation. *Drugs* 1992;**44**:554.

Ben-Yehuda O et al: Advances in therapy of autoimmune diseases. *Semin Arthritis Rheum* 1988;**17**:206.

Briggs JD: A critical review of immunosuppressive therapy. *Immunol Letts* 1991;**29**:89.

Fahey JL et al: Immune interventions in disease. *Ann Intern Med* 1987;**106**:257.

Fox DA, McCune WJ: Immunosuppressive drug therapy of systemic lupus erythematosus. *Rheum Dis Clin North Am* 1994;**20**:265.

Hazleman B: Incidence of neoplasms in patients with rheumatoid arthritis exposed to different treatment regimens. *Am J Med* 1985;**78**(suppl 1A):39.

Kahan BD, Ghobrial R: Immunosuppressive agents. *Surg Clin North Am* 1994;**74**:1029.

Marsh JW et al: Immunosuppressants. *Gastroenterol Clin North Am* 1992;**21**:679.

McCune WJ, Friedman AW: Immunosuppressive drug therapy for rheumatic disease. *Curr Opin Rheumatol* 1993;**5**:282.

Mitchell MS, Fahey JL (editors): *Immune Suppression and Modulation*, Vol 4 of: *Clinics in Immunology and Allergy.* WB Saunders, 1984.

Penn I: The occurrence of malignant tumors in immunosuppressed states. *Prog Allergy* 1986;**37**:259.

Strom TB: Immunosuppressive agents in renal transplantation. *Kidney Int* 1984;**26**:353.

Superdock KR, Helderman JH: Immunosuppressive drugs and their effects. *Semin Respir Infect* 1993;**8**:152.

Tsokos GC: Immunomodulatory treatment in patients with rheumatic diseases: Mechanisms of action. *Semin Arthritis Rheum* 1987;**17**:24.

Yunus MB: Investigational therapy in rheumatoid arthritis: A critical review. *Semin Arthritis Rheum* 1988;**17**:163.

CORTICOSTEROIDS

Auphan N et al: Immunosuppression by glucocorticoids: Inhibition of NF-κB activity through induction of IκB synthesis. *Science* 1995;**270**:286.

Claman HN: Glucocorticosteroids. I. Anti-inflammatory mechanisms. II. The clinical response. *Hosp Pract* 1983;**18**:123, 143.

Cupps TR, Fauci AS: Corticosteroid-mediated immunoregulation in man. *Immunol Rev* 1982;**65**:133.

Meulemann J, Katz P: The immunologic effects, kinetics and use of glucocorticosteroids. *Med Clin North Am* 1985;**69**:805.

Scheinman RI et al: Role of transcriptional activation of IκBα in mediation of immunosuppression by glucocorticoids. *Science* 1995;**270**:283.

Zweiman B et al: Corticosteroid effects on circulating lymphocyte subset levels in normal humans. *J Clin Immunol* 1984;**4**:151.

CYTOTOXIC DRUGS

Ahmed AR, Hombal SM: Cyclophosphamide (cytoxan). *J Am Acad Dermatol* 1984;**11**:1115.

Austin HA et al: Therapy of lupus nephritis. *N Engl J Med* 1986;**314**:614.

Berd D et al: Augmentation of the human immune response by cyclophosphamide. *Cancer Res* 1982;**42**:4862.

Boumpas D et al: Controlled trial of pulse methylprednisolone versus two regimens of pulse cyclophosphamide in severe lupus nephritis. *Lancet* 1992;**340**:741.

Clements PJ, Davis J: Cytotoxic drugs: Their clinical application to the rheumatic diseases. *Semin Arthritis Rheum* 1986;**15**:231.

Cupps TR et al: Suppression of human B lymphocytes function by cyclophosphamide. *J Immunol* 1982;**128**:2453.

Felson DT, Anderson J: Evidence for the superiority of immunosuppressive drugs and prednisone over prednisone alone in lupus nephritis. *N Engl J Med* 1984;**311**:1528.

Hoffman GS et al: Wegener granulomatosis: An analysis of 158 patients. *Ann Intern Med* 1992;**116**:488.

McCune WJ, Fox D: Intravenous cyclophosphamide therapy of severe SLE. *Rheum Dis Clin North Am* 1989;**15**:455.

McCune WJ et al: Clinical and immunologic effects of monthly administration of intravenous cyclophosphamide in severe systemic lupus erythematosus. *N Engl J Med* 1988;**318**:1423.

Moore MJ: Clinical pharmacokinetic of cyclophosphamide. *Clin Pharmacokinet* 1991;**20**:194.

Nashel DJ: Mechanisms of action and clinical applications of cytotoxic drugs in rheumatic disorders. *Med Clin North Am* 1985;**69:**817.

Turk JL, Parker D: Effect of cyclophosphamide on immunological control mechanisms. *Immunol Rev* 1982;**65:**99.

CYCLOSPORINE, TACROLIMUS, & RAPAMYCIN

Bennett WM, Norman DJ: Action and toxicity of cyclosporine. *Ann Rev Med* 1986;**37:**215.

Cohen DJ et al: Cyclosporine: A new immunosuppressive agent for organ transplantation. *Ann Intern Med* 1984;**101:**667.

Foxwell BM, Ruffel B: The mechanisms of action of cyclosporin. *Cardiol Clin* 1990;**8:**107.

Freeman DJ: Pharmacology and pharmacokinetics of cyclosporine. *Clin Biochem* 1991;**24:**9.

Harding MW, Handschumacher RE: Cyclophilin, a primary molecular target for cyclosporine. Structural and functional implications. *Transplantation* 1988;**46**(suppl 2):296.

Hess AD: Mechanisms of action of cyclosporine: Considerations for the treatment of autoimmune diseases. *Clin Immunol Immunopathol* 1993;**68:**220.

Hohman RJ, Hultsch T: Cyclosporin A: New insights for cell biologists and biochemists. *New Biol* 1990;**2:**663.

Holloran PF, Madrenas J: The mechanism of action of cyclosporin: A perspective for the 90's. *Clin Biochem* 1991;**24:**3.

Kropp KA et al: Cyclosporine versus azathioprine: A review of 200 consecutive cadaver renal transplant recipients. *J Urol* 1989;**142:**28.

Morris R: Modes of action of FK506, cyclosporin A and rapamycin. *Transplant Proc* 1994;**26:**3272.

Schreiber SL, Crabtree GR: The mechanism of action of cyclosporin A and FK506. *Immunol Today* 1992;**13:**136.

Starzl TE et al: Selective topics on FK 506 with special reference to rescue of extrahepatic whole organ grafts, transplantation of "forbidden organs," side effects, mechanisms and practical pharmacokinetics. *Transplant Proc* 1991;**23:**914.

Stein CM: Cyclosporine in the treatment of rheumatoid arthritis. *Bull Rheum Dis* 1995;**44:**1.

Thomson AW: The immunosuppressive macrolides FK-506 and rapamycin. *Immunol Lett* 1991;**29:**105.

Wiederrecht G et al: The mechanism of action of FK-506 and cyclosporin A. *Ann N Y Acad Sci* 1993;**696:**9.

PLASMAPHERESIS

Shumak KH, Rock GA: Therapeutic plasma exchange. *N Engl J Med* 1984;**310:**762.

INTRAVENOUS GAMMA GLOBULIN

Berkman SA et al: Clinical uses of intravenous immunoglobulins. *Ann Intern Med* 1990;**112:**278.

POLYCLONAL & MONOCLONAL ANTIBODIES

Alegre M-L et al: Immunomodulation of transplant rejection using monoclonal antibodies and soluble receptors. *Digest Dis Sci* 1995;**40:**58.

Chatenoud L, Bach JF: Monoclonal antibodies to CD3 as immunosuppressants. *Semin Immunol* 1990;**2:**437.

Cobbold SP: Monoclonal antibody therapy for the induction of transplantation tolerance. *Immunol Lett* 1991;**29:**117.

Cosimi AB: Clinical development of orthoclone OKT3. *Transplant Proc* 1987;**19**(suppl 1):1.

Cosimi AB: Progress in monoclonal antibodies in clinical transplantation. *Transplant Proc* 1994;**26:**1943.

Cosimi AB: Future of monoclonal antibodies in solid organ transplantation. *Digest Dis Sci* 1995;**40:**65.

Dantal J, Soulillou J-P: Use of monoclonal antibodies in human transplantation. *Curr Opin Immunol* 1991;**3:**740.

Goldstein G: Overview of the development of orthoclone OKT3: Monoclonal antibody for therapeutic use in transplantation. *Transplant Proc* 1987;**19**(suppl 1):1.

Hall BM: Therapy with monoclonal antibodies to CD4: Potential not appreciated. *Am J Kidney Dis* 1989; **14**(suppl 2):71.

Heyworth MF: Clinical experience with antilymphocyte serum. *Immunol Rev* 1982;**65:**79.

Ortho Multicenter Transplant Study Group: A randomized clinical trial of OKT3 monoclonal antibody for acute rejection of cadaveric renal transplants. *N Engl J Med* 1985;**313:**337.

Parlevliet KJ, Schellekens PTA: Monoclonal antibodies in renal transplantation: A review. *Transplant Int* 1992; **5:**234.

Steunmuler DR et al: Comparison of OKT3 with ALG for prophylaxis for patients with acute renal failure after cadaveric renal transplantation. *Transplantation* 1991; **52:**67.

Waldmann TA, Goldman CK: The multichain interleukin-2 receptor: A target for immunotherapy of patients receiving allografts. *Am J Kidney Dis* 1989;**14**(suppl 2):45.

Wood KJ: Transplantation tolerance. *Curr Opin Immunol* 1991;**3:**710.

OTHER AGENTS

Dighiero G: Potential immunological action of purine nucleoside analogues. *Drugs* 1994;**47**(suppl 6):57.

Taylor DO et al: Mycophenolate mofetil (RS-61443): Preclinical, clinical, and three-year experience in heart transplantation. *J Heart Lung Transplant* 1994;**13:**571.

59

Immunomodulators

Lawrence R. Hennessey, MD, & James R. Baker, Jr., MD

Immunomodulators are biologic response-modifying compounds that affect the immune response in either a positive or negative fashion. Although immunosuppressive drugs and some therapeutic uses of gamma globulin can be included in this definition, they are discussed at length elsewhere (see Chapter 58), as are the biologic functions of many of these agents, especially the cytokines (see Chapter 10). In contrast, the focus of this chapter is the pharmacologic and therapeutic effects of compounds that regulate or stimulate the immune response. These include a large number of compounds, which can be divided into three broad categories: general immunostimulatory agents, mostly of bacterial origin; eukaryotic source substances, such as cytokines and monoclonal antibodies, which tend to have much more specific effects; and biochemical compounds. An ever-increasing array of potential immunomodulators are being examined for therapeutic benefit in a variety of disorders, including but not limited to malignancies, immunodeficient states such as acquired immunodeficiency syndrome (AIDS), and inflammatory diseases. A number of these have reached clinical trials, and some have demonstrated considerable efficacy. Immunomodulators with currently defined actions and their clinical use are shown in Table 59–1.

COMPOUNDS DERIVED FROM BACTERIA

Bacterial compounds were among the first to be recognized as immunostimulators. Complete Freund's adjuvant (CFA), which contains mycobacterial derivatives, has long been used as an adjuvant to boost humoral immune responses in animals. Although CFA is not appropriate for human use, the attenuated mycobacterium bacillus Calmette-Guérin (BCG) has been extensively studied in the treatment of certain

malignancies. Injection of BCG into lesions of malignant melanoma has led to remission of the local tumor as well as distant metastases, although long-term survival has not in general been affected. It has also been used successfully in the treatment of bladder carcinoma via irrigation. CFA and BCG have been shown to prevent and even reverse the course of autoimmune diabetes in a murine model of this disease, but there are as yet no defined mechanisms for this effect and no data suggesting benefit in human autoimmune disorders. BCG has been shown to stimulate macrophage, T and B lymphocyte, and NK cell function and to augment interleukin-1 (IL-1) production. Various semipurified mycobacterial extracts, such as methanol extract residue, muramyl dipeptides, and several heat shock proteins, have been examined and found to perform many of the functions of the whole extract.

Certain mycobacterial heat shock proteins and other bacterial substances, such as toxins from *Staphylococcus aureus,* demonstrate "superantigen" activity; that is, they are capable of activating large numbers of T lymphocytes in a major histocompatibility complex-restricted manner. This is thought to occur as a result of binding to subset-specific conserved areas of the T-cell receptor-variable region, denoted as $V\alpha$ or $V\beta$ subsets, remote from the antigen-binding site. This polyclonal activation of certain T-cell subsets may be responsible for some of the immunomodulatory effects seen following the administration of bacterial compounds. These compounds have been reported to stimulate immune responses to certain neoplasms and may be involved in the pathogenesis of certain vasculitides and autoimmune diseases.

OK432, an extract prepared from culture medium following penicillin treatment of a strain of group A *Streptococcus pyogenes,* has been shown to augment macrophage and natural killer (NK) cell activity and has some demonstrated effect in the treatment of human head and neck, gastrointestinal, and lung tumors.

Table 59–1. Immunomodulators and their clinically defined actions, usage, and side effects.

Immunomodulator	Action	Result and Use	Side Effects
IFNα	Increase natural immune function	Antitumor activity	Flu-like syndrome, IFNα antibodies
IFNβ	Increase natural immune function	Similar to IFNα, less efficacious	Flu-like syndrome, less than IFNα
IFNγ	Increase immune responsiveness	Anti-infectious and antitumor activity	Flu-like syndrome
IL-2	Generation of activated killer cells	Antitumor activity	GI and CNS toxicity, fever
IL-4	Increase T_H2-like response	Enhance antibody responses	Promote allergic reactions (theoretical)
IL-10	Suppress T_H1 responses	Decrease cellular cytotoxicity	Promote allergic reactions (theoretical)
IL-12	Augment T_H1 responses	Increase cellular cytotoxicity, augment antitumor and infectious immunity	Unexpected mortality
Fas (CD 95)	CD8 cytotoxicity and thymic deletion	Soluble forms of ligand prevent graft rejection or autoimmunity	Unknown
GM-CSF	Augment production of WBC	Neutropenia	None
TGF-β	Increase wound healing and suppress specific immune responses	Anti-inflammatory therapy	Increased collagen production and fibrosis of multiple organs
IL-1 RA	Block IL-1 receptor binding	Prevent septic shock, allergic reactions, and wasting in cancer patients	Unknown

Abbreviations: IFN = interferon; IL = interleukin; GM-CSF = granulocyte–macrophage colony-stimulating factor; TGF = transforming growth factor; IL-1 RA = interleukin-1 receptor agonist; GI = gastrointestinal; CNS = central nervous system.

Whole or fractionated preparations of a variety of other microorganisms, including *Corynebacterium parvum, Listeria monocytogenes, Salmonella typhimurium, Brucella abortus, Pseudomonas aeruginosa,* and *Nocardia* spp., also have demonstrated immunomodulatory effects. Lipopolysaccharide from gram-negative bacteria has also been studied as an immunostimulatory compound, but the therapeutic usefulness of this preparation is limited by its toxicity.

COMPOUNDS DERIVED FROM EUKARYOTIC ORGANISMS

As knowledge of mammalian immune physiology progressed, attempts to characterize the immune function of certain organs led to the generation of crude immune tissue extracts with biologic functions. Compounds such as thymic extracts and interferons demonstrated varied immunomodulatory activities, and speculations were made regarding the potential clinical usefulness of some of these agents. Problems with obtaining adequate quantities of appropriately pure preparations limited the study of their role in the treatment of human disease, however. The advent of recombinant DNA and hybridoma technologies in the 1970s, however, allowed for the appropriate charac-

terization and production of a large number of immunoactive peptides and monoclonal antibodies. The study of the therapeutic potential of these agents is of great interest at present.

1. THYMIC HORMONES

A number of thymic peptide extracts, including thymosins, thymulin, thymopentin, thymostimulin, and thymic humoral factor, have demonstrated immunostimulatory actions. They have purported clinical benefit in a variety of viral infections, including hepatitis B, herpes zoster, and herpes labialis, as well as in chronic *Trichophyton rubrum* infection. They have also been used with limited success in patients with primary immunodeficiency states such as DiGeorge anomaly and ataxia-telangiectasia. Increased survival of patients with small-cell carcinoma of the lung has been demonstrated after administration of thymosin as an adjunct to chemotherapy. Clinical improvement in patients with rheumatoid arthritis has been reported with thymulin and thymopentin. Although increased CD4-to-CD8 T-cell ratios have been demonstrated in some asymptomatic HIV-infected individuals following treatment with thymic humoral factor, the clinical benefit of these compounds in HIV infection has not been conclusively demonstrated. The overall value of these agents in the treatment of human disease will be clarified as defined preparations of the various extracts become available.

2. CYTOKINES

Cytokines are small (<80 kd) proteins or glycoproteins that exhibit a variety of autocrine, paracrine and, in some cases, endocrine effects. They are generally subdivided into interferons, interleukins, colony-stimulating factors, and generalized growth and differentiation factors. As a group they have enormous potential for clinical use as immunomodulators and demonstrate a variety of specific as well as generalized influences on the immune system.

Interferons

Although interferons were first recognized for their effect on viral infection, their clinical usefulness as immunomodulators has been demonstrated in certain neoplastic diseases as well.

Interferon alfa (IFNα), a natural product of macrophages, has demonstrated antitumor activity in a number of neoplastic disorders. More than 90% of patients with hairy cell leukemia respond to treatment with IFNα, although most relapse shortly after treatment is discontinued. Long-term therapy, unfortunately, is often complicated by adverse effects such as chronic fatigue, and resistance occasionally develops because of the production of anti-interferon antibodies. IFNα also can induce remission in chronic myelogenous leukemia, especially if begun before the accelerated phase of the disease, and it has demonstrated benefit in multiple myeloma, non-Hodgkin's lymphoma, and cutaneous T-cell lymphoma. It also reportedly has activity against certain solid tumors, including malignant melanoma, renal cell carcinoma, and bladder and ovarian cancers. It is beneficial in the treatment of AIDS-related Kaposi's sarcoma, with a reported response rate of 25–40%, but toxicity at the high doses required for effective treatment (up to 36 million IU/day) is considerable, requiring dose reduction in up to one third of patients.

Responses to a variety of viral infections have been demonstrated with IFNα. Intralesional or topical application has led to improvement in, and in some cases resolution of, condyloma acuminatum, laryngeal papillomatosis, herpetic keratoconjunctivitis, and rhinovirus infections.

Interferon beta (IFNβ), naturally produced by fibroblasts, is not yet commercially available. Although it is somewhat less toxic than IFNα, it appears to be less efficacious as an antineoplastic drug. It may, however, be useful in the treatment of central nervous system gliomas, since it is reported to induce partial responses in 10–20% of patients.

Interferon gamma (IFNγ, immune interferon), a product of lymphocytes, also has been reported to have extensive activity in a variety of tumors and viral infections. Although it is structurally unrelated to IFNα and IFNβ, IFNγ appears to have a similar spectrum of antitumor activity. It is being used with some success as an alternative treatment in patients with AIDS-related Kaposi's sarcoma who demonstrate resistance to or intolerance of IFNα. Response to IFNγ by tumors that are resistant to the effects of IFNα (and vice versa) has been described as well. Unlike IFNα and IFNβ, IFNγ may have some applicability in the treatment of connective tissue disorders and has been shown to be effective in the treatment of lepromatous leprosy. There is evidence to support synergy between IFNα and IFNγ in the treatment of some neoplasms. Subjective improvement and increased resistance to opportunistic infections in a small number of AIDS patients treated with IFNγ has been described, but its effect on overall survival has not been demonstrated. Side effects, shared with the other interferons, include acute malaise with a "flu-like" syndrome, chronic fatigue, anorexia, and elevation of hepatic enzymes. In addition, however, IFNγ may cause lipidemia, arthralgias, hypocalcemia, and severe headaches. The most effective future use of this agent is thought to be as an adjuvant in the treatment of lymphoproliferative malignancies.

Interleukins

The interleukins are a diverse group of lymphokines, exhibiting a broad array of actions on the immune system. Many possess demonstrated or potential usefulness as therapeutic immunomodulators.

Interleukin-2 (IL-2) has been used successfully in the treatment of certain malignancies, in particular renal cell carcinoma and malignant melanoma. This is in all likelihood due to activation and proliferation of lymphocyte-activated killer (LAK) cells. Direct systemic administration of IL-2 does, however, lead to significant toxicity, including fever, chills, and edema. Severe gastrointestinal and central nervous system toxicity are also seen in most patients. Adoptive immunotherapy, involving IL-2-mediated activation of LAK cells derived from the patients' peripheral blood leukocytes, followed by readministration, has been used, and although it is less toxic than systemic IL-2 administration, it has not shown consistent efficacy in treating neoplasms.

Recently, IL-2 has been used to produce ex vivo activation of a subset of lymphocytes derived from solid tumors, known as tumor-infiltrating lymphocytes (TIL). TIL reportedly possess 50–100 times more antitumor activity than do LAK cells derived from peripheral blood, presumably because they represent a select population directed primarily against the tumor in question. Studies using this approach to immunotherapy are under way.

Interleukin-4 (IL-4), a lymphokine that is known mainly for promotion of IgE production and mast cell stimulation, also has demonstrable antitumor activity in animal models and may have some potential role in the treatment of human malignancies. Its usefulness may be limited because of the possible promotion of adverse allergic responses.

Tumor necrosis factor (TNF), a cytokine that has demonstrated considerable antitumor activity both in vitro and in vivo, has limited therapeutic potential because of its considerable systemic toxicity. Gene therapy strategies in which genes encoding TNF are introduced into TIL in an attempt to make use of the antitumor activity of this cytokine at the microenvironmental level are, however, being developed. This strategy may also prove useful in the application of IL-4 and other cytokines with antitumor activity as immunomodulators.

Interleukin-10 (IL-10), a cytokine with primarily counterregulatory properties, may be useful in the treatment of autoimmune diseases or other disorders of inflammation. It has marked antiproliferative and anti-inflammatory effects in vitro. The clinical usefulness of IL-10 is currently not well defined, however, and may be limited by its stimulatory effects on mast cells and IgE production.

Interleukin-12 (IL-12) is a cytokine with fascinating actions that has potential immunomodulatory functions. It appears to induce or augment CD8 cytotoxic responses when administered with antigen. This raises the possibility that this compound could be employed as an adjuvant to induce cytotoxic, or T_H2-like, responses to particular antigens. A T_H2 response would be useful for antitumor immunity, immunity to viruses, and in AIDS, and preliminary data in animals has suggested the effectiveness of IL-12 in some of these applications. Unfortunately, toxicity and unexpected deaths were noted in initial clinical studies. Although this may be overcome by employing different administration schedules, the potential of this compound as an immunomodulator remains unclear.

Colony-Stimulating Factors

Three cytokines with colony-stimulating properties have been studied extensively and are now being used routinely or experimentally in humans. They are erythropoietin, now used routinely to treat anemia in patients with chronic renal disease; granulocyte colony-stimulating factor (G-CSF); and granulocyte–macrophage colony-stimulating factor (GM-CSF). G-CSF hastens recovery from neutropenia in patients with nonmyelogenous malignancies who are receiving chemotherapy. GM-CSF is used to accelerate marrow recovery after autologous bone marrow transplantation. CSFs are also being explored experimentally in the treatment of leukopenia of other causes, including primary neutropenia, myelodysplasia, myeloproliferative disorders, aplastic anemia, AIDS, and the neutropenia associated with Felty's syndrome. CSFs appear to have less potential benefit in the treatment of diseases associated with increased peripheral destruction of leukocytes, such as autoimmune neutropenia or Evans' syndrome.

Growth & Differentiation Factors

Perhaps the best studied growth and differentiation factor is transforming growth factor beta (TGF-β), which has a wide range of effects on the immune response. Its uses in a variety of areas are being explored. It has potential benefit as an accelerator of wound healing and may have applications in this regard in ophthalmology, dermatology, and surgical wound healing. It is also reported to have antiproliferative and anti-inflammatory effects in vitro and may prevent postinflammatory fibrotic changes. It also markedly inhibits the IL-4-stimulated synthesis of IgE and may be clinically useful as an antiallergy drug. Other growth factors, such as epidermal growth factor, platelet-derived growth factor, and fibroblast growth factor, are being studied for potential clinical utility in wound healing and revascularization.

There is evidence to suggest that glomerulonephrosis and glomerulosclerosis may be attributable in part to deleterious effects of TGF-β, in particular the excessive accumulation of extracellular matrix proteins. This cytokine has also been suspected in the pathogenesis of systemic sclerosis. A naturally occurring proteoglycan, decorin, has been shown to bind to and effectively inactivate TGF-β and may have potential clinical utility in diseases associated with excessive TGF-β activity.

Cell-Surface Molecules

Fas (CD95, APO-1) is a molecule on the surface of target cells that induces cell suicide when it binds to its ligand on lymphoid cells. When Fas is engaged by its ligand, lymphoid cell signal transduction takes place and activates a unique set of enzymes that induce among other events, DNA fragmentation. This process, called apoptosis, appears to be a major mechanism for regulating the immune response. Fas and its ligand have structural homology to the TNF receptor and TNF, respectively, but their interaction is specific. Fas-mediated apoptosis has recently been identified as involved in a number of crucial processes in the regulation of the immune response. Fas is one of the two major pathways that mediates CD8 cytotoxicity (the other being perforin) and may be the primary mechanism in lysis of target tissues in autoimmune diseases. It also appears that Fas-induced apoptosis may be important in the thymic selection of T cells. Activated CD4/CD8, double-positive thymocytes express Fas and are sensitive to the induction of apoptosis through the interaction of Fas. Therefore Fas activation could serve as a mechanism for the negative selection of T cells in the thymus. Fas may also play a role in the maintenance of peripheral immune tolerance in that autoreactive B cells are selectively killed through Fas-mediated interactions. Most interesting is the recent observation that immunologically privileged sites may maintain this unique status through Fas-mediated inhibition of immune responses. These tissues express high levels of the Fas ligand and T cells that interact with "privileged" tissues are eliminated by the induction of apoptosis before they can mediate target cell lysis. This suggests the fascinating concept that these privileged sites are not passively hidden from the immune system but are actively involved in preventing immune damage. Thus, the interaction between Fas and Fas ligand may provide a therapeutic target for the immunotherapy of neoplasms and immunosuppressive therapy of transplantation and autoimmune disease.

3. CYTOKINE ANTAGONISTS

A great deal of interest has recently developed in the potential use of cytokine antagonists as immunomodulatory drugs. This has been due primarily to the identification and characterization of a naturally occurring interleukin-1 receptor antagonist (IL-1RA). IL-1RA is a 152-amino-acid peptide, which shares a great deal of sequence homology with both IL-1β and IL-1γ. It binds to the IL-1 receptor with similar affinity; however, it does not lead to receptor-mediated activation of target cells. IL-1RA has demonstrable anti-inflammatory activity in animal models of a variety of human diseases, many attributed at least in part to excessive production of IL-1. These include septic shock, ischemia-reperfusion injury, inflammatory bowel disease, adult respiratory distress syndrome, polyarteritis nodosa, osteoporosis, and glomerulonephritis. IL-1RA does not appear to induce immunosuppression and must be present in at least 100-fold excess over IL-1 to exert its inhibitory effects, suggesting that high doses may be needed to elicit a clinical response. Clinical trials of IL-1RA in the treatment of rheumatoid arthritis, inflammatory bowel disease, and septic shock are under way.

4. MONOCLONAL ANTIBODIES

A variety of monoclonal antibodies have been developed and proposed as potential immunomodulators, and some have been used experimentally in clinical situations. Pilot studies with murine monoclonal anti-TNF antibodies have demonstrated improvement in acute graft-versus-host disease, improved left-ventricular function in septic shock, and possible improvement in hairy cell leukemia. Benefits appeared to be transient, however, and mortality has not been affected in the limited studies performed so far. Studies in a murine model have suggested a possible role for anti-TNF antibodies in the treatment of autoimmune myocarditis, but animal studies of the efficacy of this agent in the treatment of septic shock are inconclusive.

Antiendotoxin monoclonal antibodies have been used in the treatment of gram-negative sepsis, and decreased blood levels of TNF have been documented following their administration. Data on clinical efficacy, however, are still inconclusive.

Animal studies have demonstrated immunomodulatory effects of monoclonal antibodies directed against other mediators of inflammation, including IL-6, the adhesion molecule CD11b/18, and the 55-kd receptor for TNF. The usefulness of monoclonal antibodies in the treatment of human disease is limited in many instances, however, by the development of antimurine antibodies. Future research in this area, for example the splicing of murine variable region immunoglobulin genes with human constant region genes to yield less immunogenic "hybrid" monoclonal antibodies, may render these compounds better suited to clinical use.

BIOCHEMICAL AGENTS

Primarily because of the advent of AIDS, a variety of biochemical agents have been explored as potential immunomodulators. Many of these agents, although promising in in vitro studies, unfortunately have demonstrated little benefit in vivo. Some agents, however, have shown clinical benefit in other applications.

Perhaps the best known biochemical immunomodulator is levamisole, an imidathiazole compound originally studied for its anthelmintic activity. It is immunotrophic; however, its mechanism of action is unknown and it exhibits no direct cytotoxic activity. It has little effect in immunocompetent individuals. It has been shown to reverse postviral anergy associated with measles and influenza and has some benefit in chronic infections, malignancies, and neoplastic diseases. A well-defined role for levamisole as an adjunct in the treatment of colon cancer has been established. In a study of 262 patients with Duke's class C colon cancer, addition of levamisole to 5-fluorouracil led to an increased 5-year survival rate from 37 to 49%. The use of levamisole as an adjunct in the treatment of malignant melanoma and other neoplasms is being explored.

A related imidazole drug, inosine pranobex, has been shown in two studies of HIV-infected patients to delay the progression to AIDS. Controversy exists, however, about its optimal dose, toxicity, use in combination with other drugs, and overall benefit. The compound diethyldithiocarbamate also has reported activity in the treatment of HIV infection and some cancers.

Other immunostimulatory drugs, among them polyribosinic agents, anthroguinones, and pyrimidinolones, probably act via their ability to induce the production of interferons. Aziridine derivatives, of which Imexone is perhaps the best studied, have been shown to be effective in a murine model of AIDS. A related compound, Azimexone, appears to stimulate delayed hypersensitivity in animal models; however, it paradoxically inhibits graft-versus-host responses via an unknown mechanism. Aziridine derivatives have so far shown no benefit in the treatment of cancer. These and many other agents are being evaluated for potential therapeutic benefit in a variety of other immune disorders.

REFERENCES

GENERAL

Chirigos MA: Immunomodulators: Current and future development and application. *Thymus* 1992;**19**:S7.

Hadden JW: Immunopharmacology and immunotoxicology. *Adv Exp Med Biol* 1991;**288**:1.

Hassner A, Adelman DC: Biologic response modifiers in primary immunodeficiency disorders. *Ann Intern Med* 1991;**115**:294.

Perren T, Selby P: Biological therapy. *Br Med J* 1992; **304**:1621.

CYTOKINES

Balmer CM: Clinical use of biologic response modifiers in cancer treatment: An overview. Part II. Colony stimulating factors and interleukin-2. *Drug Intell Clin Pharm* 1991;**25**:490.

Blackwell S, Crawford J: Colony-stimulating factors: Clinical applications. *Pharmacotherapy* 1992;**12**:21S.

Hom DB, Maisel RH: Angiogenic growth factors: Their effects and potential in soft tissue wound healing. *Ann Otol Rhinol Laryngol* 1992;**101**:349.

Pardoll DM et al: Molecular engineering of the antitumor response. *Bone Marrow Transplant* 1992;**9**:182S.

Rees RC: Cytokines as biologic response modifiers. *J Clin Pathol* 1992;**45**:93.

Ruocco V et al: Malignant melanoma: Biotherapeutic strategies for management with interferons. *Clin Dermatol* 1992;**9**:505.

Thompson RC et al: Interleukin-1 receptor antagonist (IL-1ra) as a probe and as a treatment for IL-1 mediated disease. *Int J Immunopharmacol* 1992;**14**:475.

CELL SURFACE MOLECULES

Clement MV, Stamenkovic I: Fas and tumor necrosis factor receptor-mediated cell death: Similarities and distinctions. *J Exp Med* 1994;**180**(2):557.

Nagata S, Suda T: Fas and Fas ligand: lpr and gld mutations. *Immunol Today* 1995;**16**(1):39.

MONOCLONAL ANTIBODIES

Herve P et al: Phase I–II trial of a monoclonal anti-tumor necrosis factor alpha antibody for the treatment of refractory severe acute graft-versus-host disease. *Blood* 1992;**79**:3362.

BIOCHEMICAL COMPOUNDS

Amery W, Bruynseels J: Levamisole, the story and the lessons. *Int J Pharmacol* 1992;**14**:481.

De Simone C et al: Inosine pranobex in the treatment of HIV infection: A review. *Int J Immunopharmacol* 1991; **13**:19S.

60

Anti-Inflammatory Drugs

James S. Goodwin, MD

The distinction between immunosuppressive and anti-inflammatory drugs is not always clear, because of the extensive interaction between the immune response and inflammation. In this chapter, drugs with anti-inflammatory activity mediated at least in part by suppression of the functions of the nonspecific inflammatory cells, especially monocytes, polymorphonuclear leukocytes, and basophils, are discussed. These drugs are effective in treating inflammation whether or not the inflammation is initiated immunologically. Drugs that primarily suppress the immune response are discussed in Chapter 58.

CORTICOSTEROIDS

Glucocorticoids are the most powerful drugs currently available for the treatment of inflammatory diseases, but their use is associated with significant toxicity (also see Chapter 58). The discovery of corticosteroids was a major advance in the treatment of inflammatory diseases. Since the first successful use in 1948 of hydrocortisone (cortisol), the principal glucocorticoid of the adrenal cortex, for suppression of the clinical manifestations of rheumatoid arthritis, numerous compounds with glucocorticoid activity have been synthesized and are presently standard therapy for many immunologic and nonimmunologic inflammatory conditions.

Pharmacology & Physiology

Corticosteroids are 21-carbon steroid hormones derived from the metabolism of cholesterol. Figure 60–1 shows the structures of the commonly used synthetic corticosteroids. The activity of corticosteroids depends on the presence of a hydroxyl group on carbon-11. Two of the most commonly used corticosteroids, cortisone and prednisone, are inactive until converted in vivo to the corresponding 11-hydroxyl compounds—cortisol and prednisolone.

The clinical potency of the various synthetic

steroids depends on their rate of absorption, concentration in target tissues, affinity for steroid receptors, and rate of metabolism and subsequent clearance. Table 60–1 shows the half-lives and relative potencies of the commonly used glucocorticoid preparations. Most are well absorbed after oral administration. Corticosteroid uptake is not usually affected by intrinsic intestinal diseases, and food intake does not influence absorption. Approximately 90% of endogenous circulating cortisol is bound with high affinity to the plasma protein corticosteroid-binding globulin. Another 5–8% is bound to albumin, a high-capacity but low-affinity reservoir for steroids. Most synthetic steroids, with the exception of prednisolone, have a low affinity for corticosteroid-binding globulin and are bound predominantly to albumin. Only the small fraction of circulating corticosteroids that are not protein-bound are free to exert a biologic action, whereas those associated with proteins are protected from metabolic degradation.

Corticosteroids are metabolized in the liver. Hydroxylation of the 4,5 double bond and ketone groups and subsequent conjugation with glucuronide or sulfate render steroids inactive and water-soluble. The kidney excretes 95% of the conjugated metabolites, and the remainder are lost in the gut. There are individual differences in the half-lives of synthetic steroids, and patients receiving those with prolonged clearance may be at increased risk for side effects from therapy. Clearance rates of corticosteroids are also affected by other drugs and disease states. Phenytoin, phenobarbital, and rifampin can increase steroid clearance by inducing hepatic-enzyme activity. Estrogen therapy and estrogen-containing oral contraceptives impair the clearance of administered steroids and may decrease the steroid requirement. In patients with liver diseases, the metabolism of corticosteroids is not significantly altered, and dose adjustments are not necessary. Dose adjustments are also generally not necessary for patients with kidney disease. Corticosteroids can lower plasma salicylate

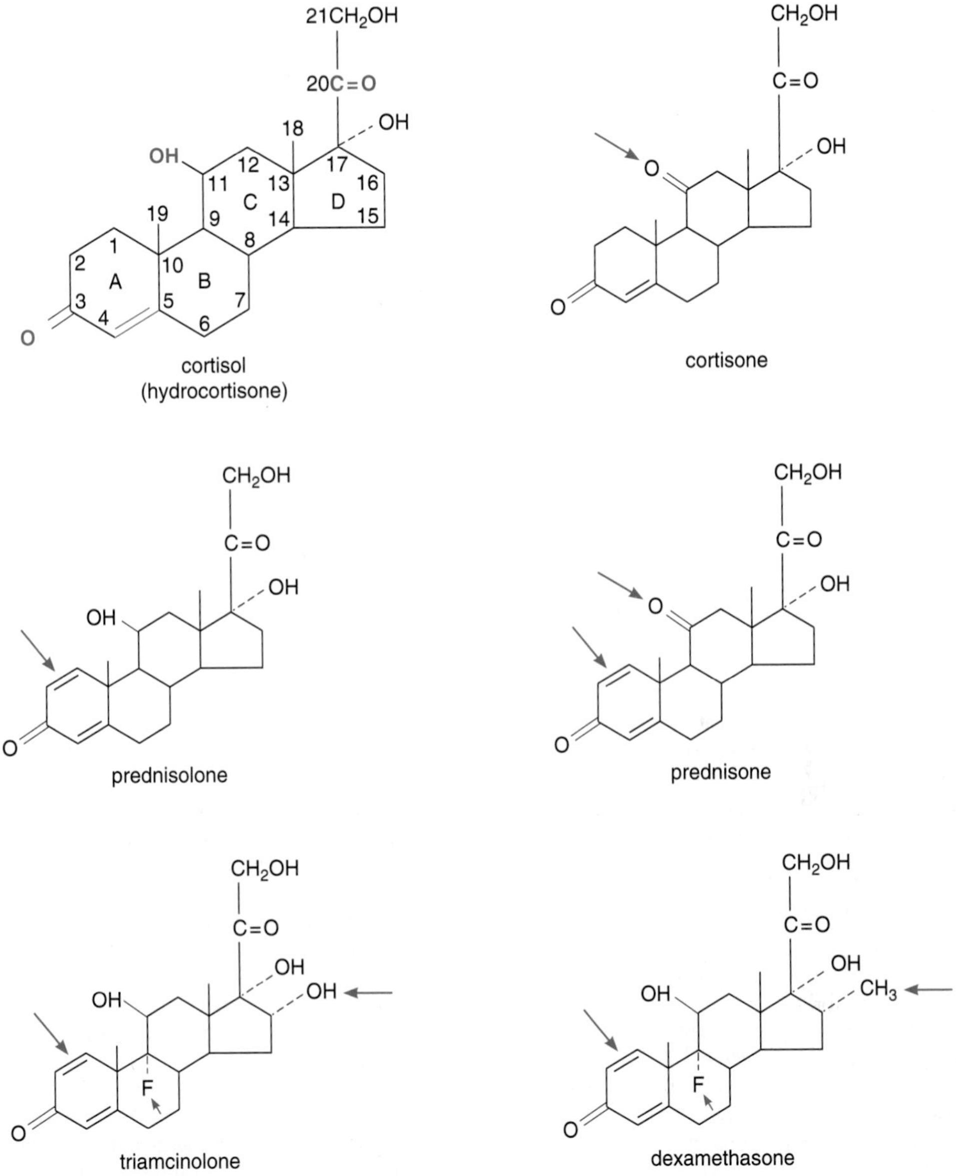

Figure 60–1. Structures of corticosteroid hormones and drugs. The arrows indicate the structural differences between cortisol and each of the other compounds.

Table 60–1. Half-life relative potency of commonly used glucocorticoids.

Glucocorticoid	Plasma Half-Life (min)	Relative Glucocorticoid Potency	Relative Mineralocorticoid Potency
Cortisol	80–120	1.0	1.0
Cortisone	80–120	0.8	0.8
Prednisone	200–210	4.0	0.8
Prednisolone	120–300	5.0	0
Triamcinolone	180–240	5.0	0
Dexamethasone	150–270	30–150	0

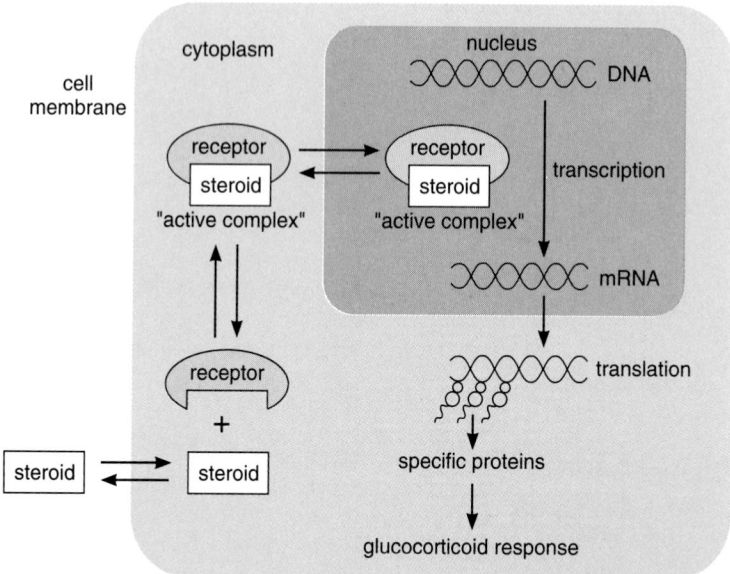

Figure 60–2. Mechanism of action of steroid hormones on a molecular level.

levels by enhancing their renal clearance. Patients on fixed-dose salicylate therapy may develop rapid increases to toxic levels of serum salicylate when glucocorticoids are withdrawn or tapered.

Mechanism of Action

All steroid hormones, including vitamin D, corticosteroids, sex hormones, and mineralocorticoid, act by binding to high-affinity receptors in the cytoplasm (Fig 60–2). The steroid–receptor complex, in turn, has a high affinity for nuclear interphase chromosomes and thus binds to chromosomal DNA. This triggers DNA transcription, with the formation of messenger RNA, leading to new protein synthesis. The specific genes transcribed and proteins produced after exposure to steroid hormones vary with the different steroid hormones and also with the target cell. Specificity of cell response is manifested in at least two ways. (1) The steroid-receptor complex binds to specific regulatory sequences, which, in turn, leads to transcription of the particular gene containing that sequence. Presumably the steroid–receptor complex binding vitamin D attaches to regulatory sequences on different genes from those used by the complex binding cortisol. (2) Only a small portion of the genome is capable of induction by steroid hormone because it is contained in an "unraveled" portion of chromatin sensitive to digestion with DNase. This unraveled portion differs depending on the cell type.

The mechanism of steroid action outlined in Figure 60–2 is consistent with the delay in appearance of the pharmacologic or physiologic effects after drug administration. Some effects of glucocorticoids and other steroids are rapid, however, implying that other mechanisms of action may also be operating.

Cells exposed to glucocorticoids synthesize and release a phospholipase A_2-inhibitory glycoprotein, now termed lipomodulin. The inhibition of phospholipase A_2 leads, in turn, to a reduction in the release of arachidonic acid, thereby slowing production of arachidonic acid metabolites. Lipomodulin appears to be a family of molecules, one of which was recently cloned and found to have potent anti-inflammatory actions. Thus, the anti-inflammatory actions of glucocorticoids may be related, at least in part, to lipomodulin-induced reduction of arachidonic acid metabolites—the prostaglandins and leukotrienes that are generated by cyclooxygenase and lipoxygenase, respectively. The role of prostaglandins and leukotrienes in mediating various aspects of the inflammatory response is discussed in Chapter 12.

Anti-Inflammatory Effects

Administration of corticosteroids results in a complex series of changes in the actions of cells involved in inflammatory reactions. After a single dose of steroids, there is a net increase in the number of circulating neutrophils, accompanied by a decrease in the margination, migration, and accumulation of neutrophils at sites of inflammation, which reduces the signs of acute inflammation and also interferes with the expression of delayed-type hypersensitivity skin reactions.

Corticosteroids also directly suppress the action of cells involved in the inflammatory response, inhibiting phagocytosis by neutrophils and monocytes, the production of degradative enzymes such as collage-

Table 60–2. Effects of glucocorticoids on molecules involved in inflammation.

Increased Production	Decreased Production
Lipomodulin	Collagenase
	Elastase
	Plasminogen activator
Cytokine receptors	Tumor necrosis factor
Neutral endopeptidase	Interleukin-1, IL-6, IL-8

nase and plasminogen activator by neutrophils and synovial lining cells, and the production of inflammatory lymphokines and monokines such as interleukin-1 and tumor necrosis factor (Table 60–2). The inhibition of these factors prevents the vasodilatation and increased vascular permeability components of the inflammatory response.

A discussion of related immunosuppressive effects of corticosteroids is in Chapter 58.

Metabolic Effects

Like other hormones, corticosteroids affect many different tissue and organ systems. At physiologic concentrations, their various metabolic effects presumably maintain normal homeostasis, but at the high concentrations used pharmacologically (or from pathologic overproduction), an accentuation of these same metabolic effects leads to target organ dysfunction.

A summary of the metabolic effects of glucocorticoids is given in Table 60–3. In general, steroids promote catabolism. They block glucose uptake by tissues; enhance protein breakdown; and decrease new

Table 60–3. Metabolic effects of glucocorticoids.

Carbohydrate metabolism
  Impairs glucose uptake and utilization by peripheral tissues.
  Increases gluconeogenesis and glycogen deposition in liver.

Lipid metabolism
  Stimulates lipolysis and increases free fatty acid levels, an effect countered by increased insulin release and gluconeogenesis.
  Increases fat deposition in truncal and facial areas.

Protein metabolism
  Inhibits synthesis and enhances breakdown of proteins in many tissues, leading to negative nitrogen balance.
  Increases plasma free amino acid levels.

Nucleic acid metabolism
  Stimulates RNA synthesis in liver, inhibits RNA synthesis in other tissues.
  Inhibits DNA synthesis in most tissues.

Fluid and electrolyte metabolism
  Mey enhance sodium retention and potassium loss independent of mineralocorticoid action.
  Increases glomerular filtration rate.

Bone and calcium metabolism
  Decreases intestinal calcium absorption.
  Decreases renal reabsorption of calcium and phosphate with resulting hypercalciuria.
  Inhibits osteoblast function.

protein synthesis in muscle, skin, bone, connective tissue, fat, and lymphoid tissue. DNA synthesis and cell proliferation in fibroblasts, lymphocytes, and adipocytes are inhibited. Chronic exposure to supraphysiologic levels of corticosteroids has a type of wasting effect, that is, loss of bone, connective tissue, and muscle and gain in water and fat.

Toxicity

The toxicities of prolonged corticosteroid therapy (listed in Table 60–4) are numerous and are the major limiting factor in the use of these agents. Susceptibility to side effects varies among patients; the reason for this is unknown. Some patients on prolonged, high-dose therapy appear to tolerate corticosteroids with few adverse effects, whereas others treated with small doses for brief intervals develop such devastating side effects as aseptic necrosis, osteoporosis, and vertebral collapse. In part, this differential sensitivity may be related to individual differences in plasma protein binding (with hypoalbuminemic patients at risk) and to variations in metabolism and clearance of synthetic steroids. Sensitivity to glucocorticoids in mice is closely linked to the H-2 histocompatibility region, and there is some evidence of analogous human leukocyte antigen (HLA) linkages in humans.

Table 60–4. Side effects of glucocorticoid therapy.

Very common and should be anticipated in all patients
  Negative calcium balance leading to osteoporosis.
  Increased appetite.
  Centripetal obesity with muscle wasting.
  Impaired wound healing.
  Increased risk of infection.
  Suppression of hypothalamic–pituitary–adrenal axis.
  Growth arrest in children.

Frequently seen
  Myopathy.
  Avascular necrosis.
  Hypertension.
  Plethora.
  Thin, fragile skin/striae/purpura.
  Edema secondary to sodium and water retention.
  Hyperlipidemia.
  Psychiatric symptoms, particularly euphoria or depression.
  Impaired glucose tolerance and diabetes.
  Posterior subcapsular cataracts.

Not very common, but important to recognize early
  Glaucoma.
  Benign intracranial hypertension.
  "Silent" intestinal perforation.
  Peptic ulcer disease (often gastric).
  Hypokalemic alkalosis.
  Hyperosmolar nonketotic coma.
  Gastric hemorrhage.

Rare
  Pancreatitis.
  Hirsutism.
  Panniculitis.
  Secondary amenorrhea.
  Impotence.
  Epidural lipomatosis.
  Allergy to synthetic steroids.

There are several useful approaches to reducing corticosteroid toxicity. One is through local application, as with topical ointments for dermatitis or administration via inhalers for asthma. Another is the use of so-called steroid-sparing drugs. These are drugs that may not have sufficient activity for use as first-line therapy but may allow a lowering of the dose of corticosteroids required to control disease activity. Drugs touted as steroid-sparing in asthma include those with demonstrable activity in other inflammatory conditions, such as dapsone, chloroquine, methotrexate, and gold. The macrolide antibiotics are "steroid-sparing" by inhibiting metabolism of corticosteroids, resulting in elevated blood levels.

ASPIRIN & OTHER NONSTEROIDAL ANTI-INFLAMMATORY DRUGS (NSAIDs)

Extracts of the willow tree (Latin, *salix*) had been used and endorsed by Hippocrates, Pliny, Galen, and other ancient practitioners for the relief of pain and fever. Later, willow bark extract (salicylate) was substituted for the more expensive and frequently unobtainable cinchona bark extract (quinine) in the treatment of pain and fever. Salicylates achieved widespread use by the end of the 19th century, when simple and inexpensive ways of synthesizing the drugs were discovered. Today 30 million lb of aspirin are consumed each year in the USA alone. Salicylates can be found in most households. Low-dose daily aspirin administration has been proven effective in the prevention of heart disease and stroke in high-risk patients, and there is increasing evidence that its chronic use is associated with a lower rate of colorectal and other cancers. In addition to the many oral formulations, salicylates are present in most skin liniments, plasters, and ointments. The newer nonsteroidal anti-inflammatory drugs (NSAIDs) are also in widespread use. Hundreds have been synthesized and dozens introduced for clinical use worldwide. As a class, NSAIDs are the most frequently prescribed medications for patients older than 65 years. Within the last several years, ibuprofen and naproxen have become available without a prescription, further contributing to the widespread consumption of NSAIDs.

Anti-Inflammatory Effects

The anti-inflammatory effects of the different NSAIDs are very similar in many experimental models, providing indirect support for the concept that they all share a single mechanism of action (discussed in the following section). NSAIDs prevent the pain, swelling, redness, and loss of function in experimental models of inflammation as diverse as sunburn and carrageenan-induced paw edema in rats. NSAID administration decreases the rate of progressive joint destruction associated with adjuvant-induced arthritis in rats. Clinically, NSAIDs have been shown to be effective in many acute and chronic inflammatory diseases, such as arthritis, tendinitis, and pericarditis, and they are analgesic, with at least some of the analgesic activities mediated by direct actions in the central nervous system.

Mechanism of Action

Since 1971, aspirin and other NSAIDs at therapeutic levels have been shown to inhibit the production of prostaglandins by inhibiting cyclooxygenase. The relative inhibiting potency in vitro of different NSAIDs generally parallels their anti-inflammatory potency in vivo. Cyclooxygenase inhibition became the in vitro screening test for new NSAIDs. More recently, two distinct cyclooxygenase molecules have been identified, termed COX-1 and COX-2. COX-1 is a constitutive enzyme found in most tissues and is responsible for the physiologic and homeostatic roles of prostaglandins. COX-2 is undetectable in most tissues under normal conditions but is rapidly inducible at sites of inflammation. Monocyte–macrophages and fibroblasts are rich in COX-2 after induction by inflammatory cytokines or endotoxins. There is approximately 60% homology between the COX-1 and COX-2 genes. All currently available NSAIDs inhibit both COX-1 and COX-2, reversibly binding at various sites in the channel leading to the enzyme's active site and thus sterically hindering the binding of arachidonic acid. Aspirin irreversibly inhibits both COX-1 and COX-2 by acetylating a serine residue in the active site. There are at least theoretical reasons to think that inhibition of COX-2 is responsible for the anti-inflammatory properties of NSAIDs, whereas COX-1 inhibition may lead to much of the toxicity. The development of highly selective COX-2 inhibitors is therefore a major goal of the pharmaceutical industry.

Prostaglandins cause vasodilation and sensitize pain receptors to other inflammatory mediators such as histamine. Prostaglandins are also involved in central control of temperature regulation and pain sensation. Other properties of NSAIDs may better explain their therapeutic anti-inflammatory effects. Inhibition of one or more lipoxygenase enzymes has been described for some NSAIDs in some in vitro systems. Also, by blocking cyclooxygenase, NSAIDs shunt arachidonic acid into metabolic pathways involving 5-, 12-, and 15-lipoxygenase, some of the products of which possess anti-inflammatory activity. NSAIDs inhibit cyclic adenosine monophosphate (AMP)-dependent protein kinase, phospholipase C, amino acid transport across cell membranes, and a variety of other membrane-associated events. The relative potency of various NSAIDs in inhibiting amino acid transport parallels their anti-inflammatory potency. All NSAIDs inhibit a variety of neutrophil and monocyte functions, such as aggregation, degranulation, and superoxide anion production, and this is not mediated via inhibition of prostaglandin production.

Table 60–5. Side effects of NSAID therapy.

Gastrointestinal
  Gastritis.
  Duodenal ulcer.
  Gastric ulcer.

Renal
  Decreased creatinine clearance.
  Acute renal failure.
  Interstitial nephritis.

Central nervous system
  Headache.
  Confusion, memory loss, personality change, especially in
    the elderly.

Toxicities not shared by all NSAIDs
  Bone marrow failure with phenylbutazone.
  Rash with meclofenamate.

Abbreviations: NSAIDs = nonsteroidal anti-inflammatory drugs.

Toxicity

The major side effects are listed in Table 60–5. Between 10 and 40% of patients in controlled trials of NSAIDs stop using the drug because of upper gastrointestinal symptoms such as pain, nausea, and vomiting. In clinical trials, approximately 1% of patients ingesting any NSAID develop upper gastrointestinal bleeding. It has been estimated that up to 25% of all hospitalizations for peptic ulcer disease are causally associated with NSAID use. Certain factors place patients at higher risk for gastrointestinal toxicity from NSAIDs (Table 60–6). NSAIDs should be avoided in these groups whenever possible. The mechanism of gastrointestinal toxicity is thought to involve three processes, two of which are secondary to cyclooxygenase inhibition: (1) Prostaglandin E is a local feedback inhibitor of hydrochloric acid secretion; (2) prostaglandin E has a cytoprotective effect on gastric mucosa independent of HCl secretion; and (3) all NSAIDs are organic acids that damage enterocyte function during absorption, uncoupling mitochondrial oxidative phosphorylation.

The rate of gastrointestinal bleeding from NSAIDs can be substantially reduced by the concurrent administration of misoprostol, a PGE_2 analogue. Most authorities recommend misoprostol if an NSAID must be administered to a patient at high risk for gastrointestinal bleeding.

The major renal complication of NSAID use is also related to cyclooxygenase inhibition. In patients with preexisting renal disease or circulatory disease resulting in decreased renal blood flow, NSAIDs tend to further reduce renal blood flow and glomerular filtration by eliminating prostaglandin-mediated compensatory mechanisms within the kidney. This becomes clinically important in some patients and can lead to total kidney failure, but it is almost always reversible on cessation of the drug. The prevalence of renal complications from NSAID is difficult to estimate, because it is too rare to be detected in most prospective, controlled clinical trials. In addition, patients most likely to experience renal toxicity because of preexisting renal or heart disease are likely to be excluded from those drug trials. Renal toxicity is rare in patients whose renal function is normal prior to the start of NSAID therapy.

Leukotriene Antagonists

A number of drugs in clinical testing block pathways of arachidonic acid metabolism other than cyclooxygenase (Fig 60–3). In addition to specific enzyme inhibitors for each of the pathways, there are also receptor antagonists for thromboxane, leukotriene B_4 (LTB_4), and the peptidoleukotrienes LTC_4, D_4, and E_4. These drugs are currently being tested for efficacy in treating diseases as diverse as asthma, psoriasis, glomerulonephritis, and inflammatory bowel disease.

COLCHICINE

Colchicine has largely been replaced in the treatment of acute gouty attacks by NSAIDs, which work quicker, are at least as efficacious, and are less toxic. It is sometimes used as an adjunctive therapy with NSAIDs in chronic or polyarticular gout and also as a prophylactic agent in low doses (0.6 mg once or twice daily) to prevent attacks.

Recently, prophylactic chronic colchicine ingestion has been found to reduce attacks of familial Mediterranean fever and to prevent the development of amyloidosis in patients with that disease. Colchicine has been reported to slow the progression of cirrhosis in patients with alcoholic liver disease.

The mechanism of action of colchicine is not completely understood. Colchicine binds to tubulin dimers, thereby preventing their polymerization to form microtubules. Microtubules are involved in many aspects of cell motion and function. The cellular target of colchicine in gout and pseudogout is the neutrophil, in which interference with microtubule formation prevents degranulation and the release of crystal-induced chemotactic factors, interleukin-1 (IL-1) and LTB_4.

GOLD, D-PENICILLAMINE, & ANTIMALARIALS

Gold, penicillamine, the antimalarial hydroxychloroquine, and perhaps also the various immunosuppressive

Table 60–6. Characteristics associated with increased risk of upper gastrointestinal bleeding with NSAIDs.

Advanced age.
History of peptic ulcer disease.
Concomitant corticosteroid use.
Concomitant anticoagulant use.
Low functional status.
Alcohol-related disease.

Abbreviations: NSAIDs = nonsteroidal anti-inflammatory drugs.

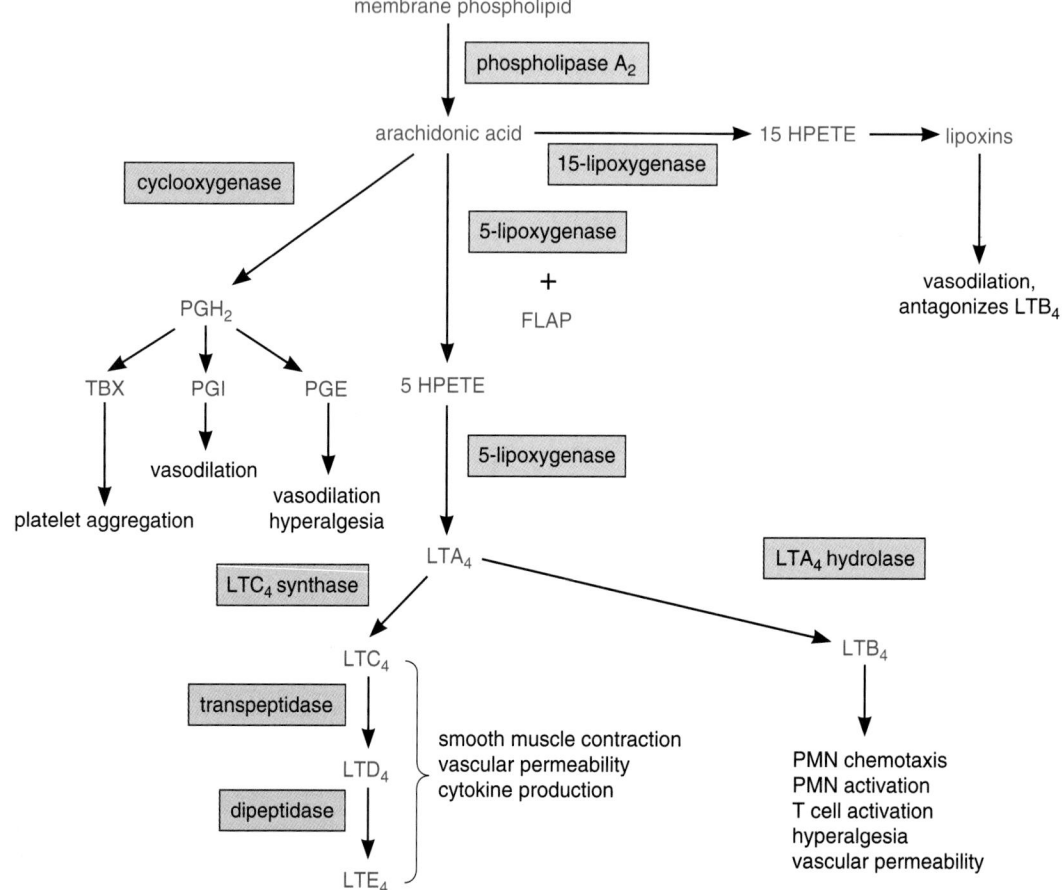

Figure 60–3. Metabolism of arachidonic acid, with contribution of metabolites to the inflammatory response.

drugs (see Chapter 58) share a number of properties when used to treat rheumatoid arthritis and other diseases. (1) These drugs require one to several months before any benefit is noted. (2) They can produce a clinical remission wherein no subjective or objective evidence of continued disease activity remains. (3) They have a narrow therapeutic spectrum. For example, gold has efficacy in rheumatoid arthritis and psoriatic arthritis but not significantly in other chronic inflammatory arthritides such as ankylosing spondylitis or systemic lupus erythematosus. (4) Many of the toxicities of the individual drugs in this class are similar. For example, gold and penicillamine can both cause rash, mouth ulcers, neutropenia, and nephritis. (5) They have little or no activity in experimental animal models of arthritis. (It is ironic that the animal models now used to screen for new treatments for arthritis would not have allowed for the discovery of the most efficacious drugs!) (6) Their mechanism of action is unknown.

In general, gold and penicillamine are considered more efficacious but also more toxic than antimalarial drugs in the treatment of rheumatoid arthritis.

Approximately 50% of patients taking gold or penicillamine stop the medication within 5 years of beginning treatment—two thirds of these because of toxicity and one third because of lack of efficacy. The major serious side effect of antimalarial drugs is retinal toxicity, which can be prevented by yearly ophthalmologic examinations.

DRUGS THAT SUPPRESS IMMEDIATE-HYPERSENSITIVITY REACTIONS

Cromolyn Sodium

Cromolyn sodium inhibits the release of mediators from mast cells, thereby blocking the tissue response and symptoms of IgE-mediated allergy. The precise mechanism of action of cromolyn sodium is unknown, but there is evidence that it interferes with calcium influx through the cell membrane. It does not interfere with the binding of IgE to mast cells nor with the interaction of antigen with the IgE bound to mast

Table 60–7. Actions of histamine at H_1 receptor sites inhibited by antihistamine.

Increased capillary permeability following histamine or antigen challenge.

Smooth muscle constriction, particularly bronchial and gastrointestinal tract.

Stimulation of sensory nerve endings, leading to pruritus and sneezing.

Secretion of exocrine glands.

Table 60–8. Commonly used antihistamines (H_1 blockers).

Classic	New Generation
Alkylamines Chlorpheniramine Dexchlorpheniramine Brompheniramine Triprolidine	Acrivastine[1,2]
Ethanolamines Diphenhydramine Dimenhydrate Clemastine Cinarrizine[2]	Ketotifen[2] Oxatomide[2]
Ethylenediamines Tripelennamine	
Piperazines Hydroxyzine Meclizine	Cetirizine[1,3]
Phenothiazines Promethazine	Mequitazine[1,2,3]
Piperidines Cyproheptadine Azatidine	Loratidine[1,3] Astemizole[1,3] Terfenadine[1] Azelastine[2]

[1] Nonsedative.
[2] Not available in the USA (as of Dec., 1995).
[3] Once-a-day dosage.

cells. Rather, it suppresses the degranulation normally triggered by the cross-linking of cell surface IgE by antigen.

Cromolyn sodium is effective only prophylactically. It is poorly absorbed after oral administration and is therefore effective only when administered topically to mucous membranes. It is available as a micronized powder in a metered-dose inhaler or as a powder for inhalation in a special dispenser for asthma, as a nasal aerosolized solution for allergic rhinitis, as eye drops for allergic conjunctivitis, and as an oral preparation for use in food allergies or for systemic mastocytosis. Nedocromil sodium is chemically unrelated but therapeutically similar to cromolyn.

The toxicity of cromolyn sodium is low and relates mostly to irritation produced by the inhaled powdered drug. It has no known utility in other inflammatory diseases.

Antihistamines

There are two classes of antihistamines, called H_1 and H_2 blockers, corresponding to two of the three types of histamine receptors found in mammalian tissues. Only H_1 blockers are considered here because H_2 blockers do not possess noticeable anti-inflammatory activity, although they are sometimes used to treat allergic diseases. The pharmacologic properties of H_1-blocking antihistamines are listed in Table 60–7.

The major therapeutic role for antihistamines is in the treatment of allergic diseases involving IgE-mediated hypersensitivity reactions. They are effective in reducing nasal and lacrimal secretions in seasonal rhinitis and conjunctivitis (hay fever). They are also effective in treating urticaria and angioedema, and they reduce pruritus associated with other dermatoses. Another major therapeutic role for antihistamines in the treatment of motion sickness and Ménière's disease.

The principal side effects of antihistamines are sedation, dryness of mucous membranes, and constipation. Several antihistamines have been developed that lack the sedative effect, probably because of their failure to penetrate the blood–brain barrier.

A large number of drugs have antihistaminic effects. The chemical classification of these drugs and representative examples are listed in Table 60–8.

Sympathomimetic (Adrenergic) Drugs

These drugs mimic the effects of sympathetic nerve stimulation. They have two general mechanisms of action: (1) stimulation of adrenergic receptors and (2) increase in the release of catecholamines from sympathetic nerve endings. Some drugs have both properties.

The sympathetic nervous system is not primarily involved in the pathogenesis of allergic disease, but in certain allergic reactions—particularly anaphylactic shock and acute asthma—the vascular and visceral effects evoke a secondary sympathomimetic response to maintain homeostasis of function in the affected organs. Sympathomimetic drugs are therefore highly effective in treating many manifestations of IgE-mediated allergy.

The diverse actions of sympathomimetic amines are explained by two classes of receptors, α and β, and their subclasses, α_1, α_2, β_1, and β_2 (Table 60–9).

α_1-Adrenergic agonists cause mucosal vasoconstriction and are widely used as nasal decongestants. Examples of such drugs are phenylephrine and phenylpropanolamine. A variety of β_2-selective bronchodilators are available for treatment of asthma. These include metaproterenol, terbutaline, albuterol, pirbuterol, isoetharine, and procaterol. Epinephrine is the drug of choice for treating anaphylaxis because it has powerful α- and β-stimulating effects necessary to counteract the systemic effects of anaphylaxis.

Methylxanthines

The methylxanthines include caffeine and theophylline. Their principal use is as central nervous system stimulants and as bronchodilators. Theophylline is poorly soluble in water and may be administered

Table 60–9. Tissue distribution and effects of different adrenergic receptors.

Receptor	Tissue Distribution	Action	Physiologic Effect
α_1	Vascular smooth muscle. Radial muscle of pupil. Trigone sphincter muscle. Pilomotor smooth muscle. Liver.	Contraction. Contraction. Contraction. Contraction. Increase gluconeogenesis.	Vasoconstriction. Dilate pupil. Inhibition of urination. Erect hair. Increase blood sugar.
α_2	Central nervous system adrenergic receptors. Platelets. Presynaptic peripheral adrenergic and cholinergic nerves. Some vascular smooth muscle. Gastrointestinal smooth muscle.	Activation. Aggregation. Inhibition of transmitter release. Contraction. Relaxation.	Diverse. Aggregation. Diverse. Vasoconstriction. Decreased motility.
β_1	Heart muscle. Coronary vessel smooth muscle. Fat cells.	Increase cyclic AMP.[1] Contraction. Increase cyclic AMP.	Increase heart rate, force of contraction, conduction velocity. Vasoconstriction. Lipolysis.
β_2	Bronchial smooth muscle. Liver. Kidney. Gastrointestinal smooth muscle.	Relaxation. Increase gluconeogenesis. Increased cyclic AMP. Relaxation.	Bronchodilation. Increased blood sugar. Increased renin secretion. Decreased motility.

Abbreviation: AMP = adenosine monophosphate.
[1] Activation of all β_1 or β_2 receptors results in increased cyclic AMP. A more distal action is listed, if known.

as a salt, such as aminophylline or oxytriphylline. Theophylline and its salts are used in treatment of chronic asthma. Side effects include nervousness, insomnia, tachycardia, ventricular arrhythmias, diuresis, anorexia, nausea, vomiting, and abdominal pain. The toxicity of theophylline is related to blood levels, which are easily obtainable in most clinical laboratories.

The mechanism of action is unknown. Methylxanthines inhibit phosphodiesterase, thereby slowing the metabolism of cyclic AMP and increasing cyclic AMP levels. Phosphodiesterase inhibition, however, requires a much higher theophylline concentration than is clinically effective for bronchodilatation. Another potential mechanism is antagonism of adenosine. Enprophylline, however, a methylxanthine and bronchodilator, reportedly is not an adenosine antagonist.

REFERENCES

GENERAL

Barnes PJ: A new approach to the treatment of asthma. *N Engl J Med* 1989;**321**:1517.

Bray MA, Morley J: *The Pharmacology of Lymphocytes.* Springer-Verlag, 1988.

McCarty DJ, Koopman WJ (editors): *Arthritis and Allied Conditions.* Lea & Febiger, 1993.

CORTICOSTEROIDS

Brann DW et al: Emerging diversities in the mechanism of action of steroid hormones. *J Steroid Biochem Molec Biol* 1995;**52**:113.

Davidson F et al: Inhibition of phospholipase A2 by "lipocortins" and calpactins. *J Biol Chem* 1987;**262**:1698.

Duval D, Freyss-Beguin M: Glucocorticoids and prostaglandin synthesis. *Prostaglandins Leukot Essent Fatty Acids* 1992;**45**:85.

Lamberts SWJ et al: Cortisol receptor resistance: The variability of its clinical presentation and response to treatment. *J Clin Endocrinol Metab* 1993;**74**:313.

Salem M et al: Perioperative glucocorticoid coverage. *Ann Surg* 1994;**219**:416.

Schleimer RP: An overview of glucocorticoid anti-inflammatory actions. *Eur J Clin Pharmacol* 1993;**45**(suppl 1):53.

NSAIDs

Bannwarth B et al: Where are peripheral analgesics acting? *Ann Rheum Dis* 1993;**52**:1.

Goodwin JS: Nonsteroidal anti-inflammatory drugs. In: *Clinical Immunology: Principles and Practice.* Rich RR (editor). Mosby, 1996, p 1959.

Hayllor J, Bjarnason I: NSAIDs, Cox-2 inhibitors, and the gut. *Lancet* 1995;**346**:521.

Henderson WR: The role of leukotrienes in inflammation. *Ann Intern Med* 1994;**121**:684.

Marcus AJ: Aspirin as prophylaxis against colorectal cancer. *N Engl J Med* 1995;**333**:656.

Patrano C: Aspirin as an antiplatelet drug. *N Engl J Med* 1994;**330**:1287.

COLCHICINE

Canaghan PG, Day RO: Risks and benefits of drugs used in the management and prevention of gout. *Drug Safety* 1994;**11**:252.

Goodwin JS, Goodwin JM: The tomato effect: Rejection of highly efficacious therapies. *JAMA* 1984;**251:**2387.

Merlini G: Treatment of primary amyloidosis. *Semin Hematol* 1995;**32:**60.

Smallwood JI, Malawigta SE: Colchicine, crystals, and neutrophil typosine phosphorylation. *J Clin Invest* 1993; **92:**1602.

GOLD & OTHER SECOND-LINE AGENTS FOR RHEUMATOID ARTHRITIS

Berlow BA et al: The effect of dapsone in steroid dependent asthma. *J Allergy Clin Immunol* 1991;**87:**710.

Felson DT et al: Use of short term efficacy/toxicity tradeoffs to select second line drugs in rheumatoid arthritis: A meta-analysis of published clinical trials. *Arthritis Rheum* 1992;**35:**1117.

Richter JA et al: Analysis of treatment terminations with gold and antimalarial compounds in rheumatoid arthritis. *J Rheumatol* 1980;**7:**153.

Thompson PW et al: Practical results of treatment with disease-modifying drugs. *Br J Rheumatol* 1985;**24:**167.

CROMOLYN SODIUM

Edwards AM: Sodium cromoglycate (Intal) as an anti-inflammatory agent for the treatment of chronic asthma. *Clin Exp Allergy* 1994;**24:**612.

ANTIHISTAMINES

Busse WW: Role of antihistamines in allergic disease. *Ann Allergy* 1994;**72:**371.

Simons FER, Simons KJ: The pharmacology and use of H₁ receptor-antagonist drugs. *N Engl J Med* 1994;**330:**1663.

SYMPATHOMIMETICS

Fanta CH et al: Treatment of acute asthma: Is combination therapy with sympathomimetics and methylxanthines indicated? *Am J Med* 1986;**80:**5.

Kemp JP: Approaches to asthma management. *Arch Intern Med* 1993;**153:**805.

Skorodin MS: Pharmacotherapy for asthma and chronic obstructive pulmonary disease. *Arch Intern Med* 1993; **153:**814.

THEOPHYLLINE

Ward AJ et al: Theophylline—An immunomodulatory role in asthma? *Am Rev Respir Dis* 1993;**147:**518.

Appendices

The CD Classification of Hematopoietic Cell Surface Markers*

Marker	Other Names	Cell Types/Lineages	Major Functions and Properties
CD1	T6	Cortical thymocytes, dendritic cells, B cells, intestinal epithelium.	Family of nonclassical MHC class I-like proteins; specialized forms of antigen presentation.
CD2	T11, sheep RBC receptor	T cells, NK cells.	Binds LFA-3 (CD58); signaling.
CD3	T3, Leu4	T lymphocytes.	Transduces signals from T-cell receptor; T-lineage marker.
CD4	T4, Leu3a	T lymphocytes, monocytes, macrophages, EBV-transformed B cells.	Coreceptor for class II MHC; marker for helper T cells; signaling; receptor for human immunodeficiency virus (HIV).
CD5	T1	T lymphocytes, some B cells.	Binds CD72; signaling; subset marker for B cells.
CD7	Leu9	T cells, NK cells, some lymphoid and myeloid precursors.	Early T-lineage marker; signaling.
CD8	T8, Leu2a	T lymphocytes.	Coreceptor for class I MHC; marker for cytotoxic T cells; signaling.
CD10	CALLA	B-cell precursors, marrow stroma.	Endopeptidase; marker for acute lymphocytic leukemia.
CD11a	LFA-1 α chain	Lymphocytes, monocytes, neutrophils, NK cells.	Integrin; binds ICAM-1 (CD54), ICAM-2, or ICAM-3; mediates leukocyte adhesion to other leukocytes or to endothelium.
CD11b	MAC-1, CR3	NK cells, monocytes, neutrophils.	Integrin; receptor for complement fragment C3bi, fibrinogen, or clotting factor X.
CD11c	CR4	NK cells, monocytes, neutrophils.	Integrin; receptor for complement fragment C3bi.
CD14	LeuM3	Monocytes.	LPS receptor.
CD15	Sialyl Lewis X	Granulocytes; some cutaneous T cells.	Oligosaccharide; bound by ELAM-1 protein on endothelial cells; T-cell homing receptor for skin.
CD16	FcγRIII	Macrophages, neutrophils, NK cells.	Low-affinity Fc receptor for IgG; lineage marker for NK cells.
CD18	LFA-1 β chain	T and B lymphocytes, monocytes, NK cells.	Integrin; binds ICAM-1 (CD54) or ICAM-2; mediates leukocyte-endothelial cell binding.
CD19	B4	B lymphocytes.	Signaling.
CD20	B1	B lymphocytes.	Signaling.
CD21	CR2, B2	B lymphocytes.	Receptor for complement fragment C3d, CD23, and EBV.
CD22		B lymphocytes.	Binds CD45RO (on T cells) or CD75 (on B cells); signaling.
CD23	FcεRII	Activated B cells, macrophages, eosinophils, thymic epithelium, platelets.	Low-affinity Fc receptor for IgE; ligand for CD21.
CD25	IL-2R α chain, Tac	Activated T and B lymphocytes, monocytes.	Low-affinity IL-2 receptor; marker for lymphocyte activation.
CD28	B7.1 (CD80) or B7.2 (CD86) proteins	Activated T lymphocytes (especially CD4 T cells), thymocytes.	Mediates costimulation of T cells by binding B7.1 (CD80) or B7.2 (CD86) proteins on activated APCs; signaling.
CD29	Integrin β1	All hematopoietic and many other cell types.	Integrin; binds to extracellular matrix components.

(continued)

* Only selected markers are listed. Certain CD designations (such as CD3) refer to heteromeric complexes of multiple polypeptide chains. Some CD proteins (such as the integrins) must associate with other proteins to mediate the functions listed here. *Abbreviations:* CALLA = common acute lymphocytic leukemia antigen; LFA = leukocyte functional antigen; MAC = membrane attack complex; NK = natural killer; EBV = Epstein-Barr virus; MHC = major histocompatibility complex; ICAM = intercellular adhesion molecules; VCAM = vascular cell adhesion molecule; IFN = interferon; TNF = tumor necrosis factor; IL = interleukin; MCSF = monocyte colony-stimulating factor; SCF = stem cell factor.

Marker	Other Names	Cell Types/Lineages	Major Functions and Properties
CD32	FCγRII	B lymphocytes, macrophages, neutrophils, eosinophils.	Medium-affinity Fc receptor for IgG complexes; signaling.
CD34		Lymph node HEV, hematopoietic stem cells, endothelium.	Sialomucin; ligand for L-selectin; vascular addressin in peripheral nodes; lineage marker for hematopoietic stem cells.
CD35	CR1	B lymphocytes, monocytes, neutrophils, some NK cells.	Receptor for complement fragments C3b and C4b.
CD38	T10	Activated lymphocytes.	Unknown.
CD40		B lymphocytes.	Mediates T cell help by binding inducible ligand (CD40L) on surface of activated T_H cells; signaling.
CD43	Leukosialin	T, B, and NK cells, monocytes.	Sialomucin ligand for ICAM-1 (CD54); deficient in Wiskott-Aldrich syndrome.
CD44	Hermes	T, B, and NK cells, monocytes.	Hyaluronate receptor; mediates leukocyte binding to other leukocytes, to endothelium, or to extracellular matrix; signaling.
CD45	Leukocyte common antigen; T200; B220 Isoforms: CD45R = 220 kd CD45RA = 205–220 kd CD45RO = 180 kd	All leukocytes.	Protein tyrosine phosphatase; multiple isoforms of extracellular domain owing to alternative RNA splicing; modulates signaling; CD45RO isoform (on T cells) binds CD22 (on B cells).
CD49d	VLA-4 α chain	T and B lymphocytes, monocytes.	Integrin; mediates leukocyte-endothelial cell interactions by binding VCAM-1.
CD54	ICAM-1	Activated lymphocytes, endothelial cells.	Binds LFA-1 or CD43; receptor for rhinoviruses and for *Plasmodium falciparum*.
CD55	Decay-accelerating factor	Many cell types.	Degrades C3 convertase on cell surfaces; prevents complement activation.
CD56	N-CAM	NK cells.	NK cell adhesion; lineage marker for NK cells.
CD58	LFA-3	Activated lymphocytes, many other cells.	Ligand for CD2.
CD62E	E-selectin	Endothelium.	Leukocyte–endothelial adhesion.
CD62L	L-selectin	Leukocytes.	Leukocyte–endothelial adhesion.
CD62P	P-selectin	Platelets, endothelium.	Leukocyte–endothelial adhesion.
CD63		Neutrophils, monocytes, platelets.	Activation marker for neutrophils and platelets.
CD64	FcγRI	Monocytes, macrophages.	High-affinity Fc receptor for IgG.
CD71	T9	Activated lymphocytes and macrophages, many proliferating cells.	Transferrin receptor.
CD72		B lymphocytes.	Ligand for CD5.
CD73	5′-Nucleotidase	Some B and T lymphocytes.	Ecto-5′-nucleotidase; may regulate nucleotide uptake.
CD74	Invariant chain	MHC class II-expressing cells.	Endocytic antigen presentation by MHC class II
CD79α,β	Ig-α, Ig-β	B lymphocytes.	Transduces signals from B-cell antigen receptor.
CD80	B7.1	B lymphocytes.	B-cell receptor for T cell CD28 (help) or CTLA-4 (inhibition).
CD86	B7.2	B lymphocytes.	B-cell receptor for T-cell CD28 (help) or CTLA-4 (inhibition).
CD89	FcαR	Leukocytes.	Fc receptor for IgA.
CD95	Fas, Apo-1	Many cell types.	Induces apoptosis on binding Fas ligand (Fas-L).
CD102	ICAM-2	Endothelial cells.	Binds LFA-1; leukocyte–endothelial adhesion.
CD106	VCAM-1	Endothelial cells.	Adhesion molecule.
CD115	c-*fms*	Monocyte–macrophages.	MCSF receptor.
CD117	c-*kit*	Hematopoietic progenitors.	SCF receptor.
CD118	IFNα,βR	Many cell types.	Receptor for type-1 interferons.
CD119	IFNγR	Monocyte–macrophages, B cells, endothelium.	Receptor for IFNγ.
CD120a,b	TNFR	Many cell types.	TNF receptor types I and II.
CD122	IL-2Rβ	NK cells, some B and T cells.	IL-2 receptor β chain.

Glossary of Symbols Used in Illustrations

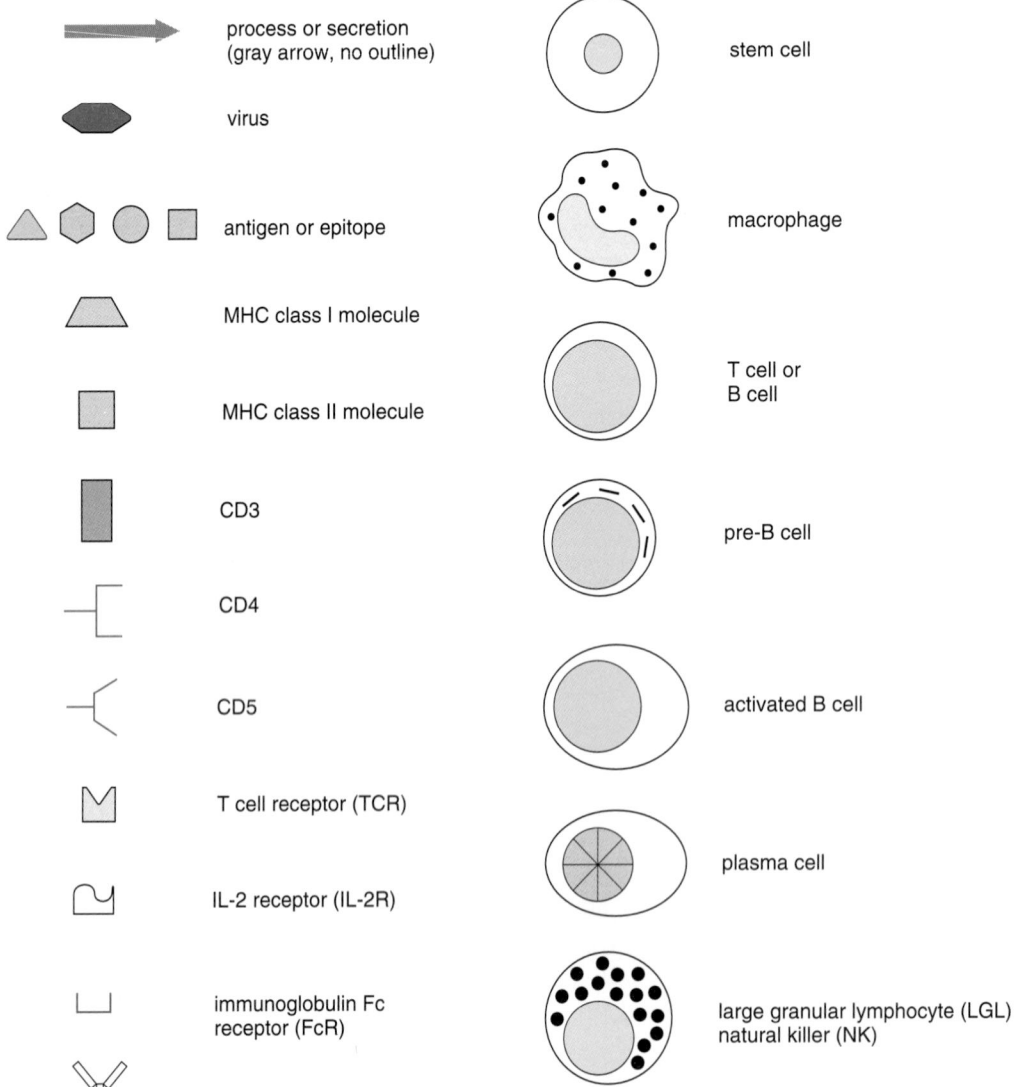

process or secretion
(gray arrow, no outline)

virus

antigen or epitope

MHC class I molecule

MHC class II molecule

CD3

CD4

CD5

T cell receptor (TCR)

IL-2 receptor (IL-2R)

immunoglobulin Fc
receptor (FcR)

immunoglobulin (Ig)

stem cell

macrophage

T cell or
B cell

pre-B cell

activated B cell

plasma cell

large granular lymphocyte (LGL)
natural killer (NK)

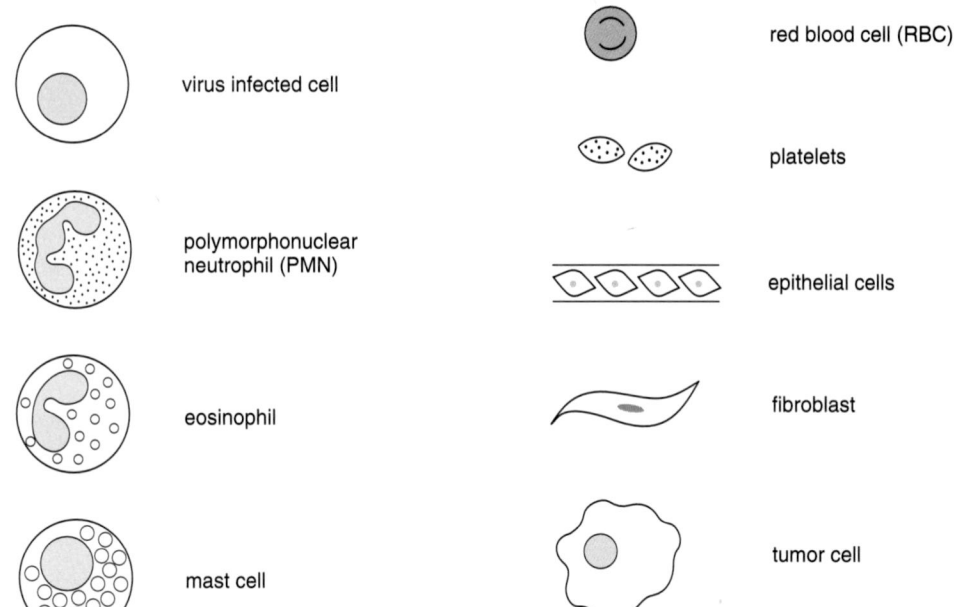

Index

Note: Page numbers followed by *t* or *f* indicate tables or figures, respectively.

α-Fetoprotein, **634**
α-Gene locus, 130–131, 131*f,* 132, 132*f*
ABO & H system, 275–276, 276*t,* 623–624
Abortion, recurrent and spontaneous, 621–622
Acanthocheilonema persians, 281
Acarus siro, 393
Acquired immune deficiency syndrome. *See* AIDS (acquired immune deficiency syndrome)
Acrosome reaction, 615
Actinobacillus actinomycetemcomitans, 542
Activation
    allergen-antibody, 379*t*
    antigen-nonspecific lymphocyte, 450
    B cell, 68
    cell death, 72
    complement system, 70, 169–170, 176–177, 177*f,* 192
    cytokine, 52
    cytolytic T lymphocyte, 68*f,* 68–69
    effector cell, 60
    helper T cell, 67–68, 68*f*
    kinin-generating system, 179–180
    lymphocyte, 44, 45*f,* 49–52, 51*f,* 51*t*
    mast cell, 185
    nonimmunologic classic pathway, 173
    phagocyte, 70
    platelet, 186
    T cell, 135–138
Activation phase of endothelial binding, 34
Active immunization, 767, 772–773, 774–781*t,* 782
Active suppression, 768
Acute disseminated encephalomyelitis, 582–583
Acute eosinophilic pneumonia, 604
Acute hepatitis B, 536
Acute inflammation, 36, 37, 182
Acute inflammatory demyelinating polyneuropathy, 583–584
Acute lymphoblastic leukemia (ALL), 662, 663*f,* 664, 821
Acute lymphocytic leukemia of childhood, 601
Acute myelogenous leukemia (AML), 820–821
Acute nephritic syndrome, 555
Acute-phase response, 28–29, 151
Acute viral bronchitis, 401–402
Acute viral hepatitis, 534
Addison's disease, 489
Adenohypophysitis, lymphocytic, 489–490
Adenosine, 188
Adenosine deaminase (ADA), 360–361, 361*f*
Adenosine monophosphate (AMP), 856
S-Adenosylhomocysteine, 360

Adhesion molecule
    antigen-presenting cells and T cell interaction, 138
    bone marrow interactions, 14–17, 16*t*
    lymphocyte binding, 61
    maturation and release of virgin lymphocyte, 118
    protein induced on activated endothelial cell, 30*t*
Adjuvant, 75, 82, 148
    antigen-nonspecific therapy, 768
    antigen-specific therapy, 767
    Complete Freund's, 846
    desensitization, 800
    mucosal, 206
Adoptive cellular immunotherapy, 637–638
Adoptive immunity, 767–768
Adrenal insufficiency, 489
Adrenergic drugs, 859, 860*t*
Adrenocorticotropic hormone (ACTH), 489
Adult immunization, 793
Adult respiratory distress syndrome (ARDS), 177, 611
Advisory Committee on Immunization Practices (A.C.I.P.), 793
Affinity chromatography, 226–227
Affinity maturation, 55, 126
African trypanosomiasis, 731–733, 733*f*
Agammaglobulinemia, X-linked, 116, 332*t,* 332–336, 333*f,* 339
Agglutination
    Bentonite flocculation test, 245
    Coombs' Test, 244–245
    direct test, 243
    inhibition of, 244
    latex fixation test, 245
    passive test, 243–244
    Rose-Waaler test, 245
Aggregate anaphylaxis, 413
Agranulocytosis, 494
AIDS (acquired immune deficiency syndrome), 435–436, 546, 596–597. *See also* HIV (human immunodeficiency virus)
    criteria for diagnosing, 753
    desensitization, 440
    expanding knowledge of human immunology, 766
    fungal disease, 706
    histoplasmosis, 716
    imexone, 851
    molecular heterogeneity of AIDS-associated lymphoma, 647, 647*t*
    Mycobacterium avium complex, 691
    syphilis, 739

AIDS-related complex (ARC), 752
Airway function test, 380, 381f
Allele and MHC protein, 86, 89t, 93
Allele-specific amplification with sequence-specific primers
   (PCR-SSP), 302, 303f
Allelic and isotypic exclusion, 117
Allergen
 activation, allergen-antibody, 379t
 allergic contact dermatitis, 426, 426t
 anaphylaxis, 412t, 412–413, 413t
 animal, 394
 arthropod, 392–394
 defining, 376
 desensitization with modified, 800
 extract, 394, 394t
 food, 394
 hypersensitivity pneumonitis, 428, 429t, 430–431
 mold, 391–392, 393f, 393t
 patch test, 382
 pollen, 391, 392f, 393
 urticaria, 417
Allergic asthma, 611
Allergic bronchopulmonary aspergillosis (ABPA), 602, 611
 asthma, 403
 cystic fibrosis, 423
 epidemiology, 421
 pathogenesis, immunologic, 421–422
Allergic contact dermatitis, 192
 allergen, 426, 426t
 clinical feature, 425–426
 defining, 425
 desensitization, 799
 diagnosis, immunologic/differential, 426, 426t
 drug allergy, 436
 epidemiology, 425
 eye disease, cell-mediated, 596
 immunologic feature, 425
 pathogenesis, immunologic, 425
 pathology, 425
 prevention, 426–427
 prognosis, 426
 treatment, 426
Allergic disease, 141
 granulomatosis of Churg and Strauss, 602t, 602–603
 immunization to ameliorate, 767
 mechanisms and classification
  effector T cell/lymphokine pathway, 379
  IgE/mast cell/mediator pathway, 377, 379t
  IgG or IgM complement/neutrophil pathway, 379
 nonatopic, 389
 rhinoconjunctivitis, 389
Allergic gastroenteropathy, 405–406
Allergic rhinitis
 clinical feature, 395
 complications, 397
 desensitization, 796, 797f
 diagnosis, immunologic/differential, 395
 epidemiology, 395
 general consideration, 394
 immunologic feature, 394
 pathogenesis, immunologic, 396
 treatment, 396–397
Allergic urticaria, 195
Allergoid, 800
Allergy. *See also* Desensitization; Drug allergy
 active immunization, 783
 allergen, 376
 asthma, 405
 atopic, 377. *See also Atop listings*

comparison with other illnesses, 376t
 defining, 376
 drug, 416
 food, 416
 general consideration, 379
 history, 379–380
 IgA deficiency, 340
 laboratory testing, 380–387
  airway function, 380, 381f
  anatomic, 382
  skin, 382–384, 383f, 383t
  tissue diagnosis, 382
  in vitro, 384, 385t
 latex, 413
 occupational, 394, 396, 401t, 428, 605
 photoallergic contact dermatitis, 427, 427t
 physical examination, 380
 susceptibility, 376–377
 transfusion reactions, 280
Allison, James, 3
Allograft monitoring, 816–819
Alloreaction, 91
Allotype variant, complement, 375
Alternative complement pathway, 173–174, 174f, 371, 558
Aluminum salts, 82
Alveolar macrophage, 606
Alveolitis, extrinsic allergic, 428–432, 429t
Alzheimer's disease, 588–589
American Society for Histocompatibility and Immunogenetics
   (ASHI), 293
Amino acid sequence variation, 440, 441t
Amino acid transport, 856
5-Aminosalicylic acid (5-ASA), 531
Amiodarone pneumonitis, 601
Amoxicillin, 440
Amphotericin B, 711, 715, 716, 720, 721
Ampicillin, 440
Amplification, types of PCR, 301–302, 303f, 304, 305–306f,
   307
Amyloidosis, 668, 669t
Amyotrophic lateral sclerosis, 588
Anabolic steroid, 374
Anaerobic bacteria, 679
Analyte, 231
Anamnestic immune response, 72
Anaphylactic reaction, 2, 419
 complement activation in inflammation, 176
 IgE-mediated inflammation, 195
 immunoglobulin, 335
Anaphylactoid reaction, 413, 414, 414t
Anaphylaxis
 allergen, 412t, 412–413, 413t
 clinical feature, 410–411
 complications and prognosis, 415–416
 defining, 409
 diagnosis, immunologic/differential, 411t, 411–412, 412t,
   414
 epidemiology, 409
 Hymenoptera venoms, 799
 pathogenesis, immunologic, 410
 pathology, 409
 prevention, 415
 treatment, 414–415
 urticaria and angioedema, 410
Anaplastic large-cell lymphoma (ALCL), 671–672
Anatomic test, 382
Ancylostoma caninum, 736
Ancylostoma duodenale, 736

Anemia
  aplastic, 501–502, 820
  immune hemolytic, 495–499, 496*t*, 498*t*
  pernicious, 533–534
Anergic B cell, 129
Anergy, 137, 254, 255*t*, 768
Anesthetic, 442
Aneurysm formation, 518
Angiitis of the central nervous system, isolated, 526
Angiocentric lymphoma, 671
Angioedema, 410, 416–418
  hereditary, 175, 180, 373–374
Angiography, 519, 519*f*
Angioimmunoblastic T cell lymphoma, 671
Angioinvasion, 706, 710–711*t*
Angiotensin-converting enzyme (ACE) inhibitor, 440, 561, 600
Anhepatic phase and liver transplantation, 811
Animal allergen, 394
Animal handler, 794
Animal sera, 785
Ankylosing spondylitis, 475–476, 592
Ann Arbor Staging Classification for Hodgkin's disease, 660
Anogenital cancer, 643–644
Anthrax, 1
Antibiotics
  asthma, 402
  Crohn's disease, 531
  drug allergy, 436
  inflammatory periodontal disease, 544
  Whipple's disease, 534
  x-linked agammaglobulinemia, 335–336
Antibody, 45. *See also* Immunoglobulin; Monoclonal antibody
  anticytoplasmic, systemic lupus erythematosus and, 460
  antierythrocyte, systemic lupus erythematosus and, 460
  antiglomerular basement membrane antibody-induced
    glomerulonephritis, 550–552, 552*f*
  antilymphocyte, 842
  antineutrophil cytoplasmic antibodies with circulating
    pattern, 522
  antineutrophil cytoplasmic antibodies with diffuse
    cytoplasmic pattern, 521
  antineutrophil cytoplasmic antibodies with perinuclear
    pattern, 519
  antinuclear, 456, 457*t*, 459
  antiphospholipid, 589
  antisperm, 615, 620–621
  β-lactam, 437–440, 438*t*
  bifunctional molecule, 95
  blocking, 798
  catalytic, 108
  cellular immunology, rebirth of, 2–3
  clinical laboratory methods for detecting
    agglutination, 243–244*t*, 243–245, 245*f*
    binder-ligand assay, 231–237, 232*f*, 234–236*f*
    comparative sensitivity of quantitative immunoassays,
      250, 251*t*
    complement assay, 245–249, 246–248*f*, 248–249*t*
    electrophoresis and immunoelectrophoresis, 216–224,
      217*t*, 218–225*f*, 224–225
    immunochemical and physicochemical methods,
      225–231, 226–227*f*, 228–229*t*, 230*f*
    immunodiffusion, 211–216, 212–215*f*
    immunohistochemical technique, 237–241*f*, 237–242,
      242*t*
    predictive value theory, 250–251, 251*t*
  Donath-Landsteiner, 499–500
  enzyme-linked, 242
  erythrocyte, coating surface of, 278*f*, 278–279
  eye disease, 591–594, 592–594*f*

  Fc receptors, 108*t*, 108–109
  herpes gestationis, 568
  host defense functions, 680, 681*t*
  immunologic therapy, 766
  influenza virus, 696
  nephritogenic antibody-antigen reaction, 549, 550*t*, 556*t*
  panel reactive, 292
  physiochemical basis of antigen-antibody binding, 78–79
  plasma cell, 67
  polyclonal, 842
  recurrent aphthous ulceration, 545
  serum, 2, 71
  syphilis, 740
  technologies, 106, 107*f*, 108
  tissue-destruction, 454
  tubulointerstitial nephritis, 559–561
Antibody (B cell) immunodeficiency disorder
  Good's syndrome, 343
  IgA deficiency, selective, 339–342
  IgM, hyper-, 339
  5-nucleotidase deficiency, 343
  selective deficiency of IgG subclasses, 342–343, 343*f*
  selective IgM deficiency, 342
  transcobalamin II deficiency, 344
  transient hypogammaglobulinemia of infancy, 336*f*,
    336–337
  variable immunodeficiency, common, 337–339
  X-linked agammaglobulinemia, 332*t*, 332–336, 333*f*
Antibody-coated erythrocytes (EA), 247
Antibody-dependent cell-mediated cytotoxicity (ADCC), 70,
  108, 144, 638, 681, 807
Antibody-mediated immune suppression (AMIS), 624–625
Antibody-mediated immunity, evaluation of, 332*t*
Anticardiolipin antibody syndrome, 509–510
Anticholinesterase drug, 587
Anticytoplasmic antibody, 460
Antiendotoxin monoclonal antibody, 850
Antierythrocyte antibody, 460
Antigen, 50, 51. *See also* Human leukocyte antigen (HLA);
    Immunogen; T cell receptor (TCR)
  active immunization, 772–773
  binding site, 97
  Celiac disease, 529
  clinical laboratory methods for detecting
    agglutination, 243–244*t*, 243–245, 245*f*
    binder-ligand assay, 231–237, 232*f*, 234–236*f*
    comparative sensitivity of quantitative immunoassays,
      250, 251*t*
    complement assay, 245–249, 246–248*f*, 248–249*t*
    electrophoresis and immunoelectrophoresis, 216–221,
      217*t*, 218–225*f*, 224–225
    immunochemical and physicochemical methods,
      225–231, 226–227*f*, 228–229*t*, 230*f*
    immunodiffusion, 211–216, 212–215*f*
    immunohistochemical technique, 237–241*f*, 237–242,
      242*t*
    monoclonal antibodies, 249–250, 250*f*, 250*t*, 251*t*
    predictive value theory, 250–251, 251*t*
  clonal organization, 63–65, 64*f*
  cross-reactivity, 481
  cytosolic pathway, 84–85
  elimination, mechanisms of, 69–70
  endocytic pathway, 83–84, 84*t*
  epidermolysis bullosa acquisita, 570
  erythrocyte, 275–279, 276*f*, 276–278*t*
  Hepatitis B, 536*f*
  histocompatibility, 3, 289
  human platelet, 503
  immunophenotypic analysis, 655*t*

Antigen *(cont.)*
　MHC proteins, 85–92, 86–90*f*
　nephritogenic antibody-antigen reaction, 549, 550*t*, 556*t*
　polysaccharide, 2
　processing and presentation, 90
　recognition, antigen-specific, 444, 445
　specialized forms of presentation, 92
　stimulation, 267, 267*t*
　superantigen, 131–132, 132*f*, 450, 682–683, 846
　T cell-independent, 120*f*, 120–121
　tumor immunology, 632–634
　World Health Organization, 286, 287*t*
Antigen-antibody complex, 192, 193
Antigenic challenge, 831–832
Antigenic shift/variation, 791
Antigen-nonspecific therapy, 768–770
Antigen-presenting cell (APC). *See also* Major
　　　histocompatibility complex (MHC)
　B cell as, 46, 92, 123*f*, 123–124
　combined T cell & B cell immunodeficiency disorder, 353
　corticosteroid, 828
　dendritic cell, 92
　graft rejection, 806, 807*f*
　high endothelial venule, 62
　immune response, 65–68, 66*f*, 68*f*
　lamina propria cell, 200
　macrophage, 41, 92
　monoclonal antibody, 842
　peripheral tolerance, 448
　Rh isoimmunization, 623
　T cell, 46–47
Antigen-specific therapy, 767–768
Antiglobulin test, 244–245, 278*f*, 278–279
Antiglomerular basement membrane antibody-induced
　　　glomerulonephritis (anti-GBM), 550–552, 552*f*, 609
Antihistamine
　allergic rhinitis, 396
　commonly used, 859, 859*t*
　H1 receptor binding, 187
　serum sickness, 421
　skin tests, allergy, 383, 384
Anti-inflammatory drug. *See also* Non-steroidal anti-
　　　inflammatory drug (NSAID)
　aspirin and other NSAIDs, 856–857, 857*t*
　colchicine, 857
　corticosteroid
　　effects, 854–855
　　mechanism of action, 854, 854*f*
　　metabolic effects, 855, 855*t*
　　pharmacology & physiology, 852, 853*f*, 853*t*, 854
　　toxicity, 855*t*, 855–856
　gold/penicillamine/antimalarial, 857–858
　immediate-hypersensitivity reactions, suppressing
　　antihistamines, 859, 859*t*
　　cromolyn sodium, 858–859
　　methylxanthine, 859–860
　　sympathomimetic drug, 859, 860*t*
Antilymphocyte antibodies, 842
Antilymphocyte globulin (ALG), 802, 805, 808, 842
Antilymphocyte serum (ALS), 842
Antimalarial drugs, 465, 857–858
Antimicrobial enzymes & binding proteins, 26*t*, 26–27, 27*f*
Antineutrophil cytoplasmic antibodies (ANCA), 533, 549
　circulating pattern, 522
　cytoplasmic pattern, 521
　perinuclear pattern, 519
　vasculitis, 562
Antinuclear antibody, 456, 457*t*, 459
Antiphospholipid antibody, 589

Antiphospholipid antibody syndrome, 622
Antiretroviral therapy, 628, 757–758, 758*t*
Antiribonucleoprotein (RNP) autoantibody, 514
Antisperm antibody, 620–621
Antithymocyte globulin (ATG), 805, 842
Antithymocyte serum (ATS), 842
Antitoxin, 2, 785
Antivenin, 785
Aphthous stomatitis, 544–545, 545*f*
Aplastic anemia, 501–502, 820
Apoptosis, 17, 22–23, 32, 40, 72, 642, 849
Aqueous epinephrine, 414
Arachidonic acid, 187–188, 188*f*, 189*f*, 856
Armed forces, 794
Arteriography, 524, 525*f*
Arteritis
　giant-cell, 522–524, 523*f*, 596
　Takayasu's, 524, 525*f*, 526
Arthritis
　hypogammaglobulinemia, 478
　juvenile, 466–468, 592
　psoriatic, 476–477
　rheumatoid, 450, 592, 830, 834
Arthropod allergen, 392–394
Arthus, Nicholas-Maurice, 419
Arthus reaction, 192, 419
Ascariasis, 737
Aspergillosis, 720–721
Aspergillus, 364, 365, 366, 403, 421–423
Aspergillus fumigatus, 421–423, 823
Aspirin
　juvenile arthritis, 468
　respiratory disease induced using, 600
　sensitivity, 399, 400
　serum sickness, 421
　ubiquitousness of, 856
　urticaria, 417
Assay
　antisperm antibody, 620–621
　B cell, 259*t*, 259–260, 260*t*
　binder-ligand, 231–237, 232*f*, 234–236*f*
　cell-mediated lympholysis, 286
　chemiluminescence, 365
　colony-forming, 13
　complement, 245–249, 246–248*f*, 248–249*t*
　disequilibrium, 232
　DNA-based, usefulness of, 317
　equilibrium, 232
　flow cytometric, 323
　functional, 247–248, 322–325
　hemolytic, 246–247
　histocompatibility and cellular, 294–297, 296*f*
　hybridization, 311–312, 312*f*
　immunoradiometric, 233
　indirect fluorescent antibody, 745
　lymphocyte clonality and gene arrangement, 313–314
　monocyte-macrophage, 269
　neutrophil microbicidal, 273
　T-cell, 257–259, 258*f*, 258*t*, 259*f*
　valid analytic range of the, 236
Asthma, 380
　allergic, 611
　allergic bronchopulmonary aspergillosis, 421
　bronchoprovocation test, 386
　cardiac, 402
　clinical feature, 398–399
　complications and prognosis, 403
　defining, 397
　diagnosis, immunologic/differential, 400–402

drug-induced respiratory disease, 599
eosinophilic pneumonia, 602
epidemiology, 398
extrinsic, 397
general consideration, 397
immunologic feature, 397
intrinsic, 397–398
kinin-generating system, 180
nonspecific trigger, 400*t*
pathogenesis, immunologic, 399–400, 400*t*
pathology, 399
treatment, 402–403
Ataxia-telangiectasia, 356*f,* 356–357, 357*f*
A *terreus,* 421
Atopic allergen, 391–394
animal, 394
arthropod, 392–394
food, 394
mold, 391–392, 393*f,* 393*t*
pollen, 391, 392*f,* 393
Atopic disease
allergic gastroenteropathy, 405–406
allergic rhinitis, 394–397
asthma, 307–403
dermatitis, 403–405, 797
keratoconjunctivitis, 591–592, 592*f*
Atopy, 799
defining, 389
etiology, 390–391
IgE-mediated inflammation, 195
immunology, 389–390
ATP-binding cassette (ABC) transporters, 84
Attenuated vaccine model, 81–82, 735
Autoantibody
crossmatching for, 294
organ-specific, 481*f,* 481*t,* 482–483
systemic lupus erythematosus, 456, 459
Autocrine effect, 67
Autoimmune disease, 93, 93*t,* 182, 340
blistering disease, 564
cancer, 644
complement deficiency, 373
genetic susceptibility, 451*t,* 451–543
helper T cell, 141
hepatitis, chronic active, 538–539
host responsiveness as component of, 453
models, 450*t*
abnormalities in lymphocyte interaction, 451
antigen-nonspecific lymphocyte activation, 450
molecular mimicry, 451
peripheral tolerance, breakdown of, 450
thymic education, failure of, 450
multifactorial pathogenesis, 450
neutropenia, 493*t,* 493–495
normal immune response: fundamental principles, 444*t*
paraneoplastic pemphigoid, 576–577
pernicious anemia, 533–534
self-tolerance, 445*t,* 445–449, 446*f,* 447*f,* 448*t*
summary, 454–455
testis and ovary, 621
tissue-destruction, mechanisms of immune-mediated, 453–454
tissue-infiltrating cells, 449
Autoimmune endocrine disease
autoantibodies, organ-specific, 481*f,* 481*t,* 482–483
mechanism of development, 480
pancreas, 487–491, 489–490*t*
thyroid, 482–487, 483–484*f,* 486*f*
Autologous transplantation, 821

Autonomic imbalance, 390
Autoradiography, 242
Autoreactive T cell, 91
Avery, O. T., 2
Avidity model of T cell selection, 134–135, 135*f*
Azathioprine, 474, 517, 526, 531, 567, 831, 832, 834, 834*f*
AZT (zidovudine), 505, 757

B7, 67, 843
B7.1/2, 138
β-Gene locus, 130–131, 131*f,* 132, 132*f*
β-Glucan, 706
β-Lactam antibody, 437–440, 438*t*
β-Lactam ring, 434, 434*f*
β-Microglobulin, 85
Babesia microti, 281, 682
Bacillus anthracis, 686
Bacillus Calmette-Guérin (BCG), 81, 692, 846
Bacillus cereus, 686
Bacteria
compounds derived from, 846–847
gram-negative, 26
immunogen, 65
neutrophil microbicidal assay, 273
normal flora, 679, 679*t*
pyogenic, 56
Bacterial disease
Bordetella pertussis, 686–687
encapsulated bacteria, 688–690
exotoxins and endotoxins, 684–685
intracellular pathogens, 690–692, 691*f*
serodiagnosis, 684
Staphylococcus aureus, 687
Streptococcus, 687
toxigenic, 685–688
Vibrio cholerae, 686
Bacteriology, 1
Bacteroides fragilis, 690
Bacteroides gingivalis, 542
Bacteroides intermedius, 542
Bare lymphocyte syndrome, 353–354
Barnard, Christiaan, 815
Basophil, 10*f,* 11, 185*t,* 186, 186*f*
atopic disease, 389
Bayliascaris procyonsis, 604
B cell, 10, 11. *See also* Antibody (B cell) immunodeficiency disorder; Combined T cell & B cell immunodeficiency disorder
activation, 45–46, 50–52, 51*f,* 52*t*
affinity chromatography, 227
affinity maturation, 55
as antigen-presenting cell, 92, 123*f,* 123–124
bystander activation, 69
cancer, 95–96
clonal organization, 63
corticosteroid, 827, 828
crossmatching by lymphocytotoxicity, 294
cyclophosphamide, 835
cyclosporin, 838
follicular, 198
follicular lymphoma, 72
generation, 115–116, 116*f*
heavy-chain class switch, 124–125, 125*f*
hematopoietic stem cells, 43
HIV (human immunodeficiency virus), 756
IgA switch differentiation, 205
immunoglobulin, 44–45, 45–46*f,* 124
immunosuppressive therapy, 832

B cell (cont.)
  laboratory tests, immunologic, 259t, 259–260, 260t, 323t, 323–324
  lymphoid follicle and germinal centers, 126f, 126–127
  malignancy, 113
  maturation and release of virgin, 117f, 117–118
  memory, 124
  mucosal immunity, 615
  neoplasms of the immune system, 657–658t, 664–670
  plasma cell, 45–46
  primary and secondary humoral response, 127t, 127–128
  protein tyrosine kinase, 49
  quantitative aspects of immune function, 71
  sarcoidosis, 605
  secondary follicle, 55
  self-tolerance, 448t, 448–449
  somatic hypermutation, 125–126
  T cell help and accessory signal, 121, 121f, 122f, 123
  T cell-independent antigen, 120f, 120–121
  T cells cooperating with, 3
  tolerance, 128f, 128–129
  tumor immunology, 635, 638
B cell antigen receptor (BCR), 118, 119f, 120
B cell growth factor-I (BCGF-I), 159
B cell stimulatory factor-I (BSF-I), 159
Bcl-2 protein, 72, 113
Bc12 protein, 22–23, 23t
Beclomethasone, 396
Beclomethasone dipropionate, 402
Behcet's disease, 475, 517, 544, 545, 596
Behring, Emil von, 2, 4, 8
Bence Jones protein, 220
Benign hypergammaglobulinemic purpura, 669
Bentonite flocculation test, 245
B hyperimmune globulin (HBIG), 810
Bias error, 233
Bile salt, 812
Biliary cirrhosis, primary, 539f, 539–540
Biliary tract. See Hepatobiliary disease
Bilineal phenotype, 652
Billingham, Rupert, 3, 4
Binder-ligand assay
  assay process, 231–233
  comparing analytic performances of different methods, 236–237
  enzymatic label, 233–235, 234–235f
  fluorometric label, 235, 235f
  radioisotopic label, 233, 234f
Biochemical agent, 850–851
Biologic response modification, 768–770
Biosynthesis, immunoglobulin, 260
Biotechnology, 640–641
Biotin-avidin system, 236, 240
Biotin-dependent carboxylase deficiency, 350–351
Biotransformation and haptenation, metabolic, 434f, 434–435, 435t
Biphenotypic phenotype, 652
Blackwater fever, 727
Black widow spider, 786t
Blastocyst, 616
Blastomycosis, 709, 711
Blistering disease, 564
Blood banking and immunohematology
  antiglobulin test, 278f, 278–279
  blood groups, 275–277, 276f, 276–277t
  component therapy, 283t, 283–284
  H & ABO systems, 275–276, 277t
  pretransfusion testing, 279
  Rh isoimmunization, 282–283

  transfusion reactions, 279t, 279–282, 281t
  type and screen, 279
Blood cell biology. See Hematopoiesis
Blood group system, 275–277, 276f, 276–277t
Blood transfusion, 804
Bone and calcium metabolism, 855t
Bone marrow
  Chédiak-Higashi syndrome, 367
  eosinophil, 183
  hematopoiesis, 9, 10f, 11–17, 14f, 15f
  immune reconstitution, 770
  neutrophil, 32
  primary lymphoid organ, 43
Bone marrow stroma, 11, 16
Bone marrow transplantation
  beginnings of, 819
  diseases treatable by, 820t
  graft-vs.-host reaction, 822t, 822–823
  indications and results, 820–821
  infection, 823–824
  neoplasms of the immune system, 660
  procedure, 821–822
  venoocclusive disease of the liver, 823
Bone transplantation
  immunosuppression, 824–825
  posttransplantation course, 824
  recovery, 825
  rejection, 824
Bordet, Jules, 2, 4, 5, 8
Bordetella pertussis, 686–687
Borrelia, 744–745
Botulism, 786t
BP 180 (BPAG2), 564, 568
BP 230 (BPAG1), 564
Bradykinin, 178–179, 281–282
Branched DNA, 312
Breast milk immunology, 207–208
Breinl, Friedrich, 2, 4
Brent, Leslie, 3, 4
Brequinar, 841
Bronchial obstruction, 414–415
Bronchiolitis, obliterative, 610
Bronchitis
  acute viral, 401–402
  chronic, 401
Bronchoprovocation test, 380, 381f, 385–387, 399, 401
Bronchospasm, 599–600
Bronchus-associated lymphoid tissue (BALT), 196
Brownian movement, 270
Brucella, 684
Brucella abortus, 691, 847
Brucella melitensis, 691
Brugia, 737
Brugia malayi, 281, 604
Bruton, Ogden, 332
Btk, 116
Buerger's disease, 526
Bullous pemphigoid, 555–557t, 564–567
  clinical feature, 566, 566f
  diagnosis, immunologic/differential, 566–567, 567t
  general consideration, 564–565
  immunologic feature, 564
  pathology, 565–566
  prognosis, 567
  treatment, 567
Burkitt's and Burkitt-like lymphoma, 113, 667
Burnet, Macfarlane, 3–5
Bystander B-cell activation, 69

C1, 478
  angioedema, hereditary, 373–374
  complement deficiency, 373
C2, 172
C3, 175f, 175–176
  angioedema, hereditary, 374
  complement deficiency, 372–373
  receptors and signal transduction, 177–178
C4, 172, 478
C5, 172, 173, 176–177, 478
C5-9, 173, 371
C6, 478
C7, 478
C8, 478
C9, 373
C4A, 373
Cadaveric transplantation, 803
Caddis fly, 394
Calcineurin, 838
Calcium ions, intracellular free, 50
Calibration, 231–232
Cancer. *See also* Neoplasms of the immune system
  active immunization, 783
  autoimmune disorders, 644
  B cell, 95–96
  biologic response modification, 768
  bladder, 836
  congenital immunodeficiency, 642t, 642–643
  cyclophosphamide, 836
  cyclosporin, 840
  HIV (human immunodeficiency virus), 645–648, 646f, 647t, 648f
  immune surveillance, 640–641
  immunocompromise, 641t, 641–642, 642t
  methotrexate, 836
  polymyositis-dermatomyositis, 474
  second tumors, 644–645
  selective IgA deficiency, 341
  skin, 840
  transplantation, 643–644
Candida, 347–350, 349f, 365, 366, 369, 546–547, 595, 597
Candida albicans, 706
Candida glabrata, 706
Candida tropicalis, 706
Candidiasis, chronic mucocutaneous, 348–350, 349f, 717–719
Capillary tube method, 270
Capnocytophaga, 542
Capping, 50
Captopril, 440
Carbohydrate-and lipid-based recognition system, 26
Carbohydrate metabolism, 855t
Carboxylase deficiency, biotin-dependent, 350–351
Carboxymethyl (CM), 226
Carcinoembryonic antigen (CEA), 633–634
Cardiac asthma, 402
Cardiac disease. *See also* Heart transplantation
  endomyocardial disease, 514
  myocardial disease, 513–514
  pericardial disease, 513
  polyarteritis nodosa, 519
Cardiomyopathy, dilated, 514
Cardiovascular response, anaphylaxis and, 410
Carrier and hapten, 78
Carrington's chronic eosinophilic pneumonia, 602, 603t
Catalytic antibody, 108
C4B, 373
C5b67 complex, 173
C8-binding protein, 178

C4-binding protein (C4bp), 175
C3b receptors, 172
C5-C8, 373
CD (cluster of differentiation), 12, 256, 257t, 653
  classification of hematopoietic cell markers, 862–863t
CD1, 92
CD2, 48, 49, 808
CD3, 67, 135, 769, 808
CD4, 3, 48, 57, 65, 91, 132, 132f, 199
  antigen-nonspecific therapy, 769
  atopy, 391
  bone marrow transplantation, 823
  cell-surface molecule, 849
  corticosteroid, 827
  drug allergy, 436
  giant-cell arteritis, 515, 523
  graft rejection, 808
  HIV (human immunodeficiency virus), 626, 627f, 628, 748, 750, 751, 754–755, 757
  human T cell leukemia virus types I and II, 763, 765
  laboratory tests, immunologic, 322
  lung transplantation, 610
  lymphocytopenia, 350
  monoclonal antibody, 843
  mucosal immunity, 614
  multiple sclerosis, 580
  pregnancy, immunity in, 620
  sarcoidosis, 605
  self-tolerance, 446
  suppressor/helper ratios, 258
  T cell, 206
  thymic hormone, 847
  trophoblast, 618
  tubulointerstitial nephritis, 561
CD4+, 49, 63, 91
CD5, 118, 259t, 323, 769
CD7, 353
CD8, 48, 57, 65, 91, 132, 132f, 823
  AIDS (acquired immune deficiency syndrome), 436
  Celiac disease, 529
  cell-surface molecule, 849
  deficiency, 352
  graft rejection, 808
  Hepatitis A, 534
  HIV (human immunodeficiency virus), 755
  Human T cell leukemia virus types I and II, 763, 765
  insulin-dependent diabetes mellitus, 488
  laboratory tests, immunologic, 322
  mucosal immunity, 614
  multiple sclerosis, 580
  Omenn syndrome, 354
  pregnancy, immunity in, 620
  self-tolerance, 446
  suppressor/helper ratios, 258
  T cell, 206
  thymic hormone, 847
  tubulointerstitial nephritis, 561
CD8+, 49, 63, 84, 91
CD10, 115, 259t, 323
CD11, 374
CD14, 26, 40, 618
CD15, 673
CD19, 115, 259t, 323, 638
CD20, 259t, 323
CD21, 118, 178, 259t
CD22, 259t, 323, 653
CD23, 118
CD25, 49

CD28, 49, 67, 137–138, 138f
  antigen-nonspecific therapy, 769
  monoclonal antibody, 843
  peripheral tolerance, 448
CD29, 49
CD30, 673
CD34, 12, 15, 61, 653, 750, 821
CD38, 12
CD40, 118
CD44, 16
CD45, 123, 136, 137f, 142, 673
CD59, 178, 374
CD95, 72
CD34+CD38−, 12
CD3 complex, 48
C diphtheriae, 686
CDK inhibitors (CDKIs), 21, 22
CD40L, 49, 69, 121, 205
CDR3, 112
CD45RO, 199
Celiac disease, 528–529, 529f
Cellcept, 812
Cell cycle, 20–22, 21f, 43–44
Cell death, 17, 22–23, 32, 40, 72
Cell isolation and lymphocytotoxicity test, 289–290
Cell-mediated eye disease
  AIDS (acquired immune deficiency syndrome), 596–597
  Behcet's disease, 596
  contact dermatitis, 596
  giant-cell arteritis, 596
  ocular sarcoidosis, 594–595
  phlyctenular keratoconjunctivitis, 596
  polyarteritis nodosa, 596
  sympathetic ophthalmia, 595–596
  Vogt-Koyanagi-Harada syndrome, 595–596
Cell-mediated hypersensitivity disease
  allergic contact dermatitis, 425–427, 426t
  hypersensitivity pneumonitis, 428–432, 429t
  photoallergic contact dermatitis, 427, 427t
  tissue-destruction, 454
Cell-mediated immunity (CMI). See also T cell
  defective, 709
  evaluation of, 354t
  explaining, 190–192, 191f, 191t
  hypogammaglobulinemia, acquired, 338
  periodontal disease, 544
  T cell as primary agent in, 46
Cell-mediated lympholysis (CML), 268, 286, 297t, 297–298
Cell proliferation & survival, 20–22, 21f
Cell-surface molecule, 849–850
Cellular assay for histocompatibility, 294–297, 296f
Cellular immunity, 2, 545
  B-lymphocyte assay, 259t, 259–260, 260t
  cytomegalovirus, 760–761
  flow cytometry, 260–264, 262–263f, 264t
  fungal disease, 708–709
  lymphocyte activation, 264–269, 265t, 266–268f, 267t
  mixed lymphocyte culture, 267–268, 268f
  monocyte-macrophage assay, 269
  natural killer cell, 268–269
  polymyositis-dermatomyositis, 473
  skin test, delayed hypersensitivity, 254–256
  syphilis, 741
  T-lymphocyte assay, 257–259, 258f, 258t, 259f
Cellular immunodeficiency disorder. See T cell
          immunodeficiency disorder
Cellular immunology, 2–3
Cellular infiltrate, 182

Cellular methods for tissue typing, 286, 294–297, 296f, 298t
Centers for Disease Control and Prevention (CDC), 783
Central nervous system (CNS). See also Neurologic disease
  isolated angiitis, 526
  polyarteritis nodosa, 519
  primary central nervous system lymphoma, 646–647, 647t
  rheumatoid arthritis, 463
  systemic lupus erythematosus, 458
  Wegener's granulomatosis, 522
Centroblast, 127
Centrocyte, 127
Cephalosporin, 439, 439t
Cestodes, 735–736
Chagas disease, 281
Chancre immunity, 740–741
Chaperon, E. A., 3
Charcot-Leyden crystal protein, 183, 184
Chase, Merrill, 2, 4
Chédiak-Higashi syndrome, 324, 367
Chemiluminescence, 272, 365
Chemistry of Antigens and Antibodies, The (Marrack), 2
Chemoattractant activity, 162
Chemokine, 34, 162–163, 163t, 188
Chemoradiotherapy, 821
Chemotactic mediator, 188
Chemotactic movement, 270
Chemotaxis, 34, 270
Chemotherapeutic agents, 601
Chemotherapy, 660
Childhood immunization, recommendations for, 792–793, 793t
Chimeric state, 809
Chlorambucil, 831, 837
2-chloro-2′-deoxyadenoside (2CDA), 841
Cholangitis, primary sclerosing, 540–541
Choledocholedochostomy, 811
Cholera, 791
Cholesterol, 706
Cholinergic anaphylactoid reaction, 413
Cholinergic urticaria, 417
Chromatography, 225–227, 226f, 227f
Chronic bronchitis, 401
Chronic demyelinating polyneuropathies, 584–585
Chronic granulomatous disease (CGD), 364–366, 365f, 366t
Chronic idiopathic eosinophilic pneumonia, 602, 603t
Chronic inflammatory infiltrate, 191
Chronic mucocutaneous candidiasis, 348–350, 349f
Chronic myelogenous leukemia (CML), 821
Chronic nonallergic rhinitis, 395
Chronic thyroiditis, 482–483, 483f, 484f
Churg-Strauss syndrome, 520, 602t, 602–603
Cicatricial pemphigoid, 568, 594
Ciliary neurotrophic factor (CNTF), 156–157
C1 inhibitor (C1INH), 174–175
Ciprofloxacin, 531
Circulating inhibitors of coagulation, 509
Cirrhosis, non-A/B hepatitis virus postnecrotic, 810
Cladotanytarsus lewisi, 394
Claman, Henry N., 3, 4
Classic complement pathway, 170f, 170–173, 171f, 371–372
Class II regulatory gene (CIITA), 354
Clinical tests. See Blood banking and immunohematology;
          Histocompatibility testing; Laboratory tests,
          immunologic; Molecular genetic techniques
Clip peptide, 89–90
Clonality, 651, 654
Clonal organization and lymphocyte, 63–65, 64f
Clonal plasma cell disorder, 667–668

Clonal selection theory, 3, 115
  anergy, 129, 445
  B cell antigen receptor, 118
  CD4 T cell, 515
  deletion, 129, 445
  restriction, 117
Cloning technology, 766
Clonorchis sinensis, 733
Clostridium botulinum, 685
Clostridium perfringens, 686
Clostridium tetani, 685
Clotting factor XI, 179, 179*f*
CMV pneumonitis, 819, 822, 823
C-Myc protein, 21–22, 50
Coagulation disorder
  anticardiolipin antibody syndrome, 509–510
  circulating inhibitors, 509
  hemophilia and Von Willebrand's disease, 508–509
Coccidioides immitis, 715
Coccidioidomycosis, 713, 715–716
Cockroach allergen, 393
Colchicine, 857
Cold agglutinin syndrome, 498
Cold urticaria, 417
Collaborative Transplant Study (CTS), 287
Collagenase, 40, 828
Collagen disorder and serum immunoglobulin levels, 217*t*
Colonoscopy, 532
Colony-forming unit (CFU), 13
Colony-stimulating factor (CSF), 12, 164*t,* 164–165, 165*t,* 495*t*
Combinatorial joining, 111
Combined heart-lung transplantation
  complications, 819
  immunosuppression and allograft monitoring, 818–819
  operative procedure, 818
  organ procurement, 818
  recipient selection, 818
  replacement for isolated lung transplantation, 817
  results, 819
Combined T cell & B cell immunodeficiency disorder
  ataxia-telangiectasia, 356*f,* 356–357, 357*f*
  bare lymphocyte syndrome, 353–354
  dwarfism and cartilage-hair hypoplasia, 360, 361*f*
  enzyme deficiency
    adenosine deaminase and nucleoside phosphorylase deficiency, 360–361, 361*f*
    X-linked lymphoproliferative syndrome, 361–362
  graft-verses-host reaction, 357–358, 358*f,* 359*f*
  Nijmegen breakage syndrome, 357
  Omenn syndrome, 354
  reticular dysgenesis, 352
  severe combined immunodeficiency, 352–353
  T cell membrane or signal defects, 353
  Wiskott-Aldrich syndrome, 354–355, 355*f*
Common acute lymphocytic leukemia antigen (CALLA), 634
Common variable immunodeficiency, 337–339
Comparative sensitivity of quantitative immunoassays, 250, 251*t*
Complementarity-determining region (CDR), 103
Complement assay, 245
  elevated complement level, 248
  fixation test, 249
  functional, 247–248
  hemolytic, 246–247
  immunoassays for components, 247
  reduced serum complement activity, 247–248
Complement deficiency
  allotype variant, 375
  alternative pathway, 371, 558

autoimmune disease, 373
C3, 372–373
classic pathway, 371–372
clinical feature, 372*t*
hereditary angioedema, 373–374
receptors and signal transduction, 374
regulatory protein, 373
Complement-dependent lymphocytotoxicity test, 290
Complement factor, 2, 27–28, 28*f,* 35, 40, 70
Complement system
  activation, 169–170, 176–177, 177*f*
  Arthus reaction, 419
  control mechanism, 174–176, 175*f*
  functions, 169
  genetic considerations, 176
  gingivitis, 544
  immune-complex formation, 192
  infection, mechanisms of immunity to, 681, 681*t*
  laboratory tests, immunologic, 325
  molecular weights and serum concentrations, 169*t*
  nomenclature, 170
  pathways of activation, 170, 170*t*
    alternative, 173–174, 174*f*
    classic, 170*f,* 170–173, 171*f*
  receptors and signal transduction, 177–178
  renal disease, 549
  rheumatic disease, 477–478
Complete blood count (CBC), 320
Complete Freund's adjuvant (CFA), 82, 846
Component therapy, 283*t,* 283–284
Computed tomographic (CT) scans, 600–601
Concomitant immunity model, 735
Condom therapy, 621
Confidence limits, 233
Congenital immunodeficiency and neoplasia, 642*t,* 642–643
Congenital thymic aplasia, 345–348, 346*f*
Conjugate vaccine, 81
Contagion concept, 1
Coombs' Test, 244–245
Coons, Albert H., 4
Corneal graft reaction, 597*f,* 597–598
Corticosteroid, 358, 402
  allergic contact dermatitis, 426
  anaphylaxis, 415
  anticardiolipin antibody syndrome, 510
  antigen-nonspecific therapy, 769–770
  antiglomerular basement membrane antibody-induced glomerulonephritis, 552
  anti-inflammatory effects, 854–855
  Behcet's disease, 517
  bullous pemphigoid, 567
  combined heart-lung transplantation, 819
  corneal graft reaction, 598
  cytokine, 843
  epidermolysis bullosa acquisita, 571
  giant-cell arteritis, 524
  heart transplantation, 816–817
  idiopathic pulmonary fibrosis, 608
  immune-complex glomerulonephritis, 558
  immunosuppressive therapy
    cellular traffic, effects on, 827–828
    clinical use, 829–830
    functional change, 828–829, 829*f*
  infertility, 621
  juvenile arthritis, 468
  kidney transplantation, 804
  mechanism of action, 854, 854*f*
  metabolic effects, 855, 855*t*
  ocular sarcoidosis, 595

Corticosteroid *(cont.)*
   pancreas transplantation, 814
   pharmacology & physiology, 852, 853f, 853t, 854
   polyarteritis nodosa, 520
   polymyositis-dermatomyositis, 474
   primary biliary cirrhosis, 540
   recurrent aphthous ulceration, 545
   rheumatoid arthritis, 465
   rheumatoid disease affecting the eye, 593
   serum sickness, 421
   Sjögren's syndrome, 470
   sympathetic ophthalmia, 596
   systemic lupus erythematosus, 461
   thrombocytopenic purpura, idiopathic, 505
   toxicity, 855t, 855–856
Corynebacterium parvum, 847
Costimulatory signal, 52, 67
Cowpox virus, 1, 81, 772
COX-1 and COX-2, 856
C1q, 177, 517
CR1, 374
CR4, 178
Craig, L., 3
C-reactive protein, 26
Creatine, 474
Crevicular fluid, 543
Crick, Francis, 3
Cricothyrotomy, 414
Crohn's disease, 530f, 530–532, 531f, 570
Cromolyn, 396, 402
Cromolyn sodium, 858–859
Cross match test, 279, 293–294, 294f
   kidney transplantation, 803
   liver transplantation, 812
   pancreas transplantation, 814–815
Cross-reacting antigen group (CREG), 292, 298, 481
Cryoglobulin, 228–229, 229t
Cryoglobulinemia, 669
Cryptococcosis, 719–720
Cryptococcus, 597
Crystal gamma counter, 232
Cumulative sum chart, 233
Cutaneous basophil hypersensitivity, 195
Cutaneous leishmaniasis, 729–730
Cutaneous test, 382–383, 383f
Cyanosis, 430
Cycle-specific drug, 831
Cyclic adenosine monophosphate (cAMP), 360, 367
Cyclin-dependent kinases (CDKs), 21
Cyclooxygenase, 856, 857
Cyclooxygenase inhibitor, 417
Cyclooxygenase product, 188
Cyclophilin, 838
Cyclophosphamide
   B and T cells reduced, 832
   bone marrow transplantation, 821
   cicatricial pemphigoid, 568
   minimal-change nephropathy, 561
   polyarteritis nodosa, 520
   properties and uses, 834t, 834–836, 835f
   Takayasu's arteritis, 526
   Wegener's granulomatosis, 522
Cyclosporin, 136, 531, 533
   bone marrow transplantation, 822
   combined heart-lung transplantation, 819
   heart transplantation, 815
   IL-2 gene, 838
   liver transplantation, 812, 813
   lung transplantation, 817
   minimal-change nephropathy, 561
   primary biliary cirrhosis, 540
   properties and uses of, 840t
   revolutionized discipline of organ transplantation, 837
   toxicity, 839f, 839–840
Cysteine proteinases, 22
Cystic fibrosis, 423
Cystitis, 836
Cytogenetic analysis, 654–656, 658–659, 659t
Cytokine. *See also* Interleukin *listings*
   activation, 52
   antagonist, 850
   antigen-nonspecific therapy, 769
   atopy, 391
   cell-surface molecule, 849–850
   chemokine, 34
   cloning technology, 766
   colony-forming assays, 13
   colony-stimulating factor, 849
   common variable immunodeficiency, 338
   corticosteroid, 843
   glycosaminoglycan, 17
   growth & differentiation factor, 849
   helper T cell activation, 67–68
   hematologic disease, 495t
   hematopoietic colony-stimulating factor, 164t, 164–165, 165t
   HSC growth promoted, 12–13
   implantation of blastocyst, 616
   inflammatory mediator, 187
   interferon, 157f, 157–158, 848
   interleukin, 848–849
   interleukin-2, 153–155, 154f, 154t
   interleukin-5, 159
   interleukin-6, 155–157, 156t
   interleukin-7, 159
   interleukin-9, 159–160
   interleukin-10, 160
   interleukin-12, 160
   interleukin-14, 160
   interleukin-15, 160
   interleukin-16, 160
   interleukin-4 and 13, 158–159
   interleukin-8 and chemokine family, 162–163, 163t
   interleukin-1 and tumor necrosis factor, 146–153, 147–149t, 152t, 153t
   lineage-specific effects of hematopoietic, 16t
   lymphoid progenitor, 43
   macrophage, 40
   multiple sclerosis, 580
   natural killer cell, 144
   overview and prospects, 166–167
   receptors and signal transduction, 17–20, 18f, 19f, 165–166, 166t
   renal disease, 550
   transforming growth factor β, 160f, 160–161
   transforming growth factor beta, 21
   trophoblast, 618
Cytolytic T lymphocyte (CTL), 67, 68f, 68–69, 141f, 141–142, 297
   Epstein-Barr virus, 763
   hepatitis B, 701, 702
   HIV (human immunodeficiency virus), 755–756
   immunopathology of infection, 682
   influenza virus, 696, 697
   respiratory syncytial virus, 699
Cytomegalovirus (CMV), 280–281, 281f, 760t, 760–761
Cytoplasmic free calcium (CA^{2+}), 136
Cytoplasmic immunoglobulin, 260

Cytoplasmic protein, 22
Cytosolic pathway, 84–85
Cytotoxic drugs, 769
  immunosuppressive therapy
    azathioprine, 834, 834*f*
    chlorambucil, 837
    clinical use, 833, 833*t*
    combining two or more drugs, 837
    cyclophosphamide, 834*f*, 834–836, 835*t*
    defining, 830
    methotrexate, 836*f*, 836–837, 837*t*
    principles forming usage of, 831–833
  polymyositis-dermatomyositis, 474
Cytotrophoblast cell, 616

Dalen-Fuchs nodule, 595
Dameshek, W., 830
Dapsone, 567
Dark zone, 127
Darwin, Charles, 1
Davaine, Casimir, 1
Davis, Mark, 3, 4
Decay-accelerating factor (DAF), 178
Decidua, 613, 616
Declining phase, 71
Decongestant, nasal, 396
Defensin, 35
Degranulation, 35, 184, 185, 271
Delay-accelerating factor (DAF), 374
Delayed-type hypersensitivity (DTH), 190–191, 254–256,
    322–323, 425, 829
Demyelinating disease
  acute disseminated encephalomyelitis, 582–583
  acute inflammatory demyelinating polyneuropathy, 583–
    584
  chronic demyelinating polyneuropathies, 584–585
  multiple sclerosis, 579–582, 580–581*f*
Dendritic cell, 92
Dental plaque, 541
Deoxy-adenosine triphosphate (ATP), 360
Deoxy-guanosine triphosphate (GTP), 360
Deoxynucleotidyl transferase (TdT), 115
Deoxyribonucleic acid. *See* DNA (deoxyribonucleic acid)
Dermatitis
  allergic contact, 192, 382, 425–427, 426*t*, 436
  atopic, 403–405, 797
  herpetiformis, 571, 572*f*, 573, 573*f*
  photoallergic contact, 427, 427*t*
Dermatologic disease, immune-mediated
  bullous pemphigoid, 555–557*t*, 564–567
  cicatricial pemphigoid, 568
  dermatitis herpetiformis, 571, 572*f*, 573, 573*f*
  epidermolysis bullosa acquisita, 570–571
  herpes gestationis, 568–570, 569*f*
  linear IgA bullous dermatosis, 573–574
  paraneoplastic pemphigus, 576–577
  pemphigus foliaceous, 574–576, 575*f*, 576*f*
  pemphigus vulgaris, 574–576, 575*f*, 576*f*
Dermatophagoides pteronyssinus, 392
Desensitization
  adverse effects, 798–799
  allergic contact dermatitis, 427
  allergic rhinitis, 396–397
  anaphylaxis, 415
  asthma, 402–403
  hypersensitivity pneumonitis, 430
  hyposensitization, 798
  indications, 799
  insulin, 441
  methods, 796–797, 797*t*
  modified allergens, 800
  monitoring, 799–800
  penicillin, 439
  sulfonamide, 440
Detection limit, 236
D *farinae*, 392
Diabetes mellitus, insulin-dependent, 487–489, 489*t*
Diacylglycerol (DAG), 50, 136
Diagnostic sensitivity, 251
Diamond, L. K., 622
Diamond-Blackfan syndrome, 502
Diapedesis, 61
Dictyocaulus filaria, 736
Dictyocaulus viviparus, 736
Didanosine, 757
Dideoxycytidine (ddC), 757
Dideoxyinosine (ddI), 757
Dietary elimination, 387
Diethylaminoethyl (DEAE), 226
Diethylcarbamazine, 604
Diethyldithiocarbamate, 850
Diffuse idiopathic skeletal hyperostosis (DISH), 475
Diffuse lymphoid tissue, 198–199, 199*f*
DiGeorge anomaly, 847
  clinical feature, 346–347
  complications and prognosis, 348
  diagnosis, immunologic/differential, 347
  general consideration, 345
  pathogenesis, immunologic, 364
  treatment, 347–348
Dihydrorhodamine (DHR), 272
Dilatation & permeability of microscopic vessels, 29*f*, 29*t*,
    29–30, 30*t*
Dilated cardiomyopathy, 514
Dimorphic fungi, 706
Dinitrochlorobenzene (DNCB), 255
Diphenylhydantoin, 601
Diphtheria, 774*t*, 786*t*
Diphtheria bacillus, 2
Diphtheria toxoid and tetanus toxoid (DPT), 686–687
Direct antiglobulin test (DAT), 278, 278*f*
Disequilibrium assay, 232
Disseminated intravascular coagulation (DIC), 150, 411
Dissociation constant (K_d), 79
DNA (deoxyribonucleic acid), 2, 3, 21. *See also* Molecular
    genetic techniques
  anti-DNA antibody and immune complex, 459–460
  antigen stimulation, 267
  ataxia-telangiectasia, 356
  branched molecule, 312
  fragmentation, 849
  Hepatitis B, 535
  histocompatibility testing, 299–300, 300*t,* 304–307, 306*f*
  mixed lymphocyte culture, 267–268
  molecular genetic analysis, 659
  neoplasms of immune system analyzed using, 654
  oncogenes and cancer, 642
  transcription, 854
  tumor immunology, 632
  vaccine, 81–82
Doherty, Peter, 3, 4
Domain, folded globular, 96–97
Dome cell, 197
Donath-Landsteiner antibody, 499–500
Donor selection/evaluation
  combined heart-lung transplantation, 818
  heart transplantation, 816
  kidney transplantation, 803–804

Dot blot hybridization, 311
Dot-blot method of SSOP, 302, 304
Double immunodiffusion, 212*f*, 212–214, 213*f*
Double-negative/positive thymocyte, 132–133
Drug allergy
   diagnosis, 436–437
   immunologic basis
      clinical feature, 436
      general consideration, 433–434
      metabolic biotransformation and haptenation, 434*f*,
         434–435, 435*t*
      other factors, 435–436
   insulin, 440–441, 441*f*
   multiple drug allergy syndrome, 441
   penicillin, 437–440, 438*t*
   pseudoallergic reaction, 441–442
   sulfonamide, 440
   treatment, 437
Drugs. *See also* Antibiotics; Anti-inflammatory drug;
        Corticosteroid; Immunosuppressive therapy;
        individual drug; Non-steroidal anti-inflammatory
        drug (NSAID); Prednisone
   adrenergic, 859, 860*t*
   allergic rhinitis, 396
   anaphylactoid reaction, 414*t*
   anaphylaxis, 412, 412*t*
   antihistamine, 187, 383, 384
   asthma, 402–403
   bone marrow transplantation, 822
   Crohn's disease, 531
   cycle-specific, 831
   eosinophilic pneumonia, drug-induced, 604, 604*t*
   haptenic, 434
   HIV (human immunodeficiency virus), 757–759
   immune-complex glomerulonephritis, 558–559
   immune hemolytic anemia, 498–499, 499*t*
   immunostimulatory, 850–851
   inflammatory response, modulation of, 770
   influenza virus, 696–697
   lung transplantation, 611
   lupus-like syndrome, 458
   minimal-change nephropathy, 561
   multiple sclerosis, 582
   myasthenia gravis, 587
   neoplasms of the immune system, 660
   neutropenia, 494
   pemphigus foliaceous, 575–576
   respiratory disease induced by, 599–602, 601*f*, 602*t*
   syphilis, 743
   ulcerative colitis, 533
   urticaria, 417
   Wegener's granulomatosis, 522
   wheal-and-flare skin reactions, nonspecific, 412*t*
Duncan's disease, 361–362
Dust, house, 393
Dwarfism and cartilage-hair hypoplasia, short-limbed, 360,
     361*f*
Dyspnea, 430

Echinococcosis, 735–736
Ectocervix, 613, 614*f*
Eczema, 355
   clinical feature, 404
   complications and prognosis, 405
   defining, 403
   diagnosis, immunologic/differential, 404
   epidemiology, 404
   general consideration, 403–404

   pathogenesis, immunologic, 405–406
   pathology, 404
   treatment, 405
Eczematous contact dermatitis, 425–427, 426*t*
Edeleman, Gerald M., 3–5
Edema, laryngeal, 414
Effector cell, 44, 49, 60, 67, 807
Effector phase in immune response, 831
Effector T cell, 379
Egg-sperm fusion, 615–616
Ehrlich, Paul, 2, 4, 8
Eikenella corrodens, 542
Ekins, F., 231
Elastase, 40
Elderly immunization, 793
Electroimmunodiffusion, 221, 224–225*f*, 225*t*
Electromyography, 474
Electrophoresis, 216–218, 218–220*f*, 221, 224*f*
Embryonic hematopoiesis, 11
Emigration, neutrophil, 33*f*, 34
Emotions and urticaria, 417
Encapsulated bacteria, 688–690
Encephalitis
   Japanese, 775*t*
   limbic, 588
   Rasmussen's, 589
Encephalomyelitis, acute disseminated, 582–583
Endocervix, 613, 614*f*
Endocrine disease. *See* Autoimmune endocrine disease
Endocytic pathway, 83–84, 84*t*
Endocytosis, receptor-mediated, 34, 35*f*
Endogenous pyrogen, 151
Endometrium, 613, 614*f*
Endomyocardial disease, 514
Endosalpinx, 613
Endothelial cell, 186–187
Endothelial responses to injury/infection, 30–31, 31*t*
Endotoxin, 682, 684–685, 688
Enterotoxin, 688
Environmental measures
   allergic rhinitis, 396
   asthma, 402
Enzymatic digestion products of immunoglobulin, 97
Enzymatic label, 233–235, 234–235*f*
Enzymatic mediator, 189
Enzyme deficiency with immunodeficiency
   adenosine deaminase and nucleoside phosphorylase,
     360–361, 361*f*
   X-linked lymphoproliferative syndrome, 361–362
Enzyme-linked antibody, 242
Enzyme-linked immunosorbent assay (ELISA), 234, 234*f*
   cestodes, 735, 736
   cross-reaction among β-lactam antibiotics, 439
   drug allergy, 437
   Hashimoto's thyroiditis, 482
   HIV (human immunodeficiency virus), 753–754
   Lyme disease, 745
   sulfonamide, 440
Enzyme-multiplied immunoassay technique (EMIT), 233, 234*f*
Eosinophil, 10*f*, 13, 159, 183–184, 184*f*
   allergic rhinitis, 395
   asthma, 398
   bullous pemphigoid, 566
   Churg-Strauss syndrome, 520
   eosinophilia, 184, 354
   inflammatory cell, 183–184, 184*f*
   Omenn syndrome, 354
Eosinophilic granuloma, 673

Eosinophilic pneumonia, 602*t*
  acute eosinophilic pneumonia, 604
  allergic granulomatosis of Churg and Strauss, 602–603
  chronic idiopathic, 602, 603*t*
  drug-induced, 604, 604*t*
  hyperosinophilic syndrome, 605
  Myalgia syndrome, 604
  parasite-induced, 604, 604*t*
  simple idiopathic pulmonary eosinophilia, 603–604
Epidermal growth factor (EGF), 616
Epidermolysis bullosa acquisita, 570–571
Epinephrine, 414, 859
Epithelioid cell, 41
Epitope
  B cell, 75–77, 76*f*, 77*f*
  conformational and linear, 77
  defining, 74
  desensitization, 800
  MHC-binding, 93
  OKT4, 353
  T cell, 79–80
Epstein-Barr virus (EBV), 23, 337
  AIDS (acquired immune deficiency syndrome), 546
  Burkitt's and Burkitt-like lymphoma, 667
  Chédiak-Higashi syndrome, 367
  clinical feature, 762
  diagnosis, differential/immunologic, 763
  Duncan's disease, 362
  immunologic features, 762*f*, 762–763, 764*f*
  immunosuppressive therapy, 674
  laboratory diagnosis of infectious mononucleosis, 762
  pathogenesis, immunologic, 761
  severe combined immunodeficiency, 353
  transfusion reactions, 281
  treatment, 763
Equilibrium assay, 232
Ergosterol, 706
E rosette-forming cell, 258–259, 259*f*
Error and quality control, 233
Erwinia, 688
Erythema nodosum, 526, 526*f*
Erythroblastosis fetalis, 622
Erythrocyte, 9, 10*f*, 11, 32
  antigen, 275–279, 276*f*, 276–277*t*, 278*f*, 279*t*
  blood component therapy, 283–284
  erythropoietin, 13
  sheep, 258–259
  spleen, 55
Erythrocyte disorder
  Diamond-Blackfan syndrome, 502
  immune hemolytic anemia, 495–499, 496*t*, 498*t*
  newborn, hemolytic disease of the, 500–501
  paroxysmal nocturnal hemoglobinuria, 501
  pure erythrocyte aplasia, 501–502
Erythroid progenitor, 10*f*
Erythropoietin (EPO), 13, 146, 495*t*
Escherichia, 688
Escherichia coli, 26, 173, 365
Estrogen therapy, 852
Eukaryotic organism
  immunomodulator
    biochemical agent, 850–851
    cytokine, 848–850
    monoclonal antibody, 850
    thymic hormone, 847–848
Euroglyphus maynei, 393
Exon, 309
Exotoxin, 684–685
Expectorant, 402–403

Exponential phase, 71
Extracellular degranulation, 38, 184
Extracellular matrix (ECM), 14, 16, 17
Extract, allergen, 394, 394*t*
Extrahepatic biliary atresia, 810
Extrinsic allergic alveolitis, 428–432, 429*t*
Extrinsic defects, phagocytic, 364
Eye disease
  antibody-mediated
    vernal/atopic keratoconjunctivitis, 591–592, 592*f*
  cell-mediated, 594–597, 596*f*
  corneal graft reaction, 597*f*, 597–598
  giant-cell arteritis, 523
  rheumatoid diseases affecting the eye, 592*f*, 592–593, 593*f*
  systemic lupus erythematosus, 458

F(ab)′2 fragment, 97
Factor H, 175
Factor I, 175
Fagraeus, Astrid, 2, 4
Fallopian tube, 613, 614*f*
False-positive/negative reaction, 255, 460
Familial cold urticaria, 417
Fasciola, 184
Fas ligand (FasL), 72, 142
Fas-mediated inhibition of immune response, 849–850
Fas protein, 72
Fc fragment, 97
Fc receptor, 35, 70, 97, 108*t*, 108–109, 121
  Arthus reaction, 419
Febrile reaction, 280
Felty's syndrome, 463
Fenner, Frank, 3, 4
Ferritin-coupled antibody, 242
Fetal hematopoiesis, 11
Fever
  Blackwater, 727
  as nonimmunologic defense against infection, 680
  relapsing, 746
Fibrin deposition, 191
Fibrinoid necrosis, 521
Fibroblasts, 157
Filarid nematode, 737
Fixation test, complement, 249
FK-binding protein (FKBP), 840
Flow cytometric assay, 323
Flow cytometry
  cell analysis, 261–262, 261–263*f*
  clinical applications, 262, 264, 264*t*
  crossmatching by lymphocytotoxicity, 294
  fluorescence-activated cell sorter, 262, 263*f*
  neutrophil, 272–273, 273*f*
Fluconazole, 715–718, 720
Fludarabine, 660
Fluid and electrolyte metabolism, 855*t*
Flunisolide, 396, 402
Fluorescein isothiocyanate (FITC), 237
Fluorescence, 237, 237*f*
Fluorescence-activated cell sorter, 262, 263*f*
Fluorescence polarization immunoassay (FPIA), 235, 235*f*
Fluorescent T *pallidum* antibody (FTA) test, 743
Fluorometric label, 235, 235*f*
Focal glomerulosclerosis, 561–562
Follicular B cell, 198
Follicular center lymphoma, 665–666
Follicular dendritic cell (FDC), 53–55, 92, 126*f*, 126–127
Follicular lymphoma, 72, 113
Follicular T cell, 197–198
Food allergen, 394, 412, 530

Forced expiratory volume, 1-second (FEV$_1$), 380, 386,
    398–399, 610
Foreignness and immunogenicity, 74
Foreign travel and immunization, 793–794
N-Formylmethionine residues, 34
Four-chain basic unit, 96–97, 97*f*
Fracastoro, Girolamo, 1
Framework region, 103
Fresh-frozen plasma (FFP), 284
Fully committed progenitor, 13
Functional assay, 247–248, 322–325
Fungal aeroallergen, 392, 394*t*
Fungal disease, 706
    forms assumed when invading host tissue, 707–710*t*
    opportunistic pathogen
        aspergillosis, 720–721
        Candidiasis, 717–719
        cryptococcosis, 719–720
        mucormycosis, 721
        pneumocystosis, 721–722
    primary pathogen
        blastomycosis, 709, 711
        coccidioidomycosis, 713, 715–716
        histoplasmosis, 716–717
        paracoccidioidomycosis, 717
    salient features of superficial/cutaneous and subcutaneous
        mycoses, 709–714*t*
Fusobacterium nucleatum, 542
Fyn, 135

Gamete intrafallopian transfer, 621
Gamma globulin, 341
Gamma-globulin fraction, 95
Gamma globulin molecules, 3
Gamma globulin peptides, 2
Ganciclovir, 821–822, 823
Gastroenteropathy, allergic, 405–406
Gastrointestinal disease, 340
    alpha heavy-chain disease, 533
    Crohn's disease, 530*f*, 530–532, 531*f*
    gluten-sensitive enteropathy, 528–529, 529*f*
    nongluten food hypersensitivity, 530
    pernicious anemia, 533–534
    ulcerative colitis, 532–533, 533*f*
    Whipple's disease, 534
Gastrointestinal system
    anaphylaxis, 411
    non-steroidal anti-inflammatory drug, 857, 857*t*
    scleroderma, 471, 472
    systemic lupus erythematosus, 458
G$_0$ (cell resting phase), 21, 43–44
Gel filtration, 226
Genes
    complement deficiency, 371
    complement system, 176
    immunoglobulin, 109–113, 109–113*f*
    leukocyte adhesion defect-type1, 368
    selective IgA deficiency, 341
Genetics. *See also* Molecular genetic techniques
    autoimmune disease, 451*t*, 451–543
    bone marrow transplantation, 820
    cytogenetic analysis, 654–656, 658–659, 659*t*
    erythrocyte antigens, 275–277, 276*f*, 276–277*t*
    oncogenes, 641–642
    pemphigus foliaceus, 574
    psoriatic arthritis, 477
    Von Willebrand's disease, 508
Gengou, Octave, 2
Genitalia, female/male, 613–615, 614*f*, 621

Germinal center, 127
Giant-cell arteritis, 515, 522–524, 523*f*, 596
Giardia lamblia, 333, 336, 339
Gingivitis, 541–544, 542*f*, 543*f*
Glomerular basement membrane (GBM), 549
Glomerulonephritis
    antiglomerular basement membrane antibody-induced,
        550–552, 552*f*
    immune-complex, 552–559, 554–556*t*, 557*f*, 558*f*
    membrane nonproliferative, 556–558*f*, 558–559
    poststreptococcal, 559, 682
Glomerulosclerosis, focal, 561–562
Glomerulus, 553
Glucagon, 80
Glucocorticoid, 20, 402, 526, 575–576, 854, 855*t. See also*
        Corticosteroid
Glucose-6-phosphate dehydrogenase deficiency (G6PD),
        366–367, 573
Glutamic acid decarboxylase (GAD), 813
Gluten, 573
Gluten-sensitive enteropathy, 528–529, 529*f*
Glycoconjugate vaccine, 81
Glycogen storage disease type 1B, 367
Glycoprotein, 34, 51
Glycosaminoglycan, 17, 18
Gold, 857–858
Gold salt, 465, 601
Goldstein, Gideon, 4
Goodpasture's syndrome, 194, 551, 601–602, 608–609, 609*f*,
        835
Good's syndrome, 343
Gordon, Jon W., 4
Gorer, P. A., 3
Graft-*vs.*-host reaction (GVH), 348, 357–358, 358*f*, 359*f*
    antigen-nonspecific therapy, 770
    bone marrow transplantation, 819–820, 822*t*, 822–823
    cyclosporin, 837
    methotrexate, 836
    polyclonal antibody, 842
    rejection, pathology of, 805–808, 806–807*f*
    severe combined immunodeficiency, 353
    transfusion reactions, 282
Graft-*vs.*-leukemia effect (GVL), 821, 823
Gram-negative rods, 688
Granular immunoglobulin, 553, 556
Granule deficiency, specific, 367
Granule types, neutrophil, 31–32
Granulocyte colony-stimulating factor (G-CSF), 364, 821, 849
    clinical applications, 495*t*
Granulocyte-macrophage colony-stimulating factor (GM-CSF),
        849
    atopy, 391
    bone marrow transplantation, 821
    clinical applications, 495*t*
    eosinophil, 184
    extracellular matrix, 17
    granulocytopenia, therapy-induced, 165
    HIV (human immunodeficiency virus), 759
    HSC growth in vitro, 12
    Jak-Stat signaling pathway, 166*t*
    neutrophils and macrophages promoted, 13, 40
    tumor cells, 637
Granulocyte-monocyte progenitor, 10*f*, 13
Granuloma, 41
Granulomatosis
    allergic angiitis, 520
    Churg and Strauss, 602*t*, 602–603
    lymphomatoid, 609–610
    Wegener's, 521*f*, 521–522, 562, 609

Granulomatous disease, chronic, 364–366, 365, 366t
Granulomatous inflammation, 191
Grave's disease, 485–487, 486f
Griscelli's syndrome, 353
Guanosine diphosphate (GDP), 20
Guanosine triphosphate (GTP), 20
Guillain-Barré syndrome, 583–584
Gut-associated lymphoid tissue (GALT), 196

H & ABO system, 275–276, 276t
Haemophilus, 81, 355, 371, 542, 688, 774t, 793
Haemophilus influenzae, 337, 342, 682, 689
Hageman factor, 179, 179f, 281–282
Hairy cell leukemia, 666–667
Hairy leukoplakia, 546
Hall, J., 597
Hand-Schüller-Christian syndrome, 673
Haplotype, 87
Hapten, 78, 231
Haptenation, metabolic transformation and, 434f, 434–435, 435t
Hashimoto's thyroiditis, 482–483, 483f, 484f
Haskins, Kathryn, 3
Hassall corpuscle, 57
Haurowitz, Felix, 2
H-chain disease, 221
Health Information for International Travel Supplement, 794
Heart
    scleroderma, 471
    systemic lupus erythematosus, 458
Heart transplantation. *See also* Combined heart-lung transplantation
    complications, 817
    donor selection, 816
    immunosuppression and allograft monitoring, 816–817
    operative procedure, 816
    organ procurement, 816
    recipient selection, 815–816
    results, 817
    tissue typing, rationale for, 288
Heavy-chain disease, 669
Heavy (H) chain
    allotypic form, 100
    B cell made up of, 44, 46f
    class switching, 124–125, 125f
    four-chain basic unit, 97–98, 98t, 100
    gene arrangement influenced, 115–117
    immunoglobulin gene, 111–112
Heidelberger, M., 2
Helicobacter pylori, 649
Helminthiasis, 391
Helper factors, 51
Hematologic disease
    coagulation, 508–510
    erythrocyte, 495–502, 496t, 498t, 499t
    leukocyte, 493t, 493–495
    neoplasms of the immune system, 674
    platelet disorders, 502–508, 503–505t
Hematopoiesis
    apoptosis, 22–23
    bone marrow, cellular interactions in, 14f, 14–17, 15f, 16t
    cell growth and differentiation, 11–14, 12f, 13f
    cell proliferation & survival, 20–22, 21f
    classes of cells produced, 9
    cytokine, 17–20, 164
    ontogeny, 11, 11f
    schematic overview, 10f
Hematopoietic colony-stimulating factor, 164t, 164–165, 165t
Hematopoietic stem cell (HSC), 9, 10f, 11, 12–13, 43

Hematopoietin receptor family, 17–19, 18f, 165
Hematuria, 555, 561
Hemoglobinuria, paroxysmal cold, 499–500
Hemoglobinuria, paroxysmal nocturnal, 501
Hemolysis, 573
Hemolytic assay, 246–247
Hemolytic disease of the newborn, 282, 500–501
Hemolytic-uremic syndrome (HUS), 507–508
Hemophilia, 508–509
Hemorrhagic Shwartzman reaction, 150
Henoch-Schönlein purpura, 516–517
Heparin TNFα, 185
Hepatic fibrosis, 836
Hepatitis
    acute viral, 534
    fulminant, 534
    transfusion reactions, 281
    viral and serologic characteristics, 535t
Hepatitis A, 534, 535t, 774t, 786t
    virus, 702–703
Hepatitis B, 534–537, 535t, 701t, 774–775t, 786–787t, 791
    antigen positive chronic active, 810
    virus, 700–702
Hepatitis B immune globulin (HBIG) vaccine, 702
Hepatitis C, 535t, 537–538, 812
Hepatitis D, 535t, 537
Hepatitis E, 535t, 538
Hepatobiliary disease, 535t
    autoimmune chronic active hepatitis, 538–539
    Hepatitis A, 534, 535t
    Hepatitis B, 534–537, 535t
    Hepatitis C, 535t, 537–538
    Hepatitis D, 535t, 537
    Hepatitis E, 535t, 538
    primary biliary cirrhosis, 539f, 539–540
    primary sclerosing cholangitis, 540–541
Hepatocellular tumors, 810
Herd immunity, 790
Hereditary angioedema, 175, 180, 373–374, 417
Herpes gestationis, 568–570, 569f
Heterodimers, 17
Heterosexual transmission of HIV, 626–627
Heterotopic transplantation, 810–811, 816
Hevea brasiliensis, 413
Heymann nephritis model of membranous glomerulonephritis, 549
High-affinity receptor (FcɛRI) for IgE, 185, 390
High endothelial venules (HEVs), 60, 61f, 61–62
High-molecular-weight kininogen (HMW), 179, 179f
High-performance liquid chromatography (HPLC), 227
High zone tolerance, 75
Hilschmann, N., 3
Hinge region, 97
Histamine, 30, 184, 187, 187t, 195
    anaphylaxis, 410, 415
Histiocyte, 38, 673–674
Histocompatibility testing, 3
    cellular assay for, 294–297, 296f
    class II HLA antigens, tissue typing by serologic methods for, 292–293
    crossmatching, 293–294, 294f
    lymphocytotoxicity test, 289–291, 290f, 291t
    molecular-biologic method, 297–307, 299–301t, 300f, 303f, 304t, 305–306f
    monoclonal antibodies to HLA antigens, 291
    rationale for tissue typing, 286–289, 287–289t
    sensitization to HLA antigen, 289
    serologic methods, 289
    sources of HLA-typing sera, 291

Histocompatibility testing *(cont.)*
  specificity of HLA antibodies, 291–292
  transplantation, 286
Histology, 1
Histoplasmosis, 716–717
Historical overview of immunization, 772, 773*t*
Hives, 416–418
HIV (human immunodeficiency virus), 334, 338, 350, 436, 546
  active immunization, 783
  cancer, 645–648, 646*f,* 647*t,* 648*f*
  clinical feature, 752*t,* 752–753
  diagnosis, differential/immunologic, 756
  epidemiology, 751–752, 752*t*
  etiology, 748–751, 749*t,* 749–750*f,* 751*t*
  general considerations, 748
  immunologic findings, 748, 754–756
  immunopathology of infection, 682
  laboratory diagnosis, 753–754
  lymphoma, 674
  prevention, 759–760
  reproductive processes, 626–628
  transfusion reactions, 281
  treatment, 757–759
  vaccine, current development of, 794
HLA. *See* Human leukocyte antigen
HLA-B27 allele, 93
HLA-DM molecule, 90
Hodgkin's disease, 647–648, 672*f,* 672–673, 673*t*
Homing receptors, 61
Homodimers, 17
Homologous restriction factor (HRF), 178, 374
Homozygous typing cell, 297, 298*t*
Horseradish peroxidase, 242
Host responsiveness as component of autoimmunity, 453
HSC. *See* Hematopoietic stem cell
Human antimouse antibodies (HAMA), 842
Human chorionic gonadotropin (HCG), 616, 620
Human herpes virus 6 (HHV-6), 765
Human immune globulin, 784–785
Human immunodeficiency virus. *See* HIV (human immunodeficiency virus)
Human leukocyte antigen (HLA), 85, 86–87, 89*f. See also* Histocompatibility testing
  autoimmune disease, 452*t,* 452–453
  autoimmune endocrine disease, 480, 480*f*
  bare lymphocyte syndrome, 354
  bone marrow transplantation, 820
  celiac disease, 529
  corneal graft reaction, 597
  dermatitis herpetiformis, 571
  graft-verses-host reaction, 359*t*
  heart transplantation, 817
  homozygosity between parents, 622
  pancreas transplantation, 813
  rheumatoid disease affecting the eye, 593
  severe combined immunodeficiency, 353
  Sjögren's syndrome, 469
  trophoblast, 618
Human platelet antigen (HPA) system, 503
Human T cell leukemia virus (HTLV), 632
Human T cell leukemia virus type I (HTLV-I), 153, 763–765
Human T cell leukemia virus type II (HTLV-II), 763–765
Humoral immune response
  B cell antigen receptor, 118, 119*f,* 120
  B cell as antigen-presenting cell, 123*f,* 123–124
  heavy-chain class switch, 124–125, 125*f*
  immunoglobulin secretion, 124
  lymphoid follicle and germinal centers, 126*f,* 126–127
  primary and secondary, 127*t,* 127–128

  somatic hypermutation, 125–126
  T cell help and accessory signal, 121, 121*f,* 122*f,* 123
  T cell-independent antigen, 120*f,* 120–121
Humoral immunity, 2, 46
HUS. *See* Hemolytic-uremic syndrome
Hyaluronic acid, 16
Hybridization assay, 311–312, 312*f*
Hybridoma, 106, 107*f,* 249, 250*f*
Hydralazine, 435, 601
Hydrogen peroxide, 272
Hydrops fetalis, 622–623
Hydroxylation, 852
Hymenoptera insect sting and anaphylaxis, 412–413, 413*t,* 415, 797, 799
Hypergammaglobulinemic purpura, benign, 669
Hyper-IgE syndrome, 339, 367–368, 368*f*
Hyper-IgM syndrome, 121
Hyperosinophilic syndrome, 605
Hypersensitivity, 2. *See also* Allergy; Cell-mediated hypersensitivity disease; Small-vessel vasculitis
  cutaneous basophil, 195
  delayed, 425
  immediate, 194, 454
  nongluten food, 530
  pneumonitis, 611
  respiratory disease, 599
Hypersensitivity pneumonitis, 425
  allergen, 428, 429*t*
  clinical feature, 430
  complications and prognosis, 431
  defining, 428
  diagnosis, immunologic/differential, 431
  epidemiology, 428
  pathogenesis, immunologic, 429–430
  pathology, 429
  prevention, 432
  treatment, 431
Hypertension, 555, 559, 561, 840
Hypervariable region, 103, 103*f,* 112
Hypochlorous acid (HOCl), 36
Hypocomplementemia, 558
Hypocomplementemic urticarial vasculitis, 517–518
Hypogammaglobulinemia, 478, 782, 787*t*
  infancy, transient, 336*f,* 336–337
Hypoparathyroidism, idiopathic, 490
Hypoproteinemia, 218
Hyposensitization, 798
Hypotension, 410
Hypothyroidism, primary, 487
Hypoxanthine phosphoribosyl transferase (HPRT), 249

Idiopathic anaphylaxis, 414
Idiopathic CD4 lymphocytopenia, 350
Idiopathic hypoparathyroidism, 490
Idiopathic pulmonary fibrosis, 606–608, 607*f,* 608*t*
Idiopathic thrombocytopenic purpura, 503–504*t,* 503–506
Idiopathic ulcerative colitis, 532–533, 533*f*
Idiopathic urticaria-angioedema, 417
Idiotype, 103
IgA, 102, 614
  anaphylaxis, 413, 415
  anti-inflammatory properties, 202
  breast milk immunology, 207–208
  corticosteroid, 828
  dermatitis herpetiformis, 571, 573
  Henoch-Schönlein purpura, 517
  hypersensitivity pneumonitis, 429
  hypogammaglobulinemia of infancy, transient, 336
  immune-complex glomerulonephritis, 556

immune exclusion, 203
immunodiffusion, 215, 216
linear IgA bullous dermatosis, 573–574
polymerization and interaction with secretory component, 201–202
proinflammatory properties, 202
proteolysis, resistance to, 202
regulation of IgA synthesis at mucosal site, 204*f*, 204–205
secretory *vs.* circulating, 203–204
selective deficiency, 339–342, 357
serum immunoglobulin levels in disease, 217*t*
structure and function, 200–201, 201*f*
transport, 202–203, 203*f*
IgD, 117, 215, 216, 360
IgE, 102. *See also Atop listings*
anaphylaxis, 409, 412
antihistamine, 859
desensitization, 798
drug allergy, 436
drug-induced respiratory disease, 599
eosinophil, 184, 185
hyper-IgE syndrome, 339, 367–368, 368*f*
hyposensitization, 798
immunosuppressive therapy, 833
inflammation, 194*f*, 194–195, 770
insulin allergy, 440, 441
nonatopic allergic disease, 389
pathway of immunologically induced inflammation, 377, 379*t*
penicillin, 437–438
serum total and disease, 389–390, 390*t*, 398, 398*f*
urticaria, 416
in vitro test for allergy, 385
wheal-and-flare reaction, 188
IgG, 101–102. *See also* Immune-complex allergic disease
affinity chromatography, 226
antiglomerular basement membrane antibody-induced glomerulonephritis, 551, 552*f*
bullous pemphigoid, 564, 566
corticosteroid, 828
cyclophosphamide, 835
drug allergy, 436
eosinophil, 184
gingivitis, 543
Hepatitis A, 534
herpes gestationis, 569
hypersensitivity pneumonitis, 429
hypogammaglobulinemia of infancy, transient, 336
immunodiffusion, 215, 216
insulin allergy, 440, 441
laboratory tests, immunologic, 324
latex fixation test, 245
paraneoplastic pemphigoid, 577
pathway of immunologically induced inflammation, 379
pemphigus foliaceous, 574
pemphigus vulgaris, 575
penicillin, 433
plasmapheresis, 841
recognition and adhesion, tests for, 270
rheumatoid disease affecting the eye, 593
selective deficiency, 342–343, 343*f*
serum immunoglobulin levels in disease, 217*t*
IgM, 102, 170. *See also* Immune-complex allergic disease
antigen-specific therapy, 768
antiglomerular basement membrane antibody-induced glomerulonephritis, 551, 552*f*
corticosteroid, 828
cyclophosphamide, 835

endotoxins and exotoxins, 685
gel filtration, 226
hypogammaglobulinemia of infancy, transient, 336
immunodeficiency with hyper-, 339
latex fixation test, 245
pathway of immunologically induced inflammation, 379
plasmapheresis, 841
rheumatoid disease affecting the eye, 593
selective deficiency, 342
serum immunoglobulin levels in disease, 217*t*
I*k*Bα, 829
Illustrations, glossary of symbols used in, 864–865
Imexone, 850
Imidathiazole, 850
Imidazole, 718
Immediate hypersensitivity, 454
Immediate phase of inflammatory response, 194, 195, 377
Immune-complex allergic disease
allergic bronchopulmonary aspergillosis, 421–423, 422*t*, 423*t*
Arthus reaction, 419
serum sickness, 420*f*, 420–421
tissue-destruction, 454
vasculitis, 514–515
Immune complexes, detection of, 229
Immune-complex glomerulonephritis
classification, 554–555*t*
clinical feature, 553, 554–555*t*, 555
complications and prognosis, 559
diagnosis, immunologic/differential, 557–558
general consideration, 552–553, 554–556*t*
immunologic feature, 552
pathogenesis, immunologic, 556–557, 558*f*
pathology, 553, 554–555*t*, 557*f*
treatment, 558–559
Immune complex-mediated inflammation, 192–194, 193*f*
Immune exclusion, 203
Immune gamma globulin for intramuscular use (IMIG), 784
Immune interferon (IFNγ), 158
Immune privilege, 72
Immune response. *See also* Autoimmune disease; Parasitic disease
atopic disease, 389–390
B cell activation, 68–69
cell death, programmed, 72
clonal organization, 63–65, 64*f*
drug allergy, 435
elimination, mechanisms of antigen, 69–70
functional properties, 63
helper T cell activation, 67–68, 68*f*
immunogen & antigen, 65, 67
inflammation, 70
localization, 70–71
modulation of, 767–770
normal immune response: fundamental principles, 444–445
antigen-specific recognition, 444
discrimination of self *vs.* nonself, 444–445
diversity of lymphocyte repertoire, 444
memory, immunologic, 445
self-limitation, 445
pathways of immunologically induced inflammation
effector T cell/lymphokine, 379
IgE/mast cell/mediator, 377, 379*t*
IgG or IgM/complement/neutrophil, 379
primary, 831
quantitative & kinetic aspects, 71–72
sequence in a, 66*f*
tumor immunology, 635–637

Immune surveillance against neoplasia, 640–641
Immune system, innate, 26, 26*t*
Immune thrombocytopenia purpura (ITP), 355
Immunity
  adoptive, 767–768
  cell-mediated, 46
  herd, 790
  humoral, 46
  phagocyte, 31–41
    monocyte-macrophage system, 38–40*t*, 38–41, 39*f*, 41*f*
    neutrophil, 31*f*, 31*t*, 31–32, 32*t*, 33*f*, 34–38, 35–37*f*, 37*t*
    soluble proteins, 25–29
    vascular & endothelial response to injury/infection, 29*f*, 29*t*, 29–31, 30*t*
Immunization
  active, 767, 772–773
    adverse reactions & risk-benefit ratio, 782
    reporting adverse effects & legal liability, 783, 784*t*
    route of, 773
    technique of, 782
    timing of primary, 773, 782
    vaccine types. *See* Vaccine
  clinical indications for
    age, 791–793, 792*t*
    antigenic shift/variation, 791
    diseases, specific, 791
    foreign travel, 793–794
    herd immunity, 790
    simultaneous immunization with multiple antigens, 793
    special populations, 794
  combined passive-active, 790
  current development, 794
  goal of, 772
  historical overview, 772, 773*t*
  passive, 767, 783
    animal sera & antitoxins, 785
    hazards, 790
    human immune globulin, 784–785
    noninfectious diseases, 785, 790
    special preparations of human immune globulin, 785
    vaccine types. *See* Vaccine
Immunoblastic lymphoma/myeloma, 674
Immunochemical and physicochemical methods, 225–231, 226–227*f*, 228–229*t*, 230*f*
Immunochemistry, 2
Immunocompromise, 641*t*, 641–642, 642*t*
Immunodeficiency disorder. *See also* Antibody (B cell) immunodeficiency disorder; Cellular immunodeficiency disorder; Combined T cell & B cell immunodeficiency disorder; Phagocyte dysfunction disease; T cell immunodeficiency disorder
  causes, 327*t*
  classification, 329*t*
  clinical features, 328*t*
  initial screening evaluation, 329*t*
  serum immunoglobulin levels in disease, 217*t*
  treatment, 330*t*
  x-linked severe combined, 154
Immunodiffusion
  double diffusion in agar, 212*f*, 212–214, 213*f*
  precipitation reaction, 211–212, 212*f*
  serum immunoglobulin levels in health and disease, 215–216
  single radial diffusion, 214*f*, 214–215
Immunodominant residues, 80
Immunoelectrophoresis, 218–221, 221*f*

Immunofixation electrophoresis, 221, 224*f*
Immunofluorescence, 2
  blistering disease, 564
  epidermolysis bullosa acquisita, 570–571
  fluorescence, 237
  method and interpretation, 238–239
  quantitative, 240, 242
  staining techniques, 239–240, 240*f*, 241*f*
Immunogen. *See also* Antigen
  adjuvant, 82
  B-cell antigen & epitope, 75–77, 76*f*, 77*f*
  contact, mode of, 75
  defining, 65, 74
  exogenous, 65, 67
  genetic constitution of host animal, 75
  immunodominant residues, 80
  physicochemical basis of antigen-antibody binding, 78*t*, 78–79
  properties, 74–75
  T cell epitope & antigen, 79–80
  thymus-independent antigen, 80
  vaccine, 80–82, 81*t*
Immunogenetics & genetic engineering, 3
Immunoglobulin (Ig), 34–35. *See also* Antibody; Ig *listings*
  anaphylactoid reaction, 335
  B cell, 44–45, 45–46*f*
  biologic activities, 100*t*, 101–102
  biosynthesis, 260
  chains, classifying constituent, 97–98, 98*t*, 100
  classes/subclasses, composition of, 98–99, 99*f*, 100*t*
  common variable immunodeficiency, 338–339
  cytoplasmic, 260
  enzymatic digestion products, 97
  four-chain basic unit, 96–97, 97*f*
  gene arrangement assay, 313–314
  genes, 109–113, 109–113*f*
  granular, 553, 556
  Job's syndrome, 368
  laboratory tests, immunologic, 324
  malignancy, B cell, 113
  membrane and secreted, 99–101
  organization and diversity, 95–96
  secretion, 124
  severe combined immunodeficiency, 353
  supergene family, 105–106, 106*t*, 165
  surface, 259–260, 260*t*
  three-dimensional structure, 103, 104*t*, 105, 105*f*
  variable region, 102–103
  X-linked agammaglobulinemia, 335
Immunohistochemical technique, 237–241*f*, 237–242, 242*t*
Immunologic therapy, 766
  antigen-nonspecific therapy, 768–770
  antigen-specific therapy, 767–768
  inflammatory response, modulation of the, 770
Immunology
  cellular immunology, rebirth of, 2–3
  drug allergy, 433
  humoral *vs.* cellular, 2
  immunogenetics & genetic engineering, 3
  molecular, 3
  Nobel prize winners, 4–5
  origin of, 1–2
  serology, 2
  time line, 3–4
  tumor immunology, 637–638
Immunomodulator, 75, 82
  bacterial compound, 846–847
  defining, 846, 847*t*

eukaryotic organism
  biochemical agent, 850–851
  cytokine, 848–850
  monoclonal antibody, 850
  thymic hormone, 847–848
Immunopathology of infection, 682–683
Immunophenotypic analysis, 653–654, 654–656*t*
Immunophilin, 838
Immunoproliferative small-intestinal disease (IPSID), 533
Immunoradiometric assay (IRMA), 233
Immunoreceptor tyrosine-based activation motif (ITAM), 120, 135
Immunorestorative therapy, 758–759
Immunostimulatory drug, 850
Immunosuppressive therapy, 576
  antilymphocyte antibodies, 842
  bone marrow transplantation, 820
  bone transplantation, 824–825
  combined heart-lung transplantation, 818–819
  corticosteroid
    cellular traffic, effects on, 827–828
    clinical use, 829–830
    functional change, 828–829, 829*f*
  crossmatching and immunosuppression, 812–813
  cyclosporin, 837–840, 838*f*, 839*f*, 840*t*
    IL-2 gene, 838
    properties and uses, 840*t*
    revolutionized discipline of organ transplantation, 837
    toxicity, 839*f*, 839–840
  cytotoxic drug
    azathioprine, 834, 834*f*
    chlorambucil, 837
    clinical use, 833, 833*t*
    combining two or more drugs, 837
    cyclophosphamide, 834*f*, 834–836, 835*t*
    defining, 830
    methotrexate, 836*f*, 836–837, 837*t*
    principles forming usage of, 831–833
  heart transplantation, 816–817
  insulin-dependent diabetes mellitus, 489
  intravenous gamma globulin, 841–842
  kidney transplantation, 804–805
  monoclonal antibody, 842–844, 843*f*
  neoplasms and hematologic proliferations, 674
  newer drugs, 841
  pancreas transplantation, 814–815
  plasmapheresis, 841
  rapamycin, 840–841
  rheumatoid arthritis, 465
  tacrolimus, 840
  warm autoimmune hemolytic anemia, 497
Immunotoxin, 106
Implantation of blastocyst, 616
Imprecision profile, 236
Indirect antiglobulin test (IAT), 278, 278*f*
Indirect fluorescent antibody assay (IFA), 745
Inducible nitric oxide synthase (iNOS), 36
Induction phase in immune response, 831
Infection
  bone marrow transplantation, 823–824
  combined heart-lung transplantation, 819
  immunologic defense
    antibody-mediated, 680, 681*t*
    complement system, 681, 681*t*
    phagocytic cell, 681, 681*t*
    T cell, 680–681
  immunopathology of, 682–683
  liver transplantation, 812

nonimmunologic defenses
  body surfaces, host defenses antibody, 678–679
  fever, 680
  inflammation, 679–680
serum immunoglobulin levels in disease, 217*t*
spleen in host defense, 682
transfusion reactions, 280–281, 281*f*
vascular & endothelial response to, 29*f*, 29*t*, 29–31, 30*t*
Infertility, 620–621
Inflammation. *See also* Anti-inflammatory drug
  chemokine, 162
  complement system, 169, 176
  defining, 70, 182, 679–680
  granulomatous, 191
  IgA, 202
  immunologic feature, 541
  mediator, 187–190
    adenosine, 188
    arachidonic acid metabolite, 187–188, 188*f*, 189*f*
    chemotactic, 188
    enzymatic, 189
    histamine, 187, 187*t*
    platelet-activating factor, 188, 190*f*
    proteoglycan, 189–190
  pathways of immunologically induced
    effector T cell/lymphokine, 379
    IgE/mast cell/mediator, 377, 379*t*
    IgG or IgM complement/neutrophil, 379
  periarticular, 462
  tissue-infiltrating cells, 449
Inflammation, acute, 36, 37
Inflammatory cell
  basophil, 186, 186*f*
  defining, 183
  endothelial cell, 186–187
  eosinophil, 183–184, 184*f*
  mast cell, 184–186, 185*f*, 185*t*
  platelet, 186
Inflammatory periodontal disease
  diagnosis, immunologic, 544
  general consideration, 541–542, 542*f*, 543*f*
  pathogenesis, immunologic, 543–544
Inflammatory response, 377
  cell-mediated immunity, 190–192, 191*f*, 191*t*
  cutaneous basophil hypersensitivity, 195
  IgE-mediated, 194*f*, 194–195
  immune complex-mediated, 192–194, 193*f*
  modulation of, 770
Influenza, 775*t*
Influenza virus
  clinical feature, 695–696
  general considerations, 694
  pathogenesis, immunologic, 696
  prevention, 697
  treatment, 696–697
  virology, 694–695, 695*t*
Ingestion, tests for, 270–271
Inhibitor of NF*k*B (I*k*B), 20
Inhibitors of coagulation, circulating, 509
Initiation and neoplasia, 641, 641*t*
Injection technique, 782, 797
Injury
  endothelial response, 30–31, 31*t*
  neutrophils, 34
  vascular response, 29*f*, 29*t*, 29–30, 30*t*
Inosine pranobex, 850
Inositol 1,4,5-trisphosphate (IP3), 50, 136
Insect venom and anaphylaxis, 412–413, 413*t*
In situ hybridization, 314

Insulin allergy, 440–441, 441f
Insulin-dependent diabetes mellitus (IDDM), 487–489, 489t
Integrin, 14–15, 374
    mediated phase of margination, 34
Intercellular adhesion molecule-1 (ICAM-1), 14, 580, 843
Interdigitating cell, 55, 92
Interferon gamma (IFN-γ), 39–40, 70, 580, 730, 806–807
Interferon (IFN), 157f, 157–158, 848
Interleukin, 12
    common variable immunodeficiency, 338
    immunomodulator, 847t, 848–849
    phenotypic deficiencies of immunoregulatory cytokine
        knockout mice, 154t
Interleukin-1β-converting enzyme (ICE), 22
Interleukin-1 (IL-1), 28, 68, 146
    family, 148–149
    membrane attack complex, 550
    nonimmunological inflammatory effects, 150–151
    properties, 147t
    receptors and signal transduction, 148–150
    target cell and actions of, 149t
Interleukin-2 (IL-2), 52, 67, 153–155, 154f, 154t
    antigen-nonspecific therapy, 769
    corticosteroid, 828
    cyclosporin, 837, 839
    hematologic disease, 495t
    HIV (human immunodeficiency virus), 750, 759
    immunomodulator, 848
    monoclonal antibody, 844
    non-T cell, 155
    phenotypic deficiencies of immunoregulatory cytokine
        knockout mice, 154t
    receptors and signal transduction, 153–154
    T cell, 154–155
    as a therapeutic agent, 155
    tumor immunology, 638
Interleukin-3 (IL-3), 12, 17, 43
    colony-stimulating factor, 164–165
    eosinophil, 184
    hematologic disease, 495t
    properties, 147t
Interleukin-4 (IL-4), 158–159
    atopy, 391
    cytokine, 849
    helper T cell, 140
    immunomodulator, 848–849
    phenotypic deficiencies of immunoregulatory cytokine
        knockout mice, 154t
    properties, 147t
Interleukin-5 (IL-5), 13, 159
    atopy, 391
    eosinophil, 184
    properties, 147t
Interleukin-6 (IL-6), 28
    family, 155–157, 156t
    hematologic disease, 495t
    properties, 147t
    trophoblast, 618
Interleukin-7 (IL-7), 159
    phenotypic deficiencies of immunoregulatory cytokine
        knockout mice, 154t
    properties, 147t
Interleukin-8 (IL-8), 162
    chemokine family, 162–163, 163t
    properties, 147t
Interleukin-9 (IL-9), 159–160
    properties, 147t
Interleukin-10 (IL-10), 160
    immunomodulator, 849

    phenotypic deficiencies of immunoregulatory cytokine
        knockout mice, 154t
    properties, 147t
    trophoblast, 618
Interleukin-11 (IL-11)
    properties, 147t
Interleukin-12 (IL-12), 82, 140, 160
    immunomodulator, 849
    properties, 147t
Interleukin-13 (IL-13), 159
    atopy, 391
    properties, 147t
Interleukin-14 (IL-14), 160
    properties, 147t
Interleukin-15 (IL-15), 160
    properties, 147t
Interleukin-16 (IL-16), 160
    properties, 147t
Interleukin-1 receptor antagonist (IL-1RA), 850
Interleukin-2R (IL-2R), 20
Intermediate-affinity (FcγRII) receptor for IgG, 184
International Lymphoma Study Group, 661
International Society for Heart and Lung Transplantation
        (ISHLT), 815, 818, 819
International Working Formulation for Clinical Use, 661
International Workshop on Human Leukocyte Differentiation
        Antigens (1983), 256
Interpolation, 231, 233
Interstitial fluid, 52–53
Intestinal T cell lymphoma, 671
Intracellular bacterial pathogen, 690–692, 691f
Intradermal route of immunization, 782
Intradermal test, 383f, 383–384
Intraepithelial lymphocyte (IEL), 198–199, 199f
Intrauterine insemination, 621
Intravenous normal pooled immunoglobulin (IVIG), 768,
        784–785, 841–842
Intrinsic disorder, phagocytic, 364
Intron, 309
Invariant chain, 89
In-vitro fertilization, 621
In vitro testing, 384, 385t, 412, 437
In vivo testing, 437
Ion-exchange chromatography, 226
Ionic compounds and anaphylactoid reaction, 413
Irradiation, total body, 821
Isoimmunization, 622–626, 624–625f
Isolated angiitis of the central nervous system, 526
Isoniazid, 601
Itraconazole, 711, 715, 717

Jak/Stat signaling pathway, 19f, 20, 166t
Japanese encephalitis, 775t
Jarisch-Herxheimer reaction, 414, 743
Jaw claudication, 523
Jenner, Edward, 1, 3, 80, 766, 772
Jennings plots, 233
Jerne, Niels, 3–5
Job's syndrome, 367–368, 368f
Joints/muscles, 457–458, 471
Jones-Mote hypersensitivity, 195
Journal of Immunology, 2
Juvenile arthritis, 466–468, 592
Juvenile periodontitis, 544

Kabat, Elvin, 2, 4
Kallikrein, 180
Kantrowitz, Adrian, 815

Kaposi's sarcoma, 644, 645–646, 753
Kaposi's sarcoma herpes virus (KSHV), 645–646
Kappa chain, 97–98
Kasai procedure, 810
Kawasaki syndrome, 785, 790, 842
k-Deleting element, 128
Kendall, Edward, 2
Keratinocyte hemidesmosomal protein, 564
Keratoconjunctivitis
   atopic/vernal, 591–592, 592*f*
   phlyctenular, 596
   vernal, 395–396
Ketoconazole, 711, 715, 717
Kidney
   scleroderma, 471
   systemic lupus erythematosus, 457–458
   tissue immunofluorescence, 460
Kidney transplantation
   ABO testing
      blood transfusion, 804
      cadaveric, 803
      crossmatching, 803
      donor selection/evaluation, 803–804
      living related donor, 802–803
      postoperative immunosuppression, 804–805
      presensitization, 803
      rejection, 805
      surgery, 804
   graft rejection, pathology of, 805–808, 806–807*f*
   tissue typing, rationale for, 287–288, 288–289*t*
Killed vaccine, 81–82, 783–785, 786–790*t*, 790
Killer cell inhibitory receptor (KIR) family, 143–144
Kinin-generating system
   activation, 179–180
   amplification and regulation, 180
   bradykinin, 178–179
   disease, 180
   low-molecular-weight kininogen, 180
   plasma inhibitors, 180
   plasma protein, 179, 179*f*
Kitasato, Shibasaburo, 2, 4
Klebs, Theodor, 2
Klebsiella, 368, 688, 689, 690
Koch, Robert, 4, 7, 772
Koch's postulates, 1
Köhler, Georges, 3–5
Kraus, Rudolf, 2, 4
Kung, Patrick, 3, 4
Kupffer cell, 38

Laboratory tests, immunologic
   antigen and antibody, 211–216, 212–215*f*
      agglutination, 243–244*t*, 243–245, 245*f*
      binder-ligand assay, 231–237, 232*f*, 234–236*f*
      comparative sensitivity of quantitative immunoassays, 250, 251*t*
      complement assay, 245–249, 246–248*f*, 248–249*t*
      electrophoresis and immunoelectrophoresis, 216–221, 217*t*, 218–225*f*, 224–225
      immunochemical and physicochemical methods, 225–231, 226–227*f*, 228–229*t*, 230*f*
      immunohistochemical technique, 237–241*f*, 237–242, 242*t*
      monoclonal antibodies, 249–250, 250*f*, 250*t*, 251*t*
      predictive value theory, 250–251, 251*t*
      separation of peripheral blood mononuclear cells, 257
   B cell, 323*t*, 323–324

cellular immunity
   B-lymphocyte assay, 259*t*, 259–260, 260*t*
   flow cytometry, 260–264, 262–263*f*, 264*t*
   lymphocyte activation, 264–269, 265*t*, 266–268*f*, 267*t*
   mixed lymphocyte culture, 267–268, 268*f*
   monocyte-macrophage assay, 269
   natural killer cell, 268–269
   neutrophil function, 269–274, 271*f*, 272–273*t*, 273*f*
   skin test, delayed hypersensitivity, 254–256
   T-lymphocyte assay, 257–259, 258*f*, 258*t*, 259*f*
   clinical utility, 320, 321*t*
   complement system, 325
   Epstein-Barr virus (EBV), 762
   HIV (human immunodeficiency virus), 753–754
   immune hemolytic anemia, 496–497
   limitations, 320
   natural killer cell, 324–325
   nonspecific, 320–321
   phagocytic cell, 325
   specific testing, 321
   T cell, 321–323, 322–323*t*
   utility, 319, 320
   variability, 319
Lactoferrin, 35, 679
Lambda chain, 97–98
Lambert-Eaton syndrome, 587
Lamina propria cell, 199*f*, 199–200
Lamivudine 2'-deoxy-3'-thiacytadine (3TC), 757
Landsteiner, Karl, 2, 4, 5, 8
Langerhans' cell, 56–57, 92
Langerhans' cell histiocytosis (LCH), 673–674
Large-cell B/T cell lymphoma, 667
Large granular lymphocyte leukemia (LGLL), 669–670
Laryngeal edema, 414
Latent phase, 71
Late phase of inflammatory response, 195, 377
Latex allergy, 413
Latex fixation test, 245
Lectin, 51
Legionella pneumophila, 691
Leishmania major, 140
Leishmaniasis, 281
   cutaneous, 729–730
   visceral, 730–731
Lens-induced uveitis, 594
Lepidoglyphus destructor, 393
Leptospirosis, 746
Letterer-Siwe syndrome, 673
Leukemia
   acute lymphoblastic, 662, 663*f*, 664, 821
   acute lymphocytic leukemia of childhood, 601
   acute myelogenous, 820–821
   adult T cell, 153
   adult T-cell leukemia-lymphoma, 670–671
   B cell chronic lymphocytic, 664
   bone marrow transplantation, 819
   chronic myelogenous, 821
   hairy cell, 666–667
   large granular lymphocyte, 669–670
   lymphoma *vs.*, 653
   marrow progenitors, 14
   prolymphocytic, 664
Leukocyte, 9, 157
   bare lymphocyte syndrome, 353–354
   corticosteroid effect on cellular traffic, 827–828
   hematologic disease, 493*t*, 493–495
Leukocyte adhesion defect-type1 (LAD-1), 368–369, 369*f*
Leukocyte adhesion defect-type2 (LAD-2), 369
Leukocyte chemotactic factor, 32, 34, 34*t*

Leukocyte functional antigen-1 (LFA-1), 118, 843
Leukocyte inhibitory factor (LIF), 156
Leukopenia, 493t, 493–495
Leukotriene antagonist, 857, 858f
Levamisole, 850
Ligand. *See also* Binder-ligand assay
  adhesion protein, 16t
  antigen, 46
  CD40, 69, 121, 205
  CD80/86, 448
  Fas, 72, 142
  glycoprotein, 34
  immunoglobulin, 45
  macrophage surface receptors, 39t
  OX40, 205
  tumor necrosis factor, 151
Ligase chain reaction (LCR), 316, 317f
Light (L) chain
  allotypic, 100
  B cell made of, 44, 46f
  four-chain basic unit, 97–98, 98t, 100
  gene arrangement influenced, 115–117
  immunoglobulin gene, 109, 111
  surrogate, 116
Light zone, 127
Limbic encephalitis, 588
Lineage, cell, 651–653, 652f, 652t
Lineage-committed progenitor, 11, 12, 12f, 13–14
Linear IgA bullous dermatosis, 573–574
Lipid metabolism, 855t
Lipids, 74
Lipomodulin, 854
Lipopolysaccharide (LPS), 26–27, 27f, 120–121, 148
Lipoxygenase product, 188
Liquid scintillation, 232
Lister, Joseph, 1
Listeria monocytogenes, 619, 691, 847
Liver disease. *See also* Hepatobiliary disease
  serum immunoglobulin levels, 217t
  venoocclusive disease, 823
Liver transplantation
  crossmatching and immunosuppression, 812–813
  indications, 809–810
  outcome, 811–812
  procedure, 810–811
  tissue typing, rationale for, 288
Living related donor transplantation, 802–803
Loa loa, 281
Loboa laboi, 706
Localization of immune response, 70–71
Löffler, Friedrich, 2
Löffler's syndrome, 603–604
Logit transformation, 232
Long-term bone marrow culture (LTBMC), 14
Long terminal repeat (LTR), 749
Low-affinity (FceRII) receptor for IGE, 184
Low-molecular-weight kininogen, 180
L-selectin, 34, 61, 118
L-tyrosine-*p*-azobenzenearsonate (ABA-Tyr), 80
Lung
  disease, occupational and environmental, 605
  injury, transfusion-related acute, 280
  rheumatoid arthritis, 462
  scleroderma, 471
  systemic lupus erythematosus, 458
  transplantation, 610–611, 817–819
Lupus-like syndrome, drug-induced, 458
Lupus syndrome, 601
Ly-49 inhibitory receptor, 143

Lyme disease, 744–746
Lymphadenopathy, 55
Lymph nodes & lymphatic circulation, 52–54f, 52–55
Lymphoblast, 50, 50f
Lymphoblastic lymphoma (LBL), 662, 663f, 664
Lymphocyte. *See also* B cell; T cell
  abnormalities in interactions, 451
  activation, 44, 45f, 49–52, 51f, 51t, 264
    antigen stimulation, 267, 267t
    cell-mediated lympholysis, 267–268, 268f
    mitogen, 260, 265t, 265–266, 266t
    natural killer cell, 268–269
  antigen-nonspecific activation, 450
  circulation & homing, 59–60f, 59–62, 61t, 62t
  clonal organization, 63–65, 64f
  cytotoxic drug, 831
  defective regulation, 404–405
  diverse repertoire, 444
  double-negative, 48
  intraepithelial, 198–199, 199f
  lymphopoiesis, 43–44
  memory, 44
  pregnancy, immunity in, 620
  production of, 11
  self-limitation, 445
  single-positive, 48
  virgin, 44, 63, 117f, 117–118
Lymphocyte-determined membrane antigen (LYDMA), 763
Lymphocyte function-associated antigen type 1 (LFA-1), 270
Lymphocytic adenohypophysitis, 489–490
Lymphocytopenia, idiopathic CD4, 350
Lymphocytotoxicity test, 289–291, 290f, 291t, 293–294
Lymphoid aggregates, mucosal, 197–198, 198f
Lymphoid follicles, 53, 54f, 55
Lymphoid organs
  lymph nodes & lymphatic circulation, 52–54f, 52–55
  spleen, 55–56, 56f
  subepithelial, 55–56, 56f
  tertiary, 62
  thymus, 57–59, 58f
Lymphoid stem cell, 10f, 43
Lymphoid tissue, diffuse, 198–199, 199f
Lymphokine, 46, 51, 146
Lymphokine-activated killer (LAK) cells, 638, 769, 848
Lymphoma
  adult T-cell leukemia-lymphoma, 670–671
  anaplastic large-cell, 671–672
  angiocentric, 671
  angioimmunoblastic T cell, 671
  Burkitt's and Burkitt-like, 113, 667
  classifying, 661, 661t, 662t
  follicular, 72, 113, 665–666
  immunoblastic, 674
  intestinal T cell, 671
  large B/T cell, 667
  leukemia vs., 653
  lymphoblastic, 662, 663f, 664
  lymphoplasmacytoid, 664–665
  mantle cell, 665
  marginal zone B cell, 666
  peripheral T cell, 671
  polymorphic, 674
  small lymphocytic, 664
Lymphomatoid granulomatosis, 609–610
Lymphopenia, 354
Lymphoplasmacytoid lymphoma, 664–665
Lymphopoiesis, 43–44
Lymphoproliferative disorder, 843
Lysis of cells/bacteria/virus, 169

Lysosome, 38, 40
Lysozyme, 26, 35

MacCleod, C. M., 2
Macrophage, 13, 38, 92. *See also* Granulocyte-macrophage
 colony-stimulating factor (GM-CSF)
 activation, 39*t,* 39–40, 40*t*
 alveolar, 606
 granuloma, 41
 spleen, 55
 tumor immunology, 635
Macropinocytosis, 84
Major histocompatibility complex (MHC), 47. *See also*
 Antigen-presenting cell (APC)
 alloreactivity & transplant rejection, 91
 antigen-specific therapy, 768
 assembly & presentation, 87–89, 90*f*
 atopy, 390
 autoimmune endocrine disease, 480
 classes of, 65
 class II chain, 89–90
 combined T cell & B cell immunodeficiency disorder, 353
 common variable immunodeficiency, 337
 complementarity, 80
 disease, 92–93
 dome cell, 197
 endocytic pathway, 69, 83–84, 84*t*
 HLA gene complex, 86–87
 interferon, 158
 interleukin-4, 159
 lamina propria cell, 200
 liver transplantation, 809
 malaria, 728
 mature B lymphocyte, 118
 mixed lymphocyte culture, 268
 multiple sclerosis, 580
 negative selection, 447
 peptide-MHC recognition by T cell, 90–91
 polymorphism, 85–86
 positive & negative selection, 91, 133–134, 447
 schematic representation, 86*f*
 self-tolerance, 446
 structures of classical, 85
 superantigen, 131–132, 132*f*
 T cell receptor, 130
 tumor immunology, 633
Mak, Tak, 3, 4
Malaria, 281, 726*f,* 726–728, 794
Malassezia, 706
Malignant histiocytosis (MH), 674
Mannose-binding protein (MBP), 26, 176
Mansonella ozzardi, 281
Mantle cell lymphoma, 665
Marginal zone B cell lymphoma, 666
Margination, 32, 33*f*
Marrack, P., 2
Marrow progenitor cell, 14–16. *See also* Bone marrow *listings*
Mast cell, 184–186, 185*f,* 185*t,* 200
 Arthus reaction, 419
 atopic disease, 389
 pathway of immunologically induced inflammation, 377,
  379*t*
Mayfly, 394
McCarty, M., 2
McDevitt, Hugh, 3, 4
M cell, 197, 197*f*
Measles, 775*t,* 788
Measles virus, 699–700
Medawar Peter, 3–5

Mediastinum, 601
Medulla, 55
Megakaryocyte, 10*f,* 11
Mek and mitosis-associated protein kinase (MAPK), 20
Membrane attack complex (MAC), 173–174, 549–550
Membrane-bound immunoglobulin, 99–100
Memory, 63
 B cell, 124
 fundamental principle of immune response, 445
 lymphocyte, 44
 T cell, 142
 thymus-independent antigen, 80
Meningococcus, 355, 775*t*
6-Mercaptopurine, 531
Metabolic biotransformation and haptenation, 434*f,* 434–435,
  435*t*
Metabolic effects of glucocorticoid, 855, 855*t*
Metchnikoff, Elie, 2–4, 7
Methotrexate, 474, 526, 601, 831, 836*f,* 836–837, 837*t*
Methylprednisolone, 559
Methylxanthine, 859–860
MHC. *See* Major histocompatibility complex
Microhemagglutination-T *pallidum* (MHA-TP) test, 743
Microparticle enzyme immunoassay (MEIA), 235
Miescher, Johann, 1
Migration inhibitory factor (MIF), 828
Milstein, Cesar, 3–5
Mimicry of complement protein, 178
Minimal-change nephropathy, 561
Mites, dust, 392–394
Mitogen, 51, 51*t,* 260, 265*t,* 265–266, 266*t*
Mitotic cycle, 831, 831*f*
Mixed antiglobulin reaction (MAR), 621
Mixed connective tissue disease, 471
Mixed lymphocyte culture (MLC), 267–268, 268*f,* 295–297,
  296*f*
Mold allergen, 391–392, 393*f,* 393*t*
Molecular-biologic method
 advent of, 3
 histocompatibility testing
  DNA typing for HLA, 299–300, 300*t*
  genetic identity determination, 307
  introduction, 297–299
  polymerase chain reaction, 301–302, 303*f,* 304, 305–306*f,*
   307
  restriction fragment-length polymorphisms, 300*f,*
   300–301
Molecular genetic technique
 cancer, 641
 gene rearrangement assay for lymphocyte clonality,
  313–314
 hybridization assay, 311–312, 312*f*
 neoplasms of the immune system, 659
 nucleic acid probes, 309–311, 311*f*
 overview and prospects, 317–318
 polymerase chain reaction, 314–316, 315–317*f*
 RNA, methods of analyzing, 317
 in situ hybridization, 314
 southern blot, 312–313, 313*f*
Molecular heterogeneity of AIDS-associated lymphoma, 647,
  647*t*
Molecular immunology, advent of, 3
Molecular mimicry, 451
Molecular size and immunogenicity, 74
Monitoring allografts, 816–819
Monitoring desensitization, 799–800
Monoclonal antibody
 eukaryotic immunomodulator, 850
 histocompatibility testing, 291

Monoclonal antibody *(cont.)*
  hybridoma, 106
  immune stimulation, 769
  immunosuppressive therapy, 842–844, 843*f*
  laboratory tests, immunologic, 249–250, 250*f,* 250*t,* 251*t,*
      325
  neoplasms of the immune system, 660
  sheep erythrocyte, 259
  technological innovation, 96
  tumor immunology, 638
Monoclonal gammopathies (MG), 217*t*
Monoclonal gammopathy of undermined significance
      (MGUS), 668
Monocyte, 10*f,* 11, 13
Monocyte colony-stimulating factor (MCSF), 146
Monocyte-macrophage system
  assay, 269
  description of, 38–40*t,* 38–41, 39*f,* 41*f*
  HIV (human immunodeficiency virus), 750, 756
  immunosuppressive therapy, 828–829
  laboratory tests, immunologic, 325
Monocytopenia, 827–828
Monokine, 146
Mucin, 15
Mucocutaneous candidiasis, chronic, 348–350, 349*f*
Mucormycosis, 721
Mucosa-associated lymphoid tissue (MALT), 56, 666
Mucosal immune system, 614*f,* 614–615
  anatomy, 196–200, 197*f*
    diffuse lymphoid tissue, 198–199, 199*f*
    lamina propria cell, 199*f,* 199–200
    lymphoid aggregates, 197–198, 198*f*
  breast milk immunology, 207–208
  IgA, 200–204, 201*f,* 203*f*
  immune exclusion, 203
  immunoglobulin other than IgA, 204
  mucosal homing, 205*f,* 205–206
  oral tolerance, 206*f,* 206–207
  regulation of IgA synthesis, 204*f,* 204–205
Multinucleated giant cell, 41
Multiple drug allergy syndrome, 441
Multiple myeloma, 667–668
Multiple sclerosis, 218
  clinical feature, 581
  diagnosis, differential/immunologic, 581
  general considerations, 579–580, 580*f*
  immunologic features, major, 579
  pathogenesis, immunologic, 580
  treatment, 582
Multipotent progenitor, 13
Mumps, 775*t*
Murray, Joseph E., 5
Muscles/joints, 457–458, 471, 473
Myalgia syndrome, 604
Myasthenia gravis, 586–587
Myasthenic syndrome, 587
Myc/Max activity, 22
Mycobacterial heat shock protein, 846
Mycobacterium avium, 753
Mycobacterium avium complex (MAC), 691
Mycobacterium bovis, 692
Mycobacterium leprae, 140, 191
Mycobacterium paratuberculosis, 530
Mycobacterium tuberculosis, 81, 191, 428, 595, 692
Mycolic acid, 74
Mycophenolate mofetil, 841
Mycoplasma pneumoniae, 682
Mycosis fungoides, 670. *See also* Fungal disease
Myelodysplasia, 820

Myelo-erythroid progenitor, 10*f*
Myeloid cell, 11, 12*f*
Myeloid progenitor, 10*f,* 11
Myeloma, immunoblastic, 674
Myeloma protein, 96
Myeloperoxidase, 36, 367
Myocardial disease
  autoimmune myocarditis, 513–514
  dilated cardiomyopathy, 514
Myocarditis, autoimmune, 513–514

NADPH (nicotinamide-ademine dinucleotide phosphate)-
    dependent oxidase, 35–36
Nasal decongestant, 396
Nasal polyposis, 395, 397, 399
Nasal provocation test, 387
National Childhood Vaccine Injury Act of 1986, 783
National Marrow Donor Program (NMDP), 820
National Organ Transplant Act of 1987, 288
Natural killer cell (NK), 10, 10*f,* 11, 43
  1.1, 140
  antibody-dependent cell-mediated cytotoxicity, 144
  antigen-nonspecific therapy, 769
  azathioprine, 834
  Behcet's disease, 475
  cellular immunity, 268–269
  cytokine produced, 144
  development and tissue distribution, 143
  killer cell inhibitory receptor family, 143–144
  laboratory tests, immunologic, 324–325
  lamina propria cell, 200
  Ly-49 inhibitory receptor, 143
  natural killing, 143
  OK432, 846
  T cell immunodeficiency disorder, 350
  tumor immunology, 635
Necator americanus, 736
Negative predictive value, 251
Negative selection, 72, 91, 133–135, 134*f,* 135*f*
  major histocompatibility complex, 447
Neisser, Albert, 1
Neisseria, 26
Neisseria gonorrhoeae, 690
Neisseria meningitidis, 690
Nematodes, 736–737
Neonatal alloimmune thrombocytopenia (NAIT), 506–507,
    625–626
Neonates with HIV, 754
Neoplasms of the immune system, 417
  acute lymphoblastic leukemia and lymphoblastic lymphoma,
      662, 663*f,* 664
  B cell, 664–670
  benign conditions mimicking or associated with, 675
  characteristics of malignant lymphoid cells
    aberrant features, 653
    clonality, 651
    leukemia *vs.* lymphoma, 653
    lineage association, 651–653, 652*f,* 652*t*
  classification of lymphomas, 661, 661*t,* 662*t*
  diagnostic approaches
    cytogenetic analysis, 654–656, 658–659, 659*t*
    DNA analysis, 654
    immunophenotypic analysis, 653–654, 654–656*t*
    integrating the data, 659–660
    molecular genetic analysis, 659
    morphologic examination, 653
  general considerations, 651
  hematologic proliferations in immunosuppressed patients,
      674

Hodgkin's disease, 672*f,* 672–673, 673*t*
mononuclear phagocytes and antigen-presenting cells,
    673–674
T cell, 670–672
therapy, 660–661
Nephelometry, 230*f,* 230–231
Nephritic factor, 558
Nephritis. *See also* Antiglomerular basement membrane
    antibody-induced glomerulonephritis (anti-GBM);
    Immune-complex glomerulonephritis
Heymann model, 549
tubulointerstitial, 559–561
Nephritogenic antibody-antigen reaction, 549, 550*t,* 556*t*
Nephrotic syndrome, 553, 555, 561
Nephrotoxicity, 839–840
Neurologic disease
Alzheimer's disease, 588–589
amyotrophic lateral sclerosis, 588
autoimmune features, 589
demyelinating, 579–585, 580–581*f,* 585*f*
limbic encephalitis, 588
neuromuscular transmission, 585–587, 586*f*
paraneoplastic cerebellar degeneration, 587–588
stroke, 589
Neuromuscular transmission, 585–587, 586*f*
Neutropenia, 364, 493*t,* 493–495
Neutrophil, 10*f,* 11, 13
Arthus reaction, 419
corticosteroid, 827
degranulation, 271
dermatitis herpetiformis, 571
fungal disease, 708–709
ingestion, test for, 270–271
intracellular killing, 271–274
    chemiluminescence, 272
    flow cytometry, 272–273, 273*f*
    microbicidal assay, 273
    nitroblue tetrazolium dye reduction test, 272
    quantitative NBT test, 272
motility, test for, 270
oxidative microbicidal pathway, 37*t*
pathway of immunologically induced inflammation, 379
polymorphonuclear, 269, 325
proteinaceous toxins, 38
recognition and adhesion, 270
renal disease, 550
Newborn, hemolytic disease of the, 500–501
Nezelof's syndrome, 352
Nicolle, Charles J., 5
Nicotinamide, 567
Nicotinamide-ademine dinucleotide phosphate (NADPH)-
    dependent oxidase, 35–36
Nijmegen breakage syndrome, 357
Nikolsky's sign, 574–575
Nippostrongylus brasiliensis, 736
Nitric oxide (NO), 36
Nitroblue tetrazolium dye reduction test (NBT), 272, 365
NK. *See* Natural killer cell
Nocardia, 847
Nonatopic allergic disease, 389
Non-Hodgkin's disease, 644, 646, 661, 661*t*
Nonlysosomal proteolytic enzymes, 828
Nonspecific testing, 320–321
Non-steroidal anti-inflammatory drug (NSAID), 856–857,
    857*t*
inflammatory response, modulation of, 770
pseudoallergic reaction, 442
Reiter's syndrome, 476
rheumatoid arthritis, 464–465

Sjögren's syndrome, 470
urticaria, 417
Northern blot technique, 317
NO secretion, 40
NSAID. *See* Non-steroidal anti-inflammatory drug
Nuclear factor kappa B (NF*k*B), 20, 829
Nuclear factor of activated T cells (NF-AT), 838
Nucleated-cell count, 821
Nucleic acid, 74
Nucleic acid metabolism, 855*t*
Nucleic acid probes, 309–311, 311*f*
Nucleoside phosphorylase, 360–361, 361*f*
5'-Nucleotidase (CD73), 118, 343
Nuttall, George H. F., 4

Obliterative bronchiolitis, 610
Occupational allergy, 394, 396, 401*t,* 605
hypersensitivity pneumonitis, 428
Ocular sarcoidosis, 594–595
OK432, 846
OKT4 epitope, 353
OKT 3 therapy, 808, 815, 842–843
2'-5' Oligoadenylate (2-5A) synthetase, 158
Oligosaccharide, 16
Omenn syndrome, 354
Onchocerca volvulus, 737
Oncogenes, 641–642
Oncogenic viruses, 632
Oncostatin M (OSM), 156
One-dimensional single/double electroimmunodiffusion,
    224–225, 225*f,* 225*t*
Oophoritis, autoimmune, 621
Opsonin, 2
immunoglobulins, 34
Opsonization
antibody binding, 45
complement system, 169
encapsulated bacteria, 688
Fc receptors, 35, 35*t,* 70, 108
immunologic defense against infection, 680
serum amyloid protein P, 26*t*
Oral candidiasis, 546–547
Oral hairy leukoplakia, 546
Oral provocative test, 397
Oral tolerance, 206*f,* 206–207
Orchitis, autoimmune, 621
Organic dust toxic syndrome (ODTS), 611
Organ procurement
combined heart-lung transplantation, 818
heart transplantation, 816
Orodental disease
AIDS (acquired immune deficiency syndrome), 546
inflammatory periodontal disease, 541–544, 542*f,* 543*f*
juvenile periodontitis, 544
oral candidiasis, 546–547
recurrent aphthous ulceration, 544–545, 545*f*
Orthotopic transplantation, 810, 816
O side chain, 26
Osler, Sir William, 456
Ostwald viscosimeter, 227
Otitis media, 397
Ouchterlony analysis, 212*f,* 212–214, 213*f*
Ovarian failure, premature, 490
Ovary, 615, 621
Overlap syndrome, 521
Owen, Ray, 2, 4
OX40, 205
Oxidizing agent, 36, 37*t*

Palpable purpura, 515
Pancreas, disorders of the endocrine
Addison's disease, 489
idiopathic hypoparathyroidism, 490
insulin-dependent diabetes mellitus, 487–489, 489*t*
lymphocytic adenohypophysitis, 489–490
ovarian failure, premature, 490
polyglandular syndrome, autoimmune, 490*t*, 490–491
Pancreas transplantation
indications, 813
islet cells, 815
outcome, 813–814
procedure, 813, 814*f*
Pancreatitis, 180
Panel reactive antibody (PRA), 292
Panniculitis, relapsing, 477–478
Paracoccidioidomycosis, 717
Paracortex, 55
Paracrine effect, 67
Paradoxic effect elicited by immunosuppressive therapy, 832
Paragonimus, 733
Paralytic poliomyelitis, 704
Paraneoplastic cerebellar degeneration, 587–588
Paraneoplastic pemphigus, 576–577
Parasite-induced eosinophilic pneumonia, 604, 604*t*
Parasitic disease
helminths, immune response to
cestodes, 735–736
nematodes, 736–737
trematodes, 733–735
protozoa, immune response to
African trypanosomiasis, 731–733, 733*f*
leishmaniasis, 729–731
malaria, 725–728, 726*f*
toxoplasmosis, 728–729
Parenchymal involvement induced by drugs, 600–601
Paroxysmal cold hemoglobinuria, 499–500
Paroxysmal nocturnal hemoglobinuria (PNH), 178, 374, 501
Partitioning methods, 232
Passive immunization, 767, 783–785, 786–790*t*, 790
Passive suppression, 768
Passive transfer of the skin test, 384
Pasteur, Louis, 1, 3, 7, 80
Patch test, 255, 382, 426, 426*t*, 437
Pauling, L., 2
Pediatric HIV-1 infection, 628
Pediculus humanus, 746
Pemphigoid
bullous, 555–557*t*, 564–567
cicatricial, 568, 594
foliaceous, 574–576, 575*f*, 576*f*
paraneoplastic, 576–577
vulgaris, 574–576, 575*f*, 576*f*, 594
Penicillamine, 465, 601, 857–858
Penicillin
biotransformation product, 434, 434*f*
cross-reactions with other β-lactam, 439
desensitization, 439
IgE, 437–438
IgG, 433
Lyme disease, 745
skin test, 438–439
Penile urethral epithelium, 614
Pentostatin, 660
Peptide antigen, 83–91, 84*t*, 86–90*f*
Peptide vaccine, 81
Peptidoglycan, 26
Peptidomannans, 706
Periarteriolar lymphoid sheath, 55

Periarticular inflammation, 462
Pericardial disease
postinfarction syndrome, 513
postpericardiotomy syndrome, 513
relapsing pericarditis, 513
Pericarditis, relapsing, 513
Perinatal transmission of HIV, 627–628
Periodontitis, 369, 541–544, 542*f*, 543*f*
juvenile, 544
Peripheral blood lymphocyte (PBL), 290
Peripheral T cell lymphoma (PTL), 671
Peripheral tolerance, 448
Pernicious anemia, 533–534
Peroxidase antiperoxidase (PAP), 242
Pertussis, 775*t*, 791
Peyer's patch, 56, 60–61, 204–205, 206*f*
Phagocyte, 70
dysfunction disease
Chédiak-Higashi syndrome, 367
chronic granulomatous disease, 364–366, 365*f*, 366*t*
evaluation, 365*t*
glucose-6-phosphate dehydrogenase deficiency, 366–367
glycogen storage disease type 1B, 367
hyper-IgE syndrome, 367–368, 368*f*
leukocyte adhesion defect-type1, 368–369, 369*f*
leukocyte adhesion defect-type2, 369
myeloperoxidase deficiency, 367
neutropenia, 364
periodontitis, 369
Shwachman syndrome, 369
specific granule deficiency, 367
Tuftsin deficiency, 369
neutrophil, 31*f*, 31*t*, 31–32, 32*t*, 33*f*, 34–38, 35–37*f*, 37*t*
Phagocytic cell, 325, 673–674, 681, 681*t*
Phagocytosis, 2, 34, 35*f*
Phagosome, 35
Phenotypic deficiencies of immunoregulatory cytokine knockout mice
colony-stimulating factor, 165*t*
interleukin, 154*t*
Phenylephrine, 859
Phenylpropanolamine, 859
Phlyctenular keratoconjunctivitis, 596
Phoshatidylosital glycan class A (PIG-A), 374
Phosphatidylinositides, 49–50
Phosphatidylinositol bis-phosphate (PIP₂), 136
Phosphoinositide glycosidic linkage, 178
Phospholipase, 854
Phospholipase C-*γ*-1, 49, 136, 137*f*
Phosphorylation, 21
Photoallergic contact dermatitis, 427, 427*t*
Photopatch test, 382, 427
Phytohemagglutinin (PHA), 297, 356, 828
Pirquet, Clemens von, 2, 4
Placenta as and immune organ, 616, 618–620
Plague, 777*t*
Plasma, 284
Plasma cell, 45–56, 124
Plasma cell myeloma, 668
Plasmacytic hyperplasia, 674
Plasmacytoma, solitary, 668
Plasma exchange, 841
Plasmapheresis, 584, 587, 841
Plasma protein, 151, 179, 179*f*
Plasmin inhibitor, 373
Plasminogen activator, 828
Plasmodium, 726–728
Plateau phase, 71
Platelet, 9, 10*f*, 186, 284

Platelet-activating factor (PAF), 188, 190*f*
  anaphylaxis, 411
Platelet-derived growth factor (PDGF), 550
Platelet disorder
  hemolytic-uremic syndrome, 507
  idiopathic thrombocytopenic purpura, 503–504*t*, 503–506
  mechanisms of destruction, 502–503, 503*t*
  neonatal alloimmune thrombocytopenia, 506–507
  posttransfusion purpura, 506
  quinine-induced immune thrombocytopenia with HUS, 508
  thrombocytopenia, drug-induced immune, 506
  thrombotic thrombocytopenic purpura, 507
Pleura, drugs causing inflammation of the, 600*t*, 601
Ploem, J., 238
Pneumococcus, 355, 777*t*
Pneumocystis carinii
  AIDS (acquired immune deficiency syndrome), 597, 753
  bone marrow transplantation, 821
  congenital thymic aplasia, 346, 347–348
  fungal disease, 706
  HIV (human immunodeficiency virus), 628
  pneumocystosis, 721–722
  severe combined immunodeficiency, 353
  short-limbed dwarfism with immunodeficiency, 360
Pneumocystosis, 721–722
Pneumonia, eosinophilic, 602*t*, 602–605, 603*f*, 604*t*
Pneumonitis
  amiodarone, 601
  CMV, 819, 822, 823
  hypersensitivity, 428–432, 429*t*, 611
Poison Control Centers, 785
Pokeweed mitogen (PWM), 260
Poliomyelitis, 704, 778*t*, 791
Poliovirus, 704
Pollen, 391, 392*f*, 393
Polyarteritis nodosa, 518*f*, 518–520, 562, 596
Polyarthritis, 335
Polychondritis, relapsing, 477
Polyclonal antibody, 842
Polyclonal B cell activator, 120
Polyglandular syndrome, autoimmune, 490*t*, 490–491
Polymerase chain reaction (PCR), 350, 537
  histocompatibility testing, 301
  HIV infection and reproductive system, 626–628
  molecular-biologic method for HLA typing
    amplification types, 301–302, 303*f*, 304, 305–306*f*, 307
    other HLA typing methods involving PCR-amplified
      products, 304, 307
    sequence-specific oligonucleotide probes, 302, 304*t*
  molecular genetic techniques, 314–316, 315–317*f*
Polymerized allergen, 800
Polymorphic hyperplasia, 674
Polymorphic lymphoma, 674
Polymorphic reticulosis, 609
Polymorphism, MHC, 85–86
Polymorphonuclear neutrophil (PMN), 269, 325
Polymyalgia rheumatica, 523
Polymyositis-dermatomyositis, 472–475, 473*f*, 513
Polyneuropathies, chronic demyelinating, 584–585
Polyneuropathy, acute inflammatory demyelinating, 583–584
Polypeptides, 74–75, 84, 87, 88
  light/heavy chain, 96–98, 100
Polysaccharide, 413
Polyserositis, 457
Porter, Rodney, 3–5
Portier, Paul, 2, 4
Positive predictive value, 251
Positive selection, 72, 91, 133–135, 134*f*, 135*f*
  major histocompatibility complex, 447

Postcapillary venules, 29
Postinfarction syndrome, 513
Postpericardiotomy syndrome, 513
Poststreptococcal glomerulonephritis, 682
Posttransfusion purpura, 506
Prausnitz-Küstner reaction, 384
Pre-B cell, 116, 116*f*, 117*f*
Precipitation reaction, 211–212, 212*f*, 232
Precipitin reaction, 2, 192
Predictive value theory, 250–251, 251*t*
Prednisone
  bone marrow transplantation, 822
  bullous pemphigoid, 567
  giant-cell arteritis, 524
  herpes gestationis, 570
  recurrent and spontaneous abortion, 622
  Takayasu's arteritis, 526
Pregnancy
  active immunization, 782
  background, 618–619
  local immunosuppression at placenta and adjacent tissues,
    619
  lymphocyte reactivity, intrinsically decreased, 620
  proposed mechanisms of altered immunity, 619
  proteins, secretion of placental, 620
  steroid hormones, secretion of placental, 619–620
Pregnancy, immunity in, 618–620
Prekallikrein, 179, 179*f*
Prelysosome, 89
Premunition, 727
Presensitization, 803
Pretransfusion testing, 279
Prevalence and predictive value, 251*t*
Primary biliary cirrhosis, 539*f*, 539–540
Primary central nervous system lymphoma, 646–647, 647*t*
Primary hypothyroidism, 487
Primary sclerosing cholangitis, 540–541
Primed lymphocyte typing (PLT), 297
Priming event, 71
Pro-B cell, 115
Procainamide, 601
Progenitor cell, hematopoietic, 821
  CD44, 16
  fully committed, 13
  granulocyte-monocyte, 10*f*, 13
  lineage-committed, 11–14, 12*f*
  marrow, 15–16
  multipotent, 13
  myelo-erythroid, 10*f*
  myeloid, 10*f*
Progesterone, 616
Progression and neoplasia, 641, 641*t*
Progressive systemic sclerosis, 470–472
Proinflammatory property, 187, 202
Prolymphocytic leukemia (PLL), 664
Promotion and neoplasia, 641, 641*t*
Prophylactic vaccine for HIV-negative people, 759
Prostaglandin, 30, 856
Prostaglandin D$_2$, 188
Proteasome, 84
Protected site concept, 176
Protein. *See also* CD *listings;* Major histocompatibility
    complex (MHC)
  A, 226
  adhesion, 16*t*, 30*t*, 118
  Bc12, 22–23, 23*t*
  Bcl-2, 72
  Bence Jones, 220
  Charcot-Leyden crystal, 183

Protein *(cont.)*
  c-myc, 21–22, 50
  control, 174–176, 175*f*
  cytoplasmic, 21–22
  Fas, 72
  FK-binding, 840
  keratinocyte hemidesmosomal, 564
  major basic, 183
  mannose binding protein, 176
  metabolism, 855*t*
  mimicry of complement, 178
  mycobacterial heat shock, 846
  myeloma, 96
  nonclassical MHC, 87
  nuclear factor of activated T cells, 838
  p53, 22, 23
  placental, secretion of, 620
  plasma, 151*t*
  proteinuria, 553, 558
  RAG-1/2, 115
  retinoblastoma, 21
  serum. *See* clinical laboratory methods for detecting *under*
      Antigens
  soluble, 25–29
  stat, 21
  transcription, 20
  tumor immunology, 633
  V/(D)/J joining, 115–116, 116*f*
  x-box-binding, 354
Proteinase inhibitor, 758
Protein tyrosine kinase (PTK) activity, 18*f,* 18–19, 49–50,
    135–136, 154
Protein tyrosine phosphatase activity, 123
Proteoglycan mediator, 189–190
Proteus, 368, 688
Protozoa, immune response to
  African trypanosomiasis, 731–733, 733*f*
  leishmaniasis, 729–731
  malaria, 725–728, 726*f*
  toxoplasmosis, 728–729
Provocative test
  bronchoprovocation, 380, 381*f,* 385–387, 399, 401
  dietary elimination, 387
  drug allergy, 437
  nasal, 387
  oral, 397
Prozone phenomenon, 212
Pseudoallergic reaction, 441–442
Pseudo-Goodpasture's syndrome, 601–602
Pseudomembranous candidiasis, 546*f,* 547
Pseudomonas, 365
Pseudomonas aeruginosa, 368, 688, 847
Pseudomonas exotoxin A, 766
Psoriatic arthritis, 476–477
Pulmonary eosinophilia
  simple idiopathic, 603–604
  tropical, 604
Pulmonary fibrosis, idiopathic, 606–608, 607*f,* 608*t*
Pulmonary vasculitis syndrome, 609*t,* 609–610
Pure erythrocyte aplasia, 501–502
Purine nucleoside analogues, 660
Pus, 37
Putnam, F., 3
Pyroglobulin, 229

Quality control, 231, 233
Quantitative immunoassay, 250, 251*t*
Quantitative immunofluorescence, 240, 242
Quartan malaria, 727

Quinine-induced immune thrombocytopenia with HUS, 508
Quinine-platelet interaction, 434

Rabies, 778–780*t,* 788
  virus, 703–704
Radiation-induced carcinogenesis, 632
Radiation therapy, 660
Radioactive counting, 232
Radioallergosorbent test (RAST), 385, 386*f,* 394, 401*t,* 422
  cross-reaction among β-lactam antibiotics, 439
  drug allergy, 437
Radioimmunoassay (RIA), 212, 231–233, 232*f*
  ultrasensitive enzymatic, 236, 236*f*
Radioisotopic label, 233, 234*f*
Random error, 233, 236
Rapamycin, 840–841
Rapid plasma reagin (RPR) circle card test, 742
Ras-dependent signaling pathway, 19*f,* 19–20, 136
Rasmussen's encephalitis, 589
Rate nephelometry, 231
Raynaud's phenomenon, 471, 472
Reagent method, limited/excess, 236–237
Receptor-editing mechanism, 128–129
Receptor-mediated endocytosis, 34, 35*f*
Receptors and signal transduction. *See also* T cell receptor
    (TCR)
  adrenergic drug, 859, 860*t*
  antiacetylcholine, 586
  antigen-specific recognition, 444
  C3b, 172
  chemokine, 162
  complement deficiency, 374
  complement system, 177–178
  cytokine, 17–20, 18*f,* 19*f,* 34, 165–166, 166*t*
  eosinophil, 184
  epidermal growth factor, 616
  Fc, 70, 97, 108*t,* 108–109, 121
  hematopoietin family, 165
  high-affinity receptor for IgE, 185, 390
  histamine, 187, 187*t*
  interleukin-1, 148–150
  interleukin-2, 153–154
  interleukin-6, 155–156
  intermediate-affinity receptor for IgG, 184
  killer cell inhibitory receptor family, 143–144
  Ly-49 inhibitory, 143
  7-transmembrane, 162
  sheep erythrocyte, 258–259
  T cell, 46
  thyroid-stimulating hormone, 485–486, 486*f*
  tumor necrosis factor, 150
Recipient selection
  combined heart-lung transplantation, 818
  heart transplantation, 815–816
Recombination signal sequence, 110*f,* 112
Recovery studies, 236
Recurrent and spontaneous abortion, 621–622
Recurrent aphthous ulceration (RAU), 544–545, 545*f*
Red blood cells. *See* Erythrocyte
Red pulp, 55
Regulatory factor deficiency, 373
Regulatory molecule, 178
Reinherz, Ellis, 4
Reiter's syndrome, 476, 592
Relapsing-fever *borreliosis,* 746
Relapsing panniculitis, 477–478
Relapsing polychondritis, 477

Renal disease
  antiglomerular basement membrane antibody-induced
      glomerulonephritis, 550–552, 552f
  classification, 550t
  focal glomerulosclerosis, 561–562
  immune-complex glomerulonephritis, 552–559, 554–556t,
      557f, 558f
  minimal-change nephropathy, 561
  nephritogenic antibody-antigen reaction, 549, 550t
  non-steroidal anti-inflammatory drug, 857
  tubulointerstitial nephritis, 559–561
  vasculitis, 562
  Wegener's granulomatosis, 521
Reproductive processes
  anatomy and immunity, 613–615, 614f
  fertilization, 615–616
  fetal tissues, immune response to, 616, 617f, 618
  HIV (human immunodeficiency virus), 626–628
  implantation, 616
  infertility, 620–621
  isoimmunization, 622–626, 624–625f
  pregnancy, immunity in, 618–620
  recurrent and spontaneous abortion, 621–622
Respiratory burst, 36, 365t
Respiratory disease
  adult respiratory distress syndrome, 611
  allergic asthma, 611
  allergic bronchopulmonary aspergillosis, 421–423, 611
  anaphylaxis, 410, 414–415
  drug-induced, 599–602, 601f, 602t
  eosinophilic pneumonias, 602t, 602–605, 603f, 604t
  Goodpasture's syndrome, 608–609, 609f
  hypersensitivity pneumonitis, 428–432, 429t, 611
  idiopathic pulmonary fibrosis, 606–608, 607f, 608t
  lung transplantation, 610–611
  occupational and environmental lung disease, 605
  pulmonary manifestation of immunodeficiency, 610
  pulmonary vasculitis syndrome, 609t, 609–610
  sarcoidosis, 605–606
  Wegener's granulomatosis, 521
Respiratory failure, 403
Respiratory syncytial virus (RSV), 697–699
Restriction enzyme, 312
Restriction fragment, 312
Restriction fragment-length polymorphisms (RFLP), 300f,
      300–301
Reticular cell, 53
Reticular dysgenesis, 352
Reticulin fibers, 53
Reticuloendothelial cell, 829
Reticulosis, polymorphic, 609
Retinoblastoma (Rb) protein, 21
Retrovirus family, 748, 749t
Revascularization and liver transplantation, 811
Reverse transcriptase PCR (RT-PCR), 317
Reverse transcriptase (RT), 632, 748, 757
Revised European-American Lymphoma (REAL)
      classification, 661, 661t
Rev-responsive element (RRE), 750
Rheumatic disease, 833t
  ankylosing spondylitis, 475–476
  Behcet's disease, 475
  complement system, 477–478
  eye, 592f, 592–593, 593f
  hypogammaglobulinemia and arthritis, 478
  juvenile arthritis, 466–468
  polymyositis-dermatomyositis, 472–475, 473f
  progressive systemic sclerosis, 470–472
  psoriatic arthritis, 476–477

Reiter's syndrome, 476
relapsing polychondritis, 477
rheumatoid arthritis, 450, 592, 830, 834
  clinical feature, 462–463
  complications and prognosis, 465
  diagnosis, differential/immunologic, 463–464
  drug treatment, 464–465
  general consideration, 461
  pathogenesis, immunologic, 461–462, 462f
  treatment, 464
Sjögren's syndrome, 468–470
systemic lupus erythematosus, 456–461, 457t, 459f
Weber-Christian disease, 477–478
Rheumatoid arthritis (RA). See rheumatoid
      arthritis under Rheumatic disease
Rheumatoid factor, 100, 245, 460
Rh immune globulin treatment, 624, 625f
Rhinitis
  allergic, 394–397
  chronic nonallergic, 395
  infectious, 395
  medicamentosa, 395
Rhinoconjunctivitis, allergic, 389
Rhinosporidium seeberi, 706
Rh isoimmunization, 282–283, 622–626, 624–625f, 785, 788t
Rhizopus arrhizus, 708
Ribonucleic acid. See RNA (ribonucleic acid)
Richet, Charles, 2, 4
Risk-benefit ratio for vaccine, 782
RNA (ribonucleic acid), 309–310, 317, 854
  hepatitis B, 700
  HIV (human immunodeficiency virus), 749–750, 757
  influenza virus, 695
  rabies virus, 703–704
  tumor immunology, 632
  virus and hepatitis, 534, 537, 538
Rose-Waaler test, 245
Rough endoplasmic reticulum (RER), 84, 87–88
Roux, P. E., 2, 4
Rubella, 780t
Rwanda, cancer in, 648

Sabin vaccine, 704
Salk vaccine, 704
Salmonella, 26, 173, 688, 753
Salmonella choleraesuis, 690–692, 691f
Salmonella enteritidis, 690–692, 691f
Salmonella typhimurium, 847
Sandwich assay, 233, 234f
Sarcoidosis, 605–606
  ocular, 594–595
Sarcomas of dendritic and interdigitating reticulum cells, 674
Scavenger receptor, 40
Schick, Bela, 4
Schick tests, 324
Schistosoma, 184
Schistosomiasis, 733–735
Schlossman, Stuart, 4
Schwartz, R., 830
Scleroderma, 470–472
Scratch test, 383
Screening serum for antibodies, 279
Secreted immunoglobulin, 100–101
Secretory immune system of the female genital tract, 613, 614f
Selectin, 15–16, 30–31, 32
Selective IgA deficiency, 357
  clinical feature, 340–341
  complications and prognosis, 342

Selective IgA deficiency *(cont.)*
 diagnosis, differential, 341
 general consideration, 339
 pathogenesis, immunologic, 339–340
 treatment, 341–342
Selective IgM deficiency, 342
Self from nonself, discrimination of, 444–445
Self-limitation and immune response, 445
Self-marker concept, 3
Self-renewing cell, 9
Self-tolerance
 B cell, 448*t,* 448–449
 Major histocompatibility complex, 446
 negative selection, 447–448
 peripheral tolerance, 448
 positive selection, 447–448
 T cell, central role of, 445–447
Septic shock, 151
Sequence-specific oligonucleotide probe (SSOP), 302, 304*t*
Serodiagnosis of bacterial disease, 684
Serodiagnosis of parasitic disease, 735, 736
Serologic methods for tissue typing, 286, 289, 292–293, 298*t*
Serology, 2
Serratia marcescens, 364, 365
Serum amyloid protein P, 26
Serum antibody, 71, 106, 278–279
Serum immunoglobulin level. *See* Laboratory tests, immunologic
Serum proteins, 214–215. *See also* clinical laboratory methods for detecting *under* Antigen
Serum sickness, 192, 194, 419–421, 420*f,* 785
Serum suppressive factor, 264, 265*t*
Serum viscosity, 227–228, 228*t*
Severe combined immunodeficiency disease (SCID), 352–353, 819, 820
Sézary syndrome, 670
Sheep erythrocyte (SRBC), 258–259
Shewhart plots, 233
Shock, anaphylactic, 2, 414, 419
Shwachman syndrome, 369
Sick building syndrome, 605
Sickle cell (SS) hemoglobin, 727
Side chain theory, 2
Signal transduction, 17–20, 19*f. See also* Receptors and signal transduction
Simian immunodeficiency virus (SIV), 749, 750
Simian papovavirus, 783
Simple idiopathic pulmonary eosinophilia, 603–604
Single immunodiffusion, 212, 214*f,* 214–215
Single-strand conformational polymorphisms (SSCP), 316
Sinopulmonary infection, 340
Sinus involvement in Wegener's granulomatosis, 521
Sjögren's syndrome, 458, 468–470, 593
Skin, 56–57, 382–384
 anaphylaxis, 411
 cancer, 643
 cutaneous test, 382–383, 383*f*
 eczematous contact dermatitis, 425–427, 426*t*
 infection, nonimmunologic defenses against, 678–679, 679*t*
 intradermal test, 383*f,* 383–384
 passive transfer, 384
 patch test, 382
 photoallergic contact dermatitis, 427, 427*t*
 polyarteritis nodosa, 519
 polymyositis-dermatomyositis, 473–474
 scleroderma, 471
 systemic lupus erythematosus, 457
 tissue immunofluorescence, 460
 Wegener's granulomatosis, 522

Skin test
 anaphylaxis, 411, 411*t*
 anesthetic, 442
 corticosteroid, 829
 delayed hypersensitivity, 254–256, 322–323
 drug allergy, 437
 leishmaniasis, 730
 penicillin, 438–439
 sulfonamide, 434
 sympathetic ophthalmia, 595
Smallpox, 780*t*
Small-vessel vasculitis, 610
 clinical feature, 515
 complications and prognosis, 516
 diagnosis, immunologic/differential, 516
 general consideration, 515
 pathology, 515, 516*f*
 syndromes associated with
  Behcet's disease, 517
  Henoch-Schönlein purpura, 516–517
  hypocomplementemic urticarial vasculitis, 517–518
 treatment, 516
Snakebite, 785, 788*t*
Sodium dodecyl sulfate-polyacrylamide gel electrophoresis (SDS-PAGE), 235
Solitary plasmacytoma, 668
Soluble protein of innate immunity, 25–29
Somatic hypermutation, 125–126
Southern blot technique, 312–313, 313*f,* 314
Specific granule deficiency, 367
Specificity of Serological Reactions, The (Landsteiner), 2
Specific testing, 321
Sperm, 615–616
Sperm-egg fusion, 615–616
Spirochetal disease
 nonvenereal treponematoses
  leptospirosis, 746
  Lyme disease, 744–746
  relapsing-fever *borreliosis,* 746
  syphilis, 739–743, 740*f,* 743*t*
Spleen, 55–56, 56*f,* 60, 682
Splenectomy, 497, 505–506, 782
Squamous cell carcinoma of the conjunctiva, 648
SRC-family kinases, 19*f,* 19–20
 SH2 domains, 20
Staphylococcus aureus, 273, 342, 365, 368–369, 687, 846
Staphylococcus epidermidis, 364, 365, 823
Starzl, Thomas, 809
Stat protein, 20
Status asthmaticus, 403
Stem cell factor (SCF), 12–13, 43, 146
Steroid, anabolic, 374
Steroid hormones, secretion of placental, 619–620
Stevens-Johnson syndrome, 436
Stiff-man syndrome, 589
Stratum functionale, 613
Streptococcus, 687
Streptococcus agalactiae, 689
Streptococcus pneumoniae, 342, 369, 688–690
Streptococcus sanguis, 545
Stroke, immunological features of, 589
Strongyloides stercoralis, 604, 736
Subepithelial lymphoid organ, 55–56, 56*f*
Subperiosteal nodule, 462
Subunit vaccine, 81
Sulfasalazine, 465, 531, 533, 601
Sulfonamide, 434, 436, 440
Superantigen, 131–132, 132*f,* 450, 682–683, 846
Supergene family, immunoglobulin, 105–106, 106*t*

Surface immunoglobulin, 259–260, 260*t*
Surgery. *See also* Transplantation
  juvenile arthritis, 468
  rheumatoid arthritis, 465
SV40, 783
Sweden, 782
Syk, 120
Symbols used in illustrations, glossary of, 864–865
Sympathetic ophthalmia, 595–596
Sympathomimetic drugs, 402, 859, 860*t*
Syncytiotrophoblast layer of the placenta, 618
Syphilis, 281
  clinical feature, 741–742
  complications and prognosis, 743
  diagnosis, differential/immunologic, 740*f*, 742*t*, 742–743
  general considerations, 739–741
  treatment, 743
Systematic necrotizing vasculitis, 518*t*
  allergic angiitis and granulomatosis, 520
  overlap syndrome, 521
  polyarteritis nodosa, 518*f*, 518–520
Systemic lupus erythematosus (SLE), 835
  anticardiolipin antibody syndrome, 510
  antiribonucleoprotein, 514
  autoimmune myocarditis, 513–514
  clinical feature, 457–458
  complication and prognosis, 461
  diagnosis, differential/immunologic, 459–460
  drug allergy, 435
  eye disease, 594
  general considerations, 456
  immune-complex glomerulonephritis, 556
  pathogenesis, immunologic, 456–457
  pathology, 457
  respiratory disease, drug-induced, 601
  treatment, 460–461
  urticaria, 417

Systemic lymphoma, 646

Tacrolimus, 812, 816, 840
Takayasu's arteritis, 524, 525*f*, 526
Talmage, David, 3, 4
TAP polypeptide, 84, 87, 88
T *cati*, 604
T cell, 10, 11. *See also* Autoimmune disease; Cell-mediated
      hypersensitivity disease; Combined T cell & B cell
      immunodeficiency disorder
  activation, 50–52, 51*f*, 52*t*
  anergic, 448
  antigen-nonspecific therapy, 769
  assay, 257–259, 258*f*, 258*t*, 259*f*
  azathioprine, 834
  B cell cooperating with, 3
  Behcet's disease, 475
  clonal organization, 63
  corticosteroid, 827, 828
  crossmatching by lymphocytotoxicity, 293–294
  cyclophosphamide, 835
  cyclosporin, 838
  cytotoxic, 68*f*, 68–69, 297
  direct contact with other cells, 47–48
  effector, 379
  epitope and antigen, 79–80
  follicular, 197–198
  graft rejection, 806–807
  help and accessory signal, 121, 121*f*, 122*f*, 123
  helper, 52, 65, 66*f*
    abnormalities in interactions, 451

  suppressor/helper ratios, 258
  T_{H1} and T_{H2} subset, 139*t*, 139–141, 140*f*
  hematopoietic stem cells, 43
  HIV (human immunodeficiency virus), 647, 755
  IgA switch differentiation, 205
  immunosuppressive therapy, 832
  independent antigen, 120*f*, 120–121
  inflammatory response, modulation of, 770
  interleukin-2, 154–155
  intravenous normal pooled immunoglobulin, 842
  laboratory tests, immunologic, 257–259, 258*f*, 258*t*, 259*f*,
        321–323, 322–323*t*
  leishmaniasis, 730
  memory, 49
  mucosal homing, 206
  mucosal immunity, 615
  neoplasms of the immune system, 670–672
  oral tolerance, 206–207
  paracortex, 55
  peptide-MHC recognition by, 90–91
  positive & negative selection, 91
  protein tyrosine kinase, 49
  receptors, 46, 52
  sarcoidosis, 605
  selection process in thymus, 57
  subset, 48, 48*t*
  surface molecule, 48, 48*t*
  thymus, 57–59
  tumor immunology, 634
  virgin, 49
  virus-infected cells, 680–681
T cell immunodeficiency disorder
  biotin-dependent carboxylase deficiency, 350–351
  CD4 lymphocytopenia, 350
  chronic mucocutaneous candidiasis, 348–350, 349*f*
  congenital thymic aplasia, 345–348, 346*f*
  natural killer cell deficiency, 350
T cell lymphocytic leukemia (T-CLL), 670
T cell receptor (TCR)
  α & β-gene locus, 130–131, 131*f*
  adhesion molecule, 138
  antigen-specific therapy, 768
  CD28, 137–138, 138*f*
  CD45, 136, 137*f*
  CD4 and CD8, 132, 132*f*
  combined T cell & B cell immunodeficiency disorder, 353
  cytolytic T cell, 141*f*, 141–142
  gene arrangement assay, 313–314
  giant-cell arteritis, 515
  intraepithelial lymphocyte, 198–199
  mediated immune response, 138–142
  memory, 142
  monoclonal antibody, 842
  recognition of antigen, 131
  signal transduction, 135–136, 136*f*, 137*f*
  stages of thymocyte development, 132–133, 133*f*
  structure of, 130, 131*f*
  superantigen interactions, 131–132, 132*f*
  transgenic mice, 207
  $\gamma\delta$ T cell, 142
Terminal deoxynucleotidyl transferase (TdT), 112
Terminal differentiation, 9–10
Tertiary lymphoid organ, 62
Testis, 615, 621
Tetanus, 780*t*, 788*t*
Tetracycline, 567, 745
Theophylline, 402
Thiazolidine ring, 434, 434*f*
Thomas, Donnall, 5

Three-dimensional structure of immunoglobulin, 103, 104*t*, 105, 105*f*
Thromboangiitis obliterans, 526
Thrombocytopenia, 355, 434
  drug-induced immune, 506
  neonatal alloimmune, 506–507, 625–626
Thrombocytopenic purpura, 790
Thrombocytopenic purpura, idiopathic, 503–504*t*, 503–506
Thrombotic thrombocytopenic purpura (TTP), 507
Thrush, 546*f*, 547
Thymic aplasia, congenital, 345–348, 346*f*
Thymic education, failure of, 450, 450*t*
Thymic hormone, 847–848
Thymocyte, 57, 58*f*, 132–133, 133*f*
Thymoma, immunodeficiency with, 343
Thymus, 43, 57–59, 58*f*
  self-tolerance, 446
Thymus-independent antigen, 80
Thyroid autoimmune disease
  chronic thyroiditis, 482–483, 483*f*, 484*f*
  Grave's disease, 485–487, 486*f*
  primary hypothyroidism, 487
  transient thyroiditis syndrome, 483–485
Thyroiditis, chronic, 482–483, 483*f*, 484*f*
Thyroiditis syndrome, transient, 483–485
Thyroid-stimulating hormone (TSH), 483, 485–486, 486*f*
Ticks and lime disease, 744
Tiselius, Arne W., 2
Tissue-destruction, mechanisms of immune-mediated, 453–454
Tissue diagnosis, 382
Tissue immunofluorescence, 460
Tissue-infiltrating cells, 449
Tissue typing. *See* Histocompatibility testing
Tolerance, B cell, 128*f*, 128–129
Tolerance, oral, 206*f*, 206–207
Tolerance, self-, 445*t*, 445–449, 446*f*, 447*f*, 448*t*
Tolypocladium inflatum Gams., 837
Tonegawa, Susumu, 3–5
Tonsil, 56–57, 60
Toxicity
  corticosteroid, 855*t*, 855–856
  cyclosporin, 839*f*, 839–840
  non-steroidal anti-inflammatory drug, 856
Toxigenic bacterial disease
  Bacillus, 686
  C *diphtheriae*, 686
  Clostridium, 685–686
  gram-negative rods, 688
Toxin neutralization, 69
Toxocara canis, 604
Toxoid vaccine, 81
Toxoplasma gondii, 281
Toxoplasmosis, 728–729
Transcobalamin II deficiency, 344
Transcription protein, 20
Transforming growth factor beta (TGFβ), 161–162
  CDK inhibitors, 21
  cell sources and effects of, 161*f*
  distant target cells, 146
  IgA synthesis at mucosal sites, 205
  oral tolerance induction *vs.* immunization and IgA production, 207
  renal disease, 550
  studies on, 849
  trophoblast, 618
Transfusion reactions, 279*t*, 279–282
  allergic, 280
  febrile, 280
  hemolytic, 280
  immunologic mechanisms of, 281–282
  infection, 280–281, 281*f*
  lung injury, 280
Transient hypogammaglobulinemia of infancy, 336*f*, 336–337
Transient thyroiditis syndrome, 483–485
Transjugular intrahepatic portasystemic shunts (TIPS), 810
7-Transmembrane receptor, 34, 162
Transplacental fetal hemorrhage, 282
Transplantation
  autologous, 821
  azathioprine, 834
  bone
    immunosuppression, 824–825
    posttransplantation course, 824
    recovery, 825
    rejection, 824
  bone marrow transplantation
    beginnings of, 819
    diseases treatable by, 820*t*
    graft-*vs.*-host reaction, 822*t*, 822–823
    indications and results, 820–821
    infection, 823–824
    procedure, 821–822
    venoocclusive disease of the liver, 823
  cancer, 643–644
  combined heart-lung transplantation
    complications, 819
    immunosuppression and allograft monitoring, 818–819
    operative procedure, 818
    organ procurement, 818
    recipient selection, 818
    replacement for isolated lung transplantation, 817
    results, 819
  future of, 825
  heart
    complications, 817
    donor selection, 816
    immunosuppression and allograft monitoring, 816–817
    operative procedure, 816
    organ procurement, 816
    recipient selection, 815–816
    results, 817
    tissue typing, rationale for, 288
  histocompatibility testing, 286
  kidney
    ABO testing, 802–805, 804–805*f*
    graft rejection, pathology of, 805–808, 806–807*f*
    tissue typing, rationale for, 287–289, 288–289*t*
  liver, 809–813
    tissue typing, rationale for, 288
  lung, 610–611
  pancreas
    crossmatching and immunosuppression, 814–815
    indications, 813
    islet cells, 815
    outcome, 813–814
    procedure, 813, 814*f*
  rejection, 91, 195
Trematode, 733–735
Trendelenberg's position, 414
Treponema pallidum, 559, 739
Treponema pallidum immobilization (TPI) test, 743
Treponema pallidum-immobilizing antibodies (TPIA), 740
T *rhodesiense*, 732
Triamcinolone acetonide, 402
Trichinella, 184
Trichinella spiralis, 736–737
Trichinosis, 736–737

Trichophyton, 595
Trichophyton rubrum, 847
Trimethoprim-sulfamethoxazole (TMP-SMZ), 436, 440, 722, 821
Triplett, R. F., 3
Tropheryma whippelii, 534
Trophoblast, 616, 617*f,* 618
Tropical pulmonary eosinophilia, 604
Trypanosoma brucei, 731
Trypanosoma cruzi, 281
Trypanosomiasis, African, 731–733, 733*f*
Tuberculin test, 384
Tuberculosis, 781*t*
Tubulointerstitial nephritis, 559–561
Tuftsin deficiency, 369
Tumor immunology
    antigens on tumor cells, 632–634
    B cell, 635
    development of tumors, 631–632
    escape from an immune response, 635–637
    immunotherapy, 637–638
    macrophage, 635
    natural killer cell, 635
    properties of tumor cells, 631*t*
    T cell, 634
Tumor-infiltrating lymphocytes (TIL), 769
Tumor necrosis factor (TNF), 147–152, 148*t,* 151*t,* 153*t*
    immunomodulator, 849
    membrane attack complex, 550
    recurrent aphthous ulceration, 545
Tumors, hepatocellular, 810
Two-by-two contingency table, 251, 251*t*
Tyan, Marvin, 3, 4
Typhoid, 781*t*
Tyrosine kinase receptor family, 18*f,* 18–19

UCLA Transplant Registry, 287
Uganda, cancer in, 648
Uhlenhuth, P., 594
Ulcerative colitis, 532–533, 533*f*
Ultrasensitive enzymatic radioimmunoassay (USERIA), 236, 236*f*
Unique tumor-specific antigen, 632, 633
United Kingdom, 782
United Network for Organ Sharing (UNOS), 288
University of Wisconsin (UW) solution, 811, 813
Urinary creatine, 474
Urine amylase, 813–814
Urticaria, 410, 416–418, 799
    allergic, 195
    pigmentosa, 417
Urticarial vasculitis, hypocomplementemic, 517–518
Uteroplacental circulation, 616, 617*f*
Utility of laboratory tests, 319, 320
Uveitis, lens-induced, 594

Vaccine, 80–82, 81*t*. *See also* Immunization
    active, 767, 772–773, 774–781*t,* 782
    age at immunization, 791–793, 792*t*
    attenuated, 1
    hepatitis B immune globulin, 702
    inactivated poliovirus, 704
    live attenuated poliovirus, 704
    passive, 81–82, 767, 783–785, 786–790*t,* 790
    prophylactic for HIV-negative people, 759
    Vaccine Adverse Event Reporting System, 783
Vaccinia, 81, 789*t*
Vagina, 613, 614*f*
Valid analytic range of the assay, 236

Variability of tests, 319
Variable immunodeficiency, common, 337–339
Variable region (VH), 97, 102–103
Variable surface glycoprotein (VSG), 732
Varicella, 781*t,* 789*t,* 791
Variolation, 1
Vascular addressin, 60–61
Vascular disease
    classification, 514, 515*t*
    giant-cell arteritis, 522–524, 523*f*
    other vasculitic syndromes
        erythema nodosum, 526, 526*f*
        isolated angiitis of the central nervous system, 526
    small-vessel vasculitis, 515–518, 516*f*
    systematic necrotizing vasculitis, 518*t,* 518–521, 519*f*
    systemic lupus erythematosus, 458
    Takayasu's arteritis, 524, 525*f,* 526
    thromboangiitis obliterans, 526
    Wegener's granulomatosis, 521*f,* 521–522
Vascular response to injury/infection, 29*f,* 29*t,* 29–30, 30*t*
Vasculitis, 193, 463. *See also* Small-vessel vasculitis; Systemic necrotizing vasculitis
    defining, 514
    immune complex-mediated, 514–515
    renal disease, 562
    urticaria, 417
Vasoactive and smooth muscle-constricting mediator, 30, 30*t,* 187*t,* 187–188, 188*f,* 189*f*
V/(D)/J joining, 111–113, 115, 116*f,* 124, 125*f,* 128*f,* 446–447
Venereal Disease Research Laboratory (VDRL), 460, 742, 743
Venoocclusive disease, 823
Vernal keratoconjunctivitis, 395–396, 591–592, 592*f*
Veterinarian, 794
Vibrio cholerae, 686
Vincristine, 505
Viral infection
    hepatitis A, 702–703
    hepatitis B, 700–702, 701*t*
    influenza virus, 694–697, 695*t,* 696*f*
    measles virus, 699–700
    poliovirus, 704
    rabies, 703–704
    respiratory syncytial virus, 697–699
Viral oncogenesis, 632
Virokine, 165–166
Viroreceptor, 165–166
Virus
    Bc12 protein family, 23
    complement system, 173
    cowpox, 1, 81
    neutralization, 69–70, 680
    T cell-mediated host defenses, 680–681
    virokine and viroreceptor, 165–166
Virus infections of immune system
    cytomegalovirus, 760*t,* 760–761
    Epstein-Barr virus, 761–763
    HIV (human immunodeficiency virus), 748–760, 749*t,* 749–750*f,* 751–753*t,* 753–755*f,* 756–759*t,* 758*f*
    human T-cell leukemia virus types I and II (HTLV-I and HTLV-II), 763–765
Visceral larva migrans, 604
Visceral leishmaniasis, 730–731
Vitamin B$_{12}$, 344, 533, 534
Vogt-Koyanagi-Harada syndrome, 595–596
Von Willebrand's disease, 508

Waldenstrom's macroglobulinemia, 664–665
Wallace, Alfred R., 1
Warm autoimmune hemolytic anemia, 497–498, 498*t*

Watson, James, 3
Weber-Christian disease, 477–478
Wegener's granulomatosis, 521*f*, 521–522, 562, 609, 835
Western blot (WB), 234–235, 235*f*, 754*t*
Wheal-and-flare reaction, 188, 383*t*, 384, 401, 412*t*
Whipple's disease, 534
White blood cell. *See Leuk* listings
White pulp, splenic, 55
Wiskott-Aldrich syndrome (WAS), 354–355, 355*f*, 819
Witmer, R., 594
World Health Organization (WHO), 286, 287*t*
Wright, Sir Almoth, 2, 4
Wuchereria, 737
Wuchereria bancrofti, 281, 604

Xanthine, 402
X-box-binding protein (RF-X), 354
X-linked agammaglobulinemia, 116, 332–336
   clinical feature, 333*f*, 333–334
   complications and prognosis, 336
   diagnosis, immunologic/differential, 334–335

   general consideration, 332–333
   immunologic feature, 332
   laboratory findings, 334
   pathogenesis, immunologic, 333
   treatment, 335–336
X-linked combined immunodeficiency, 352
X-linked infantile agammaglobulinemia, 339
X-linked lymphoproliferative syndrome (XLP), 350, 361–362
X-linked severe combined immunodeficiency (X-SCID), 154

Yalow, Berson, 231
Yalow, Rosalyn, 5, 231
Yellow fever, 781*t*, 794
Yersin, A. J. E., 2
Yersinia, 688

Zalcitabine, 757
ZAP-70, 135–136
Zidovudine (AZT), 505, 757
Zinkernagel, Rolf, 3, 4
Zone electrophoresis, 217–218, 218–220*f*